The Essential Guide to Prescription Drugs

2005 Edition

The Essential Guide to Prescription Drugs

2005 Edition

James J. Rybacki, Pharm.D.

HarperResource

An Imprint of HarperCollins*Publishers*

To Dr. Jim Long, a brilliant man and the truest colleague and friend I've ever had.

THE ESSENTIAL GUIDE TO PRESCRIPTION DRUGS 2005. Copyright © 2005, 2004, 2003, 2002, 2001 by James J. Rybacki. Copyright © 2000, 1999, 1998, 1997, 1996 by James J. Rybacki and James W. Long. Copyright © 1994 by James W. Long and James J. Rybacki. Copyright © 1977, 1980, 1982, 1985, 1987, 1988, 1989, 1990, 1991, 1992, 1993 by James W. Long. All rights reserved. Printed in the United States of America. No part of this book may be used or reproduced in any manner whatsoever without written permission except in the case of brief quotations embodied in critical articles and reviews. For information address HarperCollins Publishers Inc., 10 East 53rd Street, New York, NY 10022.

HarperCollins books may be purchased for educational, business, or sales promotional use. For information please write: Special Markets Department, HarperCollins Publishers Inc., 10 East 53rd Street, New York, NY 10022.

Designed by C. Linda Dingler

Library of Congress Catalog Card Number 87–657561
ISSN 0894–7058

ISBN 0-06-072891-4 (pbk.)   04 05 06 07 08 RRD 10 9 8 7 6 5 4 3 2 1
ISBN 0-06-072890-6   04 05 06 07 08 RRD 10 9 8 7 6 5 4 3 2 1

Contents

SECTION SIX
Tables of Medicine Information   1305

Author's Note for the 2005 Edition

Did you get the owner's manual for that body? What about the magazine article—the one that tells you exactly what to do to get better? Wouldn't it be great if it were that easy?!?

Nobody wants to be a "patient." Even the word is somehow offensive, implying a hopeless job that demands too much patience and time—the world's rarest commodities. Many patients can't even follow simple directions ("get well SOON")! Being a "patient" is a job that is thrust upon us, sometimes long-term, hopefully short-term. It often forces others to assume the role of "caregiver." Both jobs are demanding and may stretch one's limits. Either one may leave you confused, resentful, and increasingly *impatient*—not exactly the most beneficial frame of mind for setting off on a new path toward better health.

But wait. What if the illness or diagnosis that made you reach for this book could point you in a more positive direction? What if you could view this time as an opportunity to make changes that would result in better health down the road? What if you could become a *smarter* patient and this book could become an owner's manual for many, if not all, of your medicines?

There are more than 40 categories of information in each medicine profile in this edition and a new one that refers you to a new table. The new category gives you a sampling of important guidelines that involve your medicine. A crucial new feature is Table 22, which lists important national guidelines for treatment of various diseases and disorders, how to contact the national organization that created them, and where to find them on the Internet. Study after study has identified a "treatment gap" as well as an "information gap"—situations where patients never received the benefits of proven medicines and objective information. This book can help you become a smart patient and make your medicines work harder for you. This is your time to begin that journey to better health. This is an excellent place to find answers to your questions and catch up with new thinking.

I am always struck by the fact that no one teaches people how to become a patient—much less how to become a *smart patient* and recognize and then ask for the best medicines. If we start with the end in mind, we would all become the healthiest patients possible. Yet the struggle then becomes: What road do I take to get there? What questions do I ask to prevent what I can and then get on the road to recovery from what I already have? I believe a sound approach covers a six-step continuum and I encourage you to speak up:

1. What diseases or conditions am I at risk for given my family history, and what tests are currently recommended to help define the degree of risk?
2. Given the risk I face, what steps can we take to lower my risk?
3. Understanding the conditions I now have, what research (evidence base) supports the medicines I am now taking? Which national guidelines apply to me, and have they been updated since my last visit?
4. What are the goals of the medicines that I now take (or prevention steps I have undertaken)? What's a reasonable time frame to expect results from treatments or to recheck our success at prevention?
5. Given my health plan or insurance, how is information shared among the doctor's office or clinic, the pharmacy where I get my medicines, the hospital, and again my doctor's office or clinic? Often what we don't tell or share creates additional risk or blunts benefits.
6. Because the research always changes, once a year, start all over again and ask what diseases or conditions you now appear to be at risk for and ask what new studies or guidelines may impact your care.

Once you make your list of questions, mail them to your doctor ahead of time—to be added to your medical chart and ask that they be discussed at your next office visits. *Most people don't realize that the chart is the center of the universe in the office, clinic, and hospital!* Many doctors review charts the day before or the morning before YOU show up in the office. Sending your questions to your doctor ahead of time lets them THINK. Getting them on the chart also means you can start every visit after that with a check of the progress you've made. Health care as it now exists is in effect squeezing you out of the picture. Squeeze back in, become a partner with your doctor, and take your place at the center of your health care.

An office visit often results in a prescription. Does it have to? NO. A pill isn't always the answer. For example, if your cholesterol is only mildly increased and your pattern of good and bad cholesterol (particle size, etc.) is only a little out of range, your doctor may want to try diet and exercise before starting a medicine. If a medicine IS suggested, please be honest:

- Be honest about being able to afford the medicine.
- Be honest about being willing to take the medicine exactly as prescribed.
- Be honest about all of the nonprescription, prescription, and nutritional or herbal supplements that you now take.
- Be honest about how well you understand the goals of any treatment.
- Be honest in asking about when results will be checked.
- Be honest about how well your health care system talks to itself. Try to understand the relationship among the hospital, the doctor's office or clinic, your family and home, and the pharmacy or mail-order service where you actually get the medicines.

Affording medicines is one of the most daunting issues facing government and patients. There is finally a Medicare prescription drug benefit! Is it perfect? No, but it is a great start and a credit to the Bush administration that had never been accomplished by previous administrations. I hope that we also have learned from our Canadian neighbors that simply lowering the cost or providing medicines at no cost does not mean that people will take them!

Work with your doctor and national guidelines to make sure you are getting proven medicines and then plan your medicines into your day (see the Medication Map provided in Table 15). Plan your medicines into your insurance (many doctors can check if a medicine is on formulary and will be covered, while you are still in the office). Plan your medicines into your family budget (Table 21 may help). One of the most difficult things is to remember to actually take your medicines. I'm continuing to take my medicine to lower my cholesterol and am still tapping the power of my family in reminding me to take it! It's always a good idea to read about your medicines in this book and understand the mild and more serious possible side effects. Discussing these with your family will help them identify possible medicine-related problems. Finding problems early can be a lifesaver. If you are at all unsure if a new problem is related to a new or existing medicine, call your doctor. It's a good move and good medicine.

Finally: Put a date on the calendar when your medicine should help you reach the goals that you and your doctor have set! Of course the peak effect of medicines will vary, but this simple step means that you will check on progress and talk about adjusting things if your medicines aren't working as hard for you as they should. Become a smarter patient and learn how to work with your doctor, nurse, and pharmacist to give your medicines a good checkup!

As noted in each previous edition, no claim is made that all known actions, uses, side effects, adverse effects, precautions, or interactions for a drug are included in the information provided in this book. Talk to your doctor before making any changes, additions, or deletions to the medicines that you already take. This book contains information about medicines and is not medical advice. Although diligent care has been taken to ensure the accuracy of the information provided during the preparation of this revision, the continued accuracy and currentness are ever subject to change relative to the dissemination of new information derived from drug research, development, and general usage. Use this book in good health.

James Joseph Rybacki, Pharm.D.

Points for the Patient

Regardless of what you do for a living, who you know, or what you know—when you become a patient, you are no longer the same person. Dr. Jim Rybacki, the author and clinical pharmacist, talks about adherence, compliance, and concordance—the critical importance of taking medicines EXACTLY as prescribed. Jim Rybacki the patient forgets to take his once-a-day cholesterol medicine and has to involve his family in order to remember to take that single pill. Often, taking medicines becomes a lifetime endeavor. Once you've had a heart attack, you're a heart patient for life and need to keep the power of your medicines working for you!

Understanding what you are facing can be half the battle in any situation. It's important to learn as much as you can about the new disease or condition you or a loved one has and how best to manage it. Ask your doctor and pharmacist for written information, visit reputable Web sites (see Table 17) and look at Table 22 to learn about national guidelines. I try to help sort out objective information for you on my Web site, *www.medicineinfo.com*. Never be afraid to ask your nurse, doctor, or pharmacist questions about the disease or condition—you actually make their jobs easier when you help yourself. All competent health care professionals welcome the chance to help you understand your health, diseases or conditions, and medicines as they relate to their particular expertise—regardless of how busy they may be. Physicians and pharmacists are good examples. If they won't give you this critical time and these critical answers, find another physician or pharmacist who will.

We are all unique, and a critical factor in successful drug therapy is called tailoring. This means selecting each medicine for each patient and adjusting the medicine doses to each patient. In clothing, one size actually rarely fits all. In medicines, a "one dose fits all" approach can lead to perilous prescriptions. There is actually a new field called pharmacogenomics that seeks to tailor medicines to the genes that we have.

Once a medicine is prescribed, please share the responsibility for safe and effective drug treatment. Smart patients help themselves by making sure every prescriber and pharmacist who helps provide your health care is aware of all the medicines you are taking. This sounds deceptively simple—but always include prescription, nonprescription, and any herbal or nutritional support you take. Finally, there is a National Poison Control number: 1-800-222-1222. Write it down NOW where anyone can find it. Accidental poisonings unfortunately include medicines.

Don't be afraid to take another list—I've had many patients do this and welcome the complete picture. Did you know that nonprescription medicines could blunt the benefits of your prescriptions? Millions of Americans now take herbal medicines. Talk to your doctor or pharmacist BEFORE combining any herbal medicine with any other medicine. REMEMBER, herbal medicines are NOT presently approved or regulated in the same way as prescription medicines. They fall under the Dietary Supplement Health and Education Act (DSHEA) of 1994. However, as these products are more potent than ever, I believe it's time to regulate them as we do prescription medicines. They can have real benefits as well as serious interactions with prescription medicines. I've updated and broadened the possible herbal/prescription medicine interactions in the drug profiles to help protect you.

We all need to be there for our families—living in the best possible health. People do not exist alone. Your family can be a powerful resource when it comes to making your medicines work. For example, it's OK to say that you feel like you're taking too many pills. With the progress in medicines today, there are many options (for example—Caduet, a combination of a cholesterol and blood pressure medicine). Let's take a look at some specific ways to become a smarter patient.

When Your Doctor Prescribes a Drug for You

- Smart patients ALWAYS find out about the national treatment guidelines that identify proven medicines, and check to see if their medicine is in the guidelines. While there may well be good reasons for a medicine not being in the guidelines (such as being approved after the guidelines were released or not having enough study), checking the Medicine Families in the guidelines lets you see if your medicine is included.

- Take a look at Table 19 (Running a Risk: Recognizing and Regaining Control of Heart Disease Risk Factors) if you have a family history of heart disease. For other diseases or conditions, find out if risk factors can be modified to lower the chance of a repeat problem or to lessen the severity of an existing problem. For example, if you have a history of diabetes in your family and you are overweight, losing weight is one of those risk factors that you can change that can actually decrease your risk of diabetes. There is also a study (Diabetes Prevention Program) that says that lifestyle changes such as exercise as well as a medicine called metformin (Glucophage) can help PRE-VENT diabetes.

- Smart patients ALWAYS ask if there is nutritional support that may be required if a new prescription is being considered. For example: HMG CoA reductase inhibitors may deplete coenzyme Q (co-Q) in some patients. If patients begin to feel tired after starting one of the high cholesterol medicines in that class, supplementation with co-Q may help restore quality of life. Another good example are corticosteroids such as prednisone (Deltasone, Orasone, and others), which can work to weaken bones by decreasing calcium absorption. Calcium supplements and a check of bone mineral density (by DEXA or PDEXA) are advisable if prednisone or similar corticosteroids are going to be taken on an ongoing basis.

When You Get a New Diagnosis Along with a Lifestyle Change or a New Prescription

- CHANGE? Yes, change. When a new disease or condition is identified, what you are really facing is change. For example, if your cholesterol is increased, the result by itself is simply a number. When your individual family and medical history are considered, the number becomes part of a reasonable series of steps that need to be taken over a specific time frame. High cholesterol is a great example. SMART PATIENTS ALWAYS find out about specific risk factors that go along with a new diagnosis. For a closer look at where cholesterol fits in, visit Table 19 (Running a Risk: Recognizing and Regaining Control of Heart Disease Risk Factors). For people with small increases and few existing risk factors, TLC comes into play. We may think of this as tender loving care, but in the cholesterol arena, it means therapeutic lifestyle changes.
- Smart patients ALWAYS ask what the goals of any existing or new treatment are, and how long it should take to reach them. In other words, the clock is ticking. If a new medicine is prescribed, the time for that medicine to work and then be checked should be told (disclosed) to you. For example, "Here is your new prescription for cholesterol, we'll see you again in three months." While this tells you that a return visit is needed, it is an example of a prescription, not patient-centered care. A much more desirable way is: "Here is your new prescription to lower your cholesterol. It is called atorvastatin and the brand name is Lipitor. Your pharmacist will give you a printed information sheet on it. Our goal is to have Lipitor work to lower your bad cholesterol (LDL) to 100 (mg/dL) in three months. It's critical to take it at the same time every day and to never miss a day. It's okay to get a fat or lipid panel or cholesterol rechecked in about four weeks if you happen to go to a health fair—but please make sure the results are sent to me. We will also check the PATTERN of good and bad cholesterol and repeat a C-reactive protein.

This will give us the best check on how hard your medicine is working for you. Do you have any questions for me?" Now this is valuable patient-centered information!

- Smart patients ALWAYS ask what to do if goals of their medicines are not achieved in the time frame that they originally discussed with their doctor. Sometimes this means simply adjusting the dose. In any case, please do not wait until the last minute of an office visit to bring up the real reason you came to the office. While it's human nature to do this, it rarely gets the best results.

- Ask your doctor if he or she has an adherence assessment form (AAF) that can be placed in your medical chart. Explain to them that you would like to have adherence checked on every office visit and then charted (the medical term for adding it to your record) like a vital sign such as temperature.

- Sound-alike and look-alike errors are unfortunately not unusual. Smart patients protect themselves by ALWAYS asking that the prescription include both the name of the drug and the disorder for which the drug is taken. For example: Fosamax for osteoporosis or Zantac for heartburn. This helps avoid sound-alike errors. Over the phone, a person calling in Xanax may be misunderstood as saying Zantac. Zantac is for heartburn and ulcers. Xanax is for anxiety. If the disorder being treated is named on the label, it offers a second chance for a pharmacist or certified technician to discover a mistake.

- Ask your doctor to fill out the medication map from the back of this book while you're still in the office. This helps you fit the medicines realistically into your life. Taking this step may even show that a medicine being considered by your doctor might not really work out for you. The best medicine in the world does absolutely no good if you can't or won't be able to take it. Get the most from your health care dollars.

- Tell your doctor about any known drug allergies and of any prior drug-induced adverse effects. This will let the doctor check to see whether he or she has inadvertently prescribed a medicine from the same chemical family.

- Smart patients ALWAYS honestly talk about all other drugs (prescription, nonprescription, herbal, or nutritional) they are taking. Include alcohol, marijuana, and others. Remember that some herbal extracts contain the same ingredients found in prescription medicines and may lead to unforeseen toxicity, or may blunt prescription drug benefits. Interestingly, still other herbal medicines can help prescription medicines work or may even duplicate some prescription drug effects. Because of this, combining an herbal remedy with a prescription may actually require lower doses of the prescription drug. Smart patients find out about possible interactions first. Make certain you talk to your doctor before you combine ANY medicines.

- Many medicines require special precautions. Examples include avoiding certain foods, alcohol, exposure to sun, certain medicines, or even hazardous activities.

- Be sure you understand how long to take a medicine. Talk with your prescriber about this and, if applicable, when and how to stop it. A hallmark of good prescribing is that goals and time frames are set at the time a medicine is first prescribed. Unfortunately, when people take several different medicines, mistakes can be made. I see many cases where patients thought they understood what to do and actually stopped the wrong medicine in a complicated regimen.

- Ask your doctor to give you a written summary about the drug prescribed. Few people can remember all of the information and instructions that have been talked about. A concept I have pioneered is the Medication Map. Very simple, but many medicine errors are made because people forget, make incorrect combinations of medicines, mistake one pill for the other, or take medicine with food when it should not be. A Medication Map organizes all the medicines you are taking and tells you how much, when, and with what the medicines should be taken. Take the blank form from this book to your doctor or pharmacist and ask him or her to fill in the form with you. This will help you to clarify and verify pertinent information while taking the medicine itself in the best possible way. Be prepared for know-it-alls who look at the map and see only paper. Remember, the power in a doctor's office is in the chart, and this makes their chart work for you.

- Smart patients ALWAYS ask their doctor if the medicine prescribed offers the best balance of price and outcomes. This simple question will help a busy practitioner focus on his or her available choices. Remember to ask whether the dosing has been adjusted for any compromise in kidney or liver function or other chronic condition that you may have. Diseases can also "interact" with medicines.

- Many HMOs or health care insurers may not pay for some medicines. This can impact your doctor's prescribing authority and the pharmacist's ability to fill your prescription. Write the nonpayer to complain. The Patient's Bill of Rights may restore your access to the medicine that will give the best results! There is a part of the Medicare prescription drug benefit and a new concept called collaborative care where pharmacists in more than 40 states work with your doctor to make sure you reach and keep the goals of treatment.

- Smart patients tell their doctor if new symptoms develop after they start taking the drug(s) prescribed, as problems caused by medicines themselves are easily reversible if they are caught early. If you are found to have had a reaction to a medicine, ask your doctor to report the problem to the Federal Drug Administration (FDA). This reporting is critical to maintaining safe and effective medicines for everyone.

- Keep follow-up appointments with your doctor and for laboratory tests. Many drugs must be monitored closely.
- If you go to any other health care provider, tell him or her of all medications you are taking currently—prescription and nonprescription. Tell them your complete history in order to get the best possible results. Remember any herbal medicines you might be taking. Smart patients never assume that every doctor knows all the medicines that they take.
- If the prescription you got was for pain management, remember that the Joint Commission on Accreditation of Healthcare Organizations has come forth with some novel and long-overdue pain management standards. Soon you will see posters in hospital hallways that help increase awareness of your basic right to effective pain management. Pain is now the fifth vital sign. In your doctor's office, you will not see the Joint Commission, but it is perfectly acceptable to demand effective pain management!

When You Get Your Prescription Filled

- Smart patients OPEN THE BAG. This is especially valuable if you have your prescription filled in a pharmacy. Unfortunately, many people don't fully use the information that their pharmacist can provide. Many prescription bags are stapled shut, with the brief patient information sheet or even a Med Guide inside. You'll be glad if you open the bag! This gives you a chance (on a refill prescription) to see if the pills look the same as before. It is also a chance to look over the dose and make sure you know how often to take it. Make sure you understand this and ask your pharmacist questions. A few minutes reading the information about the medicine can actually save your life. If you are required or choose to use a mail-order pharmacy, once again, it is critical to check the bag and make certain that you have received the correct medicine—yet it is more difficult for you to get access to a pharmacist to confirm the medicine. The best way to go is to ask how you will have access to a pharmacist if you have medication questions. Insist on toll-free telephone numbers.
- Smart patients READ THE LABEL and auxiliary labels carefully. It's time well spent. All prescription bottles MUST be labeled with a minimum of information. Check that both the name of the drug and the disorder are specified. If these are missing, ask your pharmacist to call your doctor for permission to add them. For example, I've seen many patients who have become confused about which medicine is for what. Having a bottle for a cholesterol-lowering medicine labeled as rosuvastatin (Crestor) for cholesterol-lowering is much better than simply having the name.
- Many managed-care organizations require pill splitting. Check with your pharmacist to see if this is something you will be expected to do. If so, ask if they will split the pills for you, or if they have a pill

splitter for sale. This will help ensure that you will get an accurate dose of medicine.

- If this is a refill, check to see that the drug in the bottle is the same as the drug in your original supply. If it is not the same, ask your pharmacist to explain the difference. (Generic drug products from different manufacturers often vary in size, shape, color, etc.)

- There are more than 1,000 drug names that "look alike" in print or "sound alike" in speech. Examples: Celebrex—Celexa, cyclosporine—cycloserine, Prilosec—Prozac, Xanax—Zantac. Mistaking one drug for the other can lead to serious problems. "Sound-alikes" cause problems when a prescription is given by telephone. Listing the disorder on the prescription will help the pharmacist prevent the mistake. Many of the most often-prescribed drugs are pictured in the Color Chart insert in this book.

- Ask your pharmacist to give you printed information sheets about the drug(s) prescribed for you. Say YES if you are asked if you want counseling on your medicine! Make use of your pharmacist's training. Also ask this expert to fill out the Medication Map from the back of this book for you.

- Read the label (I'm repeating this because it is so important) and follow the directions. Some people pay more attention to a peanut butter label than they do to their prescription label. These tiny labels can help you get the most from your medicines and warn you about dosage forms that should not be altered (opened, crushed, or chewed) and about effects food may have.

- Use the same pharmacy for all of your medicines. Most pharmacies have a computer system. This can help prevent serious allergic reactions and significant drug interactions. Tell your pharmacist of all drugs (remember to include herbal remedies, megavitamins, alcohol, and nonprescription agents) you are currently taking.

Your Responsibilities—to Yourself—as a Patient

- AT LAST, there is a National Poison Control number: 1-800-222-1222. Write it down where any of your family members can find it.

- Smart patients know what the goals are for any medicine they take and how long it should take to reach those goals. If time goes by and the medicine does not help as it should, there are often many other options. Ask what your doctor wants you to do if signs and symptoms of the condition being treated return. For example—if you had a heart attack previously, ask about taking aspirin on the way to the hospital if you ever think you are having a repeat attack. Find out now!

- If you are taking more than one drug, be sure that the label of each container includes the name of the drug and the condition it treats, and know the generic, brand, and medicine family name for each of your medicines.

- Remember that foods can react with medicines. Something as simple as grapefruit juice is now known to interact with some high blood pressure medicines. The best liquid to take with most medicines is water.

- Take a moment to make sure you understand the directions for using a drug. Ask if you're not sure.
- Many nonprescription medicines were once available only by prescription. Talk with your pharmacist or physician BEFORE combining any two drugs.
- Smart patients follow medicine instructions carefully and completely. DO NOT stop an antibiotic 7 days into a 10-day prescription because you feel better. This can lead to serious illness. If you have trouble remembering to take your medications on time, ask for a dosing calendar or a weekly medication box.
- If you take medicines prescribed by more than one doctor, check the generic names for duplicate drugs with different brand names to avoid serious overdoses.
- Ask your doctor and pharmacist if he or she offers "brown-bag sessions" for your medicines. Put all the medicines you currently take into a bag and have your pharmacist review them for potency, appropriateness, and dating.
- If you are looking at a new insurance plan or HMO, ask if there is a formulary. Find out if a mail-order pharmacy must be used. If so, ask who will regularly review your medicines and how you will be able to contact a pharmacist for questions.
- If you will be using an Internet pharmacy, look at the Guidelines for Safe and Effective Drug Use in Section One of this book. Expect pharmaceutical care, not just delivery of medicine.
- Be certain all drugs you take are "in date" (have not expired).
- Effective and timely control of pain is a basic right to which you are entitled. The Agency for Health Care Policy and Research has released *Clinical Practice Guidelines,* which outline management of cancer pain but also apply to management of pain in general. Demand that your pain be respected as much as a high fever. The American Pain Society has long asked that pain become the fifth vital sign, and finally, The Joint Commission on Accreditation of Healthcare Organizations has developed an elaborate set of guidelines on pain management.
- If you are facing a terminal illness, ask whether the hospital you are considering has a palliative care program as well as a hospice program.

Suggestions for Containing the Costs of Drug Therapy

- Visit *www.helpingpatients.org.* This is a new site, which actually gives you a form to fill out, asks about your medicines and income and tells you about programs that can help you with costs. This is from the pharmaceutical manufacturers association and is something very new.
- READ TABLE 21: How to Get Your Family Help with the Cost of Medicines. As always, I've tried to include information about the

best programs, helpful tips, and balanced and objective Web sites that can help make a difference for you.

- TAKE YOUR MEDICINE IN THE RIGHT AMOUNT AT THE RIGHT TIME AND IN THE RIGHT WAY. This is a fundamental point where we fail time and time again. Unfortunately, if you skip doses, you may lose much of the possible benefit from many medicines. Additionally, your doctor could decide to add more medicine to the ones he thinks are not helping enough, further increasing your bill as well as chances for drug interactions.
- Work with your doctor to ensure an accurate diagnosis. Many signs or symptoms can be embarrassing to talk about, but your doctor needs an accurate and complete history to help make decisions about your treatment.
- Ask your doctor to prescribe the drug that is most appropriate for you, selecting the product that offers the best balance of price and outcomes. If you have several chronic diseases at the same time, what appears to be a more expensive antibiotic may give you a better outcome than a less costly one. Ask your doctor if a chosen medicine has a "cousin" in the same chemical family that may give the same results at a lower price!
- Ask your doctor or pharmacist if an acceptable generic product is available.
- If your HMO or managed care organization requires you to split pills (a present controversy), ask if they will pay for a pill splitter so that you can accomplish this accurately. If they refuse to pay for a splitter, I strongly advise you to get one yourself. Please also write to your congressperson about the managed care organization's refusal.
- Ask your doctor if there are any vitamins or minerals that you should be taking based on family history (such as folic acid to help prevent some heart attacks or calcium for osteoporosis), or even because of the medicines themselves.
- Follow your doctor's and pharmacist's advice about your prescriptions. A medicine won't do you ANY GOOD AT ALL if it stays in the bottle.
- Many HMOs and physician groups use a concept called dual-product substitution. This is a measure that I agree with. For example, some prescription products are merely different names for the same medicine (Vanceril or Beclovent; Normodyne or Trandate). It makes perfect sense that the lowest-priced brand be freely substituted for a particular prescription. Ask your doctor about this idea when he or she is writing a prescription for you.
- Ask how the HMO or physician group measures up against other groups in your area. Remember, many groups are benchmarked or measured by groups such as the National Committee on Quality Assurance (on the Web at *www.ncqa.org*, or call them at 202-955-5697).

Points for the Pharmacist

Collaborative care is finally here in nearly 40 states! While this requires some extra certification, I urge you to embrace this growing clinical opportunity. The new table on national guidelines can be a great framework to look at your customers' most common disease states and map out proven medicine strategies. As in previous years, I need to address adherence—because half the people who get a prescription fail to take it correctly. You can make a real difference by making sure that people understand how much to take, when to take it, and what to take it with. Do you encourage compliance at every initial prescription and refill? Do you call or e-mail the doctor if your patients are early or late for refills? Consider starting an adherence/compliance clinic. If you are a hospital pharmacist, find out about the American Heart Association's "Get With The Guidelines" program (for both stroke and cholesterol). They are hospital-based programs designed to identify champions in hospitals, identify patients who have had a first heart attack or stroke, and then help them get the best medicines in order to prevent a second heart attack or stroke. Learn more at *www.americanheart.org*.

Current estimates tell us that adverse drug events cost 60–100 billion dollars a year. Failure to individualize drug therapy is widespread and is something that you can help correct. Learn the current goals and time frames to achieve those goals in current objective guidelines from such organizations as the American College of Cardiology or the American Heart Association. Don't be afraid to keep your prescribers informed about goals and guidelines. Point-of-care testing, such as blood sugar and cholesterol checks (now available in the same machine), can be a valuable and compensated service. Many pharmacists are being paid for their expertise in medicines (cognitive services). There are many initiatives where you can help manage diabetes, compliance, asthma, and cholesterol problems and be reimbursed for the great help that you can give. In this book you'll find a framework for a wonderful new cognitive service: Medication Mapping. You are encouraged to copy and complete the Medication Map to show your customers how to fit their newly prescribed medicines into their lives.

Be a leader in creating connections with your hospital colleagues. The time is ripe to create inpatient to outpatient networks! Of course there will be HIPPA considerations, but it is improbable that they will be insurmountable. Talk to your customers about the importance of your new adherence program. Explain that your pharmacy works closely with physicians to get the best results from medicines. Consider a patient adherence contract and offer a small discount for great adherence. Talk to your patients and tell them that your pharmacy actually e-mails your doctor when prescriptions are filled so that he or she knows that the new medicine is being put to work! Talk to your prescribers about this new system and explain how they can be e-mailed right at the office if their patients never fill or are early or late with their prescription refills. FINALLY, there is a National Poison Control number: 1-800-222-1222. Give it to all of your customers!

I advise consumers to take the fullest advantage of their pharmacist's training and experience. Get copies of the latest clinical guidelines for any disease state management services you are offering and keep your prescribers in the loop! The Agency for Health Care Policy and Research is advocating effective and timely control of pain as a basic human right. The American Pain Society and JCAHO have made pain the fifth vital sign—and now JCAHO, the AMA, and NCQA are working together to develop quality measures (see True Breakthroughs). This is another clear opportunity for you to help in offering effective therapeutic options and superb pharmaceutical care. Call 1-800-422-6237 for more information on pain and cancer.

When You Fill a Prescription

- Clarify with the prescriber any information that is illegible, uncertain, or a potential source for erroneous interpretation—by you or the patient. Remember the Institute of Medicine data—help your customers stay alive.
- Be alert to look-alike and sound-alike drug names. This is a significant cause of dispensing errors. In accepting prescriptions by telephone, confirm the brand with the generic name as a double check. If there is still some doubt, ask the caller to spell the name of the drug.
- Include both the name of the drug and the disorder on the label (for example, Fosamax for osteoporosis) if the patient does not object, and consult with the prescribing physician when necessary. This will help (1) reduce dispensing errors caused by look-alike and sound-alike drug names and (2) prevent confusion during concurrent use of multiple drugs.
- Encourage your patients to look at the prescription label with you. Paperclip the patient drug information to the bag. Take the lead in

opening the bottle, showing the patient the medicine and making sure he or she understands how much and when to take the medicine. This also gives you a final chance to earn your place as a trusted professional.

- Check the stock bottle for accurate identification and appropriate dating. If a technician fills the prescription, be certain you open the dispensing container as well as the completed prescription and check the drug personally.

When You Counsel the Patient as You Dispense the Filled Prescription

- Always follow up on existing medicines with an adherence or compliance check. Document this in the patient record. Ask patients to tell you how they are to take or give any new medicine. Hearing THEM tell YOU about their medicines is a great way to make sure they really understand. Clarify any points of confusion or misunderstanding. Every refill is an opportunity to assess and encourage adherence. Don't fail your patients by forgetting to check the medicine itself. For those patients who have Internet access and who are at risk for heart disease—encourage them to sign up for American Heart Association programs to help patients (via patient-directed information on CAD, CHF, arrhythmia and others as appropriate). Tell them to visit *www.americanheart.org!*
- Make sure that the patient recognizes the name of the drug and the disorder being treated. A simple way to start this important dialogue is to ask, "What did your doctor tell you this medicine was going to do for you?" Explain what the drug is supposed to do and when the expected therapeutic benefits are usually realized.
- Review the details of dosing instructions: how much to take, when to take it, and for how long. It doesn't do them any good if it stays in the bottle. Begin by saying, "Tell me a little bit about how your doctor told you to take this medicine." See if your computer vendor has a module for medication maps. If not, ask the publisher for permission to use the map provided in this book. This can be a valuable cognitive service.
- If the medicine you are counseling patients about is for pain, encourage patients to view effective pain control as a basic right. If they were given a pain medicine in the hospital, they were likely visited by a pain management team.
- Talk about possible side effects or adverse effects that may occur. Try asking, "Did your doctor tell you about any possible side effects from this medicine?" Tell patients what to do if any of these occur. Encourage them to call their doctor if new signs or symptoms develop.
- Precautions are critical. This includes possible interactions with foods, beverages, drugs, or restricted activities.
- Provide written information about the drug(s) dispensed and the patient's disorder (if available).

- Clarify how best to store the medicine. Tell patients about refrigeration and avoiding the humidity of a medicine chest. If a nonchild-proof lid is dispensed, remind them to keep the drug out of reach whenever children are visiting.
- Remind patients that nonprescription (over-the-counter) drugs can interact with prescription drugs. Encourage them to call your pharmacy or their physician before combining any medicines.
- Always take a good medication history and repeat this at least every six months. On every visit, be certain to ask about new medicines and any herbal medicines or vitamins the patient may have added or may be considering.
- Encourage the patient to ask questions—at the time of dispensing and later—whenever the need arises. A good way to start this conversation is, "Now that we've talked, do you have any questions for me?" Encourage patients to call if they think of something later. This is often the case.
- Explain that drugs may not work in practice exactly as expected. Tell the patient to be alert to the possibility that a new symptom or sign *may* be drug related. If one of your patients does experience a novel adverse drug reaction, it is critical that you (or your technician/designate) call the FDA MedWatch at 1-800-332-1088.

Suggestions for Containing the Costs of Drug Therapy

- Assess and encourage compliance or adherence to medicines with every initial prescription and refill. The expense of nonadherence can be huge.
- As judgment dictates, fill the prescription with the most reasonably priced drug available—within legally possible and appropriate guidelines. Consult with the prescribing physician regarding generic substitution when feasible.
- If the patient is taking other drugs (prescribed by other physicians), look for drug duplications. Offer "brown-bag sessions" where patients can bring in all their medicines and get your expert help regarding possible problems.

Points for the Physician

I've been privileged to work side by side with many doctors. I've worked in hospitals, offices, and research. The changes in health care have been staggering and in many cases burdensome. Many practitioners view national guidelines as "cookbook medicine"—yet study after study tells us that proven medicines are not being used as often as they should. Outcomes, goals, guidelines, "prehypertension and prediabetes," benchmarking, and managed care: simple phrases that have significantly changed the way you practice medicine today. If you add closed formularies and critical paths, in some senses clinical decision making has become more focused. I hope collaborative care will be welcomed by doctors because management of medicines is a daunting task. Embracing pharmaceutical care and national guidelines creates an atmosphere of continuous improvement and is just good medicine. One of the best colleagues you can have in attaining the best results from any medicine is a fully informed patient.

Unfortunately, many patients get less than balanced information from the Web. This year Table 17 has been augmented in order to provide balanced and objective Web sites where you can feel comfortable directing patients and their families. Hospital-based programs offer a great way to get the medicines started that have the best data. Information about the "Get With The Guidelines" program (GWTG) is available at *www.americanheart.org*. GWTG is a hospital-based initiative that seeks to increase evidence-based therapy for secondary prevention of cardiovascular disease. If your patients are cared for by hospitalists after a heart attack, you may well find them returning to you with a form outlining new medicines.

Michael Weintraub, M.D., recognized the need for patient education back in 1991, when in his introduction to the *Yearbook of Drug Therapy* he stated, "In looking for trends in the medical literature, it is apparent that the need for the physician to be an educator of patients and their families is becoming greater and greater." In addition, citing an increased need for patient education, he summarized with the following opinion: "Treatment principles correctly applied by patients educated about their condition and involved in its management seem to be the wave of the future." This is clearly a description of patient-centered care. It is absolutely unacceptable that current estimates of the expense of adverse drug events and medical errors cost more than 100 billion dollars a year, more than is spent on diabetes in the United States.

Your office is probably computerized. I've been doing work to help create a seamless patient flow sheet, which I call an Adherence Assessment Form (AAF). Create your own that lists current medicines, when they were started, and their dose and interval. Send this with the patient to the hospital and insist that it is updated on discharge. Many physicians delegate care to hospitalists, and you can get the best results from them by having your AAF document augmentation of continuity of care. I wish that patients could or would use the same pharmacy, but the reality is they will shop. Make sure that your patients take or send the AAF to every pharmacy that fills prescriptions for them. Some exciting systems such as Allscripts will actually interface with office software to tell you in the exam room which medicines Jim Rybacki's insurance will pay for and what to go do next!

I've told patients to "take your medicines and take care of your family" on my Web site (*www.medicineinfo.com*). I plan to continue to encourage people to ask questions and to be partners in their health care. Don't be offended if patients bring Internet information to your office. It may be prudent to have your office staff search the Net for information on the 10 most common diagnoses that you make—and provide that data for those under your care. The good sites will tell patients that information is only to be used in conjunction with you, their doctor. I know that a six- to ten-minute patient visit can never explain all of the nuances of drug therapy. Hopefully, this book can help patients partner with you and decrease some of the calls that you get. FINALLY, there is a National Poison Control number: 1-800-222-1222. Give it to all of your patients.

When You Evaluate a Patient for Drug Therapy

- Check the current national guidelines for the top ten diagnoses you usually make. Talk to your patients about the guidelines concept and the goals you have for their treatment. This can be a great step to keep the prediabetic or prehypertensive patient from progressing down a dark and complicated road.
- Ask if the patient is currently under treatment by other health care providers or if the patient has actually gotten any prescription medicines without a prescription on the Internet.
- Ask about all drugs used currently—prescription and over-the-counter. Remember that many over-the-counter agents were once

prescription medicines. Herbal medicines are now widely used and can have beneficial as well as deleterious interactions. If some 10 billion dollars is spent each year on herbals, include a question about herbals in your routine questions. Rules about structure/function claims can be found at *http://vm.cfsan.fda.gov*. Make certain that you do not gloss over medicines they can take without ever obtaining your guidance.

- Consider a patient's history and lifestyle. Think about diseases or conditions for which the patient is at risk, and vitamins (such as folic acid for heart disease) or minerals (calcium to prevent osteoporosis and possibly reduce risk of some colon cancers) that may be used to prevent a disease or process. Rybacki's first recommendation: It is always better to prevent a disease or condition than to have to treat it. Part of NCEP ATP III actually repositions therapeutic lifestyle changes. Please also remember that some prescription medicines can negatively impact quality of life unless you recommend the appropriate nutritional support.
- Make certain that you are absolutely current. Many daily fax and e-mail services are available that can be individualized to your practice and can easily be read after your morning rounds.
- Establish the nature and severity of the disorder under consideration for drug treatment.
- Elicit significant coexisting disorders—possible absolute contraindications for certain drugs.
- Evaluate any suspected or obvious organ dysfunction—possible relative contraindications for certain drugs. When creatinine values are available, take the time to calculate creatinine clearance. Many drugs have breakpoints for adjustment of dosage at various levels of renal impairment. Even though an older patient's creatinine is within the "normal limits," his or her clearance will not be. For example, a 72-year-old, 70-kg man with a 1.4 creatinine will have a creatinine clearance of about 48.6 mL/min. This is below the level where doses or intervals of kidney (renally)-eliminated medicines must be adjusted. Hepatic disease will also impact doses or intervals for many drugs, particularly those that are highly protein-bound or heavily metabolized.
- Assess the patient's potential for adherence or nonadherence with drug therapy. Remember the expense that a given prescription presents. The most brilliant prescription choice is totally ineffective if financial considerations prevent adherence with the medicine you choose. Once-a-day dosing is much easier to remember and, combined with a dosing calendar, gets excellent results. If a complicated regimen is required, there are also pager-based systems that can give patients a "beep" with the name of the medicine and instructions for using it. Find out where your patients get their prescriptions filled and partner with the pharmacy to have adherence checked on EVERY refill. If you have an e-mail service, ask to be e-mailed if they are early or late or if they miss a refill. See if the patient's pharmacist

offers a medication mapping service. If not, map your patient's medicines yourself.

When Selecting Drugs for Therapy

- Try to match the drug's power to the patient's problem. Avoid
  overprescribing—medicinal "overkill." For example, mild to moderate stress reactions (situational anxiety-tension states) respond well
  to antianxiety drugs; they do not require antipsychotic medication.
  An uncomplicated urinary tract infection with a broadly sensitive
  single organism does not require a broad-spectrum anti-infective
  drug.
- Get a copy of the *Agency for Health Care Policy and Research Clinical
  Practice Guidelines Number 9*. The AHCPR is advocating effective
  and timely pain control as a basic human right. Increase your
  awareness of the World Health Organization Pain Ladder and the
  use of the agents that are primary analgesics and adjuvants. AHCPR
  publications are great tools to help your patients understand their
  medicine and their disease. Thanks to JCAHO, pain is now the fifth
  vital sign in your hospital.
- Always check for drug–drug, drug–food, and drug-disease interactions. Remember to take a "new" drug history periodically.
- Many new oral anti-infectives are effective against pathogens that
  historically required intravenous therapy. Although this allows you
  to avoid hospitalization, it makes the patient's adherence more
  critical.
- Consider the desired onset of drug action (immediate versus
  delayed) and the consequences or benefits of that effect.
- Choose the drug with the most favorable benefit-to-risk ratio: the
  best clinical effects with the fewest possible adverse reactions.
- When you prescribe narrow-therapeutic-window drugs that require
  periodic blood levels, be certain that blood sampling is done after
  the drug has reached its steady state (usually five half-lives). Understand which level is preferable to measure: "peak" level (as for theophylline), "trough" level (as for digoxin), and "peak and trough" for
  aminoglycosides (such as tobramycin). Many clinical pharmacists
  (the author included) will willingly calculate the best dose and interval for you and make a consultative recommendation. Remember
  that the peak-to-trough ratio can be a great indicator for true once-
  a-day dosing with oral medicines.
- Give due consideration to the patient's prior experience with other
  medicines similar to the one you are considering and prescribe
  accordingly. Prescribing a second drug from the same drug class to
  which a patient already has had an allergic reaction or adverse drug
  effect that required discontinuation of therapy or provided no therapeutic benefit is not prudent.
- Remember individual patient factors such as age, education, and cul-
  tural factors (including genetic effects on medication elimination).

- Think about the desired extent of effect (systemic or local). Some possible adverse effects can be limited by choosing an inhaled versus "pill" form.
- Set goals and time frames when you start any new medicine. Talk these over with your patient. It's amazing how many patients I see who really have no idea what their medicine is for. Frequently, dosing issues also arise, and, of course, an underdose can be just as dangerous as an overdose. If drug treatment fails after a reasonable trial with good adherence, change to a drug of another chemical class, or consider combination therapy with two medicines with different mechanisms of action. For example, if viral load decreases for a time and then increases in an AIDS patient, you MUST change treatment.
- Select the drugs you prescribe critically, utilizing independent, objective reviews of available information. The "most frequently prescribed" drug is not necessarily the best drug within its class. Slick, glossy detail pieces should always be confirmed by primary literature. Some clinical pharmacists (the author included) will provide a balanced overview of the current literature.
- Even "drugs of choice" in objective reviews can be poor choices when you consider the characteristics of individual patients. A renally compromised patient may better tolerate an "alternate drug" with dual elimination (hepatic and renal) than a "drug of choice" that is limited to renal elimination.
- Remember that possible pharmacokinetic and pharmacodynamic changes in those over 65 can lead to accumulation and excessive responses to "normal" doses and dosing intervals. In general, the possibility of side effects increases with increasing dose. Many medicines have "ceiling effects," above which dose increases act only to decrease quality of life and fail to add to therapeutic benefits.
- Be objective and discerning as you review the claims made for a newly released drug within a sizable class of drugs already available. Only a small percentage of newly approved drugs each year are classified by the FDA as truly innovative or more advantageous than similar drugs in current use. The remaining medicines are largely "me too" drugs with a limited history of use and a potential for "surprises" after a period of general use. It is best to select drugs with established records that show them to be the best in their class.

When You Issue Prescriptions in Writing or by Telephone

- When prescribing for outpatient use, slow down a little and give the pharmacist time to write. ALWAYS give both the brand and generic name, as this makes sense and can help YOU avoid a lawsuit arising from a sound-alike error. Consider the advantage of including both the name of the drug and the therapeutic indication (the patient's disorder) on the prescription label—for example, Vioxx (rofecoxib) for arthritis. Putting the disorder on the label will help (1) reduce dispensing errors caused by look-alike and sound-alike drug names and (2) prevent confusion that often occurs during concurrent use of multiple drugs, especially among the elderly: mistaken identity of drug and purpose, mistakenly altered dosing schedules, etc. Pain is now the fifth vital sign and a focus of new JCAHO guidelines. If you work in a system where inpatient care is provided by hospitalists, be aware that they will in essence be charting the outcomes of YOUR outpatient pain management.

- Respect your patients' wishes as to whether they *want* the name of the disorder written on the prescription label. If they prefer you not include it, recommend that they write it on the label themselves *after* the prescription is filled.
- Keep dosing schedules as simple as possible. Once-a-day dosing improves adherence.
- Alert the pharmacist to look-alike and sound-alike drug names. Print the drug name and generic name on written prescriptions. Spell the drug name and include the generic name when prescribing by telephone.

When Counseling Patients About Drug Therapy

- ALWAYS emphasize the critical nature of adherence. If your patients are adherence-challenged, talk about pillboxes, bottle reminders, and even pager-based systems to make sure that they will take their medicines. Briefly explain the nature of the patient's disorder and its treatment. Use language that is readily understood by the average person. I've often found clinicians using language that is barely understood by the average doctor. If you use words that are on a sixth-grade level, you'll often have a patient colleague working to achieve the goals of treatment. The patient-profiler component of the American Heart Association Web site offers patients balanced information on CAD and CHF, hypertension, arrhythmia and other conditions, repeat e-mail messages, and a real chance at continuing risk-lowering behaviors. Consider encouraging your office patients as a chance to get objective information and behavior reinforcement while they are in your office.
- Provide written information or references for educational material about the disorder. If the disorder is chronic in nature (diabetes, hypertension), explain the need to continue drug therapy indefinitely, possibly for life. It's no surprise that patients are visiting the Internet. Provide helpful Web sites (see Table 17) that give balanced information. Explain that some pharmaceutical company-provided sites may not give complete information, or may skew data to favor their products.
- Briefly explain the name and nature of the drugs you are prescribing. Again, emphasize the importance of strict adherence with the medicine. It is wise to tell the patient—in advance—about potential adverse effects. The patient who has such effects is more likely to be

understanding and forgiving if they do not come as a surprise. Talk about possible options available if the goals of therapy are not achieved in the expected time frames.

- To supplement your discussion, provide a printed document that summarizes the essential information the patient needs to use the drug(s) safely and effectively. This is comforting and will save you an amazing number of telephone calls and pages. Be sure the patient knows what to do if a dose is missed. Look at an add-on program to your office-management program that prints out relevant information for your patients to take home. Such services can provide detailed descriptions of drugs, general guidelines for drug use, and personalized instructions. Unfortunately, your patient may run into a pill-splitting reality with many medicines. Be aware of what managed-care organizations expect your patient to do. A pill splitter can be an important assurance of correct doses.
- Explain the need for follow-up visits to monitor the effects of drug treatment and the course of the disorder. If possible, empower the patient by self-testing. For example, the glycosylated hemoglobins (hemoglobin A1C) that you order and also give your diabetics better results from their medicines.
- Explain that drugs may not work in practice exactly as expected. Tell the patient to be alert to the possibility that a new symptom or sign *may* be drug related. Certainly tell the patient about probable effects and what to do about them. If one of your patients does experience a novel adverse drug reaction, it is CRITICAL that you (or your designate) call the FDA MedWatch at 1-800-332-1088.
- It is virtually impossible for the FDA to test new medicines against all multiple pill regimens. Calling MedWatch (1-800-332-1088) fulfills your voluntary obligation to Phase Four reporting and makes medication use safer for everyone. I admit that I am the one advocating mandatory reporting. Encourage the patient to call as needed regarding any aspect of drug treatment. Some of this call volume can be successfully shifted to pharmacists trained in specific disease management. Locate these pharmacy centers of excellence and work together to get the best results for your patients. Recognize the need to adjust drug selection and/or dosage regimens to accommodate individual variability.
- Give special attention to the older patient on drug therapy. The elderly (1) generally use multiple drugs concurrently and (2) are more prone to experience adverse drug effects.
- If you refer any of your patients to a specialist, be certain to take a repeat medication history when they are returned to your care. Check for duplications in medicines by cross-referencing brand or generic names.
- Every six months, ask your patients to bring in all the prescription, nonprescription, and herbal medicines that they routinely take. This kind of "brown bag session" can help you best understand all of the potential or actual interactions of therapies your patient is or will be

taking. Remember: An informed patient can be your greatest ally in optimal therapeutics and the outcomes that will be benchmarked!

Suggestions for Containing the Costs of Drug Therapy

- When you have selected the most appropriate drug, consider its cost. Look at Table 21 in this book and direct your patients to balanced and objective Web sites—including the new one from the pharmaceutical manufacturers at *www.helpingpatients.org*. While we finally have a Medicare prescription drug bill, we still need to get the most from the medicines that are prescribed. Studies performed in Canada with its socialized medicine system (see Avorn, J., in Sources) tells us that simply giving the medicines away does NOT get the best results. If the patient requests an available generic product, direct the pharmacist to dispense one with certified bioequivalence. Because of generic product variability, caution the patient to have the prescription refilled with the identical generic (same manufacturer) each time.
- Avoid polypharmacy whenever possible. Limit the number of drugs that the patient is taking concurrently to the fewest required. Do not let the cure become the disease. Medicate serious, significant disorders; discourage the use of drugs for minor, transient complaints.
- Consider carefully any requests from patients for a prescription drug they have learned about through direct-to-consumer advertising. Explain to your patients the profit motive of the producer and assure them that you will prescribe the drug that, in your judgment, is the most appropriate for them.
- When circumstances permit, use home intravenous drug therapy in preference to hospitalization. If hospitalization is required, explore IV to PO switches and medication streamlining to help appropriately decrease length of stay.
- The move toward managed care and other health care reform initiatives brings increased scrutiny to the outcomes of your therapeutic and clinical decisions. Become more familiar with the expense of various medicinal options, as well as the specific patient populations where the benefit-to-risk and cost-to-outcome ratios make the most sense. Pharmacoeconomic and disease management approaches will bring the best balance of cost and outcome.
- Work with the pharmacy your patients use to create seamless systems. Ask the pharmacy to e-mail your office if patients never fill—or are early or late—with their prescriptions. This gets you the information you need and can prompt a quick follow-up phone call from your office staff to your compliance-challenged patients. Finding out about nonadherence or noncompliance early can help prevent catastrophic events such as stroke or MI.

The Essential Guide to Prescription Drugs

2005 Edition

1

How to Use This Book

When you're sick and finally make that decision to see your doctor, it's probably one of the worst times for you to think about the medicines you take now or even that new prescription. A visit to your doctor's office can be a disconcerting experience. The reality of health care is that time has been contracted, patients may only be considered covered lives, and health care providers face severe time constraints. Becoming a smart patient means being well informed about current national guidelines that help guide treatment options. Take a good look at the new Table 22 in this edition of the guide! Please find out if you are getting proven medicines and the goals of treatment. I can help you become a partner in your health care and will always try to supplement the direction and guidance your doctor will offer about your medicines. This principle is also ascribed to on my Web site (*www.medicineinfo.com*) via the Health on the Net Principles. Just like the site, this Guide seeks to augment, NOT to replace, the role of your doctor.

Your new book is arranged into six sections. The first section offers insight into modern drug therapy and gives you helpful tips on becoming a smart patient. "True Breakthroughs in Medicines" will help identify new medicines that have gained FDA approval or that are the first new agents to treat an existing disease or condition. Section Two gives you detailed Drug Profiles covering more than 2,000 brand-name prescription drugs and nearly 400 widely used generic medicines. Selection of each drug is based on three criteria: the extent of its use, the urgency of the conditions it treats, and the volume and complexity of information essential to its proper use. You'll find that profiles are arranged alphabetically by generic name. Read carefully to be sure you have the correct medicine. Each profile is presented in the same way, and once you become familiar with the format, you'll be able to quickly find specific information on any drug. Unlike other imitators, each Essential Drug

Profile contains up to 45 helpful categories of information. Let me introduce you to the other parts of your new book:

Herbal Medicines or Minerals

Because herbal medicines are so widely used, and have seen some herbals identified as having questionable benefit to risk profiles, I've continued to broaden the section on important possible interactions between herbal and prescription medicines. Please remember that herbal products are not regulated by the FDA as medicines. They fall under the Dietary Supplement Health and Education Act (DSHEA) of 1994. Smart patients then understand that this may mean that specific products have not been well studied—others rely on borrowed science—and certainly that these products can interact with prescription medicines. For example, ephedra (see *www.fda.gov*) has been removed from the market. I've also broadened the data in your new Guide so that you'll find that I'll tell you where combinations between herbs and prescription drugs may make sense, where they do not, and of course how to talk to your doctor before you move forward. This is a very dynamic area, and I'll update this section every year! There may also be information at *www.medicineinfo.com* that can help.

Year Introduced

At first glance, this may seem trivial, but remember, the longer the drug has been in general use, the more likely all of its actions are known and the less likely ongoing use will produce new problems. This will help you identify those medicines that are more likely to be more fully understood both because they have been used for a longer time period and because they have been widely used.

Drug Class

Drug classes are like families—in fact, some of the profiles giving information about medicines from the same class have been arranged into Medication Family Profiles. Many actions, reactions, and interactions with other drugs are often shared by drugs of the same class. For example, *if you are allergic to one member of the cephalosporin family, you most likely will be allergic to a second cephalosporin. By the same logic, if a medicine in a certain class has not helped you, it is likely that a second one from the same class will do you little good*. Pay close attention to this aspect of medicines, since this is an area that often leads to problems or lack of results.

Prescription Required

Just because a medicine does not require a prescription (over-the-counter) does not mean the medicine is weak or is free from possible drug interactions. Remember, over the last 15 years there has been a great shift in medicines from prescription to nonprescription. Current examples include medicines for yeast infections, patches and gum to help you stop smoking, as well as ulcer medicines (histamine H2 blockers) that can also be used to prevent or treat heartburn. Virtually all of these medicines were previously available only by prescription. Always mention nonprescription medicine use when asked about the "medicines" you take.

Controlled Drug

The Controlled Substances Act of 1970 assigned medicines with a potential for abuse to a specific schedule in the United States. A Canadian schedule is also given when applicable. A description of the schedules of controlled drugs is found at the back of your Guide.

Available for Purchase by Generic Name

In general, costs can be reduced by buying a generic equivalent of a brand-name product. The key word is "equivalent." It is important to make sure that "bioavailability and bioequivalence"—the comparative composition, quality, and effectiveness of the generic versus the brand-name drug product—are the same if a substitution is made. Further discussion of bioavailability and bioequivalence may be found in Section Five, the Glossary of Drug-Related Terms.

Brand Names

I realize that generic or chemical names of medicines can be complicated, so brand names are given to help. Brand names are listed for the United States and for Canada (✽). A combination drug (one with more than one active ingredient) is identified by [CD] following the brand name. Be careful! In some cases THE SAME NAME used in both the United States and Canada will represent entirely different generic drugs (in a single drug product) or a significantly different mixture of generic medicines. If you travel between the two countries, make sure that the brand-name drug contains the same generic medicine(s).

Benefits versus Risks

The possible pros and cons for each drug are summarized. Capital letters emphasize the drug's principal benefits and risks, while lowercase letters are used for less critical benefits and risks. One look reveals the "comparative weights" of the two columns and gives a first impression about how a drug's benefits relate to its potential risks. This is meant to help you become more circumspect in your use of medicines—but is not to be the sole basis for deciding whether to use a drug. I find that the triad of failure to individualize drug selection and dose, failure to communicate goals of treatment, and lack of an effective system to repeatedly check, encourage, and follow up on how well people take their medicines (adherence) is the greatest weakness in current drug therapy and health care.

Principal Uses

A drug may be available as a single drug product or in combination with other drugs. The "As a Single Drug Product" section tells you the primary use(s) of the drug when it is used alone in a particular product. The "As a Combination Drug Product [CD]" section tells about the primary use(s) when an active medicine is combined with other drugs in the same pill. The uses are a consensus of the medical community and reflect current research. Where appropriate, the logic for combining certain drugs is explained.

Widely Used Guidelines That Involve This Medicine (A NEW SECTION!)

Sadly, the underuse of proven medicines continues to be a problem despite several national attempts to solve this treatment gap. In a survey of more than 1,000 women that was performed by the authors of the new update on preventing heart disease in women—only 38 percent of those women surveyed had ever been asked about heart disease by their doctors. Heart disease is the leading killer of women—how many women got proven medicines that might have prevented a first or second heart attack?

My thinking in creating this new section is to give you a sampling of reliable places (both national organization 800 number or, at least, their phone number, Web address, and current place on the Web site) where you can find national treatment guidelines that can help you figure out if you are getting proven medicines. They can also help you work with your doctor to see how the specific medicine might help you!

In the Pipeline

We all want to know the future. This section has been updated from its first appearance in the 2004 edition to try to bring you information about new diseases or conditions for which a medicine in the Guide is being studied. I'll do my best to fill you in on FDA applications that have been filed, research projects that have been publicized, or where preliminary research has been published. This section will not be present for every medicine, but will hopefully work to make you aware of progress that is being made and when results might be expected!

How This Drug Works

This section tells what a drug does to work. If a specific method of action has not been established, I will tell you about the current theory. This can be important in the sense that if you are taking two medicines that work in the same way or act on the same system, better combination therapy may be available.

Available Dosage Forms and Strengths

This gives you available manufacturers' dosage forms (tablets, capsules, elixirs, etc.) and strengths, without company identification. Dosage forms limited to hospital use are often not included. The section Dosage Forms and Strengths in the Glossary can help with those few abbreviations used to describe strengths of each dosage form.

Usual Adult Dosage Ranges

Dosing information represents a consensus by appropriate authorities and is the currently recommended standard. It is a guide showing how much of the drug can reasonably be expected to be both effective and safe. Under certain circumstances, your doctor may decide to modify the "standard" dose. Some dosage forms not covered (for example, extemporaneously made suppositories) may require different doses than those listed because of absorption at different routes.

Conditions Requiring Dosing Adjustments

Medical conditions can actually change the effect a medicine has on your body (technically called a drug-disease interaction). This fact is often missed in choosing a dose or in deciding how often a medicine should be taken (dosing interval)—and can lead to problems. For example, people over age 60 usually have an expected or "normal" age-related decline in kidney function. Throughout this book I refer to this as kidney compromise. What this means is that medicines removed by the kidneys may stay in the body longer than expected (increased half-life)—not because the kidneys are diseased but because they simply do not work as well as they used to. The real possible effect of this increased half-life is that a typically prescribed dose could in reality amount to an overdose. While the exact age when this decline starts may vary, it is critical for people at or near 60 to ask their doctors if any prescribed medicine is removed by the kidneys, and if the dose or dosing interval has been adjusted for this kidney compromise. I also include information on liver compromise (where appropriate) as well as information on other prevalent diseases or conditions that may impact dosing.

Dosing Instructions

Food and medicines can fight. Foods can actually change how much medicine gets into your body (increasing or decreasing absorption)—and this section tells you about them. Medicines can also irritate the lining of the stomach or intestines, and food can help ease this irritation. The dosing instruction section will also tell you about advisability of changing the form of the medicine itself. For example, sometimes, when medicine is urgently needed, you may have to crush the tablet or open the capsule and mix the contents with a food or beverage. On the other hand, many medicines should NEVER be crushed or altered to be taken. This information category identifies those forms of each drug that may be changed and those that should not be. A new feature of this section provides information on what to do if you forget your pill. If you are still uncertain—call your doctor. Another caveat on this: If you find yourself forgetting often, talk to your doctor and see if there is a medicine that might give the same benefits but not require so many doses! A good example is in the management of high blood pressure. Many patients may get great results from a newer medicine taken once or twice a day instead of one that has to be taken more frequently. There are also many reminder systems—including beepers—to help you take control of your disease or condition by taking your medicine right on time.

Usual Duration of Use

Many factors determine how long a medicine must be taken. This is often an area of great controversy and patient confusion. Factors such as the nature and severity of symptoms, drug form and strength, ability of the patient to respond, and use of other drugs come into play here. Some situations such as increased cholesterol or hyperlipidemia will need to be treated on an ongoing basis. It is always prudent to check results as well as problems on a regular basis. The main idea is for you and your clinician to give the medicine an appropriate amount of time to reach the goals of therapy, and to adjust the dose or even add or change the medicine if goals are not reached within the expected period of time. Where important, limitations in how long a medicine should be taken are outlined in this section.

Typical Treatment Goals and Measurements: (Outcomes and Markers)

Smart patients know the goals and actively work with their doctor to achieve them! One of the hallmarks of a good clinician lies in how well he or she sets and communicates, and then prescribes or adjusts, medicines to realize the goals of therapy. Unfortunately, I've often found this aspect of care to be sorely lacking. In order to help you understand what some reasonable expectations from treatment are, I've included typical goals, measurements, and results in ALL of this year's profiles. For example, the entries below pertain to blood sugar and cholesterol-lowering medicines that are taken by mouth.

- Blood Sugar: The general goal for blood sugar is to return it to the usual "normal" range (generally 70–120 mg/dL), while avoiding risks of excessively low blood sugar. One study (UKPDS) used a fasting plasma sugar (glucose) of less than 108 mg/dL.
- Cholesterol: The National Institutes of Health (NIH) has released ATP III—a current set of guidelines for treating people at risk for heart disease. This National Cholesterol Education Program (NCEP) effort has some changes versus the Adult Treatment Panel (ATP-2). Importantly, diabetes was added to the list of conditions that lead to increased heart disease risk. Total cholesterol targets remain at less than 200 mg/dL, but the guidelines recommend testing for the various components of

total cholesterol, such as low-density lipoproteins (LDL) and high-density lipoproteins (HDL). New designations list 100 mg/dL of LDL to be optimal (less than 70 mg/dL for very high risk people), 130–159 as borderline high, 160 mg as high, and 190 mg/dL as very high. A new focus has been placed on HDL, making the "too low" reading as 40 mg/dL for this "good" cholesterol. Because of all of these changes, instead of just a total cholesterol, ATP-3 suggests a lipid panel!

I hope that this feature on goals will let you be more involved in your health care, and will also encourage you to ask questions if the goals of your medicines are not achieved.

This Drug Should Not Be Taken If

These entries are the absolute contraindications to the use of the drug (see Contraindication in the Glossary). By consensus, these are circumstances where the medicine should NEVER be taken. Tell your doctor immediately if any information in this category applies to you.

Inform Your Physician Before Taking This Drug If

These entries tell you relative contraindications to a medicine. One way to think of this is as a relative benefit-to-risk decision. Again, tell your physician or other prescriber if these factors apply to you. For example, if you are taking a corticosteroid-type medicine and have unexplained hip or shoulder pain, it may be a sign of something more serious that should be evaluated.

Possible Side Effects

Here you can learn about natural, expected, and usually unavoidable medicine actions—the normal and anticipated consequences of taking it. This gives a realistic perspective, balancing side effects with goals of treatment. I emphasize that these are POSSIBLE side effects.

Possible Adverse Effects

These are unusual, unexpected, and infrequent drug effects that are often called adverse drug reactions or effects. These range from mild to serious. In order to more accurately define how frequently these effects happen, I've developed the following approach:

- Possible: An effect that has been documented for other drugs in the same family but not the profiled drug. Also assigned when the effect occurs in some limited patient populations and not in others.
- Case Reports: An effect that has been documented to happen, but has been seen only in isolated cases.
- Rare: An effect that is seen in less than 2 percent of patients. Another way to look at this is that 98 percent of people will take the medicine and NOT have the effect.

- Infrequent: An effect that is seen in 2 to 10 percent of patients.
- Frequent: Effects that happen in more than 10 percent of patients.

Smart patients talk to their doctor if they suspect they may be having an adverse drug effect. Serious adverse reactions may start with mild, unthreatening symptoms, and serious problems may be avoided if you call right away. It's also possible to have an adverse reaction that has not yet been reported. Don't discount an adverse effect just because it's not listed. *A properly selected drug usually has a comparatively small chance of producing serious harm.* Knowing that a drug can cause a serious adverse reaction should not deter you from using it when it has been properly selected and its use will be carefully supervised.

Author's Note: A continuation of a current feature will be found in this section where available: number of patients evaluated for safety. For example: The package insert for Plavix contains a notation: "This drug has been evaluated for safety in more than 17,500 patients at the time of this writing." I'd like you to think of this as a rough measure of how well possible adverse effects from a given medicine might be known. While adverse reactions in general tend to be underreported, a medicine that has been used in 17,500 patients is more likely to have a more fully defined group of possible adverse reactions than a drug only evaluated in 3,500 patients. I'll build more of these details into subsequent editions.

If you have had a reaction to a medicine, make sure to remember to ask that your doctor REPORT THIS REACTION. One problem with our system of medicine surveillance is that reporting of adverse effect of medicines is VOLUNTARY for health care professionals. Less than 3 percent of serious adverse reactions are reported, and this can leave the next family vulnerable to the same undesirable experience. Your doctor (or his/her staff) can call 1-800-FDA-1088 (1-800-332-1088).

Possible Effects on Sexual Function

This information is often NOT something people want to discuss, or something that patients are told about. Currently available information (often inadequate and vague) from all reliable sources is presented. Both physician and patient are well advised to discuss frankly any potential effect that drug therapy could have on sexual expression.

Adverse Effects That May Appear Similar to Natural Diseases or Disorders

Medicines can actually cause effects similar to widely diagnosed diseases or disorders. Quite often this inadvertent error is compounded by prescribing another drug to relieve the "symptoms" of the first. My father was prescribed a medicine for his "arthritis" when he was actually having an adverse effect from a medicine for his heart rhythm. For milder symptoms (e.g., nasal congestion or diarrhea from reserpine), the oversight may not be too serious. But in the case of my father, the mistake was devastating. This section tells you about this common flaw.

Natural Diseases or Disorders That May Be Activated by This Drug

Many drugs can "activate" latent disorders that may not be recognized as drug induced. If a new and seemingly unrelated disorder starts during treatment with any new medicine, ask your doctor if it may be drug related.

Possible Effects on Laboratory Tests

Most drugs have significant effects on body chemistry and organ systems. Some effects are intended and beneficial (therapeutic); others are unintended, unavoidable, and potentially harmful. Timely use of laboratory tests lets us check how well a drug is working, detect early drug toxicity, assign some lab test changes to drug and lab test interactions, and also check the course of the condition being treated.

Caution

This category gives you information on aspects of drug actions and/or drug uses that require special emphasis. Occasionally, this section may actually relate to information provided in other categories. Once again, this is an important feature this Guide offers to help you take care of your family.

Precautions for Use: Infants and Children

Doses often MUST be changed for infants and children under 12 years of age, and some drugs and/or treatment situations call for special precautions. When administering any prescription or over-the-counter drug, it is best to ask your doctor or pharmacist about needed precautions. New FDA regulations will now require study of medicines in children where the drugs are specifically used in children.

Precautions for Use: Those Over 60 Years of Age

Our bodies do not remain the same over time, and people show age at different rates and in different ways. Assessment of "age" must be based upon individual mental and physical condition, and never on years alone. Changes that accompany aging may affect the actions of the body on the drug, actions of the drug on the body—and even how well the medicine is removed. Appropriate precautions are outlined in this category.

Advisability of Use During Pregnancy: Pregnancy Category

Information about safe use of a particular drug during pregnancy was one of the most forceful concerns that led to the formal petitioning of the

Food and Drug Administration in 1975 to make sure that information was disclosed to the public. The FDA definitions of the five pregnancy categories are listed at the back of this book. The FDA does not make the initial category assignment; this is the responsibility of the manufacturer that markets the drug. The initial designation is then subject to review and modification by the FDA. The "Pregnancy Category" designations presented in each profile were determined after thorough review of pertinent literature and consultation with appropriate authorities. They are offered at this time for initial guidance only. They may not be "official" and may not have the endorsement of either the manufacturer or the FDA. If controversy exists among researchers or manufacturers, you may find more than one pregnancy category for the same medicine.

Advisability of Use if Breast-Feeding

This section tells you about effects of the drug on milk production. You will also learn if the drug goes into human milk, and the possible effects of the drug on the nursing infant. Prudent recommendations are given where appropriate. Also included are impacts of disease where appropriate.

Suggested Periodic Examinations While Taking This Drug

Getting the best results from your medicines often means that your doctor may ask you to get tests while you take the drug(s) he or she has prescribed. Which exams and when they are made depend on your past and present medical history, the nature of the condition being treated, the dose and duration of drug use, and your doctor's observations of your response. For example, checking finger-stick blood sugar and fructosamine or hemoglobin A1C while taking an oral glucose-lowering (oral hypoglycemic) medicine is critical. On the other hand, there may be many occasions when your doctor decides no examinations are necessary. Always tell your doctor about all developments you think may be drug related.

While Taking This Drug, Observe the Following:
Herbal Medicines or Minerals

Since many millions of people are taking herbal medicines as well as minerals, I think it is critical to tell you about herbs and prescription or nonprescription medicines—particularly given the action of the FDA in suspending sales of ephedra (see medications removed from the market in Table 16). I've tried to bring you timely data that tells about possible harmful combinations as well as situations where herbal medicines can actually increase beneficial effects of some prescription drugs. Complementary and beneficial use of herbal medicines may allow for lower prescription drug doses (this may be very beneficial, since it may also help you avoid side effects). Smart patients DO NOT ASSUME that because it's herbal, it's natural and will not interact with other medicines. Because new prescription drug–herbal medicine interactions are always being discovered, NEVER combine any herbal or prescription or nonprescription drug without first talking to your pharmacist and doctor. The URLs of some helpful Web sites are included in the tables near the end of this book.

While Taking This Drug, Observe the Following: Marijuana Smoking

The widespread "social" use of marijuana by virtually all age groups and the approval of medicinal smoking of marijuana in two states have led to inquiries about interactions between the active chemicals in marijuana smoke and medicines in common use. Currently available literature on the health aspects of marijuana use contains very little practical information concerning the potential for drug interactions. The limited information presented in this category of selected Drug Profiles represents those possible interactions considered likely to occur in view of the known pharmacological effects of the principal components of marijuana and of the medicine reviewed in the profile. In most instances, the interaction statements are not based on documented evidence, since very little is available. The conclusions stated—derived by logical inductive reasoning—represent the concurrence of authorities with expertise in this field. There is a well-designed study of medical marijuana use under way at the time of this writing.

While Taking This Drug, Observe the Following: Other Drugs

Medicines can fight and smart patients know this. While interactions can be a confusing and often controversial area of drug information, it is critical and is divided into five subcategories of possible interactions between drugs. Look carefully at the wording of each subcategory heading (see also Interaction in Glossary). Some of the drugs listed do not have a representative profile. If you are using one of these drugs, ask your doctor or pharmacist for help about potential interactions. A brand name (or names) that follows the generic name of an interacting drug is given as an example only. It is not intended to mean that the particular brand(s) named has interactions that are different from other brands of the same generic drug. If you are taking the generic drug, all brand names under which it is marketed MUST be considered as possible interactants. Medicines in the same or similar families may also interact.

Driving, Hazardous Activities

Clearly, medicines can change coordination and alertness. The information in this category applies not just to driving motor vehicles but to any activity of a dangerous nature, such as operating machinery, working on ladders, using power tools, and handling weapons. Your individual response and degree of reaction may vary from the way others react. Talk with your doctor or pharmacist if you take a medicine that may impair your abilities.

Aviation

Military pilots enjoy the expert guidance and surveillance provided by the flight surgeon, but no tightly structured control system exists for their civilian counterparts. The need for practical information regarding the possible effects of medicinal drugs on flight performance, however, is the same for pilots in all settings. This section can tell civilian pilots how a particular drug may affect their eligibility to fly and when it is advisable or necessary to consult a designated Aviation Medical Examiner or an FAA medical officer.

Occurrence of Unrelated Illness

Some medicines—for instance, "oral hypoglycemics" such as glipizide— require careful regulation of doses to maintain a constant drug effect within critical limits. In this section of your book, emphasis is given to those illnesses that might affect drug use. For example, if a body-wide infection were to occur, the oral hypoglycemic dose may not work and insulin injections may be temporarily required in order to maintain blood sugar in an appropriate range.

Discontinuation

How and when to stop a medicine are often as important as starting a medicine in the first place. Unfortunately, this aspect of drug use is often overlooked when a medicine is first discussed. Your doctor should always approach treatment with medicines with specific goals and time frames to reach those goals when the medicine is FIRST started, for example, reducing a blood pressure of 159/93 to 120/75 in two months using a particular medicine. Additionally, it is often mandatory that patients be fully informed on when to discontinue, when not to discontinue, and precisely how to stop use of the drug. In some cases, when one medicine is stopped, other drugs being taken at the same time may also need to be adjusted. The doctor who is primarily responsible for your overall medicine management must be kept informed of all the drugs you are taking at a given time and if and when any of them are stopped.

I believe that the remaining information categories in the Drug Profiles are self-explanatory, but I always welcome your letters and questions. My Web site is *www.medicineinfo.com.*

Section Three is called "The Leading Edge" and offers what are, in my opinion, medicines that show great promise and are just over the horizon from FDA approval. Some of these medicines may not actually be approved, but they give such significant hope that they're worth consideration. The information may let patients facing serious diseases ask to be included in scientific studies and get the medicine prior to actual approval.

Section Four is a presentation of Drug Classes arranged alphabetically by their chemical or therapeutic (generic) class. Because of chemical composition and biological activities, some drugs appear in two or more classes. For example, the drug product with the brand name Diuril will be represented by its generic name, chlorothiazide, in three drug classes: the Thiazide Diuretics (a chemical classification), the Diuretics (a drug action classification), and the Antihypertensives (a disease-oriented classification). Please use the Drug Classes to your advantage. I can't count the number of times I've seen busy physicians discover an allergy or problem with a particular medicine only to turn right around and prescribe a medicine from the same class. This section can protect you from this kind of error.

Frequently in the Drug Profiles in Section Two you are advised to "see [a particular] Drug Class." This alerts you to a possible drug contraindication, or to possible interactions with certain foods, alcohol, or other drugs. In each case, you can find the more readily recognized brand names for each drug listed generically within a drug class by looking at the appropriate Drug Profile. Timely use of these references can help you avoid many possible hazards of medication.

Section Five is a Glossary of Drug-Related Terms used throughout the book. Smart patients understand the language of medicines. The preferred use of each term is explained. Frequent references to the Glossary are made in the Drug Profiles. Use of the Glossary will help you understand how to recognize and interpret significant drug effects.

Section Six offers tables of drug and other information. The title and introductory description explain the content and purpose of each table. The tables give you another source of ready reference. I've included a Medication Map as Table 15 because it is a way for you to use your doctor's or pharmacist's expertise to arrange all of the medicines you take into a reasonable schedule. It is also something I strongly advocate that you take to the hospital with you. If a new prescription or medicine is to be given, make sure that the prescriber knows about all of the "pills" you presently take. When it's time to go home from the hospital or to leave your doctor's office, take the time to have them help you get the most from your medicines.

Table 16 identifies medicines that have been removed from the market. This may help protect you from medicines that may still be available in other countries (or on the Internet) and not available on U.S. shelves. Please use the index of brand and generic names in the back of the book. It is a single alphabetical listing that provides page references to the appropriate Drug Profile(s) for all drugs found in this book. Read the introductory explanation of the special features of this combined index.

Because of the explosion of information on the Internet, I've also updated a table that tells you the URLs of a number of Web sites that I have found to be objective and valuable (Table 17). Regard the Internet cautiously and know where to look for objective information. If you decide to buy medicines from the Net, make sure you have a prescription from your doctor and are then buying from a reputable company. Much has been heard this year about counterfeit medicines. You can actually call the National Association of Boards of Pharmacy at 847-698-6227 or visit them on the Web at *www.nabp.net* and find out if a site really does belong to a licensed pharmacy.

A clear trend in health care is the development of instruments and home test kits that can let patients themselves screen and even test and track serious illnesses. I've detailed some of the devices you are more likely to see in Table 18: Smart Patients and Home Test Kits. Work with your doctor, pharmacist, or nurse practitioner to reach an agreement on which device or test makes sense for you.

Heart disease accounts for the greatest death toll of WOMEN and MEN in the United States. How do you know if you are at risk? It is clearly a role for doctors to explain which ones apply, but I believe that it is critical that smart patients recognize risk factors and gain control of them. Table 19 will work with you to give you knowledge and power. The next step is to discuss risk factors with your doctor and figure out an individualized plan for what to do about them. The next table will also help you gain power over your heart!

One of the broadest set of national guidelines are the ones called NCEP ATP III. Let me put that in English: National Cholesterol Education Program Adult Treatment Panel, number three. The changes versus the early version NCEP ATP II are detailed on my Web site at *www.medicineinfo.com*. Table 20 describes various lifestyle changes that you can make that have been proven to help reduce risk of heart disease and stroke.

"How am I going to afford these medicines?" We all know that medicines can be very expensive when you add up the total bill on an ongoing basis. Table 21, How to Get Help with the Cost of Medicines (Programs and Web Sites), was a great new addition in 2004, and I hope it will continue be a great help while the Medicare prescription drug program continues to be phased in. In this table I've made a list of some successful strategies that are reasonable; listed the names, numbers, patient assistance programs, and other approaches to get help. You'll also find Web sites that I've found to be balanced and objective; and have identified sources that you may not have thought of—yet may be entitled to. It's very interesting that the Medicare prescription drug program will make use of some of these programs as a stopgap measure until the full program is developed. This may be one of the most useful tables in the book!

Table 22, Important National Guidelines, is a great new addition in 2005! I've created it in order to help you and your family try to figure out if you are getting proven medicines. I hope it will be a help in starting and continuing those treatments that can give you or a loved one the best chance of getting well and staying well!

2

Guidelines for Safe and Effective Drug Use; or How to Become a Smarter Patient

MEDICINES AND PHARMACY ON THE INTERNET

We all get a lot of spam e-mails—many of which offer outrageous claims and unfortunately, controlled substances without a prescription. There has been a virtual explosion of e-mails, advertisements, health claims, prescriptionless drug ordering, and even pharmacies on the Internet. While some aspects are covered in the Do and Do Not sections, I think this subject is important enough to focus on it separately. Mergers and changes in scope of service have occurred in pharmacy, as they have in other businesses. Amidst the change, there are still some common characteristics of appropriate pharmacies and medicines on the Internet. Smart patients know that at a minimum these include:

- The pharmacy site requires a prescription for a prescription medicine and provides a way for you to prove that you have one. Given the present state of the Internet, it appears prudent to stick with "known" companies. The largest current online pharmacies are *walgreens.com* and *cvs.com.*
- The site requires a medication history. This history should include allergies, current weight and height, and illnesses as well as ALL prescription and nonprescription medications and herbal or nutritional supplements you are currently taking. This ensures that you will be

15

getting appropriate pharmaceutical care (checking your medicines for interactions, errors, appropriate doses, etc.).

- Information on the site is referenced. This is critical; much of the Internet is unregulated. You should look for footnotes, endnotes, or parenthetical references or organization references placed appropriately relative to the information you have read. If such notes are not present, the information may be untrue, opinion, or inappropriately slanted. Make sure to talk to the person who prescribed any medicines for you BEFORE you make any changes based on information not provided by that prescriber—even from a well-referenced source.

- A statement disclosing how, with which references, and by whom your current prescription and any existing prescriptions will be checked for accuracy, possible drug interactions, and appropriate disease-, age-, or condition-related dosing changes. The site will also provide a way to talk to a human about questions about your medicines and possible adverse effects.

- Medicines arrive in an appropriate, labeled container that has any needed auxiliary labels on it as well. Please make sure to ask that the disease or condition being treated by the medicine is included on the label.

- Medicines can be obtained by anyone and can be shipped from anywhere. Unfortunately, not everyone has your best interests at heart. There have been a lot of news stories about counterfeit medicines— fake drugs or water substituted for expensive treatments. A real pharmacy with a board to inspect it and help ensure quality is a great idea. You can call the National Association of Boards of Pharmacy at 847-698-6227 or visit them on the Web at *www.nabp.net* to find out if a site really does belong to a licensed pharmacy.

- Information is a powerful ally when you are taking any medicine. When you look for information on a site, check to be sure that site has a date and date-revised section. This tells you that information is being reviewed and kept current.

SMART PATIENTS DO NOT

- ORDER A PRESCRIPTION MEDICINE FROM THE INTERNET WITHOUT A PRESCRIPTION. EVEN IF YOU CAN GET THE MEDICINE, YOU WON'T HAVE THE BENEFIT OF YOUR DOCTOR'S, PHARMACIST'S, OR NURSE PRACTITIONER'S TRAINING TO HELP PROTECT YOU. THIS CAN BE A PRESCRIPTION FOR DISASTER. YOU ALSO OFTEN HAVE NO WAY OF KNOWING THAT WHAT IS SUPPOSED TO BE IN THE PILL IS ACTUALLY WHAT IS THERE. COUNTERFEIT MEDICINES (PARTICULARLY EXPENSIVE FORMULATIONS) HAVE BEEN REPEATEDLY DOCUMENTED;

- automatically trust information that they get over the Internet. Appropriate information has references and at least a byline of a reputable person. If you find information that is troubling to you, talk to your doctor or pharmacist before you act on that information;

- pressure their doctor to prescribe drugs that, in his or her judgment, they do not need. A pill is not always the answer;
- blindly accept care from any provider. Ask your HMO or medical group how their results or outcomes compare to other groups in the area and the country;
- assume that all doctors know all the drugs they take. Always ask your doctor or pharmacist BEFORE combining any other medicine with medicines already prescribed;
- accept a stapled prescription bag. ALWAYS OPEN a stapled bag, check the brief patient information that may be inside the bag, and make sure you understand it. If there is a Med Guide with the prescription, read that carefully as well. While you are in the pharmacy, read the prescription label and make sure it makes sense. Look at the pills, and (especially on refill drugs) check to see that they look the same as they did before. On new prescriptions, ask that the prescription be checked to make sure it is the correct medicine;
- take prescription drugs on their own or on the advice of friends and neighbors because their symptoms are "just like theirs." Drug therapy must be individualized, based on liver and/or kidney function, medicines you currently take, and many other factors;
- offer drugs prescribed for THEM to anyone else without a physician's guidance;
- change the dose or timing of any drug without the advice of their physician (except when the drug appears to be causing adverse effects);
- leave it to a guess that they've taken their medicine. ALWAYS get a dosing calendar or make one so that you can check off each dose as you take it. There are also a huge variety of helpful technologies such as pillboxes, key fobs, phone reminders, and other great tools. Talk with your pharmacist to find out more!
- continue to take a drug that they feel is causing problems, until they are able to talk with their doctor;
- store their medicines in a bathroom medicine cabinet. This is often an area of high humidity, which can (even though the bottle is closed) enter the medicine and degrade the active drug. Select a lockable kitchen cabinet out of reach of children;
- take any drug (prescription or nonprescription) while pregnant or nursing an infant until they talk to their doctor or pharmacist. Many herbal combinations may have active ingredients similar to those found in prescription medicines;
- take any more medicines than are absolutely necessary. (The greater the number of drugs taken at the same time, the greater the likelihood of adverse effects or interactions.);
- withhold from their doctor information about previous prescription or nonprescription drug use. He or she will want to know what has helped and what has caused problems;
- take any drug in the dark. Identify every dose of medicine carefully in adequate light to be certain you are taking the intended drug;
- in general, store drugs on a bedside table. In the dark and in a sleepy

state, it's easy to get confused. Drugs for emergency use, such as nitroglycerin, are an exception. It is best to have only one such drug at the bedside for use during the night.

SMART PATIENTS DO

- visit the FDA Web site at *www.fda.gov* on a regular basis to check medicines removed from the market and other press releases. Many parts of this site are now consumer friendly. Checking your medicines to make sure you are not continuing to take a medicine that has been removed from the market (see Table 16) is prudent;
- talk with their doctor about the results or outcomes expected from any medicine being considered. Understand that taking the medicine EXACTLY as it is prescribed is critical. Missing one pill in a three-times-a-day regimen may cause you to lose the benefits of all of the medicine;
- talk with their HMO or medical group every year about how their results or outcomes compare to other providers of health care in the area and in the country. This is especially important for businesses, because the preferred provider they choose impacts the health of many people;
- ask their HMO or medical group or pharmacy what their disease management programs are and how any specific disease or condition that they may have is addressed within the scope of their disease management plan. Find out how the results or outcomes of the program compare with other programs in the area or the country;
- know the name (and correct spelling) of the drug(s) they are taking. It is best to know both the brand name and the generic name;
- understand that finding information on the Internet is often only a starting point. Make sure you openly talk to your doctor before you take any action regarding medicines because you saw something on the Net;
- open the prescription bag and the bottle WHILE THEY ARE STILL IN THE PHARMACY. This will give you a chance to best use the training and experience of your pharmacist and will also let you make sure you understand how to best take your medicine. If the prescription is a refill, make sure the pills are the same as the ones originally prescribed. If they are not, ask why;
- read the package labels of all nonprescription drugs so that they know what is in them. This is especially critical when you realize that many of these medicines have names that do not reflect all of the active compounds that are in them;
- take the medicine exactly as prescribed. If you think there will be a change in your ability to take the medicine, call your doctor before you make any change. For example, taking one dose of a medicine that should be taken three times a day often will NOT give one third of the desired effect. I've been asked this kind of question often. Taking a medicine less frequently than prescribed will often give no beneficial

effects, especially for those medicines that require a relatively constant blood level to work;

- put a dosing calendar or a reminder note on the refrigerator or near their car keys. Get a watch with an alarm and set it for the times when you need to take your medicine;
- thoroughly shake all liquid suspensions of drugs to ensure uniform distribution of ingredients;
- use a standardized measuring device for giving liquid medicines by mouth. The household "teaspoon" varies greatly in size;
- follow their doctor's advice on dietary or other measures designed to help the prescribed drugs work their best. For example, decreasing or eliminating salt when taking high blood pressure medicines may help you achieve desired drug effects with smaller doses;
- tell their anesthesiologist, surgeon, and dentist of *all* drugs they are taking, before any surgery;
- tell their doctor if they become pregnant while taking any drugs from any source;
- keep a written record of *all* drugs (prescription and nonprescription), vaccines, and herbal remedies they take during their entire pregnancy— name, dose, dates taken, and reasons for use;
- keep a written record of *all* drugs (and vaccines) to which they have become allergic or have an adverse reaction to. This should be done for each member of the family, especially the elderly or infirm;
- keep a written record of *all* drugs (and vaccines) to which their children become allergic or experience an adverse reaction to;
- fill out "Your Personal Drug Profile" (Table 14). Put the New National Poison Control Center number (1-800-222-1222) by your telephone today. The worst time to try to find an emergency number is while there is a dire need for it. Fill in the Medication Map (Table 15) and ask your doctor if the times selected and combinations of medicines are appropriate;
- tell their doctor of all known or suspected allergies, especially allergies to drugs. Be sure that allergies are a part of your medical record. People with allergies are four times more prone to drug reactions;
- call their doctor immediately they think they are having an overdose, side effect, or adverse effect from a drug;
- ask if it is safe to drive a car, operate machinery, or engage in other hazardous activities while taking the drug(s) prescribed;
- ask if it is safe to drink alcoholic beverages while taking the drug(s) prescribed. We often forget that alcohol is a drug with its own pharmacology and drug-drug interactions;
- find out if any particular foods, beverages, or other prescription or nonprescription medicines should be avoided while taking the drug(s) prescribed;
- keep all appointments for follow-up examinations or laboratory tests;
- ask for help to understand any point that confuses them. If you are concerned about remembering information or instructions for use, ask for written materials;

- throw away all outdated drugs. Couple this with an annual visit to the medicine cabinet;
- ask their doctor if a prescribed medicine offers the best balance of cost and outcomes for them;
- store all drugs out of the reach of children. This is critical for those of you with grandchildren who visit frequently.

PREVENTING ADVERSE DRUG REACTIONS

Smart patients know that it is always better to prevent a condition or disease than to have to treat it. This is especially true in the case of adverse drug reactions where the cure can become the disease. As our understanding of drug actions and reactions has expanded, we have learned that many adverse effects are, to some extent, predictable and preventable. Eleven contributing factors are now well recognized:

Previous Adverse Reaction to a Drug

People who have had an adverse drug reaction in the past are more likely to have adverse reactions to other drugs, even though the drugs are unrelated. This suggests that some people may have a genetic (inborn) predisposition to unusual or abnormal drug responses. Always tell your doctor about any history of prior adverse drug experiences.

Allergies

Some people are allergic by nature (have hay fever, asthma, eczema, hives) and are more likely to develop allergies to drugs. The allergic patient must be watched very closely when medicines are used. Known drug allergies must be written in the medical record. The patient must tell every health care provider that he or she is allergic by nature and is allergic to specific drugs. *Provide this information without waiting to be asked*. Your doctor will then be able to avoid prescribing those drugs that could provoke an allergic reaction, as well as related (cross-sensitivity) drugs.

Contraindications

Both patient and physician must strictly observe contraindications to any drug under consideration. *Absolute contraindications* include those conditions and situations that prohibit the use of the drug for any reason. *Relative contraindications* are those conditions that, in the judgment of the physician, do not preclude the use of the drug but make it essential that special care be given to its use. Often dosing adjustments, additional supportive measures, and close supervision are needed.

Precautions in Use

Patients should know any special precautions needed while taking a drug. This includes advisability of use during pregnancy or while nursing; precautions on sun exposure (or ultraviolet lamps); avoidance of extreme heat or cold; heavy physical exertion (such as with fluoroquinolone antibiotics); and so on.

Dose

It is important to take any medicine exactly as prescribed. *This is most important with drugs that have narrow margins of safety*. Even once-a-day medications should be taken at the same time of day or night to ensure the most constant blood levels. Call your doctor if nausea, vomiting, diarrhea, or other problems interfere with taking your medicine as prescribed.

Interactions

Some drugs can interact with foods (including vitamins and some herbal remedies), alcohol, and other drugs (prescription and nonprescription) to cause serious adverse effects. *The patient must be told about all likely interactants*. If, during the course of treatment, you feel you have discovered a new interaction, tell your doctor so that its full significance can be determined.

Warning Symptoms

Many drugs will cause symptoms that are early warnings of a developing adverse effect: for example, severe headaches or visual disturbances *before* a stroke in a woman taking oral contraceptives. *It is imperative that you know symptoms and signs that could be early warnings of adverse reactions*. The patient is then empowered to act in his or her own behalf by calling the doctor before taking another dose of the medicine. Adverse reactions should be reported to the FDA, following its current guidelines.

Examinations to Monitor Drug Effects

Many drugs in common use can damage vital body tissues (such as bone marrow, liver, kidney, and eye structures)—especially when these drugs are used for a long time or in high doses. Sometimes these adverse effects are not discovered until a newly approved drug has been in wide use for a long time. This damage may be reversible if found quickly. *Cooperate fully with your doctor when he or she asks for periodic exams to check for adverse drug effects*.

Advanced Age and Debility

When we age or as some disease processes progress, vital organs may not work as well and can greatly influence the body's response to drugs. These patients often poorly tolerate drugs with inherent toxic potential and frequently need smaller doses at longer intervals. *The effects of drugs on the elderly and severely ill are often unpredictable*. Great care must be taken to prevent or minimize adverse effects.

Appropriate Drug Choice

The use of any medicine is always a benefit-to-risk decision. The medication used should offer the best balance of overall cost (including lab tests) and outcomes (including quality of life). Many adverse reactions can be prevented if both physician and patient exercise good judgment and restraint.

Polypharmacy

Unfortunately, the cure can become the disease. Patients who are cared for by several physicians may end up with several drugs prescribed separately by more than one physician for different disorders—often without appropriate communication between patient and prescriber. This frequent practice can lead to serious drug–drug interactions. Every patient should routinely talk to each health care provider about all the drugs— prescription and nonprescription—that he or she may be taking. It is mandatory that each prescriber has this information before prescribing additional drugs.

DRUGS AND PEOPLE OVER 65

Smart patients know that growing older is a wonderful thing, particularly when coupled with healthy aging. It is important to realize that regardless of your health status, advancing age brings changes that can alter how you (or I) will react to medicines. For example, an impaired digestive system may interfere with drug absorption. Declines in the ability of the kidney, and in some cases the liver, to remove and to change (metabolize) drugs may lead to toxic drug levels despite a "normal" dose. We slowly lose the ability to maintain "steady state" (or homeostasis) and face increased sensitivity of many tissues to the actions of drugs, even in "normal" drug doses. This has been termed homeostenosis by some clinicians. If aging causes a decline in understanding, memory, vision, or coordination, these patients may not always use drugs safely and effectively. Adverse reactions to drugs occur three times more frequently in the older population. An unwanted drug response can change an independent older person into a confused or helpless patient. For these reasons, drug treatment in the elderly must always be accompanied by the most careful consideration of the individual's health and tolerances. Once-daily dosing may be the only viable option for an individual patient.

Guidelines for the Use of Drugs by People Over 65

- Make sure that drug treatment is needed. Many health problems of the elderly can be managed without the use of drugs. A pill isn't always the answer.
- Avoid (if possible) the use of many drugs at one time.
- Dosing schedules should be as simple as possible. Once a medicine is selected, ask your doctor if a once- or twice-a-day formulation is

available and appropriate. The balance here is convenience versus goals and time frames. For some patients, three doses a day may be required.

- Treatment with most drugs is often best started by using less-than-standard doses. Maintenance doses should be individualized and are often smaller for those over 65 years of age.
- Avoid large tablets and capsules if other dosage forms are available. Liquid forms are easier for the elderly or debilitated to swallow.
- Have all drug containers labeled with the drug name, condition being treated and directions for use in large, easy-to-read letters.
- Ask your pharmacist to package drugs in easy-to-open containers. Avoid childproof caps and stoppers (please remember this decision if grandchildren come to visit).
- Do not take any drug in the dark. Identify each dose of medicine carefully in adequate light to be certain you are taking the intended drug.
- To avoid taking the wrong drug or an extra dose, do not routinely leave medicines on a bedside table. Drugs for emergency use, such as nitroglycerin, are an exception. It is best to have only one such drug at the bedside for use during the night.
- Drug use by older people may require supervision; watch constantly to ensure safe and effective use.
- Smart patients remember the adage: "Start low, go slow, and (when appropriate) learn to say no."

Drugs Best Avoided by the Elderly Because of Increased Possibility of Adverse Reactions (many of the medicines below were found to have been inappropriately prescribed in the most recent check of medication use in this population)

antacids (high sodium)*
barbiturates*
benzodiazepines
cyclophosphamide
diethylstilbestrol
estrogens
indomethacin
(MAO) inhibitors*
oxyphenbutazone
phenacetin
phenylbutazone
(long-acting)
monoamine oxidase-
tetracyclines*

Drugs That Should Be Used by the Elderly in Reduced Dosages Until Full Effect Has Been Determined

anticoagulants (oral)*
antidepressants*
antidiabetic drugs*
antihistamines*
antihypertensives*
anti-inflammatory
  drugs*
barbiturates*
beta-blockers*
carvedilol (Coreg)
colchicine
cortisone-like drugs*
cimetidine
digitalis preparations*
diuretics* (all types)
ephedrine
epinephrine
haloperidol
isoetharine
nalidixic acid
narcotic drugs
prazosin
pseudoephedrine
quinidine
sildenafil (Viagra)
sleep inducers
  (hypnotics)*
terbutaline
thyroid preparations

*See Drug Classes, Section Four.

Drugs That May Cause Confusion and Behavioral Disturbances in the Elderly

acyclovir
albuterol
amantadine
anticholinergics*
antidepressants*
antidiabetic drugs*
antihistamines*
anti-inflammatory
  drugs*
asparaginase
atropine* (and drugs
  containing belladonna)
barbiturates*
benzodiazepines*

beta-blockers*
bromocriptine
carbamazepine
cimetidine
digitalis preparations*
diuretics*
ergoloid mesylates
famotidine
haloperidol
levodopa
meprobamate
methocarbamol
methyldopa
narcotic drugs

nizatidine
pentazocine
phenytoin
primidone
quinidine
ranitidine
reserpine
sedatives
sleep inducers (hyp-
  notics)*
thiothixene
tranquilizers (mild)*
trihexyphenidyl

Drugs That May Cause Orthostatic Hypotension in the Elderly

antidepressants*
antihypertensives*
diuretics* (all types)

neuroleptics*
phenothiazines*
sedatives

selegiline
tranquilizers (mild)*
vasodilators*

Drugs That May Cause Sluggishness, Unsteadiness, and Falling in the Elderly

barbiturates*
beta-blockers*
chlordiazepoxide
clorazepate

diazepam
diphenhydramine
flurazepam
halazepam

methyldopa
prazepam
sleep inducers
  (hypnotics)*

Drugs That May Cause Constipation and/or Retention of Urine in the Elderly

acebutolol
amantadine
amiodarone
androgens
anticholinergics*
antidepressants*
anti-parkinsonism
atropine-like drugs*

calcium
cholestyramine
epinephrine
ergoloid mesylates
famotidine
iron (some forms)
isoetharine
ketorolac

metoclopramide
narcotic drugs
phenothiazines*
ranitidine
sucralfate
terbutaline drugs*

Drugs That May Cause Loss of Bladder Control (Urinary Incontinence) in the Elderly

diuretics*
  (all types)
sedatives

sleep inducers
  (hypnotics)*
tacrine

thioridazine
tranquilizers (mild)*

*See Drug Classes, Section Four.

MEASURING DRUG LEVELS IN BLOOD
(THERAPEUTIC DRUG MONITORING)

People vary greatly in the nature and degree of their responses to medicines, and often, blood levels can help find the best dose. Frequently, the clinical response to a medicine shows that the drug is working as intended. For some drugs, however, especially those with narrow safety margins, toxic reactions may closely resemble the symptoms being treated. In many cases, the patient's expected response is not in keeping with his or her clinical condition.

By measuring blood levels at appropriate times, your doctor or clinical pharmacist can adjust dosing schedules, reduce the risk of toxicity, and achieve the best results or outcomes. These levels also tell the clinician if you've been taking your medicines as prescribed. Some medications require both a peak and trough level to ensure best results, and timing of blood sampling is critical.

In general, sampling should be avoided during the two hours after an oral dose, because during this absorption period, blood levels do not represent tissue levels of the drug, and the tissue is where many medicines actually work. The peak, or highest, level of the drug can measure several things: toxic levels within the body or how effectively bacteria are killed, for instance. The trough, or lowest, level tells how effectively a medicine is cleared from the body between doses. This can also be important, because if too much drug remains, toxicity can result, and if too little stays, it may not work well. Your doctor may also use peak-to-trough ratios to understand how often a particular medicine should be taken.

The following drugs are those most suitable for therapeutic drug monitoring. If you are using any of these on a regular basis, ask your doctor about checking blood levels. Let me remind you that these numbers are ranges where effects are usually seen, but people react differently.

Therapeutic ranges listed are not absolute fixed levels where lack of effect or toxicity definitely occur. One patient may have a therapeutic response at a level lower than the low end of the range while another won't react at all. A blood level higher than the high end of the range is not always toxic but is a level higher than desirable, and dosing changes should be made. Fortunately, most clinicians "treat the patient, not the level." Smart patients know this.

Generic Name/Brand Name	*Blood Level Range*
acetaminophen/Tylenol, etc.	10–20 mcg/mL
amikacin/Amikin	12–25 mcg/mL (peak)
	5–10 mcg/mL (trough)
amiodarone/Cordarone	0.8–2.8 mcg/mL
	(controversial—average level in supraventricular tachyarrhythmias was 1.9 mcg/mL in one study)

Generic Name/Brand Name	Blood Level Range
amitriptyline/Elavil, etc.	
(combined with nortriptyline)	120–250 ng/mL
amoxapine/Asendin	200–500 ng/mL
aspirin (other salicylates)	100–250 mcg/mL
carbamazepine/Tegretol	5–10 mcg/mL
chloramphenicol/Chloromycetin	10–25 mcg/mL
chlorpromazine/Thorazine	50–300 ng/mL
ciprofloxacin/Cipro	0.94–3.4 mcg/mL
clonazepam/Klonopin	10–50 mg/mL
cyclosporine/Sandimmune	100–150 ng/mL
desipramine/Norpramin, Pertofrane	150–300 ng/mL
digitoxin/Crystodigin	15–30 ng/mL
digoxin/Lanoxin	0.5–2.0 ng/mL (historic range)
	0.5–0.8 ng/mL (Heart failure in men, controversial drug in heart failure in women)
diltiazem/Cardizem	0.1–0.4 mcg/mL
disopyramide/Norpace	2.0–4.5 mcg/mL
doxepin/Adapin, Sinequan	100–275 mg/mL
ethosuximide/Zarontin	40–100 mcg/mL
flecainide/Tambocor	0.2–1.0 mcg/mL
flucytosine/Ancobon	50–100 mcg/mL
gentamicin/Garamycin	4.0–10 mcg/mL (peak)
	less than 2 mcg/mL (trough)
gold salts/Auranofin, etc.	1.0–2.0 mcg/mL
imipramine/Janimine, Tofranil, etc.	150–300 ng/mL
kanamycin/Kantrex	25–35 mcg/mL
lidocaine/Xylocaine, etc.	1.4–6.0 mcg/mL
lithium/Lithobid, Lithotabs, etc.	0.3–1.3 mEq/L
mephobarbital/Mebaral	1–7 mcg/mL
methotrexate/Mexate	up to 0.1 mcmol/L
methsuximide/Celontin	up to 1.0 mcg/mL
metoprolol/Lopresor	20–200 ng/mL
mexiletine/Mexitil	0.75–2.0 mcg/mL
nifedipine/Procardia	25–100 ng/mL
nortriptyline/Aventyl, Pamelor	50–150 ng/mL
(combined with amitriptyline)	125–250 ng/mL
phenobarbital/Luminal, etc.	10–25 mcg/mL
phenytoin/Dilantin	10–18 mcg/mL
primidone/Mysoline	6–12 mcg/mL
procainamide/Pronestyl	4–10 mcg/mL
(NAPA metabolite)	4–10 mcg/mL
propafenone	0.06–1 mcg/mL
propranolol/Inderal	50–100 ng/mL
protriptyline/Vivactil	70–250 ng/mL
quinidine/Quinaglute, etc.	1.0–4.0 mcg/mL
(specific to quinidine test method)	

sulfadiazine/Microsulfon	100–120 mcg/mL
sulfamethoxazole/Gantanol	90–100 mcg/mL
theophylline/Aminophylline, etc.	10–20 mcg/mL
thioridazine/Mellaril	50–300 ng/mL
tobramycin/Nebcin	4.0–10 mcg/mL (peak)
	less than 2 mcg/mL (trough)
tocainide/Tonocard	5–12 mcg/mL
trimethadione/Tridione	10–30 mcg/mL
trimethoprim/Proloprim	1–3 mcg/mL
valproic acid/Depakene	50–100 mcg/mL
vancomycin/Vancocin	30–40 mcg/mL (peak)
	5–10 mcg/mL (trough)
verapamil/Calan	0.06–0.2 mcg/mL

3

True Breakthroughs in Medicines

Every year we gain some great advances in medicines—and sometimes in the programs that help us use them to get better and longer lasting results. This section tells you about some of the best, identifies novel treatment approaches, and gives truly new uses of existing medicines. I try to distinguish between "me too" products (that may simply be an existing drug with minor chemical changes) and forward-looking advances that smart patients should know about. I believe that this section can help you make sure you are getting the very latest treatment. While this is a shorter section than previous years, some very large studies and interesting medicines are coming into their own this year. As with all medicines, the data changes on a regular basis. One way to follow up on medicines themselves is to visit the FDA Web site at *www.fda.gov* and look at the type of approval the medicine was given. A "chemical type one" designation is a new molecular entity—something that has never existed before. "Chemical type four" designations are new combinations of medicines. These two categories coupled with the latest research can help you find the latest in therapy. I also have an Update on New Medicines report on my Web site at *www.medicineinfo.com*.

ASPIRIN

For several years now, aspirin has remained on this list. Previously I put it here because it can be one of the easiest ways to help limit the damage from a heart attack, and can also make great combination therapy sense for ACS patients who are taking clopidogrel (see CURE trial in sources or at *www.medicineinfo.com*). This year I included it again because there is some emerging data showing that aspirin may help decrease breast cancer risk. Talk to your doctor to see if this makes sense for you.

DAPTOMYCIN (DAP-toe-my-sin)

Star on the Horizon

We've all heard about flesh-eating bacteria and increased resistance in bacteria. New approaches are needed. The first in an entirely new class of antibiotics (lipopeptides) has gained approval. Daptomycin, which will be known as Cidecin, is made by Cubist Pharmaceuticals. This antibiotic works against a large number (broad spectrum) of gram-positive organisms. Daptomycin also works in a unique way, by making the cell wall of the bacteria leak out vital chemicals. This medicine was recognized by the FDA and given a priority review.

FUSION INHIBITOR

Historically, all of the available HIV treatments fell into several different classes. A novel way to attack the AIDS virus was clearly needed and was discovered by Trimeris Pharmaceutical. The approach is called a fusion inhibitor—helping to keep HIV from entering cells and killing them. The first fusion inhibitor to be approved was previously known as T-20 and is now called efurvirtide (Fuseon) and is now more broadly available. I believe that the coming year will show the true colors of the first fusion inhibitor.

GET WITH THE GUIDELINES-STROKE

You'd think that prescribing medicines and having patients take them after they've suffered a stroke would be well standardized and followed. Unfortunately, this is NOT the case! The American Stroke Association has launched a new program called Get With The Guidelines (GWTG)-Stroke to address this problem. GWTG-Stroke is a hospital-based initiative seeking to help health care professionals work as teams to make sure the best medicines are started in the hospital. You can find out more by visiting *www.strokeassociation.org. More specifically, at the time of this writing, you can see the specific program at: www.strokeassociation.org/ presenter.jhtml?identifier=3002728.*

HUMAN GENOME

There are some 3 billion base pairs, and an estimated 40,000 genes in the human genome. Some 20 diseases cause more than 80 percent of deaths around the world. About 200–300 genes are responsible for these diseases. Amazingly, the human genome is now mostly known. Considering that about every three weeks we in essence get a new heart from the same set of genes, if controlling the genes becomes a reality, we can possibly knock out heart disease by knocking out the bad gene of a pair. I believe we will be hearing some interesting approaches stemming from this information in the coming year! Watch closely!

NATIONAL POISON CONTROL PHONE NUMBER

I still do not believe enough of us have this crucial number right by the phone. **Please remember**: If a loved one has taken an overdose of a medicine or toxic chemical, the last thing you want to do is search for your state's—or if you are visiting someone else, their state's—800 number for poison control. FINALLY, there is a National Poison Control number: 1-800-222-1222. PLEASE WRITE IT DOWN BY THE PHONE AND ALSO CARRY IT IN YOUR PURSE OR WALLET.

PRE-DIABETES

The breakthrough in pre-diabetes is that some sorely needed steps are being taken to acknowledge the negative contribution that being overweight makes to the entire progression from pre-diabetes to diabetes. I believe that the Bush administration (Tommy Thompson from HHS in particular) and a panel from the American Diabetes Association (ADA) and the Surgeon General have done well to create additional awareness about the relationship between diabetes and being overweight.

DRUG PROFILES

Drugs Reviewed in This Section

Included are detailed and annually updated Drug Profiles of **more than 2,000 brands** and nearly 400 drugs of major importance. The criteria are that the medicine:

1. Is used to treat or prevent a prevalent, relatively serious significant disease or disorder.

2. Is recognized by experts to be among the "best choices" in its class.

3. Has a current benefit-to-risk ratio that compares favorably with those in its class or is the only available alternative therapy for those who can't tolerate usual/first-line medicine(s).

4. May require special information and guidance for both the health care practitioner (physician, dentist, pharmacist, nurse) and the consumer (patient and family) for safe and effective use.

5. Is suitable (safe and practical) for use in an outpatient setting (home, work site, school, etc.). It can be self-administered or may require dosing by trained medical personnel (as with home intravenous therapy or free-standing cancer, emergency, or pain centers).

ACARBOSE (A KAR BOZ)

Introduced: 1996 **Class:** Alpha glucosidase inhibitor; antidiabetes agent, oral **Prescription:** USA: Yes **Controlled Drug:** USA: No; Canada: No **Available as Generic:** No
Brand Names: Glucobay, Precose, ✤Prandase

BENEFITS versus RISKS

Possible Benefits

EFFECTIVE LOWERING OF BLOOD SUGAR
DECREASES A SUDDEN RISE IN BLOOD SUGAR AFTER A MEAL
DECREASED RISK OF HIGH BLOOD PRESSURE, BLINDNESS, HEART DISEASE, OR OTHER LONG-TERM DAMAGE OF UNCONTROLLED DIABETES (WITH BETTER OR TIGHTER CONTROL OF BLOOD SUGAR)
MAY BE USED IN COMBINED TREATMENT WITH METFORMIN, INSULIN, OR A SULFONYLUREA IF NEEDED TO REACH BLOOD SUGAR CONTROL GOALS
May help PREVENT type 2 diabetes in people with pre-diabetes

Possible Risks

Gas (flatulence) and abdominal pain (often decreases over time)
Increased liver function tests
Combination use gives better results, but also increases risk of excessively low blood sugar (hypoglycemia) like other agents

---

▷ **Principal Uses**

As a Single Drug Product: Uses currently included in FDA-approved labeling: (1) Used with diet in diabetics who don't require insulin, yet don't have good (tight control of 80–120 mg/dL or as defined as acceptable by their doctor) blood sugar control with diet alone; (2) can be combined with a sulfonylurea (see Drug Classes) if diet plus acarbose or diet and sulfonylurea do not control blood sugar as well as needed; (3) can be combined with metformin or insulin if diet plus acarbose or diet plus sulfonylurea do not achieve blood sugar control goals.

Other (unlabeled) generally accepted uses: (1) Combination treatment of diabetics (type one) who require insulin; (2) the Stop-NIDDM research on 1,368 patients found that acarbose worked to delay or prevent people with pre-diabetes from developing type 2 diabetes.

How This Drug Works: By blocking the chemicals (enzymes) called intestinal alpha glucosidases and pancreatic alpha amylase, this medicine impairs starch and sucrose digestion and actually keeps sugar low after meals.

▷ **Widely Used Guidelines That Involve This Medicine (representative sample):** Please look at the section at the very beginning of this profile called "Class." Next, turn to Table 22 and you will find guidelines listed by the class involved!

Available Dosage Forms and Strengths
Tablets — 25 mg, 50 mg, 100 mg

▷ **Recommended Dosage Ranges** (Actual dose and schedule must be determined individually for each patient.)

Infants and Children: Safety and effectiveness not established in those less than 18 years old.

18 to 65 Years of Age: To start, 25 mg three times daily, taken at the start of each meal (after first bite). Dose increases are made at 4- to 8-week intervals to achieve blood sugar control while minimizing intestinal side effects (using 50 mg three times daily at the start of each meal). If response is not acceptable, patients weighing more than 132 pounds (60 kg) may be given doses up to 100 mg three times daily. Those weighing less than 60 kg should NOT be given more than 50 mg three times daily. If a dose increase doesn't give better sugar control, consider dose decrease.

Over 65 Years of Age: No specific recommendations unless kidney function is very limited, in which case a kidney specialist may be prudent.

Conditions Requiring Dosing Adjustments

Liver Function: Specific dosing changes do not appear to be needed. Enzymes found in the intestine and intestinal bacteria extensively contribute to removal of this medicine.

Kidney Function: Increases in drug levels may occur and dose decreases may be needed. Specific guidelines not available. The kidneys usually remove only about 2%.

▷ **Dosing Instructions:** Take this pill after starting to eat breakfast, lunch and dinner—after the first bite of a meal has been eaten. Dosing must be individualized. Gas (flatulence) or diarrhea is a common side effect, but often decreases over time. Limiting sucrose (read the food label) can also help.

If dose changes are made at 4- to 8-week intervals, the best sugar response and the least potential gas (flatulence) or diarrhea are realized. Often blood sugar is checked one hour after a meal (1 hr postprandial) and the dose adjusted to get the best balance of blood sugar and side effects (also avoiding too low a blood sugar). If you forget a dose but remember it while you are still eating, take it immediately. If you remember the dose just after finishing your meal, take the dose immediately (if you remember later than this, take your next dose with your next meal). Do not double doses or take acarbose between meals. Check your blood sugar as your doctor has instructed.

Usual Duration of Use: Use will be ongoing because it helps replace some of the work your pancreas no longer does. Regular use is required for good blood sugar (glucose) control. DO NOT MISS DOSES. Keeping the sugar close to normal can decrease severity or risk of problems (such as blindness, heart disease, and undesirable circulation changes) often found in diabetes.

Typical Treatment Goals and Measurements (Outcomes and Markers)

Blood Sugar: The general goal for blood sugar is to return it to the usual "normal" range (generally 80–120 mg/dL), while avoiding risks of excessively low blood sugar. One study (UKPDS) used a fasting plasma sugar (glucose) of less than 108 mg/dL. Keeping blood sugar in the normal range helps avoid complications of diabetes.

Fructosamine and Glycosylated Hemoglobin: Fructosamine levels (a measure of the past two to three weeks of blood sugar control) should be less than or equal to 310 micromoles per liter. Glycosylated hemoglobin or hemoglobin A1C (a measure of the past 2–3 months of blood sugar control) should be less than or equal to 7.0%. Some clinicians advocate less than 6.5% and there is a trend for even tighter control. Diabetes is a CHD risk equivalent in NCEP ATP 3 (see Glossary). This means that diabetics face a significant risk of heart disease. EBCT (see Glossary) may help define risk.

Possible Advantages of This Drug
May be used in combination with oral hypoglycemics (such as sulfonylureas, insulin, or metformin (see Drug Classes) to get the best control of blood sugar. Uses a different (novel) mechanism than other oral hypoglycemic drugs. Please remember—the goal is to keep the blood sugar as close to normal as possible.

▷ **This Drug Should Not Be Taken If**
- you have had an allergic reaction to it previously.
- you are in diabetic ketoacidosis.
- your history includes intestinal obstruction or you have a partial obstruction of the intestine.
- you have inflammatory bowel disease or colon ulceration.
- you have cirrhosis of the liver.
- you have an intestinal condition that may worsen (such as a megacolon or bowel obstruction) if increased gas (flatus) forms.
- you have a long-standing (chronic) intestinal disease altering digestion or your ability to absorb materials from the intestine.
- you are pregnant or are breast-feeding your infant (no data exist on use in pregnancy or breast-feeding).
- you are less than 18 years old.

▷ **Inform Your Physician Before Taking This Drug If**
- you have an infection (insulin may be required).
- you do not know what the symptoms of hypoglycemia are.
- you have a history of kidney or liver disease.
- your liver function tests (LFTs) have become known to you and they are increased.
- you will have surgery with general anesthesia.
- you forgot to tell your doctor about all the drugs you take.
- you are also taking a sulfonylurea (increased risk of excessively low blood sugar).
- you are anemic (conflicting information here, but acarbose might lower iron levels).
- you are unsure of how much or how often to take acarbose.

Possible Side Effects (natural, expected, and unavoidable drug actions)
Gas (flatulence) or diarrhea (results from bacterial action on sugars) and tends to decrease over time.

▷ **Possible Adverse Effects** (unusual, unexpected, and infrequent reactions)
If any of the following develop, consult your physician promptly for guidance.

Mild Adverse Effects
Allergic reactions: skin redness (erythema), itching (urticaria).
Sleepiness, headache, dizziness—questionable cause (may really be blood sugar control signs or symptoms).
Pain or swelling of the belly (abdomen)—frequent.
Gas (flatulence) or diarrhea—frequent (often eases over time).

Serious Adverse Effects

Erythema multiforme—case report.

Low blood sugar if combined with sulfonylureas or other anti-diabetes medicines such as insulin—possible.

Anemia—rare in clinical approval trials, but not seen in later studies.

Increased liver enzymes up to necrosis of liver tissue—case reports (case reports developed this problem in 2–8 months—with an unclear relationship to the drug). Liver toxicity can be more common in women than in men. Call your doctor if you start to have nausea, fatigue, and light colored stools or pain in the right upper part of your abdomen.

Ileus—case reports and more likely in those with prior bowel blockage history.

Abnormal lipids (increased cholesterol and triglycerides)—case report.

▷ **Possible Effects on Sexual Function:** None reported.

Possible Effects on Laboratory Tests

Glycated protein (fructosamine): trending toward normal (good effect).

Hemoglobin A1C: trending more toward normal (good effect).

Blood sugar one hour after eating (postprandial): decreased.

Serum lipids: variable effect, but usually improved.

Liver enzymes: may be increased.

CAUTION

1. This medicine itself does not cause hypoglycemia. Low sugar may result if combined with metformin, insulin, or sulfonylureas.
2. Infections may cause loss of sugar control and require temporary insulin use.
3. This medicine is part of the total management of diabetes. A properly prescribed diet and regular exercise are still required for best control of blood sugar.
4. If your kidneys fail or worsen, tell your doctor.
5. Call your doctor if you have light colored stools, nausea, and pain in the upper right part of your abdomen.

Precautions for Use

By Infants and Children: Safety and effectiveness for those under 18 not established.

By Those Over 60 Years of Age: Specific changes are not made at this time.

▷ **Advisability of Use During Pregnancy**

Pregnancy Category: B. See Pregnancy Risk Categories at the back of this book.

Animal Studies: No significant increase in birth defects in rats or rabbits.

Human Studies: Adequate studies of pregnant women are not available. Insulin is often the drug of first choice for blood sugar control in pregnancy. Ask your doctor for help.

Advisability of Use If Breast-Feeding

Presence of this drug in breast milk: Yes, in rats. No human data available. Avoid drug or refrain from nursing.

Habit-Forming Potential: None.

Effects of Overdose: Temporary gas (flatus), abdominal discomfort, and diarrhea.

Possible Effects of Long-Term Use: Beneficial effects on blood sugar, lowered risk of cardiovascular disease and of high blood pressure with better sugar control.

Suggested Periodic Examinations While Taking This Drug (at physician's discretion)

Periodic blood sugar one hour after eating.

Glycated protein (fructosamine).

Hemoglobin A1C levels.

Check for cardiovascular health as diabetes is a major risk factor for heart and blood vessel disease.

Liver function tests (transaminases)—checked every three months during the first year, then periodically thereafter. Patients taking other medicines that can be toxic to the liver should be tested more frequently.

Serum iron or iron-binding capacity prudent if anemia develops.

▷ **While Taking This Drug, Observe the Following**

Foods: Closely follow the diet your doctor has prescribed. Blood sugar control can help avoid or delay diabetes problems! Vitamin C in high dose may worsen blood sugar control.

Herbal Medicines or Minerals: Using chromium may change the way your body is able to use sugar. Some health food stores advocate vanadium as mimicking the actions of insulin, but possible toxicity and need for rigorous studies presently preclude recommending it. DHEA may change sensitivity to insulin or insulin resistance. Aloe, bitter melon, fenugreek, hawthorn, ginger, garlic, ginseng, glucomannan, guar gum, licorice, nettle, St. John's wort, and yohimbe may change blood sugar. Because these products can have an effect—talk to your doctor BEFORE combining any of these herbal medicines with acarbose. Echinacea purpurea (injectable) and blonde psyllium seed or husk should NOT be taken by people living with diabetes.

Beverages: No restrictions. May be taken with milk—mindful of the limits of the diet that your doctor has recommended.

▷ *Alcohol:* No interaction with acarbose. If you also take a sulfonylurea (see Drug Classes), alcohol can exaggerate lowering of blood sugar or cause a disulfiramlike (see Glossary) reaction.

Tobacco Smoking: No interactions expected, but I advise everyone to stop smoking.

▷ *Other Drugs*

Acarbose may ***increase*** the effects of

- insulins (see Drug Classes), further lowering blood sugar for patients who do not respond to acarbose alone (a beneficial effect when blood sugar is closely watched).
- metformin (Glucophage) may further lower blood sugar for patients who are not controlled by diet or acarbose alone (beneficial effect as above).
- sulfonylureas (see Drug Classes), causing further lowering of blood sugars (not an acarbose effect). This may be used for therapeutic benefit.
- warfarin (Coumadin)—INR testing more often is advisable.

Acarbose ***taken concurrently*** with

- activated charcoal (various) may blunt the benefits of acarbose.
- amylase (pancreatin) may blunt the benefits of acarbose.
- clofibrate (Atromid-S) may result in hypoglycemia.
- digestive enzyme products that contain amylase or lipase may result in loss of blood sugar control.
- digoxin (Lanoxin) may cause lower (subtherapeutic) blood levels of digoxin and loss of benefits (three case reports).
- disopyramide (Norpace) may result in hypoglycemia.

- fluoroquinolone antibiotics (such as ciprofloxacin-Cipro, gatifloxacin-Tequin, levofloxacin-Levaquin) may result in low blood sugar (hypoglycemia).
- high-dose aspirin or other salicylates and some NSAIDs (see Drug Classes) may result in hypoglycemia.
- monoamine oxidase (MAO) inhibitors (see Drug Classes) may increase glucose tolerance, leading to excessively low blood sugar.
- sulfonamide antibiotics (see Drug Classes) may pose an increased risk for low blood sugar (hypoglycemia).

The following drugs may *decrease* the effects of acarbose:

- adrenocorticosteroids (see Drug Classes).
- beta-blockers (see Drug Classes).
- calcium channel blockers (see Drug Classes).
- furosemide (Lasix) and bumetanide (Bumex).
- isoniazid (INH).
- nicotinic acid.
- pancreatin (or any medicines containing carbohydrate dividing enzymes such as amylase or pancreatin).
- phenytoin (Dilantin).
- rifampin (Rifadin, others).
- theophylline (Theo-Dur, others).
- thiazide diuretics (see Drug Classes).
- thyroid hormones (see Drug Classes).

▷ *Driving, Hazardous Activities:* Use caution until degree of drowsiness you may see is known.

Aviation Note: Diabetes *is a disqualification* for piloting. Consult a designated Aviation Medical Examiner.

Exposure to Sun: No restrictions.

Heavy Exercise or Exertion: Caution advised because this drug lowers peak in blood sugar after meals. Discuss dosing changes with your doctor if your exercise pattern changes.

Occurrence of Unrelated Illness: When you are sick, blood sugar control changes. Temporary use of insulin may be **required** if you are sick—such as in the case of infection.

Discontinuation: **Never** stop acarbose before calling your doctor.

ACEBUTOLOL (a se BYU toh lohl)

Introduced: 1973   **Class:** Antihypertensive, beta-adrenergic blocker, heart rhythm regulator   **Prescription:**   USA: Yes   **Controlled Drug:** USA: No; Canada: No   **Available as Generic:**   Yes

Brand Names: ✤Apo-Acebutolol, ✤Gen-Acebutolol, ✤Med-Acebutolol, ✤Monitan, ✤Rhotral, Sectral

---

BENEFITS versus RISKS

Possible Benefits	*Possible Risks*
EFFECTIVE ANTIHYPERTENSIVE (MILD–MODERATE HIGH PRESSURE) MAY BE USED ALONE OR IN COMBINATION WITH OTHER ANTIHYPERTENSIVES, ESPECIALLY DIURETICS	CONGESTIVE HEART FAILURE IN ADVANCED HEART DISEASE
MAY DECREASE DEATHS OCCURRING AFTER HEART ATTACK	Masking of low blood sugar (hypoglycemia) in diabetics
LONG-TERM USE CAN DECREASE DEATH AND HEART PROBLEMS	Rare lupus erythematosus syndrome
HELPS PREVENT ABNORMAL HEART RHYTHMS	
Because this drug also has intrinsic sympathomimetic activity it may help in patients with high cholesterol (dyslipidemia) because it avoids increases in serum triglycerides	
May be particularly useful in people with asthma or diabetes (because of heart or cardioselectivity)	

▷ **Principal Uses**

As a Single Drug Product: Uses currently included in FDA-approved labeling: (1) Treats mild to moderate high blood pressure alone or in combination; (2) used to prevent premature ventricular heartbeats and ventricular arrhythmias.

Other (unlabeled) generally accepted uses: (1) Stabilizes angina pectoris; (2) used after a heart attack to help prolong life.

How This Drug Works: It blocks sympathetic nervous system effects and slows the rate and force of the heart, reducing the extent of blood vessel contraction, expanding the walls and lowering blood pressure. Also slows nerve impulse speed through the heart, which helps ease some heart rhythm disorders.

▷ **Widely Used Guidelines That Involve This Medicine (representative sample):** Please look at the section at the very beginning of this profile called "Class." Next, turn to Table 22 and you will find guidelines listed by the class involved!

Available Dosage Forms and Strengths

Capsules — 100 mg (in Canada), 200 mg, 400 mg

Tablets — 100 mg, 200 mg, and 400 mg (in Canada)

▷ **Recommended Dosage Ranges** (Actual dose and schedule must be determined for each patient individually.)

Infants and Children: Not indicated.

18 to 65 Years of Age: High blood pressure: 200 mg a day works for some, but most patients require 400–800 mg a day, rarely 1,200 (given as 600 mg twice a day). Heart selectivity (beta one) decreases as doses increase.

Arrhythmias: 400 mg daily, as 200 mg taken morning and evening (12 hours apart as a divided dose). Increase as needed and tolerated. 600–1200 mg a day is a typical effective dose. Total dose should not exceed 1,200 mg every 24 hours (600 mg twice a day).

Angina: 600 to 1,600 mg is divided into two or three equal doses given 8 to 12 hours apart.

Over 65 Years of Age: Bioavailability (amount taken into your body) doubles because of lower liver and kidney removal. Smaller ongoing doses are needed and 800 mg a day is a **maximum.**

Conditions Requiring Dosing Adjustments

Liver Function: Used with caution in compromised liver function.

Kidney Function: Dose must be decreased by up to 75% in severe kidney failure (dicetalol metabolite can accumulate).

▷ **Dosing Instructions:** May be taken without regard to eating. Capsule may be opened when taken. NEVER stop this drug abruptly. If you forget a dose: take it right away unless it's within 4 hours of your next regular dose. If it IS within 4 hours of the next dose, just take the scheduled dose. Do NOT double doses.

Usual Duration of Use: Use on a regular schedule for 5 to 14 days may be required to see peak benefits in lowering blood pressure or stopping premature heartbeats. Long-term use determined by sustained benefit and response to a combined program (weight decrease, salt restriction, smoking cessation, etc.) in high blood pressure and response of abnormal heart rhythm. Do NOT skip doses.

Typical Treatment Goals and Measurements (Outcomes and Markers)

Blood Pressure: The RECENT guidelines (JNC VII) define normal blood pressure (BP) as **less than** 120/80. **Pre-hypertension** ranges from 120/80 to 139/89 and is intended to help your doctor encourage lifestyle changes (or in the case of people with a risk factor for high blood pressure, start treatment) much earlier—so that possible damage to blood vessels, your heart, kidneys, sexual potency, or eyes might be minimized or avoided altogether. The next two classes of high blood pressure are stage 1 hypertension: 140/90 to 159/99 and stage 2 hypertension equal to or greater than: 160/100 mm Hg. These guidelines also recommend that clinicians AND patients agree on the goals and a plan of treatment. The first-ever guidelines for blood pressure (hypertension) in African Americans recommends that MOST black patients be started on TWO antihypertensive medicines with the goal of lowering blood pressure to 130/80 for those with high risk for heart and blood vessel disease or with diabetes. For diabetics: 130/80 is the target and less than 125/75 for those who spill more than one gram of protein into their urine. Most clinicians try to achieve a BP that confers the best balance of lower cardiovascular risk and avoids the problem of too low a blood pressure. Blood pressure duration is generally increased with beneficial restriction of sodium. The goals and time frame should be discussed with you when the prescription is written. If goals are not met, it is not unusual to intensify doses or add on medicines.

Abnormal Heartbeats: The general goal is to return the heart to a normal rhythm or at least to markedly reduce the occurrence of abnormal heartbeats. In life-threatening arrhythmias, the goal is to abort the abnormal beats and return the pattern to normal. Your doctor may hook you up to a small machine and check heart rate and rhythm for a day (such as in Holter monitoring). A small heart rate and rhythm (EKG or ECG) recording device is carried around via a shoulder strap and records what the heart is doing over 24 hours. Once the recording is made, a scanning machine reviews the record, tallies abnormal heartbeats or rhythms and gives a close and extended look at how the heart is reacting or benefiting from the medicines that the patient is taking. Repeat measurements can be made if doses are changed to check the success at keeping the heart in normal sinus rhythm!

Possible Advantages of This Drug: Slows the heart less than most other beta-blocker drugs, and low doses are less likely to cause asthma attacks in asthmatics. May cause less frequent problems with blood vessels in the legs (peripheral vascular insufficiency) than non-selective beta blockers such as propranolol.

▷ **This Drug Should Not Be Taken If**
- you have had an allergic reaction to it previously.
- you are in heart failure (overt).
- you have a severely slow (bradycardia) heart rate or serious heart block (second or third degree AV).

▷ **Inform Your Physician Before Taking This Drug If**
- you have had an adverse reaction to any beta-blocker (see Drug Classes).
- you have serious heart disease or episodes of heart failure (this drug may aggravate it).
- you have disease of the mitral valve or aorta.
- you have hay fever (allergic rhinitis), asthma, chronic bronchitis, or emphysema.
- you have an overactive thyroid function (hyperthyroidism).
- you have problems with circulation to your arms and legs (peripheral vascular disease or intermittent claudication).
- you have a history of low blood sugar (hypoglycemia).
- you have impaired liver or kidney function.
- you have diabetes or myasthenia gravis.
- you take digitalis, quinidine or reserpine, or any calcium blocker (see Drug Classes).
- you will have surgery with general anesthesia.
- you do not know how much or how often to take acebutolol.
- you have not asked if the dose was adjusted for age-related kidney decline or kidney disease.

Possible Side Effects (natural, expected, and unavoidable drug actions)
Lethargy and fatigability, cold extremities—rare; slow heart rate, light-headedness in upright position (see Orthostatic Hypotension in Glossary) possible.

▷ **Possible Adverse Effects** (unusual, unexpected, and infrequent reactions)
If any of the following develop, consult your physician promptly for guidance.
Mild Adverse Effects
Allergic reactions: skin rash, itching—rare.
Fatigue—frequent.
Headache, dizziness, insomnia, fatigue, or abnormal dreams—infrequent.
Indigestion, nausea, constipation, diarrhea—infrequent.
Decreased tearing with long-term use—case reports.
Edema in the ankles—infrequent.
Increased frequency of urination or painful or nighttime urination—infrequent.
Joint and muscle discomfort—infrequent.

Serious Adverse Effects

Allergic reactions may be more severe or less responsive to epinephrine.

Mental depression or low blood sugar—rare.

Liver toxicity—case reports (may be a hypersensitivity reaction).

Chest pain, shortness of breath, precipitation of congestive heart failure—rare.

Rebound or withdrawal chest pain (angina) if this medicine is suddenly stopped—possible

Precipitation of intermittent claudication—possible in people with severe blood vessel spasm (vasospastic) disorders or severe Peripheral Artery Disease (PAD).

Bronchial asthma attack (in people with asthma)—possible, but less likely than some other beta blockers.

Positive ANA and lupus erythematosus—infrequent to frequent, up to 33%.

▷ **Possible Effects on Sexual Function:** Impotence, decreased libido, Peyronie's disease (see Glossary)—case reports to 2%.

Possible Effects on Laboratory Tests

Antinuclear antibodies (ANA) and LE cells: often positive after 3 to 6 months.

Free fatty acids (FFA): decreased.

Glucose tolerance test (GTT): decreased; abnormal tests at 60 and 120 minutes—possible.

Potassium: mild increases.

CAUTION

1. *Do not stop this drug suddenly* without the knowledge and help of your physician. Carry a note that says that you take this drug.
2. Nasal decongestants may cause sudden and SEVERE increases in blood pressure. Call your physician or pharmacist before using nasal decongestants and ask if they should ever be used.
3. Report any tendency to emotional depression.
4. This medicine may worsen preexisting kidney insufficiency.

Precautions for Use

By Infants and Children: Safety and effectiveness for those under 12 years not established. If this drug is used, watch for fainting as a sign of low blood sugar (hypoglycemia) if a meal is skipped.

By Those Over 60 Years of Age: All antihypertensive drugs used cautiously. High blood pressure should be lowered slowly, avoiding risks (such as stroke or heart attack) of excessively low blood pressure. Small doses and frequent blood pressure checks needed. The amount of medicine that gets into your body (bioavailability) from a given dose can increase by twofold in elderly people. Total daily dose should not exceed 800 mg. Watch for dizziness, falling, confusion, hallucinations, depression, or frequent urination.

▷ **Advisability of Use During Pregnancy**

Pregnancy Category: B. See Pregnancy Risk Categories at the back of this book.

Animal Studies: No significant increase in birth defects in rats or rabbits.

Human Studies: Adequate studies of pregnant women are not available.

Use this drug only if clearly needed. Ask your doctor for help.

Advisability of Use If Breast-Feeding

Presence of this drug in breast milk: Yes, and concentrated.

Avoid drug or refrain from nursing.

Habit-Forming Potential: None.

Effects of Overdose: Weakness, slow pulse, low blood pressure, fainting, cold and sweaty skin, congestive heart failure, possible coma, and convulsions.

Possible Effects of Long-Term Use: Decreased heart reserve and heart failure in some people with advanced heart disease.

Suggested Periodic Examinations While Taking This Drug (at physician's discretion)
Blood pressure checks (treated to attain goals) and heart rhythm checks.
Heart and liver function tests.
May be prudent to check for hidden Peripheral Artery Disease (PAD) by checking ankle brachial index (ABI). ABI check (see Glossary) can help find PAD early, and avoid claudication that may result if this medication is taken by someone who has PAD but does not know it.
ANA titer.

▷ **While Taking This Drug, Observe the Following**
Foods: Follow a sensible low-cardiovascular-risk diet. Avoid excessive salt intake.
Herbal Medicines or Minerals: Bitter orange, country mallow, ginseng, hawthorn, saw palmetto, ma huang (now mostly off the market), guarana (caffeine), goldenseal, yohimbe, and licorice may also cause increased blood pressure. Dong quai may block the removal of this medicine from the body leading to toxic effects with "normal" doses. St. John's wort may increase removal of this medicine from the body leading to loss of benefits despite appropriate doses. Calcium and garlic may help lower blood pressure. Ginkgo benefits in helping peripheral artery disease are as yet, unproven. Indian snakeroot has a German Commission E monograph indication for hypertension—talk to your doctor. Eleuthero root and ephedra (ma huang) should be avoided by people living with hypertension.
Beverages: No restrictions. May be taken with milk.

▷ *Alcohol:* Alcohol may exaggerate lowering of blood pressure and may increase its mild sedative effect.
Tobacco Smoking: Nicotine may reduce this drug's effectiveness and can worsen closing of bronchial tubes seen in regular smokers. I advise everyone to quit smoking.
Marijuana Smoking: Marijuana may increase blood pressure and reduce this drug's effectiveness. DO NOT COMBINE.

▷ *Other Drugs*
Acebutolol may ***increase*** the effects of
• other antihypertensive drugs, excessively lowering the blood pressure. Dose adjustments may be necessary.
• reserpine (Ser-Ap-Es, etc.), causing sedation, depression, slow heart rate, and low blood pressure.
Acebutolol ***taken concurrently*** with
• alfentanil (Alfenta) or fentanyl may result in severe slowing of the heart leading to sinus arrest. Use with great caution.
• alpha-one-adrenergic blockers (such as prazosin) may result in a severe drop in blood pressure (especially when patients stand) in response to a first dose of this medicine. Use with great caution.
• amiodarone (Cordarone) may result in severe slowing of the heart leading to sinus arrest. Use with great caution.
• calcium channel blockers such as mibefradil (Posicor) or verapamil (Calan) may lead to increased risk of abnormal heart rate or rhythm.

- clonidine (Catapres) may cause rebound high blood pressure if clonidine is withdrawn while acebutolol is still being taken.
- digoxin (Lanoxin) may change heart conduction.
- diltiazem (Cardizem) may result in increased acebutolol effects.
- fentanyl anesthesia (various) may lead to severe lowering of blood pressure.
- fluoxetine (Prozac), fluvoxamine (Luvox), paroxetine (Paxil), or venlafaxine (Effexor) may decrease removal of acebutolol from the body (not reported as yet). Caution is advised.
- insulin may cause low blood sugar (hypoglycemia).
- methyldopa (Aldomet) may lead to unexpected increases in blood pressure.
- NSAIDs (see Drug Classes) may result in decreased acebutolol benefits.
- oral antidiabetic drugs (see Drug Classes) may result in slow recovery from low blood sugar.
- ritonavir (Norvir) and perhaps other protease inhibitors may increase the metabolism of this medicine and blunt therapeutic benefits of acebutolol.

The following drugs may *decrease* the effects of acebutolol:

- indomethacin (Indocin) and some other "aspirin substitutes" (NSAIDs) can blunt acebutolol's antihypertensive effect.
- rifabutin (Mycobutin) and other drugs that may increase (induce) cytochrome P450 enzymes in the liver (the ones that help the body remove medicines like acebutolol) may result in loss of benefits of acebutolol even if every dose of acebutolol is being taken.

▷ *Driving, Hazardous Activities:* Use caution—may cause drowsiness.

Aviation Note: The use of this drug *is a disqualification* for piloting. Consult a designated Aviation Medical Examiner.

Exposure to Sun: No restrictions.

Exposure to Heat: Hot environments can exaggerate the effects of this drug.

Exposure to Cold: Elderly need to prevent hypothermia (see Glossary).

Heavy Exercise or Exertion: This drug can intensify increased blood pressure (hypertensive) response to isometric exercise. Talk to your doctor about how much and how to exercise.

Occurrence of Unrelated Illness: Fevers can lower blood pressure and require decreased doses. Nausea or vomiting may interrupt the dosing schedule. Ask your doctor for help.

Discontinuation: **DO NOT** stop the drug suddenly. Gradual dose decreases over 2–3 weeks (tapering) is needed. Stopping this medicine suddenly may lead to abnormal heart rhythm, heart attack or sudden death. Ask your doctor for help.

ACETAZOLAMIDE (a set a ZOHL a mide)

Introduced: 1953 **Class:** Anticonvulsant, antiglaucoma, diuretic, sulfonamides

Brand Names: ✤Acetazolam, Diamox, Diamox Sequels, Diamox Sustained Release

---

BENEFITS versus RISKS

Possible Benefits	*Possible Risks*
REDUCTION OF INTERNAL EYE PRESSURE in some glaucoma cases	Rare bone marrow, liver, or kidney injury
CONTROL OF ABSENCE (PETIT MAL) SEIZURES	Acidosis with long-term use—possible
	Increased risk of kidney stones
TREATMENT OF PERIODIC PARALYSIS	Tingling in the arms and legs (paresthesia)
	Paralysis—rare
REDUCES FLUID IN CONGESTIVE HEART FAILURE	Bone weakening (with long-term use)—possible
PREVENTION OR LESSENING OF SYMPTOMS OF ACUTE MOUNTAIN SICKNESS	

Author's Note: This profile has been further shortened to make room for more widely used medicines.

ACETIC ACIDS (Nonsteroidal Anti-Inflammatory Drug Family)

Diclofenac (di KLOH fen ak) **Etodolac** (e TOE doh lak) **Indomethacin** (in doh METH a sin) **Ketorolac** (KEY tor o lak) **Nabumetone** (na BYU me tohn) **Sulindac** (sul IN dak) **Tolmetin** (TOHL met in)

Introduced: 1976, 1986, 1963, 1991, 1984, 1976, 1976, respectively **Class:** Mild analgesic, NSAID **Prescription:** USA: Yes **Controlled Drug:** USA: No; Canada: No **Available as Generic:** USA: Yes, all.

Brand Names: Diclofenac, ❧Apo-Diclo, ❧Apo-Diclo SR, Arthrotec [CD], Cataflam, ❧Novo-Difenac, ❧Nu-Diclo, Voltaren, Voltaren Ophthalmic, Voltaren SR, Voltaren Timed Release, Voltaren XR; Etodolac, Lodine, Lodine XL; Indomethacin, ❧Apo-Indomethacin, Indameth, ❧Indocid, ❧Indocid-SR, ❧Indocid PDA, Indocin, Indocin-SR, ❧Novo-methacin, ❧Nu-Indo, Zendole; Ketorolac, Acular, Acular PF (ketorolac ophthalmic), ❧Apo-ketorolac, Toradol; Nabumetone, ❧Apo-Nabumetone, ❧Gen-Nabumetone ❧Novo-Nabumetone ❧Nu-Nabumetone ❧MS-Nabumetone, ❧Rhoxal-Nabumetone Relafen, Sulindac, ❧Apo-Sulin, Clinoril, ❧Novo-Sundac; Tolmetin, ❧Novo-Tolmetin, Tolectin, Tolectin DS, Tolectin 600

BENEFITS versus RISKS

Possible Benefits	*Possible Risks*
EFFECTIVE RELIEF OF MILD TO MODERATE PAIN AND INFLAMMATION	Gastrointestinal pain, ulceration, bleeding
	Liver or kidney damage
Decreased stomach (GI) problems (etodolac and Arthrotec CD form)	Fluid retention
	Bone marrow depression
	Pneumonitis (sulindac)
	Aseptic meningitis (diclofenac)
	Possible severe skin reactions (diclofenac, etodolac, nabumetone, and sulindac)

▷ **Principal Uses**

As a Single Drug Product: Uses currently included in FDA-approved labeling: (1) All of the drugs in this class except ketorolac are approved to treat osteoarthritis; (2) all of the drugs in this class except ketorolac are approved to relieve rheumatoid arthritis; (3) indomethacin, diclofenac, and sulindac are useful in ankylosing spondylitis; (4) sustained-release form of indomethacin as well as the immediate-release form of sulindac help symptoms of tendonitis, bursitis, and acute painful shoulder; (5) tolmetin eases symptoms of juvenile rheumatoid arthritis; (6) sulindac therapy is useful in acute gout; (7) ophthalmic form of diclofenac and ketorolac are useful after cataract surgery and after refractive surgery of the cornea (decreasing pain and sensitivity to light); (8) ketorolac is approved (ophthalmic form) for use in seasonal allergic conjunctivitis; (9) Arthrotec is used in patients with osteo or rheumatoid arthritis who are at high risk for damage to the stomach or intestine (gastric or duodenal ulcer risk); (10) diclofenac is used to help dysmenorrhea.

Author's Note: Because of the approval and more widespread use of other medicines in this family (acetic acid NSAIDs) that can be taken by mouth (PO) and that have a more favorable benefit to risk profile, information on ketorolac intravenous and oral has been deleted from this profile. Ophthalmic ketorolac information remains.

Other (unlabeled) generally accepted uses: (1) Diclofenac used intramuscularly is effective in acute migraine headache and kidney colic; (2) indomethacin helps reduce systemic reactions in kidney transplants and addresses low-grade neonatal intraventricular hemorrhage; (3) sulindac is effective in treating colon polyps and easing diabetic neuropathic pain; (4) NSAIDs in general have shown conflicting results in preventing colon cancer, but may have a beneficial preventive effect; (5) sulindac may be useful in lowering amounts of amniotic fluid (amnioreduction); (6) one study of 2,765 patients found NSAIDs of use in preventing decline of thinking ability in older patients; (7) indomethacin was compared to ibuprofen in infants with patent ductus arteriosus. Results of the 148-infant study found that ibuprofen offered similar benefits while causing fewer cases of decreased urine output (oliguria); (8) NSAIDS may have a beneficial effect in reducing risk of Alzheimer's (cognitive decline).

As a Combination Drug Product [CD]: Diclofenac (50 mg) is combined with misoprostol (200 mcg in the Arthrotec form) in order to help ease side effects on the stomach.

How These Drugs Work: These drugs reduce prostaglandins (and related compounds), chemicals that cause inflammation and pain. Ketorolac may offer a morphine sparing action by an unknown mechanism. Arthrotec form combines diclofenac with the prostaglandin misoprostol in order to help protect the stomach from adverse effects (irritation, ulceration). How the beneficial effects of NSAIDS are conferred in possibly decreasing risk of colon cancer and/or Alzheimer's is not known.

▷ **Widely Used Guidelines That Involve This Medicine (representative sample):** Please look at the section at the very beginning of this profile called "Class." Next, turn to Table 22 and you will find guidelines listed by the class involved!

Available Dosage Forms and Strengths
Diclofenac sodium:

Suppositories — 50 mg, 100 mg (Canada)

Tablets — 25 mg, 50 mg

Tablets-diclofenac/misoprostol — 50 mg or 75 mg diclofenac and 200 mcg misoprostol

Tablets (timed release), prolonged action — 50 mg, 75 mg, 100 mg (Canada)

Ophthalmic solution — 1 mg/1 mL

Etodolac:

Capsules — 200 mg, 300 mg

Tablets, extended-release form — 400 mg, 600 mg

Indomethacin:

Capsules — 25 mg, 50 mg, 75 mg

Gelatin capsule (Canada) — 25 mg, 50 mg

Capsules, SR (prolonged action) — 75 mg

Oral suspension — 25 mg/5 mL

Suppositories — 50 mg, 100 mg

Ketorolac:

Tablets — 10 mg

Ophthalmic solution — 3 mL, 5 mL, 10 mL (0.5%)

Injection — 10 mg (Canada), 15 mg, 30 mg

Nabumetone:

Tablets — 500 mg, 750 mg, 1000 mg (Canada)

Sulindac:

Tablets — 150 mg, 200 mg

Tolmetin:

Capsules — 400 mg, 492 mg

Gelatin capsules — 400 mg (Canada)

Tablets — 200 mg, 600 mg

▷ ## Usual Adult Dosage Ranges
Diclofenac potassium: Maximum daily dose is 200 mg.

Diclofenac sodium: 100 to 200 mg daily to start in two to five divided doses (for example: 25 mg four times a day). Reduction to the minimum effective dose is advisable. Maximum daily dose is 225 mg. The Voltaren XR form maximum dose is 100 mg twice a day. The Arthrotec form is 50 mg/200 mcg three times a day or 75 mg/200 mcg twice daily as tolerated (osteoarthritis).

Diclofenac ophthalmic: 1 drop of 1 mg per milliliter in the eye that underwent cataract surgery, four times a day, starting 24 hours AFTER surgery and continuing for 2 weeks.

Etodolac: For osteoarthritis: A starting dose of 800 to 1,200 mg is given in divided doses. The lowest effective dose is advisable, and effective treatment has been accomplished with 200 to 400 mg daily. In patients weighing less than 60 kg, the total dose in a day should not be more than 20 mg/kg.

Etodolac extended-release form (Lodine XL): Allows once-a-day dosing for many patients. Dosing range is 400 to 1,000 mg daily. Maximum dose is 1,000 mg daily. In patients weighing less than 60 kg, the total dose in a day should not be more than 20 mg/kg. Lowest effective dose should be used.

Indomethacin: For arthritis and related conditions: 25 to 50 mg two to four times daily. If needed and tolerated, dose may be increased by 25 or 50

mg per day at intervals of 1 week. For acute gout: 100 mg initially; then 50 mg three times per day until pain is relieved. Maximum daily dose is 200 mg.

Indomethacin SR form: 75 mg daily for ankylosing spondylitis or rheumatoid arthritis.

Ketorolac ophthalmic: One drop four times daily for allergic conjunctivitis.

Nabumetone: 1,000 mg daily as a single dose is given. Dose is increased as needed and tolerated to 1,500 mg daily. The lowest effective daily dose is advisable. Maximum daily dose is 2,000 mg. Some clinicians divide dosing into two equal daily doses.

Sulindac: Therapy is started with 150 to 200 mg twice daily taken 12 hours apart for ankylosing spondylitis. Maximum daily dose is 400 mg.

Tolmetin: 400 mg three times daily is started, with usual ongoing doses of 600 to 1,600 mg as needed and tolerated. Total daily dose should not exceed 1,800 mg. Children 2 years of age or older may be given 20 mg per kg of body mass orally, divided into three or four doses daily. The dose may be increased as needed and tolerated to a maximum daily dose of 30 mg per kg of body mass.

Note: Actual dose and dosing schedule must be determined for each patient individually.

Conditions Requiring Dosing Adjustments

Liver Function: These drugs are extensively metabolized in the liver. They should be used with caution in patients with liver compromise.

Kidney Function: All nonsteroidal anti-inflammatory drugs may inhibit prostaglandins and alter kidney blood flow in patients with kidney (renal) compromise. Use with caution or not at all in patients with kidney compromise.

▷ **Dosing Instructions:** Take with or following food to prevent stomach irritation. Take with a FULL GLASS of water and do not lie down for 30 minutes. Regular-release tablets may be crushed, but not extended-release forms. The regular capsules may be opened, but not prolonged-action capsules. Food increases absorption of nabumetone. Ketorolac or diclofenac ophthalmic should NOT be used while contacts are worn. If you forget a dose: Take the missed dose right away. If it is almost time to take the next dose, skip the missed dose and continue the medicine on your regular schedule. DO NOT double doses.

Usual Duration of Use: Continual use on a regular schedule for 1 to 2 weeks is usually necessary to determine drug benefit in relieving arthritic discomfort. The usual length of treatment for bursitis or tendonitis for indomethacin or sulindac is 7 to 14 days. Ketorolac oral or IV when used is only for short-term pain treatment (a MAXIMUM of 5 days regardless of the way [route] that it is taken). Ophthalmic diclofenac and ketorolac dosing is started a day after cataract surgery and used for 14 days. Long-term use of the other agents in this class requires physician supervision.

Typical Treatment Goals and Measurements (Outcomes and Markers)

Pain: Most clinicians treating pain use a device called an algometer to check your pain. This looks like a small ruler, but lets the clinician better understand your pain. The goals of treatment then relate to where the level of pain started (for example, a rating of 7 on a 0–10 scale) and what the cause of the pain was. Pain medicines may also be used together (in combination) in order to get the best result or outcome. If your pain control is not acceptable to YOU (remember, in hospitals and outpatient settings, etc., pain control is a patient right) and if after a week of arthritis pain treatment results are not acceptable, be sure to call your doctor as you may need a different medicine or combination.

Arthritis: Control of arthritis symptoms (pain, loss of mobility, decreased ability to accomplish activities of daily living) is paramount in returning patient quality of life and to checking the results (beneficial outcomes) from these medicines. Many arthritis specialists use WOMAC (see Glossary) to measure results.

▷ **These Drugs Should Not Be Taken If**
- you have had an allergic reaction to them previously.
- you are subject to asthma or nasal polyps caused by aspirin or other NSAIDS.
- you are pregnant (all NSAIDs during the last 3 months of pregnancy). Arthrotec form is category X and should never be taken in pregnancy. These medicines are not recommended if you are breast-feeding.
- you have active peptic ulcer disease or any form of gastrointestinal ulceration or bleeding.
- you have active liver disease.
- you wear contact lenses and are prescribed an ophthalmic form.
- you have severe impairment of kidney function.
- you have severe aortic narrowing (coarctation).
- you have a history of rectal bleeding or proctitis (indomethacin suppositories).
- you have porphyria (diclofenac, indomethacin).

▷ **Inform Your Physician Before Taking This Drug If**
- you are allergic to aspirin or to other aspirin substitutes.
- you have an infection.
- you have a bleeding disorder or a blood cell disorder.
- you have a history of peptic ulcer disease, Crohn's disease, ulcerative colitis, or any type of bleeding disorder.
- you have a history of epilepsy, Parkinson's disease, or mental illness (psychosis).
- you have impaired liver or kidney function.
- you have high blood pressure or a history of heart failure.
- you are taking acetaminophen, aspirin or other aspirin substitutes, or anticoagulants.

Possible Side Effects (natural, expected, and unavoidable drug actions)

Drowsiness, ringing in ears, fluid retention. ALL NSAIDS can inhibit clotting (platelet effect) and thus have an effect in prolonging bleeding time.

▷ **Possible Adverse Effects** (unusual, unexpected, and infrequent reactions)

If any of the following develop, consult your physician promptly for guidance.

Mild Adverse Effects

Allergic reactions: skin rash, hives, itching, localized swelling of face and/or extremities.

Headache—infrequent (diclofenac and nabumetone) to frequent (indomethacin).

Dizziness, feelings of detachment—infrequent.

Mouth sores, indigestion, nausea, vomiting, diarrhea—infrequent.

Ringing in the ears (tinnitus)—possible.

Temporary loss of hair (indomethacin)—case reports.

Increased urination—infrequent (etodolac).

Serious Adverse Effects
Allergic reactions: worsening of asthma, difficult breathing (bronchospasm), mouth irritation—possible.
Angioneurotic edema (nabumetone)—rare.
Blurred vision, confusion, depression—rare.
Drug fever—case report (sulindac, tolmetin).
Active peptic ulcer, with or without bleeding, colon ulcers—possible.
Liver damage with jaundice (see Glossary)—case reports.
Kidney damage with painful urination, bloody urine, reduced urine formation—rare.
Pseudoporphyria (nabumetone)—case report.
Bone marrow depression (see Glossary): fatigue, fever, sore throat, bleeding or bruising—case reports.
Thrombophlebitis—frequent (intravenous diclofenac use).
Severe skin rash (Stevens-Johnson syndrome—diclofenac, etodolac, nabumetone, sulindac)—case reports.
Fluid retention, increased blood pressure or edema—possible with all.
Congestive heart failure worsening—possible.
Peripheral neuritis (see Glossary): numbness, pain in extremities (indomethacin)—rare.
Lung fibrosis (nabumetone)—case reports.
Pancreatitis (sulindac)—rare; (indomethacin)—case reports.
Pneumonitis (sulindac)—rare; (diclofenac)—case report.
Aseptic meningitis (diclofenac)—rare.
Seizures (indomethacin only)—case reports.

▷ **Possible Effects on Sexual Function:** Enlargement and tenderness of both male and female breasts (indomethacin, sulindac)—rare.
Nonmenstrual vaginal bleeding (indomethacin)—rare.
Impotence (indomethacin, nabumetone)—rare.
Decreased libido (indomethacin)—rare.
Uterine bleeding (sulindac)—rare.

Possible Delayed Adverse Effects: Mild anemia due to "silent" blood loss from the stomach.

Adverse Effects That May Mimic Natural Diseases or Disorders
Liver reactions may suggest viral hepatitis. Pancreatitis has occurred with sulindac.

Natural Diseases or Disorders That May Be Activated by These Drugs
Peptic ulcer disease, ulcerative colitis. Borderline clotting problems. Kidney disease.

Possible Effects on Laboratory Tests
Complete blood cell counts: decreased red cells, hemoglobin, white cells, and platelets—rare.
INR (prothrombin time): increased.
Tests of platelet aggregation: decreased aggregation.
Blood lithium level: increased.
Liver function tests: increased liver enzymes (ALT/GPT, AST/GOT, and alkaline phosphatase), increased bilirubin.
Blood sugar (glucose): increased (indomethacin only)—rare.
Kidney function tests: increased blood creatinine and urea nitrogen (BUN) levels (kidney damage).
Fecal occult blood test: positive.
Urine protein (tolmetin only): may be falsely positive.

CAUTION
1. The FDA requires a warning label on all nonprescription pain (analgesic) and fever (antipyretic) products that have aspirin or other salicylates, ibuprofen, naproxen sodium, ketoprofen, or acetaminophen in them (NSAIDs) that says: ALCOHOL WARNING: IF YOU CONSUME 3 OR MORE ALCOHOLIC DRINKS EVERY DAY, ASK YOUR DOCTOR WHETHER YOU SHOULD TAKE [THE MEDICINE IN QUESTION] OR OTHER PAIN RELIEVERS/FEVER REDUCERS. [THE INGREDIENT] MAY CAUSE STOMACH BLEEDING. This is a relatively new warning intended to help protect patients from possible stomach or liver damage.
2. Dose should be limited to the smallest amount that produces reasonable improvement. Many nonprescription pain relievers also have medicines from families called NSAIDS (such as Aleve, Motrin and Nuprin). Do not combine these forms as the combination can be hard on your stomach (lead to ulceration).
3. These drugs may mask early signs of infection. Tell your doctor if you think you are developing an infection of any kind.
4. Congestive heart failure in elderly patients may be unmasked or worsened. Risk appears to increase with use of higher doses.
5. Do NOT add non-prescription or prescription NSAIDS such as aspirin, ibuprofen (Advil or Motrin), or naproxen (Aleve) while you are taking these medicines. (The adverse stomach and intestinal effects will increase).

Precautions for Use
By Infants and Children:
Diclofenac, etodolac, nabumetone, sulindac: Safety and efficacy for those under 12 years of age not established.
Indomethacin: This drug frequently impairs kidney function in infants. Fatal liver reactions are possible in children between 6 and 12 years of age; avoid the use of this drug in this age group. Note: This medicine is used in infants (patent ductus arteriosus intravenously).
Ketorolac ophthalmic: Safety and efficacy for those 3 years of age and older for seasonal allergic conjunctivitis (eases itching) is established.
Tolmetin: Safety and efficacy for those under 2 years of age not established.
By Those Over 60 Years of Age: Small doses are advisable until tolerance is determined. Watch for any signs of liver or kidney toxicity, fluid retention, dizziness, confusion, impaired memory, depression, peptic ulcer, or diarrhea, often with rectal bleeding.

▷ **Advisability of Use During Pregnancy**
Pregnancy Category: Indomethacin, diclofenac, tolmetin: B. Sulindac: B in first two trimesters. Nabumetone: C in first two trimesters. Not recommended in last trimester. Indomethacin, etodolac, nabumetone, and sulindac (D in last trimester): D. (Indomethacin is also category D if used after 34 weeks or for more than 48 hours.) Diclofenac to be avoided in late pregnancy. Arthrotec form is category X. See Pregnancy Risk Categories at the back of this book.
Animal Studies:
Indomethacin: significant toxicity and birth defects reported in mice and rats.
Diclofenac: Mouse, rat, and rabbit studies reveal toxic effects on the embryo but no birth defects.
Nabumetone, tolmetin: Rat and rabbit studies revealed no defects.

Human Studies:

Indomethacin: Adequate studies of pregnant women are not available. However, birth defects have been attributed to the use of this drug during pregnancy. The manufacturer recommends that indomethacin not be taken during pregnancy.

Diclofenac, nabumetone, sulindac, tolmetin: Adequate studies of pregnant women are not available. Avoid this drug completely during the last 3 months of pregnancy. Use it during the first 6 months only if clearly needed. Ask your doctor for guidance.

Etodolac: Adequate studies of pregnant women not available. The manufacturer advises that this drug be avoided during in late pregnancy.

Nabumetone: Fetal cardiovascular system adversely affected if used in the last trimester, so not recommended for last 3 months.

Advisability of Use If Breast-Feeding

Presence of these drugs in breast milk: Yes (all).

Avoid drugs or refrain from nursing (may have bad effects on infant's nervous system).

Habit-Forming Potential: None.

Effects of Overdose: Drowsiness, agitation, bleeding, confusion, nausea, vomiting, diarrhea, disorientation, seizures, coma.

Possible Effects of Long-Term Use: Indomethacin and tolmetin: eye changes—deposits in the cornea, alterations in the retina. Irritation of the stomach and intestine.

Suggested Periodic Examinations While Taking These Drugs (at physician's discretion)

Complete blood cell counts.

Liver and kidney function tests.

Complete eye examinations if vision is altered in any way.

Stool for hidden (occult) blood (may actually be positive from these drugs).

▷ **While Taking These Drugs, Observe the Following**

Foods: No restrictions. These medicines are taken with food to decrease stomach irritation.

Herbal Medicines or Minerals: Ginseng, ginkgo, alfalfa, clove oil, feverfew, cinchona bark, and garlic may also change clotting, so combining those herbals with these medicines is not recommended. Talk to your doctor BEFORE combining any medicines. NSAIDs may decrease feverfew effects. White willow bark (salicylates) can increase risk of stomach or intestinal adverse effects if combined. Since St. John's wort and some of these medicines may increase sensitivity to the sun, CAUTION IS ADVISED. Combined use of beta glucan and diclofenac, indomethacin, sulindac, and aspirin lead to severe reactions in lab animals (mice). Nabumetone did not appear to have severe reaction risk. Eucalyptus and skull cap may increase risk of undesirable effects on the liver. Hay flower, mistletoe herb, and white mustard seed carry German Commission E monograph indications for arthritis.

Nutritional Support: Indomethacin: Take 50 mg of vitamin C (ascorbic acid) daily.

Beverages: No restrictions. May be taken with milk.

▷ *Alcohol:* Used with caution: see FDA warning above. Alcohol can irritate the lining of the stomach. If excessive alcohol use is combined with the irritating effect of these medicines, risk of stomach and intestinal problems such as ulceration or bleeding can be increased.

Tobacco Smoking: No interactions expected. I advise everyone to quit smoking.

▷   *Other Drugs*

Medicines in this family may ***increase*** the effects of
- aminoglycoside antibiotics (amikacin, others—see Drug Classes) by increasing blood levels.
- anticoagulants such as warfarin (Coumadin) and increase the risk of bleeding; monitor INR (prothrombin time), adjust dose accordingly.
- cyclosporine (Sandimmune) and cause toxicity.
- digoxin (Lanoxin)—indomethacin only.
- eptifibatide (Integrilin) and increase risk of bleeding (benefit to risk decision).
- lithium and cause lithium toxicity (except sulindac, which may decrease lithium levels).
- methotrexate (Mexate, others) and cause toxic levels.
- phenytoin (Dilantin) because of increased drug levels.
- tacrolimus (Prograf) and increase risk of decreased kidney function.
- thrombolytics such as streptokinase or TPA.
- zidovudine (AZT) and lead to toxicity of either medicine (indomethacin).

Medications in this class may ***decrease*** the effects of
- ACE inhibitors (see Drug Classes).
- beta-blocker drugs (see Drug Classes) and reduce their antihypertensive effectiveness.
- bumetanide (Bumex).
- captopril (Capoten).
- ethacrynic acid (Edecrin).
- furosemide (Lasix) and other loop diuretics.
- thiazide diuretics (see Drug Classes).

Medications in this class ***taken concurrently*** with the following drugs may increase the risk of bleeding or serious side effects; avoid these combinations or use with great caution:
- aspirin or other NSAIDs (EVEN NONPRESCRIPTION FORMS).
- clopidogrel (Plavix).
- dicumarol.
- diflunisal (Dolobid).
- dipyridamole (Persantine).
- low-molecular-weight heparins (Lovenox, others).
- probenecid (Pro-Biosan, others).
- sulfinpyrazone (Anturane).
- valproic acid (Depakene).
- warfarin (Coumadin).

Medications in this class ***taken concurrently*** with:
- alendronate (Fosamax) may increase risk of stomach or intestinal irritation.
- colestipol and cholestyramine will reduce beneficial effects of the NSAIDs (diclofenac and sulindac).
- levofloxacin (Levaquin) and ofloxacin (Floxin) can increase risk of seizures.
- methotrexate (Mexate, others) may lead to increased methotrexate toxicity.
- ritonavir (Norvir) and other medicines that affect the cytochrome P-450 system in the liver will lead to altered blood levels of these medicines.

▷   *Driving, Hazardous Activities:* These drugs may cause drowsiness, dizziness, or impaired vision. Restrict activities as necessary.

Aviation Note: The use of these drugs ***may be a disqualification*** for piloting. Consult a designated Aviation Medical Examiner.

Exposure to Sun: Caution: Several medicines in this class have caused increased sensitivity (photosensitivity—see Glossary).

ADALIMUMAB (A dah lim you mab)

Other Name: D2E7   **Introduced:**   2003   **Class:**   Disease Modifying Antirheumatic Drug (DMARD), human monoclonal antibody to TNF alpha
Prescription: USA: Yes   **Controlled Drug:**   USA: No; Canada: No
Available as Generic: No

Brand Name: Humira

Author's Note: This treatment for rheumatoid arthritis offers the benefit of easier once every two week under the skin (subcutaneous) dosing. Current outcome measures such as quality of life, fatigue scales, acute phase reactant responses, ACR response and adverse effect profiles appear favorable at present. This is the first fully human tumor necrosis factor (TNF alpha) antibody and may be less likely to lead to allergic reactions. Information in this profile will broaden based on clinical research, once additional information is available.

ALBUTEROL (al BYU ter all)

Other Name: Salbutamol   **Introduced:**   1968   **Class:**   Antiasthmatic, bronchodilator   **Prescription:**   USA: Yes   **Controlled Drug:** USA: No; Canada: No   **Available as Generic:**   Yes

Brand Names: Accuneb, Airet, ✤Alti-Salbutamol, ✤Apo-Salvent, Combivent [CD], Diskhaler, ✤Novo-Salmol, PMS-Salbutamol, Proventil HFA, Proventil Inhaler, Proventil Repetabs, Proventil Tablets, Rotahaler, ✤Salbutamol, ✤Ventodisk Rotacaps, Ventolin HFA, Ventolin Inhaler, Ventolin Nebules, Ventolin Rotacaps, Ventolin Syrup, Ventolin Tablets, Volmax Sustained-Release Tablets, Volmax Timed-Release Tablets

BENEFITS versus RISKS	
Possible Benefits	*Possible Risks*
VERY EFFECTIVE RELIEF OF BRONCHOSPASM	Increased blood pressure or heart rate
	Fine hand tremor
FIXED DOSE COMBINATION WITH IPRATROPIUM (COMBIVENT)	Potential hyperactivity in children under twelve
HELPS WITH CHRONIC OBSTRUCTIVE PULMONARY DISEASE (COPD)	Angina in patients with coronary artery disease
	Irregular heart rhythm and fatalities—possible, with excessive use
	Paradoxical spasm of the bronchi

▷ **Principal Uses**
   As a Single Drug Product: Uses currently included in FDA-approved labeling: (1) Relieves acute bronchial asthma and reduces frequency and severity of chronic, recurrent asthmatic attacks; (2) helps prevent exercise-induced bronchospasm.
      Other (unlabeled) generally accepted uses: (1) May have a role (nebulized) where blood potassium is too high; (2) limited use in patients with premature labor—especially if the cervix is dilated less than 3 centimeters.

As a Combination Drug Product [CD]: Combivent form has 120 mcg of albuterol and 21 mcg of ipratropium per press (actuation): (1) Eases symptoms of moderate to even severe chronic obstructive pulmonary disease (COPD).

How This Drug Works: By acting on adenyl cyclase, a chemical called cyclic AMP is increased. In response to increased cyclic AMP, this drug relaxes muscle (smooth) that is found in the uterus, skeletal muscle blood vessels (vascular bed) and the bronchi. In some lung disease, albuterol also works to help the lungs move mucus and decreases chemical release from mast cells.

▷ **Widely Used Guidelines That Involve This Medicine (representative sample):** Please look at the section at the very beginning of this profile called "Class." Next, turn to Table 22 and you will find guidelines listed by the class involved!

Available Dosage Forms and Strengths
> Aerosol (actuation) — 90 mcg per press
> — 100 mcg per press (Canada)
> — 120 mcg per press
> Capsules for inhalation
> (technique is important) — 200 mcg, 400 mcg (Canada)
> Nasal inhaler (Canada) — 100 mcg/dose
> Solution for inhalation — 0.83% and 0.5%
> Rotacaps — 200 mcg
> Syrup — 2 mg/5 mL
> — 2.4 mg/5 mL
> Tablets — 2 mg, 4 mg
> Tablets, sustained release — 4 mg, 4.8 mg, 8 mg, 9.6 mg
> Tablets, timed release — 4 mg, 8 mg
> Ventodisk (Canada) — 200 mcg and 400 mcg per disk

▷ **Recommended Dosage Ranges** (Actual dose and schedule must be determined for each patient individually.)

Capsules for inhalation (Rotahaler): Dose for children more than 4 years old and for adults is to use the contents of one capsule (200 mcg) via the Rotahaler device every 4 to 6 hours.

Metered dose inhaler—Adults and children 12 or older: Two inhalations (180 mcg) repeated every 4 to 6 hours. For some patients, one inhalation every 4 hours may be enough. Taking a larger number of inhalations is not recommended. If the dose that previously worked does not provide relief, call your doctor immediately. The status of your asthma must be examined.

Author's Note: Proventil Repetabs and Volmax are FDA-approved to treat bronchospasm in patients 6 years old or older. Treatments are best checked every 3–6 months and decreased in small steps if possible.

Preventing exercise-caused asthma: Two inhalations (180 mcg of Ventolin form) 15 minutes BEFORE exercise.

Tablets (immediate release)—2 to 4 mg three to four times daily (every 8 to 6 hours).

Tablets (sustained release)—One or two tablets every 12 hours.

Do not exceed eight inhalations (720 mcg) or 32 mg (tablet form) every 24 hours. Some manufacturers limit tablets to 16 mg every 24 hours.

Conditions Requiring Dosing Adjustments
Liver Function: Low doses and caution needed in liver disease.
Kidney Function: No specific changes in dosing are available.

Heart (Coronary Artery) Disease: A maximum starting dose should be 1 mg in order to avoid chest pain (angina).

Thyroid Disease: People with low (hypoactive) thyroids may require increased doses.

▷ **Dosing Instructions:** Pill form may be taken on empty stomach or with food or milk. Nonsustained-release tablets may be crushed. Sustained-release forms should NEVER be crushed. For inhaler, follow the written instructions carefully. The Proventil inhaler should be primed FOUR TIMES before you first use it. If you have not used the Proventil inhalation aerosol for four days, please prime the aerosol twice before you use it. Do not use excessively. If you forget a dose: Use the inhaler as soon as possible. Do not double doses.

Usual Duration of Use: Do not use beyond the time necessary to stop episodes of asthma.

Typical Treatment Goals and Measurements (Outcomes and Markers)

Asthma: Short-acting beta agonists like albuterol are used to prevent or treat reversible spasms of the bronchial tubes. The peak effect happens 1 to 2 hours after dosing. Many clinicians use improved respiratory status (FEV1) to check benefits as well as no night time symptoms and ability to undertake usual activities and decreased need for hospitalizations. One center in London used measurement of peak flow (patients were asked to blow three times in quick succession into a special measuring meter) to help decide how long patients should remain in the hospital. Calculations between the first and last breath measurements were made. Patients who had a ratio of less than one were said to have a decreased peak flow (indicating inflammation) and were kept in the hospital for an additional 3 days. Patients with a ratio of more than one (acceptable peak flow and relative absence of inflammation) were successfully sent home from the hospital. In any patient, if the usual therapeutic response to this medicine is not seen, call your doctor right away.

▷ **This Drug Should Not Be Taken If**
- you have had an allergic reaction to any form of it.
- you have an irregular heart rhythm or a fast heartbeat (tachycardia—Volmax).
- you have a specific problem with the aorta (idiopathic hypertrophic subvalvular stenosis—Volmax form).
- you have an overactive thyroid (hyperthyroid).
- you are taking, or took in the past 2 weeks, any monoamine oxidase (MAO) type A inhibitor (see Drug Classes).

▷ **Inform Your Physician Before Taking This Drug If**
- you have a heart or circulatory disorder, especially high blood pressure, coronary heart disease, or aneurysms.
- you have diabetes.
- you have pheochromocytoma.
- you take any form of digitalis or any stimulant drug.
- you take other prescription or nonprescription medications that weren't discussed when albuterol was prescribed.
- you are going to have a baby (this medicine may alter contractions).
- you are unsure how much or how often to take albuterol.

Possible Side Effects (natural, expected, and unavoidable drug actions)

Aerosol: dryness or irritation of mouth/throat, altered taste.

Tablet: nervousness, palpitation, fast heart rate (tachycardia)—infrequent.

Heart effect may not be seen with nebulized albuterol.

▷ **Possible Adverse Effects** (unusual, unexpected, and infrequent reactions)
If any of the following develop, consult your physician promptly for guidance.

Mild Adverse Effects
Itching—rare.
Headache, dizziness, restlessness, insomnia—infrequent.
Fine hand tremor—frequent.
Nausea—rare.
Leg cramps, flushing of skin—rare.
Difficulty urinating—rare.
Rapid heart rate—infrequent.
Decreased platelets—possible, but not clinically significant.

Serious Adverse Effects
Hypersensitivity reaction—case report.
Heart attack—case reports after intravenous or excessive inhalation use.
Abnormal heartbeats—possible.
Chest pain (angina)—possible with higher doses in patients with coronary artery disease.
Hallucinations or convulsions (with excessive dosing)—possible.
Decreased blood potassium (hypokalemia)—possible and dose related.
High blood sugar (hyperglycemia)—possible and more likely with intravenous use.

▷ **Possible Effects on Sexual Function:** None reported.

Natural Diseases or Disorders That May Be Activated by This Drug
Latent coronary artery disease, diabetes, or high blood pressure.

Possible Effects on Laboratory Tests
Blood aldosterone: increased.
Blood HDL cholesterol level: may be slightly increased.
Blood glucose level: increased.
Blood potassium: decreased.
Blood platelets: decreased (with high doses).
Blood magnesium: one study showed doses greater than 500 mcg lowered magnesium.

CAUTION
1. This drug may be dangerous if patients increase dose and/or frequency, as it may result in rapid or irregular heart rhythm and fatalities with overuse. A July 2001 report from the Dutch Centre for Human Drug Research found that when possible, high-dose inhaled albuterol may be best given with oxygen.
2. Use of this drug by inhalation with beclomethasone aerosol (Beclovent, Vanceril) may increase the risk of fluorocarbon propellant toxicity (fluorocarbons are being phased out). Use albuterol aerosol 20 to 30 minutes before beclomethasone aerosol to reduce toxicity and enhance the penetration of beclomethasone.
3. Serious heart rhythm problems or cardiac arrest can result from excessive or prolonged inhalation.
4. In general, women have been found to have higher peak blood levels (Cmax) after oral doses than men. Therefore, women may have an increased risk of adverse effects (like lowered potassium or tremor) even with "therapeutic or usual" doses.
5. One study (see Wolfenden, L.L. in Sources) of 4,005 patients found that many patients did not accurately describe their symptoms to their doctors.

This led to patients being undertreated. Be honest with your doctor about the severity and frequency of your asthma so that the treatments can be tailored to the severity and frequency of asthma symptoms!

6. Call your doctor if you begin to increase the number of times you use this drug on a daily basis. Tolerance to the effects of this drug has been reported.

Precautions for Use

By Infants and Children: Dosing in children is often calculated on a mg per kg basis.

By Those Over 60 Years of Age: Avoid excessive and continual use. If asthma is not relieved promptly, other drugs will have to be tried. Watch for nervousness, palpitations, irregular heart rhythm, and muscle tremors. Doses of 2 mg by mouth three or four times daily are prudent.

▷ **Advisability of Use During Pregnancy**

Pregnancy Category: C. See Pregnancy Risk Categories at the back of this book.

Animal Studies: Cleft palate reported in mice.

Human Studies: Adequate studies of pregnant women are not available.

Avoid use during first 3 months if possible.

Advisability of Use If Breast-Feeding

Presence of this drug in breast milk: Yes.

Avoid drug or refrain from nursing.

Habit-Forming Potential: A few cases of dependency and abuse have been described. These may be cases of use for the effect of the propellants (propellants are changing) or the drug itself.

Effects of Overdose: Nervousness, palpitation, rapid heart rate, life-threatening arrhythmias, sweating, headache, tremor, vomiting, chest pain.

Possible Effects of Long-Term Use: Loss of effectiveness.

Suggested Periodic Examinations While Taking This Drug (at physician's discretion)

Blood pressure measurements, evaluation of heart status, frequency of bronchospasms, check on relief of symptoms at night, improved lung measurements (Peak Expiratory Flow or PEF).

▷ **While Taking This Drug, Observe the Following**

Foods: No restrictions. Because this medicine may lead to minor lowering of potassium, talk to your doctor about possible need to increase potassium in your diet (see Table 13).

Herbal Medicines or Minerals: Using St. John's wort, ma huang, ephedrine-like compounds, guarana (caffeine), or kola while taking this medicine may result in unacceptable central nervous system stimulation. Talk to your doctor and pharmacist BEFORE making any combinations. Fir or pine needle oil should NOT be used by asthmatics. Ephedra alone does carry a German Commission E monograph indication for asthma treatment. If you are allergic to plants in the Asteraceae family (aster, chrysanthemum, daisy, or ragweed), you may also be allergic to echinacea, chamomile, feverfew, and St. John's wort.

Beverages: Avoid excessive caffeine as found in coffee, tea, cola, and chocolate.

▷ *Alcohol:* No interactions expected.

Tobacco Smoking: Smoking constricts airways. I advise everyone to quit.

▷ *Other Drugs*
   Albuterol *taken concurrently* with
   - amphetamines may worsen cardiovascular side effects.
   - atomoxetine (Strattera) may worsen cardiovascular (increased blood pressure and heart rate) side effects.
   - bendroflumethiazide (Corzide, Naturetin) and other thiazide and loop diuretics (see Drug Classes) may result in additive lowering of blood potassium.
   - beta-blockers such as propranolol (Inderal) results in loss of effect of both medications.
   - digoxin (Lanoxin) may lower blood levels, but clinical importance of the 16–22% lowering from one study is unclear.
   - dopamine (Intropin) may worsen adverse effects on the heart. Avoid this combination.
   - ephedrine (Bronkaid, Tedrigen) may result in excessive heart effects.
   - ipratropium (Atrovent) can result in better (longer time) opening of the bronchi (beneficial interaction).
   - isoproterenol (Isuprel) may result in worsening of heart (cardiac) side effects.
   - monoamine oxidase (MAO) type A inhibitor drugs can cause very high blood pressure and undesirable heart stimulation.
   - pancuronium (Pavulon) or vecuronium (Norcuron) may lead to bronchospasm and delayed recovery of neuromuscular function.
   - phenylephrine (Dimetapp, Dristan, others) may worsen bad effects on the heart (adverse reaction), and the combination is not recommended.
   - phenylpropanolamine (Acutrim, Alka-Seltzer Plus, Contac, others) may worsen bad effects on the heart (adverse reaction). Do not combine.
   - pseudoephedrine (Sudafed, others) may worsen adverse heart effects. DO NOT COMBINE.
   - theophylline (Theo-Dur, others) may result in rapid removal of theophylline and loss of therapeutic theophylline effect.
   - tricyclic antidepressants (see Drug Classes) may cause a severe increase in blood pressure.

▷ *Driving, Hazardous Activities:* Use caution if excessive nervousness or dizziness occurs.
   Aviation Note: The use of this drug *is a disqualification* for piloting. Consult a designated Aviation Medical Examiner.
   Exposure to Sun: No restrictions.
   Heavy Exercise or Exertion: Use caution. Excessive exercise can cause (induce) asthma in some asthmatics.

ALENDRONATE (a LEN druh nate)

Introduced: 1996   **Class:**   Second-generation bisphosphonate, Anti-osteoporotics   **Prescription:**   USA: Yes   **Controlled Drug:**   USA: No *Available as Generic:*   No

Brand Name: Fosamax, Fosamax Once Weekly

BENEFITS versus RISKS	
Possible Benefits	*Possible Risks*
EFFECTIVE TREATMENT OF MALE AND FEMALE OSTEOPOROSIS	Esophageal irritation
INCREASE IN BONE MASS	Minor muscle pain
PREVENTION OF OSTEOPOROSIS	Flatulence
ONCE-WEEKLY TREATMENT AND/OR PREVENTION OF OSTEOPOROSIS	
DECREASED RISK OF BONE FRACTURES	
SYMPTOM RELIEF IN PAGET'S DISEASE	
PREVENTION OF POST-MENOPAUSAL OSTEOPOROSIS	
PREVENTION OF OSTEOPOROSIS IN THOSE TAKING CORTICOSTEROID-TYPE (STEROID) MEDICINES	
NEWLY APPROVED LIQUID FORM WILL BE EASIER FOR PATIENTS TO TAKE	

▷ **Principal Uses**

As a Single Drug Product: Uses currently included in FDA-approved labeling: (1) Treatment of postmenopausal osteoporosis; (2) treatment of Paget's disease; (3) prevention of postmenopausal osteoporosis; (4) prevention of osteoporosis in people who take corticosteroid-type medicines; (5) once weekly prevention or treatment of osteoporosis; (6) treatment of osteoporosis in men.

Other (unlabeled) generally accepted uses: (1) approved in Canada in combination with hormone replacement therapy (estrogen or estrogen plus progesterone) to increase positive outcomes on increased bone mass; (2) may have a role in osteoporosis sometimes seen in HIV patients (antiretroviral induced); (3) could have a role intravenously in reflex sympathetic dystrophy syndrome (RSDS); (4) early research suggests a role in early treatment of osteonecrosis (avascular necrosis of bone); (5) prevents bone loss in women who stop hormone replacement therapy (HRT).

How This Drug Works: This medicine works at the brush border of the osteoclast cell (inhibiting enzymes in the mevalonate pathway). This prevents the cell from resorbing (gobbling up) bone while the osteoblast (bone-building cell) continues to work. The end result is bone-building and decreased fracture risk.

▷ **Widely Used Guidelines That Involve This Medicine (representative sample):** Please look at the section at the very beginning of this profile called "Class." Next, turn to Table 22 and you will find guidelines listed by the class involved!

Available Dosage Forms and Strengths

Tablets — 5 mg, 10 mg, 35 mg, 40 mg, 70 mg

Oral Solution — 70 mg

▷ **Recommended Dosage Ranges** (Actual dose and schedule must be determined for each patient individually.)

Infants and Children: Efficacy and safety are not established.

18 to 65 Years of Age: Treatment of osteoporosis in women after menopause: 70 mg once a week (tablet or the new liquid/solution form) OR 10 mg taken once daily.

Osteoporosis prevention in women after menopause: 35 mg once a week OR 5 mg once daily. I strongly recommend an appropriate amount of dietary calcium and/or calcium supplementation to ensure adequate calcium every day. Discuss the need for vitamin D with your doctor. Calcium and vitamin D are critical in osteoporosis prevention and treatment.

Osteoporosis TREATMENT in women after menopause or in men: 70 mg once a week for women (can also be considered for men) OR 10 mg once daily. Calcium and vitamin D also should be added.

Prevention of glucocorticoid-induced osteoporosis: 5 mg daily in one study.

Treatment of glucocorticoid-induced osteoporosis: 5 mg once daily. In post-menopausal women who are NOT taking estrogen, the dose for this indication is 10 mg once daily.

Paget's disease: 40 mg once daily for 6 months. Repeat treatment after a 6 month evaluation period may be possible if patients relapse (increased serum alkaline phosphatase).

Over 65 Years of Age: Same as in those 18 to 65 years old.

Conditions Requiring Dosing Adjustments

Liver Function: No changes needed.

Kidney Function: Lower doses for patients with kidney compromise. Patients with creatinine clearances (see Glossary) less than 35 mL/min **should not** be given this medicine.

▷ **Dosing Instructions:** TAKE THIS MEDICINE WITH 6 TO 8 OUNCES OF TAP WATER TO GET THE BEST RESULTS. DO NOT take this drug with food or other drugs. The therapeutic benefit will be decreased. **If you are taking the new liquid form, drink two ounces** (about a fourth of a cup) of water after you drink the liquid medicine. Wait at least half an hour before eating the first food or liquids (other than plain tap water) of the day. Avoiding food or drink for more than 30 minutes lets more medicine get into your body to go to work. **DO NOT** lie down for 30 minutes (preferably an hour) after taking this drug (decreases risk of irritation of the esophagus). If you forget a dose: Take the medicine right away, unless it is nearly time for your next dose. If you are taking it once weekly, call your doctor. DO NOT double doses.

Usual Duration of Use: In Paget's disease, this medicine is used once daily for 6 months, with recheck after that. In treating osteoporosis after menopause, many doctors get a bone mineral density test (DEXA or PDEXA presently most widely used) to help decide to start therapy and then get a second test 2 years later or order certain laboratory tests to check results or outcome of therapy. Further study is needed to find the best dosing strategies in long-term (greater than 10 years) use of alendronate (cyclic or ongoing).

Typical Treatment Goals and Measurements (Outcomes and Markers)

Fracture of bone is a critical issue when bones weaken and become osteoporotic. The World Health Organization has generated guidelines that establish weak bone (osteopenia) and osteoporosis based on certain patient populations. If this medicine is being used to prevent osteoporosis, a typical strategy would be to obtain a measure of bone mineral density such as a DEXA scan. The medicine would be started based on risk factors, medicines (such as glucocorticoids) that are being taken and the results of the DEXA scan itself. Laboratory tests (such as N-telopeptides) may be tested to augment treatment decisions. Once the medicine is started, a DEXA is often rechecked in 2 years to assess the beneficial effects of this medicine. Some clinicians will also recommend check of height (height loss) as well as an earlier repeat DEXA, PDEXA, ultrasound, and/or laboratory test in patients with a family history of rapid perimenopausal bone loss. In Paget's disease, this medicine is used once daily for 6 months, with recheck after that.

Possible Advantages of This Drug

Ten–year data recently released showed that this medicine continues to improve bone mass over this extended time frame (longest clinical study of osteoporosis after menopause—see Bone, H.G. in References). This drug increases bone mass more than other available (anti-resorptive) drugs, which then decreases the risk of fractures. This medicine also helps form normal bone (microarchitecture). Alendronate also offers the adherence (taking the medicine as prescribed) benefits of once-weekly dosing in both the tablet and the NEW oral liquid form. While the role in osteonecrosis is emerging, this medicine may offer an alternative to surgical approaches. Results of the EFFECT (Efficacy of Fosamax versus Evista Comparison Trial) showed that alendronate (70 mg once a week as compared to raloxifene 60 mg once a week) favored alendronate. This study was the first head to head research and revealed significantly larger increases at the hip and spine for alendronate versus raloxifene. A head to head study of alendronate (Fosamax 70 mg a week) versus risedronate (Actonel 35 mg a week) is currently being undertaken. Alendronate was shown to protect against bone loss in women who stopped hormone replacement therapy (HRT).

▷ This Drug Should Not Be Taken If

- you are allergic to the drug or its components.
- you have a low blood calcium (hypocalcemia). Talk to your doctor.
- you have a significant kidney disease (medicine should NOT be taken if creatinine clearance less than 35 mL/min—no data).
- you are unable to sit or stand for 30 minutes after taking this medicine (increased risk of esophageal problems).
- you are pregnant or are nursing your infant.
- you have esophageal disease (abnormal esophagus) or difficulty emptying the esophagus.

▷ Inform Your Physician Before Taking This Drug If

- you have ulcers or inflammation of the duodenum.
- you have difficulty swallowing.
- you have a vitamin D deficiency.
- you have a diet poor in calcium (low calcium diet).

Possible Side Effects (natural, expected, and unavoidable drug actions)

Irritation of the esophagus and potential ulceration—rare. This effect is worsened if patients lie down soon after taking drug. Drug fever is common with intravenous use.

▷ Possible Adverse Effects (unusual, unexpected, and infrequent reactions)

If any of the following develop, consult your physician promptly for guidance.

Mild Adverse Effects
  Allergic reactions: rare skin rash or redness.
  Headache—infrequent.
  Blurred vision (possible conjunctivitis)—rare.
  Gas (flatulence), diarrhea, or constipation—infrequent (flatulence appears more likely in men in one small study).
  Pain in the muscles or skeleton (musculoskeletal)—infrequent.
  Mild calcium decrease—2% decrease (some patients at 10 mg daily).
  Mild decrease in phosphorus—up to 6%.
  Mild muscle pain—infrequent with the 10-mg dose.

Serious Adverse Effects
  Allergic reactions: none reported.
  Esophageal ulceration—rare. (Increased risk if you lie down after taking this drug. Best NOT to lie down for at least half an hour after taking this medicine.) One case report of a patient with a history of peptic ulcer disease who had stomach surgery and was also taking aspirin who developed an ulcer (anastamotic) and had mild hemorrhaging.
  Liver toxicity—one case report.
  Inflammation of the sclera (scleritis)—rare (probably idiosyncratic).

▷ **Possible Effects on Sexual Function:** None reported.

Possible Effects on Laboratory Tests
  Serum calcium or phosphorus: lowered—infrequent.
  Liver function tests: increased—rare (with intravenous form) (asymptomatic and transient).

CAUTION
  1. A "dear doctor" letter was sent out by the FDA early after alendronate approval warning of increased occurrence of esophageal ulceration. This may have been caused by patients taking the medicine with less water than directed and by patients who took the medicine and went back to bed. Take this medicine with a full glass of tap water and DO NOT LIE DOWN for 30 minutes after taking this drug.
  2. Patients who take more than 10 mg of alendronate a day may need to avoid aspirin and aspirin-containing compounds because upper gastrointestinal adverse effects may be increased in this situation if the medicines are combined (at any alendronate dose).
  3. Other causes of osteoporosis besides estrogen or aging (secondary osteoporosis) must be ruled out.
  4. Depression (long-standing) may be a risk factor for osteoporosis (probably diet related). Talk with your doctor about an osteoporosis test if depression is a problem for you.
  5. Talk to your doctor if you develop eye symptoms while taking this medicine.

Precautions for Use
  By Infants and Children: Safety and efficacy in this age group have not been established.
  By Those Over 65 Years of Age: The amount that goes into the body (bioavailability) and the places alendronate goes (disposition) are similar to those less than 65. No specific dosing changes needed. Increased sensitivity to this drug is possible.

▷ **Advisability of Use During Pregnancy**
  Pregnancy Category: C. See Pregnancy Risk Categories at the back of this book.
  Animal Studies: Studies in rats have shown toxicity to the mother as well as neonatal death following dosing of alendronate during pregnancy.

Human Studies: Adequate studies of pregnant women are not available. Avoid this medicine during pregnancy.

Advisability of Use If Breast-Feeding
Presence of this drug in breast milk: Yes in rats; unknown in humans. Avoid drug or refrain from nursing.

Habit-Forming Potential: None.

Effects of Overdose: Nausea, vomiting, hypocalcemia, and hypophosphatemia. Heartburn, ulceration of the upper gastrointestinal tract.

Possible Effects of Long-Term Use: Increased bone density and decreased fracture risk (beneficial).

Suggested Periodic Examinations While Taking This Drug (at physician's discretion)
Tests of bone mineral density (DEXA, PDEXA, ultrasound, or QCT), check of lab tests of bone loss or formation.
Blood calcium.
Measurement of height.
Assessment of any eye irritation.

▷ **While Taking This Drug, Observe the Following**
Foods: DO NOT TAKE THIS DRUG WITH FOOD.
Herbal Medicines or Minerals: Soy or other plant-derived phytoestrogens may work to complement alendronate, but have not been studied. Ipriflavone is a synthetic flavonoid currently investigational for osteoporosis (which both inhibits bone resorption by reducing osteoclast recruitment and encourages osteoblast function). Combined use with alendronate has not been studied. Use with white willow bark (salicylates) may increase stomach irritation risk.
Adequate elemental calcium and vitamin D are needed. Calcium supplements should be taken at least half an hour after taking alendronate. Effervescent calcium (resulting in a solution) may be absorbed more rapidly and help avoid problems.
Beverages: ANY liquid other than water will DECREASE the amount of alendronate that gets into your body to help you. It is critical that this medicine only be taken with 6 to 8 ounces of water.
▷ *Alcohol:* Alcohol (especially in high doses) may act as a bone-forming cell (osteoblast) poison, and excessive use is a risk factor for osteoporosis. Alcohol may also irritate the stomach lining.
Tobacco Smoking: Smoking is a risk factor for osteoporosis. STOP SMOKING.
▷ *Other Drugs*
Alendronate *taken concurrently* with
- antacids may decrease the total absorption of alendronate and decrease its therapeutic benefit.
- aspirin or aspirin-containing products or salicylates may pose an increased risk of upper gastrointestinal adverse effects if more than 10 mg of alendronate is taken daily. Although other NSAIDs (see Drug Classes) were not presented as potential problems with alendronate doses greater than 10 mg, caution is advised for this benefit to risk decision.
- calcium products (various) will blunt absorption of alendronate. Wait at least half an hour after taking alendronate to take any other medicine including a calcium supplement. Effervescent calcium forms may offer an advantage considering their speed of absorption.
- estrogens (various) taken by a few women in clinical trials did not present

problems. This combination is (both estrogen and/or estrogen plus a progestin) approved in Canada.

- foscarnet (Foscavir) may result in an additive decrease in calcium.
- magnesium (various) may increase stomach/intestine upset.
- medicines in general should NOT be taken at the same time as alendronate. Separate any dose of alendronate and any other medicine by at least half an hour.
- mesalamine or olsalazine may increase stomach/intestine upset.
- ranitidine (Zantac) (intravenous form and perhaps oral form) may double how much alendronate gets into your body. The clinical importance of this is not yet known.
- teriparatide (Forteo) may work in a beneficial way (and by a different mechanism of action) but has not yet been studied.

The following drugs may *decrease* the effects of alendronate:
- Because a small amount of alendronate gets into the body under the best conditions, take alendronate with a full 6 to 8 ounces of water. Take any other drugs at least half an hour after alendronate.

▷ *Driving, Hazardous Activities:* No specific limitations.

Aviation Note: The use of this drug is *probably not a disqualification* for piloting. Consult a designated Aviation Medical Examiner.

Exposure to Sun: No restrictions.

Heavy Exercise or Exertion: If your bone density is low, heavy aerobic exercise may not be a good idea. Discuss this with your doctor. In general, weight-bearing exercise stimulates receptors (mechanoreceptors) to release factors that result in increased bone strength.

Discontinuation: Talk with your doctor **before** stopping this medicine.

ALLOPURINOL (al oh PURE i nohl)

Introduced: 1963 **Class:** Antigout, xanthine oxidase inhibitor
Prescription: USA: Yes **Controlled Drug:** USA: No; Canada: No **Available as Generic:** USA: Yes; Canada: No

Brand Names: ✤Alloprin, ✤Apo-Allopurinol, Lopurin, ✤Novo-Purol, ✤Purinol, ✤Riva-Purinol, Zurinol, Zyloprim

<table>
<tr><td colspan="2" align="center">BENEFITS versus RISKS</td></tr>
<tr><td align="center">*Possible Benefits*</td><td align="center">*Possible Risks*</td></tr>
<tr><td>EFFECTIVE CONTROL OF GOUT
CONTROL OF HIGH BLOOD URIC
  ACID DUE TO POLYCYTHEMIA,
  LEUKEMIA, CANCER, AND
  CHEMOTHERAPY
More beneficial in patients who
  remove more than one gram of uric
  acid in a day
May have a role in restoring blood
  vessel lining cells (endothelial cell)
  function in people with diabetes
  and mild high blood pressure</td><td>Increased frequency of acute gout
  initially
Peripheral neuritis
Allergic reactions in skin, lung, blood
  vessels, and liver
Bone marrow depression
Kidney toxicity</td></tr>
</table>

▷ **Principal Uses**
  As a Single Drug Product: Uses currently included in FDA-approved labeling:
    (1) Long-term gout therapy to prevent acute gout (does not relieve sudden
    gout attacks); (2) helps prevent high blood levels of uric acid in people who
    have recurrent uric acid or calcium oxalate kidney stones, people getting
    chemotherapy or radiation for cancer or who take thiazide diuretics (see
    Drug Classes).
  Other (unlabeled) generally accepted uses: (1) May decrease pain and occur-
    rence of mouth sores in people receiving 5-fluorouracil chemotherapy; (2)
    may help prostate swelling (nonbacterial prostatitis) not caused by bacteria;
    (3) early data show benefits in blood circulation damage (ischemic tissue
    damage); (4) may help Chagas' disease; (5) appears to ease refractive
    epilepsy in children; (6) effective in combination with quinine in treating
    malaria; (7) may have a role in helping restore how well the cells lining
    blood vessels (endothelial cells) work in people with diabetes and mild high
    blood pressure (300 mg a day in a 1-month study); (8) could have a role in
    some cases of mental illness (psychosis) where patients are resistant (refrac-
    tory) to existing treatment (based on a small study of add-on allopurinol).

How This Drug Works: Works to change chemicals called purines' removal
  (metabolism) by the body. This medicine does this without changing the
  ability of the body to make purines that are important to the body. Allopurinol blocks the enzyme xanthine oxidase, thereby decreasing uric acid
  formation that is the root cause of gout. It also uses a feedback mechanism
  to block purine synthesis (requires hypoxanthine guanine phosphoribosyl-
  transferase).

▷ **Widely Used Guidelines That Involve This Medicine (representative sample):** Please look at the section at the very beginning of this profile called
  "Class." Next, turn to Table 22 and you will find guidelines listed by the
  class involved!

Available Dosage Forms and Strengths
  Tablets — 100 mg, 200 mg, 300 mg

▷ **Usual Adult Dosage Ranges:** Starts as 100 mg every 24 hours, then increased by
  100 mg every 24 hours (1 week apart) until uric acid level is normal (6 mg/dL
  or less). Usual dose is 200–300 mg every 24 hours for mild gout, and 400 to
  600 mg every 24 hours for moderate to severe gout. Daily doses of 300 mg
  or less may be taken as a single dose. Doses exceeding 300 mg daily should
  be divided into two or three equal portions. For high uric acid levels associated with cancer (to prevent uric acid nephropathy): 600–800 mg every
  24 hours, divided into three equal portions (with high water intake). Kidney stone (calcium oxalate) recurrence prevention: 200–300 mg per day.
  Extemporaneously made mouthwash: 5–6 mg/mL suspension has been
  used several times a day to prevent 5-FU stomatitis.
  **Note: Actual dosage and schedule must be determined for each patient
  individually.**

Conditions Requiring Dosing Adjustments
  Liver Function: Dose adjustment in liver compromise is not documented.
  Kidney Function: Dosing must be adjusted in kidney compromise.
  Malnutrition: Malnourished or low-protein-diet patients will not remove this
    drug normally and are at risk for toxicity. Doses must be decreased.

▷ **Dosing Instructions:** Best taken with food or milk (or a meal) to reduce stomach
  irritation. Tablet may be crushed. Drink 2 to 3 quarts (10 to 12 glasses) of

liquids daily if your doctor says it's ok (not contraindicated). If you forget a dose: Take the medicine as soon as you remember it, unless it is close to the time for the next dose—simply take the dose at the next scheduled time. Do NOT double doses.

Usual Duration of Use: Regular use for several months may be needed to prevent acute gout attacks. Ongoing use for years often needed for adequate control.

Typical Treatment Goals and Measurements (Outcomes and Markers)
  Uric Acid: Blood uric acid levels often decrease in 48 to 72 hours and may reach normal range in 1 to 3 weeks. Attacks of gout should become shorter and lessen in severity over time.

▷ **This Drug Should Not Be Taken If**
  • you have had an allergic reaction to it previously.
  • you are having an acute gout attack.

▷ **Inform Your Physician Before Taking This Drug If**
  • you have a family history of hemochromatosis.
  • you have a history of liver or kidney disease.
  • you have had a blood cell or bone marrow disorder.
  • you have a seizure or convulsive disorder (epilepsy—a slow withdrawal from this treatment is needed).
  • you take other prescription or nonprescription medications not discussed when allopurinol was prescribed.
  • you are unsure how much or how often to take allopurinol.
  • you are on a low-protein diet.
  • you do not drink very much water—talk to your doctor about this.
  • you are pregnant.

Possible Side Effects (natural, expected, and unavoidable drug actions)
  Acute gout may still occur during the first several weeks of therapy. Ask your doctor about using other medicines (such as colchicine) during this period.

▷ **Possible Adverse Effects** (unusual, unexpected, and infrequent reactions)
  If any of the following develop, consult your physician promptly for guidance.
  Mild Adverse Effects
  Allergic reactions: skin rash, hives, itching—frequent; drug fever.
  Confusion, agitation, headache, dizziness, drowsiness—rare.
  Nausea, vomiting, diarrhea, stomach cramps—rare.
  Taste disturbance—possible.
  Loss of scalp hair—rare.
  Serious Adverse Effects
  Allergic reactions: severe skin reactions—infrequent.
  High fever, chills, joint pains, swollen glands, kidney or liver damage—rare.
  Idiosyncratic reaction: catatonia, paresthesia, agitation.
  Hepatitis with or without jaundice (see Glossary): yellow eyes and skin, dark-colored urine, light-colored stools (may be part of allergy)—rare.
  Kidney damage (acute tubular necrosis or interstitial nephritis)—case reports—rare.
  Bone marrow depression (see Glossary)—rare.
  Blood vessel inflammation/damage—rare (risk increased in kidney failure and thiazide diuretic use at the same time).
  Peripheral neuritis—rare.
  Bronchospasm (part of hypersensitivity)—rare.
  Eye damage (macular), cataract formation—rare.

▷ **Possible Effects on Sexual Function:** Rare cases of bladder inflammation have been reported.

Adverse Effects That May Mimic Natural Diseases or Disorders

Toxic liver reaction may suggest viral hepatitis.

Severe skin reactions may resemble the Stevens-Johnson Syndrome (erythema multiforme). One case report of Stevens-Johnson with combined allopurinol and captopril has been made.

Possible Effects on Laboratory Tests

Complete blood cell counts: decreased red cells, hemoglobin, and platelets; increased eosinophils.

Liver function tests: increased ALT/GPT, AST/GOT, and alkaline phosphatase.

CAUTION

1. Call your doctor immediately if you develop a rash. This can be the first sign of an allergic reaction. Prompt action may avoid a more serious reaction.
2. A patient with an allopurinol allergy had cross-allergenicity and allergic reaction to acyclovir (Zovirax).
3. In the first few weeks of therapy, frequency of gout attacks may increase. These subside with ongoing therapy.
4. Drug should not be started in acute gout. It does not help.
5. Vitamin C in doses of 2 g or more daily can increase the risk of kidney stone formation during the use of allopurinol.
6. Patients with kidney function decline are more likely to have allergic reactions to this drug.
7. Frequency of rash may be increased in patients also taking a penicillin.
8. Allergic-type kidney damage can result if thiazide diuretics (see Drug Classes) are taken with allopurinol. Avoid this combination.
9. Patients on low-protein diets will not eliminate allopurinol normally. Doses must be decreased.
10. Dosing MUST be adjusted to kidney function. If you are 60 or older, "normal" declines in kidney function may require decreased doses. Talk to your doctor.

Precautions for Use

By Infants and Children: Not used in children except for increased uric acid caused by malignant growths. Watch closely for allergic skin reactions and blood cell disorders. The toxicity of azathioprine (Imuran) or mercaptopurine (Purinethol) may be increased in children receiving chemotherapy. For this kind of secondary hyperuricemia: 150 mg per day in children less than 6. Response is checked in 2 days and the dose is adjusted to response. Those 6–10 years old receive 300 mg a day with the same response check and dose changes as required.

By Those Over 60 Years of Age: Smaller starting and ongoing doses of this drug must be used (age-related decrease in kidney function).

▷ **Advisability of Use During Pregnancy**

Pregnancy Category: C. See Pregnancy Risk Categories at the back of this book.

Animal Studies: Results are conflicting and inconclusive.

Human Studies: Adequate studies of pregnant women are not available.

Avoid use of drug during the first 3 months. Use during the last 6 months only if clearly needed.

Advisability of Use If Breast-Feeding
    Presence of this drug in breast milk: Yes.
    Avoid drug or refrain from nursing.

Habit-Forming Potential: None.

Effects of Overdose: Nausea, vomiting, or diarrhea. Hypersensitivity reactions, kidney and liver function decline.

Possible Effects of Long-Term Use: Beneficial decreases in uric acid and resolution of gout symptoms.

Suggested Periodic Examinations While Taking This Drug (at physician's discretion)
    Blood uric acid levels.
    Complete blood cell counts.
    Liver and kidney function tests.
    Eye examinations (possible cataract formation or macular damage).

▷ **While Taking This Drug, Observe the Following**
    Foods: Talk to your doctor about a low-purine diet (such as avoiding liver, lentils, anchovies, etc.). A low-protein diet may increase toxicity risk if dose isn't decreased.
    Herbal Medicines or Minerals: Acerola is high in vitamin C. Inosine, like acerola, may increase uric acid levels. Aspen should be avoided in gout. Lipase may worsen gout (read the labels on all neutraceuticals). Goutweed (*Aegopodium podagraria*) does not have enough data to assess effectiveness.
    Beverages: No restrictions. May be taken with milk.
▷   *Alcohol:* Alcohol can worsen gout. Best to avoid it.
    Tobacco Smoking: No interactions expected. I advise everyone to quit smoking.
▷   *Other Drugs*
        Allopurinol may ***increase*** the effects of
        • azathioprine (Imuran) and mercaptopurine (Purinethol), making dose decreases necessary.
        • didanosine (Videx) which was noted in a case report of two patients with impaired kidneys.
        • oral anticoagulants (see Drug Classes) such as warfarin (Coumadin). INR should be checked more often.
        • theophylline (aminophylline, Elixophyllin, Theo-Dur, etc.).
        Allopurinol ***taken concurrently*** with
        • ampicillin, amoxicillin (and perhaps other penicillins) may increase the incidence of skin rash.
        • antacids containing aluminum will decrease the therapeutic effect of allopurinol.
        • captopril (Capoten) or other ACE inhibitors (see Drug Classes) can increase the likelihood of allergic reactions. CAUTION.
        • chlorpropamide (Diabinese) can cause hypoglycemia.
        • cyclophosphamide (Cytoxan, Neosar) may result in cyclophosphamide toxicity.
        • cyclosporine (Sandimmune) can cause cyclosporine toxicity.
        • iron salts may lead to excess liver iron. Avoid combining.
        • mercaptopurine (Purinethol) increases toxicity risk.
        • probenecid (Benemid, others) may increase probenecid levels.
        • tamoxifen (Nolvadex) may result in increased allopurinol levels and increased risk of liver toxicity.

- thiazide diuretics (see Drug Classes) may decrease kidney function.
- theophylline (Theo-Dur, etc.) may cause toxic theophylline levels.
- vidarabine (Vira-A) may increase risk of neurotoxicity.

▷ *Driving, Hazardous Activities:* Drowsiness may occur in some people. Use caution.

Aviation Note: The use of this drug *may be a disqualification* for piloting. Consult a designated Aviation Medical Examiner.

Exposure to Sun: No restrictions.

Discontinuation: If you have a seizure disorder, this medicine dose should be slowly decreased and then stopped.

ALOSETRON (A LOH sah trahn)

Re-Introduced: 2002   **Class:** Diarrhea predominant-Irritable Bowel Syndrome (IBS), type three serotonin receptor antagonist   **Prescription:** USA: Yes   **Controlled Drug:** USA: No; Canada: No   **Available as Generic:** No

Brand Names: Lotronex

Author's Note: This medicine was previously removed (see Table 17) from the U.S. market, but was re-approved WITH RESTRICTIONS under an sNDA. This profile will be broadened in the next edition if data warrant.

ALPRAZOLAM (al PRAY zoh lam)

Introduced: 1973, XR form 2002   **Class:** Antianxiety drug, benzodiazepines   **Prescription:** USA: Yes   **Controlled Drug:** USA: C-IV*; Canada: No   **Available as Generic:** Yes

Brand Names: Alprazolam Intensol, ✚Apo-Alpraz, ✚Med-Alprazolam, ✚Novo-Alprazol, ✚Nu-Alpraz, Xanax, Xanax XR

Warning: The brand names Xanax and Zantac are similar and can lead to serious medication errors. Xanax is alprazolam. Zantac is ranitidine, which treats peptic ulcers and heartburn. Make sure your prescription was filled correctly.

BENEFITS versus RISKS	
Possible Benefits	*Possible Risks*
RELIEF OF ANXIETY AND NERVOUS TENSION	Habit-forming potential with prolonged use
EFFECTIVE TREATMENT OF PANIC DISORDER	Minor impairment of mental functions with therapeutic doses
May have some action as an antidepressant	Tachycardia and palpitations

▷ **Principal Uses**

As a Single Drug Product: Uses currently included in FDA-approved labeling: (1) Used for short-term relief of mild to moderate anxiety and nervous tension; (2) helps relieve anxiety associated with neurosis; (3) decreases frequency and severity of panic disorder.

Other (unlabeled) generally accepted uses: (1) Can help control extreme PMS symptoms; (2) lessens a variety of types of cancer pain when given with various narcotics; (3) eases agoraphobia; (4) decreases symptoms in essential tremor; (5) decreases loudness of ear ringing in tinnitus; (6) can be helpful in alcohol withdrawal; (7) eases irritable bowel syndrome; (8) eases anxiety sometimes seen with depression; (9) helpful in reducing anticipatory vomiting from chemotherapy.

How This Drug Works: Calms by enhancing the action of the nerve transmitter gamma-aminobutyric acid (GABA), which in turn blocks higher brain centers.

▷ **Widely Used Guidelines That Involve This Medicine (representative sample):** Please look at the section at the very beginning of this profile called "Class." Next, turn to Table 22 and you will find guidelines listed by the class involved!

Available Dosage Forms and Strengths
Tablets — 0.25 mg, 0.5 mg, 1 mg, 2 mg
Tablets, extended release (XR) — 0.5 mg, 1 mg, 2 mg, 3 mg
Oral solution — 0.25 mg, 0.5 mg, 1 mg/5 mL
— 0.25 mg/2.5 mL

▷ **Usual Adult Dosage Ranges: Regular release form:** *For anxiety and nervous tension:* 0.25–0.5 mg three times daily. Maximum dose is 4 mg every 24 hours, taken in divided doses—but the lowest effective dose should be used.
For panic disorder: Initially 0.5 mg three times daily; increase dose by 1 mg every 3 to 4 days as needed and tolerated. Some patients stopped having panic attacks with 6 mg a day. Maximum daily dose is 10 mg.
For treatment of alcohol withdrawal: Dosing is variable—one source reported a mean oral daily dose to be 2.2 mg.

XR Form: 3 to 6 mg once a day. Dosing is started with 0.5 to one mg a day. Doses can be increased as needed and tolerated once every 3–4 days in steps on as much as 1 mg. Slower stepwise increase may be prudent to allow the medicine a long enough time to go to work (full pharmacodynamic effect).
Note: Actual dosage and schedule must be determined for each patient individually.

Conditions Requiring Dosing Adjustments
Liver Function: A starting dose of 0.25 mg is prudent in patients with advanced liver disease. Slow increase in dose only if needed.
Kidney Function: The manufacturer does not define specific dose reductions.
Obesity: Takes a longer time to reach final concentrations in obese people. Doses should be calculated based on ideal rather than actual body weight.
Alcoholism: Because of some of the physiological and liver changes in alcoholism, removal of drug from the body may be delayed. Lower doses/longer times (intervals) between doses are needed.

▷ **Dosing Instructions:** Regular release form may be taken on empty stomach or with food or milk. Regular release tablets may be crushed. XR form should NOT be crushed. High fat meals given up to 2 hours before a dose of this form is taken increases how much gets into your body by roughly 25%. These XR tablets are best taken once a day in the morning. Do not stop this drug abruptly if taken for more than 4 weeks (stop slowly by decreasing 0.5 mg every 3 days or longer). If you forget a dose, but have missed by less

than an hour, take the missed dose. If it is almost time for your next scheduled dose, skip the missed dose. Do NOT double doses.

Usual Duration of Use: Several days to several weeks. Continual use should not
exceed 8 weeks without evaluation by your doctor.

> **Author's Note: The National Institute of Mental Health has a current
> information page on anxiety. It can be found on the World Wide Web**
> (*www. nimh.nih.gov/healthinformation/anxietymenu.cfm*).

Typical Treatment Goals and Measurements (Outcomes and Markers)

Anxiety or panic: Goals for anxiety and panic tend to be more vague and subjective than hypertension or cholesterol. Frequently, the patient (in conjunction
with physician assessment) will largely decide if anxiety has been modified to
a successful extent. The Hamilton Depression Scale is widely used to assess
depression. In the case of panic attacks, decreased number of trips to the
hospital or ER visits may be a useful measure. In both cases, the ability of the
patient to return to normal activities is a hallmark of successful treatment.

Possible Advantages of This Drug: XR form: May allow control of anxiety with
reduced impact (pill burden) for patients.

▷ **This Drug Should Not Be Taken If**
- you have had an allergic reaction to it previously.
- you are pregnant (first 3 months).
- you have acute narrow-angle glaucoma.
- you have myasthenia gravis.

▷ **Inform Your Physician Before Taking This Drug If**
- your history includes palpitations or tachycardia (may be worsened).
- you are allergic to benzodiazepines (see Drug Classes).
- you are pregnant or planning pregnancy.
- you are breast-feeding your infant.
- you have a history of depression or serious mental illness (psychosis).
- you have a history of alcoholism or drug abuse.
- you have impaired liver or kidney function.
- you have open-angle glaucoma.
- you have a seizure disorder (epilepsy).
- you have severe chronic lung disease.
- you take other prescription or nonprescription medications that were not
  discussed when alprazolam was prescribed for you.
- you are unsure how much or how often to take alprazolam.

Possible Side Effects (natural, expected, and unavoidable drug actions)
Drowsiness, light-headedness—frequent.

▷ **Possible Adverse Effects** (unusual, unexpected, and infrequent reactions)
**If any of the following develop, consult your physician promptly for
guidance.**

Mild Adverse Effects
Allergic reactions: skin rash, hives.
Headache, dizziness, fatigue, blurred vision, dry mouth—infrequent.
Drowsiness—frequent, up to 50%.
Nausea, vomiting, constipation—infrequent.
Increased salivation—infrequent.

Serious Adverse Effects
Confusion, hallucinations, depression, excitement, agitation (paradoxical
reaction)—case reports to rare.
Tachycardia and palpitations—infrequent.

Increased liver enzymes—rare.

Increased white blood cells (leukocytosis) or decreased blood cells (pancytopenia)—case reports and of questionable causation.

Low blood pressure (hypotension)—case report.

▷ **Possible Effects on Sexual Function:** Rare but documented: inhibited female orgasm (5 mg/day); impaired ejaculation (3.5 mg/day); decreased libido, impaired erection (4.5 mg/day); altered timing and pattern of menstruation (0.75–4 mg/day).

Possible Effects on Laboratory Tests

Liver function tests: increased ALT/GPT, AST/GOT—rare and insignificant.

Urine screening tests for drug abuse: may be positive (depends upon amount of drug taken and testing method).

CAUTION

1. Do not stop taking this drug abruptly if it has been taken continually for more than 4 weeks.
2. Some nonprescription drugs with antihistamines (allergy and cold medicines, sleep aids) can cause excessive sedation.
3. This medicine is removed from the body by liver enzymes called cytochrome P450 3A4. Medicines that block this enzyme system will tend to increase alprazolam levels. Medicines that induce or increase P450 activity will tend to lower alprazolam levels and blunt effectiveness.
4. People with ongoing severe conditions such as cancer may not tolerate "typical" starting doses; 0.25 mg twice or three times a day as a starting dose is prudent. The dose may be increased as needed and tolerated.

Precautions for Use

By Infants and Children: Safety and effectiveness for those under 18 not established.

By Those Over 60 Years of Age: Starting dose should be 0.25 mg two or three times daily. Watch for excessive drowsiness, dizziness, unsteadiness, and incoordination (possible low blood pressure).

▷ **Advisability of Use During Pregnancy**

Pregnancy Category: D. See Pregnancy Risk Categories at the back of this book.

Animal Studies: Diazepam (a closely related benzodiazepine) can cause cleft palate in mice and skeletal defects in rats. No data on alprazolam.

Human Studies: Some studies suggest an association between diazepam use and cleft lip and heart deformities. Adequate studies in pregnant women are not available.

Avoid use during entire pregnancy if possible.

Advisability of Use If Breast-Feeding

Presence of this drug in breast milk: Yes.

Avoid drug or refrain from nursing.

Habit-Forming Potential: This drug can cause psychological and/or physical dependence (see Glossary), especially if used in large doses for an extended period of time.

Effects of Overdose: Marked drowsiness, weakness, feeling of drunkenness, staggering gait, tremor, stupor progressing to deep sleep or coma.

Possible Effects of Long-Term Use: Psychological and/or physical dependence.

Suggested Periodic Examinations While Taking This Drug (at physician's discretion)

None required for short-term use.

▷ **While Taking This Drug, Observe the Following**

Foods: No restrictions.

Herbal Medicines or Minerals: Kava, danshen (miltirone) and valerian may exacerbate central nervous system depression (avoid this combination). Kava is not presently recommended in Canada because of liver concerns. Kola nut, Siberian ginseng, mate, ephedra, guarana (caffeine), and ma huang may blunt the benefits of this medicine. While St. John's wort is indicated for anxiety, it is also thought to increase (induce) cytochrome P450 enzymes and will tend to blunt alprazolam effectiveness if combined with alprazolam. St. John's wort may also worsen sun sensitivity caused by alprazolam.

Beverages: Avoid excessive caffeine-containing beverages: coffee, tea, cola (counteracts effects). This drug may be taken with milk.

▷ *Alcohol:* Use with extreme caution. Alcohol may increase the sedative effects of alprazolam. Alprazolam may increase the intoxicating effects of alcohol. Avoid alcohol completely—throughout the day and night—if you find it necessary to drive or engage in any hazardous activity.

Tobacco Smoking: Heavy smoking may reduce calming. I advise quitting smoking.

Marijuana Smoking: Occasional (once or twice weekly): Increased sedative effect.

Daily: Marked increase in sedative effect.

▷ *Other Drugs*

Alprazolam may *increase* the effects of
• digoxin (Lanoxin) and cause digoxin toxicity.

Alprazolam may *decrease* the effects of
• levodopa (Sinemet, etc.) and reduce its effect in treating Parkinson's disease.

The following drugs may *increase* the effects of alprazolam:
• amprenavir (Agenerase).
• aprepitant (Emend).
• atazanavir (Reyataz).
• itraconazole or ketoconazole (azole antifungals).
• birth control pills (oral contraceptives—various kinds).
• cimetidine (Tagamet).
• delavirdine (Rescriptor).
• disulfiram (Antabuse).
• fluconazole (Diflucan).
• fluoxetine (Prozac).
• fluvoxamine (Luvox).
• isoniazid (INH, Rifamate, etc.).
• macrolide antibiotics (such as erythromycin, clarithromycin, or azithromycin—see Drug Classes).
• medicines that inhibit a liver enzyme (CYP3A4) will increase alprazolam levels (talk to your doctor and pharmacist).
• omeprazole (Prilosec).
• paroxetine (Paxil).
• propoxyphene (Darvon, etc.).
• ritonavir (Norvir) and perhaps other protease inhibitors (see Drug Classes).
• sertraline (Zoloft).
• valproic acid (Depakene).

The following drugs may *decrease* the effects of alprazolam:
• carbamazepine (Tegretol).

- rifampin (Rimactane, etc.).
- theophylline (aminophylline, Theo-Dur, etc.).

Alprazolam **taken concurrently** with

- alcohol (ethanol) will worsen coordination and mental abilities.
- benzodiazepines (see Drug Classes) can cause increased central nervous system (CNS) depression.
- buspirone (Buspar) can result in additive CNS depression.
- central nervous system active agents (see Antihistamine and Antipsychotic Drug Classes) can cause increased CNS depression.
- narcotics (morphine, etc.) cause additive CNS depression.
- medicines removed by the same cytochrome P450 3A4 enzyme (such as atorvastatin [Lipitor]) may lead to increased blood levels and added sedation.
- nefazodone (Serzone) may double the blood level.
- tricyclic and other kinds of antidepressants (see Drug Classes) results in additional CNS depression.

▷ *Driving, Hazardous Activities:* This drug can impair mental alertness, judgment, physical coordination, and reaction time. Avoid hazardous activities accordingly.

Aviation Note: The use of this drug **is a disqualification** for piloting. Consult a designated Aviation Medical Examiner.

Exposure to Sun: Use caution; rare photosensitivity reports (see Glossary).

Discontinuation: If this drug has been taken for an extended period of time, do not stop it abruptly. Various withdrawal schedules have been developed. Some clinicians decrease by 0.5 mg every three days. Another schedule uses dose reductions of 1 mg per week until a total daily dose of 4 mg is reached; by 0.5 mg per week until a total daily dose of 2 mg is reached; and then by 0.25 mg per week thereafter. Ask your doctor for help.

AMANTADINE (a MAN ta deen)

Introduced: 1966 **Class:** Anti-Parkinsonism, antiviral **Prescription:** USA: Yes **Controlled Drug:** USA: No; Canada: No **Available as Generic:** USA: Yes; Canada: Yes
Brand Names: Antadine, Symadine, Symmetrel

BENEFITS versus RISKS

Possible Benefits	*Possible Risks*
Partial relief of rigidity, tremor, and impaired motion in all forms of parkinsonism	Skin rashes, mild to severe
	Confusion, hallucinations
	Rare congestive heart failure
Combination treatment of hepatitis C that has failed to respond to interferon	Increased risk of prostatism (see Glossary)
Possible role in helping autism and other developmental disorders	Abnormally low white blood cell counts
Prevention and treatment of respiratory infections caused by influenza type A viruses*	

▷ **Principal Uses**

As a Single Drug Product: Uses currently included in FDA-approved labeling: (1) Treats all forms of parkinsonism; (2) prevents or treats respiratory tract infections caused by influenza type A virus (rimantadine is the drug of first choice because of amantadine's more frequent CNS side effects); (3) eases movement problems caused by some phenothiazine type medicines (drug-induced extrapyramidal symptoms).

Other (unlabeled) generally accepted uses: (1) Role in managing behavioral problems in brain injuries, autism, others; (2) some success reversing symptoms of mild dementia; (3) eases some resistant myoclonic or absence seizures; (4) may help bed-wetting (enuresis) in children; (5) may ease fatigue in multiple sclerosis (MS) patients; (6) may give increased responses as part of combination therapy of hepatitis C—in both initial therapy and in interferon-resistant cases.

How This Drug Works: It increases a nerve transmitter (dopamine) in some nerve centers and reduces muscular rigidity, tremor, and impaired movement associated with Parkinsonism. May help some dyskinesias by blocking glutamate transmission in the globus pallidus. Helps wearing off or dyskinesia with advancing disease. By keeping the influenza from entering cells, it prevents the flu.

▷ **Widely Used Guidelines That Involve This Medicine (representative sample):** Please look at the section at the very beginning of this profile called "Class." Next, turn to Table 22 and you will find guidelines listed by the class involved!

Available Dosage Forms and Strengths
Capsules (gelatin and softgel) — 100 mg
Syrup — 50 mg/5 mL
Tablet — 100 mg

▷ **Usual Adult Dosage Ranges**

Anti-Parkinsonism: 100 mg once daily (for patients getting high doses of other antiparkinson medicines or who have serious sickness in addition to Parkinson's. Other patients take 100 mg twice daily. Some patients may benefit from up to 400 mg daily. In general, many clinicians keep the total daily dose at 300 mg.

Antiviral: 200 mg once daily or 100 mg every 12 hours such as in flu (influenza) treatment. Dividing the total dose can help prevent side effects involving the central nervous system (CNS). (Hepatitis C cases with interferon alfa 2a for 12 months used 200 mg once daily.)

Children 1 to 9 years old: Treatment of type A flu: The CDC recommends 5 mg per kg per day up to 150 mg per day in order to prevent the flu, but decrease amantadine toxicity risk. This preventive "treatment" is best continued for 10 days after the exposure happened. The manufacturer gives a dosing range of: 4.4 to 8.8 mg per kg of body mass per day, up to a maximum of 150 mg once daily.

Children 10 and older: for those less than 40 kg, the CDC recommends 5 mg per kg per day (regardless of age). For those more than 40 kg, 100 mg twice daily is recommended.

Fatigue in multiple sclerosis: 100 mg two times a day for adults.

Note: Actual dose and schedule must be determined for each patient individually.

Conditions Requiring Dosing Adjustments

Liver Function: No dosing changes currently thought to be needed.

Kidney Function: Must be carefully adjusted to blood levels in people with kidney problems. Those with creatinine clearances of 30–50 mL/min should receive 100 mg daily. Those with 15–29 clearance should receive 100 mg every other day. Those with clearances less than 15 should receive 200 mg once a week.

Epilepsy: Doses of 200 mg/day should be avoided, as seizure risk may increase.

▷ **Dosing Instructions:** May be taken with or following meals. Can open the capsule to take it. If you forget a dose: Take the missed dose right away. If it is almost time to take the next dose, skip the missed dose and continue the medicine on your regular schedule. DO NOT double doses. If effectiveness is lost, the medicine can be gradually reduced (tapered) to zero and then restarted.

Usual Duration of Use: Use on a regular schedule for up to 2 weeks usually needed to see best effect in relieving Parkinson's symptoms. Long-term use (months to years) requires periodic check of response and dose changes. May allow for some levodopa decreases, but benefits may only last 6 months. See your doctor on a regular basis. Following exposure to influenza type A, protection requires continual daily doses for at least 10 days. During influenza epidemics, this drug may be given for 6 to 8 weeks.

Typical Treatment Goals and Measurements (Outcomes and Markers)

Parkinson's: The general goal is to ease movement problems and to allow for lowering of the levodopa dose. Benefits may be limited to about 6 months and therapy will then need to be adjusted.

Influenza (flu): Lessens the severity and length of time for the flu. PLEASE NOTE that a flu shot (or the nasal spray "shot") is still the best way to deal with (PREVENT) the flu.

▷ **This Drug Should Not Be Taken If**

- you have had an allergic reaction to it previously.

▷ **Inform Your Physician Before Taking This Drug If**

- you have any type of seizure disorder.
- you have a history of a serious emotional or mental disorder.
- you have a history of heart disease, especially previous heart failure.
- you have impaired liver or kidney function.
- you have a history of lowering of blood pressure when you stand (orthostatic hypotension).
- you have a history of peptic ulcer disease.
- you have eczema or recurring eczema-like skin rashes.
- you are taking any drugs for emotional or mental disorders.
- you have angle closure glaucoma.
- you have a history of low white blood cell counts.
- you are unsure how much or how often to take this medicine.

Possible Side Effects (natural, expected, and unavoidable drug actions)

Light-headedness, dizziness, weakness, feeling faint (see Orthostatic Hypotension in Glossary). Dry mouth, constipation. Reddish-blue pattern or patchy skin discoloration on your legs or feet (livedo reticularis—transient and unimportant).

▷ **Possible Adverse Effects** (unusual, unexpected, and infrequent reactions)

If any of the following develop, consult your physician promptly for guidance.

Mild Adverse Effects
>   Allergic reaction: skin rash.
>   Headache, nervousness, irritability, inability to concentrate, insomnia, night-
>   mares—rare to infrequent.
>   Unsteadiness, visual disturbances, slurred speech—infrequent.
>   Swelling (fluid retention) (arms, feet, or ankles)—case report.
>   Difficulty breathing—possible.
>   Urine retention—rare.
>   Loss of appetite, nausea, vomiting—infrequent.

Serious Adverse Effects
>   Allergic reaction: severe eczema-like skin rashes.
>   Idiosyncratic reactions: confusion, depression, hallucinations, aggression—
>   case reports to rare.
>   Neuroleptic malignant syndrome (NMS)—case reports when the medicine is
>   stopped.
>   Increased seizure activity in epileptics—possible.
>   Congestive heart failure—rare.
>   Aggravation of prostatism (see Glossary)—possible.
>   SIADH (see Glossary)—case reports.
>   Elevated liver function tests—rare.
>   Low white blood cell counts: fever, sore throat, infection—rare.
>   Catatonia or seizures (if abruptly stopped).
>   Myasthenia gravis—case reports.

▷ **Possible Effects on Sexual Function:** None reported.

Adverse Effects That May Mimic Natural Diseases or Disorders
>   Mood changes, confusion, or hallucinations may suggest a psychotic disor-
>   der.
>   Swelling of the legs and feet may suggest (but not necessarily indicate) heart,
>   liver, or kidney disorder.

Natural Diseases or Disorders That May Be Activated by This Drug
>   Latent epilepsy, incipient congestive heart failure.

Possible Effects on Laboratory Tests
>   Liver function tests: increased (AST/GOT, alkaline phosphatase).
>   Kidney function tests: brief increase—blood urea nitrogen (BUN).

CAUTION
>   1. NARROW margin of safety. Maximum dose is 400 mg in 24 hours. Watch
>   for adverse effects with doses over 200 mg a day.
>   2. Initial anti-Parkinsonism benefit may last 3 to 6 months. If this happens,
>   ask your doctor if a new drug or dose is needed.
>   3. May increase susceptibility to German measles. Avoid exposure to active
>   German measles.
>   4. Watch for early signs of congestive heart failure: shortness of breath on
>   exertion or during the night, mild cough, swelling of feet or ankles.
>   Report these promptly to your doctor.
>   5. May increase risk of seizures in people with epilepsy.
>   6. If you have been taking this medicine to help Parkinson's disease—do not
>   stop it abruptly. Abruptly stopping this medicine may lead to Parkinson-
>   ian type crisis.

Precautions for Use
>   *By Infants and Children:* Safety and effectiveness for those under 18 not
>   established.

By Those Over 60 Years of Age: Confusion, delirium, hallucinations, and disorderly conduct may develop. Prostatism may be aggravated.

▷ **Advisability of Use During Pregnancy**
Pregnancy Category: C. See Pregnancy Risk Categories at the back of this book.
Animal Studies: Birth defects reported in rat studies; no defects reported in rabbit studies.
Human Studies: Adequate studies of pregnant women are not available. Single case of heart lesions. Ask your doctor for help.

Advisability of Use If Breast-Feeding
Presence of this drug in breast milk: Yes.
Nursing infant may develop skin rash, vomiting, or urine retention. Avoid drug or refrain from nursing.

Habit-Forming Potential: This drug has a potential for abuse because of its ability to cause euphoria, hallucinations, and feelings of detachment.

Effects of Overdose: Hyperactivity, disorientation, confusion, visual hallucinations, aggressive behavior, severe toxic psychosis, seizures, heart rhythm disturbances, drop in blood pressure.

Possible Effects of Long-Term Use: Livedo reticularis (see "Possible Side Effects" on page 77). Congestive heart failure in predisposed people.

Suggested Periodic Examinations While Taking This Drug (at physician's discretion)
White blood cell counts.
Liver and kidney function tests.
Evaluation of heart function.

▷ **While Taking This Drug, Observe the Following**
Foods: No restrictions.
Herbal Medicines or Minerals: Calabar bean (chop nut, Fabia, ordeal nut, others) is unsafe when taken by mouth (physostigmine is the active ingredient) and should never be taken by people with Parkinson's disease. Betel nut contains cholinergic compounds—will lower anticholinergic effect of amantadine, hence the combination is not recommended. Kava kava may block the effectiveness of amantadine. Health Canada has told their citizens not to take kava. Echinacea purpurea should be avoided by those with multiple sclerosis.
Beverages: No restrictions. May be taken with milk.
▷ *Alcohol:* May impair mental function, lower blood pressure excessively.
Tobacco Smoking: No interactions expected. I advise everyone to quit smoking.
Marijuana Smoking: Added drowsiness.
▷ *Other Drugs*
Amantadine may *increase* the effects of
- atropine-like drugs used to treat Parkinsonism, especially benztropine (Cogentin), orphenadrine (Disipal) and trihexyphenidyl (Artane). Amantadine can increase results, but if doses are too large, these drugs (taken with amantadine) may cause confusion, delirium, hallucinations, and nightmares.
- levodopa (Dopar, Larodopa, Sinemet, etc.) can enhance results. Combination use with levodopa finds most clinicians limiting amantadine dose to 100 mg once or twice daily while they increase the levodopa dose to best patient results. Patients should be observed for sudden mental disturbances and doses adjusted accordingly.

The following drugs may *increase* the effects of amantadine:
- amphetamine and amphetamine-like stimulant drugs may cause excessive stimulation and adverse behavioral effects.
- hydrochlorothiazide with triamterene may increase the blood level of amantadine and cause toxicity.

Amantadine *taken concurrently* with
- cotrimoxazole may increase risk of CNS stimulation or arrhythmias.
- hydrochlorothiazide (Dyazide, Esidrix, others) may increase risk of amantadine toxicity.
- sulfamethoxazole may increase risk of CNS stimulation or arrhythmia.
- triamterene may increase risk of CNS toxicity.
- trimethoprim may increase risk of CNS toxicity.
- zotepine (Nipolept) may decrease amantadine benefits.

▷ *Driving, Hazardous Activities:* May cause drowsiness, dizziness, blurred vision, or confusion. If these drug effects occur, avoid hazardous activities.
Aviation Note: The use of this drug *may be a disqualification* for piloting. Consult a designated Aviation Medical Examiner.
Exposure to Sun: No restrictions.
Exposure to Cold: Use caution. Excessive chilling may enhance the development of livedo reticularis (see "Possible Side Effects" on page 77).
Discontinuation: When used to treat Parkinsonism, this drug should not be stopped abruptly (slowly tapering is prudent). Sudden discontinuation may cause an acute Parkinsonian crisis and cases of delirium or catatonia have been described. When treating influenza A infections, drug is continued for 48 hours *after* symptoms stop.

AMILORIDE (a MIL oh ride)

Introduced: 1967 **Class:** "Water pill" (Diuretic), potassium sparing diuretic **Prescription:** USA: Yes **Controlled Drug:** USA: No; Canada: No **Available as Generic:** Yes

Brand Names: ✤Apo-Amilzide, Midamor, ✤Moduret [CD], Moduretic [CD], ✤Novamilor [CD], ✤Nu-Amilzide [CD], ✤Riva-Amilzide [CD]

BENEFITS versus RISKS	
Possible Benefits	*Possible Risks*
EFFECTIVE DIURETIC WITH DECREASED POTASSIUM LOSS	ABNORMALLY HIGH BLOOD POTASSIUM WITH EXCESSIVE USE
	Rare heart arrhythmias
	Rare kidney toxicity
	Rare liver toxicity

▷ **Principal Uses**
As a Single Drug Product: Uses currently included in FDA-approved labeling: (1) Removes excessive fluid (edema) seen in congestive heart failure; (2) treats high blood pressure, especially those prone to low potassium; (3) thiazide-caused low blood potassium (hypokalemia).
As a Combination Drug Product [CD]: Combined with other thiazide diuretics to prevent excess potassium loss.

Other (unlabeled) generally accepted uses: (1) May be able to help dissolve kidney stones in patients unable to tolerate surgery; (2) can help correct increased urination that occurs in patients taking lithium; (3) can help prevent lowered magnesium and potassium seen in patients who are given amphotericin B for serious fungal infections.

How This Drug Works: This drug promotes loss of sodium and water from the body and potassium retention by altering kidney enzymes that control urine formation.

▷ **Widely Used Guidelines That Involve This Medicine (representative sample):** Please look at the section at the very beginning of this profile called "Class." Next, turn to Table 22 and you will find guidelines listed by the class involved!

Available Dosage Forms and Strengths
>Tablets — 5 mg
>Combination Tablets — 5 mg amiloride and 50 mg hydrochlorothiazide

▷ **Usual Adult Dosage Ranges:** One 5-mg dose a day, preferably in the morning. May increase up to 15 mg daily as needed and tolerated. Should not exceed 20 mg every 24 hours.
Note: Actual dose and schedule must be determined for each patient individually.

Conditions Requiring Dosing Adjustments
Liver Function: Extreme caution in patients with severe liver disease.
Kidney Function: Should NOT be used in patients who can't make urine or who have acute kidney failure or creatinine clearance less than 50 mL/min.

▷ **Dosing Instructions:** Best taken when you wake up, with food. Tablet may be crushed for administration. If you forget a dose: Take the medicine right away, unless it is nearly time for your next dose, then omit the missed dose and take the medicine when it was next scheduled. DO NOT double doses. Once excess fluid is removed, use may be intermittent in some patients.

Usual Duration of Use: Ongoing long-term use to treat high blood pressure. Some clinicians use this medicine as needed (PRN) to remove abnormal fluid accumulation. Use every other day also minimizes imbalance of sodium and potassium.

Typical Treatment Goals and Measurements (Outcomes and Markers)
Blood Pressure: The current guidelines (JNC VII) define normal blood pressure (BP) as **less than** 120/80. **Pre-hypertension:** ranges from 120/80 to 139/89 and is intended to help your doctor encourage lifestyle changes (or in the case of people with a risk factor for high blood pressure, start treatment) much earlier—so that possible damage to blood vessels, your heart, kidneys, sexual potency, or eyes might be minimized or avoided altogether. The next two classes of high blood pressure are stage 1 hypertension: 140/90 to 159/99 and stage 2 hypertension equal to or greater than 160/100 mm Hg. These guidelines also recommend that clinicians **and** patients agree on the goals and a plan of treatment. The first-ever guidelines for blood pressure (hypertension) in African Americans recommends that MOST black patients be started on TWO antihypertensive medicines with the goal of lowering blood pressure to 130/80 for those with high risk for heart and blood vessel disease or with diabetes. For diabetics: 130/80 is the target and less than 125/75 for those who spill more than one gram of protein into their urine. Most clinicians try to achieve a BP that confers the

best balance of lower cardiovascular risk and avoids the problem of too low a blood pressure. Blood pressure duration is generally increased with beneficial restriction of sodium. The goals and time frame should be discussed with you when the prescription is written.

▷ **This Drug Should Not Be Taken If**
- you have had an allergic reaction to it before.
- your blood potassium level is greater than 5.5 mEq per liter and/or your serum creatinine is more than 1.5 mg/dL and your blood urea nitrogen (BUN) is more than 30 mg/dL (talk to your doctor about this).
- you have diabetic nerve damage (diabetic nephropathy).
- your kidneys are not making urine (anuria).

▷ **Inform Your Physician Before Taking This Drug If**
- you are allergic to any similar drug.
- you have diabetes or glaucoma.
- you have reason to believe that minerals such as potassium or chloride (electrolytes) are out of balance in your body.
- you have kidney disease or impaired kidney function.
- you take a different diuretic, blood pressure drug, digitalis, or lithium.
- you don't know how much to take or how often to take it.

Possible Side Effects (natural, expected, and unavoidable drug actions)
Abnormally high blood potassium level—infrequent.
Abnormally low blood sodium level, dehydration, decreased blood magnesium, constipation—possible.
Dizziness on standing (orthostatic hypotension)—possible.

▷ **Possible Adverse Effects** (unusual, unexpected, and infrequent reactions)
If any of the following develop, consult your physician promptly for guidance.
Mild Adverse Effects
Allergic reactions: skin rash, itching—rare.
Headache—infrequent.
Dizziness, weakness, fatigue, numbness and tingling—case reports (related to electrolyte problems).
Dry mouth, nausea, vomiting, stomach pains, diarrhea—infrequent.
Decreased ability to taste salt, bad taste—possible.
Loss of scalp hair—rare.
Serious Adverse Effects
Idiosyncratic reactions: joint and muscle pains.
Liver or kidney toxicity—rare.
Abnormally low sodium or high potassium—possible.
Increased internal eye pressure (of concern in glaucoma)—rare.
Depression, visual disturbances, ringing in ears, tremors—infrequent.
Bone marrow depression—rare (questionable cause).
Palpitations and arrhythmias—rare.
Decreased circulation to the legs (with combination furosemide use)—case reports.

▷ **Possible Effects on Sexual Function:** Does not appear to be a present side effect.

Adverse Effects That May Mimic Natural Diseases or Disorders
Nervousness, confusion, or depression may mimic spontaneous mental disorder.

Natural Diseases or Disorders That May Be Activated by This Drug
Preexisting peptic ulcer, latent glaucoma.

Possible Effects on Laboratory Tests
Blood cholesterol level: decreased.
Blood creatinine level: increased with long-term use.
Blood potassium level: possibly increased.
Blood uric acid level: decreased with long-term use.
Blood sodium level: possibly decreased.

CAUTION
1. Do **NOT** take potassium supplements or eat more high-potassium foods.
2. More frequent potassium levels are needed if you take digitalis compounds.
3. Do not stop this drug abruptly unless your doctor says you must.

Precautions for Use
By Infants and Children: Oral dosing with 0.625 mg per kg of body mass daily has been used to promote water loss (diuresis) in young patients weighing from 6 to 20 kg.
By Those Over 60 Years of Age: Declines in kidney function may make it likely that you will retain potassium. Limit use of this drug to periods of 2 to 3 weeks if possible. The dose MUST be reduced. May cause too much water loss, possible increased tendency of the blood to clot, and increased risk of clots (thrombosis, heart attack, stroke).

▷ **Advisability of Use During Pregnancy**
Pregnancy Category: B. See Pregnancy Risk Categories at the back of this book.
Animal Studies: No birth defects reported.
Human Studies: Adequate studies of pregnant women are not available.
Use only if clearly needed.

Advisability of Use If Breast-Feeding
Presence of this drug in breast milk: Unknown, but probably present.
This drug may suppress milk production. Avoid drug if possible. If use is necessary, watch nursing infant closely and stop drug or nursing if adverse effects develop.

Habit-Forming Potential: None.

Effects of Overdose: Thirst, drowsiness, fatigue, weakness, nausea, vomiting, confusion, numbness and tingling of face and extremities, irregular heart rhythm, shortness of breath.

Suggested Periodic Examinations While Taking This Drug (at physician's discretion)
Complete blood counts.
Blood levels of sodium, potassium, magnesium, and chloride.
Kidney function tests.
Easing of edema.

▷ **While Taking This Drug, Observe the Following**
Foods: Avoid excessive salt restriction and high-potassium foods. Taking this drug with food may help nausea and stomach upset.
Herbal Medicines or Minerals: Ginseng, bitter orange, country mallow, eleuthero root, guarana (high caffeine dose), hawthorn, saw palmetto, ma huang (now off the market), goldenseal, and licorice may cause increased blood pressure—blunting the beneficial effects of this medicine. Arginine (a medicine

used to treat metabolic alkalosis but also found as supplements) has led to severe increases in potassium in some patients who had previously (and recently) been given spironolactone. Licorice may also increase hypokalemia risk. Couch grass may worsen edema due to heart or kidney problems. Indian snakeroot, calcium, and garlic may help lower blood pressure. Talk to your doctor and pharmacist BEFORE adding any herbal medicines.

Beverages: Caffeine may increase blood pressure. Talk to your doctor about consumption. May be taken with milk.

▷ *Alcohol:* Use caution. Alcohol can exaggerate the blood-pressure-lowering effect of this drug and cause orthostatic hypotension (see Glossary).

Tobacco Smoking: No interactions expected. I advise everyone to quit smoking.

▷ *Other Drugs*

Amiloride may ***increase*** the effects of
- other blood-pressure-lowering drugs. Dose decreases may be needed.

Amiloride may ***decrease*** the effects of
- digoxin (Lanoxin, etc.) and reduce its effect in treating heart failure.

Amiloride ***taken concurrently*** with
- ACE inhibitors (see Drug Classes) such as benazepril or angiotensin II antagonists (valsartan [Diovan], etc.) may result in abnormally high blood potassium.
- arginine (various) may cause extreme and life-threatening potassium increases.
- chlorpropamide (Diabinese) may lead to excessively low blood sodium.
- cyclosporine (Sandimmune, others) may cause excessively high potassium levels.
- digoxin (Lanoxin) may decrease benefits (positive inotropic effect) of digoxin.
- dofetilide (Tikosyn) may cause serious irregular heartbeats. Combine only with great caution and careful patient monitoring.
- lithium (Lithobid) may cause lithium toxicity.
- metformin (Glucophage) may increase Glucophage levels and increase lactic acidosis (cationic drug interaction) or excessively lowered blood sugar (hypoglycemia) risk.
- NSAIDs (see Drug Classes) may decrease therapeutic effect.
- potassium supplements may result in extremely elevated blood potassium levels.
- quinidine (Quinaglute, others) may prolong the QRS interval and increase risk of abnormal heartbeats.
- spironolactone (Aldactone, Aldactazide) or triamterene (Dyrenium, Dyazide) may cause dangerous potassium levels. Avoid combining.
- tacrolimus (Prograf) may cause excessive potassium levels. Increased potassium checks are prudent.
- triamterene (Dyazide) may cause excessively high potassium levels and should not be combined.
- valsartan (Diovan) may cause excessively high potassium levels. Caution and more frequent checks of potassium are needed if this combination is undertaken.

▷ *Driving, Hazardous Activities:* May cause drowsiness, dizziness, and orthostatic hypotension. If these drug effects occur, avoid hazardous activities.

Aviation Note: The use of this drug ***may be a disqualification*** for piloting. Consult a designated Aviation Medical Examiner.

Exposure to Sun: No restrictions.

Exposure to Heat: Caution is advised. Excessive sweating can cause water, sodium and potassium imbalance. Hot environments can cause lowering of blood pressure.

Occurrence of Unrelated Illness: Call your doctor if you contract an illness causing vomiting or diarrhea.

Discontinuation: With high doses or prolonged use, withdraw this drug gradually. Excessive potassium loss may occur with sudden withdrawal.

AMINOPHYLLINE (am in OFF i lin)

Other Name: Theophylline ethylenediamine

Introduced: 1910 **Class:** Antiasthmatic, bronchodilator, xanthines
Prescription: USA: Yes **Controlled Drug:** USA: No; Canada: No
Available as Generic: Yes

Brand Names: Aminophyllin, Mudrane [CD], Mudrane GG [CD], ✤Palaron, Phyllocontin, Somophyllin, ✤Somophyllin-12, Truphylline

Author's Note: This drug is actually (79%) theophylline. See the theophylline profile for further details.

AMIODARONE (AM EE oh dur ohn)

Introduced: 1986 **Class:** Heart rhythm regulator (Antiarrhythmic), Class III agent **Prescription:** USA: Yes **Controlled Drug:** USA: No; Canada: No **Available as Generic:** Yes

Brand Names: Cordarone, ✤Alti-Amiodarone, Braxan, ✤Gen-Amiodarone, ✤Med-Amiodarone, ✤Novo-Amiodarone, Pacerone

<table>
<tr><td colspan="2" align="center">BENEFITS versus RISKS</td></tr>
<tr><td align="center">Possible Benefits</td><td align="center">Possible Risks</td></tr>
<tr><td>EFFECTIVE TREATMENT OF SELECTED LIFE-THREATENING HEART RHYTHM DISORDERS</td><td>SIGNIFICANT LIVER ENZYME (CYP3A) DRUG INTERACTIONS</td></tr>
<tr><td>TREATMENT OF ATRIAL FIBRILLATION (LOW MEDICINE DOSE)</td><td>LUNG (PULMONARY) TOXICITY
SLOWED HEART RATE (BRADYCARDIA)</td></tr>
<tr><td>PREVENTION OF ATRIAL FIBRILLATION RECURRENCE (LOW DOSE)</td><td>Some isolated cases of arrhythmia worsening
Tingling in the extremities (peripheral neuropathy)</td></tr>
<tr><td>BENEFICIAL EFFECTS ON HEART FAILURE</td><td>Liver toxicity
Changes in thyroid gland function (hypo or hyper)</td></tr>
<tr><td>INTRAVENOUS USE OF GREAT BENEFIT (NEWER DATA) IN CARDIAC ARREST AND IN ADVANCED CARDIAC LIFE SUPPORT (ACLS) WHEN CARDIAC ARREST HAS RESULTED FROM (SECONDARY TO) VENTRICULAR ARRHYTHMIA</td><td>Heart conduction or rhythm abnormalities
Microdeposits in the eye (cornea)
Very long half-life</td></tr>
<tr><td>EFFECTIVE IN TREATING VENTRICULAR ARRHYTHMIAS AND FAST HEART RATE (TACHYCARDIA) THAT HAS FAILED TO RESPOND (REFRACTORY) TO OTHER AGENTS
Very long half-life</td><td></td></tr>
</table>

▷ **Principal Uses**

As a Single Drug Product: Uses currently included in FDA-approved labeling: (1) Treats abnormal rhythms in the heart ventricles (life-threatening ventricular arrhythmias such as recurrent hemodynamically unstable ventricular tachycardia).

Other (unlabeled) generally accepted uses: (1) Chest pain (angina pectoris); (2) suppression of abnormal heart rhythms in severe congestive heart failure (CHF) and may ease CHF itself; (3) effective in treating ventricular arrhythmias seen in heart inflammation patients (myocarditis) caused by Chagas' disease; (4) supraventricular arrhythmias (such as atrial fibrillation); (5) treats drug-induced (sotalol) Torsade de Pointes; (6) survivors of sudden heart attack (acute myocardial infarction) who have frequent or repetitive premature ventricular depolarizations (VPDs) may benefit from amiodarone therapy; (7) prevented repeat (recurrent) atrial fibrillation better than propafenone or sotalol in the Canadian CTAF study.

How This Drug Works: Originally classified as a class three antiarrhythmic. Appears to work on the complete spectrum (blocks the sodium channel, slows heart rate, and impedes the AV node by blocking beta-adrenergic receptors as well as calcium channels) of classes. It also lengthens ventricular and atrial repolarization time by inhibiting the potassium channel.

These effects help restore normal heart rate and rhythm. Amiodarone also decreases cytokines (such as interleukin 6 or IL-6), which may explain its benefits in heart failure. Prior TNF alpha data does not appear to be explanatory of benefits.

▷ **Widely Used Guidelines That Involve This Medicine (representative sample):** Please look at the section at the very beginning of this profile called "Class." Next, turn to Table 22 and you will find guidelines listed by the class involved!

Available Dosage Forms and Strengths
   Injection — 50 mg/mL
      Tablet — 200 mg, 400 mg

▷ **Usual Adult Dosage Ranges:** *Supraventricular arrhythmias:* Oral dosing has been started at 600–1,200 mg daily for one to two weeks, and then lowered (tapered) to 400–600 mg daily for one to three weeks and then lowered further to the lowest possible ongoing (maintenance) dose. The typical blood (serum) level in patients who have been successfully treated was 1.9 micrograms per milliliter and the median dose was 200 mg a day in one study. One Canadian study used 10 mg/kg per day for at least 14 days which was followed by 300 mg a day for 4 weeks, then 200 mg a day. Additional studies are needed. Some patients over 60 years old have gained control of their atrial fibrillation using 100 mg a day.

Ventricular arrhythmias: Oral doses are 800–1,600 mg per day as a loading dose for one to three weeks or longer (based on how well the heart rhythm problem responds), and then doses are gradually lowered to no more than 400 mg a day. Some European clinicians use generally lower ongoing doses. In the ALIVE trial, intravenous doses of 5 mg/kg were given versus 1.5 mg/kg of lidocaine. In hemodynamically unstable ventricular tachycardia or ventricular fibrillation, the manufacturer recommends loading doses as above. Giving the medicine with meals in divided doses if more than 1,000 mg is required is recommended. Once the heart rhythm is under control, doses can often then be lowered to 600–800 mg a day for a month, then to 400–600 mg a day. Ongoing doses are then given once or twice a day depending on patient response.

   Note: Actual dose and schedule must be determined for each patient individually.

Conditions Requiring Dosing Adjustments
Liver Function: Dosing hasn't been studied in liver failure, but since there is extensive liver metabolism, decreased doses and use of blood levels to guide dosing appear prudent in liver compromise. The medicine is also removed in the bile. Talk to your doctor if you have a block or periodic block in your bile duct (such as a gallstone) and this medicine is being considered.

Kidney Function: Dosing changes do NOT appear to be needed.

▷ **Dosing Instructions:** Tablets should be swallowed whole and may be taken with or following food to reduce stomach irritation. If you forget to take a dose: omit that dose and continue with the next scheduled dose. If you forget to take it for two or more days—call your doctor.

Usual Duration of Use: Regular use for 10 days may be required (with oral dosing) to begin to help ventricular tachycardia, but may take three to six weeks. Several months may be required to see the peak benefits. Long-term use requires supervision and ongoing evaluation by your doctor.

Typical Treatment Goals and Measurements (Outcomes and Markers)

Abnormal heartbeats: The general goal is to return the heart to a normal rhythm or at least to markedly reduce the occurrence of abnormal heartbeats. In life-threatening arrhythmias, the goal is to abort the abnormal beats and return the pattern to normal. Some increase in the QT interval (10–15% corrected for rate) may be seen when loading doses are being used, but is generally not a reliable prediction of serum amiodarone or desmethylamiodarone levels. Checks of ongoing success may involve placement of adhesive-backed temporary electrodes on the skin in several positions around the heart. A small heart rate and rhythm (EKG or ECG) recording device is carried around via a shoulder strap and records what the heart is doing over 24 hours. Once the recording is made, a scanning machine reviews the record, tallies abnormal heartbeats or rhythms and gives a good report on how the heart is benefiting from the medicines that the patient is taking. Repeat measurements can be made if doses are changed! In cases where the heart stops (cardiac arrest) this medicine was nearly two times as effective as lidocaine (see ALIVE trial in sources).

Possible Advantages of This Drug: Other antiarrhythmics such as quinidine and procainamide can be associated with development of antinuclear antibodies (ANA). One study showed that amiodarone does NOT induce ANA. Because of its broad mechanism of action, amiodarone may be effective where other antiarrhythmics fail. Has additional direct beneficial effects on heart failure that other heart rhythm modifiers do not have. A sub-study of the Atrial Fibrillation follow-up Investigation of Rhythm Management (AFFIRM) showed that amiodarone is the most effective medicine at keeping patients in normal sinus rhythm, helping them avoid cardioversion, staying alive, and staying on the same medicine.

▷ **This Drug Should Not Be Taken If**
- you had an allergic reaction to amiodarone or similar drugs (also related to a thyroid hormone).
- you have second-degree or third-degree AV block (and do not have a pacemaker).
- you have "sick sinus" syndrome or severe heart slowing (sinus bradycardia—talk with your doctor).
- you are in heart (cardiogenic) shock.

▷ **Inform Your Physician Before Taking This Drug If**
- you have had unfavorable reactions to antiarrhythmic drugs.
- you have heart disease, especially "heart block."
- you have a history of heart attack, heart muscle changes (cardiomegaly), slow heartbeat, or low blood pressure (especially with intravenous dosing).
- you have had a heart attack.
- you have impaired liver function.
- you have low blood platelets.
- your vision is impaired (this drug may cause microdeposits on the cornea).
- your blood electrolytes (such as potassium or magnesium) are not in balance.
- you have lung disease (pulmonary dysfunction).
- you live or will travel to a place where your heart rhythm cannot be checked (this medicine can help abnormal heartbeats, but may also worsen them and this must be checked when treatment is started).
- the left ventricle of your heart does not work correctly (left ventricular dysfunction).

- you have thyroid problems (hypo or hyper thyroidism).
- your job requires you to work outside in the sun or you already take other medicines that can increase sun sensitivity.

Possible Side Effects (natural, expected, and unavoidable drug actions)
Inflammation of the vein (with intravenous use)—possible.
Asymptomatic microdeposits in the cornea—frequent with long-term (more than six months) use.

▷ **Possible Adverse Effects** (unusual, unexpected, and infrequent reactions)
If any of the following develop, consult your physician promptly for guidance.
Mild Adverse Effects
Allergic reactions: skin rash, itching—case reports.
Blue-gray skin discoloration—rare to frequent (also sun sensitivity—see below).
Hair loss (alopecia)—rare to infrequent.
Headache, tiredness, or sleep disturbances—rare-infrequent.
Movement problems (incoordination-ataxia), fatigue, dizziness—infrequent.
Lowered blood pressure (more common with the intravenous form)—up to frequent.
Swelling of the epididymis (epididymitis)—infrequent.
Increased serum creatinine—possible.
Cholesterol changes (increased in one study and lowered in another)—possible.
Increased liver function tests—infrequent to frequent (should be clinically monitored and dose lowered or medicine stopped if persistent).
Loss of appetite, taste disturbances, indigestion, nausea, vomiting—infrequent to frequent (usually responds to dosing adjustment or dividing).
Increased creatinine—case reports (usually happens during first six months of treatment).
Serious Adverse Effects
Allergic reaction—toxic epidermal necrolysis (TEN)—case report.
Neuropathy—frequent.
Abnormal thyroid function (hypo or hyper)—rare to frequent (may happen within one to 73 months).
Abnormal heart rhythm (such as excessive heart slowing-bradycardia)—infrequent.
Torsades de pointes—rare.
Lung toxicity (pulmonary)—rare to frequent (includes fatal cases).
High blood sugar (glucose)—rare (not seen in a small later study).
Abnormal blood sodium (syndrome of inappropriate antidiuretic hormone-SIADH)-case reports.
Abnormal movement (possible neurotoxic reaction)—may be frequent and may relate to large loading doses or ongoing doses more than 600 mg.
Jaundice (see Glossary) or liver toxicity—infrequent.
Optic neuritis, corneal changes—rare.
Abnormally low blood platelets, anemia, and pancytopenia—case reports-rare.

▷ **Possible Effects on Sexual Function:** Impotence or loss of libido—case reports.
Swelling and tenderness of male breast tissue (gynecomastia)—case report.

Adverse Effects That May Mimic Natural Diseases or Disorders
Reversible jaundice may suggest viral hepatitis. Abnormal heart rhythms may mimic slow (brady) arrhythmias from other causes.

Natural Diseases or Disorders That May Be Activated by This Drug
Abnormal heart rhythms, abnormal thyroid function, epididymal swelling may mimic infectious epididymitis.

Possible Effects on Laboratory Tests
Blood platelets: rarely decreased.
Liver function tests: increased liver enzymes (ALT/GPT, AST/GOT, and alkaline phosphatase), increased bilirubin.
Abnormally low sodium (SIADH)—case reports.
Blood urea nitrogen (BUN)—increased.
Increased or decreased thyroid function.

CAUTION
1. Thorough heart exam (including electrocardiogram) is critical prior to using this drug.
2. Periodic heart exams are needed to follow drug responses. Some people may have heart rhythm or function declines. Close monitoring of heart rate, rhythm and overall performance is essential.
3. Dose must be individualized. Do not change your dose without your doctor's supervision.
4. Talk with your doctor about signs and symptoms of thyroid function changes. This medicine contains iodine; consequently protein-bound iodine (PBI) testing will NOT detect thyroid problems.
5. Do not take any other antiarrhythmic drug while taking this drug unless directed to do so by your doctor.

Precautions for Use
By Infants and Children: In pediatric patients, amiodarone is given on a mg-per-kg-of-body-mass basis. Dose is then divided into equal doses, given at times determined by patient response. Some patients from one to four years old will receive 10 to 20 mg per kg of body mass per day, divided into equal doses and given every six hours. Initial use of this drug requires hospitalization and supervision by a qualified pediatrician.
By Those Over 60 Years of Age: Watch closely for light-headedness, dizziness, unsteadiness and tendency to fall. Older patients may be more susceptible to problems from heart slowing and should be closely followed once this medicine is started.

▷ **Advisability of Use During Pregnancy**
Pregnancy Category: D. See Pregnancy Risk Categories at the back of this book.
Animal Studies: Can cause thyroid changes, maternal and embryo death in rabbits given 10 mg per kg or greater.
Human Studies: Adequate studies of pregnant women are not available. This medicine should be used only if the potential benefit outweighs fetal risk.

Advisability of Use If Breast-Feeding
Presence of this drug in breast milk: Yes.
Refrain from nursing.

Habit-Forming Potential: None.

Effects of Overdose: Extremely slow heart rate (bradycardia), excessively low blood pressure, heart block (AV) and possibly cardiogenic shock as well as liver toxicity.

Possible Effects of Long-Term Use: Microdeposits in the cornea of the eye.

Suggested Periodic Examinations While Taking This Drug (at physician's discretion)

Liver function tests BEFORE starting treatment and every six months thereafter.

Electrocardiograms.

Complete blood counts.

Blood levels.

Vision checks periodically throughout therapy.

▷ **While Taking This Drug, Observe the Following**

Foods: No restrictions. Food may actually help avoid upset stomach.

Herbal Medicines or Minerals: Using St. John's wort, ma huang or ephedra (now off the market), guarana, bitter orange, country mallow or kola while taking this medicine may result in unacceptable heart stimulation. Belladonna, henbane, *Scopolia*, pheasant's eye extract or lily-of-the-valley, or squill powdered extracts should NOT be taken if you have abnormal heart rhythms. Eucalyptus and skull cap may increase liver toxicity risk. Since St. John's wort and amiodarone may increase sun sensitivity, the combination is NOT advised. Pyridoxine may increase risk of phototoxicity.

Beverages: Your doctor may ask you to restrict caffeine intake. May be taken with milk.

▷ *Alcohol:* Use caution. Alcohol can increase the blood-pressure-lowering effects and may have an undesirable effect on heart rhythm in high doses.

Tobacco Smoking: Nicotine can irritate the heart, reducing effectiveness. I advise everyone to quit smoking.

▷ *Other Drugs*

Amiodarone may ***increase*** the effects of

- antihypertensive drugs and cause excessive lowering of blood pressure.
- atropine-like drugs (see Drug Classes).
- cyclosporine (Sandimmune, others) can lead to cyclosporine toxicity if cyclosporine doses are not lowered.
- digoxin (Lanoxin) by increasing blood level.
- procainamide (Procan SR, others) and NAPA.
- warfarin (Coumadin, etc.); check INR (prothrombin times) more often, and adjust dosing.

Amiodarone ***taken concurrently*** with

- amprenavir (Agenerase), indinavir (Crixivan), ritonavir (Norvir), and perhaps other protease inhibitors (see Drug Classes) may increase amiodarone blood levels and lead to toxicity.
- beta blockers (see Drug Classes) may result in abnormally low heart rates or sinus arrest. Extreme caution is advised.
- calcium channel blockers (see Drug Classes) should be avoided in patients with partial block (AV) or sick sinus syndrome.
- cimetidine (Tagamet) can increase amiodarone levels.
- cisapride (Propulsid) may lead to serious heart rhythm problems. DO NOT COMBINE.
- clonazepam (Klonopin) caused clonazepam toxicity in one case report. Caution is advised.
- digoxin (Lanoxin) can cause digoxin toxicity.
- disopyramide (Norpace) can prolong QT interval and lead to abnormal heart rhythms.
- dofetilide (Tikosyn) can lead to heart toxicity.
- dolasetron (Anzemet) can lead to heart toxicity.
- fentanyl (Actiq, Duragesic) may lead to low blood pressure, slow heart rate and lowered ability of the heart to work (cardiac output).

- flecainide (Tambocor) may allow lower flecainide dose to get the same effect.
- gatifloxacin (Tequin), levofloxacin (Levaquin), sparfloxacin (Zagam), and other quinolone antibiotics (see drug classes) may result in abnormal QT intervals and lead to abnormal heart rhythms. DO NOT COMBINE.
- halofantrine (Halfan) can lead to heart toxicity.
- ibutilide (Corvert) can lead to excessively refractory ventricles and atria of the heart.
- indinavir (Crixivan) can lead to amiodarone toxicity.
- insulin or oral antidiabetic drugs (see Drug Classes) may result in blunted blood sugar benefits.
- lidocaine (various) may lead to lidocaine toxicity. Extreme caution is advised.
- methotrexate (Rheumatrex, others) increases risk of methotrexate toxicity. Extreme caution is advised.
- mexiletine (Mexitil) may result in abnormal heart beats. Caution is advised.
- moxifloxacin (Avelox) may result in abnormal heart beats. DO NOT COMBINE.
- nelfinavir (Viracept) may result in amiodarone toxicity. DO NOT COMBINE.
- phenytoin (Dilantin) or fosphenytoin (Cerebyx) can result in phenytoin, phosphenytoin, and amiodarone toxicity.
- propafenone (Rythmol) may lead to propafenone toxicity. Reduced propafenone doses may be needed.
- quinidine can cause increases in quinidine levels.
- ritonavir (Norvir) may increase amiodarone levels and could result in abnormal heart beats. DO NOT COMBINE.
- sotalol (Betapace) may result in increased risk of abnormal heart rhythms because of prolongation of the QT interval. This combination is NOT recommended.
- verapamil (Calan, others) can precipitate or worsen congestive heart failure.
- ziprasidone (Geodon) may prolong the QT interval. DO NOT combine.

The following drugs may ***decrease*** the effects of amiodarone:

- cholestyramine (Questran, others) by increasing removal (enterohepatic elimination) of amiodarone.
- rifabutin (Mycobutin).
- rifampin (Rimactane, Rifadin).

▷ *Driving, Hazardous Activities:* May cause dizziness or blurred vision. Limit activities as needed.

Aviation Note: The use of this drug ***may be a disqualification*** for piloting. Consult a designated Aviation Medical Examiner.

Exposure to Sun: Use caution. This drug causes photosensitization (see Glossary).

Exposure to Heat: Use caution. The use of this drug in hot environments may increase the risk of heatstroke.

Occurrence of Unrelated Illness: Vomiting, diarrhea, or dehydration can affect this drug's action adversely. Report such developments promptly.

Discontinuation: This drug should not be stopped abruptly after long-term use. Ask your doctor for help regarding gradual dose reduction.

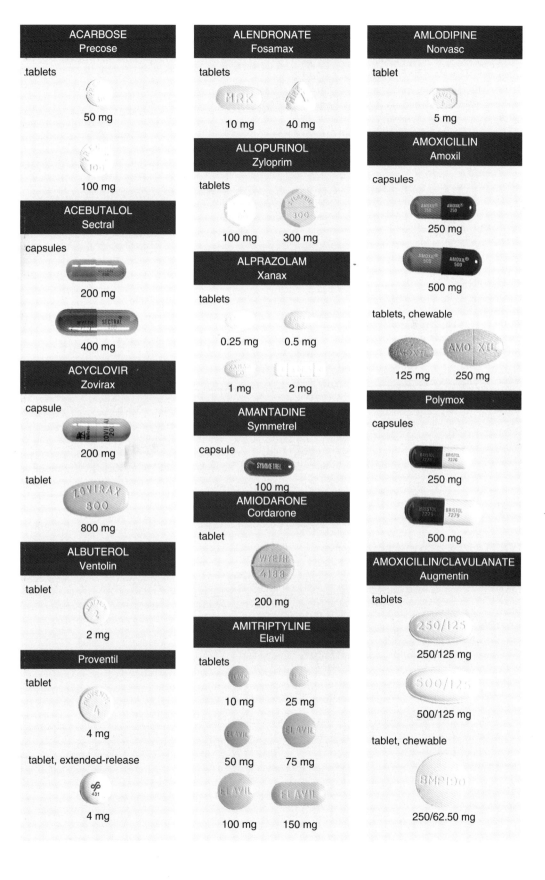

ACARBOSE
Precose

tablets

50 mg

100 mg

ACEBUTALOL
Sectral

capsules

200 mg

400 mg

ACYCLOVIR
Zovirax

capsule

200 mg

tablet

800 mg

ALBUTEROL
Ventolin

tablet

2 mg

Proventil

tablet

4 mg

tablet, extended-release

4 mg

ALENDRONATE
Fosamax

tablets

10 mg   40 mg

ALLOPURINOL
Zyloprim

tablets

100 mg   300 mg

ALPRAZOLAM
Xanax

tablets

0.25 mg   0.5 mg

1 mg   2 mg

AMANTADINE
Symmetrel

capsule

100 mg

AMIODARONE
Cordarone

tablet

200 mg

AMITRIPTYLINE
Elavil

tablets

10 mg   25 mg

50 mg   75 mg

100 mg   150 mg

AMLODIPINE
Norvasc

tablet

5 mg

AMOXICILLIN
Amoxil

capsules

250 mg

500 mg

tablets, chewable

125 mg   250 mg

Polymox

capsules

250 mg

500 mg

AMOXICILLIN/CLAVULANATE
Augmentin

tablets

250/125 mg

500/125 mg

tablet, chewable

250/62.50 mg

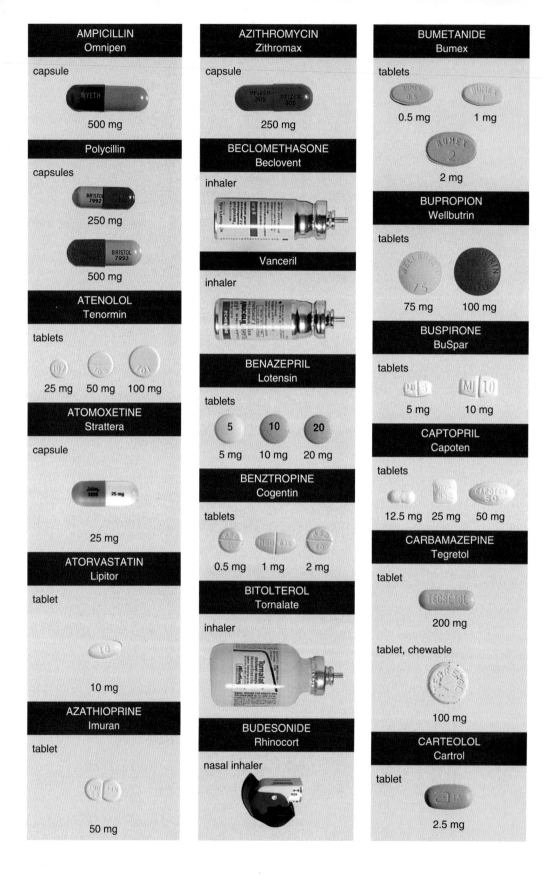

AMPICILLIN
Omnipen

capsule
500 mg

Polycillin

capsules
250 mg
500 mg

ATENOLOL
Tenormin

tablets
25 mg   50 mg   100 mg

ATOMOXETINE
Strattera

capsule
25 mg

ATORVASTATIN
Lipitor

tablet
10 mg

AZATHIOPRINE
Imuran

tablet
50 mg

AZITHROMYCIN
Zithromax

capsule
250 mg

BECLOMETHASONE
Beclovent

inhaler

Vanceril

inhaler

BENAZEPRIL
Lotensin

tablets
5 mg   10 mg   20 mg

BENZTROPINE
Cogentin

tablets
0.5 mg   1 mg   2 mg

BITOLTEROL
Tornalate

inhaler

BUDESONIDE
Rhinocort

nasal inhaler

BUMETANIDE
Bumex

tablets
0.5 mg   1 mg
2 mg

BUPROPION
Wellbutrin

tablets
75 mg   100 mg

BUSPIRONE
BuSpar

tablets
5 mg   10 mg

CAPTOPRIL
Capoten

tablets
12.5 mg   25 mg   50 mg

CARBAMAZEPINE
Tegretol

tablet
200 mg

tablet, chewable
100 mg

CARTEOLOL
Cartrol

tablet
2.5 mg

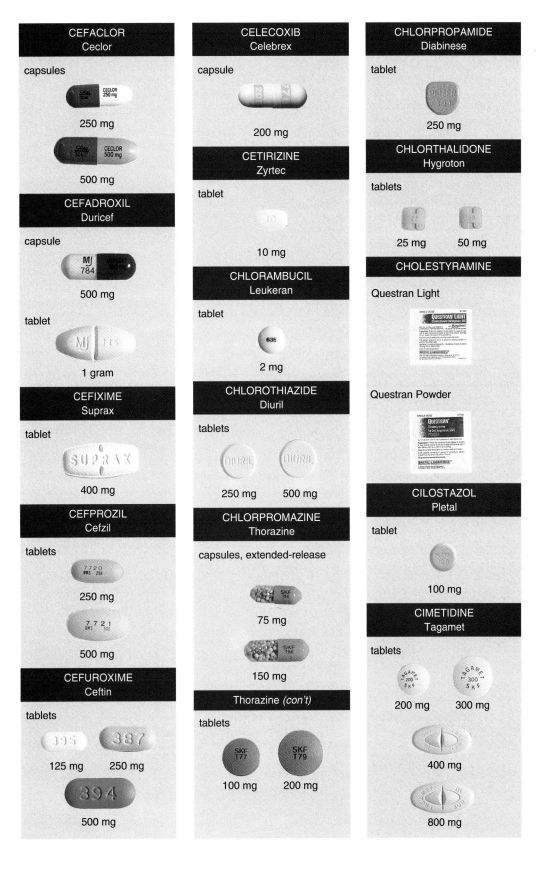

CEFACLOR
Ceclor

capsules

250 mg

500 mg

CEFADROXIL
Duricef

capsule

500 mg

tablet

1 gram

CEFIXIME
Suprax

tablet

SUPRAX

400 mg

CEFPROZIL
Cefzil

tablets

250 mg

500 mg

CEFUROXIME
Ceftin

tablets

125 mg   250 mg

500 mg

CELECOXIB
Celebrex

capsule

200 mg

CETIRIZINE
Zyrtec

tablet

10 mg

CHLORAMBUCIL
Leukeran

tablet

2 mg

CHLOROTHIAZIDE
Diuril

tablets

250 mg   500 mg

CHLORPROMAZINE
Thorazine

capsules, extended-release

75 mg

150 mg

Thorazine *(con't)*

tablets

100 mg   200 mg

CHLORPROPAMIDE
Diabinese

tablet

250 mg

CHLORTHALIDONE
Hygroton

tablets

25 mg   50 mg

CHOLESTYRAMINE

Questran Light

Questran Powder

CILOSTAZOL
Pletal

tablet

100 mg

CIMETIDINE
Tagamet

tablets

200 mg   300 mg

400 mg

800 mg

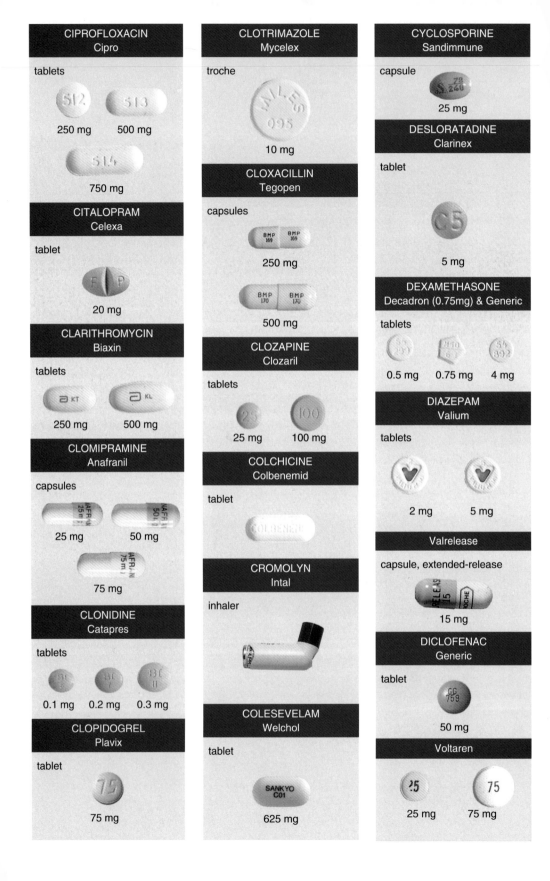

CIPROFLOXACIN
Cipro

tablets

250 mg   500 mg

750 mg

CITALOPRAM
Celexa

tablet

20 mg

CLARITHROMYCIN
Biaxin

tablets

250 mg   500 mg

CLOMIPRAMINE
Anafranil

capsules

25 mg   50 mg

75 mg

CLONIDINE
Catapres

tablets

0.1 mg   0.2 mg   0.3 mg

CLOPIDOGREL
Plavix

tablet

75 mg

CLOTRIMAZOLE
Mycelex

troche

10 mg

CLOXACILLIN
Tegopen

capsules

250 mg

500 mg

CLOZAPINE
Clozaril

tablets

25 mg   100 mg

COLCHICINE
Colbenemid

tablet

CROMOLYN
Intal

inhaler

COLESEVELAM
Welchol

tablet

625 mg

CYCLOSPORINE
Sandimmune

capsule

25 mg

DESLORATADINE
Clarinex

tablet

5 mg

DEXAMETHASONE
Decadron (0.75mg) & Generic

tablets

0.5 mg   0.75 mg   4 mg

DIAZEPAM
Valium

tablets

2 mg   5 mg

Valrelease

capsule, extended-release

15 mg

DICLOFENAC
Generic

tablet

50 mg

Voltaren

25 mg   75 mg

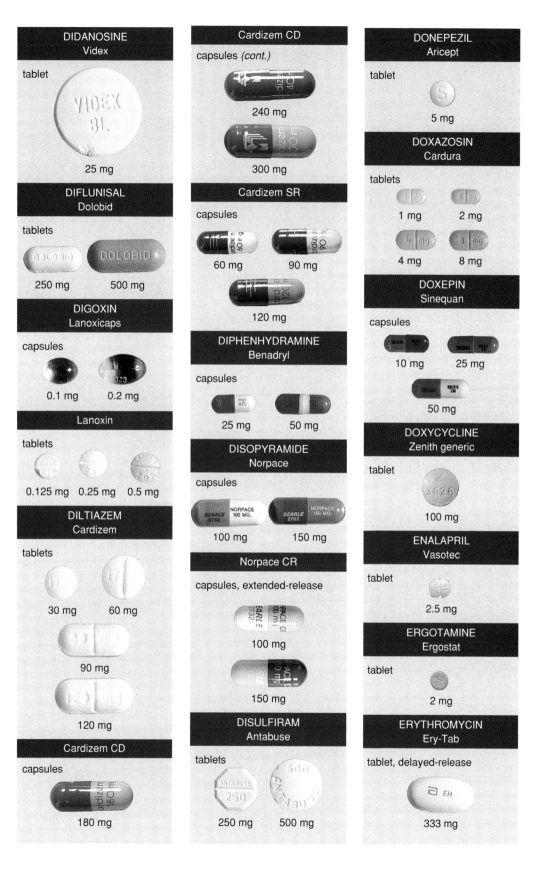

DIDANOSINE
Videx

tablet

25 mg

DIFLUNISAL
Dolobid

tablets

250 mg   500 mg

DIGOXIN
Lanoxicaps

capsules

0.1 mg   0.2 mg

Lanoxin

tablets

0.125 mg   0.25 mg   0.5 mg

DILTIAZEM
Cardizem

tablets

30 mg   60 mg

90 mg

120 mg

Cardizem CD

capsules

180 mg

Cardizem CD

capsules *(cont.)*

240 mg

300 mg

Cardizem SR

capsules

60 mg   90 mg

120 mg

DIPHENHYDRAMINE
Benadryl

capsules

25 mg   50 mg

DISOPYRAMIDE
Norpace

capsules

100 mg   150 mg

Norpace CR

capsules, extended-release

100 mg

150 mg

DISULFIRAM
Antabuse

tablets

250 mg   500 mg

DONEPEZIL
Aricept

tablet

5 mg

DOXAZOSIN
Cardura

tablets

1 mg   2 mg

4 mg   8 mg

DOXEPIN
Sinequan

capsules

10 mg   25 mg

50 mg

DOXYCYCLINE
Zenith generic

tablet

100 mg

ENALAPRIL
Vasotec

tablet

2.5 mg

ERGOTAMINE
Ergostat

tablet

2 mg

ERYTHROMYCIN
Ery-Tab

tablet, delayed-release

333 mg

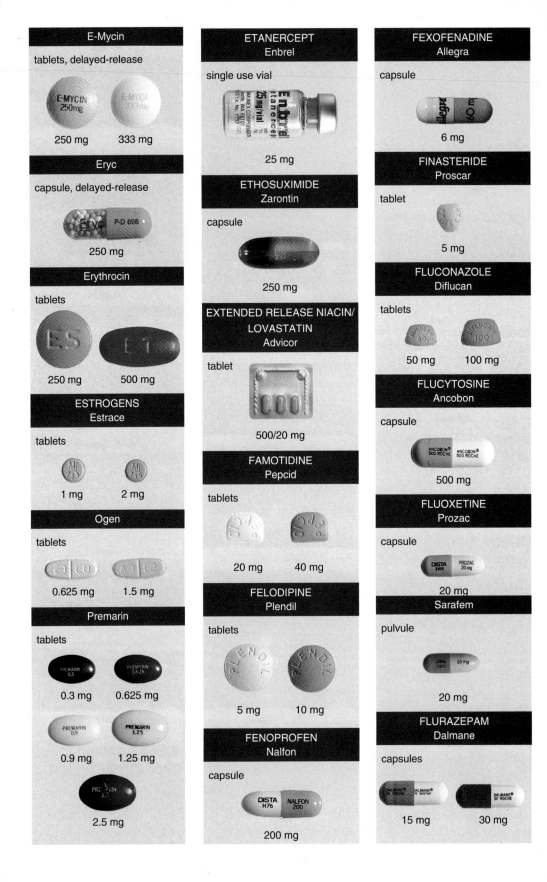

E-Mycin

tablets, delayed-release

250 mg   333 mg

Eryc

capsule, delayed-release

250 mg

Erythrocin

tablets

250 mg   500 mg

ESTROGENS
Estrace

tablets

1 mg   2 mg

Ogen

tablets

0.625 mg   1.5 mg

Premarin

tablets

0.3 mg   0.625 mg

0.9 mg   1.25 mg

2.5 mg

ETANERCEPT
Enbrel

single use vial

25 mg

ETHOSUXIMIDE
Zarontin

capsule

250 mg

**EXTENDED RELEASE NIACIN/
LOVASTATIN**
Advicor

tablet

500/20 mg

FAMOTIDINE
Pepcid

tablets

20 mg   40 mg

FELODIPINE
Plendil

tablets

5 mg   10 mg

FENOPROFEN
Nalfon

capsule

200 mg

FEXOFENADINE
Allegra

capsule

6 mg

FINASTERIDE
Proscar

tablet

5 mg

FLUCONAZOLE
Diflucan

tablets

50 mg   100 mg

FLUCYTOSINE
Ancobon

capsule

500 mg

FLUOXETINE
Prozac

capsule

20 mg

Sarafem

pulvule

20 mg

FLURAZEPAM
Dalmane

capsules

15 mg   30 mg

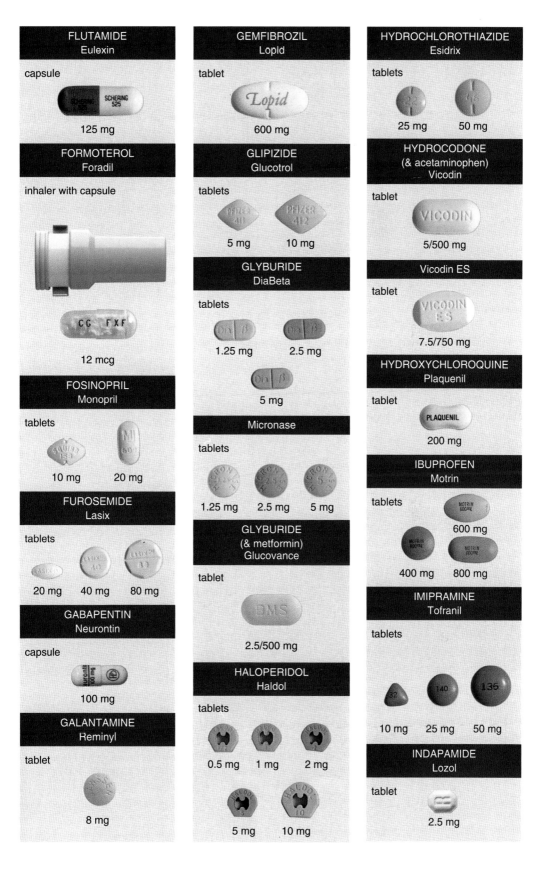

FLUTAMIDE	GEMFIBROZIL	HYDROCHLOROTHIAZIDE
Eulexin	Lopid	Esidrix

FLUTAMIDE
Eulexin

capsule

125 mg

FORMOTEROL
Foradil

inhaler with capsule

12 mcg

FOSINOPRIL
Monopril

tablets

10 mg   20 mg

FUROSEMIDE
Lasix

tablets

20 mg   40 mg   80 mg

GABAPENTIN
Neurontin

capsule

100 mg

GALANTAMINE
Reminyl

tablet

8 mg

GEMFIBROZIL
Lopid

tablet

600 mg

GLIPIZIDE
Glucotrol

tablets

5 mg   10 mg

GLYBURIDE
DiaBeta

tablets

1.25 mg   2.5 mg

5 mg

Micronase

tablets

1.25 mg   2.5 mg   5 mg

GLYBURIDE
(& metformin)
Glucovance

tablet

2.5/500 mg

HALOPERIDOL
Haldol

tablets

0.5 mg   1 mg   2 mg

5 mg   10 mg

HYDROCHLOROTHIAZIDE
Esidrix

tablets

25 mg   50 mg

HYDROCODONE
(& acetaminophen)
Vicodin

tablet

5/500 mg

Vicodin ES

tablet

7.5/750 mg

HYDROXYCHLOROQUINE
Plaquenil

tablet

200 mg

IBUPROFEN
Motrin

tablets

600 mg

400 mg   800 mg

IMIPRAMINE
Tofranil

tablets

10 mg   25 mg   50 mg

INDAPAMIDE
Lozol

tablet

2.5 mg

INDINAVIR
Crixivan

capsule

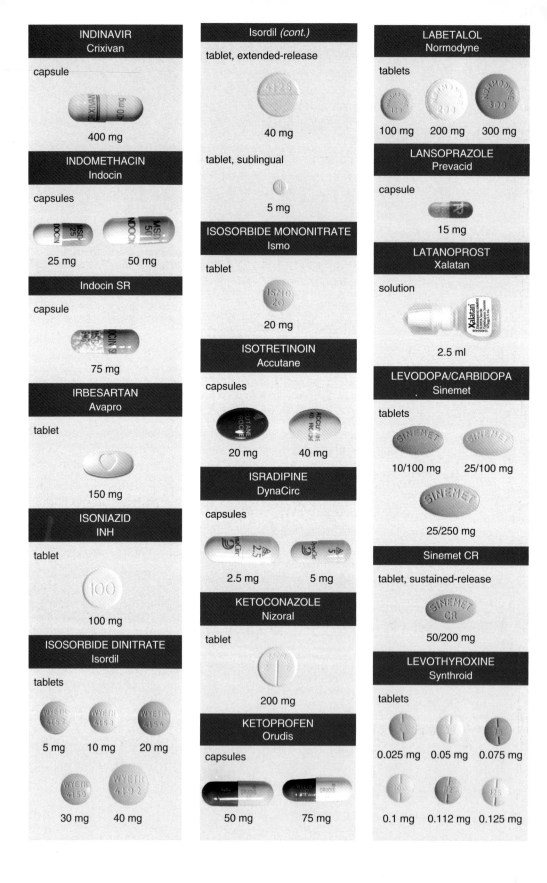

400 mg

INDOMETHACIN
Indocin

capsules

25 mg   50 mg

Indocin SR

capsule

75 mg

IRBESARTAN
Avapro

tablet

150 mg

ISONIAZID
INH

tablet

100 mg

ISOSORBIDE DINITRATE
Isordil

tablets

5 mg   10 mg   20 mg

30 mg   40 mg

Isordil *(cont.)*

tablet, extended-release

40 mg

tablet, sublingual

5 mg

ISOSORBIDE MONONITRATE
Ismo

tablet

20 mg

ISOTRETINOIN
Accutane

capsules

20 mg   40 mg

ISRADIPINE
DynaCirc

capsules

2.5 mg   5 mg

KETOCONAZOLE
Nizoral

tablet

200 mg

KETOPROFEN
Orudis

capsules

50 mg   75 mg

LABETALOL
Normodyne

tablets

100 mg   200 mg   300 mg

LANSOPRAZOLE
Prevacid

capsule

15 mg

LATANOPROST
Xalatan

solution

2.5 ml

LEVODOPA/CARBIDOPA
Sinemet

tablets

10/100 mg   25/100 mg

25/250 mg

Sinemet CR

tablet, sustained-release

50/200 mg

LEVOTHYROXINE
Synthroid

tablets

0.025 mg   0.05 mg   0.075 mg

0.1 mg   0.112 mg   0.125 mg

Synthroid
tablets *(cont.)*

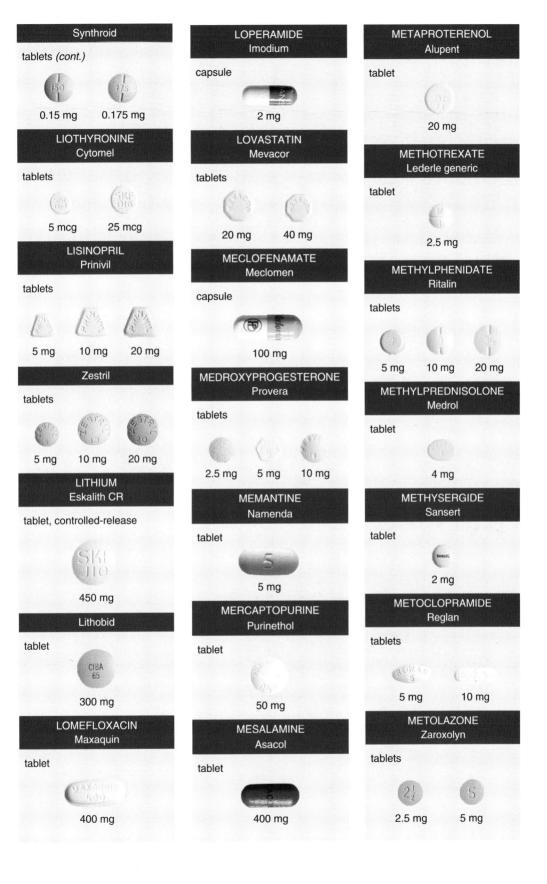

0.15 mg   0.175 mg

LIOTHYRONINE
Cytomel

tablets

5 mcg   25 mcg

LISINOPRIL
Prinivil

tablets

5 mg   10 mg   20 mg

Zestril

tablets

5 mg   10 mg   20 mg

LITHIUM
Eskalith CR

tablet, controlled-release

450 mg

Lithobid

tablet

300 mg

LOMEFLOXACIN
Maxaquin

tablet

400 mg

LOPERAMIDE
Imodium

capsule

2 mg

LOVASTATIN
Mevacor

tablets

20 mg   40 mg

MECLOFENAMATE
Meclomen

capsule

100 mg

MEDROXYPROGESTERONE
Provera

tablets

2.5 mg   5 mg   10 mg

MEMANTINE
Namenda

tablet

5 mg

MERCAPTOPURINE
Purinethol

tablet

50 mg

MESALAMINE
Asacol

tablet

400 mg

METAPROTERENOL
Alupent

tablet

20 mg

METHOTREXATE
Lederle generic

tablet

2.5 mg

METHYLPHENIDATE
Ritalin

tablets

5 mg   10 mg   20 mg

METHYLPREDNISOLONE
Medrol

tablet

4 mg

METHYSERGIDE
Sansert

tablet

2 mg

METOCLOPRAMIDE
Reglan

tablets

5 mg   10 mg

METOLAZONE
Zaroxolyn

tablets

2.5 mg   5 mg

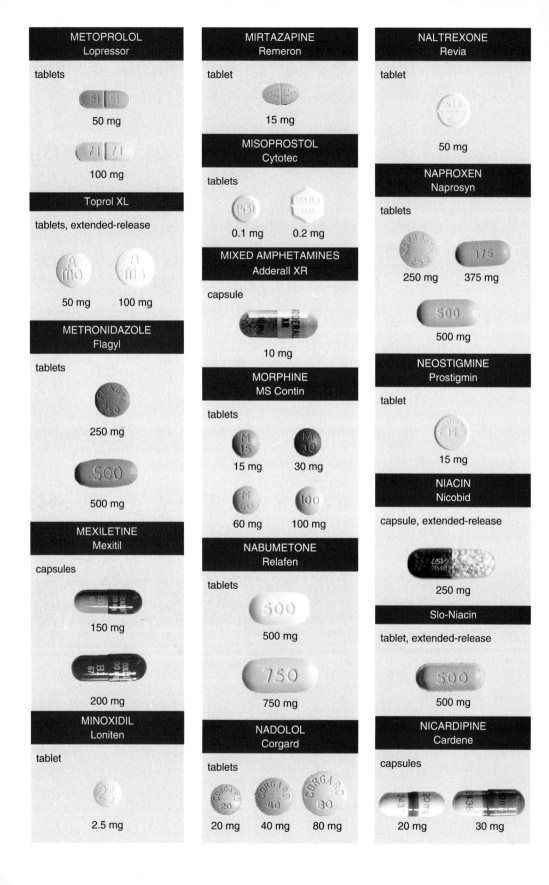

METOPROLOL
Lopressor

tablets

50 mg

100 mg

Toprol XL

tablets, extended-release

50 mg   100 mg

METRONIDAZOLE
Flagyl

tablets

250 mg

500 mg

MEXILETINE
Mexitil

capsules

150 mg

200 mg

MINOXIDIL
Loniten

tablet

2.5 mg

MIRTAZAPINE
Remeron

tablet

15 mg

MISOPROSTOL
Cytotec

tablets

0.1 mg   0.2 mg

MIXED AMPHETAMINES
Adderall XR

capsule

10 mg

MORPHINE
MS Contin

tablets

15 mg   30 mg

60 mg   100 mg

NABUMETONE
Relafen

tablets

500 mg

750 mg

NADOLOL
Corgard

tablets

20 mg   40 mg   80 mg

NALTREXONE
Revia

tablet

50 mg

NAPROXEN
Naprosyn

tablets

250 mg   375 mg

500 mg

NEOSTIGMINE
Prostigmin

tablet

15 mg

NIACIN
Nicobid

capsule, extended-release

250 mg

Slo-Niacin

tablet, extended-release

500 mg

NICARDIPINE
Cardene

capsules

20 mg   30 mg

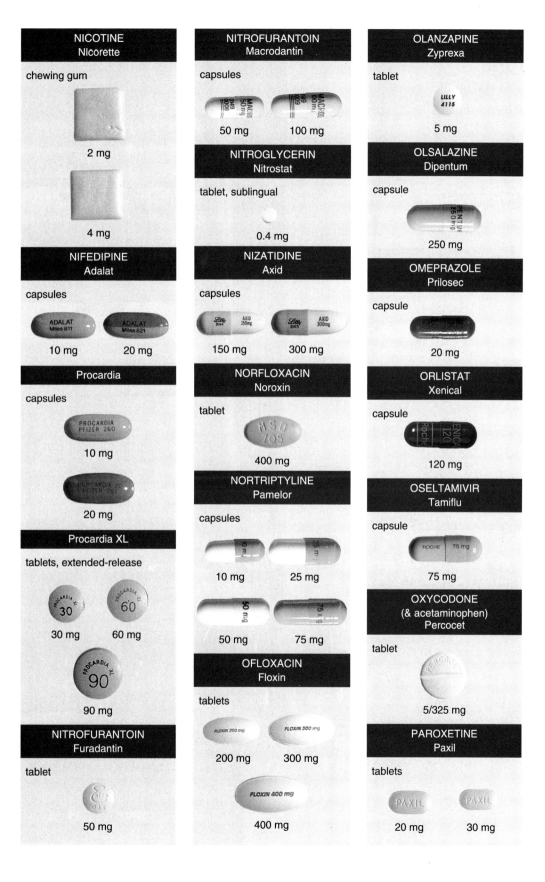

NICOTINE
Nicorette

chewing gum

2 mg

4 mg

NIFEDIPINE
Adalat

capsules

10 mg   20 mg

Procardia

capsules

10 mg

20 mg

Procardia XL

tablets, extended-release

30 mg   60 mg

90 mg

NITROFURANTOIN
Furadantin

tablet

50 mg

NITROFURANTOIN
Macrodantin

capsules

50 mg   100 mg

NITROGLYCERIN
Nitrostat

tablet, sublingual

0.4 mg

NIZATIDINE
Axid

capsules

150 mg   300 mg

NORFLOXACIN
Noroxin

tablet

400 mg

NORTRIPTYLINE
Pamelor

capsules

10 mg   25 mg

50 mg   75 mg

OFLOXACIN
Floxin

tablets

200 mg   300 mg

400 mg

OLANZAPINE
Zyprexa

tablet

5 mg

OLSALAZINE
Dipentum

capsule

250 mg

OMEPRAZOLE
Prilosec

capsule

20 mg

ORLISTAT
Xenical

capsule

120 mg

OSELTAMIVIR
Tamiflu

capsule

75 mg

OXYCODONE
(& acetaminophen)
Percocet

tablet

5/325 mg

PAROXETINE
Paxil

tablets

20 mg   30 mg

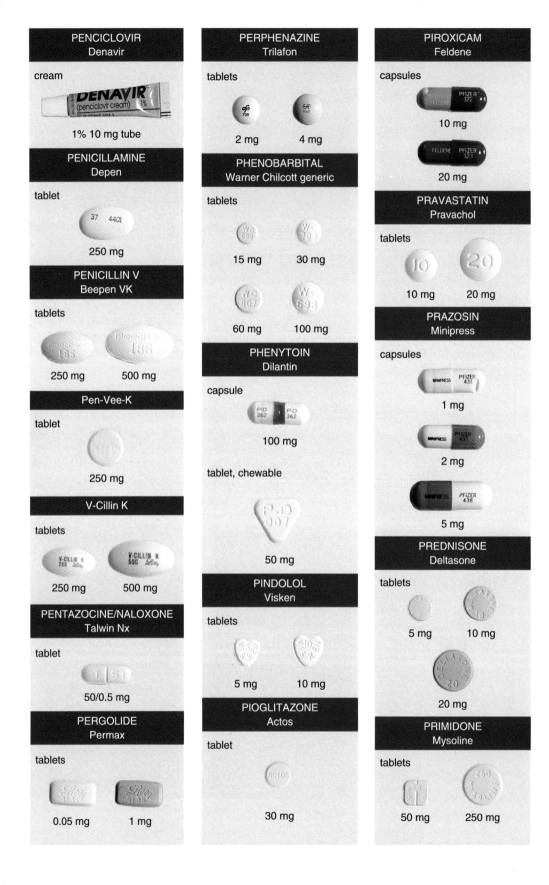

PENCICLOVIR
Denavir

cream

1% 10 mg tube

PENICILLAMINE
Depen

tablet

250 mg

PENICILLIN V
Beepen VK

tablets

250 mg   500 mg

Pen-Vee-K

tablet

250 mg

V-Cillin K

tablets

250 mg   500 mg

PENTAZOCINE/NALOXONE
Talwin Nx

tablet

50/0.5 mg

PERGOLIDE
Permax

tablets

0.05 mg   1 mg

PERPHENAZINE
Trilafon

tablets

2 mg   4 mg

PHENOBARBITAL
Warner Chilcott generic

tablets

15 mg   30 mg

60 mg   100 mg

PHENYTOIN
Dilantin

capsule

100 mg

tablet, chewable

50 mg

PINDOLOL
Visken

tablets

5 mg   10 mg

PIOGLITAZONE
Actos

tablet

30 mg

PIROXICAM
Feldene

capsules

10 mg

20 mg

PRAVASTATIN
Pravachol

tablets

10 mg   20 mg

PRAZOSIN
Minipress

capsules

1 mg

2 mg

5 mg

PREDNISONE
Deltasone

tablets

5 mg   10 mg

20 mg

PRIMIDONE
Mysoline

tablets

50 mg   250 mg

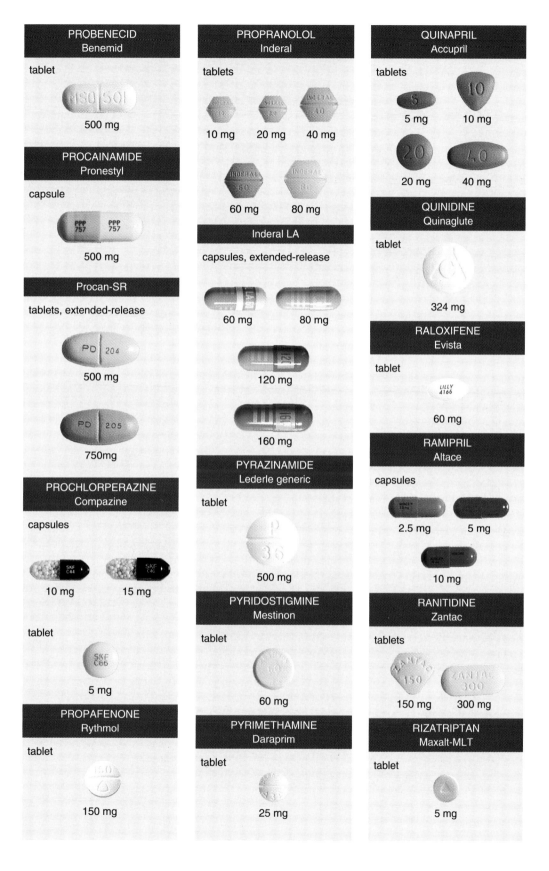

PROBENECID
Benemid

tablet

500 mg

PROCAINAMIDE
Pronestyl

capsule

500 mg

Procan-SR

tablets, extended-release

500 mg

750mg

PROCHLORPERAZINE
Compazine

capsules

10 mg   15 mg

tablet

5 mg

PROPAFENONE
Rythmol

tablet

150 mg

PROPRANOLOL
Inderal

tablets

10 mg   20 mg   40 mg

60 mg   80 mg

Inderal LA

capsules, extended-release

60 mg   80 mg

120 mg

160 mg

PYRAZINAMIDE
Lederle generic

tablet

500 mg

PYRIDOSTIGMINE
Mestinon

tablet

60 mg

PYRIMETHAMINE
Daraprim

tablet

25 mg

QUINAPRIL
Accupril

tablets

5 mg   10 mg

20 mg   40 mg

QUINIDINE
Quinaglute

tablet

324 mg

RALOXIFENE
Evista

tablet

60 mg

RAMIPRIL
Altace

capsules

2.5 mg   5 mg

10 mg

RANITIDINE
Zantac

tablets

150 mg   300 mg

RIZATRIPTAN
Maxalt-MLT

tablet

5 mg

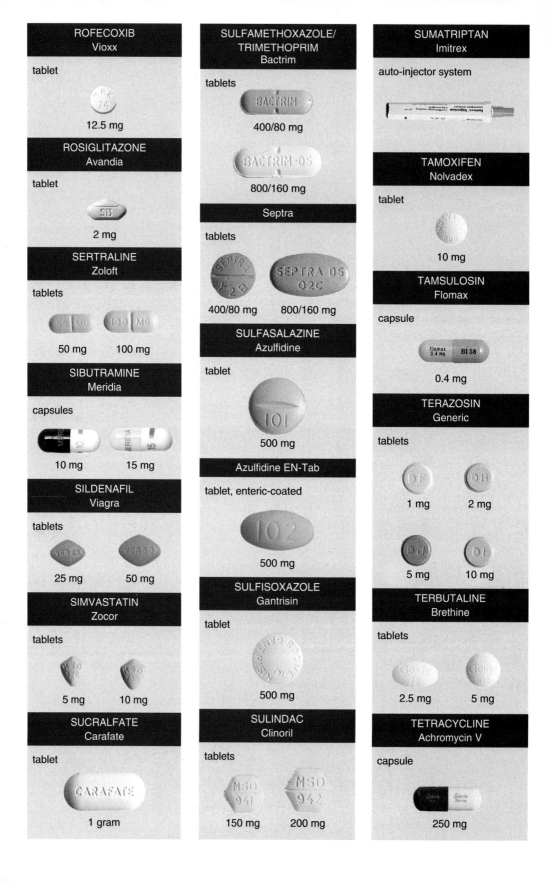

ROFECOXIB
Vioxx

tablet

12.5 mg

ROSIGLITAZONE
Avandia

tablet

2 mg

SERTRALINE
Zoloft

tablets

50 mg   100 mg

SIBUTRAMINE
Meridia

capsules

10 mg   15 mg

SILDENAFIL
Viagra

tablets

25 mg   50 mg

SIMVASTATIN
Zocor

tablets

5 mg   10 mg

SUCRALFATE
Carafate

tablet

1 gram

**SULFAMETHOXAZOLE/
TRIMETHOPRIM**
Bactrim

tablets

400/80 mg

800/160 mg

Septra

tablets

400/80 mg   800/160 mg

SULFASALAZINE
Azulfidine

tablet

500 mg

Azulfidine EN-Tab

tablet, enteric-coated

500 mg

SULFISOXAZOLE
Gantrisin

tablet

500 mg

SULINDAC
Clinoril

tablets

150 mg   200 mg

SUMATRIPTAN
Imitrex

auto-injector system

TAMOXIFEN
Nolvadex

tablet

10 mg

TAMSULOSIN
Flomax

capsule

0.4 mg

TERAZOSIN
Generic

tablets

1 mg   2 mg

5 mg   10 mg

TERBUTALINE
Brethine

tablets

2.5 mg   5 mg

TETRACYCLINE
Achromycin V

capsule

250 mg

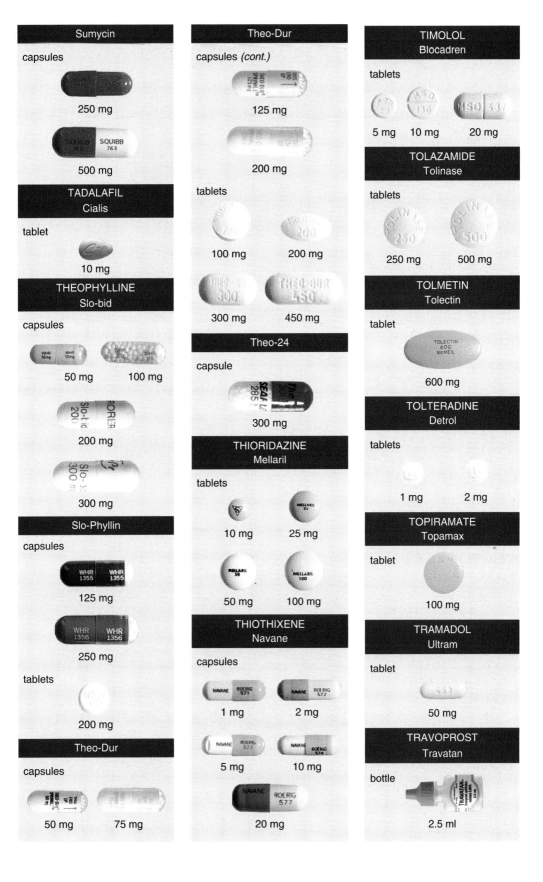

Sumycin

capsules

250 mg

500 mg

TADALAFIL
Cialis

tablet

10 mg

THEOPHYLLINE
Slo-bid

capsules

50 mg   100 mg

200 mg

300 mg

Slo-Phyllin

capsules

125 mg

250 mg

tablets

200 mg

Theo-Dur

capsules

50 mg   75 mg

Theo-Dur

capsules *(cont.)*

125 mg

200 mg

tablets

100 mg   200 mg

300 mg   450 mg

Theo-24

capsule

300 mg

THIORIDAZINE
Mellaril

tablets

10 mg   25 mg

50 mg   100 mg

THIOTHIXENE
Navane

capsules

1 mg   2 mg

5 mg   10 mg

20 mg

TIMOLOL
Blocadren

tablets

5 mg   10 mg   20 mg

TOLAZAMIDE
Tolinase

tablets

250 mg   500 mg

TOLMETIN
Tolectin

tablet

600 mg

TOLTERADINE
Detrol

tablets

1 mg   2 mg

TOPIRAMATE
Topamax

tablet

100 mg

TRAMADOL
Ultram

tablet

50 mg

TRAVOPROST
Travatan

bottle

2.5 ml

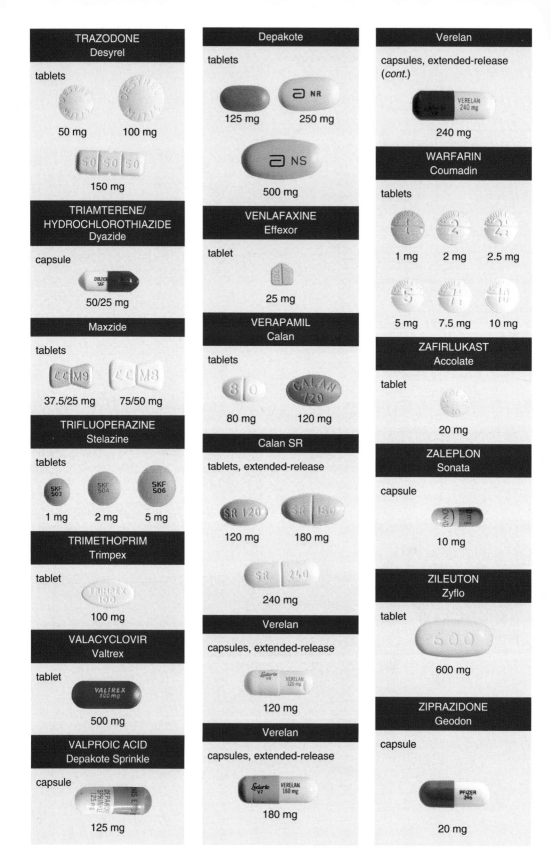

TRAZODONE
Desyrel

tablets

50 mg   100 mg

150 mg

**TRIAMTERENE/
HYDROCHLOROTHIAZIDE**
Dyazide

capsule

50/25 mg

Maxzide

tablets

37.5/25 mg   75/50 mg

TRIFLUOPERAZINE
Stelazine

tablets

1 mg   2 mg   5 mg

TRIMETHOPRIM
Trimpex

tablet

100 mg

VALACYCLOVIR
Valtrex

tablet

500 mg

VALPROIC ACID
Depakote Sprinkle

capsule

125 mg

Depakote

tablets

125 mg   250 mg

500 mg

VENLAFAXINE
Effexor

tablet

25 mg

VERAPAMIL
Calan

tablets

80 mg   120 mg

Calan SR

tablets, extended-release

120 mg   180 mg

240 mg

Verelan

capsules, extended-release

120 mg

Verelan

capsules, extended-release

180 mg

Verelan

capsules, extended-release
(*cont.*)

240 mg

WARFARIN
Coumadin

tablets

1 mg   2 mg   2.5 mg

5 mg   7.5 mg   10 mg

ZAFIRLUKAST
Accolate

tablet

20 mg

ZALEPLON
Sonata

capsule

10 mg

ZILEUTON
Zyflo

tablet

600 mg

ZIPRAZIDONE
Geodon

capsule

20 mg

AMITRIPTYLINE (a mee TRIP ti leen)

Introduced: 1961 **Class:** Antidepressant **Prescription:** USA:
Yes **Controlled Drug:** USA: No; Canada: No **Available as Generic:**
Yes

Brand Names: Amitid, Amitril, ✦Apo-Amitriptyline, ✦Elatrol, Elavil,
✦Elavil Plus [CD], Emitrip, Endep, Enovil, ✦Entrafon-Plus [CD], Etrafon
[CD], ✦Etrafon-A [CD], ✦Etrafon-D [CD], Etrafon-Forte [CD], ✦Levate,
✦Novo-Triptyn, PMS-Levazine [CD], Limbitrol [CD], SK-Amitriptyline,
✦Triavil [CD]

BENEFITS versus RISKS

Possible Benefits	*Possible Risks*
EFFECTIVE RELIEF OF ENDOGENOUS DEPRESSION	ADVERSE BEHAVIORAL EFFECTS: Confusion, disorientation, hallucinations
Additive (adjunctive) therapy in some pain syndromes (such as peripheral neuropathic pain or pain after herpes infections—post-herpetic neuralgia)	CONVERSION OF DEPRESSION TO MANIA in manic-depressive disorders
	Irregular heart rhythms—possible Blood cell abnormalities—rare

---

▷ **Principal Uses**

As a Single Drug Product: Uses currently included in FDA-approved labeling:
(1) Eases symptoms of spontaneous (endogenous) depression; (2) helps
depression resistant (refractory) to a single medicine.

Other (unlabeled) generally accepted uses: (1) Additive (adjuvant) therapy in
chronic pain/pain syndromes (such as peripheral neuropathic pain); (2)
eases agitation; (3) helps diabetic nerve (neuropathy) pain; (4) is an alternative in intractable hiccups; (5) combined with other medicines to ease
the pain of postherpetic neuralgia; (6) some benefit easing pain of chronic
vulvar burning (vulvodynia); (7) used in fish (ciguatera) poisoning.

As a Combination Drug Product [CD]: Combined with chlordiazepoxide to relieve
anxiety and depression. Also available in combination with perphenazine, a
phenothiazine, to relieve severe agitation that may occur with depression.

How This Drug Works: Eases depression by restoring normal levels of two nerve
impulse chemicals (norepinephrine and serotonin).

▷ **Widely Used Guidelines That Involve This Medicine (representative sample):** Please look at the section at the very beginning of this profile called
"Class." Next, turn to Table 22 and you will find guidelines listed by the
class involved!

Available Dosage Forms and Strengths

Injection — 10 mg/mL

Oral suspension — 10 mg/5 mL

Tablets — 10 mg, 25 mg, 50 mg, 75 mg, 100 mg, 150 mg

▷ **Usual Adult Dosage Ranges:** Intramuscular injection is given as 80 to 120 mg
per day divided into four doses. Switch to oral form made as soon as possible. Oral dosing starts with 25 mg two to three times daily. May be
increased cautiously as needed/tolerated by 10 to 25 mg daily at intervals
of 1 week with dose increases usually made later in the day or at bedtime.

Usual ongoing dose is 50 to 100 mg daily. Total dose should not exceed 150 mg daily outside of the hospital (where 200–300 mg doses have occasionally been given). Once the best dose is found, it may be taken at bedtime as one dose. Some clinicians start with 50 mg at bedtime.

Note: Actual dose and schedule must be determined for each patient individually.

Conditions Requiring Dosing Adjustments

Liver Function: Specific guidelines not available; however, low doses and a check of blood levels are prudent.

Kidney Function: Lower doses and blood level checks are needed with kidney failure (18% of drug is removed this way).

▷ **Dosing Instructions:** May be taken without regard to meals. Immediate-release form tablets may be crushed to take it. DO NOT CRUSH SUSTAINED-RELEASE form (available in Great Britain). If you forget a dose: Take the medicine right away, unless it is nearly time for your next dose. If you only take one dose at bedtime, don't take the missed dose in the morning, skip the missed dose and take the next dose right on schedule. DO NOT double doses.

Usual Duration of Use: Some benefit in depression in 1 to 2 weeks, but peak benefit may take 30 days or longer. Some clinicians quicken the onset of tricyclic antidepressants like amitriptyline by adding thyroid supplements. This benefit seems to particularly work well in women. Long-term use of antidepressants should not exceed 6 months without follow-up evaluation. In a set of guidelines issued by the American College of Physicians, older and newer antidepressants were found to give equal results in treating depression, but the general characteristics were different. Older medicines were found to generally have more frequent constipation, dizziness, dry mouth, blurred vision, and tremors while newer medicines caused more diarrhea, headache, and nausea. The importance here is that many options are available and possible side effects can be somewhat tailored to try to avoid overlap. Start (onset) of benefits in pain management may happen more quickly than in depression.

Typical Treatment Goals and Measurements (Outcomes and Markers)

Depression: The general goal: to lessen the degree and severity of depression, letting patients return to their daily lives. Specific measures of depression involve testing or inventories (such as the Hamilton Depression Inventory) and can be valuable in helping check benefits from this medicine.

Pain syndromes: The general goal: to decrease pain to a manageable level. Pain should be appropriately checked (assessed), and progress defined based on lowering of overall pain level and improved quality of life. A PQRSTBG (see Glossary) and patient goal assessment should be made and rechecked.

▷ **This Drug Should Not Be Taken If**
- you are allergic to any of the brand names listed above.
- you are taking, or have taken within the past 14 days, any monoamine oxidase (MAO) type A inhibitor drug (see Drug Classes) or are taking cisapride.
- you are recovering from a recent heart attack (MI or myocardial infarction).
- you are pregnant.

▷ **Inform Your Physician Before Taking This Drug If**
- you have a history of diabetes, epilepsy (or other seizure disorder), glaucoma, heart disease, prostate gland enlargement (or urinary outflow problems), or overactive thyroid function.

- you will have surgery with general anesthesia.
- you have heart-induced chest pain (angina pectoris).
- you have a rapid heart rate that occurs spontaneously (paroxysmal tachycardia).
- you have narrow-angle glaucoma.
- you are unsure how much or how often to take this drug.
- you have a history of schizophrenia—this drug may worsen any paranoia.
- you have a history of prostate or sexual problems.
- you have a liver or kidney disorder.
- you have a blood cell disorder.
- you have a history of intestinal block (ileus).

Possible Side Effects (natural, expected, and unavoidable drug actions)
Drowsiness, blurred vision, dry mouth, constipation, impaired urination.

▷ **Possible Adverse Effects** (unusual, unexpected, and infrequent reactions)
If any of the following develop, consult your physician promptly for guidance.

Mild Adverse Effects
Allergic reactions: skin rash, hives, swelling of face or tongue, drug fever (see Glossary).
Headache, dizziness, weakness, fainting, unsteady gait, tremors—infrequent.
Ringing in the ears (tinnitus)—reported with other medicines in the same family.
Peculiar taste, irritation of tongue or mouth, nausea, indigestion—rare to infrequent.
Fluctuation of blood sugar levels—possible.
Increased dental cavities (caries)—increased risk.
Restlessness, nightmares—rare.
Change in the ability to perceive tones—case report.

Serious Adverse Effects
Allergic reactions: hepatitis (see Glossary).
Idiosyncratic reactions: neuroleptic malignant syndrome (see Glossary).
Confusion or hallucinations—may be more likely in older patients and with higher doses.
Bowel obstruction (ileus)—rare.
SIADH (see Glossary)—rare.
Excessively low blood pressure (hypotension)—possible.
Seizures—rare.
Severe eye or other movement problems—case reports.
Heart palpitation and irregular rhythm—rare and more likely with increasing doses or overdose.
Bone marrow depression (see Glossary): fatigue, weakness, fever, sore throat, abnormal bleeding or bruising—rare.
A lupus erythematosus–like syndrome has been reported.
Peripheral neuritis (see Glossary): numbness, tingling, pain, loss of arm or leg strength—possible.
Parkinson-like disorders (see Glossary): often mild and infrequent—more likely in the elderly.
Liver toxicity—rare.
Serotonin syndrome—possible.
Worsening of paranoid psychosis in schizophrenic patients—possible.

▷ **Possible Effects on Sexual Function:**
Decreased libido—rare.

Increased libido (possible antidepressant effect), inhibited female orgasm, inhibited ejaculation—case reports.

Male and female breast enlargement, milk production, swelling of testicles, impotence—case reports.

These effects usually disappear within 2 to 10 days after discontinuation of the drug.

Adverse Effects That May Mimic Natural Diseases or Disorders
Liver toxicity may suggest viral hepatitis.

Natural Diseases or Disorders That May Be Activated by This Drug
Latent diabetes, epilepsy, glaucoma, impaired urination due to prostate gland enlargement.

Possible Effects on Laboratory Tests
Complete blood counts: decreased white cells and platelets; increased eosinophils.

Liver function tests: increased ALT/GPT, AST/GOT, alkaline phosphatase, increased bilirubin.

Blood glucose levels: increased or decreased (fluctuations).

CAUTION
1. Make sure you make follow-up visits to your doctor.
2. Best to withhold this drug if electroconvulsive therapy (ECT, "shock" treatment) is to be used.

Precautions for Use
By Infants and Children: Safety and effectiveness for those under 12 years old not established.

By Those Over 60 Years of Age: During the first 2 weeks watch for confusion, agitation, forgetfulness, delusions, and hallucinations. Decreased dose or stopping the drug may be needed. Unsteadiness may predispose to falling and injury. May worsen impaired urination seen with prostate gland enlargement (prostatism).

▷ Advisability of Use During Pregnancy
Pregnancy Category: C. See Pregnancy Risk Categories at the back of this book.

Animal Studies: Skull deformities reported in rabbits.

Human Studies: There have been reports of developmental delays, limb deformities, and central nervous system (CNS) problems in infants whose mothers had taken amitriptyline during pregnancy. Adequate studies of pregnant women are not available.

Use during pregnancy is a benefit-to-risk decision.

Advisability of Use If Breast-Feeding
Presence of this drug in breast milk: Yes.

One source says this medicine is NOT compatible with breast-feeding. Product insert notes levels of up to 151 ng/mL in breast milk—yet undetectable levels in the infant serum. Best to talk to your doctor about the benefits versus risks of breast feeding if you are taking this medicine.

Habit-Forming Potential: If prolonged therapy has been given, stopping this medicine suddenly can lead to headache, nausea, and weakness (malaise). Rare reports of hypomania or mania have been made 2 to 7 days after stopping therapy with tricyclic antidepressants.

Effects of Overdose: Confusion, hallucinations, marked drowsiness, heart palpitations, dilated pupils, tremors, stupor, deep sleep, coma, convulsions.

Suggested Periodic Examinations While Taking This Drug (at physician's discretion)

Complete blood cell counts.

Liver function tests.

Serial blood pressure readings and electrocardiograms.

▷ **While Taking This Drug, Observe the Following**

Foods: Excessive vitamin C can blunt therapeutic benefit of this drug. May also increase appetite and cause excessive weight gain.

Herbal Medicines or Minerals: Since amitriptyline and St. John's wort may act to increase serotonin, the combination is not advised. St. John's wort also increases sun sensitivity. Since part of the way ginseng works may be as a MAO inhibitor, do not combine with amitriptyline. Indian snake-root, kava kava, and yohimbe are also best avoided while taking this medicine.

Beverages: No restrictions. May be taken with milk.

▷ *Alcohol:* Even modest amounts of alcohol can lead to blackouts. Discuss any alcohol use with your doctor as this combination can markedly increase the intoxicating effects of alcohol and brain function depression. Many clinicians advise avoiding alcohol.

Tobacco Smoking: May hasten the removal of this drug from your body. I advise you to quit smoking.

▷ *Other Drugs*

Amitriptyline may ***increase*** the effects of

- albuterol or other direct sympathomimetic drugs (amphetamines, epinephrine).
- antihistamines (such as diphenhydramine—Benadryl, others), which can increase the risk of urinary retention, chronic glaucoma, and bowel obstruction (ileus). This is especially problematic in the elderly.
- atropine-like drugs (see Drug Classes).
- cimetidine (Tagamet).
- disulfiram (Antabuse), which can worsen the disulfiram effect if alcohol is consumed, but may also lead to decreased mental status.

Amitriptyline may ***decrease*** the effects of

- clonidine (Catapres).
- guanethidine (Ismelin).
- guanfacine (Tenex).
- methyldopa, which can result in reduced amitriptyline and/or methyldopa benefits.

Amitriptyline ***taken concurrently*** with

- amphetamines can cause excessive amitriptyline responses.
- amprenavir (Agenerase), ritonavir (Norvir), and perhaps other protease inhibitors (see Drug Classes) can lead to amitriptyline toxicity.
- anticoagulants such as warfarin (Coumadin) may cause an increased risk of bleeding.
- baclofen (Lioresal) may lead to muscle weakness and memory loss.
- bepridil (Vascor) can lead to heart rhythm problems. DO NOT COMBINE.
- carbamazepine (Tegretol) may decrease the blood level of amitriptyline.
- cisapride (Propulsid) can lead to heart rhythm problems. DO NOT COMBINE.
- diazepam (Valium) and perhaps other benzodiazepines (see Drug Classes) can result in additive loss of psychomotor skills.
- dofetilide (Tikosyn) can lead to heart rhythm problems. DO NOT COMBINE.
- enflurane (various) may increase seizure risk. DO NOT COMBINE.
- epinephrine may cause an increased risk of rapid heart rate and high blood pressure.

- estrogens (see Drug Classes) may increase amitriptyline drug levels.
- ethanol (alcohol) may give additive central nervous system toxicity.
- fluconazole (Diflucan) can result in very high levels of amitriptyline.
- fluoxetine (Prozac) can result in very high levels of amitriptyline.
- fluvoxamine (Luvox) can result in very high levels of amitriptyline.
- gatifloxacin (Tequin), grepafloxacin (Raxar), moxifloxacin (Avelox), or sparfloxacin (Zagam) may result in heart toxicity—DO NOT COMBINE.
- ibutilide (Corvert) may result in abnormal heart rhythms. DO NOT COMBINE.
- meperidine (Demerol) worsens breathing (respiratory) depression risk.
- monoamine oxidase (MAO) type A inhibitor drugs may cause high fever, delirium, and convulsions (see Drug Classes).
- phenytoin (Dilantin) or fosphenytoin (Cerebyx) can lead to amitriptyline toxicity.
- potassium (various) may lead to ulceration from potassium as amitriptyline may slow the intestine.
- propafenone (Rhythmol) can result in increased antidepressant blood levels and possible toxicity (sedation, dry mouth, difficulty urinating, etc.).
- quinidine (Quinaglute, etc.) can result in increased antidepressant blood levels.
- S-adenosylmethionine (SAMe) may lead to serotonin syndrome. Combination is not recommended.
- salmeterol (Serevent) should be used with great care because of increased cardiovascular risk (changes in blood pressure, pulse, and electrocardiograms or EKGs).
- sertraline (Zoloft) can lead to heart rhythm problems. DO NOT COMBINE.
- thyroid preparations may impair heart rhythm and function, but may also help depression when used in combination. Ask your doctor for help with time frames for results in making depression better, adjustment of thyroid dose, and checks for changes in heart rhythm.
- tramadol (Ultram) may increase risk of seizures. This combination is not advised.
- venlafaxine (Effexor) can result in very high levels of amitriptyline.
- verapamil (Calan, others) can result in very high levels of amitriptyline.
- warfarin (Coumadin) may lead to increased bleeding risk. More frequent INRs are prudent.

▷ *Driving, Hazardous Activities:* This drug may impair mental alertness, judgment, physical coordination, and reaction time. Avoid hazardous activities.

Aviation Note: The use of this drug ***is a disqualification*** for piloting. Consult a designated Aviation Medical Examiner.

Exposure to Sun: This drug may cause photosensitivity (see Glossary).

Exposure to Heat: May inhibit sweating and impair the body's adaptation to hot environments, increasing risk of heatstroke. Avoid saunas.

Exposure to Cold: Older patients should avoid prolonged cold exposure (conducive to hypothermia—see Glossary).

Discontinuation: It is best to stop this drug gradually. Abrupt withdrawal after long-term use can cause a withdrawal syndrome (headache, malaise, and nausea).

AMLODIPINE (am LOH di peen)

Introduced: 1986 **Class:** Anti-anginal, antihypertensive, calcium channel blocker **Prescription:** USA: Yes **Controlled Drug:** USA: No; Canada: No **Available as Generic:** No

Brand Names: Lotrel [CD], Norvasc

Controversies in Medicine: Medicines in this class have had many conflicting reports. Amlodipine got the first FDA approval to treat high blood pressure or angina in those with congestive heart failure. Some data appear to show that amlodipine lowers the risk of stroke or heart attack in people with coronary artery disease. CCBs are currently second-line agents for high blood pressure according to the JNC VII (see Glossary).

```
BENEFITS versus RISKS

      Possible Benefits                    Possible Risks
EFFECTIVE PREVENTION OF           DOSE-RELATED CHANGES IN
  BOTH MAJOR TYPES OF ANGINA        HEART RHYTHM
EFFECTIVE TREATMENT OF            Peripheral edema (fluid retention in
  HYPERTENSION                       feet and ankles)
                                  Dose-related palpitations
                                  Other medicines in the same family
                                    have rare concern about depression,
                                    memory loss, or malignancy
```

▷ **Principal Uses**

As a Single Drug Product: Uses currently included in FDA-approved labeling: (1) Treats angina pectoris due to spontaneous coronary artery spasm (Prinzmetal's variant angina) that is not associated with exertion; (2) classical angina-of-effort (caused by "hardening" or atherosclerosis of coronary arteries) in people who don't respond or can't tolerate nitrates or beta-blockers; (3) mild to moderate hypertension.

Other (unlabeled) generally accepted uses: (1) May keep early atherosclerotic lesions from getting worse; (2) can help stop premature labor; (3) helps some symptoms in cases of lung (pulmonary) hypertension; (4) can work to lower blood pressure and decrease the amount of protein in the urine (microalbuminuria) of diabetics; (5) may ease silent myocardial ischemia in combination with a beta blocker; (6) some limited use in preventing migraines.

As a Combination Drug Product [CD]: In combination with benazepril offers the benefits of an ACE inhibitor and a calcium channel blocker.

How This Drug Works: This drug blocks normal passage of calcium through cell walls, inhibiting coronary artery and peripheral arteriole narrowing. As a result, this drug

- prevents spontaneous coronary artery spasm (Prinzmetal's angina).
- decreases heart rate and contraction force in exertion, making effort-induced angina less likely.
- opens contracted peripheral arterial walls, lowering blood pressure. (Also lessens heart work and helps prevent angina.)

May also offer dual receptor binding characteristics. The combination form (Lotrel) adds the benefits of inhibiting angiotensin converting enzyme (ACE) via the active benazeprilat form.

▷ **Widely Used Guidelines That Involve This Medicine (representative sample):** Please look at the section at the very beginning of this profile called "Class." Next, turn to Table 22 and you will find guidelines listed by the class involved!

Available Dosage Forms and Strengths
Lotrel capsules — 2.5/10 mg, 5/10 mg, and 5/20 mg
Tablets — 2.5 mg, 5 mg, 10 mg

▷ **Recommended Dosage Ranges** (Actual dose and schedule must be determined for each patient individually.)
Infants and Children: Dosage not established.
12 to 65 Years of Age: High blood pressure: 2.5 to 10 mg daily, in a single dose. The fixed combination (Lotrel form) is usually given as one to two capsules a day. In older (or frail patients) some clinicians limit the dose of the amlodipine component to 2.5 mg a day.
Chronic angina: 5 to 10 mg daily; 10 mg may improve exercise ability in stable angina patients.
Congestive heart failure: 5 mg once daily for 2 weeks with increase to 10 mg as needed and tolerated.
Over 65 Years of Age: Lower doses (2.5 mg for high blood pressure and 5 mg for angina) are prudent and effective.

Conditions Requiring Dosing Adjustments
Liver Function: Patients with damaged livers started on a daily 2.5-mg dose for high blood pressure, 5 mg for angina. Then dosing may be slowly increased as needed or tolerated.
Kidney Function: No adjustment in dosing is needed.
Low Protein or Starvation: This drug is moved around the body by a protein called albumin. If protein is low, in liver failure or starvation, increased effect may be seen with "normal" doses. Start therapy with low doses. Increase only if needed or tolerated.

▷ **Dosing Instructions:** May be taken with or following food to reduce stomach irritation. The tablet may be crushed. If you forget a dose: Take the medicine right away, unless it is nearly time for your next dose, then omit the missed dose and take the medicine when it was next scheduled. DO NOT double doses.

Usual Duration of Use: Regular use for 2 to 4 weeks often needed to see benefit in reducing angina frequency or severity of angina and in high blood pressure control. Best to use the lowest dose that works for long-term use (months to years). Periodic evaluation by your doctor is needed.

Typical Treatment Goals and Measurements (Outcomes and Markers)
Blood Pressure: Current guidelines (JNC VII) define normal blood pressure (BP) as **less than** 120/80. **Pre-hypertension is** from 120/80 to 139/89 and is intended to help your doctor encourage lifestyle changes (or in the case of people with a risk factor for high blood pressure, start treatment) much earlier—so that possible damage to blood vessels, your heart, kidneys, sexual potency, or eyes might be minimized or avoided altogether. The next two classes of high blood pressure are stage 1 hypertension: 140/90 to 159/99 and stage 2 hypertension equal to or greater than: 160/100 mm Hg. These guidelines also recommend that clinicians work with their patients to agree on the goals and a plan of treatment. The first-ever guidelines for blood pressure (hypertension) in African Americans recommends that MOST black patients be started on TWO antihypertensive medicines with

the goal of lowering blood pressure to 130/80 for those with high risk for heart and blood vessel disease or with diabetes. The American Diabetes Association recommends 130/80 as the target for people living with diabetes and less than 125/75 for those who spill more than one gram of protein into their urine. Most clinicians try to achieve a BP that confers the best balance of lower cardiovascular risk and avoids the problem of too low a blood pressure. Blood pressure duration is generally increased with beneficial restriction of sodium. The goals and time frame should be discussed with you when the prescription is written. If goals are not met, it is not unusual to intensify doses or add on medicines.

Possible Advantages of This Drug

Slow onset and prolonged effect, allowing effective once-a-day treatment for both angina and high blood pressure. The combination form offers two distinct mechanisms of action to help lower blood pressure.

▷ This Drug Should Not Be Taken If

- you have had an allergic reaction to it previously.
- you have active liver disease.
- you have low blood pressure—systolic below 90 mm Hg.
- your left heart ventricle doesn't work well (dysfunctional).

▷ Inform Your Physician Before Taking This Drug If

- you have had a bad reaction to any calcium blocker.
- you take digitalis or a beta-blocker (see Drug Classes).
- you are taking any drugs that lower blood pressure.
- you have had congestive heart failure, heart attack, or stroke.
- you have a contracted or narrowed (stenosed) aorta.
- you are subject to disturbances of heart rhythm.
- you have a history of drug-induced liver damage.
- you develop a rash or other skin reaction while taking this medicine.
- you are unsure how much or how often to take this drug.
- you have circulation problems in your hands.
- you have muscular dystrophy.

Possible Side Effects (natural, expected, and unavoidable drug actions)

Swelling of feet and ankles, flushing (4.5% in women and 1.5% in men) and sensation of warmth.

Impaired sense of smell.

▷ Possible Adverse Effects (unusual, unexpected, and infrequent reactions)

If any of the following develop, consult your physician promptly for guidance.

Mild Adverse Effects

Allergic reaction: skin rash (call your doctor, as persistent rashes may become serious).

Headache (up to 12%), dizziness (dose related)—infrequent.

Fatigue, nausea, or constipation—infrequent.

Dose-related palpitations, low dose—rare; 10 mg—infrequent.

Overgrowth of the gums (gingival hyperplasia)—up to 40% with drugs in the same class.

Increased urge to urinate at night—rare.

Visual changes (eye pain, double vision)—rare.

Ringing in the ears (tinnitus)—rare.

Cough, muscle pain—infrequent.

Dose-related flushing (4.5% in women and 1.5% in men)—infrequent.

Elevated liver enzymes (may be a hypersensitivity, usually resolves)—rare.

Serious Adverse Effects

   Allergic reactions: exfoliative dermatitis—very rare.
   Idiosyncratic reactions: Parkinson-like symptoms—case report.
   Dose-dependent edema (up to 6.2% in those over 65)—infrequent.
   Exfoliative dermatitis or erythema multiforme—rare.
   Agranulocytosis (only other medicines in this class)—case reports.
   Rebound angina—if drug is abruptly stopped—possible.
   Difficulty breathing (dyspnea)—infrequent (up to 15% in the PRAISE trial as pulmonary edema).

▷ **Possible Effects on Sexual Function:** Sexual dysfunction (both men and women)—1–2%.
   Swelling and tenderness of male breast tissue (gynecomastia)—case report.

Adverse Effects That May Mimic Natural Diseases or Disorders
   An allergic rash and swelling of the legs may resemble erysipelas.

Possible Effects on Laboratory Tests
   Liver function tests: transient increases in liver enzymes.

CAUTION
   1. Make sure all your health care providers know you take this drug. List this drug on a card in your purse or wallet.
   2. Nitroglycerin or other nitrate drugs can be used as needed to ease acute angina pain. If your attacks become more frequent or intense, call your doctor promptly.

Precautions for Use
   By Infants and Children: Safety and effectiveness for use by those under 12 not established.
   By Those Over 60 Years of Age: May be more likely to be weak, dizzy, or faint or fall. Be careful to prevent injury. Low starting doses are prudent.

▷ **Advisability of Use During Pregnancy**
   Pregnancy Category: C. See Pregnancy Risk Categories at the back of this book.
   Animal Studies: No information available.
   Human Studies: Adequate studies of pregnant women are not available.
   Avoid this drug during the first 3 months. Use during the last 6 months only if clearly needed. Ask your physician for guidance.

Advisability of Use If Breast-Feeding
   Presence of this drug in breast milk: Unknown.
   Avoid drug or refrain from nursing.

Habit-Forming Potential: None.

Effects of Overdose: Weakness, fainting, fast pulse, low blood pressure, slow heartbeat, metabolic acidosis, low potassium and calcium, sinus arrest, heart attack, seizures.

Possible Effects of Long-Term Use: Possible overgrowth of the gums.

Suggested Periodic Examinations While Taking This Drug (at physician's discretion)
   Heart function tests: electrocardiograms; blood pressure check while supine, sitting, and standing.

▷ **While Taking This Drug, Observe the Following**
   Foods: This medicine is increased by grapefruit or grapefruit juice. Avoid eating grapefruit for an hour after taking this medicine. Avoid excessive salt intake.

Herbal Medicines or Minerals: Ginseng, bitter orange, country mallow, peppermint oil, eleuthero root, hawthorn, saw palmetto, ma huang (now off the market), guarana, goldenseal, and licorice may cause increased blood pressure. Indian snakeroot, calcium, and garlic may help lower blood pressure. Ask your doctor if calcium and/or garlic makes sense for you. St. John's wort may increase sun sensitivity and because of its effect on liver enzymes, may also decrease drug benefits in controlling blood pressure. Talk to your doctor BEFORE adding any herbal medicines.

Beverages: See foods above. May be taken with milk.

▷ *Alcohol:* Use caution. Alcohol may exaggerate the drop in blood pressure.

Tobacco Smoking: Nicotine may reduce the effectiveness of this drug. I advise everyone to quit smoking.

Marijuana Smoking: Possible reduced effectiveness of this drug; mild to moderate increase in angina; possible changes in electrocardiogram, confusing interpretation.

▷ *Other Drugs*

Amlodipine ***taken concurrently*** with

- adenosine (Adenocard) may cause extended problems with slow heart rate.
- amiodarone (Cordarone) may worsen AV block or cause further slowing of the heart in partial atrioventricular (AV) block or sick sinus syndrome.
- azole antifungals (such as fluconazole [Diflucan] or itraconazole [Sporanox]) and imidazoles (see Drug Classes) such as ketoconazole (Nizoral) may lead to toxic amlodipine blood levels.
- beta-blocker drugs or digitalis preparations (see Drug Classes) may cause heart rate and rhythm problems.
- cyclosporine (Sandimmune) causes increased cyclosporine blood levels and increased risk of toxicity.
- delavirdine (Rescriptor) may cause increased amlodipine levels and toxicity.
- dofetilide (Tikosyn) may cause dofetilide toxicity.
- medicines that inhibit cytochrome P450 3A4 will increase amlodipine blood levels and those that induce 3A4 will decrease amlodipine blood levels.
- NSAIDs or oral anticoagulants such as Coumadin (warfarin—see Drug Classes) may lead to increased risk of bleeding in the gastrointestinal (GI) tract.
- quinupristin/dalfopristin (Synercid) may cause extended amlodipine effects or toxicity.
- rifampin (Rifater, others) may result in decreased therapeutic benefit of amlodipine.
- ritonavir (Norvir) and probably other protease inhibitors (see Drug Classes) may lead to amlodipine toxicity.

The following drug may ***increase*** the effects of amlodipine

- cimetidine (Tagamet).

▷ *Driving, Hazardous Activities:* This drug may cause dizziness. Restrict activities as necessary.

Aviation Note: Coronary artery disease ***is a disqualification*** for piloting. Consult a designated Aviation Medical Examiner.

Exposure to Sun: Four case reports of phototoxicity have been made. Caution is advised.

Exposure to Heat: Caution is advised. Hot environments can exaggerate the blood-pressure-lowering effects of this drug. Observe for light-headedness or weakness.

Heavy Exercise or Exertion: This drug may improve your ability to be more active without resulting angina pain. Use caution.

Discontinuation: Do not stop this drug abruptly—gradual withdrawal is often prudent. Watch for development of rebound angina.

AMOXAPINE (a MOX a peen)

Introduced: 1970   **Class:** Antidepressant   **Prescription:** USA: Yes   **Controlled Drug:** USA: No; Canada: No   **Available as Generic:** Yes

Brand Name: Asendin

BENEFITS versus RISKS	
Possible Benefits	*Possible Risks*
EFFECTIVE RELIEF OF PRIMARY DEPRESSIONS: ENDOGENOUS, NEUROTIC, REACTIVE	ADVERSE BEHAVIORAL EFFECTS: CONFUSION, DELUSIONS, DISORIENTATION, HALLUCINATIONS CONVERSION OF DEPRESSION TO MANIA IN MANIC-DEPRESSIVE DISORDERS Rare blood cell abnormalities Rare movement disorders Rare seizures Rare liver toxicity

Author's Note: Since use of this medicine has declined in favor of newer medicines, the information in this profile has been shortened.

AMOXICILLIN (a mox i SIL in)

AMOXICILLIN/CLAVULANATE (a mox i SIL in/KLAV yu lan ayt)

AMPHETAMINE/DEXTROAMPHETAMINE (Am FET ah meen/DEX troh am FET ah meen)

Introduced: 1996 (immediate release), 2002 (XR form)   **Class:** Amphetamine-like drug, anti–attention deficit disorder drug   **Prescription:** USA: Yes   **Controlled Drug:** USA: C-II*; Canada: Yes   **Available as Generic:** USA: No; Canada: No

Brand Names: Adderall, Adderall XR

BENEFITS versus RISKS

Possible Benefits	*Possible Risks*
USEFUL IN ATTENTION DEFICIT HYPERACTIVITY DISORDER (ADHD)	POTENTIAL FOR SERIOUS PSYCHOLOGICAL DEPENDENCE (by mouth (oral) dosing versus intravenous reaches brain levels slowly and appears to be more likely to avoid this effect)
XR FORM OFFERS ONCE-DAILY DOSING	SUPPRESSION OF GROWTH IN CHILDHOOD (recovers when medicine is stopped)
	Abnormal behavior

▷ **Principal Uses**

As a Single Drug Product: Uses currently included in FDA-approved labeling: Treats (1) attention deficit hyperactivity disorder in childhood.

Other (unlabeled) generally accepted uses: (1) Profile will focus on ADHD for this edition.

How This Drug Works: The exact way (mechanism of action) that amphetamines work in ADHD is not clearly defined. Activates the brain stem, improves alertness and concentration, increases learning ability and attention span. A study in *Science* found that levels of the nerve transmitter serotonin are increased by this medicine, restoring a proper balance between serotonin and other brain chemicals.

▷ **Widely Used Guidelines That Involve This Medicine (representative sample):** Please look at the section at the very beginning of this profile called "Class." Next, turn to Table 22 and you will find guidelines listed by the class involved!

Available Dosage Forms and Strengths

Capsules, extended release (Adderall XR)—5 mg, 10 mg, 15 mg, 20 mg, 25 mg, and 30 mg

Author's Note: Each capsule contains varying amounts of a mixture of amphetamines. For example: The 5 mg capsule has dextroamphetamine saccharate: 1.25 mg; amphetamine aspartate monohydrate: 1.25 mg; dextroamphetamine sulfate: 1.25 mg; amphetamine sulfate: 1.25 mg.

Tablets (immediate release)—5 mg, 7.5 mg, 10 mg, 12.5 mg, 15 mg, and 30 mg

▷ **Recommended Dosage Ranges:** *Attention deficit hyperactivity disorder:* Immediate release tablet form: NOT recommended for children less than 3. For 3–5 year olds: 2.5 mg a day is given in the morning, with dosing increased as needed and tolerated to the beneficial response desired. For those 6 or older: Dosing is started at 5 mg once or twice daily. Doses are then increased at needed and tolerated in 5 mg steps to the desired response at weekly intervals. Rare to require more than 40 mg daily. XR form: Not studied in those less than 6 years old: For those 6 or older: Dosing is started with 10 mg daily given in the morning. Dosing is adjusted as needed and tolerated to desired response. Doses more than 30 mg have not been studied.

Note: Actual dose and schedule must be determined for each patient individually.

Conditions Requiring Dosing Adjustments

Liver Function: Used with caution and prudent to decrease dose in liver disease.

Kidney Function: No changes currently thought to be needed.

▷ **Dosing Instructions:** The regular tablet may be crushed. Food does not change absorption, but a high fat meal will mean that the medicine stays in the body longer than usual. The prolonged-action capsule may be opened and taken with applesauce or similar food. Best to take this in the morning if you only take it once a day. Taking it close to bedtime can lead to problems falling asleep. If you forget a dose: take the missed dose as soon as you remember it, unless it's nearly time for your next dose—if that is the case, skip the missed dose and take the next dose right on schedule. Talk with your doctor and pharmacist if you find yourself missing doses.

Usual Duration of Use: Regular use for 3 to 4 weeks determines benefits in easing ADHD. If there is no improvement after this time, the drug should be stopped. Long-term use (months to years) requires supervision by your doctor.

Typical Treatment Goals and Measurements (Outcomes and Markers)

Attention Deficit: The general goal is to achieve the ability to "stay on task." This medicine can also help decrease impulsiveness and increase socially appropriate behavior. Specific measures of cognitive function, motor performance, and educational tasking may help assess response. Treatment guidelines from AHCPR and DSM-IV criteria from the American Psychiatric Association are widely used. The American Academy of Pediatricians has an important set of guidelines. Please remember that these are guidelines and therapy must still be individualized. The guidelines can be found at *www.pediatrics.org* (see also Sources and American Academy of Pediatrics).

▷ **This Drug Should Not Be Taken If**
- you have had an allergic reaction to it previously.
- you have glaucoma.
- you have symptomatic heart and blood vessel disease (cardiovascular), advanced arteriosclerosis or moderate to severe high blood pressure (hypertension).
- you have excessive activity of your thyroid (hyperthyroidism).
- you have taken a monoamine oxidase inhibitor (MAOI—see Drug Classes) in the last 14 days.
- you have Tourette's syndrome or experience tics while using this medicine.
- you are experiencing a period of severe anxiety, nervous tension, or emotional depression.

▷ **Inform Your Physician Before Taking This Drug If**
- you have a history of mental illness.
- you have a seizure disorder.
- you have a history of abnormal heartbeats.

Possible Side Effects (natural, expected, and unavoidable drug actions)

Nervousness, excitement, euphoria, insomnia. Dry mouth. Reduced appetite/weight loss, anorexia. Growth suppression (stopping the medicine in the summer is used to allow a growth spurt). Slight increase in heart rate.

▷ **Possible Adverse Effects** (unusual, unexpected, and infrequent reactions)

If any of the following develop, consult your physician promptly for guidance.

Mild Adverse Effects

Allergic reactions: skin rash, hives, drug fever—possible.

Headache, dizziness, increased blood pressure, rapid and forceful heart palpitation—infrequent.

Nausea, abdominal discomfort—infrequent.

Stuttering and hallucinations—case reports.

Serious Adverse Effects

Allergic reactions: possible.

Idiosyncratic reactions: abnormal patterns of behavior (labile emotions, psychosis)—case reports.

Movement disorder (dyskinesia)—rare.

Excessive temperature (hyperthermia)—rare.

Liver toxicity—case report for a similar medicine (methylphenidate).

Precipitation of Tourette's syndrome—case reports.

▷ **Possible Effects on Sexual Function:** Impotence or changes in libido.

Natural Diseases or Disorders That May Be Activated by This Drug

Latent epilepsy. Increased eye pressure unmasking glaucoma.

Possible Effects on Laboratory Tests

Liver function tests: possible increase with liver toxicity.

Plasma or urine corticosteroid levels: can be significantly increased.

CAUTION

1. This drug should be used ONLY AFTER a careful assessment by a qualified specialist is made. True attention deficit disorder requires careful assessment to differentiate it from behavior problems arising from family tensions or other conditions that do not require methylphenidate therapy.
2. Careful dose adjustments on an individual basis are mandatory.
3. Paradoxical reactions (see Glossary) can occur, causing aggravation of initial symptoms for which this drug was prescribed.
4. Drug testing screens for amphetamines will be positive—indicating the use of this medicine versus the abuse of medicine that these tests typically screen for. If illicit use of amphetamine or similar substances is also undertaken, levels will be higher than predicted.
5. Where possible, periodic interruptions of therapy should be made in order to check ongoing need for this medicine.

Precautions for Use

By Infants and Children: Safety and effectiveness for those less than 6 years of age are not established for the XR form. During long-term use, monitor the child for normal growth and development.

▷ **Advisability of Use During Pregnancy**

Pregnancy Category: C. See Pregnancy Risk Categories at the back of this book.

Animal Studies: No birth defects found in mouse studies.

Human Studies: Adequate studies of pregnant women are not available.

Ask your doctor for guidance.

Advisability of Use If Breast-Feeding

Presence of this drug in breast milk: Unsafe.

Avoid drug or refrain from nursing.

Habit-Forming Potential: This drug can produce tolerance and cause serious psychological dependence (see Glossary), a potentially dangerous characteristic of amphetaminelike drugs (see Drug Classes). Caution is needed. If you start to feel like the medicine is not working, call your doctor.

Effects of Overdose: Headache, vomiting, agitation, tremors, dry mouth, fever, confusion, hallucinations, seizures, coma.

Possible Effects of Long-Term Use: Suppression of growth (in weight and/or height) occurs. Many patients are taken off the drug during summer vacations.

Suggested Periodic Examinations While Taking This Drug (at physician's discretion)
Blood pressure measurements.
Height and weight.
Follow-up evaluation for beneficial effects of treatment.

▷ **While Taking This Drug, Observe the Following**
Herbal Medicines or Minerals: Using St. John's wort, guarana, mate, ma huang (no longer on the market for weight loss), bitter orange, country mallow, or kola while taking this medicine may result in unacceptable central nervous system stimulation.
Beverages: This drug may be taken with milk.
▷ *Alcohol:* Not expected to apply to children.
Tobacco Smoking: No interactions expected. I advise everyone to quit smoking.
▷ *Other Drugs*
Amphetamine/dextroamphetamine may ***increase*** the effects of
• meperidine (Demerol).
• norepinephrine (various).
• tricyclic antidepressants (see Drug Classes) and enhance their toxic effects.
Amphetamine/dextroamphetamine may ***decrease*** the effects of
• antihistamines (the drowsiness side effect).
• guanethidine (Ismelin) and impair its ability to lower blood pressure.
Amphetamine/dextroamphetamine ***taken concurrently*** with
• adrenergic blockers will have beneficial effects inhibited by amphetamines.
• alkalinizers such as sodium bicarbonate and some thiazide diuretics will lead to increased blood levels and possible toxicity.
• anticonvulsants (such as phenobarbital, fosphenytoin, or phenytoin) may delay absorption of the anticonvulsant.
• blood or urine acidifiers will increase removal of this medicine, lower the blood levels of amphetamine/dextroamphetamine and blunt the therapeutic benefits.
• blood pressure medicines (see drug classes for Beta Blockers, ACE inhibitors, other antihypertensives) may blunt the therapeutic benefits in controlling blood pressure. (A non-stimulant such as atomoxetine is a better choice in hypertensive patients).
• ethosuximide (Zarontin) will delay absorption of ethosuximide.
• haloperidol (Haldol) will lead to a blunting of the beneficial effect of amphetamines.
• lithium (Lithobid, others) may inhibit the stimulant effect of amphetamines.
• monoamine oxidase (MAO) type A inhibitors (see Drug Classes) may cause a significant rise in blood pressure; avoid the concurrent use of these drugs.
• morphine may be used to great therapeutic benefit to increase alertness, especially if high doses of morphine must be used.
• propoxyphene (Darvon, others) if taken in overdose amount may lead to increased central nervous system stimulation if combined with amphetamine/dextroamphetine potentially leading to fatal seizures.
• tricyclic antidepressants (see Drug Classes) may result in undesirable increases in blood pressure or worsening of cardiovascular effects.

▷ *Driving, Hazardous Activities:* This drug may cause dizziness or drowsiness. Restrict activities as necessary.

Aviation Note: The use of this drug **is a disqualification** for piloting. Consult a designated Aviation Medical Examiner.

Exposure to Sun: No restrictions.

Discontinuation: If the drug has been taken for a long time, do not stop it abruptly. Talk to your doctor about how to slowly decrease doses.

AMPICILLIN (am pi SIL in)

Please see the penicillin family profile for further information on amoxicillin, amoxicillin/clavulanate, or ampicillin.

ANAKINRA (ANN ah kin rah)

Other Names: Recombinant human interleukin-1 receptor antagonist. RhIL-1ra

Introduced: 2002   **Class:** Interleukin-1 receptor antagonist   **Prescription:** USA: Yes   **Controlled Drug:** USA: No; Canada: No   **Available as Generic:** No

Brand Name: Kineret

BENEFITS versus RISKS	
Possible Benefits	*Possible Risks*
USEFUL IN RHEUMATOID ARTHRITIS	INFECTIONS CAUSED BY IMMUNOSUPPRESSION FROM THE MEDICINE ITSELF
HAS A ROLE IN JUVENILE RHEUMATOID ARTHRITIS (ORPHAN DRUG)	Injection site reactions (usually mild)
CAN BE USED IN COMBINATION WITH METHOTREXATE	Possible development of antibodies
PREVENTION OF DISEASE PROGRESSION	Should NOT be started in people with active infections or lowered white blood cell counts
MAY GIVE A RESPONSE WHERE OTHER AGENTS HAVE FAILED	

▷ **Principal Uses**

As a Single Drug Product: Uses currently included in FDA-approved labeling: (1) Approved for treatment (alone or in combination with non-TNF therapies) of moderate to severe rheumatoid arthritis (RA) in people over 18, where one or more Disease Modifying Antirheumatic Drug (DMARD—see Glossary) has failed.

Other (unlabeled) generally accepted uses: (1) May have a role in graft-versus-host disease.

How This Drug Works: Binds competitively with two kinds of interleukin-1 receptors in the body (type 1 and 2). The effect of this binding is that the cellular responses that would have been seen from natural interleukin-1 alpha and beta is at least partially blocked.

▷ **Widely Used Guidelines That Involve This Medicine (representative sample):** Please look at the section at the very beginning of this profile called

"Class." Next, turn to Table 22 and you will find guidelines listed by the class involved!

Available Dosage Forms and Strengths

Injection — 100 mg/mL in a 1 mL prefilled syringe.

▷ **Recommended Dosage Ranges** (Actual dose and schedule must be determined for each patient individually.)

Infants and Children: Not studied in children.

Usual Adult Dosage Ranges: For rheumatoid arthritis (adults 18 and older): 100 mg injected under the skin (subcutaneously), once a day. (Remember to change or rotate where you inject.)

Conditions Requiring Dosing Adjustments

Liver Function: No changes needed, as only small amounts are removed via the liver or gall bladder.

Kidney Function: Removal of anakinra from plasma is decreased 70–75% in people with creatinine clearance (see Glossary) less than 30 mL/min, but no guidelines for dosing changes are available as yet.

▷ **Dosing Instructions:** It is very important that you understand how to inject this drug under the skin (subcutaneously) and NOT intravenously. Please ask your doctor or pharmacist if you do not understand. Please also remember to change (rotate) where you inject (the injection site), and inject it at the same time every day (helps keep blood levels about the same). Combination use with TNF-type therapies has not yet been studied. Talk to your doctor before injecting anakinra if you have an infection. If you forget a dose: Take the missed dose right away, unless it is nearly time for your next dose—if that is the case, skip the missed dose and take the next dose right on schedule. Call your doctor if you find yourself missing doses.

Usual Duration of Use: Use on a regular schedule determines benefit. In rheumatoid arthritis this drug usually goes to work in 1 to 3 weeks. Ongoing use (months to years) requires physician supervision and checks of ACR scores.

Typical Treatment Goals and Measurements (Outcomes and Markers):

Arthritis: Control of arthritis symptoms (pain, loss of mobility, decreased ability to accomplish activities of daily living, range of motion, etc.) is paramount in returning patient quality of life and to checking the results (beneficial outcomes) from this medicine. The American College of Rheumatology has a set of criteria for positive results in treating rheumatoid arthritis (you may hear this referred to as ACR 20, 50, or 70). Many arthritis management or pain centers use interdisciplinary teams (physicians from several specialties, nurses, physician's assistants, physical and occupational therapists, pharmacotherapists, psychotherapists, social workers, and others) to get the best results. Specific mobility goals are often set by the physician and administered by a physical/occupational therapist. The arthritis foundation has additional information at *www.arthritis.org*.

Possible Advantages of This Drug Uses: A novel mechanism (against interleukin-1) to fight rheumatoid arthritis. May give relief where other agents have failed.

▷ **This Drug Should Not Be Taken If**

- you have had an allergic reaction to it or to proteins that come from a bacteria called *E. coli*.
- you currently have an active infection.

▷ **Inform Your Physician Before Taking This Drug If**
   - you have moderate to severe kidney (renal) compromise (removal of the medicine will be lowered by up to 75%).
   - you develop a new infection while taking this medicine.
   - you have recently received a live virus vaccine.
   - you have a white blood cell count less than 2,000 (ask your doctor about leukopenia).
   - you have a disease or condition that weakens your immune system (are immunosuppressed).
   - you are pregnant or planning pregnancy in the near future.
   - you are breast-feeding your infant.
   - you are taking a tumor necrosis blocking agent (not studied yet).
   - you have a history of allergies to other medicines.

Possible Side Effects (natural, expected, and unavoidable drug actions)
   Report such developments to your physician promptly.
   Discomfort at the injection site.

▷ **Possible Adverse Effects** (unusual, unexpected, and infrequent reactions)
   If any of the following develop, consult your physician promptly for guidance.
   Mild Adverse Effects
   Allergic reaction: skin rash at the injection site—possible.
   Headache—frequent.
   Sinusitis—up to 7% in clinical trials.
   Nausea—may be frequent.
   Serious Adverse Effects
   Allergic reactions—possible.
   Lowering of a specific kind of white blood cell (neutrophil)—neutropenia—rare.
   Infections—may be frequent.

▷ **Possible Effects on Sexual Function:** None reported.

Possible Delayed Adverse Effects: Possible development of anti-anakinra antibodies. Long-term effects on response and benefits from anakinra are not fully understood.

Possible Effects on Laboratory Tests
   Anti-anakinra antibodies: positive.

CAUTION
   1. This drug must be followed carefully by a qualified physician.
   2. Make certain you understand how to inject this medicine under the skin.
   3. Live-virus vaccines should be avoided during use of this drug. Live-virus vaccines could actually produce infection rather than stimulate an immune response.
   5. The manufacturer advises against using this medicine if you have an active infection.
   6. Patients should be followed closely if they develop an infection while taking this medicine, and treatment should be STOPPED in patients with serious infections or sepsis.

Precautions for Use
   By Those Over 60 Years of Age: Specific changes are not indicated at present.

▷ **Advisability of Use During Pregnancy**
   Pregnancy Category: B. See Pregnancy Risk Categories at the back of this book.
   Human Studies: Adequate studies are NOT available.

Talk to your doctor about benefits versus risks of use.

Advisability of Use If Breast-Feeding
Presence of this drug in breast milk: Unknown.
Avoid drug or refrain from nursing.

Habit-Forming Potential: None.

Effects of Overdose: Symptomatic management indicated.

Possible Effects of Long-Term Use: Positive anti-anakinra antibodies—significance not presently known.

Suggested Periodic Examinations While Taking This Drug (at physician's discretion)
Beneficial response to the medicine (ACR criteria).
Sedimentation rate (ESR) and rheumatoid factor or C-reactive protein.
If used in congestive heart failure, tests of heart function and symptom-free walking time.

▷ **While Taking This Drug, Observe the Following**
Foods: No specific recommendations.
Herbal Medicines or Minerals: There is NO DATA on combined use of this drug with glucosamine or hay flower, mistletoe herb, or white mustard seed. Echinacea may actually blunt the immune response if used on an ongoing basis, and therefore combination is not advisable. Talk to your doctor before combining any herbal medicine with anakinra.
Beverages: No restrictions.
▷ *Alcohol:* No specific recommendations.
Tobacco Smoking: No interactions expected. I advise everyone to quit smoking.
Marijuana Smoking: May impair immunity.
▷ *Other Drugs*
Anakinra **taken concurrently** with
• medicines that blunt the immune system may lead to additive immune system depression if combined with etanercept.
• TNF blocking agents (such as etanercept (Enbrel) or infliximab (Remicade) has not been well studied, but may lead to increased risk of infection.
• yellow fever, pneumococcal, smallpox, or any other live vaccine may result in decreased immune response to the vaccine as well as possible transmission of the infection BY the vaccine.
▷ *Driving, Hazardous Activities:* No restrictions.
Aviation Note: The use of this drug is **probably not a disqualification** for piloting, but the condition being treated may be. Consult a designated Aviation Medical Examiner.
Exposure to Sun: No restrictions.
Occurrence of Unrelated Illness: Call your doctor to report any sign of infection.
Discontinuation: No specific recommendations. Ask your doctor before stopping any drug for any reason.
Special Storage Instructions: Keep this medicine in the refrigerator, but do not freeze it.

ANASTROZOLE (Ann AZ troh zoal)

Other Names: ZD 1033, ICID1033

Introduced: 2002   **Class:** Aromatase inhibitor, selective aromatase inhibitor, cancer chemotherapy antagonist   **Prescription:** USA: Yes
Controlled Drug: USA: No; Canada: No   **Available as Generic:** No
Brand Name: Arimidex

BENEFITS versus RISKS

Possible Benefits	*Possible Risks*
FIRST-LINE TREATMENT OF BREAST CANCER IN POST-MENOPAUSAL WOMEN SECOND-LINE TREATMENT OF ADVANCED BREAST CANCER IN WOMEN WHO HAVE HAD A RELAPSE OF BREAST CANCER AFTER HAVING BEEN TREATED FIRST WITH TAMOXIFEN	BLOOD CLOTS (thromboembolic events)—less than 4.1%
	HOT FLASHES (FLUSHES)
	JOINT OR BONE PAIN
	Increased risk of bone fracture
	Fluid buildup (edema)
MORE FAVORABLE RESULTS AND SIDE EFFECT PROFILE THAN TAMOXIFEN IN WOMEN AFTER MENOPAUSE (hormone sensitive early breast cancer)	

▷ **Principal Uses**

> *As a Single Drug Product:* Uses currently included in FDA-approved labeling: (1) Approved for first-line treatment of postmenopausal women who have early breast cancer that is hormone receptor positive or receptor unknown cancer which is either advanced on a local basis or is metastatic; (2) second-line treatment for women with advanced breast cancer that has continued to grow (progressed) after having first been treated with tamoxifen.
>
> Other (unlabeled) generally accepted uses: Not defined as yet. One case report or use in severe endometriosis.
>
> **Author's Note: Data presented from the ATAC (Arimidex, Tamoxifen Alone or in Combination) study was presented in Barcelona, Spain. The study, which involved more than 9,000 women showed that anastrozole outperformed tamoxifen (lower occurrence of hot flushes, blood clots, and cancer of the uterus) and also showed a 58% lower risk in development of a new tumor in the other breast. The company received fast-track designation by the FDA for approval for use in early breast cancer.**

How This Drug Works: This medicine works to lower estrogen levels in women after menopause by interfering with the conversion of androstenedione to estrone in peripheral tissues. This is accomplished by blocking an enzyme called aromatase.

▷ **Widely Used Guidelines That Involve This Medicine (representative sample):** Please look at the section at the very beginning of this profile called

"Class." Next, turn to Table 22 and you will find guidelines listed by the class involved!

Available Dosage Forms and Strengths

Tablets — 1 mg

▷ **Usual Adult Dosage Ranges:** *Breast cancer or advanced breast cancer in women after menopause:* One mg is given once daily. In first-line treatment of advanced breast cancer, the treatment is continued until the tumor progresses.

Note: Actual dose and schedule must be determined for each patient individually.

Conditions Requiring Dosing Adjustments

Liver Function: Doses may accumulate in mild to moderate liver disease, however no dosing changes are yet defined.

Kidney Function: Dose decreases are not thought to be needed in kidney disease (only 10% is removed that way).

▷ **Dosing Instructions:** The tablet may be crushed and taken either on an empty stomach or with food. If you forget a dose: Take the missed dose as soon as you remember it, unless it's nearly time for your next dose—if that is the case, skip the missed dose and take the next dose right on schedule. DO NOT double up on doses. Talk with your doctor if you find yourself missing doses—there are effective phone-based and other systems to help you remember your medicine.

Usual Duration of Use: Use on a regular schedule for 2 weeks usually finds the peak response. The ideal (optimal) length of treatment is not fully defined (approval was based on study of patients for a median two and a half years). Ongoing use (months to years) requires physician supervision and periodic evaluation.

Typical Treatment Goals and Measurements (Outcomes and Markers)

Breast cancer: Treatment of existing cancer seeks to attain a complete remission. The minimum goal is to shrink (regress) the size of the tumor and decrease the probability of spread. Talk to your doctor about the goals of treatment when this medicine is prescribed.

▷ **This Drug Should Not Be Taken If**
- you had a serious allergic or adverse reaction to it before.
- you are pregnant.

▷ **Inform Your Physician Before Taking This Drug If**
- you have a history of pulmonary embolism.
- you have a history of stroke or blood clots.
- you have a history of edema.
- you have impaired liver function.
- you have high cholesterol.
- you plan to have surgery in the near future.

Possible Side Effects (natural, expected, and unavoidable drug actions)
Hot flashes—frequent.
Fluid retention (edema), weight gain.

▷ **Possible Adverse Effects** (unusual, unexpected, and infrequent reactions)
If any of the following develop, consult your physician promptly for guidance.
Mild Adverse Effects
Allergic reaction: skin rash.
Sweating—infrequent.

Joint pain (arthralgia) or arthritis—frequent.
Increased cholesterol—infrequent.
Headache, dizziness, drowsiness, fatigue, insomnia—infrequent.
Nausea, vomiting, diarrhea—frequent.
Urinary tract infection, vaginal dryness—infrequent.

Serious Adverse Effects
Osteoporosis—infrequent (talk to your doctor about steps to prevent this).
Development of clots (thromboembolic disease)—increased risk.
Depression—may be frequent.
Liver toxicity—rare.

▷ **Possible Effects on Sexual Function:** Vaginal dryness may lead to discomfort during intercourse. A lubricant may be prudent.

Possible Effects on Laboratory Tests
Liver function tests: increased liver enzyme (AST/GOT).
Cholesterol: may be increased.

CAUTION
1. This medicine is presently used ONLY used after menopause.
2. Case reports of undesirable lipid changes (increased cholesterol) have been made. Periodic checks are prudent.

▷ **Advisability of Use During Pregnancy**
Pregnancy Category: **D.** See Pregnancy Risk Categories at the back of this book.
Animal Studies: No birth defects due to this drug reported.
Human Studies: Adequate studies of pregnant women are not available.
It should not be used during pregnancy.

Advisability of Use If Breast-Feeding
Presence of this drug in breast milk: Unknown.
Avoid drug or refrain from nursing.

Habit-Forming Potential: None.

Effects of Overdose: Severe extension of the pharmacological effects.

Possible Effects of Long-Term Use: Osteoporosis.

Suggested Periodic Examinations While Taking This Drug (at physician's discretion)
Measurement of bone mineral density.
Check of Hamilton Depression scale.

▷ **While Taking This Drug, Observe the Following**
Foods: Food appears to change how much medicine gets into your body, but the maker of this drug has not supplied any specific guidelines.
Herbal Medicines or Minerals: Some patients use echinacea to attempt to boost their immune systems. Unfortunately, use of echinacea is not recommended in people with damaged immune systems. This herb may also actually weaken any immune system if it is used too often or for too long a time. Black cohosh's estrogenic effects may have an undesirable effect—do not combine. Talk to your doctor to find out about further research and BEFORE combining any herbal or neutraceutical product with this medicine.
Beverages: No restrictions. May be taken with milk.
▷ *Alcohol:* No interactions expected.
Tobacco Smoking: No interactions expected. I advise everyone to quit smoking.
Marijuana Smoking: Animal Studies show an increased suppression of the immune system; significance in humans is not known.

▷ *Other Drugs*

The following drugs may *decrease* the effects of anastrozole:
- estrogens.
- oral contraceptives (those that contain estrogens).

Anastrozole *taken concurrently* with
- tamoxifen (Nolvadex) is not recommended by the manufacturer (lowers anastrozole blood levels).

▷ *Driving, Hazardous Activities:* This drug may cause dizziness or drowsiness. Restrict activities as necessary.

Aviation Note: The use of this drug *may be a disqualification* for piloting. Consult a designated Aviation Medical Examiner.

Exposure to Sun: No restrictions.

ANGIOTENSIN CONVERTING ENZYME (ACE) INHIBITOR FAMILY

Benazepril   (ben AY ze pril)   **Captopril**   (KAP toh pril)   **Enalapril** (e NAL a pril)   **Fosinopril**   (Foh SIN oh pril)   **Lisinopril**   (li SIN oh pril)   **Quinapril**   (KWIN a pril)   **Ramipril**   (RAH mi pril)

Other Names: ACEIs

Introduced: 1985, 1979, 1981, 1986, 1988, 1984, 1985, respectively **Class:**   ACE   inhibitor,   antihypertensive   **Prescription:**   USA: Yes **Controlled Drug:**   USA: No; Canada: No   **Available as Generic:**   Yes (captopril, enalapril, lisinopril)

Brand Names: Benazepril: Lotensin, Lotensin HCT [CD], Lotrel [CD], Captopril: Acediur [CD], ✤Alti-Captopril, ✤Apo-Capto, Capoten, Capozide [CD], ✤Novo-Captopril, ✤Nu-Capto, ✤Syn-Captopril, Enalapril: Lexxel [CD], ✤Vaseretic (also in U.S.) [CD], Vasotec, Fosinopril: ✤Lin-Fosinopril, Monopril, Monopril HCT, Lisinopril: Prinivil, Prinzide [CD], Zestoretic [CD], Zestril, Quinapril: Accupril, Accuretic, Ramipril: Altace, ✤Ramace, ✤Altace Plus Felodipine [CD]

Author's Note: Ramipril (Altace) plus felodipine is available as a combination product in Canada only. Perindopril (Aceon), moexipril (Univasc), moexipril/hydrochlorothiazide (Uniretic), trandolapril (Mavik), and trandolapril/verapamil (Tarka) information will be added to this profile in future editions if differential benefits emerge from clinical studies. Data from a study in the British Medical Journal found that combination of ramipril (Altace) plus a water pill (thiazide diuretic) used by patients who had previous transient ischemic attacks (TIAs) or strokes helped prevent a first or a repeat stroke. The interesting finding was that for some patients, the protective benefits happened even though blood pressure was reduced only slightly.

BENEFITS versus RISKS

Possible Benefits	*Possible Risks*
RAMIPRIL HAS DATA SHOWING THAT IT CAN DECREASE THE RISK OF HEART ATTACK AND STROKE (lowered cardiovascular events by 22% in the HOPE trial; lisinopril also approved for use after heart attack)	Impaired white blood cell production—rare (not for ramipril)
	Bone marrow depression—rare (not for ramipril)
	Allergic swelling of face, tongue, throat, vocal cords—possible
EFFECTIVE CONTROL OF MILD TO SEVERE HIGH BLOOD PRESSURE	Kidney damage—rare (enalapril, lisinopril, quinapril, and ramipril lower risk)
USEFUL ADJUNCTIVE TREATMENT FOR CONGESTIVE HEART FAILURE	Liver damage—rare (not for ramipril)
MAY DECREASE RISK OF KIDNEY PROBLEMS IN DIABETICS TAKING INSULIN (CAPTOPRIL)	
MAY REDUCE RISK OF DEATH AND/OR CONGESTIVE HEART FAILURE AFTER HEART ATTACK (several ACES are approved for this)	
MAY BE DRUGS OF FIRST CHOICE FOR PATIENTS WITH HIGH BLOOD PRESSURE WHO EXERCISE	
COMBINATION USE OF PERINDOPRIL WITH INDAPAMIDE REDUCED RISK OF RECURRENT STROKE BY NEARLY HALF IN ONE STUDY	
USE OF RAMIPRIL AND A THIAZIDE DIURETIC LOWERED STROKE RISK BY 32% AND FATAL STROKE RISK BY 61%	
LISINOPRIL HAS BEEN SHOWN TO REDUCE THE FREQUENCY, SEVERITY, AND DURATION OF MIGRAINES	
Quinapril has been shown to stimulate growth of new blood vessels in laboratory animals	

▷ **Principal Uses**

As Single Drug Products: Uses currently included in FDA-approved labeling: (1) Treats all degrees of high blood pressure; (2) helps prevent death after heart attacks (Ramipril, Lisinopril); (3) used in advanced heart failure; (4) used in diabetics who have kidney problems (decreases or controls amount of protein in urine); (5) helps people live longer (improves survival) in cases of congestive heart failure; (6) Ramipril approved to lower risk of heart and blood vessel disease (cardiovascular) in people with coronary artery disease, stroke, diabetes or peripheral vascular disease who have one or more risk factors (for example—high cholesterol or blood pressure); (7) captopril used if undesirable increases in red blood cells happen after a kidney transplant.

Author's Note: Enalapril was studied in the ABCD trial and was found to control blood pressure and also decrease risk of heart attack in people living with diabetes. Follow-up research is pending.

Other (unlabeled) generally accepted uses: (1) Helps relieve symptoms of cystinuria (captopril); (2) may ease rheumatoid arthritis symptoms (captopril or enalapril); (3) can help Raynaud's phenomenon symptoms (captopril); (4) enalapril and lisinopril help prevent migraines (prophylaxis); (5) enalapril and quinapril may be helpful in aortic regurgitation; (6) helps treat increased blood pressure resulting from blood vessel problems in the kidneys (renovascular hypertension) in people who can't have angioplasty or surgery; (7) combination use of indapamide with perindopril (Aceon) reduced risk of repeat stroke by nearly 50% in one study. A study (see Bosch, J. in Sources) undertaken in England found that use of ramipril plus a thiazide diuretic lowered risk for all strokes by 32% and for fatal strokes by 61%. These benefits occurred despite small lowering of blood pressure. Both studies will probably lead to use of ramipril and a thiazide to help prevent first or repeat strokes in patients at risk for stroke. The goal then of therapy will focus on stroke prevention rather than lowering of blood pressure; (8) lisinopril lowered the percentage of people who had retinopathy (retinopathy score) increases in the EUCLID research.

Author's Note: One large study found that patients using captopril had similar low rates of nonfatal and fatal heart (cardiovascular) events to patients taking beta-blockers or diuretics. Another study showed that fosinopril cut the risk of heart attack or stroke by 51% in people who have high blood pressure and diabetes.

As Combination Drug Products [CD]: In combination with hydrochlorothiazide, captopril, enalapril, fosinopril, lisinopril, and benazepril offer the benefits of an ACE inhibitor and a diuretic. Benazepril has also been combined with amlodipine, a calcium channel blocker (Lotrel form).

How These Drugs Work: By blocking an enzyme system (angiotensin converting enzyme or ACE), these drugs relax arterial walls and lower pressure. This decreases the work a heart has to do and improves performance. Benefits after heart attack come from blunting reaction to catecholamines, scavenging free-radicals and increasing prostacyclin or bradykinin. Some members of this class must be converted by the liver to the active drug form. Combined therapy with diuretics helps ease fluid load. Combination with a calcium channel blocker works by blocking calcium channels and acts primarily on peripheral circulation to lower blood pressure. Amlodipine offers the further advantage of getting into the body well (bioavailability) and increased binding when blood flow is compromised (ischemic conditions and low pH). Ramipril plus a thiazide may help prevent strokes by acting in decreasing plaque rupturing, blood vessel blockage, lowered proliferation of smooth muscle in blood vessels, and through encouraging fibrin degradation (fibrinolysis).

▷ **Widely Used Guidelines That Involve This Medicine (representative sample):** Please look at the section at the very beginning of this profile called "Class." Next, turn to Table 22 and you will find guidelines listed by the class involved!

Available Dosage Forms and Strengths
Benazepril:

Capsules — 2.5 mg of amlodipine with 10 mg of benazepril, 5 mg of amlodipine with 10 mg of benazepril and 5 mg of amlodipine with 20 mg of benazepril (Lotrel form)

Tablets — 5 mg, 10 mg, 20 mg, 40 mg (Lotensin)

Captopril:

Tablets — 6.25 mg, 12.5 mg, 25 mg, 50 mg, 100 mg

Tablet, combination (Capozide) — 25 or 50 mg captopril with 15 or 25 mg of hydrochlorothiazide

Enalapril:

Injection — 1.25 mg/mL

Tablets — 2.5 mg, 5 mg, 10 mg, 20 mg

Tablets (Vaseretic) — 10 mg enalapril and 25 mg of hydrochlorothiazide

Fosinopril:

Tablets — 5 mg, 10 mg, 20 mg, 40 mg

Lisinopril:

Tablets — 2.5 mg, 5 mg, 10 mg, 20 mg, 30 mg, 40 mg

Tablet, combination — 20 mg lisinopril with 12.5 or
(Prinzide, Zestoretic)   25 mg of hydrochlorothiazide

Quinapril:

Tablets — 5 mg, 10 mg, 20 mg, 40 mg

Tablet, combination (Accuretic) — 10 or 20 mg of quinapril with 12.5 or 25 mg of hydrochlorothiazide

Ramipril:

Capsules (gelcaps in Canada) — 1.25 mg, 2.5 mg, 5 mg, 10 mg

▷ **Usual Dosage Ranges for Infants and Children**

Captopril: One study used a starting dose of 0.01 to 0.25 mg per kg of body mass every 12 hours in infants; 0.05 to 0.5 mg per kg of body mass three times daily has been used in older children. Maximum dose is 2 mg/kg per dose up to three times a day.

Enalapril: Malignant Hypertension: 0.625–1.25 mg per dose, given every 6 hours. Maximum dose is 5 mg every 6 hours intravenously. In hypertension 0.08 mg per kg of body weight daily.

Quinapril, benazepril, ramipril, fosinopril, and lisinopril: Dosage not established in infants and children.

▷ **Usual Adult Dosage Ranges**

For high blood pressure:

Captopril: 25 mg two or three times daily for 1–2 weeks. If pressure goals are not met—dose may be increased to 50 mg three times daily if needed. If blood pressure still not acceptable, a diuretic (low dose similar to 25 mg of hydrochlorothiazide) or change to a combination form may be needed. Maximum daily dose is 450 mg.

Enalapril (if not also taking a diuretic): 5 mg once daily starting dose. Usual ongoing dose is 10 to 40 mg daily in a single dose or divided into two equal doses. Total daily dose should not exceed 40 mg if kidney function is impaired. If pressure goals are not met by enalapril alone, a diuretic can be added (pill burden is decreased by fixed dose combinations).

Fosinopril (18 to 60 years of age): For hypertension, initially 10 mg once daily. Usual maintenance dose is 20 to 40 mg daily taken in a single dose. Total daily dosage should not exceed 80 mg.

Quinapril, benazepril, lisinopril (12 to 60 years of age): 10 mg once daily for those not taking a diuretic; 5 mg once daily if taking a diuretic. Usual ongoing dose is 20 to 40 mg daily, taken in a single dose. If once-a-day dosing does not give stable blood pressure control over the day, divide the dose equally into morning and evening doses. Some studies have found better blood pressure control despite some data for full 24 hour coverage for some ACE inhibitors.

Ramipril: Initially 2.5 mg once daily for 2 to 4 weeks. Usual ongoing dose is 2.5 to 20 mg daily in a single dose or two divided doses. If taking diuretics, either stop diuretic for 3 days before starting this drug or begin treatment with 1.25 mg of this drug.

For congestive heart failure (CHF):

Captopril: A test dose of 6.25 to 12.5 mg three times a day is used by some clinicians to reduce risk of undesirably low blood pressure. If needed and tolerated, doses of 25 mg three times daily are started.

Enalapril: 2.5 to 10 mg once or twice daily. Usually combined with other medications. Maximum is 40 mg daily.

Fosinopril: Starting doses of 5 mg (especially for dehydrated patients or those who have kidney failure) to 10 mg have been recommended. Some studies have used once-daily dosing. Dosing must be individualized.

Ramipril: Test dose of 1.25 mg, then a dose of 2.5 to 5 mg twice a day.

To decrease cardiovascular risk:

Ramipril: Starting dose 2.5 mg a day, followed by 5 to 10 mg daily.

After a heart attack:

Captopril: A test dose of 6.25 mg is given to see if excessive lowering of the blood pressure occurs. Test usually delayed until 3 days after heart attack. If the test is tolerated, 12.5 mg is given three times a day. This dose is then increased toward a goal blood pressure or an ongoing dose of 50 mg three times a day.

Enalapril: Test dose of 2.5 mg (24 hours after a heart attack), followed by 2.5 mg twice a day, with increase (titration) to 20 mg as quickly as tolerated (in the EDEN study).

Lisinopril (when hemodynamically stable): Often a test dose of 5 mg may be given within 24 hours after symptoms started. If this dose is tolerated, a repeat dose is given 24 hours later and then increased to 10 mg a day. Therapy continues for at least 6 weeks, but may be ongoing.

Ramipril: 10 mg a day started within 24 hours has been used. Protocol driven systems have used 1.25 mg to start, then 2.5 mg given 12 hours later, followed by daily interval increases to 10 mg once a day.

Diabetic kidney problems (nephropathy) and eye problems (retinopathy):

Captopril: Success has been achieved with 50 mg twice daily in two large studies. The manufacturer suggests a starting dose of 25 mg three times a day.

Over 60 Years of Age:

Captopril: Dosing interval is adjusted to any age-related decrease in creatinine clearance or glomerular filtration rate. The initial change (cut point) is from 75 to 35 mL/minute: dose every 12 to 24 hours. Dosing is started once a day and increased as needed and tolerated.

Enalapril: Same as in younger patients, with dosing corrected for age-related decline in kidney function.

Benazepril: Same as 12 to 60 years of age, if kidney function is normal. If kidney function is significantly impaired, reduce dose by 50%. Total daily maximum is 40 mg in those with impaired kidneys.

Fosinopril: Same as 18 to 60 years of age, but these patients may be more sensitive to fosinopril. Smaller and more gradual dose increases are prudent as needed and tolerated.

Lisinopril: Exercise tolerance was improved by 2.5 to 20 mg daily. Any needed dose increases should be made at longer intervals between adjustments.

Quinapril: Same as 12 to 60 years of age, if kidney function is normal. If kidney function is significantly impaired, reduce dose by 50%. The total daily dose should not exceed 40 mg.

Ramipril: Small doses are advisable until tolerance has been determined. Sudden and excessive lowering of blood pressure can predispose to stroke or heart attack in those with impaired brain circulation or coronary artery heart disease.

Note: Actual dose and schedule must be determined for each patient individually.

Conditions Requiring Dosing Adjustments

Liver Function:

Captopril: Must be used with extreme caution and started at a lower dose in liver failure.

Enalapril: In patients with liver compromise, the dose may need to be **increased** because less of the drug is activated.

Fosinopril: Is a prodrug and is changed into fosinoprilat (the active form) by the liver. Use with caution and in lower doses by patients with liver compromise.

Quinapril, benazepril and lisinopril: The liver is minimally involved in removing these drugs.

Ramipril: Close monitoring for adverse effects is prudent.

Kidney Function:

Benazepril: For people with creatinine clearances of less than 30 mL/min, or serum creatinine greater than 3 mg/dL (ask your doctor), the starting dose should be 5 mg once daily.

Captopril: Increased blood level and risk of adverse effects (low blood counts and protein in the urine) if used in kidney failure. **Must** decrease dose according to decreases in creatinine clearance. The lowest effective dose must be used.

Enalapril: Patients with mild to moderate kidney failure can be given 5 mg/day. In severe kidney failure, maximum dose is 2.5 mg/day.

Fosinopril: This drug undergoes liver and bile (dual hepatobiliary) and kidney (renal) elimination. Patients with renal compromise (especially those with renal artery stenosis) should start on a decreased dose, with slow dose increases if needed.

Lisinopril: Patients with moderate kidney failure should be started on 5 mg daily. In severe kidney failure, the patient can take 2.5 mg of lisinopril daily. This drug is contraindicated in kidney blood flow problems (renal artery stenosis). Combination (with hydrochlorothiazide) drugs (fixed dose products) should NOT be used in kidney failure as loop (see Drug Classes) diuretics are more effective.

Quinapril: Patients with mild kidney failure can take 10 mg daily. Those with moderate kidney failure should take 5 mg daily. In severe kidney failure, 2.5 mg per day may be taken. If needed and tolerated, dose increases should only be made every 2 weeks.

Ramipril: For patients with moderate kidney failure or creatinine values of greater than 2.5 mg/dL, 1.25 mg of ramipril can be taken daily.

Diabetes:

Enalapril: Patients with diabetes with decreased creatinine clearance and protein in the urine (proteinuria) should be given decreased doses.

▷ **Dosing Instructions**

Captopril: Best taken on empty stomach, 1 hour before meals.

Enalapril, quinapril, benazepril, ramipril, fosinopril, and lisinopril: May be taken without regard to food. All ACE drugs should be taken at the same time each day, and all ACE tablets at the time of this writing may be crushed if needed to make them easier to take. If extended-release forms are present when you read this profile—talk to your doctor and pharmacist before crushing any dosage form. If you forget a dose: Take the medicine right away, unless it is nearly time for your next dose, then skip or omit the missed dose and take the medicine when it was next scheduled. DO NOT double doses.

Usual Duration of Use: Several weeks of use on a regular schedule may be required to see best benefits in lowering high blood pressure and for other uses. Use in treating high blood pressure is often a partnership for life for taking control of high blood pressure and when used in kidney disease. Reach the goal and stay on target!

Typical Treatment Goals and Measurements (Outcomes and Markers)

Blood Pressure: Current guidelines (JNC VII) define normal blood pressure (BP) as **less than** 120/80. **Pre-hypertension:** ranges from 120/80 to 139/89 and is intended to help your doctor encourage lifestyle changes (or in the case of people with a risk factor for high blood pressure, start treatment) much earlier—so that possible damage to blood vessels, your heart, kidneys, sexual potency, or eyes might be minimized or avoided altogether. The next two classes of high blood pressure are stage 1 hypertension: 140/90 to 159/99 and stage 2 hypertension equal to or greater than: 160/100 mm Hg. These guidelines also recommend that clinicians work with their patients to agree on the goals and a plan of treatment. The first-ever guidelines for blood pressure (hypertension) in African Americans recommends that MOST black patients be started on TWO antihypertensive medicines with the goal of lowering blood pressure to 130/80 for those with high risk for heart and blood vessel disease or with diabetes. The American Diabetes Association recommends 130/80 as the target for people living with diabetes and less than 125/75 for those who spill more than one gram of protein into their urine. Most clinicians try to achieve a BP that confers the best balance of lower cardiovascular risk and avoids the problem of too low a blood pressure. Blood pressure duration is generally increased with beneficial restriction of sodium. The goals and time frame should be discussed with you when the prescription is written. If goals are not met, it is not unusual to intensify doses or add on medicines.

Stroke Prevention: Combination use of ramipril and a thiazide diuretic for patients at high risk for stroke (even those with normal blood pressure) will not use the typical blood pressure goals outlined above. The goal of the combination is to prevent the frequency of TIAs (see Glossary) and non-fatal or fatal stoke.

Possible Advantages of These Drugs

Quinapril, benazepril, ramipril, fosinopril, and lisinopril control blood pressure effectively with one daily dose with relatively low incidence of adverse effects (ramipril at present has the most favorable data). No adverse influence on asthma, cholesterol blood levels, or diabetes. Sudden withdrawal does not result in a rapid increase in blood pressure. Fosinopril can decrease total cholesterol by 10% in patients with both high blood pressure and protein in the urine.

Captopril has a special chemical (sulfhydryl group) at its active site. This may help it ease intolerance to nitrates. Lisinopril and captopril DO NOT require activation by the liver to work. They may be drugs of choice in situations where an ACE inhibitor is desirable and liver compromise is also present. Quinapril goes into tissues well and may have a future role in treating or preventing problems (dysfunction) of the lining (endothelium) of blood vessels. Quinapril also has some laboratory data showing it to be able to stimulate growth of new blood vessels in laboratory animals. The Joint National Committee number seven (see JNC VII in Glossary) advocates ACE inhibitors as preferred medicines in diabetics with high blood pressure who have protein in their urine.

Ramipril has important and robust data to show it decreases risk of heart attack and stroke! The HOPE trial showed ramipril to decrease risk of death from any heart (cardiovascular) event by 25%, nonfatal heart attack by 20% and nonfatal stroke by 32%. This is remarkable by itself, yet dramatic when coupled with a 30% lowering of development of diabetes and kidney disease in people living with diabetes.

ACE inhibitors in general are drugs of first choice in African Americans who are at risk for or who have kidney (renal) problems (dysfunction). The African American Study of Kidney Disease and Hypertension research showed that African Americans with nephrosclerosis and hypertension who took ramipril (Altace) were found to have a 41% lower risk of end-stage kidney disease and death than those taking amlodipine (a calcium channel blocker). An analysis (meta analysis) of existing studies (see Shekelle in Sources and the AIRE, CONSENSUS, SAVE, SMILE, SOLVD, and TRACE studies) found that ACE inhibitors benefit most patients with heart failure.

▷ **These Drugs Should Not Be Taken If**
- you have had an allergic reaction to them.
- you develop swelling of the tongue, face, or throat while taking this drug or with a previous ACE inhibitor (angioedema). Call your doctor immediately if this effect starts while taking this medicine.
- you are pregnant (last 6 months especially).
- you currently have a blood cell or bone marrow disorder.
- you have an abnormally high level of blood potassium (talk to your doctor).

▷ **Inform Your Physician Before Taking These Drugs If**
- you develop swelling of the tongue, face, or throat while taking this drug. Call your doctor immediately.
- you are planning pregnancy or to breast-feed your child.
- you have kidney disease or impaired kidney function.
- you have had an allergic reaction while undergoing desensitization for bee stings (ask your doctor).
- you have scleroderma or systemic lupus erythematosus.
- you have any form of heart or liver disease.
- you have diabetes.
- you have an elevated potassium level.
- you have a blood cell disorder.

- you take other antihypertensives, diuretics, nitrates, allopurinol (Zyloprim), Indocin, or potassium supplements.
- you will have surgery with general anesthesia.
- you have renal artery or aortic stenosis (ask your doctor).
- you are taking medicines that suppress the immune system.
- you are unsure how much to take or how often to take it.

Possible Side Effects (natural, expected, and unavoidable drug actions)

Dizziness, light-headedness, fainting (excessive drop in blood pressure). Increased heart rate on standing (captopril).

Scalded mouth sensation for some class members.

Impaired sense of smell—case reports for enalapril.

Nausea or constipation, increased blood potassium—all rare.

Cough—rare to infrequent (captopril, enalapril [highest withdrawal rate at 10%], fosinopril 2–10%. Lisinopril 3.5%, quinapril 1–4%, ramipril 3–12% [greatest with delapril and least with quinapril and less than 5% overall] may start in as little as a day or up to 10 months).

▷ **Possible Adverse Effects** (unusual, unexpected and infrequent reactions)

If any of the following develop, consult your physician promptly for guidance.

Mild Adverse Effects

Allergic reactions: skin rash, psoriasis—rare to infrequent.

Swelling of face, hands, or feet; fever—rare.

Ringing in the ears (tinnitus)—lisinopril—rare.

Lost or altered (metallic or salty) taste, mouth or tongue sores—case reports.

Hair loss—captopril—possible.

Headache—infrequent–relatively frequent.

Nightmares, joint pain—rare.

Increased temperature (hyperthermia)—case reports (captopril).

Low blood sugar—case reports (idiosyncratic?—and limited clinical effect)—captopril and enalapril.

Rapid heart rate on standing—case reports.

Serious Adverse Effects

Allergic reactions: swelling (angioedema) of face, tongue, and/or vocal cords—rare; can be life-threatening—case reports.

Bone marrow depression (neutropenia, anemia, aplastic anemia): weakness, fever, sore throat, bleeding or bruising—rare (infrequent in kidney failure and collagen vascular disease) (not reported for ramipril).

Hemolytic or aplastic anemia—case reports (not for ramipril).

Kidney damage: water retention (edema)—case reports to rare (first 8 months usually for captopril).

Elevated blood potassium (hyperkalemia)—case reports.

Rare fluid formation around the heart (pericarditis)—case reports (captopril).

Hallucinations—rare (captopril, quinapril, and enalapril).

Stevens-Johnson syndrome, lupus erythematosus, or other serious skin conditions (some members of this class)—rare.

Pancreatitis—case reports with some members of this class.

Liver damage (with or without jaundice)—rare but may be fulminant (lisinopril) and has been seen in as little as 5 days and up to 3 years after starting treatment (watch for dark urine, clay colored stools, yellow eyes or skin, and abdominal pain or tenderness).

▷ **Possible Effects on Sexual Function:** Decreased male libido—rare (captopril, lisinopril, and perindopril). Impotence. Swelling and tenderness of male breast tissue (gynecomastia)—rare (enalapril and captopril). Vulvovaginal itching-case report for enalapril.

Possible Effects on Laboratory Tests

Complete blood counts: decreased red cells, hemoglobin, white cells, and platelets; increased eosinophils.

Blood antinuclear antibodies (ANA): increased (captopril, lisinopril, quinapril).

Blood cholesterol (decreased—fosinopril) and triglycerides: decreased (benazepril).

Blood sodium level: decreased.

Blood urea nitrogen level (BUN): increased.

Blood uric acid level: may be increased (ramipril).

Insulin sensitivity: increased—captopril.

Blood potassium level: may be increased.

Liver function tests: increased liver enzymes (alkaline phosphatase, AST/GOT, LDH), increased bilirubin—possible.

Urine ketone tests: false positive results with Keto-Diastix and Chemstrip-6 (captopril).

Blood sugar (glucose): decreased—case reports (captopril, enalapril).

Venereal Disease Research Laboratory (VDRL): rare false-positive results (captopril).

Digoxin blood level: may read falsely low with fosinopril.

IgA deficiency: case report captopril.

CAUTION

1. If possible, may be best to stop all other antihypertensive drugs (especially diuretics) for 1 week before starting these medicines.
2. **Tell your doctor immediately if you become pregnant.** These drugs should not be taken after the first 3 months of pregnancy.
3. **Report promptly** any signs of infection (fever, sore throat) and any indications of water retention (weight gain, swollen feet or ankles).
4. Many salt substitutes contain potassium; ask your doctor before using.
5. Laboratory tests are needed (see below) **before taking these medicines.**
6. The FDA has started to evaluate blood levels of ACE inhibitors (trough to peak ratios—T/P—see Glossary) to check how these medicines should be taken. Talk to your doctor about this.
7. One observational epidemiologic study found that ACE inhibitors were often prescribed in lower than recommended doses and were also underused. Check your ACE inhibitor dose, and ask if an ACE inhibitor is appropriate if you are NOT currently taking one.
8. High blood pressure rarely has symptoms. If this medicine is controlling your blood pressure, STAY ON IT—even if you never felt sick from your prior high blood pressure.

Precautions for Use

By Infants and Children: Benazepril, fosinopril, lisinopril, quinapril, and ramipril: Safety and effectiveness not established.

By Those Over 60 Years of Age: Smaller starting doses advisable. Sudden or excessive lowering of blood pressure can cause stroke or heart attack.

▷ **Advisability of Use During Pregnancy**

Pregnancy Category: C during the first 3 months; **D during the last 6 months** (last two trimesters). See Pregnancy Risk Categories at the back of this book.

Animal Studies: Birth defects found in some animals for some ACE inhibitors.

Human Studies: The use of ACE inhibitor drugs during the last 6 months of pregnancy is known to possibly cause very serious injury and possible death to the fetus; skull and limb malformations, lung defects, and kidney failure have been reported in over 50 cases (captopril) worldwide.

Avoid these drugs completely during the last 6 months. During the first 3 months of pregnancy, use this drug only if clearly needed. Ask your doctor for guidance.

Advisability of Use If Breast-Feeding

Presence of this drug in breast milk: Yes, in small amounts (captopril, enalapril, and ramipril); benazepril—in very small amounts; lisinopril, quinapril, fosinopril—unknown.

Monitor nursing infant closely, and discontinue drug or nursing if adverse effects develop. Breast-feeding while taking ramipril is not recommended. Breast-feeding with benazepril and enalapril is probably safe, but fixed dose combinations with hydrochlorothiazide and amlodipine (such as Lotensin HCT or Lotrel) are NOT recommended.

Habit-Forming Potential: None.

Effects of Overdose: Excessive drop in blood pressure—light-headedness, dizziness, fainting.

Possible Effects of Long-Term Use: Gradual increase in blood potassium level, cough.

Suggested Periodic Examinations While Taking These Drugs (at physician's discretion)

Before drug is started: complete blood cell count, urine analysis, creatinine BUN and electrolytes.

Once started: Blood counts during the first 3 months, then periodically. Congestive heart failure patients may need more frequent testing. Urine protein prudent every month for the first 9 months, then periodically. Periodic blood potassium tests. ANA titer for some ACEs. Blood pressure goals should be checked and results evaluated.

▷ **While Taking This Drug, Observe the Following**

Foods: Talk to your doctor about salt intake.

Herbal Medicines or Minerals: Ginseng, bitter orange, country mallow, hawthorn, guarana, saw palmetto, ma huang (contraindicated in hypertension and now removed from the market), goldenseal, and licorice may also cause increased blood pressure. Excessive caffeine from coffee, mate, or guarana may also increase blood pressure. Calcium and garlic may help lower blood pressure. One case report of excessively low zinc in a (polycystic kidney) patient for captopril. Talk with your doctor before combining any herbal medicine with your current prescriptions.

Nutritional Support: **Do not** take potassium supplements unless directed by your doctor. Case reports of zinc deficiency have been made (captopril). Large amounts of garlic, soy, and calcium may lower blood pressure. A small study by Hong at Sungkyukwan University in Seoul found that use of 256 mg of iron daily over a 4-week treatment period found all of the treatment group had cough improved with three patients nearly stopping this adverse effect. Further research is needed. Talk to your doctor to find out if additional research has been done, if this iron benefit only applies to patients with low iron or if a consensus has developed that rational use of iron while avoiding iron side effects makes sense for you.

Beverages: Grapefruit juice may increase amlodipine in the Lotrel form. May be taken with milk or water.

▷ *Alcohol:* Alcohol can further lower blood pressure. Use with caution.

Tobacco Smoking: Smoking can certainly irritate the airways and since these medicines can also lead to cough, smoking is not advisable. I advise everyone to quit smoking.

▷ *Other Drugs*

These medicines *taken concurrently* with

- allopurinol (Zyloprim) may increase risk of serious skin reactions.
- azathioprine (Imuran) may result in severe anemia.
- capsaicin (Zostrix, others) may increase risk of cough.
- clomipramine (Anafranil, others) may result in clomipramine toxicity and confusion, mood changes and irritability. Lower doses may be required if these medicines are combined.
- cyclosporine (Sandimmune) may result in kidney failure that takes a while to appear (delayed acute renal dysfunction).
- dalfopristin (Synercid) may result in increased amlodipine levels with Lotrel form.
- erythropoietin (various) may result in lowered erythropoietin benefits and require a higher dose to reach the same hematocrit.
- fluconazole and any imidazole or triazole antifungal (itraconazole and ketoconazole) may increase amlodipine levels with the Lotrel form.
- iron (various) may result in decreased ACE inhibitor absorption and blunted benefits. Separate dosing by 1 to 2 hours.
- interferons (alpha and beta) may greatly increase risk of blood problems with some members of this class. Monitor blood counts if combination must be used (captopril, lisinopril, quinapril, benazepril—case reports).
- lithium (Lithobid, others) may result in toxic blood lithium levels and **toxicity.**
- loop diuretics (such as Lasix or Bumex; see Drug Classes) may cause excessively low blood pressure on standing (postural hypotension) but may also be therapeutically needed.
- metformin (Glucophage) lead to high potassium levels and lactic acidosis in a diabetic patient with kidney compromise who combined metformin and enalapril.
- nesiritide (Natrecor) may increase risk of excessively low blood pressure (hypotension).
- oral hypoglycemic agents (glyburide—Glynase, others) may result in decreased insulin resistance and the need to decrease the dose of the oral hypoglycemic agent (enalapril only).
- pergolide (Permax, others) has a single case report of hypotension with lisinopril—caution is advised.
- phenothiazines (see Drug Classes) may result in postural hypotension.
- potassium preparations (K-Lyte, Slow-K, etc.) will increase blood potassium with risk of serious heart rhythm disturbances.
- potassium-sparing diuretics—amiloride (Moduretic), spironolactone (Aldactazide), triamterene (Dyazide)—may increase blood levels of potassium with risk of serious heart rhythm disturbances.
- quinupristin (Synercid) may result in increased amlodipine levels with Lotrel form.
- rifampin (Rifadin) or rifabutin (Mycobutin) may cause decreased therapeutic benefit from enalapril.
- saquinavir (Invirase) may result in increased amlodipine levels with Lotrel form.
- thiazide diuretics (hydrochlorothiazide, others) may result (especially

in older people) in increased levels of enalaprilat (the active medicine) and increased reduction in blood pressure. May be used to therapeutic benefit.
- cotrimoxazole (trimethoprim component; Bactrim, Trimpex, others) may increase blood potassium (risk of serious heart rhythm disturbances).

The following drugs may *decrease* the effects of these medicines:
- antacids—by decreasing captopril (and perhaps other ACEs) absorption. Separate doses by 2 hours.
- COX-II inhibitors (celecoxib, rofecoxib and valdecoxib).
- ibuprofen (Motrin), indomethacin (Indocin), or other NSAIDs (see Drug Classes).
- naloxone (Narcan).
- salicylates (aspirin, etc.) or other NSAIDs (see Drug Classes).

▷ *Driving, Hazardous Activities:* Usually no restrictions. Be aware of possible drops in blood pressure with resultant dizziness or faintness.

Aviation Note: The use of these drugs *may be a disqualification* for piloting. Consult a designated Aviation Medical Examiner.

Exposure to Sun: Caution is advised. Some drugs in this class can cause photo-sensitivity (captopril, enalapril, moexipril, ramipril, and trandolapril).

Exposure to Heat: Caution is advised. Excessive perspiring may drop blood pressure.

Occurrence of Unrelated Illness: Call your doctor to report any disorder causing vomiting or diarrhea. Fluid and chemical imbalances must be corrected as soon as possible.

Discontinuation: Captopril, lisinopril, quinapril, fosinopril, and benazepril have been stopped abruptly without causing a sudden increase in blood pressure (though not recommended). Ask your doctor before stopping any drug for any reason.

ANGIOTENSIN II RECEPTOR ANTAGONIST FAMILY

Candesartan   (KAN da sar tan)   **Eprosartan**   (Eh PRO sar tan)
Irbesartan   (Ir BAH sar tan)   **Losartan**   (LOW sar tan)   **Telmisartan**
(TELL mih sar tan)   **Valsartan**   (VAL sar tan)

Other Names: ARBs

Introduced: 1998, 1999, 1997, 1995, 1998, 1997, respectively   **Class:** Angiotensin II antagonists (ARBs)   **Prescription:**   USA: Yes   **Controlled Drug**   USA: No; Canada: No   **Available as Generic:** USA: irbesartan and hydrochlorothiazide Yes, others No; Canada: No

Brand Names: *Candesartan:* Atacand, Atacand HCT [CD]; *Eprosartan:* Teveten; *Irbesartan:* Avapro, Avalide [CD]; *Losartan:* Cozaar, Hyzaar [CD]; *Telmisartan:* Micardis, Micardis HCT [CD]; *Valsartan:* Diovan, Diovan HCT [CD]

Author's Note: Information in this profile will be broadened in subsequent editions to include data on eprosartan and telmisartan if the data warrant inclusion. One early study showed that using eprosartan WITH an ACE inhibitor reduced blood pressure (diastolic—the bottom blood pressure number) in people with chronic heart failure—yet did NOT increase heart rate as an undesirable effect. Emerging information on combination use of ACE inhibitors (ACEIs) and ARBs in people with compromised kidneys appears to have increased benefits. Some data shows that two of the

medicines in this family did not work as well as in African Americans as other high blood pressure medicines. One study (see Mancia in Sources) found that irbesartan (Avapro) lowered blood pressure to a greater degree than valsartan in people with high blood pressure. An additional head to head trial found that maximum doses of candesartan lowered blood pressure to a greater degree than did losartan. A recent approval for losartan gives it FDA approval to prevent stroke.

BENEFITS versus RISKS	
Possible Benefits	*Possible Risks*
EFFECTIVE CONTROL OF HIGH BLOOD PRESSURE	Increased liver function tests (all except irbesartan)
DECREASED NUMBER OF DEATHS FROM CONGESTIVE HEART FAILURE (LOSARTAN)	
USE IN (LOSARTAN) PEOPLE LIVING WITH DIABETES TO HELP THEIR KIDNEYS (NEPHROPATHY)	
DECREASED RISK OF STROKE, HEART ATTACK, AND DEATH IN SERIOUSLY ILL HEART PATIENTS (LOSARTAN)	
LOSARTAN IS FDA APPROVED TO PREVENT STROKE IN PATIENTS WITH HIGH BLOOD PRESSURE AND LEFT-SIDED HEART ENLARGEMENT	
DECREASED RISK OF NEW ONSET DIABETES (BY 25% IN THE LIFE STUDY-LOSARTAN)	
Decreased cough side effect versus ACE inhibitors	
Candesartan increases insulin sensitivity	

▷ **Principal Uses**

As a Single Drug Product: Uses currently included in FDA-approved labeling: (1) Treatment of high blood pressure; (2) decreases abnormal size of the left ventricle (left ventricular hypertrophy) (losartan); (3) candesartan works to increase insulin sensitivity; (4) losartan, irbesartan approved in type 2 diabetics with a specific kidney problem (nephropathy); (5) losartan is approved to prevent stroke in people with high blood pressure and left sided heart enlargement (left ventricular hypertrophy), (6) valsartan approved for use in congestive heart failure (CHF).

Author's Note: The JNC VI (see Glossary) report placed use of these medicines as appropriate in patients who have indications for ACE therapy but do not tolerate those medicines (such as intolerable ACE inhibitor–induced cough). JNC VII on equal ground with ACEs. The International Society for Hypertension recommended this class of medicines as first-line treatment in patients with heart failure. Some

early data show some reversal of fibrosis in animals treated with losartan. Because of trials such as LIFE (see Dahlof in Sources), where there were clear data from a large study showing decreased heart attack, stroke, death, and diabetes risk with use of losartan, I expect that losartan will have much broader use.

Other (unlabeled) generally accepted uses: (1) The ELITE study compared losartan to an ACE inhibitor (in patients over 65 with ejection fraction mean of 30%) and found a significant decrease in deaths for any reason (all-cause death) in treating congestive heart failure; (2) congestive heart failure (CHF); (3) excessive protein excretion in diabetic patients (nephropathy); (4) one study of hypertensive men with sexual dysfunction found improved sexual satisfaction and erections (erectile function) after 12 weeks of losartan treatment; (4) may have a role in helping prevent migraine headaches; (5) losartan may work to ease sexual dysfunction; (6) irbesartan in combination with amiodarone was more effective in easing atrial fibrillation than amiodarone alone in one small study.

As Combination Drug Products [CD]: These medicines have been combined with hydrochlorothiazide in fixed-dose forms. These drugs complement each other, making the combination a more effective blood pressure approach if control is not achieved with initial therapy.

How These Drugs Work: They block the effects of angiotensin II by binding to a specific site (the AT1 receptor). This helps the blood vessels stay open and lowers blood pressure. These drugs and some of their metabolites also block aldosterone, something of benefit in congestive heart failure. When combined with hydrochlorothiazide, these medicines have the added benefit of removing excessive accumulation of body water.

▷ **Widely Used Guidelines That Involve This Medicine (representative sample):** Please look at the section at the very beginning of this profile called "Class." Next, turn to Table 22 and you will find guidelines listed by the class involved!

Available Dosage Forms and Strengths

Candesartan:

> Tablet — 4 mg, 8 mg, 16 mg and 32 mg
> Tablet (*Atacand HCT*) — candesartan 16mg or 32 mg and hydrochlorothiazide (HCTZ) 12.5 mg

Irbesartan:

> Tablet — 75 mg, 150 mg, 300 mg
> Tablet (*Avalide* irbesartan and HCTZ) — irbesartan 150 or 300 mg and HCTZ 12.5 mg

Losartan:

> Tablet — 25 mg, 50 mg, 100 mg
> Tablet (*Hyzaar*) — losartan 50 mg and HCTZ 12.5 mg
> Tablet (*Hyzaar*) — losartan 100 mg and HCTZ 25 mg

Valsartan:

> Tablet — 80 mg and 160 mg
> Tablet (*Diovan HCT*) — valsartan 80 mg and HCTZ 12.5 mg
> — valsartan 160 mg and HCTZ 12.5 mg
> — valsartan 160 mg and HCTZ 25 mg

▷ **Recommended Dosage Ranges** (Actual dose and schedule must be determined for each patient individually.)

Infants and Children: Not recommended for use in this age group.

18 to 60 Years of Age:

High blood pressure (hypertension):

Candesartan: Starting dose of 16 mg A DAY in patients who have normal blood volume (normovolemic). Hypovolemic patients are given lower starting doses. Total dose can be divided into two doses and given twice a day or given in a single dose. Some European countries use lower starting doses in all patients and a maximum of 8 mg. Doses may be increased as needed and tolerated to 32 mg once daily.

Irbesartan: Starting dose of 150 mg daily. This dose may be increased as needed and tolerated to 300 mg daily. A starting dose of 75 mg daily is used in people also taking hydrochlorothiazide.

Losartan: A starting dose of 50 mg daily is used. If the blood pressure response is not sufficient, the same dose may be divided into two equal doses and given twice daily. The dose may also be increased as needed and tolerated and taken in two divided doses daily. The maximum daily dose is 100 mg. In people who are hypovolemic or who are on water pills (diuretics), the starting dose is 25 mg. Peak effects may not be seen for 3 to 6 weeks once dosing changes are made. Maximum daily doses are lower in those taking diuretics and hypovolemics.

Valsartan: Starting dose is 80 mg daily. Dosing may be increased to 160 mg, then a maximum of 320 mg once daily as needed and tolerated. Many clinicians will change to a combination HCTZ form if goals are not met with a 160-mg dose of the single-ingredient product.

Over 60 Years of Age:

Candesartan: No initial dose change needed, but some older patients may be more sensitive than younger ones.

Irbesartan: No age-related changes needed.

Losartan: Patients who are dehydrated or have a decreased intravascular volume should take 25 mg once daily as a starting dose.

Valsartan: No clinically relevant changes.

Author's Note: Combination forms containing hydrochlorothiazide (HCTZ) are used only after target goals for blood pressure are not met with the ARB alone. Dosing is then usually started with the lowest available combination dose and increased as needed and tolerated. Hydrochlorothiazide (HCTZ) side effects may be a mixture of rare dose-independent (such as pancreatitis) and dose-dependent problems (such as excessive lowering of potassium, which is largely avoided using low-HCTZ forms).

Diabetic Nephropathy:

Irbesartan: 300 mg once a day (in type 2 diabetics).

Losartan: 50 mg once a day (in type 2 diabetics). Dose can be increased as needed and tolerated to 100 mg daily.

Congestive Heart Failure:

Valsartan: 40 mg twice a day. Dose can be increased as needed and tolerated to 80–160 mg twice daily.

Conditions Requiring Dosing Adjustments

Liver Function:

Candesartan: No changes in mild liver compromise. Some European clinicians start at 2 mg daily.

Irbesartan: No changes needed.

Losartan: This drug is extensively changed (metabolized) in the liver to an active metabolite. The starting dose should be 25 mg. Dosing is then increased as needed and tolerated at weekly intervals. The fixed-dose drug Hyzaar should not be used by patients with liver failure.

Valsartan: Maximum starting dose is 80 mg in mild to moderate liver failure. Drug has not been used in severe liver failure.

Kidney Function:

Candesartan: No change in starting dose in mild kidney compromise.

Irbesartan: No changes needed.

Losartan: No dosing changes appear to be needed. The fixed-dose combination Hyzaar should not be used by patients with creatinine clearances (see Glossary) less than 30 mL/min.

Valsartan: Some clinical trials started dosing at 40 mg daily with increase to 80 mg after 28 days as needed and tolerated.

▷ **Dosing Instructions:** Food slows the absorption of losartan and valsartan but does not decrease the total absorption. Irbesartan and candesartan can be taken with or without food. If you forget a dose: take it right away unless it's nearly time for your next regular dose. If it is nearly dosing time, just take the scheduled dose. DO NOT double doses.

Usual Duration of Use: Regular use for 3 to 4 weeks is usually needed to determine peak effectiveness in controlling high blood pressure. Long-term use (months to years) requires periodic evaluation of response and dose adjustment. See your doctor on a regular basis and stay on target with pressure goals!

Typical Treatment Goals and Measurements (Outcomes and Markers)

Blood Pressure: The (JNC VII) guidelines define normal blood pressure (BP) as **less than** 120/80. **Pre-hypertension:** ranges from 120/80 to 139/89 and is intended to help your doctor encourage lifestyle changes (or in the case of people with a risk factor for high blood pressure, start treatment) much earlier—so that possible damage to blood vessels, your heart, kidneys, sexual potency, or eyes might be minimized or avoided altogether. The next two classes of high blood pressure are stage 1 hypertension: 140/90 to 159/99 and stage 2 hypertension equal to or greater than: 160/100 mm Hg. Guidelines recommend that clinicians work with their patients to agree on the goals and a plan of treatment. The first-ever guidelines for blood pressure (hypertension) in African Americans recommends that MOST black patients be started on TWO antihypertensive medicines: goal of lowering blood pressure to 130/80 for those with high risk for heart and blood vessel disease or with diabetes. For diabetics: 130/80 as the general target and less than 125/75 for those who spill more than one gram of protein into their urine. Most clinicians try to reach a BP that gives the best balance of lower heart and blood vessel risk and avoids the problem of too low a blood pressure. The goals and time frame should be discussed with you when the prescription is written. If goals are not met, it is not unusual to intensify doses or add on medicines.

Possible Advantages of These Drugs

A different mechanism of action in treating high blood pressure than diuretics or beta blockers. Lower rate of cough side effect than ACE inhibitors. Candesartan has NOT been associated with dry cough in any clinical trial. Once-daily dosing can improve patient compliance. Irbesartan: dosing changes NOT needed in those over 60 or in people with kidney or liver disease. Candesartan: The cytochrome P-450 system is NOT involved in removal of the medicine. Candesartan appears to avoid dry cough side effect and also works to increase sensitivity to insulin, making it a preferred agent for patients with high blood pressure who also have insulin resistance. Irbesartan appears to avoid potential of liver damage. Losartan has critically important data showing decreased risk of heart attack, stroke, diabetes and death in seriously ill heart patients. The LIFE study compared patients with left ventricular hypertrophy taking losartan versus atenolol (a beta blocker) with positive results. One small head to head trial of mild to moderate hypertension found that irbesartan/HCTZ (Avalide) was better at lowering blood pressure than losartan/HCTZ (Hyzaar). Irbesartan has shown a most favorable duration of action of angiotensin II inhibition versus losartan or valsartan. Once a day dosing helps people take their medicines well (adherence)! If migraine prevention data holds up, this could be a great use for these medicines as they are better tolerated than some other drugs currently used to prevent migraines.

▷ **These Drugs Should Not Be Taken If**
- you had an allergic reaction to them previously (note: HCTZ combinations should also be avoided by people with sulfonamide allergies).
- you have stenosis of the kidney arteries on both sides (bilateral) renal artery stenosis (candesartan).
- you have primary hyperaldosteronism (candesartan).
- you are pregnant.

▷ **Inform Your Physician Before Taking These Drugs If**
- you have a history of liver or kidney disease.
- you have a history of circulation problems in the brain.
- you are breast-feeding your infant.
- you have a history of lupus erythematosus (losartan).
- you have a history of aspirin or penicillin allergy (losartan).
- you have a history of disease in the blood vessels that supply the heart (coronary artery disease) or aortic or mitral valve stenosis or stenosis of one kidney artery.
- you have abnormal heart rhythms (cardiac).
- you develop swelling of the face, glottis, or tongue (angioedema). Call your doctor immediately.
- you are taking a diuretic (doses will need to be lowered).
- you are going to have general anesthesia (these medicines require more careful use of induction agents to avoid excessive lowering of the blood pressure.

Possible Side Effects (natural, expected, and unavoidable drug actions) Taste disorders.
Candesartan may cause flushing and/or excessive sweating in some patients.
Headache is possible with any of these medicines—though less than placebo for some.
First-dose excessive lowering of blood pressure is probably possible with all of these medicines (reported first for losartan).

▷ **Possible Adverse Effects** (unusual, unexpected, and infrequent reactions)
If any of the following develop, consult your physician promptly for guidance.
Mild Adverse Effects
Allergic reaction: skin rash.
Dizziness, headache, or sleep disturbances—infrequent.

Taste disorders—case reports for losartan.

Fatigue or muscle cramps—infrequent.

Nose bleed—case reports for candesartan and valsartan (questionable causation).

Cough—possible for some members (up to 3.4% losartan, 2.8% irbesartan, 0.8% valsartan and not reported with candesartan in clinical trials).

Diarrhea—infrequent.

Serious Adverse Effects

Allergic reactions: not defined.

Swelling of the face and lips (angioedema)—case reports for losartan, valsartan, and irbesartan probably possible for all.

Migraine headaches—rare.

Gout—rare and of questionable cause (losartan).

Liver toxicity—case reports (irbesartan, losartan, valsartan).

Kidney toxicity—possible (see Caution).

Pancreatitis—case reports for losartan.

Dose-related increase in blood potassium (hyperkalemia).

Anemia—case reports, minimal clinical significance (candesartan, losartan, valsartan).

Neutropenia—rare (valsartan).

Movement problem (ataxia)—rare (valsartan).

▷ **Possible Effects on Sexual Function:** Decreased libido, impotence—both rare (losartan and valsartan).

Possible Delayed Adverse Effects: None reported.

▷ **Adverse Effects That May Mimic Natural Diseases or Disorders**

Increases in liver function tests may mimic infectious hepatitis (candesartan, irbesartan, losartan, and valsartan).

Natural Diseases or Disorders That May Be Activated by These Drugs: None reported.

Possible Effects on Laboratory Tests

Losartan, irbesartan, candesartan, and valsartan: Liver function tests: increased.

Potassium level: may be increased.

Increased kidney function tests: creatinine possible with candesartan, irbesartan, losartan, and valsartan.

CAUTION

1. Goals are set in the current approach to antihypertensive therapy. If the blood pressure lowering goals are not met in a reasonable amount of time, dosing changes and/or new medicines must be started.

2. Patients with low renin levels (often the case in African American patients) may get a lessened benefit from these medicines.

3. These drugs should not be taken during pregnancy. Losartan manufacturer says to stop it once pregnancy is identified.

4. Case reports of kidney problems emphasized the need for periodic checking of kidney function and withdrawal of therapy if kidney problems (dysfunction) begin.

5. Losartan undergoes a significant change (first pass effect) in the liver. Because of this activation to the active medicine, inhibitors of the liver enzyme system (CYP 3A4) such as grapefruit juice may block conversion to active drug and blunt the effectiveness of the medicine.

Precautions for Use

By Infants and Children: Safety and effectiveness for use by those under 18 years of age have not been established.

By Those Over 60 Years of Age: People in this age group may be more sensitive to the effects of medicines that lower blood pressure. Lower starting doses are indicated for patients who are dehydrated.

▷ **Advisability of Use During Pregnancy**

Pregnancy Category: C in the first 3 months, **D in the fourth month through birth.** See Pregnancy Risk Categories at the back of this book.

Animal Studies: Rat studies have produced kidney toxicity and death in fetuses.

Human Studies: Information from adequate studies of pregnant women is not available.

If pregnancy is detected, these medicines should be stopped as soon as possible.

Advisability of Use If Breast-Feeding

Presence of this drug in breast milk: Unknown, but expected (losartan and valsartan), yes in rats (candesartan and irbesartan).

Avoid drug or refrain from nursing.

Habit-Forming Potential: None.

Effects of Overdose: Severe decreases in blood pressure and dizziness. Possible increased or decreased heart rate.

Possible Effects of Long-Term Use: Not defined.

Suggested Periodic Examinations While Taking This Drug (at physician's discretion)

Periodic checks of blood pressure (high blood pressure is treated to a target lowering of blood pressure and should be kept there).

Liver function tests (irbesartan, losartan, and valsartan). May be prudent for all these medicines as they are structurally similar.

Kidney function tests when starting and at two and four weeks into treatment. Some clinicians also check kidney function after any dose increases as well. Case reporting advocated immediate withdrawal of ARB treatment if kidney (renal) impairment starts while taking an ARB.

▷ **While Taking This Drug, Observe the Following**

Foods: Follow the diet that your doctor has prescribed. Grapefruit may blunt the benefits of losartan, and further research is required to define the clinical significance of this.

Herbal Medicines or Minerals: Ginseng, bitter orange, country mallow, eleuthro root, guarana, hawthorn, saw palmetto, ma huang (now off the market), goldenseal, yohimbe, and licorice may also increase blood pressure. Calcium and garlic may help lower blood pressure and could be part of complementary care. Use of calcium to excess (7.5 to 10 grams) with combination thiazide diuretics can lead to excessive calcium levels. Talk to your doctor about how much calcium to take. Indian snakeroot has a German Commission E monograph indication for hypertension—talk to your doctor. St. John's wort can cause sun sensitivity. Since some of these medicines can cause sun sensitivity also—caution is advised. Because some members of this family (losartan, irbesartan, and valsartan) and kava kava have had recent case reports of adverse effects on the liver, the combination should be voided.

Nutritional Support: Specific measures are not indicated.

Beverages: Avoid excessive caffeine intake. Grapefruit juice may blunt losartan benefits.

▷ *Alcohol:* Alcohol may intensify the blood pressure lowering effects of this medicine. Ask your doctor for guidance.

Tobacco Smoking: No interactions expected. I advise everyone to quit smoking.

Marijuana Smoking: May increase the blood pressure lowering effects of this drug.

▷ *Other Drugs*

These medicines **taken concurrently** with

- ACE inhibitors (see Drug Classes) when combined with CD HCTZ forms may lead to severe first-dose lowering of blood pressure (hypotension). Low-dose ACE and caution are critical—yet the combination is also therapeutically useful.
- corticosteroids (methylprednisolone, others—see Drug Classes) may lead to excessive loss of potassium when used with the HCTZ combination forms of these medicines. Caution is advised.
- fluconazole (Diflucan) may blunt clinical benefits of losartan by blocking conversion to an active chemical. If these medicines are combined—watch for changes in therapeutic benefits.
- hydrochlorothiazide (various) may increase clinical benefits (redundant with CD forms unless extra fluid loss desired and HCTZ dose less than maximum).
- lithium (Lithobid, others) (case reports for some HCTZ combinations) resulted in lithium toxicity. Caution is advised.
- moxonidine (Cynt, available in Germany) may result in additive lowering of blood pressure.
- rifampin (various) may lower losartan blood levels. Blood pressure should be checked and dosing adjusted as needed.
- ritonavir (Norvir) may change losartan blood levels.

Losartan and valsartan **taken concurrently** with

- amiloride, spironolactone, and triamterene (potassium-sparing diuretics) may lead to undesirable increases in potassium.

Candesartan **taken concurrently** with

- insulin and perhaps other oral hypoglycemic agents may increase response to insulin or oral agents because of increased insulin sensitivity. This may be used to clinical advantage.

Losartan **taken concurrently** with

- inhibitors of cytochrome P450 3A4 may blunt therapeutic benefits of this medicine by blocking an activation step to the active medicines. Examples to be avoided are use with grapefruit juice, erythromycin, and antifungal agents such as ketoconazole.

▷ *Driving, Hazardous Activities:* These drugs may cause confusion or dizziness. Restrict activities as necessary.

Aviation Note: The use of these drugs **may be a disqualification** for piloting. Consult a designated Aviation Medical Examiner.

Exposure to Sun: Caution is advised. Isolated cases of photosensitivity have been reported.

Exposure to Heat: Caution: Excessive sweating (perspiration) may lead to dehydration and an excessive blood pressure lowering effect of these drugs.

Discontinuation: Talk with your doctor before stopping these medicines for any reason.

ANTI-ALZHEIMER'S DRUG FAMILY

Donepezil   (DON ep a zill)   **Rivastigmine**   (REEVA stig meen)
Tacrine   (TA kreen)   **Galantamine**   (GAH lan tah meen)

Introduced: 1993, 2000, 1996, 2001   **Class:**   Acetylcholinesterase inhibitor, anti-Alzheimer's drug, nicotinic acid receptor blocker (galantamine only)   **Prescription:**   USA: Yes   **Controlled Drug:**   USA: No; Canada: No   **Available as Generic:**   USA: Pending for donepezil at the time of this writing, No for others

Brand Names: *Donepezil:* Aricept; *Rivastigmine:* Exelon; *Tacrine:* Cognex; *Galantamine:* Reminyl

Author's Note: Information on rivastigmine will not be broadened in this edition. CAUTION: In Canada felodipine, a calcium channel blocker, carries the brand name Renedil. Because this is so similar sounding a name, errors may occur during a telephone prescription. Memantine (Namenda) will appear in a separate profile because of its different way of working and indication for moderate to severe Alzheimer's.

BENEFITS versus RISKS

Possible Benefits	*Possible Risks*
IMPROVEMENT OF MEMORY IN MILD TO MODERATE ALZHEIMER'S DISEASE	LIVER TOXICITY (TACRINE-dose related)
IMPROVEMENT OF SYMPTOMS IN MILD TO MODERATE ALZHEIMER'S DISEASE	Nausea (A CAUTION FOR RIVASTIGMINE)
MILD TO MODERATE ALZHEIMER'S PATIENTS CONTINUED TO BENEFIT FROM SUSTAINED TREATMENT FOR MORE THAN ONE YEAR (DONEPEZIL)	Dizziness
WORKS ON ACETYLCHOLINESTERASE AND ALLOSTERIC NICOTINIC RECEPTORS (GALANTAMINE ONLY)	
ONCE-DAILY DOSING (DONEPEZIL) MAKES IT EASIER FOR CAREGIVERS AND PATIENTS TO KEEP TAKING THE MEDICINE	
GALANTAMINE WAS RECENTLY FOUND TO BE USEFUL IN PEOPLE WHO HAVE CEREBROVASCULAR DISEASE	
Galantamine is available as an oral solution	
Donepezil was shown to work to fight sleepiness from morphine in a small study of cancer patients	

▷ **Principal Uses**

As a Single Drug Product: Uses currently included in FDA-approved labeling: Treats mild to moderate Alzheimer's disease symptoms (all these medicines).

Other (unlabeled) generally accepted uses: (1) Donepezil may have a role in people who have memory problems after brain injuries; (2) galantamine works in people with cerebrovascular disease; (3) donepezil had moderate benefits in fighting sleepiness (sedation) in a small study of cancer patients who were taking morphine.

How These Drugs Work: Alzheimer's disease is thought to be caused by a loss of nerve cells that make a nerve transmitter (acetylcholine). Donepezil and tacrine act to increase levels of a neurotransmitter (acetylcholine) in the brain. Galantamine also works to increase levels of acetylcholine and has been found to have activity at nicotinic acid receptors as well.

▷ **Widely Used Guidelines That Involve This Medicine (representative sample):** Please look at the section at the very beginning of this profile called "Class." Next, turn to Table 22 and you will find guidelines listed by the class involved!

Available Dosage Forms and Strengths

Donepezil:
>   Tablets — 5 mg, 10 mg

Galantamine:
>   Oral solution — 4 mg per mL
>   Tablets — 4 mg, 8 mg and 12 mg

Tacrine:
>   Capsules — 10 mg, 20 mg, 30 mg, 40 mg

▷ **Recommended Dosage Ranges** (Actual dosage and schedule must be determined for each patient individually.)

Infants and Children: No data are available on use of these drugs in infants and children.

18 to 60 Years of Age:

Donepezil: Start with 5 mg once daily at bedtime, and keep at this dose for 6 weeks. As needed and tolerated increase to 10 mg. The 10-mg dose has had increased GI side effects.

Tacrine: Start at 10 mg four times a day (between meals). This can be increased at 4-week intervals if needed and tolerated. Maximum daily dose is 160 mg.

Galantamine: Dosing is usually started at 4 mg twice a day. If this dose is well tolerated, the dose should be increased to 8 mg twice a day. An additional increase to 12 mg twice a day should be attempted only after an additional 4 weeks at the 8 mg dose has been found to be tolerated. One placebo compared trial found that an ongoing (maintenance) dose of 24–32 mg had generally better results on thinking than lower doses.

Over 60 Years of Age: Same as 18 to 60 years of age.

Conditions Requiring Dosing Adjustments

Liver Function:

Donepezil: Lower doses and blood levels prudent in liver disease.

Tacrine: Not used at all with previous liver toxicity (bilirubin more than 3 mg per dL) and used with caution in liver compromise.

Galantamine: Not used at all in severe liver disease (Child-Pugh 10–15) and used with caution, with more time between dose increases and a maximum 16 mg dose in moderate in liver compromise (Child-Pugh score of 7–9).

Kidney Function: Dose decreases in kidney compromise not now indicated for donepezil or tacrine. Galantamine should NOT be used in people with creatinine clearance (see Glossary) less than or equal to 9 mL/min. In mild kidney compromise (renal function decline), dose increases should be made slowly and with great care.

▷ **Dosing Instructions:** The donepezil tablet may be crushed and is not affected by food. The tacrine capsule may be opened and best taken 1 hour before meals. Food decreases tacrine body levels by 30 to 40%. Liver function tests should be checked while this medicine is being taken. Galantamine is best taken with milk or food (morning and evening meals often works well). The oral liquid form of galantamine should be measured in a dose cup or measuring spoon. If you forget a dose: take it right away unless it's nearly time for your next regular dose. If it IS nearly time, just take the scheduled dose. DO NOT double doses.

Usual Duration of Use: Regular use for 3 to 4 weeks may be needed to see improvement from these medicines. Dose increases are made at 4- to 6-week intervals. Long-term use (months to years) requires periodic evaluation of response and dose. If benefits do not occur within 6 weeks, patients or family members should talk with the prescriber about stopping these drugs. Research shows that donepezil benefits continue for more than a year with regular use.

Typical Treatment Goals and Measurements (Outcomes and Markers)

Thinking and cognition: Improvement in the Mini-Mental State Examination (sMMSE), Alzheimer's Disease Assessment Scale (ADAS-cog) and/or global function using the Clinician Interview Based Assessment of Change. Assessments should be made periodically as benefits from these medicines will decay over time.

Possible Advantages of These Drugs

Improvement of memory and other symptoms of mild to moderate Alzheimer's with fewer side effects than other agents. Donepezil has a more favorable side effect profile than tacrine, offers once-a-day dosing and also avoids liver damage. Donepezil benefits continue for more than 140 weeks with regular use. Galantamine has Alzheimer's improvement data for 52 weeks (newer medicine) and is available in an oral solution form. Recent data showed galantamine helps in cerebrovascular disease. Galantamine also has data that shows effectiveness in people who were previously given different acetylcholinesterase inhibitors.

Currently a "Drug of Choice"

Donepezil is preferred for treatment of symptoms in mild to moderate Alzheimer's disease. Galantamine is preferred in people with cerebrovascular disease, but may become the preferred agent as additional studies are completed.

▷ **These Drugs Should Not Be Taken If**

Donepezil:
- you have had an allergic reaction to it previously.

Tacrine:
- you have had an allergic reaction to it previously.
- you have bronchial asthma.
- you had tacrine liver toxicity and bilirubin levels greater than 3 mg/dL.
- you have an overly active thyroid (hyperthyroidism).
- you have peptic ulcer disease.
- you have an intestinal or urinary tract obstruction.

Galantamine:
- you have had an allergic reaction to it previously.
- your liver or kidneys are severely impaired.

▷ **Inform Your Physician Before Taking These Drugs If**
- you have a history of seizure disorder.
- you have had liver disease.
- you have a history of peptic ulcer disease.
- you have a slow heartbeat (bradycardia), abnormal electrical conduction in your heart (AV conduction defect), or excessively low blood pressure.
- you take an NSAID (see Drug Classes).
- you take muscle relaxants.
- you have glaucoma (angle closure).
- you have asthma.
- you are pregnant.
- you are anemic or have low blood platelets.
- you will be having surgery (donepezil may enhance some muscle relaxants).

Possible Side Effects (natural, expected, and unavoidable drug actions)

Symptoms of cholinergic excess (abdominal upset, agitation). Weight loss—up to 11% in one galantamine study. Indigestion (dyspepsia) is the most common adverse effect of galantamine.

▷ **Possible Adverse Effects** (unusual, unexpected, and infrequent reactions)

If any of the following develop, consult your physician promptly for guidance.

Mild Adverse Effects

Allergic reactions: skin rash, itching.

Increased sweating—rare.

Increased salivation—may be frequent with galantamine.

Increased urination—infrequent.

Muscle aches—infrequent.

Pisa syndrome (abnormal body posturing)—case reports (donepezil).

Abnormal dreams—possible (donepezil).

Insomnia—frequent (galantamine).

Increased risk of passing out or syncope (galantamine—dose related)—possible.

Lowered blood pressure—possible.

Nausea/vomiting, diarrhea, decreased appetite—infrequent to frequent (dose dependent with donepezil).

Dizziness, confusion, insomnia—infrequent to frequent (frequent with galantamine).

Serious Adverse Effects

Allergic reactions: anaphylactoid reactions.

Dose-related increase in liver function tests (starts 6 to 8 weeks after therapy begins)—frequent (tacrine only).

Hallucinations—case report (tacrine).

Inner ear problems—rare (tacrine).

Purpura—infrequent (tacrine).

Aggravation of asthma in asthmatics, bronchospasm or pulmonary edema—possible (increased acetylcholine because of the way that these medicines work).

Severe decrease in white blood cells—one tacrine case report.

Anemia or low blood platelets—infrequent (donepezil).

Slow heart rate (bradycardia) or abnormal rhythm—possible to rare. Seizures—case reports (tacrine).

▷ **Possible Effects on Sexual Function:** Very rare effect of causing lactation (tacrine). Donepezil has had case reports of INCREASED libido.

Possible Delayed Adverse Effects: Liver toxicity (tacrine only), rash, low white blood cell count (tacrine only).

Adverse Effects That May Mimic Natural Diseases or Disorders
Liver toxicity of tacrine may mimic acute hepatitis.

Natural Diseases or Disorders That May Be Activated by These Drugs
Tacrine, galantamine, and donepezil may worsen bronchial asthma, precipitate seizures (may be dose-related), and could exacerbate peptic ulcer disease because of their mechanism of action.

Possible Effects on Laboratory Tests
Tacrine:
Liver function tests: increased SGOT, SGPT, and CPK.
Complete blood count: decreased white blood cells.
Donepezil: decreased hematocrit or platelets.

CAUTION
1. These drugs should **NOT** be stopped abruptly. Sudden decline in thinking may happen (acute deterioration of cognitive abilities).
2. Changes in color of stools (light or very black—tacrine) should be promptly reported to your doctor.
3. These drugs do **NOT** alter the course of Alzheimer's disease. Over time, benefits may be lost.
4. The dose of tacrine **must** be lowered by 40 mg per day if liver function tests (transaminases) rise three to five times the upper normal value.
5. Females achieve 50% higher tacrine blood levels than men. Dose-related side effects may occur sooner (with lower doses) in women than in men. Beneficial doses may be lower for women than men.
6. Donepezil shows benefits for more than 140 weeks with regular ongoing use. Interruption of therapy is NOT appropriate for that time span.
7. Galantamine is removed by two widely used liver enzymes (cytochrome P-450 2D6 and 3A4). Medicines that inhibit these enzymes will increase blood levels of galantamine, which may lead to toxic effects—requiring galantamine dosing decreases while or if the medicines are combined. Because galantamine is derived from daffodils—talk to your doctor if you are allergic to daffodils.

Precautions for Use
By Infants and Children: Safety and effectiveness for those under 18 years of age not established.
By Those Over 60 Years of Age: No specific changes are presently indicated.

▷ **Advisability of Use During Pregnancy**
Pregnancy Category: B for galantamine, C for donepezil and tacrine. See Pregnancy Risk Categories at the back of this book.
Animal Studies: Data not available.
Human Studies: Adequate studies of pregnant women are not available. Consult your doctor.

Advisability of Use If Breast-Feeding
Presence of these drugs in breast milk: Unknown.
Monitor nursing infant closely, and discontinue drug or nursing if adverse effects develop.

Habit-Forming Potential: None.

Effects of Overdose: May precipitate a cholinergic crisis—severe nausea and vomiting, slow heartbeat, low blood pressure, extreme muscle weakness, collapse, and convulsions.

Suggested Periodic Examinations While Taking These Drugs (at physician's discretion)

Assessment of mental status: periodically—check benefits or loss of benefits as Alzheimer's progresses.

For tacrine, liver function tests should be checked every other week for the first 16 weeks of treatment, then every 3 months ongoing if the same dose is used. If medicine is stopped for more than 4 weeks, the liver tests should be repeated again on the same schedule.

Tacrine and donepezil patients need complete blood counts periodically or if symptoms of low blood count occur.

Homocysteine levels.

▷ **While Taking These Drugs, Observe the Following**

Foods: Tacrine is best NOT taken with food. Donepezil is not affected by food. Galantamine is best taken WITH FOOD. Homocysteine appears to have a role in dementia. Current data shows that people with high homocysteine levels are twice as likely to develop Alzheimer's or some form of dementia. A check of homocysteine levels and certainly augmented B vitamins is prudent and good complimentary care. The NIH is planning a large study to look at the effect of using folic acid, vitamin B_{12}, and vitamin B_6 to decrease homocysteine and the rate of thinking (cognitive) decline in Alzheimer's patients.

Herbal Medicines or Minerals: Data from appropriate scientific studies about combination of these medicines with ginkgo biloba is not available and cannot be recommended. A well-designed study of ginkgo biloba DID show it to be effective in mild to moderate Alzheimer's. Because galantamine is derived from daffodils, talk to your doctor if you have a daffodil allergy before taking this medicine. Herbal products with possible effects on the liver (such as kava kava, skull cap, and others) are not advisable.

Beverages: No restrictions.

▷ *Alcohol:* Occasional small amounts of alcohol are okay. Frequent use may worsen memory problems and affect the liver.

Tobacco Smoking: No interactions expected. I advise everyone to quit smoking.

Marijuana Smoking: Additive dizziness may occur.

▷ *Other Drugs*

These medicines may ***increase*** the effects of
- bethanechol (Duvoid, others).
- theophylline (Theo-Dur, others) by doubling the drug level (reported for tacrine).
- succinylcholine (Anectine, others).

These medicines may ***decrease*** the effects of
- anticholinergic medications (see Drug Classes).

The following drug may ***increase*** the effects of tacrine and galantamine:
- cimetidine (Tagamet).

These medicines ***taken concurrently*** with
- carbamazepine (Tegretol), dexamethasone, phenobarbital, fosphenytoin (Cerebyx), phenytoin (Dilantin), or rifampin (Rifater, others) may decrease therapeutic benefits of the anti-Alzheimer drugs.
- dexamethasone (various) may blunt donepezil benefits.

- erythromycin (various) or paroxetine (Paxil) increases blood levels of these medicines. Caution and close patient follow up for signs or symptoms of dose excess is needed.
- ibuprofen (Motrin, others) was associated with delirium in one case report on tacrine.
- ketoconazole, quinidine, and perhaps ritonavir (Norvir) or other protease inhibitors (see Drug Classes) may lead to increased risk of donepezil or tacrine toxicity (decreased removal by two liver enzymes. Caution and close patient follow up is advised.
- medicines removed by cytochrome P-450 enzymes (2D6 and 3A4) or that inhibit those enzymes may lead to toxic levels of all of these medicines. Caution is advised.
- NSAIDs (see Drug Classes) may cause additive stomach upset.
- riluzole (Rilutek) may increase risk of tacrine toxicity (both drugs removed by P450 1A2).

▷ *Driving, Hazardous Activities:* These drugs may cause confusion or dizziness. Restrict activities as necessary.

Aviation Note: The use of these drugs ***may be a disqualification*** for piloting. See a designated Aviation Medical Examiner.

Exposure to Sun: No restrictions.

Exposure to Heat: Increased sweating may occur rarely with tacrine. The combination of increased sweating and hot environments may lead to more rapid dehydration.

Discontinuation: These drugs should NOT be abruptly stopped. Some adverse effects are dose related and may abate if the dose is decreased. Slow withdrawal of the drug is indicated if it is not tolerated. A discontinuation syndrome has been reported for donepezil.

ANTI-LEUKOTRIENE FAMILY

Montelukast: (mon TELL oo cast) **Zafirlukast** (zah FUR lew kast) **Zileuton** (ZEYE loo ton)

Introduced: 1998, 1996, 1997 **Class:** Antiasthmatic, anti-leukotriene, 5-lipoxygenase inhibitor (zileuton) **Prescription:** USA: Yes **Controlled Drug:** USA: No; Canada: No **Available as Generic:** No

Brand Names: *Montelukast:* Singulair; *Zafirlukast:* Accolate; *Zileuton:* Zyflo

---

BENEFITS versus RISKS	
Possible Benefits	*Possible Risks*
EFFECTIVE PREVENTION AND CHRONIC TREATMENT OF BRONCHIAL ASTHMA	Headache
	Nausea
	Liver enzyme increase
TREATS HAY FEVER (montelukast)	
May have a role in treating bronchospasm caused by exercise (montelukast, zafirlukast)	
May have a role in preventing or treating allergies to cats (zafirlukast)	

▷ **Principal Uses**

As a Single Drug Product: Uses currently included in FDA-approved labeling: (1) Prevent recurrence of asthmatic episodes; (2) chronically treat asthmatic episodes; (3) zafirlukast is approved to prevent and for long-term treatment of asthma in patients 5 years old or older; (4) montelukast is approved to prevent and treat ongoing asthma in adults and in pediatric patients who are 2 years old or older as well as for use in preventing asthma induced by exercise; (5) montelukast approved for allergic rhinitis.

Other (unlabeled) generally accepted uses: (1) montelukast and zafirlukast may have a role in preventing spasm of the bronchi caused by exercise; (2) zileuton may have a role in preventing allergic rhinitis or aspirin-sensitive asthma; (3) zafirlukast combined with loratadine yielded superb results in treating hay fever symptoms in a study of 458 patients; (4) zafirlukast may help prevent allergic reactions to cats; (5) montelukast could have a role in preventing migraines; (6) montelukast eases delayed pressure urticaria; (7) leukotrienes in general would be expected to have steroid sparing effects in asthma and may have a role in psoriasis.

How These Drugs Work: Zafirlukast and montelukast work by blocking (leukotriene receptor antagonist) action of chemicals called leukotrienes (slow-reacting substances of anaphylaxis). Zileuton works by blocking creation of (leukotriene pathway inhibitor) leukotrienes themselves. By inhibiting action or formation of leukotrienes, all medicines help keep the airways open.

▷ **Widely Used Guidelines That Involve This Medicine (representative sample):** Please look at the section at the very beginning of this profile called "Class." Next, turn to Table 22 and you will find guidelines listed by the class involved!

Available Dosage Forms and Strengths

Montelukast:
Chewable tablets — 4 mg and 5 mg
Tablet — 10 mg

Zafirlukast:
Tablet — 10 mg and 20 mg

Zileuton:
Tablet — 600 mg

▷ **Recommended Dosage Ranges** (Actual dosage and schedule must be determined for each patient individually.)

Children 12 to 23 months:
Montelukast only: One 4-mg packet of oral granules or one 4 mg chewable tablet in the evening.

Children 2 to 5:
Montelukast only: One 4-mg chewable tablet in the evening.

Children 5 to 11:
Zafirlukast: 10 mg in the morning and evening.

Children 6 to 14:
Montelukast only: One 5-mg chewable tablet in the evening.

People 12 to 60 Years of Age:
Zafirlukast: 20 mg twice daily.
Zileuton: 600 mg four times a day.

People 15 to 60 years of age:
Montelukast: 10 mg once a day, taken in the evening.

Over 60 Years of Age:
   Montelukast: No difference in safety or efficacy, but increased sensitivity to the drug can't yet be ruled out.
   Zafirlukast: Maximum blood level can be twice that of younger patients. Prudent to lower doses, but specific guidelines have not been developed. Package insert notes that using typical dose did not result in adverse effects in clinical trials.
   Zileuton: Same as those for 12 to 60 years old.
   Author's Note: These medicines may be continued during an acute worsening (exacerbation) of asthma, but are not to be used to treat a sudden (acute) asthma attack.

Conditions Requiring Dosing Adjustments
   Liver Function:
   Montelukast has NOT been studied in liver compromise, but is removed by liver (CYP450 3A4, 2C9, and 2A6) therefore lower doses may be prudent.
   Zafirlukast stays in the body up to 60% longer in patients with alcoholic cirrhosis. Lower doses and blood levels appear prudent.
   Zileuton should not be given if active liver disease is present.
   Kidney Function: Dosage changes not needed for the medicines in this class.

▷ **Dosing Instructions:** Montelukast should be taken in the evening. Zafirlukast should be taken on an empty stomach, 1 hour before or 2 hours after a meal. Zileuton may be given with or without food. It's important to note that these medicines are NOT to be used to stop a sudden (acute) asthma attack, but are usually continued during exacerbation (worsening) of asthma if they have already been started. If you forget a dose: take it right away unless it's nearly time for your next regular dose. If it IS nearly time, just take the scheduled dose. DO NOT double doses.

Usual Duration of Use: Both zafirlukast and zileuton start to work in half an hour. Montelukast peaks and also starts to work in 3–4 hours. It lasts for 24 hours. Zafirlukast significantly relaxes bronchi in 30 minutes, and lasts for 12 hours after a typical dose. Zileuton peaks in 2–4 hours, and with multiple doses may last up to 7 days. Ongoing use requires periodic follow-up with your doctor.

Typical Treatment Goals and Measurements (Outcomes and Markers)
   Asthma: The frequency of asthma attacks as well as the severity of asthma attacks that occur (such as those requiring an emergency department visit) are a benchmark of effectiveness. Pulmonary function tests such as FEV1 are valuable measures to assess response. Some clinicians also use the number of times a rescue inhaler must be used as well as daily and night (nocturnal) symptom scores as clinical fine points. Prednisone dose decreases (physician supervised) may also indicate that the medicine is working. Goals should be communicated and checked.

Possible Advantages of These Drugs
   A completely new mechanism of action in preventing asthma and some allergic reactions. Once-daily dosing can improve how well people take these medicines (patient adherence or compliance).

▷ **These Drugs Should Not Be Taken If**
   • you have had an allergic reaction to one of the medicines in this family.
   • you have active liver disease or increased liver enzymes (transaminases) greater than three times the upper normal limit (zileuton).

▷ **Inform Your Physician Before Taking These Drugs If**
- you have a liver disease (montelukast or zafirlukast).
- you are having a sudden (acute) asthma attack.
- you are a child less than 12 years old (zafirlukast).
- you are taking warfarin (zafirlukast).
- you have impaired kidney function (zafirlukast or zileuton).
- you drink large amounts of alcohol (zileuton).
- you develop a rash, tingling of the arms or legs, flu-like symptoms, or sinusitis.
- you are pregnant or are breast-feeding your baby.

Possible Side Effects (natural, expected, and unavoidable drug actions)
Not defined at present.

▷ **Possible Adverse Effects** (unusual, unexpected, and infrequent reactions)
If any of the following develop, consult your physician promptly for guidance.

Mild Adverse Effects
Allergic reactions: skin rash, hives.
Headache—frequent (montelukast, zafirlukast).
Fatigue, weakness—infrequent.
Dizziness—rare for zafirlukast, infrequent for zileuton.
Nausea or abdominal pain—infrequent.
Muscle pain—rare for zafirlukast, infrequent for zileuton.

Serious Adverse Effects
Allergic reactions: possible.
Idiosyncratic reactions: drug-induced lupus erythematosus—case reports.
Liver toxicity (increased enzyme tests)—rare for zafirlukast, less frequent for montelukast, infrequent for zileuton.
Decreases in steroid doses may be followed by onset of Churg-Strauss syndrome (montelukast and zafirlukast, possibly zileuton)—rare.

▷ **Possible Effects on Sexual Function:** None reported.

Natural Diseases or Disorders That May Be Activated by These Drugs: Since all three medicines may increase liver enzymes, hidden (subclinical) liver problems may be activated.

Possible Effects on Laboratory Tests
Liver function tests (SGPT, SGOT, LDH): may be increased.

CAUTION
1. The chewable montelukast tablet has phenylalanine (0.842 mg per 5-mg tablet). People with phenylketonuria (PKU) must be advised.
2. Talk with your doctor about continuing other asthma drugs once you start one of these medicines.
3. Since these medicines can affect the liver, it is critical that you have lab tests of liver function as your doctor orders them.
4. One case report of drug fever for zafirlukast.
6. All these medicines may be rare causes of Churg-Strauss syndrome. Call your doctor if you develop a rash, tingling of the arms or legs, flu-like symptoms, or sinusitis.
7. One study (see Wolfenden, L.L. in Sources) of 4,005 patients found that many patients did not accurately describe their symptoms to their doctors. This lead to patients being under treated. Be honest with your doctor about the severity and frequency of your asthma so that the treatments can be tailored to the severity and frequency of asthma symptoms!

Precautions for Use

By Children: Make certain that these medicines are taken in the amount and for the number of times they are ordered.

By Those Over 65 Years of Age: Zafirlukast goes to higher peak blood levels and remains in the body longer in those over 65, so smaller starting doses are indicated. Montelukast and zileuton are not changed by age.

▷ **Advisability of Use During Pregnancy**

Pregnancy Category: Montelukast and zafirlukast: B; zileuton: C. See Pregnancy Risk Categories at the back of this book.

Animal Studies: Montelukast—no teratogenicity at 320 times the maximum human dose in rats. Zafirlukast—no teratogenicity up to 160 times maximum recommended human dose given to mice. Zileuton—adverse effects were seen in rats given 18 times the typical human dose.

Human Studies: Adequate studies of pregnant women are not available. Ask your doctor for guidance.

Advisability of Use If Breast-Feeding

Presence of this drug in breast milk: Yes (zafirlukast); unknown (montelukast [but yes in rats], zileuton).

Avoid drug or refrain from nursing.

Habit-Forming Potential: None.

Effects of Overdose: No overdose experience in humans for montelukast (900 mg a day was given for a week in one study without any adverse effects) or zafirlukast. Zileuton overdose experience is limited. One patient received 6.6 to 9.0 g of zileuton, which caused vomiting, but recovered without ill effects.

Possible Effects of Long-Term Use: Possible increased liver enzymes.

Suggested Periodic Examinations While Taking This Drug (at physician's discretion)

Periodic liver function tests, lung (pulmonary) function tests.

▷ **While Taking This Drug, Observe the Following**

Foods: Zafirlukast should be taken on an empty stomach; no restrictions for montelukast or zileuton.

Herbal Medicines or Minerals: Using St. John's wort with zafirlukast or montelukast may cause a problem as St. John's wort has known interactions with CYP 3A4 and 2C9—the enzymes that remove zafirlukast and probably montelukast and zileuton. Fir or pine needle oil should NOT be used by asthmatics. Ephedra alone does carry a German Commission E monograph indication for asthma treatment. Talk to your doctor as this has not been studied with leukotriene inhibitors. If you are allergic to plants in the Asteraceae family (aster, chrysanthemum, daisy, or ragweed), you may also be allergic to echinacea, chamomile, feverfew, and St. John's wort.

Beverages: No restrictions.

▷ *Alcohol:* May worsen drowsiness.

Tobacco Smoking: Smoking may lower levels of zileuton and is NOT advisable for anyone, least of all people living with asthma. I advise everyone to quit smoking.

Marijuana Smoking: May cause additive drowsiness.

▷ *Other Drugs*

These medicines *taken concurrently* with

- aspirin (various brands) may cause zafirlukast toxicity.
- astemizole (Hismanal—no longer on the U.S. market) may lead to heart toxicity with zileuton.

- beta-blocker drugs (see Drug Classes) may cause beta-blocker toxicity if combined with zileuton.
- dofetilide (Tikosyn) may increase dofetilide blood levels if taken with zafirlukast.
- erythromycin (E-Mycin, etc.) may decrease zafirlukast's benefits.
- phenobarbital (various) may lower montelukast blood levels.
- prednisone (montelukast report only) lead to severe accumulation of fluid (peripheral edema) in one patient. Close patient follow up and caution is prudent. The other members of this class may be corticosteroid sparing.
- propranolol (Inderal) and perhaps other beta-blockers (see Drug Classes) cause excessive/undesirable beta blockage.
- rifampin (Rifater) may lower montelukast blood levels.
- terfenadine (Seldane—no longer on the U.S. market) may decrease zafirlukast blood levels and its therapeutic benefits. Zileuton may decrease terfenadine (and perhaps other similarly structured minimally sedating antihistamine levels) and lead to toxicity. DO NOT combine.
- theophylline (Theo-Dur, others) may decrease zafirlukast blood levels and its therapeutic benefits. Zileuton may result in doubling of theophylline levels and require reduced theophylline doses.
- warfarin (Coumadin) may lead to increased risk of bleeding (zafirlukast and zileuton). More frequent INRs are needed.

▷ *Driving, Hazardous Activities:* These drugs may cause dizziness. Restrict activities as necessary.

Aviation Note: The use of these drugs **may be a disqualification** for piloting. Consult a designated Aviation Medical Examiner.

Exposure to Sun: No restrictions.

Discontinuation: Do not stop these medicines without first talking with your doctor.

APREPITANT (AH prep in tant)

Introduced: 2003   **Class:**   Antiemetic; Neurokinin-1 (NK-1 receptor blocker)   **Prescription:**   USA: Yes   **Controlled Drug:**   USA: No; Canada: No   **Available as Generic:**   USA: No; Canada: No

Brand Name: Emend

Author's Note: This medicine is the latest addition to the families of medicines that can help stop vomiting. Information in this profile will be broadened as clinical study results and comparative data warrant.

ARIPIPRAZOLE (AIR ih pip rah zohl)

Introduced: 2002   **Class:**   Antipsychotic; Atypical antipsychotic agent, dopamine system stabilizer; partial agonist   **Prescription:**   USA: Yes   **Controlled Drug:**   USA: No; Canada: No   **Available as Generic:**   USA: No; Canada: No

Brand Name: Abilify

As a Single Drug Product: Uses currently included in FDA-approved labeling: (1) Treatment of schizophrenia.

Other (unlabeled) generally accepted uses: (1) A well-designed clinical trial presented at the American Psychiatric meeting found rapid onset of benefit (as soon as day four) in treating sudden (acute) bipolar mania using 30 mg of aripiprazole a day, with the option to decrease to 15 mg daily. Patients showed improved Young Mania Rating Scale (Y-MRS) results and improved Clinical Global Impression-Bipolar Disorder (CGI-BP), Positive and Negative Syndrome Scaled (PANSS)-total (PANNSS-total) as well as the PANSS hostility subscale.

Author's Note: The FDA now requires warnings for ALL atypical antipsychotic medicines which describe an increased risk of problems with blood sugar (risk of hyperglycemia and diabetes) when patients are taking these medicines. Information in this profile will be broadened in the next edition as clinical data warrant.

ASPIRIN* (AS pir in)

Other Names: acetylsalicylic acid, ASA

Introduced: 1899 **Class:** Analgesics, mild; antiplatelet, antipyretic, NSAIDs, salicylates **Prescription:** USA: No **Controlled Drug:** USA: No; Canada: No **Available as Generic:** Yes

Brand Names: Added Strength Analgesic Pain Reliever, Adult Strength Pain Reliever [CD], Aggrenox [CD], Alka-Seltzer Effervescent Pain Reliever and Antacid [CD], Alka-Seltzer Night Time [CD], Alka-Seltzer Plus [CD], Alka-Seltzer Plus Cold [CD], Anacin [CD], Anacin Maximum Strength [CD], ✤Anacin w/Codeine [CD], ✤Ancasal, APC [CD], APC w/Codeine [CD], ✤APO-ASA, Arthritis Pain Formula [CD], Arthritis Strength Bufferin, A.S.A. Enseals, ✤Asasantine [CD], Ascriptin [CD], Ascriptin A/D [CD], Aspergum, ✤Aspirin,* Aspirin PROTECT, Asprimox, ✤Astrin, Axotal [CD], Azdone [CD], Bayer Aspirin, Bayer Children's Chewable Aspirin, Bayer Enteric Aspirin, Bayer Back & Body Pain, Bayer Plus, Bayer PM Extra Strength, BC Powder, Buffaprin, Bufferin [CD], Bufferin Arthritis Strength [CD], Bufferin Extra Strength [CD], Bufferin w/Codeine [CD], Cama Arthritis Pain Reliever [CD], Cardioprin, Carisoprodol Compound [CD], Cope [CD], Coricidin [CD], ✤Coryphen, ✤Coryphen-Codeine [CD], ✤C2 Buffered [CD], Darvon Compound [CD], Direct Formulary Aspirin, ✤Dristan [CD], Easprin, Ecotrin, 8-Hour Bayer, Empirin, Empirin w/Codeine No. 2, 4 [CD], ✤Entrophen, Excedrin [CD], Excedrin Extra Strength Geltabs [CD], Excedrin Migraine* [CD], Fiorinal [CD], ✤Fiorinal-C [Q],-C [h] [CD], Fiorinal w/Codeine [CD], Genacote, Genprin, Goody's Headache Powder [CD], Halprin, Hepto [CD], Lortab ASA [CD], Low Dose Adult Chewable Aspirin, Marnal [CD], Maximum Bayer Aspirin, Measurin, Midol Caplets [CD], Momentum [CD], Norgesic [CD], Norgesic Forte [CD], Norwich Aspirin, ✤Novasen, Orphenadrine [CD], PAP w/Codeine [CD], Percodan [CD], Percodan-Demi [CD], ✤Phenaphen [CD], ✤Phenaphen No. 2, 3, 4 [CD], Pravigard PAC [CD], Propoxyphene Compound [CD], ✤Riphen-10, Robaxisal [CD], ✤Robaxisal-C [CD], Roxiprin [CD], ✤692 [CD], SK-65 Compound [CD], Soma Compound [CD], St. Joseph Children's Aspirin, ✤Supasa, Synalgos [CD], Synalgos-DC [CD], Talwin Compound [CD], Talwin Compound-50 [CD], ✤Tecnal Tablet [CD], ✤Triaphen-10, ✤217 [CD], ✤217 Strong [CD], ✤292 [CD], Vanquish [CD], Verin, Wesprin, Zorprin

---

BENEFITS versus RISKS

| EFFECTIVE RELIEF OF MILD TO MODERATE PAIN AND INFLAMMATION | *Possible Risks* |

EFFECTIVE RELIEF OF MILD TO
  MODERATE PAIN AND
  INFLAMMATION
REDUCTION OF FEVER
PREVENTION OF BLOOD CLOTS
PREVENTION OF HEART ATTACK
  (a benefit when satisfactory blood
  pressure control has been achieved
  prior to starting aspirin)
PREVENTION OF STROKE
PREVENTION OF COLON CANCER
ACTS TO LIMIT THE SIZE AND
  SEVERITY OF HEART ATTACKS
  ONCE THEY HAVE STARTED
TREATMENT OF MIGRAINE HEAD-
  ACHES (EXCEDRIN MIGRAINE
  ONLY)
PREVENTION OF COLON CANCER
  (COLORECTAL ADENOMAS) IN
  PEOPLE WITH PREVIOUS
  COLORECTAL CANCER
PREVENTION OF STROKE IN
  PEOPLE WITH ATRIAL
  FIBRILLATION
PREVENTION OF ADVERSE
  OUTCOMES IN ACUTE
  CORONARY SYNDROME
PATIENTS WHEN COMBINED
  WITH CLOPIDOGREL (PLAVIX)
May have a role in preventing breast
  cancer (talk to your doctor)

Possible Risks
Stomach irritation, bleeding, and/or
  ulceration
Decreased numbers of white blood
  cells and platelets
Hemolytic anemia—rare
Liver toxicity—rare
Bronchospasm in asthmatics—possible
Ringing in the ears (tinnitus) possible
  as toxicity sign
Hemorrhagic strokes—case
  reports/increased risk
Full-dose use (not low-dose) carries
  an increased risk of hospitalization
  for congestive heart failure in the el-
  derly (NSAIDs as a class effect)

▷ **Principal Uses**

As a Single Drug Product: Uses currently included in FDA-approved labeling: (1) Relieves mild to moderate pain and eases symptoms in conditions causing inflammation or high fever. Treats musculoskeletal disorders, especially acute and chronic arthritis, as well as painful menstruation (dysmenorrhea). Used selectively to: (2) reduce risk of first heart attack; (3) reduce the risk of repeat heart attack; (4) prevent platelet embolism to the brain (in men); (5) reduce risk of clots (thromboembolism) after heart attack and in people with artificial heart valves and after hip surgery (see Blood Platelets in Glossary); (6) help prevent a second stroke in people who have had a stroke; (7) help prevent strokes in people with transient ischemic attack (TIA) history; (8) help prevent migraine headaches (Excedrin Migraine only); (9) treat TIA in women and men; (10) treat sudden heart attack (acute myocardial infarction or AMI) in men and women; (11) decrease risk of heart attack in patients with unstable angina or NSTEMI; (12) treat pleurisy associated with systemic lupus erythematosus; (13) used in some patients after coronary angioplasty; (14) used in combination with clopidogrel (Plavix) in some patients with acute coronary syndromes (see CURE trial reference and unstable angina).

Other (unlabeled) generally accepted uses: (1) Long-term use may decrease the risk of colon polyps or colon cancer in women AND MEN. Recent data also shows benefits in preventing colorectal adenomas in people who have already had colon or rectal cancer; (2) may limit size and severity of a heart attack if aspirin is taken immediately after symptoms are recognized and is continued for at least 30 days after the heart attack; (3) can help reduce flushing caused by niacin; (4) used after carotid artery surgery (endarterectomy) to prevent TIA or stroke; (5) general data supporting NSAID use and decreased Alzheimer's risk; (6) one 1999 study found that low dose (100 mg) of aspirin given 8 hours after waking or at bedtime worked to decrease blood pressure in women at risk for gestational hypertension or preeclampsia; (7) used in some atrial fibrillation patients (intolerant of anticoagulant treatment) to help prevent strokes; (8) ADA recommendation for prevention strategy for people living with diabetes who are also at risk for cardiovascular disease; (9) a survey of 14,000 women appears to show that long-term aspirin use may decrease risk of lung cancer; (10) may have a role in preventing breast cancer (see Terry, MB in Sources).

As a Combination Drug Product [CD]: Frequently combined with other mild or strong analgesic drugs to enhance pain relief. Also combined with antihistamines and decongestants in many cold preparations to relieve headache and general discomfort. Aggrenox combines 200 mg of dipyridamole with 25 mg of aspirin. Pravigard PAC combines the benefits of the "statin" medicine (HMG-CoA reductase inhibitor) called pravastatin or Pravachol with aspirin in a variety of doses.

How This Drug Works: Reduces prostaglandins, chemicals involved in the production of inflammation and pain. By modifying the temperature-regulating center in the brain, dilating blood vessels and increasing sweating, aspirin reduces fever. Works on blood clotting elements called platelets to inactivate prostaglandin G/H synthase. This inactivation leads to almost complete suppression of platelet ability to make thromboxanes. By preventing the production of thromboxane in blood platelets, aspirin inhibits formation of blood clots.

▷ **Widely Used Guidelines That Involve This Medicine (representative sample):** Please look at the section at the very beginning of this profile called "Class." Next, turn to Table 22 and you will find guidelines listed by the class involved!

Available Dosage Forms and Strengths

Capsules, enteric coated — 500 mg

Capsules, enteric-coated granules — 325 mg

Gum tablets — 227.5 mg

Suppositories — 60 mg, 120 mg, 125 mg, 130 mg, 195 mg, 200 mg, 300 mg, 325 mg, 600 mg, 650 mg, 1.2 g

Tablets — 65 mg, 81 mg, 165 mg, 325 mg, 496 mg, 500 mg

Tablets, chewable — 81 mg

Tablets, enteric coated — 81 mg, 165 mg, 325 mg, 500 mg, 650 mg, 975 mg

Tablets, prolonged action — 80 mg (Canada), 650 mg, 800 mg, 975 mg

▷ **Usual Adult Dosage Ranges:** *In men or women having a heart attack:* One (325 mg) nonenteric-coated aspirin (then call 911). If only enteric-coated aspirin is available, it should be chewed in order to make it enter the body faster. Aspirin is then continued for 30 days after the heart attack. Some studies have continued it for up to 2 years.

In stroke: 50–325 mg showed a benefit in the CAST study.

In preventing transient ischemic attacks (TIA): 325–900 mg a day has been used. Low-dose treatment of TIA has used 50–325 mg. For the Aggrenox combination form: Prevention of stroke in people who have had transient brain blood flow problems (ischemia) or those who have suffered an ischemic stroke from a clot (thrombosis)—one capsule in the morning and in the evening has been used.

For pain or fever: 325 to 650 mg every 4 hours and as needed for fever (ongoing pain or fever use should be medically supervised).

Arthritis (and related conditions): 3,600 to 5,400 mg daily in divided doses.

Prevention of blood clots: 80–162 mg daily or every other day. Low-dose, long-term daily aspirin may also decrease risk of colon cancer or heart attacks. FDA advocates 75–325 mg daily for unstable angina or a previous heart attack to reduce risk of death or another heart attack. The U.S. Preventive Services Task Force recommends that clinicians consider low-dose aspirin use in patients who are 40 or older who have significantly increased risk of heart attack (myocardial infarction or MI) and who are not contraindicated low-dose aspirin. A phenomenon called **aspirin resistance** has been described in several studies. The practical implication of this research is that some patients may be more resistant to the beneficial effects of aspirin in preventing blood clots than others. Some clinicians use tests of how well blood elements called platelets clump (aggregate), while others advocate urine tests (see Eikelboom, J.W. in Sources) in order to check results from aspirin and to adjust dosing. Once resistance is found, the added power of higher aspirin doses or of another added medicine may be required.

Note: For long-term use, actual dosage and schedule must be determined for each patient individually.

Conditions Requiring Dosing Adjustments

Liver Function: This medicine should be avoided in severe liver disease.

Kidney Function: Avoided or used with caution in patients with kidney problems. NOT to be used in severe (creatinine clearance less than 10 mL/min) kidney failure.

Glucose-6-Phosphate Dehydrogenase (G6PD) Deficiency: May cause destruction of red blood cells in patients with G6PD deficiency.

▷ **Dosing Instructions:** Take with food, milk or a full glass of water to reduce stomach upset. Regular tablets may be crushed and capsules opened for administration. Enteric-coated tablets, prolonged-action tablets, A.S.A. Enseals, Cama tablets, and Ecotrin tablets should not be crushed. If you forget a dose: take it right away unless it's nearly time for your next regular dose. Aggrenox capsules SHOULD NOT be chewed. If it IS nearly time, just take the scheduled dose. DO NOT double dose.

Usual Duration of Use: Short-term use is recommended—3 to 5 days for fever or cold symptoms. Daily use should not exceed 10 days without physician supervision. Use on a regular schedule for 1 week usually needed to see benefit in relieving chronic arthritis symptoms. Response must be evaluated and dose adjusted in long-term use. Ongoing use for prevention of heart attack, colon cancer, or stroke REQUIRES ongoing supervision by your doctor, even though aspirin is not a prescription drug.

Typical Treatment Goals and Measurements (Outcomes and Markers)
> *Pain:* Most clinicians treating pain use a device called an algometer to check
> your pain. This looks like a small ruler, but lets the clinician better under-
> stand your pain. The goals of treatment then relate to where the level of
> pain started (for example, a rating of 7 on a zero to ten scale) and what
> the cause of the pain was. Pain medicines may also be used together (in
> combination) in order to get the best result or outcome. If your pain con-
> trol is not acceptable to YOU after a week of arthritis pain treatment, be
> sure to call your doctor as you may need a different medicine or combi-
> nation.
>
> *Cardiovascular disorders (strokes and heart attacks):* The clear marker here is
> prevention of a first or second stroke or heart attack. Measures of 11-
> dehydro thromboxane B2 in the urine (see Eikelboom in Sources) and use
> of the PFA-100 may help define people who have more clotting propensity
> to overcome or who activate their platelets by a pathway different than
> cyclooxygenase (such as Thrombin). These tests may help identify "aspirin
> resistant patients."

Possible Advantages of This Drug: Inexpensive medicine that treats a wide
variety of conditions and can also help prevent heart attacks, colon cancer, and strokes. A recent study found that one baby aspirin (81 mg) daily
decreased risk of a first heart attack in high risk, otherwise healthy
patients. Your doctor should decide if this makes sense for you. Bayer
Back & Body Pain has a Micro-coating (Toleraid) that makes it more easily
swallowed.

▷ **This Drug Should Not Be Taken If**
  • you have had an allergic reaction to any form of aspirin.
  • you have a history of urticaria/angioedema or spasm of the bronchi with
    rhinoconjunctivitis with aspirin, other NSAID or selective COX II inhibitor
    (adults who developed nasal polyps, asthma, chronic rhinitis, or ongoing
    angioedema or urticaria make these reactions more likely).
  • you have any type of bleeding disorder (such as hemophilia).
  • you have active peptic ulcer disease.
  • you are a child or even teenager with a viral infection (use in viral illnesses
    in those populations increases the risk of Reye's syndrome—see Glossary).
  • it smells like vinegar. This indicates decomposition of aspirin.

▷ **Inform Your Physician Before Taking This Drug If**
  • you are taking any anticoagulant drug or have a history of blood clotting
    difficulties (such as low vitamin K or prothrombin).
  • you are taking a COX II inhibitor and this medicine is prescribed.
  • you are taking oral antidiabetic drugs.
  • you have a history of peptic ulcer (FDA advisory committee notes that peo-
    ple who take 3 or more alcohol containing drinks a day, increased risk of
    stomach bleeding occurs).
  • you have gout.
  • you have lupus erythematosus.
  • you are pregnant (particularly third trimester) or planning pregnancy.
  • you have asthma, carditis, or nasal polyps.
  • you plan to have surgery of any kind (used in different doses before some
    kinds of surgery and not at all before others).
  • you take prescription or nonprescription medications not discussed when
    aspirin was recommended for you.

- you are unsure how much to take or how often to take it.
- you have a history of liver or kidney problems.
- you have low glucose-6-phosphate dehydrogenase (G6PD).
- you drink three or more alcoholic drinks a day (see Caution).

Possible Side Effects (natural, expected, and unavoidable drug actions)
Mild drowsiness in sensitive patients.
Interference with usual blood clotting.

▷ **Possible Adverse Effects** (unusual, unexpected, and infrequent reactions)
If any of the following develop, consult your physician promptly for guidance.

Mild Adverse Effects
Allergic reactions: skin rash, hives, nasal discharge (resembling hay fever), nasal polyps.
Stomach irritation, heartburn, nausea, vomiting, constipation—infrequent to frequent.
Ringing in the ears (tinnitus)—a sign of excessive doses or dose sensitivity-call your doctor if this happens (see serious adverse effects)—possible.
Lowering of the blood sugar—rare.

Serious Adverse Effects
Allergic reactions: acute anaphylactic reaction (see Glossary), allergic destruction of blood platelets (see Glossary) and bruising—rare.
Idiosyncratic reactions: hemolytic anemia (see Glossary)—rare.
Stevens-Johnson syndrome—possible.
Hemorrhagic stroke in some populations—case reports.
Erosion of stomach lining, with silent bleeding—may be dose and frequency related.
Activation of peptic ulcer, with or without hemorrhage—frequent with long-term non-enteric-coated use.
Bone marrow depression (see Glossary): fatigue, weakness, fever, sore throat, abnormal bleeding or bruising—possible.
Hepatitis with jaundice (see Glossary): yellow skin and eyes, dark-colored urine, light-colored stool—possible, especially with daily use of more than 2 grams (2,000 mg)—dose related.
Hearing toxicity (ototoxicity, tinnitus)—more common with higher doses and long-term use.
Kidney function decline—possible in kidney failure patients who depend on prostaglandins for their kidneys to work.
Bronchospasm when used in patients with nasal polyps, asthma—possible.
May worsen angina attacks (Prinzmetal's) and increase their frequency—possible.
Reye's syndrome if used during viral illness—DO NOT USE in children or teenagers with viral illnesses.

▷ **Possible Effects on Sexual Function:** None reported.

Adverse Effects That May Mimic Natural Diseases or Disorders: Liver damage may suggest viral hepatitis or reveal (unmask) low-level (subclinical) liver disease. May lead to decline in kidney function in people with borderline kidney disease.

Possible Effects on Laboratory Tests
Complete blood counts: decreased red cells, hemoglobin, white cells, and platelets.
Bleeding time: prolonged.
INR (prothrombin time): increased by large doses; decreased by small doses.

Blood glucose level: decreased.
Blood uric acid level: increased by small doses; decreased by large doses.
Liver function tests: increased ALT/GPT, AST/GOT, alkaline phosphatase.
Thyroid function tests: increased T3 uptake, free T3, and free T4; decreased
  TSH, T3, T4, and free thyroxine index (FTI).
Urine sugar tests: false positive with Clinitest or Benedict's solution.
Fecal occult blood test: positive with large doses of aspirin.

CAUTION

1. The FDA now requires a warning noting that people who have three or more alcoholic drinks a day may have increased risk of stomach bleeding if they also use aspirin (problems may also occur with lower alcohol use).

2. **Aspirin is a drug.** We tend to have an unrealistic sense of its safety and its potential for adverse effects. TALK TO YOUR DOCTOR TO SEE IF BENEFITS OUTWEIGH RISKS OF REGULAR ASPIRIN USE. A meta-analysis of 55,462 patients and 16 clinical trials found an increased risk of stroke (12 strokes for every 10,000 patients). The study concluded that benefits may outweigh risks for many people. Talk to your doctor.

3. Talk to your doctor about dosing of aspirin BEFORE you take it and also before undertaking any ongoing use of aspirin.

4. An outcome study of 5,499 men found that the risk of stroke with aspirin treatment related to blood pressure. One conclusion is that blood pressure should be satisfactorily controlled BEFORE aspirin therapy for prevention of CHD is started.

5. Remember that aspirin can
   • cause new illnesses.
   • complicate existing illnesses.
   • complicate pregnancy.
   • complicate surgery.
   • interact unfavorably with other drugs.
   • When a health care professional asks, "Are you taking any drugs?" the answer is "yes" if you are taking aspirin. This also applies to *any* nonprescription drug you may be taking (see Over-the-Counter Drugs in the Glossary).

6. Some patients may be "aspirin resistant." This term is used to help identify people who still have platelets that clump to their usual extent, despite appropriate low-dose aspirin treatment.
   • **Controversies in Medicine: Some clinicians think that aspirin will remove some of the benefits of ACE inhibitors (see Drug Classes) if these two medicines are taken together.**
   • Aspirin tends to be underused in people with diabetes and in patients with coronary artery disease (one study found only 26% use), others even less. If you are living with diabetes, or have coronary artery disease, ask your doctor if aspirin makes sense for you.

7. A study by MacDonald (see Sources) found that ibuprofen (not diclofenac, acetaminophen, or rofecoxib) can inhibit beneficial (cardio-protective) effects of aspirin. His conclusion was that aspirin should be taken two hours before ibuprofen so that aspirin can go to work first. Other clinicians recommended avoiding ongoing use of ibuprofen in patients receiving aspirin for heart protection.

Precautions for Use

By Infants and Children: Reye's syndrome (brain and liver damage in children, often fatal) can follow flu or chickenpox in children and teenagers. Some reports suggest that the use of aspirin by children with flu or chickenpox can increase the risk of developing this complication. Consult your physician before giving aspirin to a child or teenager with chickenpox, flu, or similar infection.

Usual dosage schedule for children (Up to 2 years of age—consult physician):

    2 to 4 years of age — 160 mg/4 hours, up to 5 doses/24 hours.

    4 to 6 years of age — 240 mg/4 hours, up to 5 doses/24 hours.

    6 to 9 years of age — 320 mg/4 hours, up to 5 doses/24 hours.

    9 to 11 years of age — 400 mg/4 hours, up to 5 doses/24 hours.

    11 to 12 years of age — 480 mg/4 hours, up to 5 doses/24 hours.

Do not exceed 5 days of continual use without talking to your doctor. Give all doses with food, milk or a full glass of water.

By Those Over 60 Years of Age: Watch for signs of high blood level: irritability, ringing in the ears, deafness, confusion, nausea or stomach upset. Aspirin can cause serious stomach bleeding. This can occur as "silent" bleeding of small amounts over a long time. Sudden hemorrhage can occur, even without a history of stomach ulcer. Watch for gray- to black-colored stools, an indication of stomach bleeding.

▷ Advisability of Use During Pregnancy

Pregnancy Category: C/D. See Pregnancy Risk Categories at the back of this book.

Animal Studies: Significant birth defects due to this drug have been reported.

Human Studies: Information from studies of pregnant women indicates no increased risk of birth defects in 32,164 pregnancies exposed to aspirin. Studies show, however, that the regular use of aspirin during pregnancy is often detrimental to the health of the mother and the welfare of the fetus. Anemia, hemorrhage before and after delivery and an increased incidence of stillbirths and newborn deaths have been reported. There are data that support use of aspirin in low doses to prevent toxemia of pregnancy in some women with a history of this problem.

Ask your doctor for help. Avoid aspirin altogether during the last 3 months unless your doctor prescribes it.

Advisability of Use If Breast-Feeding

Presence of this drug in breast milk: Yes.

Avoid drug or refrain from nursing.

Habit-Forming Potential: Extended high-dose use may cause a psychological dependence (see Glossary).

Effects of Overdose: Stomach distress, nausea, vomiting, ringing in the ears, dizziness, impaired hearing, blood chemistry imbalance, stupor, fever, deep and rapid breathing, twitching, delirium, shock, hallucinations, convulsions.

Possible Effects of Long-Term Use

A form of psychological dependence (see Glossary). Anemia due to chronic blood loss from erosion of stomach lining. The development of stomach ulcer. The development of "aspirin allergy"—nasal discharge, nasal polyps, asthma. Kidney damage. Prolonged bleeding time, critical in the event of injury or surgery.

Suggested Periodic Examinations While Taking This Drug (at physician's discretion)

Complete blood cell counts.

Kidney function tests and urine analyses.

Liver function tests.

▷ **While Taking This Drug, Observe the Following**

Foods: May decrease the total amount of aspirin per dose that is absorbed.

Herbal Medicines or Minerals: Many herbal medicines may interact with aspirin. Examples include evening primrose oil (EPO), ginkgo, garlic, ginger, ginseng, guggul, skull cap and feverfew. St. John's wort may increase sensitivity to the sun, and caution is advised as additive sensitivity may develop. White willow bark contains salicylates. Adding products that contain that herb add additional aspirin and are not advised. Talk to your doctor and pharmacist before adding any herbal products.

Nutritional Support: Do not take large doses of vitamin C while taking aspirin regularly.

Beverages: No restrictions. May be taken with milk.

▷ *Alcohol:* Use of alcohol and aspirin at the same time may increase risk of stomach damage and may prolong bleeding time (see cautions).

Tobacco Smoking: No interactions expected. I advise everyone to quit smoking.

▷ *Other Drugs*

Aspirin may *increase* the effects of
- adrenocortical steroids (see Drug Classes), leading to additive stomach irritation and possible bleeding.
- insulin (various brands including insulin lispro) and require dosage adjustment when more than 650 mg of aspirin is taken daily.
- heparin and cause abnormal bleeding.
- methotrexate and increase its toxic effects.
- oral anticoagulants (see Drug Classes) such as low-molecular-weight heparins (see Drug Classes) and warfarin (Coumadin) and cause abnormal bleeding.
- oral antidiabetic drugs (see Drug Classes) and cause hypoglycemia. Dosage adjustments are often necessary—particularly with first-generation agents.
- ticlodipine (Ticlid) may increase bleeding risk. Careful monitoring of blood counts is prudent.
- tiludronate (Skelid) by increasing blood levels by 50%.
- thrombolytics such as TPA and reteplase (Retavase). Careful monitoring is advised if these medicines are combined.
- valproic acid (Depakene).

Aspirin may *decrease* the effects of
- ACE inhibitors—since vein opening or vasodilator prostaglandins may account for some of the ACE beneficial effects and aspirin inhibits prostaglandins, aspirin may blunt ACE inhibitor benefits. Still, many clinicians feel that the benefits of aspirin and ACE use after a heart attack outweigh any blunting effect.
- beta-adrenergic-blocking drugs (see Drug Classes).
- captopril (Capoten).
- enalapril (Vasotec) by decreasing enalapril's beneficial increase in heart (cardiac) output.
- furosemide (Lasix).
- other NSAIDs (see Drug Classes).
- phenytoin (Dilantin) and fosphenytoin (Cerebyx) by decreasing phenytoin or fosphenytoin blood levels (high aspirin doses).
- probenecid (Benemid) and reduce its effectiveness in the treatment of gout—with aspirin doses of less than 2 g every 24 hours.
- spironolactone (Aldactazide, Aldactone, others) and reduce its diuretic effect.
- sulfinpyrazone (Anturane) and reduce its effectiveness in the treatment of gout—with aspirin doses of less than 2 g every 24 hours.

- tiludronate (Skelid) by decreasing the amount getting into the body.

Aspirin *taken concurrently* with

- alendronate (Fosamax) or other bisphosphonates (tiludronate or Skelid or risedronate or Actonel) may result in increased risk of stomach upset/diarrhea and decreases bisphosphonate.
- capsaicin (Zostrix and others) increases risk of bleeding.
- celecoxib (Celebrex), etoricoxib (investigational), rofecoxib (Vioxx), or valdecoxib (Bextra) (see Cox II Inhibitors in Drug Classes) increases risk of stomach ulcers. Benefits versus risks of low dose (such as 81 mg) aspirin in combination may favor benefits in many patients. Talk to your doctor.
- cilostazol (Pletal) changed platelet clumping (aggregation) in one study but the clinical significance of the change found is unknown. Caution is prudent.
- clopidogrel (Plavix) is a benefit-to-risk decision because of increased risk of bleeding. Talk to your doctor to see if the benefits (see CURE trial above) of combining aspirin and clopidogrel outweigh any increased bleeding risk.
- cortisone-like drugs (see Drug Classes) increases risk of stomach ulcers.
- diltiazem (Cardizem) may result in increased risk of bleeding.
- eptifibatide (Integrilin) increases risk of bleeding.
- high blood pressure (antihypertensive) medicines may blunt their therapeutic benefit, especially those that are diuretics such as furosemide (Lasix), spironolactone, or thiazides (see Drug Classes).
- ibuprofen (Motrin, others) may result in blunting of cardioprotective effects of aspirin. If mini-dose aspirin is being taken, the aspirin should be taken two hours BEFORE the ibuprofen. Ongoing use of ibuprofen in patients using aspirin for heart protective benefits should probably be avoided until further data are available.
- intrauterine devices (IUDs) may result in decreased IUD effectiveness.
- lithium (Lithobid) may increase lithium blood levels.
- low-molecular-weight heparins (Lovenox, Fragmin, others) increases the risk of bleeding.
- methotrexate (Mexate) may cause toxicity.
- niacin (various) may BENEFICIALLY decrease flushing from niacin.
- quinidine (Quinaglute, others) may increase risk of bleeding.
- tirofiban (Aggrastat) may increase bleeding risk. Careful monitoring of blood counts is prudent.
- valproic acid (Depakote) may cause toxic blood levels.
- varicella vaccine (Varivax) may result in Reye's syndrome. **Avoid aspirin and other salicylates for 6 weeks following Varivax inoculation**.
- verapamil (Calan, others) may cause increased bleeding risk.
- zafirlukast (Accolate) may increase zafirlukast blood levels and increase adverse effects.

The following drugs may *increase* the effects of aspirin:

- acetazolamide (Diamox).
- cimetidine (Tagamet).
- para-aminobenzoic acid (Pabalate).

The following drugs may *decrease* the effects of aspirin:

- antacids, with regular continual use.
- cholestyramine (Questran, others)—will decrease the amount of aspirin that goes to work; separate doses by 30 minutes.
- cortisone-like drugs (see Drug Classes).
- urinary alkalinizers (sodium bicarbonate, sodium citrate).

▷ *Driving, Hazardous Activities:* No restrictions or precautions.

Aviation Note: It is advisable to watch for mild drowsiness and restrict activities accordingly.

Exposure to Sun: Use caution, may cause photosensitivity.

Discontinuation: Aspirin should be stopped 1 week before some kinds of surgery. There are some data for use of low-dose aspirin in some cases (such as in carotid endarterectomy).

ATAZANAVIR (at ah ZAN ah veer)

Introduced: 2004 **Class:** Anti-viral, Anti-HIV, antiviral **Prescription:** USA: Yes **Controlled Drug:** USA: No; Canada: No **Available as Generic:** Yes

Brand Names: Reyataz

Author's Note: Please see the protease inhibitor family profile for further preliminary information on this medicine. It is the first once a day medicine in this family.

ATENOLOL (a TEN oh lohl)

Introduced: 1973 **Class:** Anti-anginal, antihypertensive, beta-adrenergic blocker **Prescription:** USA: Yes **Controlled Drug:** USA: No; Canada: No **Available as Generic:** Yes

Brand Names: ♣Apo-Atenolol, ♣Novo-Atenolol, ♣Nu-Atenolol,♣PMS-Atenolol, Tenoretic [CD], Tenormin

---

BENEFITS versus RISKS	
Possible Benefits	*Possible Risks*
EFFECTIVE ANTI-ANGINAL DRUG in the management of effort-induced angina	CONGESTIVE HEART FAILURE in advanced heart disease
EFFECTIVE, WELL-TOLERATED ANTIHYPERTENSIVE in mild to moderate high blood pressure	Worsening of angina in coronary heart disease (abrupt withdrawal)
DECREASES RISK OF DYING AFTER A HEART ATTACK	May lead to low blood sugar in type one diabetics
DECREASES RISK OF PROBLEMS (MORBIDITY) AFTER A HEART ATTACK	Masking of low blood sugar (hypoglycemia) in drug-treated diabetes
HELPS PREVENT MIGRAINE HEADACHES	May provoke bronchial asthma in people with asthma when used in high doses
Probable role in decreasing risk of death (morbidity) or problems (morbidity) when taken before bypass (CABG) surgery	

▷ **Principal Uses**

As a Single Drug Product: Uses currently included in FDA-approved labeling: (1) Treats classical, effort-induced angina pectoris; (2) used for mild to moderately severe high blood pressure (may be used alone or in combination with other antihypertensive drugs, such as diuretics); (3) used following heart attacks to prolong life, help decrease risk of a second heart attack, decrease the size of the heart attack, and reduce risk of abnormal heartbeats.

Other (unlabeled) generally accepted uses: (1) Can help people with stage fright; (2) may have a role in preventing migraine headaches; (3) can have an adjunctive role in alcohol withdrawal; (4) helps congestive heart failure when used with fosinopril (Monopril); (5) taken before and after surgery, this drug can help maintain blood flow to the heart and decrease death; (6) decreases preeclampsia in women at risk for this; (7) a May 2002 study from Duke (see Ferguso, et al. in Sources) found that people who get beta blockers before heart bypass surgery (CABG) have better results than those who do not take those medicines.

As a Combination Drug Product [CD]: Used in combination with a thiazide diuretic (chlorthalidone) to combine the benefits of a beta-blocker with the excess-fluid-losing properties of a thiazide. This attacks high blood pressure using two different mechanisms.

How This Drug Works: It blocks some actions of the sympathetic nervous system, reducing heart rate and contraction force and reducing oxygen needs as the heart works, and it reduces blood vessel contraction, resulting in opening and lowering of blood pressure. Combination with a "water pill" or diuretic removes excess fluid.

▷ **Widely Used Guidelines That Involve This Medicine (representative sample):** Please look at the section at the very beginning of this profile called "Class." Next, turn to Table 22 and you will find guidelines listed by the class involved!

Available Dosage Forms and Strengths
Injection — 5 mg/10 mL
Tablets — 25 mg, 50 mg, 100 mg
Tablets, combination — 50 mg, 100 mg of atenolol with 25 mg of chlorthalidone

▷ **Usual Adult Dosage Ranges**
Hypertension: Initially 50 mg once daily. Dose may be increased gradually at intervals of 7 to 10 days as needed and tolerated up to 100 mg every 24 hours. The usual maintenance dose is 50 to 100 mg every 24 hours. The total dose should not exceed 100 mg every 24 hours.

Angina: Starting dose is 50 mg once daily. May be gradually increased at 7- to 10-day intervals as needed and tolerated up to 100 mg every 24 hours. Usual ongoing dose is 50 to 100 mg every 24 hours. Some patients require 200 mg daily.

After a heart attack (post-MI): Within 12 hours after the attack, 5 mg of this drug is given via a vein (intravenously). This is followed by a second 5-mg intravenous dose 10 minutes later. Twelve hours after the second intravenous dose, 50 mg is given orally, followed by a second 50 mg 12 hours later. Oral dosing is continued at 100 mg orally for the next 10 days. Talk to your doctor about ongoing use to help prevent a repeat heart attack.

Note: Actual dose and schedule must be determined for each patient individually.

Conditions Requiring Dosing Adjustments
Liver Function: No decreases needed (liver has a small removal role).
Kidney Function: The dose must be decreased, with 25 mg a day as a maximum dose in some people.

▷ **Dosing Instructions:** Food decreases the amount of drug that gets into your body by up to 20%. Better taken on an empty stomach. Tablet may be crushed to take it. **DO NOT** stop this drug abruptly. If you forget a dose: take it right away unless it's within 8 hours of your next regular dose. If it IS within 8 hours of the next dose, just take the scheduled dose. DO NOT double doses.

Usual Duration of Use: Regular use for 3 to 7 days usually needed to see this drug's benefits in lowering blood pressure. Peak benefits may take two weeks. Meeting blood pressure goals will decide long-term use. Medicines are often coupled to an overall program of weight reduction, salt restriction, smoking cessation, etc. May take 3 months for peak chest pain benefits. Use after a heart attack to help prevent a repeat heart attack is ongoing. See your doctor regularly.

Typical Treatment Goals and Measurements (Outcomes and Markers)
  Blood Pressure: Guidelines (JNC VII) define normal blood pressure (BP) as **less than** 120/80. **Pre-hypertension:** ranges from 120/80 to 139/89 and is intended to help your doctor encourage lifestyle changes (or in the case of people with a risk factor for high blood pressure, start treatment) much earlier—so that possible damage to blood vessels, your heart, kidneys, sexual potency, or eyes might be minimized or avoided altogether. The next two classes of high blood pressure are stage 1 hypertension: 140/90 to 159/99 and stage 2 hypertension equal to or greater than: 160/100 mm Hg. These guidelines also recommend that clinicians work with their patients to agree on the goals and a plan of treatment. The first-ever guidelines for blood pressure (hypertension) in African Americans recommends that MOST black patients be started on TWO antihypertensive medicines with the goal of lowering blood pressure to 130/80 for those with high risk for heart and blood vessel disease or with diabetes. The goal then for diabetics: 130/80 as the target and less than 125/75 for those who spill more than one gram of protein into their urine. Most clinicians try to achieve a BP that confers the best balance of lower cardiovascular risk and avoids the problem of too low a blood pressure. Blood pressure control is generally increased with beneficial restriction of sodium. If goals are not met, it is not unusual to intensify doses or add on medicines.

Possible Advantages of This Drug: Least likely of all beta-blocker drugs to cause central nervous system adverse effects: confusion, hallucinations, nervousness, nightmares. This medicine (unlike metoprolol or propranolol) has minimal involvement using the liver for removal from the body. May be a drug of choice in patients with liver compromise who require a beta blocker.

▷ **This Drug Should Not Be Taken If**
  • you have had an allergic reaction to it previously.
  • you are in heart failure (overt).
  • you have an abnormally slow heart rate or a serious form of heart block.
  • you are taking, or have taken within the past 14 days, any monoamine oxidase (MAO) type A inhibitor drug (see Drug Classes).
  • you are in cardiogenic shock.

▷ **Inform Your Physician Before Taking This Drug If**
  • you've had beta-blocker adverse reactions (see Drug Classes).
  • you have a history of serious heart disease, with or without episodes of heart failure.

- you have a history of hay fever (allergic rhinitis), asthma, chronic bronchitis, chronic obstructive pulmonary disease (COPD), or emphysema.
- you have been taking clonidine.
- you have a history of overactive thyroid function (hyperthyroidism).
- you have low blood sugar (hypoglycemia) or diabetes—may hide some symptoms of hypoglycemia.
- you have impaired liver or kidney function.
- you have diabetes or myasthenia gravis.
- you take digitalis, quinidine, reserpine, or any calcium blocker (see Drug Classes).
- you take clonidine (atenolol should be stopped a few days before stopping clonidine).
- you will have surgery with general anesthesia.
- you take prescription or nonprescription drugs not discussed when atenolol was prescribed.
- you are unsure how much or how often to take this drug.

Possible Side Effects (natural, expected, and unavoidable drug actions)

Lethargy, fatigability, cold extremities, slow heart rate, light-headedness in upright position (see Orthostatic Hypotension in Glossary)—all reported during treatment.

▷ **Possible Adverse Effects** (unusual, unexpected, and infrequent reactions)

If any of the following develop, consult your physician promptly for guidance.

Mild Adverse Effects

Allergic reactions: skin rash, itching.

Headache, abnormal dreams—infrequent.

Dizziness, tiredness, or depression—rare to frequent.

Indigestion, nausea, diarrhea—infrequent.

Joint and muscle discomfort, fluid retention (edema)—possible.

Serious Adverse Effects

Allergic reactions: may contribute to seriousness and refractory allergic reactions.

Chest pain, shortness of breath, can lead to congestive heart failure—rare.

May lead to an asthma attack (in asthmatic people)—possible.

Angina or rebound hypertension—if abruptly stopped.

Difficulty walking (intermittent claudication)—controversial.

Psychosis—case reports.

Systemic lupus erythematosus—case reports.

▷ **Possible Effects on Sexual Function:** Decreased libido and impaired potency (50 to 100 mg per day). This drug is less likely to cause lowered ability to achieve a completely firm penis (reduced erectile capacity) than most drugs of its class. Impotence—rare.

Possible Effects on Laboratory Tests

Blood cholesterol, LDL and VLDL cholesterol levels: no effect with doses of 50 mg/day; increased with doses of 100 mg/day.

ANA titer: increased.

Blood triglyceride levels: no effect with doses of 50 mg/day; increased with doses of 100 mg/day.

Blood HDL cholesterol levels: no effect with doses of 50 mg/day; decreased with doses of 100 mg/day.

CAUTION
1. Control your high blood pressure for life! Even though it usually does not have any signs or symptoms, high blood pressure does damage. Control your pressure and take your medicine. Visit *www.americanheart.org* for more information.
2. ***DO NOT stop this drug suddenly*** without the guidance of your doctor. Carry a note in your purse or wallet that says you take this drug.
3. Talk to your doctor or pharmacist BEFORE using nasal spray or pill decongestants. These may cause sudden increases in blood pressure when combined with beta-blocker drugs.
4. Report any tendency to emotional depression to your doctor.

Precautions for Use
By Infants and Children: Safety and effectiveness by those under 12 years of age not established. However, if this drug is used, watch for development of low blood sugar (hypoglycemia), especially if meals are skipped.
By Those Over 60 Years of Age: Proceed ***cautiously*** with all antihypertensive drugs. High blood pressure should be reduced slowly, avoiding excessively low blood pressure. Small doses and frequent blood pressure checks are needed. Sudden and excessive decrease in blood pressure can predispose to stroke or heart attack. Watch for dizziness, unsteadiness, tendency to fall, confusion, hallucinations, depression, or urinary frequency.

▷ **Advisability of Use During Pregnancy**
Pregnancy Category: **D.** See Pregnancy Risk Categories at the back of this book.
Animal Studies: Increased resorptions of embryo and fetus reported in rats, but no birth defects.
Human Studies: Adequate studies of pregnant women are not available, but the drug has caused fetal harm. This drug has been used during the last 3 months of pregnancy; however, fetal growth may be slowed and the child may be born with low blood pressure and temperature.
Ask your doctor for guidance.

Advisability of Use If Breast-Feeding
Presence of this drug in breast milk: Yes.
Avoid drug if possible. If drug is necessary, observe nursing infant for slow heart rate and indications of low blood sugar.

Habit-Forming Potential: None.

Effects of Overdose: Weakness, slow pulse, low blood pressure, fainting, cold sweaty skin, congestive heart failure, coma, and convulsions.

Possible Effects of Long-Term Use: Reduced heart reserve or heart failure in some people with advanced heart disease.

Suggested Periodic Examinations While Taking This Drug (at physician's discretion)
Measurements of blood pressure (checks at health fairs or pharmacies are a great idea).
Evaluation of heart function.
ANA titer.

▷ **While Taking This Drug, Observe the Following**
Foods: Can decrease total atenolol absorption by 20%. Best to avoid excessive salt intake.
Herbal Medicines or Minerals: Ginseng, guarana, bitter orange, country mallow, hawthorn, saw palmetto, ma huang (removed from the market), goldenseal, yohimbe, and licorice may cause increased blood pressure. Calcium

and garlic may help lower blood pressure. Indian snakeroot has a German Commission E monograph indication for hypertension—talk to your doctor. Eleuthero root and ephedra should be avoided by people living with hypertension.

Beverages: No restrictions. May be taken with milk.

▷ *Alcohol:* Use caution. Alcohol may exaggerate this drug's ability to lower blood pressure and may increase its mild sedative effect.

Tobacco Smoking: Nicotine may reduce this drug's effectiveness. I advise everyone to quit smoking.

▷ *Other Drugs*

Atenolol may ***increase*** the effects of

- other antihypertensive drugs and cause excessive lowering of blood pressure. Dosage adjustments may be necessary.
- reserpine (Ser-Ap-Es, etc.) and cause sedation, depression, slowing of heart rate, and lowering of blood pressure.

Atenolol ***taken concurrently*** with

- amiodarone (Cordarone) may result in cardiac arrest.
- ampicillin or bacampicillin may result in lower blood levels of atenolol.
- calcium (various) may result in ***large decreases*** in atenolol blood levels.
- calcium channel blockers (dihydropyridine forms—various) may result in heart impairment or severe lowering of blood pressure. Caution is advised with this combination, but it may have good therapeutic use.
- clonidine (Catapres) requires close monitoring for rebound high blood pressure if clonidine is stopped while atenolol is still being taken.
- digoxin (Lanoxin) may result in very slow heart rates.
- dolasetron (Anzemet) may result in slow heart beat, low blood pressure, or headache from accumulation of a metabolite of dolasetron.
- fentanyl anesthesia (various) may cause excessive lowering of the blood pressure.
- insulin requires close monitoring to avoid undetected hypoglycemia (see Glossary).
- oral antidiabetic drugs (see Drug Classes) may result in prolonged low blood sugar.
- phenothiazines (see Drug Classes) may increase the effects of both agents and result in phenothiazine toxicity or excessively low blood pressure.
- quinidine (Quinaglute) may cause additive lowering of the blood pressure.
- ritodrine (Yutopar) may blunt ritodrine benefits.
- verapamil can result in undesirable slowing of the heart rate and excessively low blood pressure.

The following drugs may ***decrease*** the effects of atenolol:

- antacids—decrease atenolol absorption.
- aspirin (various).
- indomethacin (Indocin), and possibly other "aspirin substitutes," or NSAIDs, which may impair atenolol's blood pressure lowering (antihypertensive) effect.

▷ *Driving, Hazardous Activities:* Use caution until the full extent of drowsiness, lethargy and blood pressure change has been determined.

Aviation Note: The use of this drug is ***a disqualification*** for piloting. Consult a designated Aviation Medical Examiner.

Exposure to Sun: No restrictions.

Exposure to Heat: Caution is advised. Hot environments can lower blood pressure and exaggerate the effects of this drug.

Exposure to Cold: Caution is advised. Can enhance the circulatory deficiency that may occur with this drug. The elderly should be careful to prevent hypothermia (see Glossary).

Heavy Exercise or Exertion: Avoid exertion that causes light-headedness, excessive fatigue or muscle cramping. This drug may worsen the blood pressure response to isometric exercise.

Occurrence of Unrelated Illness: Fever can lower blood pressure and require a decreased dose. Nausea or vomiting may interrupt the dosing schedule. Ask your physician for help.

Discontinuation: Avoid stopping this drug suddenly. If possible, gradual reduction of dose over a period of 2 to 3 weeks is recommended. During such reduction, physical activity is best kept to a minimum. Ask your doctor for help.

ATOMOXETINE (a TOM oh seteen)

Introduced: 2003 **Class:** Norepinephrine reuptake inhibitor, anti-attention-deficit-disorder drug **Prescription:** USA: Yes **Controlled Drug:** USA: No; Canada: No **Available as Generic:** USA: No; Canada: No

Brand Names: Strattera

BENEFITS versus RISKS	
Possible Benefits	*Possible Risks*
EFFECTIVE IN ATTENTION DEFICIT HYPERACTIVITY	ANOREXIA Sleepiness
May be useful in some cases of depression	Insomnia

▷ **Principal Uses**

As a Single Drug Product: Uses currently included in FDA-approved labeling: Treats (1) Attention deficit hyperactivity disorder (ADHD).

Other (unlabeled) generally accepted uses: (1) May treat mild to moderate depression.

Author's Note: This medicine is NOT a cure for ADHD. Some sources estimate that about 60% of people with ADHD in childhood will also have it as an adult. The largest study in adults with ADHD was presented at the June 2003 American Psychiatric Association meeting. The study involved 31 sites and showed very strong outcomes.

How This Drug Works: The medicine acts as a selective (presynaptic) norepinephrine reuptake inhibitor. Changes in this nerve transmitter are thought to help control impulsivity, hyperactivity, and augments being inattentive.

▷ **Widely Used Guidelines That Involve This Medicine (representative sample):** Please look at the section at the very beginning of this profile called "Class." Next, turn to Table 22 and you will find guidelines listed by the class involved!

Available Dosage Forms and Strengths

Capsules — 10 mg, 18 mg, 25 mg, 40 mg, and 60 mg

▷ **Recommended Dosage Ranges:**

Attention deficit disorder: Pediatric dosing: *Children over 6 years old or adolescents weighing less than 70 kg (154 pounds):* are given 0.5 mg per kg per day.

This dose is then increased after three days to a goal dose of 1.2 mg per kg. The 1.2 mg per kg dose can be given as a single dose in the morning or as equally divided doses given in the morning and late afternoon or early evening. The total dose in children and adolescents should NOT exceed 1.4 mg per kg or 100 mg (whichever is less).

Children over 6 years old, adolescents **or adults** *weighing more than 70 kg (154 pounds):* The starting dose is 40 mg. This initial dose is increased after at least three days to 80 mg. The 80 mg dose can be given as a single dose in the morning or as two equally divided doses—one in the morning and one in the late afternoon or early evening. After 14 to 28 days, the dose may be increased (if outcome goals are not met) as needed and as tolerated to 100 mg. 100 mg is the maximum dose. SEE CYP 2D6 dosing instructions in Caution and While Taking this Drug sections below.

Note: Actual dose and schedule must be determined for each patient individually.

Conditions Requiring Dosing Adjustments

Liver Function: People with moderate (Child-Pugh class B) liver (hepatic) compromise should be given 50% of the usual initial and goal (target) doses. Those with severe (Child-Pugh class C) liver compromise should have the initial and target doses decreased by 25%.

Kidney Function: No dosing changes thought required.

▷ **Dosing Instructions:** The capsules SHOULD NOT be broken or sprinkled on food (take whole, and don't crush or alter). It is best to take medicines with a full glass of water. If you forget a dose: Take the missed dose as soon as you remember it, unless it's nearly time for your next dose—if that is the case, skip the missed dose and take the next dose right on schedule. Talk with your doctor if you find yourself missing doses.

Usual Duration of Use: Regular use for one week in children and in 2 weeks is adults usually determines benefits in improving ADHD. If there is no improvement 4 weeks with use of methylphenidate, the manufacturer recommends discontinuation. There is not presently such a recommendation for atomoxetine, and discontinuation will be a clinician decision. Long-term need for treatment of ADHD is generally acknowledged, however, benefits of therapy using this medicine for longer than 9 weeks and safety for more than a year have not been studied. Ongoing use requires supervision by your doctor.

Typical Treatment Goals and Measurements (Outcomes and Markers)

Attention Deficit: The general goal is to achieve the ability to "stay on task." This medicine can also help decrease impulsiveness and socially appropriate behavior. Specific measures of cognitive function, motor performance and educational tasking may help assess response. Treatment guidelines from AHCPR and DSM-IV criteria from the American Psychiatric Association are widely used. The American Academy of Pediatricians has an important set of guidelines. Please remember that these are guidelines and therapy must still be individualized. The guidelines can be found at www.pediatrics.org (see also sources and American Academy of Pediatrics and the clinical practice guidelines on Treatment of the School-Aged Child With Attention-Deficit/Hyperactivity Disorder). Additional information is available at the American Academy of Child and Adolescent Psychiatry at *www.aacap.org*. Clinical trials used the Attention-Deficit hyperactivity Disorder rating Scale (ADHDrs) to check results of treatment. In adults, the Conners' Adult ADHD Rating Scale (CAARS) is often used.

Possible Advantages of This Drug: The first non-stimulant medicine to be approved to treat ADHD.

▷ **This Drug Should Not Be Taken If**
  • you have had an allergic reaction to it previously.
  • you have taken a monoamine oxidase inhibitor (MAOI-see Drug Classes) in the last 14 days.
  • you have narrow angle glaucoma and this medicine has been prescribed for you (causes pupil dilation—mydriasis).

▷ **Inform Your Physician Before Taking This Drug If**
  • you are experiencing a period of severe anxiety, nervous tension, or emotional depression.
  • you have a seizure disorder or bipolar disorder.
  • you have a history of abnormal heartbeats, heart disease or fast heart rate (tachycardia).
  • you have high blood pressure, angina, or epilepsy.
  • you are less than 6 years old (not studied).

Possible Side Effects (natural, expected, and unavoidable drug actions)
  Anxiety or insomnia. Reduced appetite (7–12%), weight loss. Growth should be monitored during ongoing use (there are no data on atomoxetine effects on growth). Slight increase in heart rate and/or blood pressure. Dilation of the pupil of the eye (mydriasis).

▷ **Possible Adverse Effects** (unusual, unexpected, and infrequent reactions)
  If any of the following develop, consult your physician promptly for guidance.
  Mild Adverse Effects
  Allergic reactions: skin rash, hives—possible.
  Sleepiness and dizziness (may be dose related)—possible.
  Headache—possible.
  Nausea or vomiting—infrequent.
  Urinary retention—infrequent (adults).
  Serious Adverse Effects
  Allergic reactions: possible.
  Palpitations or chest pain—rare.

▷ **Possible Effects on Sexual Function:** Decreased libido, ejaculatory problems. Painful or difficult menstruation (dysmenorrhea)—infrequent.

Natural Diseases or Disorders That May Be Activated by This Drug
  Because this medicine can dilate the pupil, it should not be used in narrow angle glaucoma.

Possible Effects on Laboratory Tests
  Not defined at present.

CAUTION
  1. This drug should be used ONLY AFTER a careful assessment by a qualified specialist is made. True attention deficit disorder requires careful assessment to differentiate it from behavior problems arising from family tensions or other conditions that do not require atomoxetine therapy.
  2. Some people remove this medicine from their bodies poorly (are poor metabolizers found in about 7% of the population). A lower dose may be prudent.
  3. The American Academy of Pediatricians has an important set of guidelines. Please remember that these are guidelines and therapy must still be

individualized. The guidelines can be found at *www.pediatrics.org* (see also Sources and American Academy of Pediatrics).

4. Careful dose adjustments on an individual basis are mandatory.

Precautions for Use

By Infants and Children: Safety and effectiveness for those under 6 years of age are not established. See Poor Metabolizer note above. If methylphenidate is not beneficial in managing an attention deficit disorder after a trial of 1 month, it should be stopped. Specific guidelines for this medicine are not established and are a clinical judgment. During ongoing use, monitor the child for ongoing benefits.

By Those Over 60 Years of Age: Not studied in this population.

▷ **Advisability of Use During Pregnancy**

Pregnancy Category: C. See Pregnancy Risk Categories at the back of this book.

Animal Studies: No birth defects found in mouse studies.

Human Studies: Adequate studies of pregnant women are not available. Ask your doctor for guidance.

Advisability of Use If Breast-Feeding

Presence of this drug in breast milk: Unknown in humans, yes in rats. Avoid drug or refrain from nursing.

Habit-Forming Potential: This drug is NOT a stimulant type medicine or amphetaminelike drug like methylphenidate (Ritalin). The abuse potential of atomoxetine has not been established.

Effects of Overdose: Experience with more than twice the maximum daily dose is not present. Headache, vomiting, and other extensions of expected increased norepinephrine levels would drive symptoms and management.

Possible Effects of Long-Term Use: Not fully defined.

Suggested Periodic Examinations While Taking This Drug (at physician's discretion)

Blood pressure and pulse measurements.

Height and weight.

Follow up evaluation for beneficial effects of treatment.

▷ **While Taking This Drug, Observe the Following**

Herbal Medicines or Minerals: Using St. John's wort, guarana, ma huang (now off the market), or kola while taking this medicine may result in unacceptable central nervous system stimulation.

Beverages: Avoid beverages prepared from meat or meat extracts. This drug may be taken with milk.

▷ *Alcohol:* Avoid beer, Chianti wines, and vermouth (may have high tyramine contents).

Tobacco Smoking: No interactions expected. I advise everyone to quit smoking.

▷ *Other Drugs*

Atomoxetine may *increase* the effects of

• albuterol (and other beta two agonists—see Drug Classes) and enhance their actions on the heart and blood vessels (cardiovascular system). Combined with caution

Atomoxetine *taken concurrently* with

• medicines that increase CYP 2D6 enzyme levels in the liver will blunt atomoxetine benefits. Medicines that decrease or inhibit CYP 2D6 (such as paroxetine—Paxil, fluoxetine—Prozac or quinidine—Quinaglute, others) may lead to toxic atomoxetine levels.

- monoamine oxidase (MAO) type A inhibitors (see Drug Classes) may cause a significant rise in blood pressure; avoid the concurrent use of these drugs.

▷ *Driving, Hazardous Activities:* This drug may cause dizziness or drowsiness. Restrict activities as necessary.

Aviation Note: The use of this drug **may be a disqualification** for piloting. Consult a designated Aviation Medical Examiner.

Exposure to Sun: No restrictions.

Discontinuation: A specific withdrawal syndrome has NOT been identified as yet. Talk to your doctor if you are considering stopping it for any reason.

ATORVASTATIN (a TOR va stat in)

Introduced: 1996 **Class:** Cholesterol-lowering agent, HMG-CoA reductase inhibitor **Prescription:** USA: Yes **Controlled Drug:** USA: No; Canada: No **Available as Generic:** No
Brand Name: Caduet [CD], Lipitor

```
BENEFITS versus RISKS
```

Possible Benefits	*Possible Risks*
REDUCTION OF TOTAL AND LDL CHOLESTEROL	Drug-induced hepatitis (without jaundice)—rare
DECREASED TRIGLYCERIDES	Drug-induced myositis (muscle inflammation)—rare
INCREASES HDL-C (GOOD CHOLESTEROL) IN PEOPLE WITH PRIMARY HYPER-CHOLESTEROLEMIA AND MIXED DYSLIPIDEMIA	Decreased coenzyme Q10
	Possible easing of benefit over time
MAY LOWER THE RISK OF REPEATED PROBLEMS (ISCHEMIC EVENTS) ONCE A PATIENT HAS HAD A SUDDEN CORONORY SYNDROME	
BENEFICIAL EFFECT ON C-REACTIVE PROTEIN LEVELS	
BENEFICIAL EFFECT ON THE PATTERN OF UNDESIRABLE CHOLESTEROL	
Newly approved to prevent heart attack, angina, or risk of heart (coronary) revascularization	

▷ **Principal Uses**

As a Single Drug Product: Uses currently included in FDA-approved labeling: (1) Treats high blood cholesterol (in people with Types IIa and IIb hypercholesterolemia) due to increased fractions of low-density lipoprotein (LDL) cholesterol; (2) also works in primary dysbetalipoproteinemia (Fredrickson Type III) and in patients with elevated serum triglycerides (Fredrickson Type IV). Used in conjunction with a cholesterol-lowering diet. Should not be used until an adequate trial of nondrug methods has proved to be ineffective. NCEP ATP 3 (see Glossary) recognizes therapeutic lifestyle changes (TLC) as very important; (3) also helps familial hypercholesterolemia; (4) approved to increase HDL-C (good cholesterol) in people with primary hypercholesterolemia and mixed dyslipidemia.

Other (unlabeled) generally accepted uses: (1) a *New England Journal of Medicine* study found that atorvastatin was as effective as getting an angioplasty when it was used to treat stable heart (coronary) artery disease; (2) prevention of coronary heart disease; (3) treats abnormal fat (lipid) changes caused by protease inhibitors; (4) may help prevent bone loss (osteoporosis) in type two diabetics and osteoporosis in general; (5) may help prevent clogging (restenosis) of tubes (stents) placed in coronary arteries; (6) starting atorvastatin quickly after a sudden coronary problem (see acute coronary syndromes in Glossary) may help lower the risk of circulatory events (recurrent ischemic events) based on results of the MIRACL trial; (7) ongoing use may help lower the risk of dementia (such as Alzheimer's disease); (8) one case-control study found a 20% reduction in cancer risk by "statin type" medicines. Further research is needed.

As a Combination Drug Product [CD]: Used in combination with a calcium channel blocker (amlodipine) in the Caduet form for people with abnormal cholesterol who also have high blood pressure. This attacks two different problems with the same pill.

How This Drug Works: Blocks a liver enzyme that starts making cholesterol. Lowers low-density lipoproteins (LDL), the cholesterol fraction thought to increase risk of coronary heart disease. Since the amount of cholesterol is reduced in the liver, the VLDL fraction may also be decreased. There is a growing body of evidence that "statins" also have beneficial changes on what is in the blood, blood flow and even the blood vessel walls themselves (some of this may account for benefits in decreasing Alzheimer's risk). Specific compounds or effects of platelet derived growth factor (PDGF), undesirable blood clotting via thrombin-antithrombin III, thrombomodulin, and other chemicals may be beneficially lowered or effects mitigated by statins.

▷ **Widely Used Guidelines That Involve This Medicine (representative sample):** Please look at the section at the very beginning of this profile called "Class." Next, turn to Table 22 and you will find guidelines listed by the class involved!

Available Dosage Forms and Strengths
    Tablets — 10 mg, 20 mg, 40 mg, 80 mg

▷ **Recommended Dosage Ranges** (Actual dosage and schedule must be determined for each patient individually.)

Infants and Children: Data are not available.

18 to 65 Years of Age:
    Cholesterol management: Patients are started on a typical low cholesterol diet (see *www.americanheart.org*). Atorvastatin dosing is started with 10 mg once daily. Patients who require more than a 45% decrease in LDL can be started at 40 mg once a day. The starting dose is increased (dose intensified) as needed and tolerated to a maximum of 80 mg daily. Lipid levels best rechecked within 2 to 4 weeks of starting or changing the dose. Some clinicians are studying weekly divided dosing, but conclusions are not yet made. A large study of people hospitalized after Acute Coronary Syndrome (ACS) compared 80 mg of atorvastatin to 40 mg of pravastatin and found that the 80 mg of atorvastatin gave greater protection against death or

major heart and blood vessel events than using the lower medicine dose (see Cannon, CP in Sources).

Acute Coronary Syndromes: (based on MIRACL data): 80 mg once a day is started 24–96 hours after the patient goes into the hospital (along with other medicines such as aspirin, beta blockers, nitrates, and heparin).

Over 65 Years of Age: Some research shows that usual doses may result in higher levels than seen in younger patients. It appears prudent that the lowest dose (10 mg) should be used and LDL-C levels be checked to guide any dose increases. Dose increases must be made after weighing the benefits and risks, mindful that any given dose may result in a higher than expected blood level.

Conditions Requiring Dosing Adjustments

Liver Function: Caution should be used in patients with liver compromise. In those with liver damage caused by alcohol, removal from the body has been prolonged. A 10-mg dose appears prudent. Like other HMG-CoA medicines, atorvastatin should not be given during active liver disease.

Kidney Function: The manufacturer does not recommend dosing changes.

▷ **Dosing Instructions:** The tablet may be crushed or split. Better taken on an empty stomach. Since cholesterol is made at the fastest rate between midnight and 5 a.m., many clinicians advise patients to take such medicines at bedtime. If you forget a dose, take it immediately unless it is almost time for your next dose. If your next dose is shortly due, skip the missed dose and just take the next scheduled dose. DO NOT double doses.

Usual Duration of Use: Use on a regular schedule for 2 to 4 weeks usually determines the effectiveness of this drug in reducing blood levels of total and LDL-C cholesterol. Increases in good cholesterol (HDL) may take longer. Use is usually ongoing. Long-term use (months to years) requires periodic physician evaluation and follow-up.

Typical Treatment Goals and Measurements (Outcomes and Markers)

Cholesterol: Current guidelines (National Cholesterol Education Program or NCEP) acknowledge diabetes as one of the conditions that increases risk of heart disease, modifying risk factors, therapeutic lifestyle changes (TLC), and recommending routine testing for all of the cholesterol fractions (lipoprotein profile) versus total cholesterol alone. Goals are: a total cholesterol of 200 mg/dL, and optimal bad cholesterol (LDL) of less than 100 mg/dL. Less than 70 mg/dL (see Grundy, S.M. in Sources) is a reasonable optional goal for very high risk patients (such as diabetics with acute coronary syndromes, etc.). 130–159 mg/dL as borderline high, 160 mg/dL as high and 190 mg/dL as very high. Did you know that there are at least five different kinds of "good cholesterol" or HDL? The "too low" measure for HDL is still 40 mg/dL, but in order to learn more about cholesterol types some doctors are starting to order lipid panels. There are at least seven different kinds of "bad cholesterol." The new panels tell doctors about the kinds of cholesterol that your body makes. This is important because some kinds (small dense particles) tend to stick to blood vessels (are highly atherogenic). Take your medicine to reach your goals! Two additional tests you will hear about will be electron beam computed tomography (EBCT) and CRP. EBCT is an important tool used in conjunction with laboratory studies. Findings show that even patients who meet cholesterol goals (particularly females over 55) can still be at significant cardiovascular risk. EBCT then defines risk by giving a calcium score and a "virtual tour" of the coronary arteries. C Reactive Protein or CRP is a relatively new and apparently independent predictor of heart disease risk. A large study (see Ridker, P.M. in

Sources) found that CRP predicted heart disease risk independently of bad cholesterol (low density lipoprotein). Talk to your doctor about this laboratory test and ask about current guidelines for who should be tested (see Pearson, T.A. in Sources).

Possible Advantages of This Drug: Studies indicate that drugs of this class (HMG-CoA reductase inhibitors) are more effective and better tolerated than other drugs currently available for reducing total and LDL-C cholesterol. Atorvastatin decreased LDL by up to 51% in one study. Another study showed this medicine to be as effective as angioplasty when used to treat coronary artery disease that is stable. This medicine is easily split, although pill splitting—certainly forced pill splitting is an area of controversy. At the time of this writing, the price is the same for a 20 or 80 mg tablet. Splitting tablets (get a pill splitter for accuracy) can lower costs a lot. One short-term outcome study of changing other statins to this medicine (therapeutic interchange of atorvastatin for simvastatin or pravastatin) found that both significant lowering of LDL and cost savings occurred.

This Drug Should Not Be Taken If
- you have had an allergic reaction to it previously.
- you have active liver disease or increased liver function tests that are unexplained.
- you are pregnant or are breast-feeding your infant.

Inform Your Physician Before Taking This Drug If
- you have previously taken and have not tolerated other drugs in this class such as: lovastatin (Mevacor), simvastatin (Zocor) (see Drug Classes).
- you have liver disease or impaired liver function.
- you have kidney disease.
- you are not using any method of birth control or you are planning pregnancy.
- you regularly consume substantial amounts of alcohol.
- you develop unexplained muscle weakness, pain, or tenderness.
- you have any type of chronic muscular disorder.
- goals were set by another doctor and have not been met using this medicine.

Possible Side Effects (natural, expected, and unavoidable drug actions)
None with usual doses.

Possible Adverse Effects (unusual, unexpected, and infrequent reactions)
If any of the following develop, consult your physician promptly for guidance.
Mild Adverse Effects
Allergic reaction: skin rash—infrequent.
Headache—infrequent to frequent, rare drowsiness.
Vision changes—case report.
Flu-like syndrome—infrequent.
Reversible hair loss (alopecia)—case report.
Diarrhea, constipation or gas (flatulence)—infrequent.
Muscle pain (myalgia)—infrequent with 20-mg dose (tell your doctor right away if this happens).
Serious Adverse Effects
Allergic reactions: not reported as yet.
Neuropathy—reported for a different member of this class.
Marked and persistent abnormal liver function tests (with or without jaundice)—case reports to rare.

Lowered blood platelets (thrombocytopenia)—rare.

Acute myositis (muscle pain and tenderness)—rare to infrequent with 10- to 80-mg doses.

Rhabdomyolysis with sudden kidney failure—rare with HMG-CoA medicines.

Roughly sixty cases of short-term memory loss (atorvastatin [23], pravastatin [1] and simvastatin [36] have been made.

Possible Effects on Sexual Function: Case reports of impotence.

Possible Delayed Adverse Effects: Increased liver enzymes. Decreased coenzyme Q10 (co-Q10 or ubiquinone).

Natural Diseases or Disorders That May Be Activated by This Drug
Latent liver disease.

Possible Effects on Laboratory Tests
Blood total cholesterol, LDL cholesterol and triglyceride levels: decreased. HDL: increased.

CAUTION
1. If pregnancy occurs while taking this drug, stop drug immediately and call your doctor.
2. Report promptly any development of unexplained muscle pain or tenderness, especially if accompanied by fever or weakness (malaise).
3. Report promptly the development of altered or impaired vision so that appropriate evaluation can be made.
4. If liver enzymes (ALT or AST) increase to more than three times the upper limit of normal and persist, the dose should be lowered and/or the medicine should be stopped.
5. A chart review showed a trend of peak benefit in lowering LDL. Some 220 days after peak benefits were achieved, an increase in LDL of about 15% and plateau of benefit. One source concluded that this may represent a tachyphylaxis.

Precautions for Use
By Infants and Children: Safety and effectiveness for those under 18 years of age not established.
By Those Over 60 Years of Age: Blood levels for those over 65 may be higher than those reached by the same dose in younger people.

▷ **Advisability of Use During Pregnancy**
Pregnancy Category: X. See Pregnancy Risk Categories at the back of this book.
Animal Studies: Rat studies reveal decreased pup survival and maturity with high-dose studies.
Human Studies: Adequate studies of pregnant women are not available.
This drug should be avoided during entire pregnancy.

Advisability of Use If Breast-Feeding
Presence of this drug in breast milk: Yes, in rats; expected in humans.
Avoid drug or refrain from nursing.

Habit-Forming Potential: None.

Effects of Overdose: Increased indigestion, stomach distress, nausea, diarrhea with other HMG-CoA medicines.

Possible Effects of Long-Term Use: Abnormal liver function tests. Decreased coenzyme Q10 (co-Q10 or ubiquinone). Loss of beneficial effects—reported with some statin type medicines.

Suggested Periodic Examinations While Taking This Drug (at physician's discretion)

Blood cholesterol studies: total cholesterol, HDL and LDL fractions. This may be especially important with this medicine as one retrospective chart review appeared to show a tachyphylaxis.

Liver function tests before treatment, at 12 weeks (the same for any dose increases) and then semiannually (every 6 months) thereafter. If the ALT or AST increases to more than three times the upper limit of normal and persist, the dose should be lowered and or the drug stopped. Ask your doctor for guidance.

Checks of the pattern of HDL and LDL (cholesterol subtypes). This helps the clinician determine how well cholesterol is being taken back to the liver (reverse cholesterol transport by HDL) and how likely the cholesterol that your body makes is to stick to blood vessels (small particles are highly atherogenic).

C-reactive Protein (CRP).

Author's Note: A related medicine called cerivastatin (Baycol) was removed from the market because of liver changes. At the time of this writing, the FDA has not asked for more frequent checks of liver function for atorvastatin.

Electron beam computed tomography (EBCT) can help predict silent ischemia and other problems with blood vessels that supply the heart itself. This also may help define the results (outcomes) you are getting from this medicine.

▷ **While Taking This Drug, Observe the Following**

Foods: Follow a standard low-cholesterol diet. Your doctor may also recommend some specific foods such as increased vegetables or functional foods such as Benecol. Three well-designed studies found that both in women and men and before and after a heart attack, people who ate more fish (2–4 servings a week) appeared to avoid heart disease. Additionally putting supplements containing Omega 3 polyunsaturated fatty acids (PUFA) into the diet also appeared to protect against abnormal heart rhythms and sudden death from heart attack. Increasing oat bran in the diet may be of additional help in lowering cholesterol, but can decrease the amount of medicine that gets into your body. Take oat bran two hours before atorvastatin or four to six hours after. Your doctor may also recommend increasing B vitamins. See Tables 19 and 20 about lifestyle changes and risk factors you can fix!

Herbal Medicines or Minerals: No data exist from well-designed clinical studies about garlic and atorvastatin combinations and cannot presently be recommended. Additionally, garlic may inhibit blood clotting (platelet) aggregation—something to consider if you are already taking a platelet inhibitor. The FDA has allowed one dietary supplement called Cholestin to continue to be sold. This preparation actually contains lovastatin. Since use of two HMG-CoA inhibitors may increase risk of rhabdomyolysis or myopathy, the combination is NOT advised. Some products containing plant sterols (Benecol) may be useful as complementary care. Soy (milk, tofu, etc.) contains phytoestrogens that have led to an FDA-approved health claim for reducing risk of heart disease (if they have at least 6.25 grams of soy protein per serving). Substituting soy for some of the meat in your diet can help avoid cardiovascular problems. Lastly, because atorvastatin can deplete coenzyme Q10, supplementation may be needed. Policosanol (a supplement derived from sugar cane) has not been studied with atorvastatin, but does lower cholesterol. Talk to your doctor before adding any supplements.

Beverages: DO NOT take this medicine with grapefruit juice. Excessive blood levels and increased risk of muscle damage may occur. May be taken with water or milk.

▷ *Alcohol:* Excessive alcohol not recommended.

Tobacco Smoking: No interactions expected. I advise everyone to quit smoking.

▷ *Other Drugs*

Atorvastatin may ***increase*** the effects of

- clofibrate (Atromid-S) and other fibric acid derivatives—has been associated with increased risk of muscle damage (rhabdomyolysis).

Atorvastatin ***taken concurrently*** with

- amprenavir (Agenerase) and ritonavir (Norvir), saquinavir (Invirase), atazanavir (Reyataz) and perhaps other protease inhibitors may increase atorvastatin levels and the risk of muscle damage (myopathy).
- antacids decreases the amount of atorvastatin that gets into your body.
- azole antifungals (such as itraconazole or Sporanox) may increase the risk for muscle damage (myopathy).
- birth control pills (oral contraceptives) may increase the levels of the contraceptives (certain kinds) and may increase risk of adverse effects.
- clopidogrel (Plavix) may blunt the benefits of clopidogrel. This is a new drug interaction. The degree of clinical effect of this interaction is not presently known. Some later data appears to call this interaction into question. In any case, it appears prudent that testing of platelet aggregation be undertaken if these medicines must be combined. If this is not possible, pravastatin (Pravachol) or rosuvastatin (Crestor) should be considered as they do not use the same liver pathway.
- colesevelam (Welchol) results in better lowering of LDL-C.
- colestipol (Colestid) results in lowered atorvastatin blood levels, but better lowering of LDL-C.
- cyclosporine (Sandimmune) may increase the risk for myopathy.
- digoxin (Lanoxin, others) can increase digoxin levels (and possibly lead to toxic effects).
- erythromycin (and perhaps other macrolide antibiotics) may increase the risk for myopathy.
- ezetimibe (Zetia) increases beneficial effects on cholesterol.
- fluconazole (Diflucan) or itraconazole (Sporanox) or ketoconazole (Nizoral) will increase risk of myopathy. Extreme caution is advised.
- fosphenytoin (Cerebyx) and phenytoin (Dilantin) may blunt atorvastatin therapeutic effects.
- gemfibrozil (Lopid) may increase the risk of muscle damage (myopathy).
- medicines that change cytochrome P450 3A4 (inhibitors will increase atorvastatin levels and inducers will blunt atorvastatin therapeutic effects).
- nefazodone (Serzone) may lead to atorvastatin toxicity.
- niacin (various) may increase the risk for myopathy. Niacin may also increase homocysteine levels—a risk factor for heart disease.
- oral contraceptive (norethindrone and ethinyl estradiol) level increases are likely. Increased monitoring for adverse effects is prudent.
- quinupristin/dalfopristin (Synercid) may increase the risk for myopathy by increasing atorvastatin blood levels.

▷ *Driving, Hazardous Activities:* This drug may cause drowsiness. Restrict activities as necessary.

Aviation Note: The use of this drug ***may be a disqualification*** for piloting. Consult a designated Aviation Medical Examiner.

Exposure to Sun: No restrictions.

Occurrence of Unrelated Illness: Call your doctor if another physician (such as a specialist) diagnoses a sudden liver problem.

Discontinuation: Do not stop this drug without your doctor's knowledge and help. There may be a significant increase in blood cholesterol levels if this medicine is stopped. Patients who have acute coronary syndromes or ACS (such as unstable angina, heart attack [non-p; Q-wave myocardial infarction], and Q-wave myocardial infarction) were reviewed as part of the Platelet Receptor Inhibitor in Ischemic Syndrome Management (PRISM) study. It was found that pretreatment with statin type medicines (HMG-CoA reductase inhibitors such as the medicine in this profile) significantly lowered risk during the first 30 days after ACS symptoms started. Talk with your doctor BEFORE stopping any statin type medicine.

AURANOFIN (aw RAY noh fin)

Introduced: 1976   **Class:**   Antiarthritic   **Prescription:**   USA: Yes   **Controlled Drug:**   USA: No; Canada: No   **Available as Generic:** Yes

Brand Name: Ridaura

BENEFITS versus RISKS	
Possible Benefits	*Possible Risks*
REDUCTION OF JOINT PAIN, TENDERNESS, AND SWELLING IN ACTIVE, SEVERE RHEUMATOID ARTHRITIS	SIGNIFICANTLY REDUCED LEVELS OF RED AND WHITE BLOOD CELLS AND BLOOD PLATELETS
Effective when taken by mouth	LIVER DAMAGE WITH JAUNDICE
	Diarrhea
	Ulcerative colitis
	Skin rash
	Mouth sores
	Kidney toxicity (protein in the urine)
	Lung damage

Author's Note: Given the FDA approval of DMARDS (see Glossary), this profile has been shortened to make room for more widely used medicines.

AZATHIOPRINE (ay za THI oh preen)

Introduced: 1965   **Class:**   Antiarthritic, immunosuppressive   **Prescription:**   USA: Yes   **Controlled Drug:** USA: No; Canada: No   **Available as Generic:**   Yes

Brand Name: Imuran, ✚Med-azathioprine, ✚Riva-azathioprine

```
┌─────────────────────────────────────────────────────────────┐
│                    BENEFITS versus RISKS                      │
│     Possible Benefits                    Possible Risks       │
│ PREVENTION OF REJECTION IN      UNACCEPTABLE ADVERSE          │
│   KIDNEY (RENAL) TRANSPLANT       EFFECTS IN 15% OF USERS     │
│ Reduction of joint pain in active,  REDUCED LEVELS OF WHITE   │
│   severe, resistant rheumatoid      BLOOD CELLS               │
│   arthritis                       REDUCED LEVELS OF RED BLOOD │
│                                     CELLS AND PLATELETS       │
│                                   LIVER DAMAGE WITH JAUNDICE  │
│                                   POSSIBLE INCREASED RISK OF  │
│                                     MALIGNANCY                │
└─────────────────────────────────────────────────────────────┘
```

▷ **Principal Uses**
   As a Single Drug Product: Uses currently included in FDA-approved labeling:
   (1) Helps prevent transplanted kidney rejection (adjunctive use); (2) also
   used in active, severe rheumatoid arthritis (in adults) failing conventional
   treatment.
   Other (unlabeled) generally accepted uses: (1) Used to treat actinic dermatitis.

How This Drug Works: It impairs metabolism of purines, DNA, and RNA. This
   blunts the immune reaction responsible for rheumatoid arthritis, lupus,
   and erythematosus.

▷ **Widely Used Guidelines That Involve This Medicine (representative sample):** Please look at the section at the very beginning of this profile called
   "Class." Next, turn to Table 22 and you will find guidelines listed by the
   class involved!

Available Dosage Forms and Strengths
   Injection — 100 mg per 20-mL vial
   Tablets — 50 mg

▷ **Usual Adult Dosage Ranges:** *As immunosuppressant:* 3–5 mg per kg of body
   mass daily, 1 to 3 days before transplantation surgery; for ongoing postoperative use—1–3 mg per kg of body mass daily, but the amount needed to
   have minimal toxicity yet prevent rejection will vary from patient to
   patient. Careful follow up is required.

▷ **While Taking This Drug, Observe the Following**
   Foods: No restrictions and may help stomach upset.
   Herbal Medicines or Minerals: Some patients use echinacea to attempt to boost
   their immune systems. Unfortunately, use of echinacea is not recommended
   in people with damaged immune systems. This herb may also actually
   weaken any immune system if it is used too often or for too long a time.
   Beverages: No restrictions. May be taken with milk.
▷ *Alcohol:* No interactions expected, but excessive drinking will also blunt the
   immune system.
   Tobacco Smoking: No interactions expected. I advise everyone to quit smoking.
   Marijuana Smoking: May contain infectious agents (such as toxoplasmosis)
   which may be more likely to cause infections in a person with a blunted
   immune system.
▷ *Other Drugs*
   Azathioprine may ***decrease*** the effects of
   • certain muscle relaxants (gallamine, pancuronium, tubocurarine) and
     make it necessary to increase their dosage.
   • oral anticoagulants (warfarin, etc.) and requires increased doses.

The following drug may *increase* the effects of azathioprine:
- allopurinol (Zyloprim)—may increase its activity and toxicity and make it necessary to reduce its dosage.

Azathioprine *taken concurrently* with
- ACE inhibitors (see Drug Classes) such as captopril or enalapril may cause severe white blood cell count lowering or anemia.
- cotrimoxazole (Bactrim, others) can cause severe lowering of white blood cell counts.
- cyclosporine (Sandimmune, others) may lead to decreased cyclosporine levels, requiring more frequent blood level checks and dosing adjustments.
- prednisolone will result in lower prednisolone blood levels and risk of decreased therapeutic benefit.
- vaccines (live—various) may result in abnormal patient responses to the vaccines and risk of infection by the live vaccine itself.
- warfarin (Coumadin) may result in decreased anticoagulant effectiveness.

▷ *Driving, Hazardous Activities:* No restrictions.
Aviation Note: The use of this drug *may be a disqualification* for piloting. Consult a designated Aviation Medical Examiner.
Exposure to Sun: No restrictions.
Discontinuation: A gradual reduction in dosage is preferable. Consult your physician for a withdrawal schedule.
Author's Note: Information in this profile has been truncated to make room for more widely used medicines.

AZITHROMYCIN (a zith roh MY sin)

See the macrolide antibiotics profile for further information.

BACAMPICILLIN (bak am pi SIL in)

See the penicillins profile for further information.

BECLOMETHASONE (be kloh METH a sohn)

Introduced: 1976 **Class:** Antiasthmatic, cortisonelike drugs **Prescription:** USA: Yes **Controlled Drug:** USA: No; Canada: No **Available as Generic:** No

Brand Names: ✽Apo-Beclomethasone-AQ, ✽Beclodisk, ✽Beclóforte, Beclovent, ✽Beclovent Rotacaps, ✽Beclovent Rotahaler, Beconase AQ Nasal Spray, Beconase Nasal Inhaler, ✽Med-Beclomethasone-AQ, ✽Nu-Beclomethasone, ✽Propaderm, ✽Propaderm-C, QVAR, Vancenase AQ Nasal Spray, Vancenase Nasal Inhaler, Vanceril

```
┌─────────────────────────────────────────────────────────────────┐
│                      BENEFITS versus RISKS                        │
│       Possible Benefits                    Possible Risks         │
│  EFFECTIVE RELIEF OF ALLERGIC       FUNGUS INFECTIONS OF THE      │
│     RHINITIS                           MOUTH AND THROAT           │
│  EFFECTIVE CONTROL OF SEVERE,       Localized areas of "allergic" │
│     CHRONIC ASTHMA                     pneumonia                  │
│  HELPS PREVENT NASAL POYLPS         Changes in lining of the nose │
│                                        (nasal mucosa)             │
│                                     Increased cataract risk       │
│                                     Possible osteoporosis         │
└─────────────────────────────────────────────────────────────────┘
```

▷ **Principal Uses**

As a Single Drug Product: Uses currently included in FDA-approved labeling: (1) Bronchial asthma in people who don't have sufficient response to bronchodilators and need cortisone-like drugs for asthma control; (2) prevents nasal polyp return after surgical removal; (3) treats seasonal and perennial rhinitis in children and adults (AQ nasal forms).

Other (unlabeled) generally accepted uses: (1) Helps lung disease (bronchopulmonary dysplasia) allowing smaller daily prednisone doses; (2) helps hoarseness seen in LE and juvenile rheumatoid arthritis.

How This Drug Works: It increases cyclic AMP, thus increasing epinephrine, which opens bronchial tubes and fights asthma. Also reduces local lung inflammation in the respiratory tract.

▷ **Widely Used Guidelines That Involve This Medicine (representative sample):** Please look at the section at the very beginning of this profile called "Class." Next, turn to Table 22 and you will find guidelines listed by the class involved!

Available Dosage Forms and Strengths

Inhalant — 17 g (50 mcg)
Nasal inhaler — 16.8 g (42 or 82 mcg each)
Nasal spray — 0.042%, 42 mcg and 84 mcg per spray (52 mcg in Canada)
Oral inhaler — 16.8 g (200 doses of 42 mcg each, 50 mcg in Canada)
Rotacaps (Canada) — 100- and 200-mcg capsules
Topical lotion (Canada) — 0.025%

▷ **Usual Adult Dosage Ranges**

Infants and Children: Data are not available for infants. Children 6–12 years old may receive: Nasal spray—one (42 mcg) dose in each nostril twice a day. Oral inhalation (42 mcg)—one to two inhalations, three or four times a day depending on the response. Some clinicians use 4 inhalations twice daily. Oral inhalation (double strength—84 mcg)—2 inhalations twice a day. Maximum is 5 inhalations (420 mcg for Vanceril Double Strength).

18 to 65 Years of Age: Nasal spray—one to two sprays (42–84 mcg) in each nostril twice daily. Oral inhaler (double strength)—two inhalations (of 84 mcg) twice daily. For severe asthma—6 to 8 inhalations daily. Nasal polyp prevention after surgery: 42 or 84 mcg in each nostril twice a day (Beconase AQ form).

Those Over 65 Years of Age: Doses similar to those in younger patients have been effective and safe. In some cases, oral-steroid-dependent patients have been able to slowly taper and then stop oral steroids while taking beclomethasone.

Note: Actual dose and schedule must be determined for each patient individually.

Conditions Requiring Dosing Adjustments

Liver Function: Use with caution in patients with liver compromise.

Kidney Function: No adjustments in dosing expected to be needed.

▷ **Dosing Instructions:** May be used without regard to eating. Instructions are supplied with this product—read them carefully in order to get the most benefit from this medicine. Shake the inhaler well before you use it. Rinse the mouth and throat (gargle) with water thoroughly after each inhalation. If you forget a dose: Use the inhaler as soon as possible. DO NOT double doses.

Usual Duration of Use: Regular use for 1 to 3 weeks is usually needed to see this drug's effectiveness in relieving severe, chronic allergic rhinitis and in controlling severe, chronic asthma. Up to 2 weeks may be needed to relieve rhinitis by nasal inhalation. If signs and symptoms have not improved in 21 days, beclomethasone should be discontinued. Long-term use must be physician-supervised. See your doctor regularly.

Typical Treatment Goals and Measurements (Outcomes and Markers)

Asthma: This medicine is NOT useful in a sudden asthma attack, but is used to decrease the severity and frequency of attacks. Some clinicians also use the number of times a rescue inhaler is used as another clinical benchmark. FEV1 (a lung function test) is widely used to check results when available. While using this medicine—call your doctor immediately if it becomes less beneficial (helps less than it used to).

Possible Advantages of This Drug: Inhaled beclomethasone does not suppress or causes minimal suppression of the HPA axis versus medicines such as fluticasone (which causes greater suppression than other agents).

Currently a "Drug of Choice"

The "nose" (intranasal) form is a first choice in allergic rhinitis.

▷ **This Drug Should Not Be Taken If**
- you have had an allergic reaction to any form of this drug.
- you are having severe acute asthma or status asthmaticus (requires more intense and prompt treatment).
- other antiasthmatic drugs can control your asthma that are not related to cortisone.
- you have a form of nonallergic bronchitis with asthmatic features.

▷ **Inform Your Physician Before Taking This Drug If**
- you take or recently took any cortisone-related drug (including ACTH by injection) for any reason (see Drug Classes).
- you have a history of tuberculosis of the lungs.
- you have chronic bronchitis or bronchiectasis.
- you think you have an active infection of any kind, especially a respiratory infection.
- you have recently been exposed to chickenpox or other viral illnesses.
- you are prone to nosebleeds (epistaxis) (nasal forms).
- you are unsure how much to take or how often to take this drug.

Possible Side Effects (natural, expected, and unavoidable drug actions)

Fungus infections (thrush) of the mouth and throat. Headache. Changes in ability to taste.

▷ **Possible Adverse Effects** (unusual, unexpected, and infrequent reactions)
  If any of the following develop, consult your physician promptly for guidance.
  Mild Adverse Effects
  Allergic reaction: skin rash—rare.
  Dryness of mouth, hoarseness, sore throat, cough—possible.
  Nosebleeds (epistaxis)—infrequent.
  May decrease growth rate in children—possible.
  Serious Adverse Effects
  Allergic reaction: localized areas of "allergic" pneumonitis (lung inflammation), angioedema-possible.
  Bronchospasm, asthmatic wheezing—rare.
  Shrinking of the nasal tissues (nasal atrophy)—possible.
  Yeast infections (up to 41%)—frequent.
  Severe chicken pox—case reports with intranasal form.
  Increased risk of cataracts with long-term (chronic) use—possible.
  Suppression of the adrenal gland (HFA axis)—possible in sensitive individuals.
  Increased pressure in the head (pseudotumor cerebri)—possible.
  Osteoporosis (any corticosteroid can cause this)—possible.

▷ **Possible Effects on Sexual Function:** None reported.

Natural Diseases or Disorders That May Be Activated by This Drug
  Cortisone-related drugs having systemic effects impair immunity and lead to reactivation of "healed" or dormant tuberculosis. People with a history of tuberculosis must be watched closely while using this drug.

Possible Effects on Laboratory Tests
  Blood cortisol levels: decreased.
  Bone mineral density: possibly decreased with chronic use although much less likely than with systemic forms.

CAUTION
  1. This drug should not be relied upon for immediate relief of acute asthma.
  2. If you required cortisone-like drugs *before* starting this inhaler, you may again require a cortisone-like drug if you are injured, have an infection or need surgery.
  3. If severe asthma returns while using this drug, call your doctor immediately. Cortisone-like drugs may be required.
  4. Carry an ID card saying that you have used (if true) cortisone-related drugs in the past year.
  5. Wait 5 to 10 minutes after using a bronchodilator inhaler such as epinephrine, isoetharine or isoproterenol (which should be used first) before this drug. This permits greater penetration of beclomethasone into the lung. The time between inhalations also reduces risk of adverse propellant effects.
  6. This drug does NOT replace systemic steroids, but may allow dosage decreases in some patients.
  7. If this drug is used long-term, a bone mineral density test before treatment and every two years is prudent.
  8. Unlike other corticosteroids, reports of osteonecrosis (avascular necrosis or aseptic necrosis) have not been made for this medicine. Caution is prudent, and patients should report any unexplained joint (such as knee, hip, or shoulder) pain to their doctor.

Precautions for Use

By *Infants and Children:* Safety and effectiveness for use of the nasal inhaler or oral inhaler by those under 6 years of age has not been established. Maximum daily dose in children 6 to 12 years of age varies with the products being used.

By *Those Over 60 Years of Age:* People with bronchiectasis should be watched closely for the development of lung infections.

▷ **Advisability of Use During Pregnancy**

Pregnancy Category: C. See Pregnancy Risk Categories at the back of this book.

Animal Studies: Mouse, rat, and rabbit studies reveal significant birth defects due to this drug.

Human Studies: Adequate studies of pregnant women are not available.

Avoid drug during the first 3 months. Use infrequently and only as clearly needed during the last 6 months.

Advisability of Use If Breast-Feeding

Presence of this drug in breast milk: Probably yes.

Avoid drug or refrain from nursing.

Habit-Forming Potential: With recommended dosage, a state of functional dependence (see Glossary) is not likely to develop. There have been a small number of cases reported where the aerosol was abused for the fluorocarbon propellants.

Effects of Overdose: Indications of cortisone excess (due to systemic absorption)—fluid retention, flushing of the face, stomach irritation, nervousness.

Suggested Periodic Examinations While Taking This Drug (at physician's discretion)

Inspection of nose, mouth, and throat for fungus infection.

Inspection of the nose tissues for abnormal nose changes (nasal atrophy).

Assessment of adrenal function in people using cortisone-related drugs for an extended time prior to this drug.

Lung X-ray if a prior history of tuberculosis.

Measures of bone mineral density (DEXA or PDEXA) and cataract check.

▷ **While Taking This Drug, Observe the Following**

Foods: No specific restrictions beyond those advised by your physician.

Herbal Medicines or Minerals: Fir or pine needle oil should NOT be used by asthmatics. Ephedra alone does carry a German Commission E monograph indication for asthma treatment. If you are allergic to plants in the Asteraceae family (aster, chrysanthemum, daisy, or ragweed), you may also be allergic to echinacea, chamomile, feverfew, and St. John's wort. Talk to your doctor BEFORE adding it to any medicines that you already take.

Beverages: No specific restrictions.

▷ *Alcohol:* No interactions expected.

Tobacco Smoking: Smoking can reduce the benefits of this drug. I advise everyone to quit smoking.

▷ *Other Drugs*

The following drugs may *increase* the effects of beclomethasone:

• some antiepileptic medicines such as phenytoin (Dilantin)—may increase risk of osteoporosis.

• flunisolide (Nasalide).

• inhalant bronchodilators—epinephrine, isoetharine, isoproterenol.

• oral bronchodilators—aminophylline, ephedrine, terbutaline, theophylline, etc.

Beclomethasone *taken concurrently* with
* alendronate (Fosamax) helps prevent steroid-induced osteoporosis.

▷ *Driving, Hazardous Activities:* No restrictions.

Aviation Note: The use of this drug and the disorder for which this drug is prescribed *may be disqualifications* for piloting. Consult a designated Aviation Medical Examiner.

Exposure to Sun: No restrictions.

Occurrence of Unrelated Illness: Acute infections, serious injuries, and surgery can create an urgent need for cortisone-related drugs. Call your doctor immediately in the event of new illness or injury.

Discontinuation: If this drug has made it possible to reduce or stop ongoing cortisonelike drugs, do not stop this drug abruptly. If you must stop this drug, call your doctor. You may need to resume cortisone medicines.

Special Storage Instructions: Store at room temperature. Avoid exposure to temperatures above 120 degrees F (49 degrees C). Do not store or use this inhaler near heat or open flame. Protect from light.

BENAZEPRIL (ben AY ze pril)

Class: ACE inhibitor, antihypertensive

Please see the new angiotensin converting enzyme (ACE) inhibitor family profile for more information.

BENZTROPINE (BENZ troh peen)

Introduced: 1954   **Class:**   Anti-Parkinsonism, atropine-like drugs
Prescription: USA: Yes   **Controlled Drug:**   USA: No; Canada: No
Available as Generic: USA: Yes; Canada: Yes

Brand Names: ♣Apo-Benztropine, ♣Bensylate, Cogentin ♣PMS Benztropine

---

BENEFITS versus RISKS

Possible Benefits	*Possible Risks*
PARTIAL RELIEF OF SYMPTOMS OF PARKINSON'S DISEASE RELIEF OF DRUG-INDUCED EXTRAPYRAMIDAL REACTIONS	Atropine-like side effects: blurred vision, dry mouth, constipation, impaired urination Toxic psychosis—rare Tardive dyskinesia—rare

---

▷ **Principal Uses**

As a Single Drug Product: Uses currently included in FDA-approved labeling: (1) Used in combination to treat all types of Parkinsonism (if relief is inadequate supplemental medicines are used); (2) controls Parkinsonian reactions from many antipsychotic drugs; (3) eases Parkinsonian symptoms after encephalitis.

Other (unlabeled) generally accepted uses: (1) helps sweating caused by other drugs (such as venlafaxine); (2) can help drooling (sialorrhea) in developmentally disabled patients.

Author's Note: Some clinicians are using higher-dose vitamin E for decreasing Parkinsonian symptoms seen with some antipsychotic medicines. Some use it in combination with benztropine.

How This Drug Works: Restores a more normal balance of two brain chemicals (acetylcholine and dopamine), thereby decreasing Parkinsonism symptoms.

▷ **Widely Used Guidelines That Involve This Medicine (representative sample):** Please look at the section at the very beginning of this profile called "Class." Next, turn to Table 22 and you will find guidelines listed by the class involved!

Available Dosage Forms and Strengths
   Injection — 1 mg/mL, 2 mg/mL
   Tablets — 0.5 mg, 1 mg, 2 mg

▷ **Usual Adult Dosage Ranges:** *For Parkinson's disease:* 1–2 mg daily, taken in a single dose by mouth at bedtime. *For drug-induced Parkinsonian (extrapyramidal) reactions:* 1 to 4 mg once or twice a day. The total daily dose should not exceed 6 mg. *For Parkinson's symptoms after encephalitis:* Starting doses of 2 mg/day are used. May then be increased as needed or tolerated to 4 to 6 mg per day.
   Note: Actual dosage and schedule must be determined for each patient individually.

Conditions Requiring Dosing Adjustments
   Liver Function: Use with **Caution** in patients with impaired liver function.
   Kidney Function: **Caution:** Decreased kidney function may lead to an increased blood level and an increased risk of adverse effects.

▷ **Dosing Instructions:** May be taken with or following food to reduce stomach irritation. Tablet may be crushed. If you forget a dose, take the missed dose as soon as possible. If it is nearly time for your next dose, skip the missed dose and continue benztropine on its regular schedule. DO NOT double doses.

Usual Duration of Use: Regular use for 2 to 4 weeks usually needed to see peak benefit relieving symptoms of Parkinsonism. Long-term use (months to years) requires physician supervision.

Typical Treatment Goals and Measurements (Outcomes and Markers)
   Parkinson's: This medicine helps treat symptoms of Parkinson's disease, but does NOT halt its progression and combination therapy is often required. Usual goals are to decrease symptom severity and improve quality of life. Regular physician assessment is required as symptoms change or exacerbate.

▷ **This Drug Should Not Be Taken If**
   • you have had an allergic reaction to it.
   • you are a child under 3 years of age.
   • you have tardive dyskinesia.
   • you have narrow-angle glaucoma (untreated).

▷ **Inform Your Physician Before Taking This Drug If**
   • you have had an unfavorable reaction to atropine or atropine-like drugs.
   • you have glaucoma or myasthenia gravis.
   • you have heart disease or high blood pressure.
   • you have a history of liver or kidney disease.
   • you have difficulty emptying the urinary bladder, especially if due to an enlarged prostate gland.

- you are taking, or took in the past 2 weeks, any monoamine oxidase (MAO) type A inhibitor (see Drug Classes).
- you take prescription or nonprescription medicines not discussed when benztropine was prescribed for you.
- you are unsure how much to take or how often to take it.
- you will be exposed to extreme heat for extended periods, such as some iron smelters or those who must work outdoors in tropical climates.
- you have a history of bowel obstructions.

Possible Side Effects (natural, expected, and unavoidable drug actions)

> Nervousness, blurring of vision, dryness of mouth, constipation, impaired urination. (These often subside as drug use continues.) Heat intolerance.

▷ **Possible Adverse Effects** (unusual, unexpected, and infrequent reactions)

> **If any of the following develop, consult your physician promptly for guidance.**

Mild Adverse Effects

> Allergic reaction: skin rashes—rare.
> Headache, dizziness, drowsiness, muscle cramps—possible.
> Indigestion, nausea, vomiting—reported.
> Fast heart rate (tachycardia)—infrequent.
> Memory problems—possible.

Serious Adverse Effects

> Idiosyncratic reactions: abnormal behavior, confusion, delusions, hallucinations, toxic psychosis—case reports.
> Tardive dyskinesia—case reports.
> Dystonia—rare.
> Bowel obstruction—case reports.
> Abnormal temperature (hyperthermia)—case reports.

▷ **Possible Effects on Sexual Function:** Reversal of male impotence due to the use of fluphenazine (a phenothiazine antipsychotic drug).

> Male infertility (0.5 to 6 mg per day).
> May help treat priapism.

Natural Diseases or Disorders That May Be Activated by This Drug

> Latent glaucoma, latent myasthenia gravis.

Possible Effects on Laboratory Tests

> Prolactin: may be increased (especially if taken with haloperidol).

CAUTION

1. Many over-the-counter (OTC) drugs for allergies, colds, and coughs should NOT be combined with benztropine. Ask your doctor or pharmacist for help.
2. This drug may aggravate tardive dyskinesia (see Glossary). Ask your physician for guidance.
3. If you exercise or use a sauna or hot tub, caution is advised as this medicine will make you less able to sweat and your body may overheat.
4. If you develop a rash while taking this medicine, talk to your doctor (medicine should be discontinued if the dose is lowered and the rash continues).

Precautions for Use

By Infants and Children: Safety and effectiveness for those under 3 years of age not established. Children are especially susceptible to the atropine-like effects.

By Those Over 60 Years of Age: Small starting doses are prudent. Increased risk of confusion, nightmares, hallucinations, increased internal eye pressure (glaucoma), and impaired urination associated with prostate gland enlargement (prostatism).

▷ **Advisability of Use During Pregnancy**

Pregnancy Category: C. See Pregnancy Risk Categories at the back of this book.

Animal Studies: No data available.

Human Studies: Adequate studies of pregnant women are not available.

Avoid use if possible, especially close to delivery. This drug can impair the infant's intestinal tract following birth.

Advisability of Use If Breast-Feeding

Presence of this drug in breast milk: Unknown.

Ask your doctor for help.

Habit-Forming Potential: Occasional reports of anti-Parkinsonian drug abuse have been made. Sudden withdrawal of benztropine may lead to craving, restlessness, nervousness, and depression. Propranolol (20–80 mg three times daily) or diazepam (Valium, others) has been used to ease these symptoms.

Effects of Overdose: Weakness; drowsiness; stupor; impaired vision; rapid pulse; excitement; confusion; hallucinations; dry; hot skin; skin rash; dilated pupils.

Possible Effects of Long-Term Use: Increased internal eye pressure—possible glaucoma, especially in the elderly.

Suggested Periodic Examinations While Taking This Drug (at physician's discretion)

Measurement of internal eye pressure at regular intervals. Check of continued effectiveness of the drug itself.

▷ **While Taking This Drug, Observe the Following**

Foods: No restrictions.

Herbal Medicines or Minerals: See marijuana below. Additionally, talk to your doctor BEFORE adding any herbs to any medicines that you already take. Phenylalanine (200–500 mg daily) has been used by some clinicians to ease Parkinson's. Calabar bean (chop nut or ordeal bean) and octacosanol should be AVOIDED by people living with Parkinson's. Betel nut may impair benztropine benefits.

Beverages: No restrictions.

▷ *Alcohol:* Use caution. Alcohol may increase the sedative effects.

Tobacco Smoking: No interactions expected, but I advise everyone to quit smoking.

Marijuana Smoking: May increase heart rate to unacceptable levels. Avoid completely if this increased heart rate will be a problem for you.

▷ *Other Drugs*

Benztropine may *decrease* the effects of

• phenothiazines (Haloperidol, Thorazine, others).

The following drugs may *increase* the effects of benztropine:

• antihistamines may add to the dryness of mouth and throat.

• monoamine oxidase (MAO) type A inhibitor drugs may intensify all effects of this drug (see Drug Classes).

• tricyclic antidepressants (Elavil, etc.) may add to eye effects and further increase internal eye pressure (dangerous in glaucoma).

Benztropine *taken concurrently* with

• amantadine (Symmetrel) may cause increased confusion and possible hallucinations.

- belladonna (contains atropine, L-hyoscyamine and scopolamine) may cause increased risk of excessive anticholinergic side effects such as weakness, confusion and possible hallucinations.
- clozapine (Clozaril) can cause increased risk of elevated temperatures, neurological adverse effects and bowel obstruction (ileus).
- procainamide (Procanbid, etc.) may increase risk of heart conduction problems.

▷ *Driving, Hazardous Activities:* Drowsiness and dizziness may occur. Avoid hazardous activities until full effects and tolerance have been determined.

Aviation Note: The use of this drug **is a disqualification** for piloting. Consult a designated Aviation Medical Examiner.

Exposure to Sun: No restrictions.

Exposure to Heat: Use caution. This drug may reduce sweating, cause an increase in body temperature and increase risk of heatstroke.

Heavy Exercise or Exertion: Use caution. Avoid in hot environments.

Discontinuation: Do not stop this drug abruptly. Ask your doctor how to reduce the dose gradually.

BETAXOLOL (be TAX oh lohl)

Introduced: 1983 **Class:** Antihypertensive, beta-adrenergic blocker
Prescription: USA: Yes **Controlled Drug:** USA: No; Canada: No
Available as Generic: Yes (ophthalmic)

Brand Names: Betoptic, Betoptic-Pilo [CD], Betoptic-S, Kerlone, ✚Novo-Betaxolol

BENEFITS versus RISKS	
Possible Benefits	*Possible Risks*
EFFECTIVE, WELL-TOLERATED ANTIHYPERTENSIVE IN MILD TO MODERATE HIGH BLOOD PRESSURE	CONGESTIVE HEART FAILURE in advanced heart disease
EFFECTIVE TREATMENT OF CHRONIC, OPEN-ANGLE GLAUCOMA	Worsening of angina in coronary heart disease (abrupt withdrawal)
PROLONGATION OF LIFE AFTER HEART ATTACK	Masking of low blood sugar (hypoglycemia) in diabetes
TREATMENT OF EYE (OCULAR) HYPERTENSION	Provocation of bronchial asthma (with high doses)
	Rare anemia and low blood platelets (above risks for systemic form)

▷ **Principal Uses**

As a Single Drug Product: Uses currently included in FDA-approved labeling: Used to treat (1) mild to moderate high blood pressure (alone or combined with other antihypertensive drugs, such as diuretics); (2) chronic open-angle glaucoma (eyedrops); (3) ocular hypertension (ophthalmic forms); (4) Betoptic-Pilo—reduces elevated eye pressure in primary open-angle glaucoma who have failed Betoptic-S therapy.

Other (unlabeled) generally accepted uses: (1) The oral form may help decrease death (mortality) from a heart attack; (2) helps decrease incidence and severity of chest pain (angina); (3) can ease aggressive behavior or movement disorders in some psychiatric patients; (4) can treat selected cases of stuttering.

How This Drug Works: By blocking some sympathetic nervous system actions, it reduces heart rate and contraction force, lowers blood ejection pressure and reduces oxygen needed by the heart. Relaxes blood vessel walls, resulting in expansion and lower blood pressure. Reduces internal eye pressure.

▷ **Widely Used Guidelines That Involve This Medicine (representative sample):** Please look at the section at the very beginning of this profile called "Class." Next, turn to Table 22 and you will find guidelines listed by the class involved!

Available Dosage Forms and Strengths
Eyedrops (solution) — 2.8 mg/mL, 5.0 mg/mL, 5.6 mg/mL
Eyedrops (suspension) — 0.25%
— 0.25%/1.75% (Betoptic-Pilo)
Tablets — 10 mg, 20 mg

▷ **Usual Adult Dosage Ranges:**
Hypertension: Initially 10 mg once daily. Dose may be increased at intervals of 7 to 14 days as needed and tolerated up to 20 mg every 24 hours. Usual ongoing dose is 10 to 15 mg daily. Some people tolerate 40 mg, but had no further blood pressure effects. Total maximum is 20 mg daily.
For use in glaucoma: One or two drops of the 2.8 mg/mL solution or one drop of the 5.6 mg/mL twice daily.
Betoptic-Pilo (betaxolol/pilocarpine) used to lower eye pressure in primary open-angle glaucoma when Betoptic-S: Follow doctor and label instructions.
Note: Actual dose and schedule must be determined for each patient individually.

Conditions Requiring Dosing Adjustments
Liver Function: Use with caution; this drug is metabolized in the liver. Dose decreases not routinely needed.
Kidney Function: Starting dose is 5 mg. The dose is increased as needed and tolerated by 5 mg every 2 weeks for a maximum of 20 mg daily.

▷ **Dosing Instructions:** May be taken without regard to eating. The tablet may be crushed. Do not stop this drug abruptly. If you forget a dose: take it right away unless it's within 8 hours of your next regular dose. If it IS within 8 hours of the next dose, just take the scheduled dose. DO NOT double doses. Wash your hands with water and soap BEFORE using the eye drops. Talk to your doctor about how to use the drops. Ophthalmic suspension should be re-suspended (see package instructions) before instilling it in your eye. Many ophthalmologists want patients to use their index finger to pull out the lower eye lid to form a pocket, then drop the required number of drops into the pocket.

Usual Duration of Use: Regular use for 10 to 14 days usually needed to see this drug's effectiveness in lowering blood pressure. Long-term use determined by success in lowering blood pressure and response to overall treatment program (weight reduction, salt restriction, smoking cessation, etc.). See your doctor regularly. Use for glaucoma will be ongoing and may take two weeks to reach its maximum benefit.

Typical Treatment Goals and Measurements (Outcomes and Markers)

Blood Pressure: Guidelines (JNC VII) define normal blood pressure (BP) as **less than** 120/80 and **pre-hypertension** ranges from 120/80 to 139/89 and is intended to help your doctor encourage lifestyle changes (or in the case of people with a risk factor for high blood pressure, start treatment) much earlier—so that possible damage to blood vessels, your heart, kidneys, sexual potency, or eyes might be minimized or avoided altogether. Stage 1 hypertension: 140/90 to 159/99. Stage 2 hypertension equal to or greater than: 160/100 mm Hg. These guidelines also recommend that clinicians work with their patients to agree on the goals and a plan of treatment. The first-ever guidelines for blood pressure (hypertension) in African Americans recommends that MOST black patients be started on TWO antihypertensive medicines with the goal of lowering blood pressure to 130/80 for those with high risk for heart and blood vessel disease or with diabetes. The general target for diabetics is 130/80 and less than 125/75 for those who spill more than one gram of protein into their urine. Most clinicians try to achieve a BP that confers the best balance of lower cardiovascular risk and avoids the problem of too low a blood pressure. Blood pressure duration is generally increased with beneficial restriction of sodium. If goals are not met, it is not unusual to intensify doses or add on medicines.

Glaucoma: Return of eye pressure (intraocular pressure) to normal and avoidance of consequences of increased pressure. If this medicine does not work well enough by itself, combination treatment is typical.

Possible Advantages of This Drug: Usually effective and well-tolerated with a single dose daily, which is easier to remember to take. Twice-daily dosing for glaucoma also enhances taking the medicine (adherence). Suspension form may be better tolerated than the solution form.

▷ **This Drug Should Not Be Taken If**
- you have had an allergic reaction to it previously.
- you have heart (overt) failure or cardiogenic shock.
- you have an abnormally slow heart rate (bradycardia) or a serious heart block (second or third degree).
- you take, or took in the past 14 days, any monoamine oxidase (MAO) type A inhibitor (see Drug Classes).

▷ **Inform Your Physician Before Taking This Drug If**
- you have had an adverse reaction to any beta-blocker (see Drug Classes).
- you have serious heart disease or episodes of heart failure.
- you have a history of hay fever (allergic rhinitis), asthma, chronic bronchitis, or emphysema. Some drugs in this class are contraindicated in asthmatics.
- you have overactive thyroid function (hyperthyroidism).
- you have a history of low blood sugar (hypoglycemia) or diabetes.
- you have impaired liver or kidney function.
- you have narrowing of the vessels in your legs or arms (peripheral vascular disease). Discuss this with your doctor.
- you have myasthenia gravis.
- you take digitalis, quinidine or reserpine, or any calcium blocker drug (see Drug Classes).
- you will have surgery with general anesthesia.
- you take prescription or nonprescription medications not discussed when betaxolol was prescribed for you.

Possible Side Effects (natural, expected, and unavoidable drug actions)

Lethargy, fatigue (up to 10%), cold extremities—rare; slow heart rate, light-headedness in upright position (see Orthostatic Hypotension in Glossary), rebound hypertension if drug is stopped suddenly.

Possible Adverse Effects (unusual, unexpected, and infrequent reactions)

If any of the following develop, consult your physician promptly for guidance.

Mild Adverse Effects

Allergic reactions: skin rash, itching—rare.

Hair loss—case reports (even with ophthalmic use).

Headache (up to 15%)—frequent.

Dizziness, fatigue—infrequent.

Insomnia or abnormal dreams—infrequent.

Indigestion, nausea, diarrhea—infrequent.

Joint and muscle discomfort—infrequent.

Fluid retention (edema)—rare.

Difficulty breathing—infrequent.

Serious Adverse Effects

Allergic reactions: may make allergic reactions more difficult to treat (refractory to epinephrine).

Mental depression or anxiety—rare.

Increased blood sugar (hyperglycemia) in non-insulin-dependent diabetics—possible.

Chest pain, shortness of breath, congestive heart failure—rare.

Induction of bronchial asthma (in asthmatic patients)—possible.

Low blood platelets and anemia—rare.

Systemic Lupus erythematosus—case report.

Angina (if pill form abruptly stopped).

Slow heart rate (bradycardia)—infrequent.

Intermittent problems walking (intermittent claudication)—possible.

Heart attack (myocardial infarction)—rare.

Author's Note: Adverse effects from eye drops happen rarely versus "pill" form.

▷ **Possible Effects on Sexual Function:** Decreased libido, impotence—rare and less frequent than other medicines in this class.

Altered menstrual patterns (reported rarely with other medicines in this class)—possible.

Adverse Effects That May Mimic Natural Diseases or Disorders

Reduced blood flow to extremities may mimic Raynaud's disease (see Glossary).

Possible Effects on Laboratory Tests

Glaucoma-screening test (measurement of internal eye pressure): pressure is decreased (false low or normal value).

Antinuclear antibodies (ANA) test: case report.

Blood potassium: slightly increased.

Blood platelet counts and hemoglobin: decreased—rare.

Blood glucose: increased in non-insulin-dependent diabetics.

CAUTION

1. Do not stop this drug suddenly without calling your doctor. Always carry a note with you that says you are taking this drug.

2. Ask your physician or pharmacist before using nasal decongestants. These can cause sudden increases in blood pressure when combined with beta-blocker drugs.

3. Levobetaxolol (Betaxon) is NOT the same medicine as betaxolol.
4. Report any tendency to emotional depression.
5. Eye (ophthalmic) form may cause additive effects on blood pressure if taken with the pill form.

Precautions for Use

By Infants and Children: Safety and effectiveness for those less than 12 years of age not established.

By Those Over 60 Years of Age: Caution: High blood pressure should be slowly reduced, avoiding risks associated with excessively low blood pressure. Treatment should be started with 5 mg daily and blood pressure checked often. Sudden, rapid and excessive reduction of blood pressure can cause stroke or heart attack. Total daily dosage should not exceed 10 to 15 mg. Watch for dizziness, unsteadiness, tendency to fall, confusion, hallucinations, depression, or urinary frequency. This age group is more prone to develop excessively slow heart rates and hypothermia.

▷ **Advisability of Use During Pregnancy**

Pregnancy Category: C. C/**D** from one researcher. See Pregnancy Risk Categories at the back of this book.

Animal Studies: Rat studies reveal increased resorptions of embryo and fetus, retarded growth and development of newborn, and mild skeletal defects.

Human Studies: Adequate studies of pregnant women are not available.

Avoid use of drug during the first 3 months if possible. Avoid use during labor and delivery because of the possible effects on the newborn infant.

Advisability of Use If Breast-Feeding

Presence of this drug in breast milk: Yes.

Avoid drug if possible. If drug is necessary, observe nursing infant for slow heart rate and indications of low blood sugar.

Habit-Forming Potential: None.

Effects of Overdose: Weakness, slow pulse, low blood pressure, fainting, cold and sweaty skin, congestive heart failure, possible coma, and convulsions.

Possible Effects of Long-Term Use: Reduced heart reserve and eventual heart failure in susceptible individuals with advanced heart disease. Case reports of carpal tunnel syndrome with some medicines in this family.

Suggested Periodic Examinations While Taking This Drug (at physician's discretion)

Measurements of blood pressure.

Evaluation of heart function. Checks of intraocular pressure (ophthalmic use).

▷ **While Taking This Drug, Observe the Following**

Foods: No restrictions. Avoid excessive salt intake.

Herbal Medicines or Minerals: Ginseng, bitter orange, country mallow, hawthorn, saw palmetto, ma huang (now off the market), goldenseal, yohimbe, and licorice may increase blood pressure. Calcium and garlic may help lower blood pressure. Indian snakeroot has a German Commission E monograph indication for hypertension—talk to your doctor. Eleuthero root and ephedra should be avoided by people living with hypertension. Belladonna, ephedra, henbane leaf, and scopolia root should be avoided by people living with glaucoma. Dong Quai may lead to higher than expected blood levels. St. John's wort may lower blood levels and blunt therapeutic benefits.

Beverages: No restrictions. May be taken with milk.

▷ *Alcohol:* Use with caution. Alcohol may exaggerate oral form lowering of blood pressure and may increase its mild sedative effect.

Tobacco Smoking: Nicotine may reduce this drug's effectiveness. High drug doses worsen bronchial constriction caused by regular smoking. I advise everyone to quit smoking.

▷ *Other Drugs*

Betaxolol may *increase* the effects of
- other antihypertensive drugs and cause excessive lowering of blood pressure. Dosage decreases may be necessary.
- reserpine (Ser-Ap-Es, etc.) and cause sedation, depression, slowing of heart rate and lowering of blood pressure (light-headedness, fainting).
- verapamil and cause additive risk of congestive heart failure and slow heart rate (bradycardia).

Betaxolol *taken concurrently* with
- amiodarone (Cordarone) may result in extremely slow heart rate and arrest.
- calcium channel blockers (Diltiazem, etc. or other dihydropyridine forms) may severely lower blood pressure.
- clonidine (Catapres) requires close monitoring for rebound high blood pressure if clonidine is stopped while betaxolol is still being taken.
- digoxin (Lanoxin) may prolong AV conduction time and digoxin toxicity.
- fluoroquinolone (see Drug Classes) antibiotics may cause an increase in betaxolol blood levels and lead to toxicity.
- fluvoxamine (Luvox) may cause excessive slowing of the heart and very low blood pressure.
- insulin requires close supervision to avoid hidden hypoglycemia (see Glossary).
- methyldopa (various) may lead to an exaggerated hypertensive response to stress.
- oral antidiabetic (hypoglycemic) drugs (see Drug Classes) may prolong recovery from low blood sugars.
- phenothiazines (see Drug Classes) may result in additive blood pressure lowering effects.
- rifabutin (Mycobutin) may decrease betaxolol benefits.
- ritonavir (Norvir) and perhaps other protease inhibitors (see Drug Classes) may decrease betaxolol benefits.
- venlafaxine (Effexor) may cause excessive slowing of the heart and very low blood pressure.
- zileuton (Zyflo) may cause excessive blood pressure lowering.

The following drugs may *decrease* the effects of betaxolol:
- indomethacin (Indocin) and possibly other "aspirin substitutes," or NSAIDs, may impair betaxolol's antihypertensive effect.

▷ *Driving, Hazardous Activities:* Use caution until the full extent of drowsiness, lethargy, and blood pressure change has been determined.

Aviation Note: The use of this drug *is a disqualification* for piloting. Consult a designated Aviation Medical Examiner.

Exposure to Sun: No restrictions.

Exposure to Heat: Caution is advised. Hot environments can lower blood pressure and exaggerate the effects of this drug.

Exposure to Cold: Caution is advised. Cold environments can enhance the circulatory deficiency in the extremities that may occur with this drug. The elderly should be careful to prevent hypothermia (see Glossary).

Heavy Exercise or Exertion: Talk with your doctor about an exercise program that is right for you, mindful of this medicine and your physical condition.

Occurrence of Unrelated Illness: Fever can lower blood pressure and require dosing changes. Nausea or vomiting may interrupt dosing. Ask your doctor for help.

Discontinuation: DO NOT stop this drug suddenly. Gradual physician-supervised dose reduction over 2 to 3 weeks is recommended.

BITOLTEROL (bi TOHL ter ohl)

Introduced: 1985   **Class:**   Antiasthmatic, bronchodilator   **Prescription:**   Yes   **Controlled Drug:**   No   **Available as Generic:** No

Brand Name: Tornalate

Author's Note: This medicine is no longer available in the inhaler form. The information in this profile has been truncated to make room for more widely used medicines.

BROMOCRIPTINE (broh moh KRIP teen)

Introduced: 1975   **Class:**   Anti-Parkinsonism,   ergot   derivative   **Prescription:**   USA: Yes   **Controlled Drug:**   USA: No; Canada: No   **Available as Generic:**   No

Brand Names: Normatine, Parlodel

Author's Note: This profile has been shortened to make room for more widely used medicines.

BUDESONIDE (byou DES oh nyde)

Introduced: 1994 (Rhinocort), 1997 (Turbuhaler)   **Class:**   Antiasthmatic, cortisonelike drugs   **Prescription:**   USA: Yes   **Controlled Drug:** USA: No; Canada: No   **Available as Generic:**   No

Brand Names: ♣Entocort, Entocort EC, ♣Gen-Budesonide-AQ, Pulmicort, ♣Pulmicort Nebuamp, Pulmicort Respules and Turbuhaler, Rhinocort Aqua, Rhinocort Turbuhaler

```
┌─────────────────────────────────────────────────────────────────┐
│                    BENEFITS versus RISKS                          │
│     Possible Benefits              Possible Risks                 │
│ EFFECTIVE RELIEF OF ALLERGIC     FUNGUS INFECTIONS OF THE         │
│   RHINITIS                         MOUTH AND THROAT               │
│ EFFECTIVE CONTROL OF ASTHMA      Changes in lining of the nose (nasal │
│ TENDS TO HAVE MORE LOCAL           mucosa)                        │
│   THAN SYSTEMIC EFFECTS          Increased cataract risk          │
│   (HIGH RATIO)                   Osteoporosis risk                │
│ THE ENTOCORT EC FORM IS                                           │
│   SPECIFICALLY APPROVED TO                                        │
│   TREAT SUDDEN (ACUTE) FLARE                                      │
│   UPS OF CROHN'S DISEASE                                          │
│   WHILE AVOIDING MANY                                             │
│   SYSTEMIC EFFECTS OF OTHER                                       │
│   STEROIDS                                                        │
└─────────────────────────────────────────────────────────────────┘
```

▷ **Principal Uses**

As a Single Drug Product: Uses currently included in FDA-approved labeling: (1) Ongoing treatment of bronchial asthma in people who don't have sufficient response to bronchodilators and need cortisone-like drugs for asthma control; (2) treats seasonal and perennial rhinitis in children and adults (nasal form); (3) Entocort EC form is a form taken by mouth specifically for mild to moderate Crohn's disease that effects the ileum or ascending colon.

Other (unlabeled) generally accepted uses: (1) Eases nasal polyps (nasal polyposis).

How This Drug Works: It reduces inflammation (arachidonic acid pathway) and decreases response to immediate and delayed hypersensitivity. Also reduces local lung inflammation in the respiratory tract. The Entocort EC form is released in the small intestine and ascending colon where is works to decrease inflammation. Systemic effects are minimized because it next goes to the liver where it is transformed.

▷ **Widely Used Guidelines That Involve This Medicine (representative sample):** Please look at the section at the very beginning of this profile called "Class." Next, turn to Table 22 and you will find guidelines listed by the class involved!

Available Dosage Forms and Strengths

Enteric Capsules (EC) — 3 mg

Nasal inhaler — 7 g (32 mcg per press)

Nasal spray — 200-dose canister (50 mcg per dose) (Canada)

Oral inhaler — 200 doses of 1 or 4 mg per mL

Spacer form — same as above (200 doses of 1 or 4 mg per mL)

Turbuhaler — 200 mcg (100 and 400 mcg in Canada)

▷ **Recommended Dosage Ranges**

Infants and Children:

Seasonal rhinitis (children 6 or older): Pressurized nasal inhaler—two inhalations in each nostril twice a day, morning and evening, or 4 inhalations in each nostril in the morning (256 mcg maximum).

Perennial allergic rhinitis: Same dose, but see Caution section.

Seasonal and perennial rhinitis (for those 12 or older): Nonaerosol pump nasal spray—one puff (50 mcg) in each nostril twice daily. This may be increased to 2 puffs twice daily if required (256 mcg maximum).

Asthma: Oral inhalation form (in those more than 6 and based on prior treatment): (a) Bronchodilators alone—200 mcg twice a day; (b) inhaled corticosteroids—200 mcg twice daily; (c) oral corticosteroids—400 mcg twice daily. Children under 12 years old are given one puff or 0.2 mg twice a day with a maximum of 2 puffs a day (0.8 mg). Some clinicians use 400 mcg per square meter.

> **Author's Note: Use in pediatrics may slow a child's rate of growth, although current data shows that they reach normal adult height.**

Adults:

Seasonal rhinitis: Non-aerosol pump spray form—one puff (equals 50 mcg) in each nostril twice a day. Dosing can be increased to 2 puffs in each nostril twice daily if needed and tolerated. The effect should be checked in 3 to 7 days and the medicine stopped in 3 weeks if an adequate response isn't achieved.

Perennial rhinitis: Same dose as seasonal rhinitis, but see Caution section. Once adequate benefits have been seen, the dose is then slowly decreased to the lowest dose that works. If symptoms return while doses are being lowered, the dose may be increased back to the starting dose (briefly) and then decreased back to the dose that worked before the symptoms returned.

Asthma (use in is based on prior treatment): Oral inhaler—people receiving (a) bronchodilators alone—200–400 mcg twice a day; (b) inhaled corticosteroids—200–400 mcg twice daily; (c) oral corticosteroids—400–800 mcg twice daily. If asthma has been controlled by corticosteroids taken by mouth, the budesonide inhaler must be used at the same time as the oral corticosteroids for about 1 week. After a week, the oral corticosteroid can be SLOWLY tapered. The patient should be closely watched for the return of asthma or other effects (see Caution section).

Crohn's disease (Entocort EC form): Used for sudden (acute) flare ups of Crohn's disease that involves the ileum or ascending colon: Three capsules taken once a day in the morning for up to eight weeks. Dosing is decreased (tapered) to 6 mg a day for 14 days before it is stopped.

Those Over 65 Years of Age: Doses similar to those used in younger patients have been effective and safe.

> **Note: Actual dose and schedule must be determined for each patient individually.**

Conditions Requiring Dosing Adjustments

Liver Function: Use with caution in patients with liver compromise. This drug may stay in the body longer in people with liver damage, and lower doses appear prudent. The Entocort EC form is rapidly transformed (metabolized) in the liver, but was not studied in severe liver dysfunction and can not be recommended in that population.

Kidney Function: No adjustments in dosing appear to be required.

▷ **Dosing Instructions:** May be used without regard to eating. Rinse the mouth and throat (gargle) with water thoroughly after each inhalation. If you forget a dose: Use the inhaler or spray as soon as possible. DO NOT double doses. Entocort EC form should NOT be crushed, chewed, or altered.

Usual Duration of Use: Regular use for 1 to 2 weeks is often needed to see the best response from the oral inhalation form in asthma, but Pulmicort form may work in a day in some patients. The nasal inhalation form may go to work in 3–7 days. This is why results are checked after 3–7 days and at 3 weeks. If acceptable relief isn't seen in 3 weeks, the drug should be stopped.

Once relief is achieved, the dose should be decreased at 2- to 4-week intervals to the minimum effective dose. Long-term use must be physician-supervised. See your doctor regularly. For Entocort EC form, dosing is continued for up to eight weeks. A repeat episode of active Crohn's can be treated with a repeat eight-week course.

Typical Treatment Goals and Measurements (Outcomes and Markers)

Asthma: Frequency and severity of asthma attacks should ease. Some clinicians also use decreased frequency of rescue inhaler use as a further clinical indicator. It is critical that this medicine is used regularly to get the best results. An additional goal of therapy is to use the lowest effective dose. Some people keep their improvements when doses are lowered, while others relapse. Those with a less than 2-fold improvement in airway response and people who stay in the moderate to severe asthma range despite high budesonide doses may be more likely to relapse. If the usual benefit is not realized, call your doctor.

Allergic rhinitis: Symptoms such as itchy, runny nose, sore throat, and post-nasal drip should all ease once this medicine begins to work. Because there may be some seasonality to the pollen or molds that can cause rhinitis, talk to your doctor about exactly how you should use this medicine.

Crohn's Disease: Flare ups involving the ileum or ascending colon are brought under control.

Possible Advantages of This Drug

Turbuhaler form avoids pressurized metered dose inhaler CFCs as well as increased amount of drug in the lung. Intranasal form causes less depression of free cortisol. Inhaled forms cause less of a systemic effect than the same medicine taken by mouth. Medicines in this class are considered first-line treatment by many clinicians in allergic rhinitis because they slow (attenuate) early-phase reactions and suppress late-phase allergic reactions (they may also cost less). In asthma, inhaled steroids have been recommended in revised guidelines for those with more than infrequent or mild asthma. Entocort EC form releases the active drug in the small intestine and part of the colon (ascending) and eases inflammation. The drug is subsequently quickly transformed (metabolized) in the liver so that only a small amount goes out the whole body (systemic circulation).

▷ This Drug Should Not Be Taken If

- you have had an allergic reaction to any form of this drug.
- you are having severe acute asthma or status asthmaticus (requires intense treatment for prompt relief).
- other antiasthmatic drugs can control your asthma that are not related to cortisone.
- your asthma requires cortisone-like drugs infrequently for control.

▷ Inform Your Physician Before Taking This Drug If

- you take or recently took any cortisone-related drug (including ACTH by injection) for any reason (see Drug Classes).
- you have a history of tuberculosis of the lungs.
- you have chronic bronchitis or bronchiectasis.
- you think you have an active infection of any kind, especially a respiratory infection or herpes of the eye.
- you have recently been exposed to chickenpox or other viral illnesses.
- you are prone to nosebleeds (epistaxis) or have nose ulcers or have had nose surgery (nasal forms).

- you are unsure how much to take or how often to take this drug.
- you are a child and your growth rate has not been checked.

Possible Side Effects (natural, expected, and unavoidable drug actions)
Author's Note: The Entocort EC form is released in the intestines and quickly deactivated in the liver. Because very little drug actually reached the general circulation (systemic), whole body effects such as suppression of the adrenal gland, acne, moon face, and other changes are minimized or absent.
Fungus infections (thrush) of the mouth and throat. Voice changes (dysphonia).
Suppression of the adrenal glands—possible.
Stinging of nasal tissues (nasal form)—possible.

▷ **Possible Adverse Effects** (unusual, unexpected, and infrequent reactions)
If any of the following develop, consult your physician promptly for guidance.
Mild Adverse Effects
Allergic reaction: skin rash (contact dermatitis)—infrequent.
Headache—frequent (oral inhalation).
Dryness of mouth, hoarseness, sore throat, cough—possible.
Nosebleeds (epistaxis)—infrequent.
Weight gain—infrequent.
Serious Adverse Effects
Allergic reaction: localized areas of "allergic" pneumonitis (lung inflammation), immediate type hypersensitivity reactions.
Bronchospasm, asthmatic wheezing—rare.
Behavioral changes—case reports.
Nose perforation (septal)—rare.
Hyperglycemia (dose related)—case report.
Increased susceptibility to chickenpox—possible.
Growth slowing (growth retardation)—possible.
Increased risk of cataracts with long-term (chronic) use.
Osteoporosis (any corticosteroid can cause this)—possible.

▷ **Possible Effects on Sexual Function:** None reported.

Natural Diseases or Disorders That May Be Activated by This Drug
Cortisone-related drugs having systemic effects impair immunity and lead to reactivation of "healed" or dormant tuberculosis. People with a history of tuberculosis must be watched closely while using this drug.

Possible Effects on Laboratory Tests
Blood cortisol levels: decreased.
HDL and blood sugar may increase.
Bone mineral density: may be decreased with chronic use.

CAUTION
1. The substance (sorbitan trioleate) that one form of this medicine is delivered in (vehicle) may cause symptoms that are like rhinitis. Doses early in treatment may suppress these symptoms, and they may slowly come back once the dose is lowered. If this occurs and the dose can't be lowered, other treatment may be needed.
2. The maker of the pressurized nasal inhaler uses the amount of drug released from the nasal adapter (32 mcg) to determine the dose. The nasal inhaler actually releases 50 mcg.

3. Use in people with asthma REQUIRES regular use to get the best results. Please do not skip doses.
4. This drug should not be relied upon for immediate relief of acute asthma.
5. The inhaled powder form does not prevent asthma precipitated by exercise.
6. If you required cortisone-like drugs before starting this inhaler, you may again require a cortisone-like drug if you are injured, have an infection or need surgery. Extreme care must be taken if you are being changed from corticosteroids that work in the whole body (systemically active) to this medicine.
7. If severe asthma returns while using this drug, call your doctor immediately. Cortisone-like drugs may be required.
8. Carry a personal ID card saying that you have used (if true) cortisone-related drugs in the past year.
9. This drug may allow dosage decreases in some patients.
10. If this medicine is to be used long-term, a bone mineral density test before treatment and every 2 years is prudent.
11. Entocort EC form should NOT be used for ongoing (chronic) therapy. DO NOT drink grapefruit juice while this form is being taken.
12. Unlike other corticosteroids, reports of osteonecrosis (avascular necrosis or aseptic necrosis) have not been made for this medicine. Caution is prudent, and patients should report any unexplained joint (such as knee, hip or shoulder) pain to their doctor.

Precautions for Use

By Infants and Children: Safety and effectiveness as described above. Children may be more susceptible to adverse effects of this drug and should be watched closely.

By Those Over 60 Years of Age: People with bronchiectasis should be watched closely for the development of lung infections.

▷ **Advisability of Use During Pregnancy**

Pregnancy Category: C. See Pregnancy Risk Categories at the back of this book.
Animal Studies: Mouse, rat, and rabbit studies reveal significant birth defects due to this drug.
Human Studies: Adequate studies of pregnant women are not available.
Talk with your doctor.

Advisability of Use If Breast-Feeding

Presence of this drug in breast milk: Amount not determined.
Controversial. Discontinue nursing or the medicine. Discuss this with your doctor.

Habit-Forming Potential: With recommended dosage, a state of functional dependence (see Glossary) is not likely to develop.

Effects of Overdose: Indications of cortisone excess (due to systemic absorption)—fluid retention, flushing of the face, stomach irritation, nervousness.

Suggested Periodic Examinations While Taking This Drug (at physician's discretion)
Inspection of nose, mouth, and throat for fungus infection.
Inspection of the nose tissues for damage.
Assessment of adrenal function in people using cortisone-related drugs for an extended time prior to this drug.

Lung X-ray if a prior history of tuberculosis.

Measures of bone mineral density (DEXA, ultrasound, or PDEXA) and cataract check.

▷ **While Taking This Drug, Observe the Following**

Foods: Follow specific restrictions advised by your physician. Grapefruit can change the ability of the body to remove this medicine—DO NOT eat this—particularly with the Entocort EC form.

Herbal Medicines or Minerals: Fir or pine needle oil should NOT be used by asthmatics. Ephedra alone does carry a German Commission E monograph indication for asthma treatment. If you are allergic to plants in the Asteraceae family (aster, chrysanthemum, daisy, or ragweed), you may also be allergic to echinacea, chamomile, feverfew, and St. John's wort. Taking added calcium and vitamin D while taking this medicine is prudent. Talk to your doctor BEFORE adding any herbals to this medicine.

Beverages: Avoid grapefruit juice as it increases blood levels of the non-EC form and will also increase the chance of whole body effects of even the EC form. DO NOT drink grapefruit juice while taking this medicine.

▷ *Alcohol:* No interactions expected.

Tobacco Smoking: Smoking can reduce the benefits of this drug. I advise everyone to quit smoking.

▷ *Other Drugs*

The following drugs may *increase* the effects of budesonide:
- some antiepileptic medicines such as phenytoin (Dilantin) may increase risk of osteoporosis.
- inhalant bronchodilators—epinephrine, isoetharine, isoproterenol.
- methylphenidate (Ritalin) may cause increased growth suppression.
- oral bronchodilators—aminophylline, ephedrine, terbutaline, theophylline, etc.

Budesonide *taken concurrently* with:
- amiodarone (Cordarone) may cause increased risk of Cushing's syndrome (because of liver enzyme-CYP450 3A4 inhibition). Careful clinical follow-up is needed.
- bupropion (Wellbutrin or Zyban) may increase risk of seizures. Smaller doses, gradual dose increases and caution is advised.
- ketoconazole (Nizoral), itraconazole, erythromycin, ritonavir, and other inhibitors of CYP450 3A4 may cause increased budesonide levels. Caution is advised.

▷ *Driving, Hazardous Activities:* No restrictions.

Aviation Note: The use of this drug and the disorder for which this drug is prescribed *may be disqualifications* for piloting. Consult a designated Aviation Medical Examiner.

Exposure to Sun: No restrictions.

Occurrence of Unrelated Illness: Acute infections, serious injuries, and surgery can create an urgent need for cortisone-related drugs. Call your doctor immediately in the event of new illness or injury.

Discontinuation: If this drug has made it possible to reduce or stop ongoing cortisonelike drugs, *do not* stop this drug abruptly. If you must stop this drug, call your doctor. You may need to resume cortisone medicines. The Entocort EC form is lowered (tapered) to 6 mg daily for 14 days before it is stopped.

BUMETANIDE (byu MET a nide)

Introduced: 1983 **Class:** Diuretic **Prescription:** USA: Yes; Canada: No **Controlled Drug:** USA: No **Available as Generic:** Yes

Brand Names: Bumex, Burinex

BENEFITS versus RISKS

Possible Benefits	*Possible Risks*
POTENT, EFFECTIVE DIURETIC BY MOUTH OR INJECTION	ABNORMALLY LOW BLOOD POTASSIUM with excessive use
TREATS CONGESTIVE HEART FAILURE, HIGH BLOOD PRESSURE, AND FLUID BUILD UP IN KIDNEY FAILURE	Decreased magnesium with chronic therapy
	Blood disorders—rare
	Possible bone weakening with prolonged use

▷ **Principal Uses**

As a Single Drug Product: Uses currently included in FDA-approved labeling: (1) Removes fluid excess in patients with congestive heart failure, kidney or liver disease; (2) eases edema in people who fail to respond to or will not tolerate furosemide (Lasix).

Other (unlabeled) generally accepted uses: (1) Used as an adjunct to other therapy in high blood pressure (hypertension); (2) can help older people decrease the number of times they must get up at night to urinate (nocturia); (3) eases the amount of fluid that can build up in the lungs (pulmonary edema).

In the Pipeline: The Health and Human Services secretary has identified a group of medicines to be tested for use in children. Bumetanide was on that list of the 12 highest priority medicines to be studied in children (find out more at *www.hhs.gov*).

How This Drug Works: Increases removal of salt and water from the body (through increased urine production). Reduces sodium and amount of fluid in the blood.

▷ **Widely Used Guidelines That Involve This Medicine (representative sample):** Please look at the section at the very beginning of this profile called "Class." Next, turn to Table 22 and you will find guidelines listed by the class involved!

Available Dosage Forms and Strengths
Injection — 0.25 mg/mL (2-mL ampules)
Tablets — 0.5 mg, 1 mg, 2 mg

▷ **Usual Adult Dosage Ranges:** 0.5 to 2 mg daily, usually taken in the morning as a single dose. If needed, an additional second or third dose may be taken later in the day at 4- to 5-hour intervals. The total daily dose should not exceed 10 mg. Ongoing (maintenance) doses should be given intermittently (every other day) and typically have been the safest way to control edema.

Note: Actual dose and schedule must be determined for each patient individually.

Conditions Requiring Dosing Adjustments

Liver Function: Rapid body fluid removal can cause a coma in liver failure patients. Use of loop diuretics only done under close medical supervision (hospital or outpatient care center).

Kidney Function: NOT recommended for use in progressive renal failure.

▷ **Dosing Instructions:** May be crushed when taken and given with or following food to reduce stomach irritation. If you forget a dose: take it right away unless it's nearly time for your next regular dose. If it IS nearly time for the next dose, just take the scheduled dose. DO NOT double doses.

Usual Duration of Use: Two to three days of regular use often needed to see peak effect relieving fluid buildup (edema). Once peak benefit is realized, intermittent use reduces risk of sodium, potassium, magnesium, and water imbalance. Long-term use requires supervision by your doctor.

Typical Treatment Goals and Measurements (Outcomes and Markers)

Blood Pressure: Guidelines (JNC VII) define normal blood pressure (BP) as **less than** 120/80 and **pre-hypertension** as 120/80 to 139/89. This new range is intended to help doctors encourage lifestyle changes (or in the case of people with a risk factor for high blood pressure, start treatment) much earlier—so that damage to blood vessels, heart, kidneys, sexual potency, or eyes might be minimized or avoided altogether. Stage 1 hypertension is 140/90 to 159/99 and stage 2 hypertension equal to or greater than: 160/100 mm Hg. These guidelines also recommend that clinicians work with their patients to agree on the goals and a plan of treatment. The first-ever guidelines for blood pressure (hypertension) in African Americans recommends that MOST black patients be started on TWO antihypertensive medicines with the goal of lowering blood pressure to 130/80 for those with high risk for heart and blood vessel disease or with diabetes. The American Diabetes Association also recommends 130/80 as the target for diabetics and less than 125/75 for those who spill more than one gram of protein into their urine. Most clinicians try to achieve a BP that confers the best balance of lower cardiovascular risk and avoids the problem of too low a blood pressure. Blood pressure duration is generally increased with beneficial restriction of sodium. If goals are not met, it is not unusual to intensify doses or add on medicines.

Congestive heart failure: Used to remove excessive fluid which builds up in the body. Typical treatment markers include resolution of ankle swelling and increased output of fluid (diuresis).

Possible Advantages of This Drug

Diuretic effect is usually complete in 4 hours; diuretic effect of furosemide usually lasts from 6 to 8 hours. Hearing impairment (ototoxicity) is probably less than that with furosemide (Lasix).

▷ **This Drug Should Not Be Taken If**
- you have had an allergic reaction to sulfonamides or to bumetanide.
- coma caused by liver failure is present (a point for caregivers).
- severe electrolyte or fluid imbalance.
- you have developed a marked increase in creatinine or blood urea nitrogen (BUN) while taking this drug.
- your kidneys are unable to produce adequate urine (oliguria).

▷ **Inform Your Physician Before Taking This Drug If**
- you are allergic to any form of sulfa drug.
- you are pregnant or planning pregnancy.
- you have a blood disorder.

- you have impaired liver or kidney function.
- you have diabetes, a diabetic tendency, or a history of gout.
- you have impaired hearing or develop hearing loss during therapy.
- you have low blood platelets.
- you are taking: cortisone, digitalis, oral antidiabetic drugs, insulin, probenecid (Benemid), indomethacin (Indocin), lithium, or aminoglycoside antibiotics.
- you will have surgery with general anesthesia.
- you are unsure how much to take or how often to take it.

Possible Side Effects (natural, expected, and unavoidable drug actions)
Light-headedness on arising from sitting or lying position (see Orthostatic Hypotension in Glossary).
Hearing impairment (ototoxicity)—rare.
Increase in level of blood sugar, affecting control of diabetes.
Increase in level of blood uric acid, affecting control of gout.
Decreased blood potassium and sodium with muscle weakness and cramping.
Decreased blood magnesium. Increased calcium loss in the urine (calciuria).

▷ **Possible Adverse Effects** (unusual, unexpected, and infrequent reactions)
If any of the following develop, consult your physician promptly for guidance.
Mild Adverse Effects
Allergic reactions: skin rashes, hives, itching.
Headache, dizziness, vertigo, fatigue, weakness, sweating, earache—rare.
Nausea, vomiting, stomach pain, diarrhea—infrequent.
Breast nipple tenderness, joint and muscle pains or cramps—rare.
Serious Adverse Effects
Serious skin rash (Stevens-Johnson Syndrome)—case reports.
Liver coma (in preexisting liver disease)—possible.
Abnormally low magnesium, potassium, and sodium (electrolytes): possible with long-term or high-dose use—rare to frequent.
Low white blood cells and platelets (leukopenia and thrombocytopenia)—rare.
Kidney failure—rare.
Pseudoporphyuria—case report.
Pancreatitis—case reports.
Elevated blood glucose—infrequent.
Lung fibrosis—case reports.
Hearing toxicity (ototoxicity)—rare.

▷ **Possible Effects on Sexual Function:** Difficulty maintaining an erection; premature ejaculation (0.5 to 2 mg daily)—rare.
Male breast enlargement and tenderness (gynecomastia)—case reports.

Natural Diseases or Disorders That May Be Activated by This Drug
Latent diabetes, gout.

Possible Effects on Laboratory Tests
White blood cell counts: increased—usual; decreased—rare.
Blood platelets: decreased.
Blood sugar (glucose): increased.
Blood lithium or uric acid levels: increased.
Blood potassium, magnesium or chloride: decreased.

CAUTION
1. High doses can cause excessive excretion of water, sodium, and potassium, with loss of appetite, nausea, weakness, confusion, and profound

drop in blood pressure (circulatory collapse). Magnesium may also be lost and should be checked and replaced as needed.

2. May cause digitalis toxicity by depleting potassium. If you are taking a digitalis preparation (digitoxin, digoxin), ensure an adequate intake of high-potassium foods.

3. People with cirrhosis of the liver must never increase their dose unless told to do so by their doctor. Excess dosing can cause liver coma.

4. People who take lithium may experience lithium toxicity.

5. Use with aminoglycoside antibiotics may increase risk of ear problems (ototoxicity).

Precautions for Use

By Infants and Children: Safety and effectiveness for those under 18 years of age not established.

By Those Over 60 Years of Age: Small starting doses are advisable. You may be more susceptible to the development of impaired thinking, orthostatic hypotension, potassium loss, and elevation of blood sugar. Overdose and prolonged use can cause excessive loss of body water, thickening of the blood, and an increased risk of blood clots, stroke, heart attack, or thrombophlebitis.

▷ **Advisability of Use During Pregnancy**

Pregnancy Category: C, **D** by one researcher. See Pregnancy Risk Categories at the back of this book.

Animal Studies: Ten times the maximum therapeutic human dose caused bone defects in rabbits.

Human Studies: Adequate studies of pregnant women are not available.

Only used in pregnancy if a very serious complication of pregnancy occurs for which this drug is significantly beneficial.

Advisability of Use If Breast-Feeding

Presence of this drug in breast milk: Unknown.

Avoid drug or refrain from nursing.

Habit-Forming Potential: None.

Effects of Overdose: Weakness, lethargy, dizziness, confusion, nausea, vomiting, muscle cramps, thirst, electrolyte disturbances, drowsiness progressing to deep sleep or coma, weak and rapid pulse.

Possible Effects of Long-Term Use: Impaired balance of water, magnesium, salt, and potassium in blood and body tissues. Dehydration with possible increased blood viscosity and potential for abnormal clotting. Increased blood sugar in some patients. Osteoporosis due to increased calcium loss in the urine.

Suggested Periodic Examinations While Taking This Drug (at physician's discretion)

Complete blood counts.

Blood levels of sodium, potassium, magnesium, chloride, sugar, uric acid.

Liver and kidney function tests.

Bone mineral density tests (with long term use).

▷ **While Taking This Drug, Observe the Following**

Foods: Salt restriction and a high-potassium diet may be needed. Ask your doctor. See Table 13, High-Potassium Foods.

Herbal Medicines or Minerals: Ginseng, hawthorn, bitter orange, country mallow, saw palmetto, ma huang (no longer on the market), goldenseal, guarana, and licorice may cause increased blood pressure. Calcium and garlic may help lower blood pressure. Dandelion root has diuretic properties. Talk to your doctor BEFORE combining any herbals with this medicine.

Beverages: No restrictions unless directed by your doctor. May be taken with milk.

▷   *Alcohol:* Alcohol can exaggerate the blood pressure lowering effect of this drug and cause orthostatic hypotension (see Glossary).

Tobacco Smoking: No interactions expected. I advise everyone to quit smoking.

▷   *Other Drugs*

Bumetanide may ***increase*** the effects of:

- antihypertensive drugs. Careful decreases in dose are needed to prevent excessive lowering of the blood pressure.

Bumetanide ***taken concurrently*** with:

- ACE inhibitors (see Drug Classes) may result in severe lowering of blood pressure on standing (postural or orthostatic hypotension).
- aminoglycoside antibiotics (amikacin, gentamicin, kanamycin, neomycin, streptomycin, tobramycin, viomycin) increases the risk of hearing loss (ototoxicity).
- cephalosporins (see Drug Classes) may increase risk of kidney toxicity.
- cortisone-related drugs may cause excessive potassium loss and also blunted therapeutic benefits.
- digitalis-related drugs (digoxin-Lanoxin, others—see Drug Classes) requires very careful monitoring to prevent serious disturbances of heart rhythm.
- lithium (Lithobid, others) may increase lithium toxicity risk.

The following drugs may ***decrease*** the effects of bumetanide:

- indomethacin (Indocin) or other NSAIDs (see Drug Classes) may reduce its diuretic effect.

▷   *Driving, Hazardous Activities:* Caution: Varying degrees of dizziness, weakness, or orthostatic hypotension (see Glossary) may occur.

Aviation Note: The use of this drug ***may be a disqualification*** for piloting. Consult a designated Aviation Medical Examiner.

Exposure to Sun: No restrictions.

Occurrence of Unrelated Illness: Report vomiting or diarrhea promptly to your doctor.

Discontinuation: It may be advisable to stop this drug 5 to 7 days before major surgery. Ask your doctor for help.

BUPROPION (byu PROH pee on)

Other Name: Amfebutamone   **Introduced:**   1986   **Class:**   Antidepressant   **Prescription:**   USA: Yes **Controlled Drug:**   USA: No; Canada: No   **Available as Generic:**   USA: Yes

Brand Names: Wellbutrin, Wellbutrin SR, Wellbutrin XL, Zyban

BENEFITS versus RISKS	
Possible Benefits	*Possible Risks*

BENEFITS versus RISKS

Possible Benefits

EFFECTIVE IN SMOKING
CESSATION (ZYBAN)
EFFECTIVE TREATMENT OF
MAJOR DEPRESSIVE
DISORDERS
SEXUAL DESIRE MAY BE
INCREASED IN SOME PEOPLE
AND USED IN TREATMENT
MAY HELP ADHD IN ADULTS
Offers a different class than tricyclic,
MAO, or SSRI antidepressants

Possible Risks

DRUG-INDUCED SEIZURES—RARE
Excessive mental stimulation:
excitement, anxiety, confusion,
hallucinations, insomnia
Conversion of depression to mania in
manic-depressive disorders
57 case reports of people who smoked
and who took Zyban and died have
been made in the United Kingdom
(reports contained both seizures
and heart attacks)

▷ **Principal Uses**
As a Single Drug Product: Uses currently included in FDA-approved labeling:
(1) Helps smokers quit smoking (Zyban); (2) treatment of major depressive
disorders.
Other (unlabeled) generally accepted uses: (1) May ease chronic fatigue syndrome symptoms; (2) can reduce cocaine craving when combined with
psychotherapy; (3) drug of choice in people who have significant weight
gain while taking tricyclic antidepressants; (4) can help some cases of low
back pain not responding to other agents; (5) increased sexual desire in
77% of patients in one study; (6) an Alabama Veterans Affairs medical center study found this drug to be effective in post-traumatic stress disorder;
(7) works to help people stop using smokeless tobacco; (8) is an alternative
to stimulant-type medicines to treat attention deficit hyperactivity disorder
(ADHD) based on one cohort study with variable dosing (both in children
and in adults); (8) useful in chronic fatigue syndrome; (9) eases periodic
limb movement disorder.

How This Drug Works: Bupropion increases levels of two nerve transmitters
(norepinephrine and dopamine). It is biochemically unique and works differently from other antidepressants (may be a benefit if other medicines
have failed). How it works in quitting smoking is unknown.

▷ **Widely Used Guidelines That Involve This Medicine (representative sample):** Please look at the section at the very beginning of this profile called
"Class." Next, turn to Table 22 and you will find guidelines listed by the
class involved!

Available Dosage Forms and Strengths
Tablets, immediate release — 75 mg, 100 mg
Tablets, extended release — 150 mg and 300 mg
Tablets, sustained release — 50 mg (Canada), 100 mg, 150 mg,
200 mg
Zyban Tablets, sustained release only — 150 mg

▷ **Recommended Dosage Ranges** (Actual dose and schedule must be determined
for each patient individually.)
Infants and Children: Dosage not established for those under 18 years of age.
18 to 60 Years of Age:
Depression: For first 3 days, 100 mg in the morning and evening. On the
fourth day, dose may be increased to 100 mg in the morning, at noon, and
in the evening; total daily dose of 300 mg. This schedule of 100 mg, three

times daily, 6 hours apart, is used for 3 to 4 weeks. If needed and beneficial, dose may be slowly increased to a maximum of 450 mg daily. Increases should not exceed 100 mg per day in a period of 3 days. No single dose should exceed 150 mg. If daily dose is 450 mg, take 150 mg in the morning, then 100 mg every 4 hours for three more doses. The lowest effective dose should be used. Drug should be stopped if significant improvement is not seen after a trial of 450 mg daily. Doses higher than 450 mg daily may only increase risk of seizures. For the sustained release (SR) form, the starting dose is 150 mg in the morning. For the extended release (XL form), the starting dose its 150 mg in the morning. If the dose is tolerated by the patient after 4 days of treatment, the dose can be increased to the typical dose of 300 mg a day. If no improvement is seen after several weeks, a further increase to 450 mg is possible. If a switch from the immediate release or even the sustained release TO THE EXTENDED RELEASE FORM is a goal: the same total daily dose is given where possible. For example, people getting 100 mg three times a day of the immediate release form can be changed over to ONE of the 300 mg extended release form tablets once a day to treat depression.

Smoking cessation: 150 mg once a day for 3 days, then 150 mg twice daily for 7 to 12 weeks. If progress has not been made in 7 weeks, talk with your doctor. Combination strategies with use of this medicine and a nicotine patch (transdermal) have been undertaken. Talk to your doctor before starting this combination.

ADHD in adults: 100 to 200 mg of the SR form twice daily.

Over 60 Years of Age: Same as 18 to 60 years of age.

Conditions Requiring Dosing Adjustments

Liver Function: Lower dosages and caution in monitoring should be used.

Kidney Function: Not specifically studied in Zyban form; however, prudent to decrease the dose in people with damaged kidneys or who develop kidney damage while taking this drug.

Dosing Instructions: May be taken with food to reduce stomach upset. Best to swallow the tablet whole, not chewing or crushing it; this drug has a bitter taste and a local numbing effect on the lining of the mouth. Sustained or extended-release forms should never be crushed or altered. If you forget a dose (and you take the regular-release tablets): Take the medicine right away, unless it is nearly time for your next dose. When this medicine is being used to help stop smoking, it takes about a week to achieve needed blood levels. The medicine should be started while the patient is still smoking and a quit date decided on by both patient and doctor in the second week. For the sustained or extended-release forms: If you miss a dose, don't take the missed dose, simply take the next scheduled dose. DO NOT double doses. Call your doctor if you miss more than one dose. Some doctors use combined therapy with bupropion and nicotine "patches" (transdermals).

Usual Duration of Use: Regular use for 3–4 weeks needed to realize benefits in depression. Long-term use (months to years) requires periodic evaluation of response and dose. Some clinical guidelines suggest that 4–9 months of treatment should continue after the symptoms of depression go away. Some clinicians use lower ongoing doses to prevent depression. People who take their medicine regularly are least likely to have a recurrence.

For use in quitting smoking: Use for 7–12 weeks (although likelihood of quitting decreases if little progress occurs after 7 weeks). Some cases of success where 300 mg was used for 6 months have been reported. ADHD treatment continues into adulthood for many (some studies indicate 60%) patients. See your doctor regularly.

Typical Treatment Goals and Measurements (Outcomes and Markers)

Depression: The general goal: to help lessen the degree and severity of depression, letting patients return to their daily lives. In a set of guidelines issued by the American College of Physicians, older and newer antidepressants were found to give equal results in treating depression. Older medicines were found to generally have more frequent constipation, dizziness, dry mouth, blurred vision, and tremors while newer medicines caused more diarrhea, headache and nausea. The importance here is that many options are available and possible side effects can be somewhat tailored to try to avoid overlap. Activities of living (ADLs) and interest level can help tell patients when the medicine is starting to show benefits. The Hamilton Depression Scale is a useful measure of success in depression treatment for clinicians.

Smoking Cessation: The general goal: to stop smoking. Combination with a "quit smoking" course and/or support group can increase beneficial results.

▷ **Possible Advantages of This Drug**

Causes less atropinelike side effects: blurred vision, dry mouth, constipation, or impaired urination than other antidepressants. Does not cause sedation or orthostatic hypotension (see Glossary). Some clinicians use it for add on therapy for existing depression treatments. May cause **weight loss** instead of weight gain like other antidepressants. Avoids stimulant effects possible with stimulant type medicine for ADHD such as methylphenidate (Ritalin). Once daily dosing of XL form encouraged adherence.

▷ **This Drug Should Not Be Taken If**

- you have had an allergic reaction to it previously.
- you have a history of anorexia nervosa or bulimia (may be associated with increased seizure risk).
- you have a seizure disorder of any kind (while not a disorder, this includes people who have recently had to suddenly stop sedatives [such as Valium—diazepam] or alcohol).
- you are taking, or took in the past 14 days, any monoamine oxidase (MAO) type A inhibitor (see Drug Classes).

▷ **Inform Your Physician Before Taking This Drug If**

- you have had any adverse effects from antidepressant drugs.
- you are pregnant or planning pregnancy.
- you are breast-feeding your infant.
- you have a history of mental illness, head injury, or brain tumor.
- you have a history of alcoholism or drug abuse.
- you have any kind of heart disease, especially a recent heart attack.
- you have impaired liver or kidney function.
- you take prescription or nonprescription drugs not discussed when bupropion was prescribed for you.
- you take other medicines that can make seizures more likely.

Possible Side Effects (natural, expected, and unavoidable drug actions)

Nervousness, anxiety, confusion, insomnia (may be frequent), tremor.

Weight loss of more than 5 pounds—frequent (19–28% depending on the product).

▷ **Possible Adverse Effects** (unusual, unexpected, and infrequent reactions)

If any of the following develop, consult your physician promptly for guidance.

Mild Adverse Effects
   Allergic reactions: skin rash, itching—rare to infrequent.
   Headache, dizziness, tremor (dose related), agitation (9.7% more than
      placebo), or blurred vision (4.3% more than placebo)—infrequent.
   Agitation—common.
   Vivid dreaming—possible (more likely with higher doses).
   Indigestion, nausea and vomiting, constipation—infrequent.
   Dry mouth or edema—frequent.
   Taste disorders (taste perversion)—infrequent and may be dose related.
   Excessive sweating (diaphoresis)—frequent.
   Bruising (ecchymosis)—possible (prudent to tell your doctor if this happens).
   Ringing in the ears (tinnitus)—possible.
   Palpitations—frequent.
   Increased blood pressure—possible to infrequent.
Serious Adverse Effects
   Drug-induced seizures—rare, more common with high doses (roughly 0.4%
      with 400 mg a day of Wellbutrin SR).
   Change of depression to mania in manic-depressive disorders—possible.
   Psychosis in patients with psychotic predisposition—possible.
   Migraine headache—may be common.
   Increased blood pressure (hypertension)—infrequent but may be significant
      In people who had high blood pressure before starting bupropion.
   Decreased (leukopenia) or increased (leukocytosis) white blood cell counts
      or low platelets—case reports.
   Liver toxicity—case reports.
   Rhabdomyolysis—case report.
   Movement disorders—possible, but not causally proven.
   Heart attack/arrhythmia—case reports (in the United Kingdom—238 reports
      of chest pain and 134 cases of chest tightness were reported—call your
      doctor if you have these signs or symptoms).
▷ **Possible Effects on Sexual Function:** A study at the University of Alabama
   found 77% of patients experienced **increased** sexual desire. Clitoral pri-
   apism was reported in one case report.
   Impotence—infrequent; however, another study reported a decrease in sex-
      ual dysfunction when patients were switched from fluoxetine (Prozac) to
      bupropion.
   Altered menstruation up to 3.6% more than placebo in clinical trials—
      infrequent.

Possible Delayed Adverse Effects: Tardive dyskinesia.

Natural Diseases or Disorders That May Be Activated by This Drug
   Latent epilepsy, latent psychosis, manic phase of bipolar affective disorder.

Possible Effects on Laboratory Tests
   White blood cell or platelet counts: increased or decreased.

CAUTION
   1. Take exactly the amount prescribed; rapid dose increases can cause
      seizures. Watch closely for excessive stimulation.
   2. Ask your doctor or pharmacist BEFORE taking any other prescription or
      nonprescription drug.
   2. Do not take any monoamine oxidase (MAO) type A inhibitor while taking
      this drug (see Drug Classes). If you have taken a MAO inhibitor, wait 2
      weeks before starting bupropion
   3. 57 case reports of people who smoked and who also took Zyban and died

have been made in the United Kingdom (reports contained both seizures and heart attacks).

4. The FDA has required makers of antidepressants such as bupropion to alert healthcare professionals to the fact that children and adults with major depression may develop worsening depression or suicidal thoughts and behavior whether they take medicine for depression or do not take it. Patients should be carefully followed for such clinical worsening (particularly when treatment is started or doses are increased or decreased).

Precautions for Use

By Infants and Children: Safety and effectiveness for those under 18 years of age not established.

By Those Over 60 Years of Age: Age-related liver or kidney function decline may require dose decreases.

▷ **Advisability of Use During Pregnancy**

Pregnancy Category: B. See Pregnancy Risk Categories at the back of this book.

Animal Studies: Rat and rabbit studies reveal no significant birth defects.

Human Studies: Adequate studies of pregnant women are not available.

Use this drug only if clearly needed. Ask your doctor for help. A pregnancy registry has been established at 888-825-5249. Encourage your doctor to register you if you have taken this medicine while pregnant.

Advisability of Use If Breast-Feeding

Presence of this drug in breast milk: Yes.

Avoid drug or refrain from nursing.

Habit-Forming Potential: Remote with use of recommended doses. Slight potential for abuse by those who abuse stimulant drugs.

Effects of Overdose: Headache, agitation, confusion, hallucinations, seizures, loss of consciousness.

Possible Effects of Long-Term Use: Not reported.

Suggested Periodic Examinations While Taking This Drug (at physician's discretion)

Liver and/or kidney function tests as appropriate. Check of weight and blood pressure.

▷ **While Taking This Drug, Observe the Following**

Foods: No restrictions.

Herbal Medicines or Minerals: Ginseng, ma huang (no longer on the market), yohimbe, and St. John's wort may interact with antidepressants, so combining those herbals with this medicine is not recommended.

Beverages: No restrictions. May be taken with milk.

▷ *Alcohol:* Avoid completely. Alcohol may predispose to the development of seizures.

Tobacco Smoking: I advise everyone to quit smoking.

Marijuana Smoking: Avoid completely; it may lead to psychotic behavior.

▷ *Other Drugs*

The following drugs *taken concurrently* with bupropion may *increase* the risk of major seizures:

• antidepressants (tricyclic) or other bupropion-containing medicines.
• clozapine (Clozaril).
• fluoxetine (Prozac).
• guanfacine (Tenex).
• haloperidol (Haldol).
• lithium (Lithobid, others).

- loxapine (Loxitane).
- maprotiline (Ludiomil).
- molindone (Moban).
- phenothiazines (see Drug Classes).
- thioxanthenes (see Xanthine Drug Class).
- trazodone (Desyrel).

Bupropion *taken concurrently* with
- carbamazepine (Tegretol) may result in lowered carbamazepine levels.
- cimetidine (Tagamet) may lead to increased bupropion levels.
- flecainide (Tambocor) may lead to increased flecainide levels (interference with P450 2D6). The manufacturer suggests that flecainide doses be used at the lower end of the dose range if these medicines are combined. Flecainide blood levels are prudent.
- levodopa results in increased nausea, restlessness and tremor.
- MAO inhibitors (see Drug Classes) can lead to sudden toxicity. Do not combine.
- metoprolol (Toprol XL, others) can lead to toxicity. Lower metoprolol doses are prudent.
- phenobarbital may result in decreased levels.
- phenytoin (Dilantin) or fosphenytoin (Cerebyx) may result in decreased phenytoin or fosphenytoin levels.
- propafenone (Rythmol) can lead to toxicity. Lower propafenone doses and blood levels are prudent.
- risperidone (Risperdal), sertraline (Zoloft) and other medicines removed from the body by P450 2D6 may lead to increased blood levels of the medicine removed by P450 2D6. Lower doses and careful patient follow-up are prudent if these medicines are combined.
- ritonavir (Norvir) and probably other protease inhibitors may lead to increased blood levels of bupropion and toxicity—DO NOT COMBINE.
- zolpidem (Ambien) may lead to hallucinations.

▷ *Driving, Hazardous Activities:* This drug may cause dizziness, drowsiness or seizures. Restrict activities as necessary.

Aviation Note: The use of this drug *is a disqualification* for piloting. Consult a designated Aviation Medical Examiner.

Exposure to Sun: No restrictions.

Discontinuation: Do not stop this drug abruptly. Ask your doctor for help.

BUSPIRONE (byu SPI rohn)

Introduced: 1979 **Class:** Antianxiety drug **Prescription:** USA: Yes **Controlled Drug:** USA: No; Canada: No **Available as Generic:** Yes

Brand Names: ✤Apo-buspirone, Buspar, Buspar Dividose, ✤Buspirex, ✤Med-buspirone, ✤Buspirex, Censpar, Sorbon

```
                    BENEFITS versus RISKS
        Possible Benefits                    Possible Risks
EFFECTIVE RELIEF OF MILD TO        Mild dizziness, faintness, or
   MODERATE ANXIETY                   headache—uncommon
DECREASED RISK OF SEDATION         Tachycardia—rare
   OR DEPENDENCE THAN OTHER         Restlessness, depression, tremor, or
   AGENTS                             rigidity (with high doses)—rare
```

▷ **Principal Uses**

As a Single Drug Product: Uses currently included in FDA-approved labeling: (1) Relieves mild to moderate anxiety and nervous tension (useful in elderly, alcoholics and addiction-prone people because of its lack of significant sedative effects or abuse potential); (2) helps control self-injurious behaviors or aggression in developmentally disabled adults.

Other (unlabeled) generally accepted uses: (1) May reduce alcohol craving in alcoholics; (2) can help aggression or hyperactivity in people living with autism; (3) may decrease symptoms in obsessive-compulsive disorder; (4) can help in sexual dysfunction in people with generalized anxiety disorder; (5) may help decrease smoking urge in smokers; (6) can help prevent chronic tension headaches and migraines; (7) some data with success in treatment resistant depression and for those with anxiety and depression; (8) may have a role in preventing (prophylaxis) of migraines; (9) could have a role in easing post-traumatic stress disorder.

How This Drug Works: Changes brain chemicals (dopamine, norepinephrine, serotonin), resulting in a calming effect. Decreases actions of serotonin using nerve cells (neurons) in part of the brain (nuclei raphe). Also a partial agonist at serotonin reuptake sites (5HT1A).

▷ **Widely Used Guidelines That Involve This Medicine (representative sample):** Please look at the section at the very beginning of this profile called "Class." Next, turn to Table 22 and you will find guidelines listed by the class involved!

Available Dosage Forms and Strengths

Tablets — 5 mg, 10 mg, 15 mg, 30 mg
Tablets scored (Dividose) — 15 mg, 30 mg

▷ **Usual Adult Dosage Ranges:** Initially 7.5 mg twice daily; if needed, dose can be increased by 5 mg/day every 2 or 3 days as needed and tolerated. Some patients respond well to total daily doses of 20–30 mg which are divided into two or three equal doses. Maximum daily dose is 60 mg.

Note: Actual dose and schedule must be determined for each patient individually.

Conditions Requiring Dosing Adjustments

Liver Function: Doses should be decreased in people with compromised livers. The manufacturer does NOT support use in people with compromised liver function.

Kidney Function: One study based on kinetics suggested a the dose should be lowered to 25–50% of normal dose in people with mild to severe kidney compromise. The manufacturer does NOT recommend this medicine for people with severely impaired kidneys.

▷ **Dosing Instructions:** The tablet may be crushed and taken without regard to food—however, it is best to always take it with or without food in order to help keep blood levels steady. DO NOT take this medicine with grapefruit juice—take it with water. If you forget a dose, but have missed by less than an hour, take the missed dose. If it is almost time for your next scheduled dose, skip the missed dose and simply take the next scheduled dose. DO NOT double doses. Some researchers have reported this medicine to be equal to diazepam (Valium) in treating anxiety. If this medicine is meant to replace previous benzodiazepine use such as diazepam, the benzodiazepine should be slowly withdrawn (tapered) before the buspirone is started (avoids withdrawal problems).

Usual Duration of Use: Regular use for 7 to 14 days may be needed to see full benefit in relieving anxiety and nervous tension. Continual use should not exceed 8 weeks without evaluation by your doctor.

Author's Note: The National Institute of Mental Health has a good information page on anxiety, and anxious reactions to terrorism. It can be found on the World Wide Web (*www.nimh.nih.gov/healthinformation/anxietymenu.cfm*).

Typical Treatment Goals and Measurements (Outcomes and Markers)

Anxiety or panic: Goals for anxiety and panic tend to be more vague and subjective than hypertension or cholesterol. Frequently, the patient (in conjunction with physician assessment) will largely decide if anxiety has been modified to a successful extent. In the case of panic attacks, decreased number of trips to the hospital or emergency department visits may be a useful measure. In both cases, the ability of the patient to return to normal activities is a hallmark of successful treatment. The Hamilton Anxiety Scale is used by many physicians.

Possible Advantages of This Drug: Relieves anxiety or tension without severe sedation or impaired thinking. Low abuse potential compared to benzodiazepines. May be a drug of choice in patients prone to getting addicted and also in people with lung disease.

▷ **This Drug Should Not Be Taken If**
  • you have had an allergic reaction to this medicine.
  • you take, or took in the last 2 weeks, a MAO inhibitor (see Drug Classes). May increase blood pressure.

▷ **Inform Your Physician Before Taking This Drug If**
  • you take other drugs that affect the brain or nervous system: tranquilizers, sedatives, hypnotics, analgesics, narcotics, antidepressants, antipsychotic drugs, anticonvulsants, or anti-Parkinsonism drugs.
  • you have impaired liver or kidney function.
  • you take fluoxetine (Prozac) for depression.
  • you are prone to fast heart rate (tachycardia).

Possible Side Effects (natural, expected, and unavoidable drug actions)
Mild drowsiness (less than with benzodiazepines) (may be more likely with higher doses up to 8%)—infrequent; lethargy is possible. Infrequent dry mouth. Case reports of bed-wetting (enuresis).

▷ **Possible Adverse Effects** (unusual, unexpected, and infrequent reactions)
If any of the following develop, consult your physician promptly for guidance.
Mild Adverse Effects
Headache, faintness, paradoxical excitement—infrequent.
Nervousness—infrequent.
Dizziness—infrequent.
Tingling and touch sensation changes (paresthesias)—rare.

Insomnia and dream disturbances, racing thoughts, or depression—possible.
Increased blood pressure—case reports.
Nausea—infrequent.
Serious Adverse Effects
Tachycardia or palpitations—infrequent but greater than seen with diazepam.
With high doses: dysphoria, restlessness, rigidity, tremors—possible (may be
  more likely with high doses).
Movement disorders—case reports.
Apnea increases (in some patients with sleep apnea)—possible.

▷ **Possible Effects on Sexual Function:** Difficult or absent orgasm—case report.
  May increase prolactin; however, no cases of male breast tenderness or
  enlargement have been reported. One case of painful and sustained erection (priapism).

Possible Effects on Laboratory Tests
  Growth hormone: Conflicting increases or lack of effect on growth hormone
  levels.
  Blood prolactin levels: dose-related increase.
  May or may not change (increase delta or theta waves) on the EEG.

CAUTION
  1. This drug is reported to have very mild sedative effects and no abuse
     potential; however, it should be used with caution and only when clearly
     needed. Actual dysphoria has been reported with higher doses and may
     preclude its recreational use.
  2. Best to take this medicine the same way (with or without food) to help
     keep the blood levels steady.

Precautions for Use
  By Infants and Children: Safety and effectiveness for those under 18 years of
  age not established.
  By Those Over 60 Years of Age: Expected to be tolerated much better than benzodiazepines and barbiturates. Watch for increased dizziness or weakness
  and avoid falls.

▷ **Advisability of Use During Pregnancy**
  Pregnancy Category: B. See Pregnancy Risk Categories at the back of this
  book.
  Animal Studies: No birth defects found in rat and rabbit studies.
  Human Studies: Adequate studies of pregnant women are not available.
  Discuss any use of this drug during pregnancy with your doctor.

Advisability of Use If Breast-Feeding
  Presence of this drug in breast milk: Excreted in rat milk; probably also in
  humans.
  Avoid drug or refrain from nursing.

Habit-Forming Potential: Does not appear to cause addiction; however, more
  studies are needed. Higher doses result in a dysphoric reaction, which may
  keep it from becoming a drug involved in recreational use.

Effects of Overdose: Drowsiness, fatigue, nausea, dysphoria, tingling sensations
  (paresthesias), and a rare chance of seizures.

Possible Effects of Long-Term Use: None reported.

Suggested Periodic Examinations While Taking This Drug (at physician's discretion)
  Periodic check of heart rate and of course, success in controlling anxiety.

▷ **While Taking This Drug, Observe the Following**

Foods: No restrictions; taking with food may result in a clinically insignificant increase in absorption of this drug.

Herbal Medicines or Minerals: Hawthorn, bitter orange, guarana, and ephedra (no longer on the market) may react antagonistically to buspirone. Avoid those medicines. One case report of a problem with combined therapy with ginkgo (multiple medicines). Valerian may interact additively (drowsiness) and has not been recommended because of liver toxicity concerns. Hops, Indian snakeroot, passionflower herb, and St. John's wort carry German Commission E monograph indications for anxiety. Indian snakeroot and kava kava (not recommended in Canada because of liver problems) are contraindicated in depression and well-designed studies in anxiety combined with this medicine are not available. Talk to your doctor BEFORE you take any herbal medicine with buspirone.

Beverages: No restrictions.

▷ *Alcohol:* Milder problems than diazepam (Valium), but avoid the combination.

Tobacco Smoking: No interactions expected. I advise everyone to quit smoking.

Marijuana Smoking: Additive increase in drowsiness.

▷ *Other Drugs:*

Buspirone ***taken concurrently*** with

- citalopram (Celexa) may result in serotonin syndrome. This combination is not advisable.
- clozapine (Clozaril) may result in serious lowering of blood sugar and stomach bleeding.
- diazepam (Valium) may increase risk of headache, dizziness, and nausea.
- diltiazem (Cardizem, etc) may increase buspirone drug concentrations. Watch for increased drowsiness—lower buspirone doses may be needed.
- dofetilide (Tikosyn) may increase blood levels of dofetilide and risk of adverse effects. If this combination must be used, low doses of dofetilide and careful patient follow-up are critical.
- erythromycin (various) may increase blood levels of buspirone and risk of adverse effects.
- fluoxetine (Prozac) may increase underlying anxiety or mental disorder such as obsessive-compulsive disorder. Combination is best avoided, but if deemed clinically necessary, patients should be closely watched for worsening of symptoms.
- fluvoxamine (Luvox) resulted in serious slowing of the heart (bradycardia) in one case report (peak buspirone level was doubled). A later trial in healthy volunteers found elevated blood levels, but no clinical changes. Caution is advised.
- itraconazole (and perhaps other similar antifungals) may increase blood levels of buspirone and risk of adverse effects.
- MAO inhibitors (see Drug Classes) such as phenelzine (Nardil) may result in large blood pressure increases. DO NOT COMBINE.
- narcotics such as oxycodone (Percodan) may result in additive sedation and potential decreases in breathing (respiratory depression).
- nefazodone (Serzone) may increase blood levels of buspirone and risk of adverse effects. If this combination must be used, low doses of buspirone and careful patient follow-up are critical.
- paroxetine (Paxil) may increase blood levels of buspirone and risk of adverse effects. If this combination must be used, lower doses of buspirone and careful patient follow-up are critical.

- rifampin (Rifater, others) may decrease buspirone blood levels. If this combination must be used, buspirone doses may need to be increased.
- trazodone (Desyrel) may lead to liver toxicity. Liver tests should be obtained regularly if the two drugs are combined.
- venlafaxine (Effexor) may lead to decreased buspirone benefits or venlafaxine toxicity.
- verapamil (Calan, etc) may increase blood levels of buspirone and risk of adverse effects.

▷ *Driving, Hazardous Activities:* This drug may cause dizziness, faintness, or fatigue. Restrict activities as necessary.

Aviation Note: The use of this drug *may be a disqualification* for piloting. Consult a designated Aviation Medical Examiner.

Exposure to Sun: No restrictions.

CALCITONIN (kal si TOH nin)

Other Names: Salcatonin, thyrocalcitonin

Introduced: 1977, 1995 (nasal spray form) **Class:** Anti-osteoporotic, hormone **Prescription:** USA: Yes **Controlled Drug:** USA: No; Canada: No **Available as Generic:** USA: Yes (one injectable form); Canada: No

Brand Names: Calcimar, Cibacalcin, Miacalcin Injection, Miacalcin Nasal Spray

---

BENEFITS versus RISKS

Possible Benefits	*Possible Risks*
PARTIAL RELIEF OF SYMPTOMS OF PAGET'S DISEASE OF BONE	Nausea (with or without vomiting)
NASAL FORM CAN INCREASE BONE MASS	Allergic reactions
Effective adjunctive treatment of postmenopausal osteoporosis	
Effective adjunctive treatment of abnormally high blood calcium levels (associated with malignant disease)	

Author's Note: Information in this profile has been shortened to make room for more widely used medicines.

CAPECITABINE (CAP eh sit ah been)

Introduced: 2001 for colon cancer **Class:** Antineoplastic **Prescription:** USA: Yes **Controlled Drug:** USA: No; Canada: No **Available as Generic:** No

Brand Names: Xeloda

Available Dosage Forms and Strengths
Tablets — 150 mg and 500 mg
Tablets, chewable — 100 mg, 200 mg

Author's Note: Information in this profile will be further broadened in the next edition, if clinical data warrant. This medicine was first approved for treatment of breast cancer, and now has been approved for treatment of metastatic colorectal cancer. This first treatment for such cancers to be available taken by mouth (oral), capecitabine is changed (metabolized) into 5-fluorouracil in the body. Capecitabine causes fewer mouth ulcers and less diarrhea and nausea, but seems to cause pain and swelling of the hands and feet more frequently than other therapies. Information in this profile will be broadened further when more specific information becomes available. An excellent and evidence based review of cancer treatments is available from *www.cancer.gov/cancerinfo/pdq/ treatment/colon/HealthProfessional.*

CAPTOPRIL (KAP toh pril)

Introduced: 1979   **Class:**   ACE inhibitor, antihypertensive
Please see the new angiotensin converting enzyme (ACE) inhibitor family profile for more information.

CARBAMAZEPINE (kar ba MAZ e peen)

Introduced: 1962   **Class:**   Anticonvulsant, antineuralgic, pain syndrome modifier, mood stabilizer   **Prescription:**   USA: Yes   **Controlled Drug:**   USA: No; Canada: No   **Available as Generic:**   Yes
Brand Names: ❦Apo-Carbamazepine, Carbitrol Extended Release, ❦ Dom-carbamazepine-CR, Epitol, ❦Gen-Carbamazepine CR, ❦Mazepine, ❦Novo-Carbamaz, ❦PMS Carbamazepine, Taro-carbamazepine CR, Tegretol, Tegretol Chewable Tablet, ❦Tegretol-CR, Tegretol-XR

BENEFITS versus RISKS

Possible Benefits	*Possible Risks*
RELIEF OF PAIN IN TRIGEMINAL NEURALGIA	BONE MARROW DEPRESSION (reduced formation of all blood cells)—RARE
EFFECTIVE CONTROL OF CERTAIN TYPES OF EPILEPTIC SEIZURES	Liver damage with jaundice—rare
EFFECTIVE IN SUDDEN ONSET AND IN PREVENTING BIPOLAR DISORDER	
Relief of pain in some rare forms of nerve pain (neuralgia)	

▷ **Principal Uses**

As a Single Drug Product: Uses currently included in FDA-approved labeling: (1) pain relief in true trigeminal neuralgia (tic douloureux) or glossopharyngeal neuralgia; (2) for control of several types of epilepsy (grand mal, tonic-clonic, psychomotor/temporal lobe, complex partial and mixed seizure patterns as well as infantile spasms or myoclonic-astatic seizures). Precise diagnosis and careful management are mandatory.

Other (unlabeled) generally accepted uses: Beneficial in (1) bipolar affective disorders; (2) schizoaffective disorders; (3) resistant schizophrenia; (4) post-traumatic stress disorder; (5) tabes dorsalis; (6) diabetic neuropathy; (7) hemifacial spasm; (8) cocaine withdrawal; (9) aggression in some Alzheimer's patients; (10) helping hiccups and belching associated with flutter of the diaphragm; (11) treating nerve problems from thiamine deficiency; (12) has a role in pain that occurs when an arm or leg is amputated (phantom limb pain) and pain associated with depression; (13) easing a perceived repetitive ear noise called clicking tinnitus; (14) case reports of being helpful in people having difficulty making purposeful movements even though they have normal coordination and muscle power (apraxia).

How This Drug Works: Reduces impulses at certain nerve terminals and relieves pain (of trigeminal neuralgia). Also reduces excitability of nerve fibers in the brain, decreasing likelihood, frequency, and severity of seizures.

▷ **Widely Used Guidelines That Involve This Medicine (representative sample):** Please look at the section at the very beginning of this profile called "Class." Next, turn to Table 22 and you will find guidelines listed by the class involved!

Available Dosage Forms and Strengths
Oral suspension — 100 mg/5 mL, 200 mg/5 mL
Tablets — 200 mg (400 mg in Canada)
Tablets, chewable — 100 mg, 200 mg
Tablets, controlled release — 200 mg, 400 mg
Tablets, extended release — 100 mg, 200 mg, 300 mg, 400 mg

▷ **Recommended Dosage Ranges:**
Epilepsy: Initially 200 mg every 12 hours (regular or extended-release tablets). Suspension is started at 100 mg four times a day. Dose may be increased at weekly intervals by 200 mg daily as needed and tolerated and as guided by drug levels. The dose is given twice daily for the extended-release tablets (in general, extended-release forms are given in the same total daily dose—but are given less often). The regular release tablets are given three times daily. Because suspensions give higher peak blood levels in the body, they are generally given in smaller, more frequent doses. Total daily dosage should generally not exceed 1,200 mg, but rare uses of 1,600 mg have been required.
Migraine prevention (prophylaxis): 10–20 mg per kg of body weight per day separated into two equal daily doses has been used.
Trigeminal neuralgia: 50 mg of the suspension four times daily or 100 mg twice daily (tablets or extended release form). Dose is then increased as needed and tolerated to 400–800 mg daily with a 1,200 mg maximum. Every three months you and your doctor should try to lower the dose to the minimum dose that works (minimum effective dose) and to discontinue the medicine.
Bipolar disorder: Required doses have been in the 2,000–3,000 mg a day, but most people respond to 600–1,600 mg a day. Patients who go from mania to depression quickly (rapid cycling patients) may need 1,000–2,000 mg a day to help ease the swings in mood.
Infants and Children: Children under age 6 are given 10–20 mg per kg of body mass. This dose is divided into two to three equal doses and is given two to three times daily. The suspension dosing is the same daily dose divided into 4 equal doses given four times daily. Increased as needed or tolerated based on clinical response and blood levels, with a maximum dose of 35 mg/kg/day. Children over 12 are given 200 mg twice daily or 100 mg of the suspension four times daily. The dose can then be increased by 200 mg

a day after a week, as needed and tolerated—guided by blood levels and clinical response. The typical dose that works is in the range of 17–25 mg/kg/day. Maximum is 1,000 mg or lower.

Note: Actual dosage and schedule must be determined for each patient individually. Dosing must be guided by blood levels.

Conditions Requiring Dosing Adjustments

Liver Function: Use with extreme caution, in lower doses and closely watched. Should NOT be used in active liver disease or in worsened liver compromise.

Kidney Function: May be toxic to kidneys. Used with caution.

Heart Attack: Changes in blood distribution (perfusion) and protein binding may give much higher than expected blood levels. More frequent lab tests are needed to guide dosing and avoid toxicity.

▷ **Dosing Instructions:** Take at same time each day, with or following food to reduce stomach irritation. Regular-release tablet may be crushed for administration. Extended-release tablet should not be altered or taken if they are broken. The suspension SHOULD NOT be given at the same time as other medicines or diluents. The suspension will generally give higher peak levels than an equal dose of a tablet form. Patients changed from the tablet to the suspension may be asked to take the same number of milligrams a day, but to take smaller doses more often. If you forget a dose: Take the medicine as soon as you remember it, unless it is close to the time for the next dose—simply take the dose at the next scheduled time. DO NOT double doses. Call your doctor if you miss more than one dose.

Usual Duration of Use: Regular use for 3 months may be needed to see effect in easing of trigeminal neuralgia. Longer periods, with dose changes, may be required for control of epileptic seizures. Careful evaluation of tolerance and response should be made every 3 months during long-term treatment. Every three months, the minimum effective dose should be tried to be found and/or the medicine attempted to be stopped if it is being used to treat trigeminal neuralgia.

Typical Treatment Goals and Measurements (Outcomes and Markers)

Seizures: The general goal for this medicine is effective seizure control. Neurologists tend to define effective on a case-by-case basis depending on the seizure type and patient factors.

Currently a "Drug of Choice"

For patients with partial seizures (without or with secondary generalization).

▷ **This Drug Should Not Be Taken If**
- you have had an allergic reaction to it previously.
- you have active liver disease.
- you currently have a blood cell or bone marrow disorder.
- you currently take, or have taken within the past 14 days, a monoamine oxidase (MAO) type A inhibitor (see Drug Classes).

▷ **Inform Your Physician Before Taking This Drug If**
- you have had an allergic reaction to any tricyclic antidepressant drug (see Drug Classes).
- you have taken this drug in the past.
- you have had any blood or bone marrow disorder, especially drug induced.
- you have a history of liver or kidney disease.
- you have depression or other mental disorder.
- you have had vein inflammation and blood clots (thrombophlebitis).
- you have high blood pressure, heart disease, increased eye pressure, or glaucoma.

- you take more than two alcoholic drinks a day.
- you take prescription or nonprescription drugs not discussed when carba-mazepine was prescribed for you.
- you are unsure how much to take or how often to take it.
- you are pregnant or are breast-feeding your baby.

Possible Side Effects (natural, expected, and unavoidable drug actions)
Dry mouth and throat, constipation, impaired urination.

▷ **Possible Adverse Effects** (unusual, unexpected, and infrequent reactions)
  If any of the following develop, consult your physician promptly for guidance.
  Mild Adverse Effects
  Allergic reactions: skin rash, hives, itching, drug fever—rare to infrequent.
  Idiosyncratic reactions (cough or shortness of breath)—possible.
  Dizziness, drowsiness, unsteadiness—may be frequent when therapy is started (often eases).
  Fatigue, blurred vision, confusion—infrequent.
  Exaggerated hearing, ringing in ears—case reports.
  Loss of appetite, nausea, vomiting, indigestion, diarrhea—may be frequent when starting therapy.
  Hair loss—case reports.
  Decreased sense of taste—possible.
  Aching of muscles and joints, leg cramps—case reports.
  Serious Adverse Effects
  Allergic reactions: severe dermatitis with peeling of skin (including toxic epidermal necrolysis-TEN and Stevens Johnson Syndrome), irritation of mouth and tongue, swelling of lymph glands—case reports.
  Idiosyncratic reactions: lung inflammation (pneumonitis), may also be an aseptic meningitis mechanism.
  Agranulocytosis may also be idiosyncratic—case reports.
  Pure red cell aplasia—case reports.
  Lowering of white blood cells (leukopenia): may be up to 10%—infrequent.
  Aplastic anemia—rare.
  Abnormally low blood platelets—thrombocytopenia (clotting elements on blood)—rare, but tends to happen 2–3 weeks after the medicine is started.
  Low thyroid hormones—rare.
  Bone marrow depression (see Glossary) (agranulocytosis, hemolytic or aplastic anemia) or thrombocytopenia: fatigue, weakness, fever, sore throat, abnormal bleeding, or bruising—case reports.
  Pseudolymphoma or systemic lupus erythematosus—case reports.
  Abnormal heartbeats—case reports.
  Aggravation of disease of the coronary arteries (CAD)—possible.
  Liver damage with jaundice (see Glossary): yellow eyes or skin, dark-colored urine, light-colored stools—case reports.
  Kidney damage or porphyria—case reports.
  Mental depression or agitation/psychosis or paradoxical increase in seizures—case reports.
  Abnormally elevated urine output (SIADH)—case reports.
  Neuroleptic malignant syndrome—case reports.
  Abnormal movement and muscle contractions—case reports.
  Pancreatitis—case reports.
  Retinopathy, visual hallucinations, peripheral neuritis (see Glossary)—case reports.

Vitamin D deficiency (especially if other risk factors are present). This may lead to osteoporosis.

▷ **Possible Effects on Sexual Function:**

Decreased libido and/or impotence—case reports.

Possible male infertility.

This drug is used to control hypersexuality (exaggerated sexual behavior) that can result from injury to the temporal lobe of the brain.

Adverse Effects That May Mimic Natural Diseases or Disorders

Liver reactions may suggest viral hepatitis. Lung reactions may suggest interstitial pneumonitis. SLE syndrome mimics SLE.

Natural Diseases or Disorders That May Be Activated by This Drug

Latent psychosis, systemic lupus erythematosus, osteoporosis, heart disease (see homocysteine note below).

Possible Effects on Laboratory Tests

Complete blood cell: decreased red cells, hemoglobin, white cells, and platelets; increased eosinophils, increased white cells.

Blood calcium level: decreased.

Blood sodium: may be lowered in SIADH.

INR (prothrombin time): decreased.

Thyroid hormones: decreased blood levels.

Blood urea nitrogen level (BUN): increased.

Liver function tests: increased liver enzymes (ALT/GPT, AST/GOT, and alkaline phosphatase), increased bilirubin.

Urine pregnancy tests: false negative or inconclusive results with Prepurex, Predictor, Gonavislide, Pregnosticon.

ANA: positive if SLE effect begins.

CAUTION

1. This drug should be used only after less toxic drugs have failed.
2. *Before* the first dose is taken, blood cell counts, liver function tests and kidney function tests should be obtained.
3. Careful periodic testing for blood cell or bone marrow toxicity is *mandatory*.
4. *This drug should not be used* to prevent recurrence of trigeminal neuralgia when it is in remission.
5. *Do not stop this drug suddenly* if it is being used to control seizures.
6. If exposed to humidity, tablet hardens, resulting in poor absorption and erratic control of seizures. Store in a cool, dry place; avoid bathrooms. Try a locking kitchen cabinet.
7. Case reports have been made about an allergic (atypical cross-sensitivity) reaction in people who are allergic to phenytoin who are given carbamazepine. Talk to your doctor if you have this allergy and carbamazepine is prescribed for you.
8. If you are prescribed the suspension, usually the same total dose is given, but smaller and more frequent doses are used because the suspension gives a higher peak level.
9. Because of some carbamazepine caused (drug induced) lowering of pyridoxal 5-phosphate and folate, homocysteine levels are increased with this therapy. See foods below.
10. There are reports of people who are allergic to oxcarbazepine also being allergic to carbamazepine (25–30%). This can also happen with phenytoin as noted in number 7 above.
11. Grapefruit and grapefruit juice can lead to toxicity from this medicine.

Do not eat grapefruit or drink grapefruit juice while taking this medicine.

Precautions for Use

By Infants and Children: Careful testing of blood production and liver and kidney function must be performed regularly. This drug can reduce the effectiveness of other anticonvulsant drugs. Blood levels of all anticonvulsant drugs should be checked if this drug is added to the treatment program.

By Those Over 60 Years of Age: Can cause confusion and agitation. Watch for aggravation of glaucoma, coronary artery disease (angina), or prostatism (see Glossary).

▷ Advisability of Use During Pregnancy

Pregnancy Category: **D.** See Pregnancy Risk Categories at the back of this book.
Animal Studies: Rat studies reveal significant birth defects.
Human Studies: Adequate studies of pregnant women are not available.
Avoid completely during the first 3 months. Use during the last 6 months only if clearly needed.

Advisability of Use If Breast-Feeding

Presence of this drug in breast milk: Yes.
Levels in breast milk appear to be 24 to almost 70% of the mother's plasma level. Discuss avoiding drug or refrain from nursing with your doctor.

Habit-Forming Potential: None.

Effects of Overdose: Dizziness, drowsiness, disorientation, tremor, involuntary movements, nausea, vomiting, flushed skin, dilated pupils, stupor progressing to coma, cardiac arrest.

Possible Effects of Long-Term Use: Water retention (edema), impaired liver function, possible jaundice, possible osteoporosis.

Suggested Periodic Examinations While Taking This Drug (at physician's discretion)

Complete blood counts weekly during the first 3 months and then monthly.
Liver and kidney function tests.
Eye examinations.
Serum iron levels.
Blood levels of the medicine.
Thyroid hormone levels.
Bone mineral density tests (for osteoporosis) and/or check of height.
Homocysteine levels.

▷ While Taking This Drug, Observe the Following

Foods: DO NOT eat grapefruit or drink the juice while taking this medicine. There may be a minor increase in absorption if taken with food. Because of drug effects on B vitamins, homocysteine levels are prudent and supplementation with B vitamins while this drug is being taken is also prudent.

Herbal Medicines or Minerals: Using kola, guarana, bitter orange, country mallow, or ma huang (no longer on the market) may result in unacceptable central nervous system stimulation. Valerian and kava kava (not recommended in Canada) may interact to increase drowsiness. St. John's wort may increase carbamazepine blood levels and also cause increased sun sensitivity—caution is advised. Some ginkgo products (depending on the amount of 4-o-methylpyridoxine in them) may increase risk of seizures.

Beverages: DO NOT drink grapefruit juice while taking this medicine. May be taken with milk.

▷ *Alcohol:* Avoid alcohol, unless your doctor approves alcohol use.

Tobacco Smoking: No interactions expected. I advise everyone to quit smoking.

▷ *Other Drugs*

Carbamazepine may *increase* the effects of
- medicines that increase heart block such at adenosine (Adenocard). Where possible, carbamazepine should not be given until adenosine has cleared from the body (roughly 4.32 or 5 half-lives, which is 4 days).
- sedatives, tranquilizers, hypnotics and narcotics, and enhance their sedative effects.
- voriconazole (Vfend) and lead to much higher than expected blood levels.

Carbamazepine may *decrease* the effects of
- adrenocortical steroids (see Drug Classes).
- alprazolam (Xanax).
- amprenavir (Agenerase).
- antidepressants (see Drug Classes).
- bupropion (Wellbutrin, Zyban).
- caspofungin (Cancidas).
- corticosteroids (such as prednisone or cortisone; see Drug Classes).
- cyclosporine (Sandimmune).
- doxycycline (Doxy-II, Vibramycin, etc).
- felodipine (Plendil).
- haloperidol (Haldol) or other phenothiazines.
- imatinib (Gleevec).
- isradipine (DynaCirc).
- lamotrigine (Lamictal).
- methylphenidate (Ritalin, others).
- midazolam (Versed).
- nelfinavir (Viracept).
- olanzapine (Zyprexa).
- quetiapine (Seroquel).
- sirolimus (Rapamune) blood levels and dosing adjusted to blood sirolimus levels is prudent.
- tacrolimus (Prograf) blood levels and dosing adjusted to tacrolimus levels is prudent.
- tetracyclines (see Drug Classes).
- tramadol (Ultram) and cause loss of tramadol efficacy.
- valproic acid (Depakene, etc).
- vincristin (Oncovin).
- warfarin (Coumadin). Increased frequency of INR testing is indicated.

Carbamazepine *taken concurrently* with
- acetaminophen (Tylenol, others) may increase risk of acetaminophen liver toxicity.
- activated charcoal (various) will bind this drug and lower benefits.
- birth control pills (oral contraceptives) may lower blood levels of the birth control pills and result in pregnancy.
- chlorpromazine (Thorazine) solution may form a rubbery orange precipitate that is passed in the stool. DO NOT combine.
- cisplatin (Platinol, others).
- clozapine (Clozaril) may result in serious bone marrow suppression.
- delavirdine (Rescriptor) may lower trough levels of delavirdine.
- doxorubicin (Doxil, others).
- felbamate (Felbatol) may result in decreased carbamazepine levels and seizures.

- itraconazole (Sporanox) may cause loss of itraconazole benefits.
- ketorolac (Toradol) may blunt carbamazepine benefits.
- lithium (Lithobid, others) may cause serious neurological problems: confusion, drowsiness, weakness, unsteadiness, tremors, and twitching.
- monoamine oxidase (MAO) type A inhibitor drugs (see Drug Classes) may cause severe toxic reactions.
- N-acetylcysteine (various) may blunt seizure control.
- phenytoin (Dilantin, etc) and fosphenytoin (Cerebyx) may cause unpredictable fluctuations of blood levels of both drugs and impair seizure control.
- primidone (Mysoline) may blunt carbamazepine effectiveness.
- sildenafil (Viagra) may result in changes in blood levels.
- terfenadine (Seldane), and perhaps other nonsedating antihistamines, may result in carbamazepine toxicity.
- theophylline (Theo-Dur, etc) may reduce the effects of both drugs.
- thioridazine (Mellaril) solution may form a rubbery orange precipitate that is passed in the stool. DO NOT combine.

The following drugs may *increase* the effects of carbamazepine:
- cimetidine (Tagamet).
- danazol (Danocrine).
- diltiazem (Cardizem)—and perhaps other calcium channel blockers.
- flu shots (influenza vaccine).
- fluoxetine (Prozac); may lead to toxicity.
- fluvoxamine (Luvox); may result in toxicity.
- isoniazid (INH).
- ketoconazole (Nizoral) and fluconazole (Diflucan).
- macrolide antibiotics—erythromycins, clarithromycin, or troleandomycin (not azithromycin).
- nefazodone (Serzone).
- nicotinamide (nicotinic acid amide).
- omeprazole (Prilosec).
- propoxyphene (Darvon, Darvocet, etc).
- quinupristin/dalfopristin (Synercid) may lead to increased blood levels of carbamazepine and toxicity. Blood levels are prudent and carbamazepine dose decreases may be required.
- rifampin (Rifampicin) may result in toxicity.
- ritonavir (Norvir) and perhaps other protease inhibitors such as amprenavir (Agenerase) (see Drug Classes).
- verapamil (Calan, Isoptin).

▷ *Driving, Hazardous Activities:* Can cause dizziness, drowsiness, or blurred vision. Adjust activities.

Aviation Note: The use of this drug *is a disqualification* for piloting. Consult a designated Aviation Medical Examiner.

Exposure to Sun: This drug can cause photosensitivity (see Glossary). Use caution until sensitivity to sun is known.

Heavy Exercise or Exertion: Use caution if you have coronary artery disease. Can intensify angina and reduce tolerance for physical activity.

Occurrence of Unrelated Illness: You MUST tell all health care providers that you take this drug.

Discontinuation: If treating trigeminal neuralgia, attempts to reduce the maintenance dose or to stop this drug are needed every 3 months. If used to control epilepsy, this drug *must not be stopped abruptly*.

Special Storage Instructions: Store tablets in a cool, dry place. Protect from humid conditions (**DO NOT store in a bathroom medicine cabinet**) as humidity can decrease potency of both brand or generic forms to a serious degree (significant percentage degradation of drug).

CARTEOLOL (KAR tee oh lohl)

Introduced: 1983   **Class:** Antihypertensive, beta-adrenergic blocker
Prescription: USA: Yes   **Controlled Drug:** USA: No; Canada: No
Available as Generic: Yes (ophthalmic)
Brand Names: Cartrol, Ocupress, Occupress

BENEFITS versus RISKS	
Possible Benefits	*Possible Risks*
EFFECTIVE, WELL-TOLERATED ANTIHYPERTENSIVE	Congestive heart failure worsening (in some patients)
EFFECTIVE GLAUCOMA TREATMENT	Worsening of angina in coronary heart disease (abrupt withdrawal)
Prevention of angina	Possible masking of low blood sugar (hypoglycemia) in drug-treated type 2 diabetics
May help prevent complications and left ventricle damage after a heart attack	Provocation of asthma in asthmatics
May help prevent tolerance to nitrates	

▷ **Principal Uses**
As a Single Drug Product: Uses currently included in FDA-approved labeling: (1) Treats mild to moderate high blood pressure, alone or in combination with other drugs, such as diuretics; (2) helps lower eye (intraocular) pressure in people with glaucoma or increased eye pressure (ocular hypertension).
Other (unlabeled) generally accepted uses: (1) Increases amount of exercise that can be performed before angina occurs; (2) can help decrease aggressive behavior; (3) decreases risk of abnormal heart rhythms; (4) has shown benefits after heart attacks—preserving left heart ventricle function and preventing second heart attacks; (5) may help lessen panic attacks.

How This Drug Works: Blocks certain actions of the sympathetic nervous system. Reduces the heart rate and contraction force, lowering ejection pressure of blood leaving the heart. Reduces extent of blood vessel wall contraction, relaxing the walls, and lowering blood pressure. Reduces elevated eye pressure (intraocular) and relieves glaucoma symptoms.

▷ **Widely Used Guidelines That Involve This Medicine (representative sample):** Please look at the section at the very beginning of this profile called "Class." Next, turn to Table 22 and you will find guidelines listed by the class involved!

Available Dosage Forms and Strengths
Ophthalmic solution — 5 mL, 10 mL (1%)
Tablets — 2.5 mg, 5 mg

▷ **Usual Adult Dosage Ranges:** *High blood pressure (hypertension):* Starts with 2.5 mg daily (by itself or combined with a water pill or diuretic) once a day. If needed because blood pressure goals are not reached, the dose can be gradually (peak benefits from a given dose may take several days up to several weeks) increased to 5 or 10 mg a day. This medicine has a maximum dose effect (ceiling effect), and doses above 10 mg are not likely to give added benefit in controlling high blood pressure—yet may increase how often side effects happen.

For angina: A wide range of effective doses from 2.5 to a maximum of 60 mg has been used. Most commonly, 20–40 mg once a day has been reported to control pressure for many patients.

For glaucoma or eye (ocular) hypertension: One drop in the affected eye or eyes two times a day.

Note: Actual dose and schedule must be determined for each patient individually.

Conditions Requiring Dosing Adjustments

Liver Function: Liver does play a role in removing this medicine, but how much of a role is not defined. Decreased doses are probably needed in severe liver failure.

Kidney Function: Dosing interval **MUST** be decreased in kidney compromise. For example, in severe compromise (creatinine clearance less than 10), 5 mg is given every 48 to 72 hours.

▷ **Dosing Instructions:** Tablet may be crushed and taken without regard to eating. Do not stop this drug abruptly. If you forget a dose: take it right away unless it's nearly time for your next daily dose. If it IS within 8 hours of the regular dose, skip the missed dose and just take the scheduled dose. DO NOT double doses. It is important to wash your hands BEFORE using the eye drops. Make sure you understand how your doctor wants you to place (instill) the eye drops. Your vision may be cloudy or blurry for a little while after you place the eye drops in the eyes.

Usual Duration of Use: Regular use for up to 3 weeks may be needed to see effectiveness in lowering blood pressure, and the medicine should be given this reasonable therapeutic trial before it is discontinued or dose escalated. Long-term use (months to years) is determined by lowering of blood pressure and response to a overall program (weight reduction, salt restriction, smoking cessation, etc). See your doctor on a regular basis. For the eye drops, use is usually ongoing with follow up checks of eye pressure (intraocular pressure or IOP) helping decide additional therapy or dose adjustments.

Typical Treatment Goals and Measurements (Outcomes and Markers)

Blood Pressure: Guidelines (JNC VII) define normal blood pressure (BP) as **less than** 120/80 and **pre-hypertension** as 120/80 to 139/89. This new range is intended to help doctors encourage lifestyle changes (or in the case of people with a risk factor for high blood pressure, start treatment) much earlier—so that damage to blood vessels, your heart, kidneys, sexual potency, or eyes might be minimized or avoided altogether. Stage 1 hypertension is 140/90 to 159/99 and stage 2 hypertension equal to or greater than: 160/100 mm Hg. These guidelines also recommend that clinicians work with their patients to agree on the goals and a plan of treatment. The first-ever guidelines for blood pressure (hypertension) in African Americans recommends that MOST black patients be started on TWO antihypertensive medicines with the goal of lowering blood pressure to 130/80 for those with high risk for heart and blood vessel disease or with diabetes. The American Diabetes Association also recommends 130/80 as the target for diabetics and less than 125/75 for those who spill more than one gram of protein into their urine. Most clinicians try to achieve a BP that confers the best balance of lower cardiovascular risk and avoids the problem of too low a blood pressure. Blood pressure duration is generally increased with beneficial restriction of sodium. If goals are not met, it is not unusual to intensify doses or add on medicines.

Possible Advantages of This Drug: Adequate control of blood pressure with a single daily dose helps adherence or compliance. Causes less slowing of the heart rate than most other beta-blocker drugs.

▷ **This Drug Should Not Be Taken If**
- you have bronchial asthma and/or obstructive lung (pulmonary) disease.
- you have had an allergic reaction to it previously.
- you have congestive heart failure (overt) or are in shock of heart origin (cardiogenic shock).
- you have an abnormally slow heart rate (bradycardia) or a serious heart block (second- or third-degree AV).

▷ **Inform Your Physician Before Taking This Drug If**
- you have had an adverse reaction to any beta blocker (see Drug Classes).
- you have serious heart disease or episodes of heart failure.
- you have had hay fever (allergic rhinitis), asthma, chronic bronchitis, or emphysema.
- you have a history of overactive thyroid function (hyperthyroidism).
- you have a history of low blood sugar (hypoglycemia), diabetes (particularly type 1), or myasthenia gravis.
- you have impaired liver or kidney function.
- you have a circulation problem (Raynaud's phenomenon, claudication, pains in legs).
- you take any form of digitalis, quinidine or reserpine, or any calcium blocker drug (see Drug Classes).
- you will have surgery with general anesthesia.

Possible Side Effects (natural, expected, and unavoidable drug actions)
Lethargy and fatigability, cold extremities, slow heart rate. Rebound angina if this medicine is stopped abruptly. Short-term itching or eye tearing with the ophthalmic drops—frequent.

▷ **Possible Adverse Effects** (unusual, unexpected, and infrequent reactions)
If any of the following develop, consult your physician promptly for guidance.
Mild Adverse Effects
Allergic reactions: skin rash—rare.
Headache, dizziness, nervousness, drowsiness—infrequent to frequent.
Indigestion, nausea, vomiting, constipation, diarrhea—infrequent.
Slight increase in blood potassium—possible.
Cough, wheezing or sinusitis—rare.
Joint and muscle discomfort, numbness of fingers or toes—rare.
Carpal tunnel syndrome—case reports with other medicines in this class.
Episodic difficulty walking (intermittent claudication with peripheral vascular disease)—possible.
Tearing and irritation (with eye use)—infrequent to frequent.
Serious Adverse Effects
Mental depression—possible, but less likely than some other beta blockers.
Chest pain, irregular heartbeat, shortness of breath; can cause congestive heart failure—possible.
Induction of bronchial asthma (in asthmatic patients)—possible.
Aggravation of myasthenia gravis—possible.
May hide symptoms of low blood sugar.

▷ **Possible Effects on Sexual Function:** Decreased libido, impotence—case reports.

Adverse Effects That May Mimic Natural Diseases or Disorders
Decreased extremity blood flow may mimic Raynaud's phenomenon (see Glossary).

Natural Diseases or Disorders That May Be Activated by This Drug
Raynaud's disease, intermittent claudication, myasthenia gravis.

Possible Effects on Laboratory Tests
Blood creatine kinase level: increased.
Blood potassium: slight increase.

CAUTION
1. ***Do not stop this drug suddenly*** without the knowledge of your doctor. Carry a note that says you are taking this drug.
2. Ask your physician or pharmacist before using nasal decongestants. These can cause sudden increases in blood pressure when combined with beta-blocker drugs.
3. Report any new tendency to emotional depression.
4. Use of the eye (ophthalmic) form may lead to additive lowering of blood pressure with other beta blockers.

Precautions for Use
By Infants and Children: Safety and effectiveness by those under 12 years of age not established.
By Those Over 60 Years of Age: **Caution:** Unacceptably high blood pressure should be reduced without creating excessively low blood pressure. Small doses and frequent blood pressure checks are needed. Sudden/excessive blood pressure lowering can cause stroke or heart attack. Watch for dizziness, confusion, depression, or urinary frequency.

▷ **Advisability of Use During Pregnancy**
Pregnancy Category: C. See Pregnancy Risk Categories at the back of this book.
Animal Studies: No birth defects found in rat or rabbit studies.
Human Studies: Adequate studies of pregnant women are not available.
Use this drug only if clearly needed. Ask your physician for guidance.

Advisability of Use If Breast-Feeding
Presence of this drug in breast milk: Unknown in humans; yes in animals.
Avoid drug or refrain from nursing.

Habit-Forming Potential: None.

Effects of Overdose: Weakness, slow pulse, low blood pressure, fainting, cold and sweaty skin, congestive heart failure, possible coma, and convulsions.

Possible Effects of Long-Term Use: Reduced heart reserve and eventual heart failure in susceptible individuals with advanced heart disease.

Suggested Periodic Examinations While Taking This Drug (at physician's discretion)
Measurements of blood pressure (treated to pressure goal within a set time frame).
Evaluation of heart function. Recheck of eye pressure.

▷ **While Taking This Drug, Observe the Following**
Foods: No specific restrictions, but losing weight can help meet blood pressure goals. Avoid excessive salt intake.
Herbal Medicines or Minerals: Ginseng, guarana, bitter orange, country mallow, hawthorn, saw palmetto, ma huang (no longer on the market), goldenseal,

yohimbe, and licorice may cause increased blood pressure. St. John's wort can change liver removal of medicines and is not recommended for people taking beta blockers. Calcium and garlic may help lower blood pressure, and the dose has to be individualized with a standardized extract. Dong quai can change the removal of medicines by the liver—caution is advised for excessive lowering of blood pressure. Ginger, vanadium, and nettle may also change blood sugar, an effect that may be hidden by some of the actions of this medicine. Indian snakeroot has a German Commission E monograph indication for hypertension—talk to your doctor. Eleuthero root and ephedra should be avoided by people living with hypertension. Talk to your doctor BEFORE adding any herbals.

Beverages: No restrictions. May be taken with milk.

▷ *Alcohol:* Use caution. Alcohol may exaggerate blood pressure lowering and also increase its mild sedative effect.

Tobacco Smoking: Nicotine may reduce benefits in treating high blood pressure. High doses may worsen bronchial constriction caused by regular smoking. I advise everyone to quit smoking.

▷ *Other Drugs*

Carteolol may ***increase*** the effects of

- other antihypertensive drugs and cause excessive lowering of the blood pressure. Dosage adjustments may be necessary.
- reserpine (Ser-Ap-Es, etc) and cause sedation, depression, slowing of the heart rate, and low blood pressure. This combination is best avoided.
- theophyllines (aminophylline, dyphylline, oxtriphylline, etc).
- verapamil (Calan, Isoptin) and cause excessive depression of heart function; monitor this combination closely.

Carteolol ***taken concurrently*** with

- amiodarone (Cordarone) may cause severe slowing of the heart and sinus arrest. Do not combine these agents.
- clonidine (Catapres) requires close monitoring for rebound high blood pressure if clonidine is stopped while carteolol is still being taken. Severe rebound hypertension may occur.
- digoxin (Lanoxin) may lead to abnormal heart conduction. Caution is prudent.
- diltiazem (Cardizem) and other dihydropyridine type calcium channel blockers (like verapamil) may be very helpful in patients with normal heart function, but may result in AV conduction problems.
- epinephrine (Adrenalin, etc) may cause sudden rise in blood pressure followed by slowing of the heart rate. Avoid this combination.
- ergot preparations (ergotamine, methysergide, etc) may enhance serious ergot-induced constriction of peripheral circulation.
- fluoxetine (Prozac) may result in dangerous slowing of the heart or dangerously low blood pressure.
- fluvoxamine (Luvox) may result in dangerous slowing of the heart or dangerously low blood pressure.
- insulin requires close monitoring to avoid hypoglycemia (see Glossary).
- nifedipine (and perhaps other dihydroperidine calcium channel blockers) may result in excessive lowering of the blood pressure.
- oral antidiabetic drugs (see Drug Classes) may cause prolonged recovery from hypoglycemia should it occur.
- phenothiazines (see Drug Classes) can cause increased effects of both drugs.
- rifabutin (Mycobutin) may reduce carteolol's effectiveness.

- ritodrine (Yutopar) may block Yutopar actions. Maker of ritodrine does NOT recommend this combination.
- sibutramine (Meridia) may lead to increases in blood pressure.
- venlafaxine (Effexor) may lead to toxicity from either drug.
- zileuton (Zyflo) may result in increased toxicity risk from carteolol. Caution is advised.

The following drugs may *decrease* the effects of carteolol:
- indomethacin (Indocin), and possibly other "aspirin substitutes" or NSAIDs, and may impair carteolol's antihypertensive effect.

▷ *Driving, Hazardous Activities:* Use caution until the full extent of fatigue, dizziness, and blood pressure change have been determined.

Aviation Note: The use of this drug *is a disqualification* for piloting. Consult a designated Aviation Medical Examiner.

Exposure to Sun: No restrictions.

Exposure to Heat: Caution is advised. Hot environments can lower the blood pressure and exaggerate the effects of this drug.

Exposure to Cold: Caution is advised. The elderly should take precautions to prevent hypothermia (see Glossary).

Heavy Exercise or Exertion: Avoid exertion that produces light-headedness, excessive fatigue, or muscle cramping.

Occurrence of Unrelated Illness: Fever can lower blood pressure and require decreased doses. Illnesses that cause nausea or vomiting may interrupt the regular dosage schedule. Ask your physician for guidance.

Discontinuation: **DO NOT STOP this drug suddenly**. If possible, gradual reduction of dose over a period of 2 to 3 weeks is recommended. Ask your physician for help.

CARVEDILOL (KAR vi die lohl)

Introduced: 1997   **Class:**   Alpha adrenergic blocker, antihypertensive, beta-adrenergic blocker   **Prescription:**   USA: Yes   **Controlled Drug:** USA: No; Canada: No   **Available as Generic:**   No

Brand Names: Coreg, ✤Dilatrend, ✤Eucardic, ✤Proreg

BENEFITS versus RISKS

Possible Benefits	*Possible Risks*
EFFECTIVE, WELL-TOLERATED ANTIHYPERTENSIVE	Worsening of heart failure (often responds to dose changes)
IMPROVES CONGESTIVE HEART FAILURE (mild–severe)	Slow heartbeat
CONFERS SIGNIFICANT SURVIVAL BENEFITS IN PATIENTS WITH ADVANCED CONGESTIVE HEART FAILURE	Masking of low blood sugar (hypoglycemia) in drug-treated diabetics (possible)
DECREASES RISK OF DEATH IN HEART ATTACK PATIENTS WITH HEARTS THAT DO NOT WORK PROPERLY (IMPAIRED CARDIAC FUNCTION)	Provocation of asthma in asthmatics
WORKS ON TWO KINDS OF BETA RECEPTORS (B1 AND B2) AND ALPHA [ALPHA 1]) RECEPTORS	
COMET TRIAL (SEE BELOW) SHOWED SIGNIFICANT LOWERING OF ALL-CAUSE MORTALITY (DEATH) AND DEATH FROM HEART AND BLOOD VESSEL DISEASE VERSUS METOPROLOL	

▷ **Principal Uses**

As a Single Drug Product: Uses currently included in FDA-approved labeling: (1) Treats mild to moderate high blood pressure, alone or in combination with other drugs; (2) improves congestive heart failure or CHF (one of two beta blockers along with metoprolol XL form approved for CHF). Approved for mild to severe CHF; (3) lowers risk of death (23%) in heart attack victims who have hearts that no longer have their usual heart function (impaired cardiac function).

Other unlabeled, generally accepted uses: (1) Eases frequency and severity of angina; (2) may help prevent loss of benefits from nitroglycerin (nitrate tolerance) when that medicine is used to ease angina pain; (3) may be of help in people with increased blood pressure in the liver blood circulation that stems from liver disease (portal hypertension).

Author's note: The COMET (Carvedilol or Metoprolol European Trial) was the first study to make a head to head (drug to drug) comparison of two beta blockers in people with ongoing (chronic) heart failure (CHF) and looked at the effect of the two medicines on survival. CARVEDILOL showed a significant preferential lowering of death from heart and blood vessel disease (cardiovascular mortality) as well as all-cause mortality versus another beta blocker called metoprolol.

How This Drug Works: Blocks certain actions of the sympathetic nervous system and:
- reduces the heart rate and contraction force, lowering ejection pressure of blood leaving the heart.
- reduces extent of blood vessel wall contraction, relaxing the walls and lowering blood pressure.

- after a heart attack, works to prevent inappropriate changes (remodeling) in the left ventricle, prevent repeat heart attacks and also appears to help decrease the size of the heart attack (infarct size in animals).

Carvedilol also is able to open (dilate) blood vessels in the periphery because of alpha-1 receptor blockade. This medicine acts as an antioxidant and inhibits programmed cell death, benefiting blood vessel lining (endothelial) function.

▷ **Widely Used Guidelines That Involve This Medicine (representative sample):** Please look at the section at the very beginning of this profile called "Class." Next, turn to Table 22 and you will find guidelines listed by the class involved!

Available Dosage Forms and Strengths
Tablets — 3.125, 6.25, 12.5, 25 mg
Tablets — 25 mg, 50 mg (Dilatrend in Canada)

▷ **Usual Adult Dosage Ranges**
For high blood pressure (hypertension): Starts with 6.25 mg twice daily. Dose may be increased to 12.5 mg twice daily and then to 25 mg twice daily at intervals of 2 weeks, as needed and tolerated. This medicine should be taken with food in order to decrease the risk of postural hypotension (see Glossary).
For angina: 25 to 50 mg twice a day (benefits are dose related).
For congestive heart failure: 3.125 mg twice a day. After 2 weeks, this dose may be increased to 6.25 mg twice daily as needed and tolerated. The dose can be subsequently doubled every 14 days to a maximum of 25 mg twice daily (for those less than 85 kg) or to 50 mg twice daily for people weighing more than 85 kg. When the dose is changed, patients should be watched for dizziness (for 2 hours after the first dose at the new level). Carvedilol should be taken with food to slow the speed at which it enters the body (see note in dosing instructions below regarding heart failure).
Note: Actual dose and schedule must be determined for each patient individually.

Conditions Requiring Dosing Adjustments
Liver Function: Twenty percent of the usual dose is given in people with cirrhosis of the liver. Carvedilol should NOT be used in severe liver failure.
Kidney Function: No changes thought to be needed.

▷ **Dosing Instructions:** Tablet may be crushed. Doses should be taken with food in order to decrease the risk of abnormally low blood pressure when standing up (orthostatic hypotension). Do not stop this drug abruptly. When the medicine is used in congestive heart failure, if the heart failure worsens—water pill doses (diuretics) should be increased and the dose of carvedilol not increased any further until the situation stabilizes. Talk to your doctor about how he or she wants you to manage this. If you forget a dose, take it right away unless it's nearly time for your next dose. If it is nearly time, just take the scheduled dose. DO NOT double doses.

Usual Duration of Use: Regular use brings the best results in lowering blood pressure. DO NOT SKIP DOSES. This medicine may reach its peak benefit with the first dose. Long-term use (months to years) is determined by lowering of blood pressure and response to an overall program (weight reduction, salt restriction, smoking cessation, etc). See your doctor on a regular basis.

Typical Treatment Goals and Measurements (Outcomes and Markers)
Blood Pressure: Guidelines (JNC VII) define normal blood pressure (BP) as **less than** 120/80 and **pre-hypertension** as 120/80 to 139/89. This new range is

intended to help doctors encourage lifestyle changes (or in the case of people with a risk factor for high blood pressure, start treatment) much earlier—so that damage to blood vessels, your heart, kidneys, sexual potency, or eyes might be minimized or avoided altogether. Stage 1 hypertension is 140/90 to 159/99 and stage 2 hypertension equal to or greater than: 160/100 mm Hg. These guidelines also recommend that clinicians work with their patients to agree on the goals and a plan of treatment. The first-ever guidelines for blood pressure (hypertension) in African Americans recommends that MOST black patients be started on TWO antihypertensive medicines with the goal of lowering blood pressure to 130/80 for those with high risk for heart and blood vessel disease or with diabetes. The American Diabetes Association also recommends 130/80 as the target for diabetics and less than 125/75 for those who spill more than one gram of protein into their urine. Most clinicians try to achieve a BP that confers the best balance of lower cardiovascular risk and avoids the problem of too low a blood pressure. Blood pressure duration is generally increased with beneficial restriction of sodium. If goals are not met, it is not unusual to intensify doses or add on medicines.

Possible Advantages of This Drug

Works on two kinds of beta receptors and alpha receptors as well. May reach its peak benefit with the first dose. The COMET trial showed a significant benefit for this medicine in decreasing death and death from heart and blood vessel disease. Carvedilol may have a more desirable effect on insulin sensitivity than other beta blockers.

▷ This Drug Should Not Be Taken If

- you have bronchial asthma and/or obstructive lung (pulmonary) disease.
- you have had an allergic reaction to it previously.
- you have sick sinus syndrome (ask your doctor).
- you have decompensated heart failure (NYHA Class four).
- you have a severely slow heart rate (bradycardia) or a serious heart block (second or third degree).

▷ Inform Your Physician Before Taking This Drug If

- you have had an adverse reaction to any beta blocker (see Drug Classes).
- you have serious heart disease or episodes of heart failure.
- you have had hay fever (allergic rhinitis), asthma, chronic bronchitis, or emphysema.
- you have a history of overactive thyroid function (hyperthyroidism).
- you have pheochromocytoma.
- you have a history of low blood sugar (hypoglycemia), diabetes, or myasthenia gravis.
- you have impaired liver or kidney function.
- you have a circulation problem (Raynaud's phenomenon, claudication pains in legs).
- you have low blood platelets.
- you take any form of digitalis, quinidine, or reserpine, or any calcium blocker drug (see Drug Classes).
- you will have surgery with general anesthesia.

Possible Side Effects (natural, expected, and unavoidable drug actions)

Lethargy and fatigability, cold extremities, slow heart rate, light-headedness in upright position (see Orthostatic Hypotension in Glossary)—rare when treating hypertension, infrequent when treating congestive heart failure. Rebound hypertension if this medicine is stopped abruptly.

Dizziness—frequent in congestive heart failure.

▷ **Possible Adverse Effects** (unusual, unexpected, and infrequent reactions)
If any of the following develop, consult your physician promptly for guidance.

Mild Adverse Effects
Allergic reaction: skin rash—rare.
Headache, dizziness, nervousness, drowsiness—infrequent to frequent.
Indigestion, nausea, vomiting, constipation, diarrhea—infrequent.
Urination at night (nocturia) or difficulty urinating—reported with other beta blockers.
Cough, wheezing, or sinusitis—reported with other beta blockers.
Episodic difficulty walking (intermittent claudication with peripheral vascular disease)—possible.
Muscle aches or back pain—case reports.
Visual changes—infrequent.

Serious Adverse Effects
Allergic reactions: One case report of Stevens-Johnson syndrome.
Lowering of blood platelets—rare and questionable cause.
Slow heartbeat (bradycardia)—possible with higher doses.
Fainting (syncope)—possible.
Edema (dependent and peripheral)—rare in hypertension and infrequent in CHF.
Increased blood sugar—possible.
May hide symptoms of low blood sugar.
Chest pain, irregular heartbeat, shortness of breath; can cause congestive heart failure—possible.
Induction of bronchial asthma (in asthmatic patients)—possible.
Liver toxicity (hepatotoxicity)—infrequent.
Aggravation of myasthenia gravis—possible.
Resistance to epinephrine in hypersensitivity or other similar treatment—possible.

▷ **Possible Effects on Sexual Function:** Impotence—case reports with other beta blockers. This rare effect is less common with heart selectivity and low fat (lipid) solubility.

Adverse Effects That May Mimic Natural Diseases or Disorders
Decreased extremity blood flow may mimic Raynaud's phenomenon (see Glossary).

Natural Diseases or Disorders That May Be Activated by This Drug
Intermittent claudication, diabetes.

Possible Effects on Laboratory Tests
Blood sugar: increased or decreased in diabetics.

CAUTION
• ***Do not stop this drug suddenly*** without the knowledge of your doctor (may cause dangerous increases in blood pressure or angina). Carry a note that says you are taking this drug.
• Ask your physician or pharmacist before using nasal decongestants. These can cause sudden increases in blood pressure when combined with beta-blocker drugs.
• May worsen positional blood pressure lowering (postural hypotension) in the elderly.
• Report any new tendency to emotional depression.
• Because dizziness is a common side effect, make sure you know the extent

and severity of this possible effect before undertaking activities that may be hazardous.

Precautions for Use

By Infants and Children: Safety and effectiveness in children not established.

By Those Over 60 Years of Age: **Caution:** Unacceptably high blood pressure should be reduced without creating excessively low blood pressure. Small doses and frequent blood pressure checks are needed.

Sudden/excessive blood pressure lowering can cause stroke or heart attack. Watch for dizziness, confusion, depression, or urinary frequency.

▷ **Advisability of Use During Pregnancy**

Pregnancy Category: C. See Pregnancy Risk Categories at the back of this book.

Animal Studies: No birth defects found in rat or rabbit studies.

Human Studies: Adequate studies of pregnant women are not available.

Use this drug only if clearly needed. Ask your physician for guidance.

Advisability of Use If Breast-Feeding

Presence of this drug in breast milk: Unknown in humans, but expected (large volume of distribution and is fat soluble or lipophillic).

Avoid drug or refrain from nursing.

Habit-Forming Potential: None.

Effects of Overdose: Weakness, slow pulse, low blood pressure, fainting, cold and sweaty skin, congestive heart failure, possible coma, and convulsions.

Possible Effects of Long-Term Use: Not defined.

Suggested Periodic Examinations While Taking This Drug (at physician's discretion): Measurements of blood pressure and treatment to goals within a set time frame, blood sugar, periodic evaluation liver, heart, and visual function.

▷ **While Taking This Drug, Observe the Following**

Foods: No restrictions. Avoid excessive salt intake.

Herbal Medicines or Minerals: Ginseng, guarana, bitter orange, country mallow. hawthorn, saw palmetto, ma huang (no longer on the market), goldenseal, yohimbe, and licorice may cause increased blood pressure. St. John's wort can change liver removal of medicines and is not recommended for people taking beta blockers. Calcium and garlic may help lower blood pressure, and the dose has to be individualized with a standardized extract. Dong quai can change the removal of medicines by the liver—caution is advised for excessive lowering of blood pressure. Ginger, vanadium, and nettle may also change blood sugar, an effect that may be hidden by some of the actions of this medicine. Indian snakeroot has a German Commission E monograph indication for hypertension—talk to your doctor. Eleuthero root and ephedra should be avoided by people living with hypertension. Talk to your doctor BEFORE adding any herbals.

Beverages: No restrictions. May be taken with milk.

▷ *Alcohol:* Use caution. Alcohol may exaggerate blood pressure lowering and also increase its mild sedative effect.

Tobacco Smoking: Nicotine may reduce benefits in treating high blood pressure. High doses may worsen bronchial constriction caused by regular smoking. I advise everyone to quit smoking.

▷ *Other Drugs*

Carvedilol may **increase** the effects of

• cyclosporine (Sandimmune, others) requiring cyclosporine dose decreases.

- other antihypertensive drugs, and cause excessive lowering of the blood pressure. Dosage adjustments may be necessary.
- reserpine (Ser-Ap-Es, etc), and cause sedation, depression, slowing of the heart rate, and low blood pressure. This combination is best avoided.
- verapamil (Calan, Isoptin), can cause excessive depression of heart function; monitor this combination closely.

Carvedilol *taken concurrently* with

- amiodarone (Cordarone) may cause severe slowing of the heart and sinus arrest. Do not combine this agent.
- cimetidine (Tagamet) may lead to excessive levels of carvedilol and possible toxic effects.
- clonidine (Catapres) requires close monitoring for rebound high blood pressure if clonidine is stopped while carvedilol is still being taken. Severe rebound hypertension may occur.
- digoxin (Lanoxin) may lead to abnormal heart conduction and increased blood digoxin levels. Caution is prudent. A small study in children from 14 days to 8 years old found that this combination slowed the removal of digoxin by 50%. Lower doses and more frequent blood levels are prudent if this combination must be used—particularly in children.
- diltiazem (Cardizem) (like verapamil) may be very helpful in patients with normal heart function, but may result in AV conduction problems.
- epinephrine (Adrenalin, etc) may cause sudden rise in blood pressure followed by slowing of the heart rate. Avoid this combination.
- insulin requires close monitoring to avoid hypoglycemia (see Glossary).
- medicines that increase CYP 2D6 or 2C9 will blunt carvedilol benefits while those that inhibit those liver enzymes will increase effects of carvedilol.
- nifedipine (dihydroperidine) may result in excessive lowering of the blood pressure.
- oral antidiabetic drugs (see Drug Classes) may cause prolonged recovery from hypoglycemia should it occur.
- rifabutin (Mycobutin) may reduce carvedilol's effectiveness.
- ritodrine (Yutopar) may block Yutopar actions. Maker of ritodrine does NOT recommend this combination.
- sibutramine (Meridia) may lead to increases in blood pressure.
- zileuton (Zyflo) may result in increased toxicity risk from carvedilol. Caution is advised.

The following drugs may *decrease* the effects of carvedilol:

- indomethacin (Indocin), and possibly other "aspirin substitutes" or NSAIDs, may impair carvedilol's antihypertensive effect.

▷ *Driving, Hazardous Activities:* Use caution until the full extent of fatigue, dizziness, and blood pressure change has been determined. Dizziness is more common in congestive heart failure patients.

Aviation Note: The use of this drug *is a disqualification* for piloting. Consult a designated Aviation Medical Examiner.

Exposure to Sun: No restrictions.

Exposure to Heat: Caution is advised. Hot environments can lower the blood pressure and exaggerate the effects of this drug.

Exposure to Cold: Caution is advised. The elderly should take precautions to prevent hypothermia (see Glossary).

Heavy Exercise or Exertion: Avoid exertion that produces light-headedness, excessive fatigue, or muscle cramping.

Occurrence of Unrelated Illness: Fever can lower blood pressure and require decreased doses. Illnesses that cause nausea or vomiting may interrupt the regular dosage schedule. Ask your physician for guidance.

Discontinuation: **DO NOT STOP this drug suddenly.** If possible, gradual reduction of dose over a period of 2 to 3 weeks is recommended. Ask your physician for help.

CEPHALOSPORIN ANTIBIOTIC FAMILY
(SEF a low spoar in)

Cefaclor   (SEF a klor)   **Cefadroxil**   (SEF a drox il)   **Cefixime** (SE fix eem)   **Cefprozil**   (SEF proh zil)   **Ceftriaxone**   (SEF try ax own)   **Cefuroxime**   (SEF yur ox eem)   **Cephalexin**   (SEF ah lex in) **Loracarbef**   (lor ah KAR bef)

Introduced: 1979, 1977, 1986, 1991, 1984, 1974, 1969, 1992, respectively **Class:**   Antibiotics, cephalosporins   **Prescription:**   USA: Yes   **Controlled Drugs:**   USA: No; Canada: No   **Available as Generic:**   *Cefaclor:* yes; *Cefadroxil:* yes; *Cefixime:* no; *Cefprozil:* no; *Ceftriaxone:* no; *Cefuroxime:* yes; *Cephalexin:* yes; *Loracarbef:* no

Brand Names: *Cefaclor:* Ceclor; *Cefadroxil:* Duricef, Ultracef; *Cefixime:* Suprax; *Cefprozil:* Cefzil; *Ceftriaxone:* Rocephin; *Cefuroxime:* Ceftin, Kefurox, Zinacef; *Cephalexin:* ♣Apo-Cephalex, Cefanex, ♣Ceporex, Keflet, Keflex, Keftab, ♣Novo-Lexin, ♣Nu-Cephalex; *Loracarbef:* Lorabid

BENEFITS versus RISKS	
Possible Benefits	*Possible Risks*
EFFECTIVE TREATMENT OF INFECTIONS DUE TO SUSCEPTIBLE MICRO-ORGANISMS	ALLERGIC REACTIONS, MILD TO SEVERE (MAY ALSO BE SEEN IN THOSE ALLERGIC TO PENICILLIN)
HOME INTRAVENOUS TREATMENT OF SERIOUS INFECTIONS (ceftriaxone)	Drug-induced colitis—rare Superinfections (see Glossary)
ONE-INJECTION TREATMENT OF SOME CHILDHOOD EAR INFECTIONS	Low white blood cell or platelet counts (cefixime or ceftriaxone)— rare Anemia (ceftriaxone)—rare

▷ **Principal Uses**

As a Single Drug Product: Uses currently included in FDA-approved labeling: (1) To treat some infections of the skin and skin structures, the upper and lower respiratory tract (including middle ear infections—ceftriaxone has a one-dose indication for bacterial otitis media—and "strep" throat), some urinary tract and some postoperative wound infections; (2) treatment of advanced Lyme disease (stage 2 or 3) via home intravenous (home IV) services (ceftriaxone); (3) treatment of serious bone infections (osteomyelitis) via home IV; (4) treatment of gonorrhea (cefuroxime).

Other unlabeled, generally accepted uses: (1) May have an alternative role in helping prevent rheumatic fever if the bacteria are resistant to erythromycin (cefaclor); (2) may help treat resistant cervical infections (cefixime); (3) part of combination treatment of Whipple's disease (cefixime); (4) treats sexual assault cases and chancroid (ceftriaxone); (5) used in *Shigella* infections;

(6) used to change from an intravenous medicine to one taken by mouth in order to shorten hospital stays and preserve results (cefuroxime).

How These Drugs Work: These drugs destroy susceptible infecting bacteria by interfering with their ability to produce new protective cell walls as they multiply and grow.

▷ **Widely Used Guidelines That Involve This Medicine (representative sample):** Please look at the section at the very beginning of this profile called "Class." Next, turn to Table 22 and you will find guidelines listed by the class involved!

Available Dosage Forms and Strengths

Cefaclor:
　　　　Capsules — 250 mg, 500 mg
　　Oral suspension — 125 mg, 187 mg, 250 mg, 375 mg/5 mL

Cefadroxil:
　　　　Capsules — 500 mg, 1,000 mg
　Gelatin capsules (Canada) — 500 mg
　　Oral suspension — 125 mg, 250 mg, 500 mg/5 mL
　　　　Tablets — 1,000 mg (1 g)

Cefixime:
　　Oral suspension — 100 mg/5 mL
　　　　Tablets — 200 mg, 400 mg

Cefprozil:
　　Oral suspension — 125 mg, 250 mg/5 mL
　　　　Tablets — 250 mg, 500 mg

Ceftriaxone:
　　250 mg of Rocephin — Boxes of 1 or 10 vial(s)
　　500 mg of Rocephin — Boxes of 1 or 10 vial(s)
　　1 g of Rocephin — Boxes of 1 or 10 vial(s) or piggyback bottles of 10
　　2 g of Rocephin — Boxes of 10 vials, or piggyback bottles of 10
　　10 g of Rocephin — Box of one 1 g or 2 g ADD-Vantage packaging

Cefuroxime:
　　Intravenous — 750 mg/10 mL
　　　　— 750 mg/50 mL
　　　　— 750 mg/100 mL
　　　　— 1.5 g/100 mL
　　　　— 1.5 g/50 mL
　　　　— 1.5 g/20 mL
　　　　— 7.5 g/127 mL
　　Oral suspension — 125 mg/5 mL, 250 mg/5 mL
　　　　Tablets — 125 mg, 250 mg, 500 mg

Cephalexin:
　　　　Capsules — 250 mg, 500 mg
　　Oral suspension — 125 mg, 250 mg/5 mL
　　Pediatric oral suspension — 100 mg/mL
　　　　Tablets — 250 mg, 500 mg, 1,000 mg (1 g)

Loracarbef:
　　　　Capsules — 200 mg and 400 mg
　　Oral suspension — 100 mg or 200 mg/5 mL

▷ **Recommended Dosage Ranges**

Cefaclor: For FDA labeled uses. 250 mg every 8 hours for susceptible infections, up to 500 mg every 8 hours for severe infections. Maximum daily dose is 2 g (2,000 mg).

Cefadroxil: Skin infections—500 mg every 12 hours, or 1 g daily. "Strep" throat—500 mg every 12 hours for 10 days. Urinary tract infections—500 mg to 1 g every 12 hours, or 1 to 2 g daily. Maximum daily dose 6 g (6,000 mg).

Cefixime: 400 mg daily, taken as a single dose or as 200 mg every 12 hours. For treatment of multidrug-resistant *Salmonella*—20 mg per kg of body mass per day in equal doses every 12 hours, for at least 12 days. Uncomplicated gonorrhea—400 to 800 mg as a single dose.

Cefuroxime: See general dosing below. Blood levels in pregnancy are up to 50% lower than in non-pregnant females. Dosing in pregnancy should be adjusted to achieve the usual peak to MIC ratio needed to kill the infecting organism.

Cephalexin: 250 to 500 mg every 6 hours. Total daily dose should not exceed 4 g.

Loracarbef: 200–400 mg every 12 hours for 7–14 days depending on the infection being treated.

Infants and Children:

Cefaclor: 20 to 40 mg per kg of body mass per day is given in divided doses every 8 hours. Maximum dose is 1 g (1,000 mg) daily.

Cefadroxil: 30 mg per kg of body mass per day, given in divided doses every 12 hours.

Cefixime (for children over 6 months of age): 8 mg per kg of body mass per day, all in one dose or divided into two doses.

Cefprozil: For otitis media (6 months to 12 years of age)—15 mg per kg of body mass every 12 hours, for 10 days.

Ceftriaxone: For neonates and children less than 12 for treatment of serious infections caused by susceptible organisms (other than CNS infections such as meningitis)—50–75 mg per kg of body mass per day, given in two equally divided doses 12 hours apart (not to exceed 2 g daily). Some clinicians use 50 mg per kg of body weight per day for neonates 1 week old or younger; neonates older than 1 week and weighing 2 kg or less also receive 50 mg per kg of body mass per day; neonates older than 1 week and weighing more than 2 kg receive 50–75 mg per kg of body mass per day.

For meningitis (caused by susceptible organisms)—the dose for neonates and children 12 or younger is 100 mg per kg of body mass (no more than 4 grams or 4,000 mg) daily, divided into two equal doses given every 12 hours. The American Academy of Pediatrics suggests 80–100 mg per kg of body mass be given once daily or in two equally divided doses every 12 hours for children older than 1 month. Because the once-daily regimen is relatively new, I suggest that the 12-hour regimen be used. For serious CNS disease—children can be treated with 75–100 mg per kg of body mass IV daily for 21 days.

For heart (cardiac disease)—children can be given 75–100 mg per kg of body mass per day IV. Treatment of serious Lyme arthritis, cardiac or neurologic complications of early or late (stage 2 or 3) Lyme disease: Arthritis: 75–100 mg per kg of body mass per day IV. One recent article advocated a single dose of ceftriaxone for some childhood ear infections. For otitis media: 75–100 mg per kg of body mass per day, in four divided doses.

Cefuroxime: Oral (for children over 2)—125 mg twice a day, 250 mg twice daily for treatment of otitis media. Intravenous—Those over 3 months should be given 50 to 100 mg per kg of body mass per day, divided every 6 to 8 hours. Maximum dose is 4 g.

Cephalexin: 25 to 50 mg per kg of body mass per day in two to four divided doses. Maximum dose is 4 g (4,000 mg).

Loracarbef: For ear infection (otitis media)—30 mg per kg per day given in equal doses, taken every 12 hours for 10 days (suspension only—capsules should NOT be substituted for suspension).

12 to 60 Years of Age:

Cefprozil: Pharyngitis or tonsillitis—500 mg every 24 hours (once daily), for 10 days. Acute or chronic bronchitis—500 mg every 12 hours, for 10 days. Bacterial pneumonia—250 mg three times a day for 14 days. Skin or skin structure infections—250 to 500 mg every 12 to 24 hours, for 10 days.

Ceftriaxone: For most infections (caused by susceptible organisms)—1–2 g daily or in equally divided doses two times a day depending on the type and severity of the infection. Children over 12 are given the adult dose. Some clinicians use 4 g daily in CNS infections in adults. This is the maximum adult dosage recommended by the manufacturer. Uncomplicated gonorrhea caused by penicillinase-producing strains of *Neisseria gonorrhea* (PPNG) or non-penicillinase-producing strains—Single IM 250-mg dose. Disseminated gonococcal infection should be treated by 1 g of ceftriaxone IV or IM once a day for 7 days. Acute sexually transmitted epididymitis in adults—Single 250-mg IM dose, followed by 7 days of oral tetracycline or erythromycin. For treatment of acute pelvic inflammatory disease (PID)—Single 250-mg IM dose, followed by 100 mg of oral doxycycline two times a day for 10–14 days. Treatment of serious Lyme arthritis, cardiac or neurologic complications of early or late (stage 2 or 3) Lyme disease: Arthritis—2 g IV daily. Serious CNS disease—2 g IV daily for 21 days. Cardiac disease—2 g IV per day for 21 days.

Cefuroxime: Oral—250 to 500 mg every 12 hours. Total daily dosage should not exceed 4 g. Intravenous—750 mg to 1.5 g every 8 hours.

Over 60 Years of Age:

Cefprozil: No specific age-related changes. Decreased dose in kidney failure.

Ceftriaxone: No specific changes needed.

Loracarbef: Same as adult dose unless kidney function has declined.

Note: Actual dosage and schedule must be determined for each patient individually for ALL of these medicines.

Conditions Requiring Dosing Adjustments

Liver Function:

Cefaclor, cefixime, cefprozil, cefuroxime, cephalexin, or loracarbef: No changes in dosing needed at present.

Cefadroxil: The liver is involved to a minimal degree. No dosing changes anticipated in liver compromise.

Ceftriaxone: Patients with both liver and kidney problems should have blood levels checked and a maximum dose of 2 g given.

Kidney Function:

Cefaclor: 40–80% eliminated by the kidney. For creatinine clearances (CrCl) of 10–50 mL/min, 50–100% of the usual dose at the normal interval is used. For creatinine clearances of less than 10 mL/min, 50% of the usual dose at the usual time is given.

Cefadroxil: With creatinine clearances of 10–50 mL/min, use the usual doses every 12–24 hours. For CrCl less than 10 mL/min, usual doses are given every 24–48 hours.

Cefixime: Dose **must be decreased** in mild to moderate kidney problems. In severe failure, a single dose every 48 hours is often used.

Cefprozil: With severe kidney failure, **half** the dose can be given at the usual time.

Ceftriaxone: Patients with kidney compromise must be carefully followed for adverse effects.

Cefuroxime: 750 mg once daily for most kidney compromise. Dose must be repeated after dialysis, as this medicine is dialyzable.

Cephalexin: For creatinine clearances of 10–50 mL/min, usual dose every 6 hours. For creatinine clearances less than 10 mL/min, usual dose every 8–12 hours.

Loracarbef: Usual dose for CrCl 50 mL/minute or greater. If the CrCl is 10–49 mL/min half the usual dose is given at the usual time.

Phenylketonuria (PKU): Cefprozil only: The suspension has 28 mg of phenylalanine in every 5 mL. This may preclude use of this drug in these patients.

▷ **Dosing Instructions:** May be taken on an empty stomach or with food if stomach upset occurs. Loracarbef must be taken on an empty stomach. Capsule (cefaclor, cefadroxil) may be opened and tablet forms crushed. Cefuroxime tablet can give a bitter taste that lingers. Shake suspension forms well before measuring dose (use a measured dose cup or calibrated dose measure). Intravenous forms should be brought to room temperature if they are refrigerated. Take the full course prescribed. If you forget a dose: Take the missed dose as soon as you remember it, and take any remaining doses for the day at evenly spaced time periods. If you miss more than one dose, please call your doctor.

Usual Duration of Use: Regular use for 3–5 days is usually needed to see effectiveness of these drugs in controlling the infection. Response varies with the infection. Treatment time will vary from 1 week (for some minor infections) to 6 weeks (as in some bone infections). Some cases **require 10–14 consecutive days** of treatment to prevent rheumatic fever. Follow your doctor's instructions carefully as many want you to call them if symptoms worsen or fever persists for 24–48 hours after you start these medicines.

Typical Treatment Goals and Measurements (Outcomes and Markers)

Infections: The most commonly used measures of serious infections are white blood cell counts and differentials (the kind of blood cells that occur most often in your blood) and temperature. Many clinicians look for positive changes in 24–48 hours. NEVER stop an antibiotic because you start to feel better. For many infections, a full 14 days is REQUIRED to kill the bacteria. The goals and time frame (see peak benefits above) should be discussed with you when the prescription is written.

Possible Advantages of These Drugs

One-time dosing (injection) of ceftriaxone guarantees that the medicine will be taken (adherence) by children with one kind of ear infection (acute otitis media).

These Drugs Should Not Be Taken If
- you are allergic to any cephalosporin (see Drug Classes).
- you have pseudomembranous colitis.

▷ **Inform Your Physician Before Taking These Drugs If**
- you have a history of allergy to any penicillin (see Drug Classes).
- you have a history of regional enteritis or ulcerative colitis.
- you have impaired kidney function.
- you have a history of blood clotting disorders.
- you have a history of low platelets or white blood cell count (cefprozil, cefixime, or ceftriaxone).

Possible Side Effects (natural, expected, and unavoidable drug actions)
Superinfections (see Glossary).

▷ **Possible Adverse Effects** (unusual, unexpected, and infrequent reactions)
If any of the following develop, consult your physician promptly for guidance.

Mild Adverse Effects
Allergic reactions: skin rash, itching, hives.
Nausea and vomiting or mild diarrhea—most common adverse effects.
Sore mouth or tongue—possible.
Mild and reversible decrease in white blood cells (neutrophils) (cefaclor).
Confusion, nervousness, insomnia, dizziness—rare.

Serious Adverse Effects
Allergic reactions: drug fever (see Glossary), anaphylactic reaction (see Glossary), Stevens-Johnson Syndrome—rare.
Idiosyncratic reactions: lowered white blood cell counts or platelets (cefixime, ceftriaxone, cefuroxime)—rare and idiosyncratic (cephalexin).
Extended time for blood to clot (reported with chronic use of other second- or third-generation cephalosporins in debilitated patients and for loracarbef)—case reports to rare.
Genital itching (may represent a fungus superinfection)—possible.
Serum sickness (itching, joint pain and irritated swellings)—rare.
Increased blood urea nitrogen (BUN) or serum creatinine—rare.
Gallbladder concretions (ceftriaxone)—rare.
Severe diarrhea may be drug-induced colitis—rare.
Increases in liver enzymes (cefadroxil and loracarbef) and jaundice (cholestatic) (cefaclor)—rare.

▷ **Possible Effects on Sexual Function:** None reported.

Adverse Effects That May Mimic Natural Diseases or Disorders
Skin rash and fever may resemble measles.

Possible Effects on Laboratory Tests
Blood platelet counts: decreased—rare (see above).
INR: may be increased (cefixime, ceftriaxone)—rare.
PTT: extended (cefprozil)—rare.
Liver enzymes: increased (cefaclor, cefuroxime, cefprozil, ceftriaxone)—rare.
BUN and creatinine: increased (cefaclor, cefprozil, cefuroxime, ceftriaxone)—rare.
White blood cell counts: decreased (cefprozil, cefixime, cefuroxime, ceftriaxone, cephalexin, loracarbef)—rare.
A specific kind of white blood cell increased (eosinophils): loracarbef-rare.

CAUTION
- ***Do not stop these drugs*** without the knowledge of your doctor (may cause dangerous bacterial resistance).
- Some drugs in this class can cause a false-positive test result for urine sugar when using Clinitest tablets, Benedict's solution, or Fehling's solution, but not with Tes-Tape.
- Cefuroxime suspension and tablets DO NOT get into the body to the same extent (bioavailability). They should not be substituted on a mg of ingredient to mg of ingredient basis.

Precautions for Use
By Infants and Children: Not recommended for use in infants less than 1 month old (cefaclor) or 1 year old (cephalexin). The maximal dose in children should not exceed 1 g every 24 hours (cefaclor). Dosing of other medicines

in this class is based on weight. Follow the dosing instructions exactly. Safety and effectiveness for those under 6 months not established (cefixime, cefprozil).

By Those Over 60 Years of Age: Dosage must be carefully individualized and based upon evaluation of kidney function. Natural changes in the skin may predispose to severe and prolonged itching reactions in the genital and anal regions. Such reactions should be reported promptly. The natural decline in kidney function often requires a decrease in dose and achieves the same effect as a larger dose (all but ceftriaxone).

▷ **Advisability of Use During Pregnancy**

Pregnancy Category: B. See Pregnancy Risk Categories at the back of this book.

Animal Studies: No birth defects reported.

Human Studies: Information from adequate studies of pregnant women is not available.

Generally considered to be safe. Ask your physician for guidance. See dosing in pregnancy above for cefuroxime.

Advisability of Use If Breast-Feeding

Presence of these drugs in breast milk: Yes, in small amounts (cefaclor, cefadroxil, ceftriaxone, cefuroxime, and cephalexin); unknown (cefixime, cefprozil, and loracarbef).

Ask your doctor for advice.

Habit-Forming Potential: None.

Effects of Overdose: Nausea, vomiting, stomach cramps, and/or diarrhea.

Possible Effects of Long-Term Use: Superinfections (see Glossary).

Suggested Periodic Examinations While Taking These Drugs (at physician's discretion)

Complete blood cell counts.

Liver enzymes.

INR or PTT (for some of these medicines).

BUN and creatinine with long-term therapy.

▷ **While Taking These Drugs, Observe the Following**

Foods: Delays the absorption of these drugs and may result in decreased antibiotic effect: cefaclor and loracarbef—take these 1 hour before or 2 hours after eating. No restrictions: cefadroxil, cefprozil, cefixime, ceftriaxone, cefuroxime, or cephalexin.

Herbal Medicines or Minerals: Echinacea: Some patients use echinacea to attempt to boost their immune systems. Unfortunately, use of echinacea is not recommended in people with damaged immune systems. This herb may also actually weaken any immune system if it is used too often or for too long a time. Do NOT take mistletoe herb, oak bark or F.C. of marshmallow root, and licorice.

Beverages: No restrictions. May be taken with milk.

▷ *Alcohol:* Ceftriaxone: May cause severe nausea and vomiting.

Others: No interactions expected, but large amounts of alcohol may blunt the immune system.

Tobacco Smoking: No interactions expected. I advise everyone to quit smoking.

▷ *Other Drugs*

These medicines *taken concurrently* with

- any aminoglycoside antibiotic (see Drug Classes) may result in increased kidney (renal) toxicity.

- anticoagulants (blood thinners) such as heparin or warfarin (Coumadin) may have anticoagulant effects increased by some medicines in this class.
- birth control pills (oral contraceptives) may result in **decreased effectiveness** in preventing conception and pregnancy.
- cholestyramine may decrease cephalexin (and perhaps other drugs in this class) absorption and blunt the beneficial effects in fighting infection.
- cyclosporine (Sandimmune, others) may lead to cyclosporine toxicity with some members of this family. More frequent cyclosporine levels are prudent.
- live typhoid vaccine (Vivotif Berna) may blunt the response to the vaccine if taken with some of these medicines. Separate the last dose of antibiotic and vaccination by 24 hours.
- loop diuretics such as ethacrynic acid may result in increased risk of kidney toxicity.
- nilvadipine (Escor) may increase cephalosporin blood levels.
- probenecid (Benemid) will slow the elimination of these drugs, resulting in higher blood levels and prolonged effect.

▷ *Driving, Hazardous Activities:* Usually no restrictions.

Aviation Note: The use of these drugs *may be a disqualification* for piloting. Consult a designated Aviation Medical Examiner.

Exposure to Sun: No restrictions.

Special Storage Instructions: Oral suspension should be kept at room temperature (cefixime or loracarbef). Oral suspensions should be refrigerated (cefaclor, cefadroxil, cefprozil, cephalexin, ceftriaxone IV form). Cefuroxime may be stored at room temperature or in the refrigerator.

Observe the Following Expiration Times: Do not take the oral suspension of this drug if it is older than 14 days (cefaclor, cefadroxil, cefprozil, cephalexin, or loracarbef) or 10 days (cefuroxime).

CERIVASTATIN (SIR iv a sta tin)

Brand Name: Baycol

Author's Note: This medicine was voluntarily removed from the market (see Table 16 for more information).

CHLORAMBUCIL (klor AM byu sil)

Introduced: 1974   **Class:**   Anticancer, immunosuppressant   **Prescription:**   USA: Yes   **Controlled Drug:**   USA: No; Canada: No   **Available as Generic:**   USA: No; Canada: No

Brand Names: Leukeran, ✤Alti-Chlorambucil

BENEFITS versus RISKS

Possible Benefits	*Possible Risks*
EFFECTIVE PALLIATIVE TREATMENT FOR CHRONIC LYMPHOCYTIC LEUKEMIA	BONE MARROW DEPRESSION (see Glossary)
EFFECTIVE PALLIATIVE TREATMENT FOR HODGKIN'S DISEASE AND OTHER LYMPHOMAS	INCREASED SUSCEPTIBILITY TO INFECTIONS
	CENTRAL NERVOUS SYSTEM TOXICITY
Immunosuppression of nephrotic syndrome	Male and female sterility
Immunosuppression of rheumatoid arthritis	Drug-induced liver or lung damage
	Development of secondary cancers

▷ **Principal Uses**

As a Single Drug Product: Uses currently included in FDA-approved labeling: Treats (1) chronic lymphocytic leukemia; (2) Hodgkin's lymphoma and other malignant lymphomas.

Other (unlabeled) generally accepted uses: (1) Hairy cell leukemia; (2) multiple myeloma; (3) Letterer-Siwe disease; (4) nephrotic syndrome; (5) ovarian cancer; (6) combined with methylprednisolone in one study to stabilize kidney disease of unknown cause (idiopathic membranous nephropathy); (7) case reports of combination treatment with corticosteroids in Sjögren's syndrome.

How This Drug Works: This drug blocks genetic activity (impairs DNA and RNA) and inhibits production of essential proteins. This kills cancerous cells.

▷ **Widely Used Guidelines That Involve This Medicine (representative sample):** Please look at the section at the very beginning of this profile called "Class." Next, turn to Table 22 and you will find guidelines listed by the class involved!

Available Dosage Forms and Strengths

Tablets — 2 mg, 5 mg

▷ **Usual Adult Dosage Ranges:** *For leukemia and lymphoma:* Dosing is started with 0.1 to 0.2 milligrams per kilogram of body weight per day (4–10 mg per day for an average sized patient). Those with chronic lymphocytic leukemia often only need 0.1 mg/kg/day which is given all at one time. This dosing is continued for three to six weeks. Dosing is carefully adjusted according to individual patient reaction and is lowered once the white blood cell count abruptly falls. Some clinicians use twice weekly or once a month dosing schedules. Such interrupted dosing schedules usually start with one dose of 0.4 mg/kg, and dosing is increased by 0.1 mg per kg until desired control of white blood cells (lymphocytes) or toxicity is seen. After this, following doses are adjusted to result in mild blood (hematologic) toxicity. Many clinicians think that this kind of intermittent or pulse dosing is safer.

For immunosuppression: 0.1–0.2 mg/kg of body mass daily, given in a single dose, then adjusted (titrated) based on response and toxicity.

Note: Actual dose and schedule must be determined for each patient individually. Strategies for combination use tend to evolve based on emerging research.

Conditions Requiring Dosing Adjustments
> *Liver Function:* Can cause liver damage. Use with extreme caution in liver compromise. Extensively changed (metabolized) by the liver.
>
> *Kidney Function:* Can cause bladder inflammation; caution is advised in cases of compromised urine outflow.

▷ **Dosing Instructions:** Best to swallow the tablet whole—do NOT crush it. May be taken with food; however, food may decrease absorption by up to 20%. See your doctor if vomiting prevents you from taking chlorambucil. It is best to drink 6–8 glasses of water a day while you are taking this medicine. If you forget a dose: Take the dose immediately, unless it is nearly time for your next dose—then skip the missed dose and take the next dose on schedule. DO NOT DOUBLE DOSES. If you miss more than one dose, call your doctor. Remember to ask about needed vaccinations, timing of vaccinations and vaccinations to avoid BEFORE dosing is started.

Usual Duration of Use: Regular use for 3 to 4 weeks is usually required to see benefits in controlling leukemia or lymphoma. See dosing above and comment on pulse dosing. Repeat laboratory studies (such as complete blood counts or CBCs, uric acid, and perhaps bone marrow aspirations will help guide both results and dosing adjustments.

Typical Treatment Goals and Measurements (Outcomes and Markers)
> *Leukemia (chronic lymphocytic):* Many clinicians use lowering of lymphocyte count and easing of lymph swelling (lymphadenopathy) as markers of response to treatment. Pulse dosing is a balance of toxicity and beneficial outcomes.

▷ **This Drug Should Not Be Taken If**
- you have had an allergic reaction or no benefit from it previously.
- you currently have an uncontrolled infection.

▷ **Inform Your Physician Before Taking This Drug If**
- you are allergic to melphalan (Alkeran).
- you are pregnant, planning pregnancy, or breast-feeding.
- you have had bone marrow depression or blood cell disorders.
- you had full-course radiation therapy less than 4 weeks ago.
- you have a history of gout or urate kidney stones.
- you develop a skin reaction while taking this drug.
- you have a seizure disorder of any kind.
- you have a history of porphyria.
- you have impaired liver or kidney function.
- you have had cancer chemotherapy or radiation therapy.
- you are taking drugs that can impair your immunity.
- you had or recently were exposed to chickenpox or herpes zoster.

Possible Side Effects (natural, expected, and unavoidable drug actions)
> Decreased white blood cell and platelet counts. Decreased immunity; susceptibility to infections. Increased blood levels of uric acid, formation of kidney stones. Nausea, vomiting, or diarrhea.

▷ **Possible Adverse Effects** (unusual, unexpected, and infrequent reactions)
> **If any of the following develop, consult your physician promptly for guidance.**
>
> *Mild Adverse Effects*
> Allergic reactions: skin rash, itching, drug fever (see Glossary)—rare.
> Mouth and lip sores, nausea, vomiting—infrequent.
>
> *Serious Adverse Effects*
> Allergic reactions: drug-induced hepatitis with jaundice—case reports.

Delayed allergic reaction erythema multiforme, TEN and Stevens-Johnson Syndrome.

Cataract formation with high-dose usage—case reports.

Blindness—case reports.

Central nervous system toxicity: agitation, confusion, hallucinations, twitching, seizures, tremors, paralysis—case reports.

Peripheral neuritis (see Glossary), movement disorders (ataxia)—possible.

Lung damage (pulmonary fibrosis): cough, shortness of breath—case reports.

Bone marrow damage, aplastic anemia (see Glossary)—possible (dose-related and can be dose limiting).

Leukemia (may depend on dose and length of treatment)—possible.

Liver damage (hepatotoxicity and jaundice)—case reports.

Severe skin damage (toxic epidermal necrolysis-TEN)—case reports.

▷ **Possible Effects on Sexual Function:** Can inhibit reproduction: stops sperm production (male sterility); alters menstrual patterns (amenorrhea, others), blocks ovulation and menstruation (female sterility)—possible.

Possible Delayed Adverse Effects

Severe bone marrow depression (even after drug is stopped). Secondary cancers (especially leukemia) have been reported. Lung damage (pulmonary fibrosis). Delayed allergic reaction.

Adverse Effects That May Mimic Natural Diseases or Disorders

Drug-induced seizures may suggest epilepsy. Drug-induced jaundice may suggest viral hepatitis.

Natural Diseases or Disorders That May Be Activated by This Drug

Gout, urate kidney stones, porphyria, latent epilepsy.

Possible Effects on Laboratory Tests

Complete blood counts: decreased red cells, hemoglobin, white cells, and platelets.

Bone marrow: normalization of bone marrow prep.

Blood uric acid level: increased.

Liver function tests: increased liver enzymes (ALT/GPT, AST/GOT), increased bilirubin, increased icterus index.

Sperm counts: decreased or absent.

CAUTION

1. Long-term, ongoing use has been replaced by pulse dosing. Use of this drug in noncancerous conditions requires extreme caution. Risks include permanent sterility, lung damage and the development of secondary cancers. It should only be used where less toxic medicines have failed.
2. Periodic check for leukemia is appropriate.
3. Four weeks should pass after a full course of radiation therapy or chemotherapy before chlorambucil is started.
4. Have dental work prior starting drug. Bone marrow depression could lead to gum infection, bleeding and delayed healing.
5. If gout develops, allopurinol is the drug of choice for chlorambucil-caused gout symptoms.
6. Both killed or live virus vaccines will not work while you take this drug. Live virus vaccines may actually cause infection. It may take 3 months to a year for the immune system to recover after stopping this or similar drugs. People in close contact with chlorambucil patients should not get oral poliovirus vaccine. This eliminates risk of accidental exposure.

7. Immediately report: Infection, unusual bruising or bleeding, excessive fatigue, tremors or muscle twitching, trouble walking, loss of appetite with nausea or vomiting. The lowering of white blood cells (neutrophils) may continue for 10 days after the last dose of this medicine.
8. It is advisable to avoid pregnancy while taking this drug. A nonhormonal method of contraception is recommended. Call your doctor promptly if you think pregnancy has occurred.
9. High-dose treatment increases risk of seizures.

Precautions for Use

By Infants and Children: Dosage schedules and treatment monitoring should be supervised by a qualified pediatrician. Children with nephrotic syndrome can be more prone to drug-induced seizures.

By Those Over 60 Years of Age: Watch for central nervous system toxicity.

▷ **Advisability of Use During Pregnancy**

Pregnancy Category: **D.** See Pregnancy Risk Categories at the back of this book.

Animal Studies: Rat studies reveal drug-associated defects of the nervous system, palate, skeleton, and urogenital system.

Human Studies: Adequate studies of pregnant women are not available. There are two known cases of an infant born with an absent kidney and ureter following exposure to this drug during early pregnancy.

If possible, this drug should be avoided during pregnancy, especially the first 3 months. A nonhormonal contraceptive is generally advisable during treatment with this and similar drugs.

Advisability of Use If Breast-Feeding

Presence of this drug in breast milk: Unknown.

Avoid drug or refrain from nursing.

Habit-Forming Potential: None.

Effects of Overdose: Fatigue, weakness, fever, sore throat, bruising, agitation, unstable gait, bone marrow depression, seizures.

Possible Effects of Long-Term Use: Permanent sterility, secondary cancers (leukemia), lung damage (pulmonary fibrosis).

Suggested Periodic Examinations While Taking This Drug (at physician's discretion)

Before drug treatment and periodically during drug use: Complete blood counts, uric acid levels, liver function tests. Sperm counts in men.

▷ **While Taking This Drug, Observe the Following**

Foods: No restrictions.

Herbal Medicines or Minerals: Echinacea: Some patients use echinacea to attempt to boost their immune systems. Unfortunately, use of echinacea is not recommended in people with damaged immune systems. This herb may also actually weaken any immune system if it is used too often or for too long a time.

Beverages: No restrictions. May be taken with milk. Drinking 2 to 3 quarts of liquids daily can reduce kidney stone risk. Ask your doctor.

▷　*Alcohol:* Use with caution. Avoid if platelet counts are low and there is a risk of stomach bleeding.

Tobacco Smoking: No interactions expected. I advise everyone to quit smoking.

Marijuana Smoking: Best avoided. Increases risk of central nervous system toxicity. Some fungal infections (toxoplasmosis) may be contracted from marijuana itself if the immune system is weak.

▷ *Other Drugs*
Chlorambucil *taken concurrently* with
- amphotericin B (Abelcet) may increase risk of bronchial spasm, low blood pressure and kidney (nephrotoxicity) toxicity.
- antidepressant or antipsychotic (neuroleptic) drugs requires careful monitoring; these drugs lower the seizure threshold and increase the risk of chlorambucil-induced seizures.
- aspirin may increase the risk of bruising or bleeding; the platelet-reduction effects of chlorambucil and the antiplatelet action of aspirin are additive. Avoid aspirin while taking chlorambucil.
- other immunosuppressant drugs can increase the risk of infection and the development of secondary cancers.
- tramadol (Ultram) may increase risk of seizures.
- live virus vaccines (such as MMWR) may result in overwhelming infections.

▷ *Driving, Hazardous Activities:* This drug may cause nervous agitation, confusion, hallucinations or seizures. Restrict activities as necessary.
Aviation Note: The use of this drug *may be a disqualification* for piloting. Consult a designated Aviation Medical Examiner.
Exposure to Sun: No restrictions.
Discontinuation: Many factors will determine when and how this drug should be stopped. Follow your doctor's advice to get the best results.

CHLORAMPHENICOL (KLOR am fen ih coll)

Introduced: 1947 **Class:** Antibiotic **Prescription:** USA: Yes
Controlled Drug: USA: No; Canada: No **Available as Generic:** USA: Yes; Canada: No

Brand Names: Ak-Chlor, Chloracol, Chlorofair, Chloromycetin, Chloroptic, Chloroptic SOP, Econochlor, ✤Elase-Chloromycetin, I-Chlor, ✤Isopto Fenicol, ✤Minims, ✤Nova-Phenicol, ✤Novochlorocap, ✤Ocu-Chlor, Ophthochlor, ✤Ophtho-Chloram, Ophthocort, ✤PMS-Chloramphenicol, ✤Sopamycetin, ✤Sopamycetin/HC

BENEFITS versus RISKS

Possible Benefits	*Possible Risks*
VERY EFFECTIVE TREATMENT OF INFECTIONS DUE TO SUSCEPTIBLE MICROORGANISMS	BONE MARROW DEPRESSION APLASTIC ANEMIA (see Glossary) Peripheral neuritis (see Glossary) Liver damage, jaundice

---

Author's Note: Risks are largely as defined for systemic use, not for ophthalmic use.

▷ **Principal Uses**
As a Single Drug Product: Uses currently included in FDA-approved labeling: (1) Very effective in a broad spectrum of serious infections—however, because of serious toxicity (fatal aplastic anemia), it is now reserved for life-threatening infections (such as meningitis) caused by resistant organisms and for infections in people who cannot tolerate other appropriate anti-infective drugs; (2) used in eye (intraocular) infections.

▷ **Widely Used Guidelines That Involve This Medicine (representative sample):** Please look at the section at the very beginning of this profile called "Class." Next, turn to Table 22 and you will find guidelines listed by the class involved!

Available Dosage Forms and Strengths
Previously available capsules and oral suspensions are no longer made.
Cream — 1%
Eye/ear solutions — 0.5%
Eye ointment — 1%
Injection — 100 mg/mL
Ophthalmic/otic suspension — 2 mg/mL

▷ **Usual Adult Dosage Ranges:** Ophthalmic: Chloramphenicol plus hydrocortisone suspension or solution is given as two drops to the affected eye every 3 hours day and night for 48 hours. After this, the time between doses is usually lengthened and therapy continued until 48 hours after the eye appears normal.

Note: Actual dose and schedule must be determined for each patient individually.

Author's Note: Because use of this medicine is largely limited to ophthalmic use, this profile has been shortened to make room for more widely used medicines.

CHLOROQUINE (KLOR oh kwin)

Introduced: 1964 **Class:** Amebecide, antimalarial **Prescription:**
USA: Yes **Controlled Drug:** USA: No; Canada: No **Available as**
Generic: USA: Yes; Canada: No

Brand Names: Aralen, Kronofed-A-JR, ❧Novo-Chloroquine

Warning: The brand names Aralen and Arlidin are similar and can be mistaken for each other; this can lead to serious medication errors. These names represent very different drugs. Verify that you are taking the correct drug.

BENEFITS versus RISKS	
Possible Benefits	*Possible Risks*
EFFECTIVE PREVENTION AND TREATMENT OF CERTAIN FORMS OF MALARIA	INFREQUENT BUT SERIOUS DAMAGE OF CORNEAL AND RETINAL EYE TISSUES
EFFECTIVE COMBINATION TREATMENT OF SOME FORMS OF AMEBIC INFECTION	RARE BUT SERIOUS BONE MARROW DEPRESSION; aplastic anemia, deficient white blood cells, and platelets
Possibly effective in palindromic rheumatism	Heart muscle damage—rare
Possibly effective in short-term treatment of systemic lupus erythematosus	Ear damage; hearing loss, ringing in ears—rare
Can be of help in refractory Rheumatoid arthritis	Eye damage—rare

Author's Note: Because this medicine is not as widely used as other medicines, this profile has been shortened to make room for more widely

used drugs. Newer combination data for this medicine combined with azithromycin (Zithromax) lead to 96% of malaria patients being symptom free.

CHLOROTHIAZIDE (klor oh THI a zide)

Please see the thiazide diuretic family profile.

CHLORPROMAZINE (klor PROH ma zeen)

Introduced: 1952 **Class:** Antipsychotic, phenothiazines, strong tranquilizer **Prescription:** USA: Yes **Controlled Drug:** USA: No; Canada: No **Available as Generic:** Yes

Brand Names: ✿Chlorpromanyl, ✿Largactil, ✿Novochlorpromazine, Ormazine, Thora-Dex, Thorazine, Thorazine SR

```
┌─────────────────────────────────────────────────────────────┐
│                   BENEFITS versus RISKS                       │
│      Possible Benefits              Possible Risks            │
│ EFFECTIVE CONTROL OF ACUTE     Toxic effects on the brain with long-│
│   MENTAL DISORDERS               term use—rare but possible    │
│ Beneficial effects on thinking, mood,  Liver damage with jaundice—rare │
│   and behavior                 Rare blood disorders: hemolytic │
│ Moderately effective control of nausea   anemia, abnormally low white │
│   and vomiting                   blood cell count              │
│                                Eye toxicity                    │
└─────────────────────────────────────────────────────────────┘
```

▷ **Principal Uses**
  As a Single Drug Product: Uses currently included in FDA-approved labeling: (1) Treats acute and chronic psychotic disorders such as agitated depression, schizophrenia and mania; (2) can be used for presurgical anxiety; (3) helps reduce symptoms in porphyrias and tetanus; (4) is used to stop prolonged hiccups; (5) lessens or stops vomiting caused by toxic chemotherapy or a potent drug used to treat fungal infections (amphotericin B).
  Author's Note: The information in this profile has been shortened to make room for more widely used medicines.

CHLORPROPAMIDE (klor PROH pa mide)

Introduced: 1958 **Class:** Antidiabetic, sulfonylureas **Prescription:** USA: Yes **Controlled Drug:** USA: No; Canada: No **Available as Generic:** Yes

Brand Names: ✿Apo-Chlorpropamide, ✿Chloronase, Diabinese, Glucamide

---

BENEFITS versus RISKS

Possible Benefits	*Possible Risks*
Helps in regulating blood sugar in non-insulin-dependent diabetes (adjunctive to appropriate diet and weight control)	HYPOGLYCEMIA, severe and prolonged
	Allergic skin reactions (some severe)
	Water retention
Tight blood sugar control may avoid or delay blood vessel, heart, nerve, and vision damage possible with uncontrolled increase in blood sugar	Liver damage or blood cell and bone marrow disorders—rare

---

Author's Note: The information in this profile has been shortened to make room for more widely used medicines.

CHLORTHALIDONE (klor THAL i dohn)

Please see the thiazide diuretics family profile.

CHOLESTYRAMINE (koh LES tir a meen)

Introduced: 1959 **Class:** Anticholesterol **Prescription:** USA: Yes **Controlled Drug:** USA: No; Canada: No **Available as Generic:** USA: No; Canada: No

Brand Names: Questran, Questran Light, ✤Novo-Cholamine, ✤Novo-Cholamine Light, Prevalite

Author's Note: Questran and Questran Light were proposed to the FDA to be changed from prescription to nonprescription status. Approval was not granted.

BENEFITS versus RISKS

Possible Benefits	*Possible Risks*
EFFECTIVE REDUCTION OF TOTAL CHOLESTEROL AND LOW-DENSITY CHOLESTEROL IN TYPE IIA CHOLESTEROL DISORDERS	Constipation (may be severe)
	Reduced absorption of fat-soluble vitamins (A, D, E, K), folic acid, and niacin
Reduction of total cholesterol and LDL cholesterol	May increase triglycerides
EFFECTIVE RELIEF OF ITCHING associated with biliary obstruction	Reduced formation of prothrombin with possible bleeding
Effective binding of medicines in some drug overdoses	
Helps remove leflunomide (Arava) in patients desiring pregnancy	

▷ **Principal Uses**

As a Single Drug Product: Uses currently included in FDA-approved labeling:
(1) Reduces high blood levels of total cholesterol and low-density (LDL)

cholesterol in Type IIa cholesterol disorders; (2) relieves itching due to the deposit of bile acids in the skin associated with partial biliary obstruction; (3) reduces risk of heart disease in type II hyperlipoproteinemia; (4) reduces progression of disease in coronary arteries in people with type II hyperlipoproteinemia.

Other (unlabeled) generally accepted uses: (1) Because leflunomide (Arava) stays in the body for a very long time, cholestyramine has been used by some clinicians to help remove the medicine in patients desiring to become pregnant or who are having problems with the drug; (2) may help biliary fistulas and skin irritations seen in colostomy; (3) helps lower thyroid hormone levels if too much thyroid hormone is given; (4) treats cholesterol ester storage disease (CESD); (5) treats relapses of resistant diarrhea (pseudomembranous colitis); (6) eases diarrhea caused by quinidine.

Author's Note: Information in this profile has been shortened to make room for more widely used medicines.

CILOSTAZOL (SIGH low stay zahl)

Introduced: 1999   **Class:**   Blood flow agent, phosphodiesterase (type III) inhibitor   **Prescription:**   USA: Yes   **Controlled Drug:**   USA: No; Canada: No   **Available as Generic:**   No
Brand Name: Pletal

BENEFITS versus RISKS	
Possible Benefits	*Possible Risks*
IMPROVED BLOOD FLOW IN PERIPHERAL ARTERIAL DISEASE	Worsening of congestive heart failure (CHF) (never to be used in CHF)
REDUCES PAIN OF INTERMITTENT CLAUDICATION	Palpitation
DATA FROM A STUDY OF 1,052 PATIENTS FOUND A SIGNIFICANT RELATIVE RISK REDUCTION (41.7%) IN RECURRENT STROKES	Diarrhea
	Headache
Some increase in force of contraction of the heart	
May have a role in improving function of blood vessel linings in smokers	

▷ **Principal Uses**

As a Single Drug Product: Uses currently included in FDA-approved labeling: Used in people who have pain on walking (intermittent claudication) to help improve how far they can walk without pain.

Other (unlabeled) generally accepted uses: (1) May be used as part of combination treatment of problems in small vessels (microangiopathic hemolytic anemia) in graft-versus-host disease; (2) could have a role in angioplasty (percutaneous transluminal coronary) in helping keep the blood vessel from having problems after the procedure (post procedure re-stenosis); (3) May have a role in preventing repeat (recurrent) strokes in people who have suffered a first stroke; (4) appears to improve blood vessel function (by improving how well the lining or endothelium works) in people who smoke.

How This Drug Works: Acts as a selective inhibitor (type three) of phosphodiesterase. Works to keep platelets from clumping directed by arachidonic acid, epinephrine, thromboxane A2, platelet activating factor, ADP or collagen. Works to dilate the bronchi and decreases thrombomodulin in diabetics. Works to prevent repeat blockage of coronary arteries in dogs after a clot buster (thrombolytic) has been used (unknown in humans). Improves blood vessel response (vasodilation) by an unknown mechanism that probably involves the lining (endothelium) of blood vessels in smokers.

▷ **Widely Used Guidelines That Involve This Medicine (representative sample):** Please look at the section at the very beginning of this profile called "Class." Next, turn to Table 22 and you will find guidelines listed by the class involved!

Available Dosage Forms and Strengths
Tablets — 50 mg, 100 mg

▷ **Usual Adult Dosage Ranges:** *Intermittent claudication:* 100 mg twice daily, taken half an hour before or two hours after breakfast and dinner.
Preventing a second stroke: One study used 100 mg twice daily and appeared to provide nearly a 42% decrease in repeat (recurrent) strokes.
Note: Actual dose and schedule must be determined for each patient individually.

Conditions Requiring Dosing Adjustments
Liver Function: No apparent changes in mild liver impairment. This drug has NOT been studied in moderate to severe liver impairment. Used with caution and patients closely monitored.
Kidney Function: No changes thought to be needed.

▷ **Dosing Instructions:** Take cilostazol at the same time each day, one half hour before or two hours after breakfast and dinner. It is taken this way because food (especially a high-fat meal) INCREASES the amount that gets into your body. If you forget a dose: Take it as soon as you remember it, unless it's nearly time for your next dose, then simply take the next scheduled dose. DO NOT double doses.

Usual Duration of Use: Regular use for 2–4 weeks may show benefits, but up to 12 weeks may be required to see the full benefit of cilostazol in preventing or delaying intermittent claudication pain when walking. Long-term use (months to years) requires follow-up with your doctor and checks of progression of blood vessel problems.

Typical Treatment Goals and Measurements (Outcomes and Markers)
Claudication: Many clinicians use distance a patient can walk without leg pain as a way to standardize response. Another measure is absence of leg pain. Ankle/brachial index (ABI) is used to check peripheral artery disease or PVD (normal value is more than one, and less than 0.9 suggests PVD). Roughly a third (33%) of people with PVD have intermittent claudication (see McDermott, M.M. et al. in Sources).

Possible Advantages of This Drug
Works on both blood vessel (vascular) beds and on heart function. Keeps platelets from clumping and may also have good effects on blood lipoproteins which adversely effect blood vessels. Good cholesterol (HDL) has been increased in some patients.

▷ **This Drug Should Not Be Taken If**
- you have had an allergic reaction to it previously.
- you have an active hemorrhage.
- you have congestive heart failure.

▷ **Inform Your Physician Before Taking This Drug If**
- you have impaired liver or kidney function.
- you have low blood pressure or arrhythmias.
- you get migraines.
- you are pregnant.
- you have a bleeding problem or low blood platelets.
- you smoke tobacco.
- you are taking any antihypertensive drugs, antiplatelet medicines, or anti-coagulants or medicines that change liver enzyme levels (CYP 3A4 or CYP 2C19) or block them (see drug interactions below).

Possible Side Effects (natural, expected, and unavoidable drug actions)
Prolonged bleeding time (one investigator).

▷ **Possible Adverse Effects** (unusual, unexpected, and infrequent reactions)
If any of the following develop, consult your physician promptly for guidance.

Mild Adverse Effects
Allergic reaction: Skin rash.
Headache (mild to severe)—frequent.
Dizziness or vertigo—rare to infrequent.
Flushing of the face—infrequent.
Runny nose—infrequent to frequent.
Edema (peripheral)—infrequent.
Back pain or muscle aches—infrequent.
Nausea—infrequent.
Diarrhea—infrequent to frequent.
Palpitations or fast heart rate—possible to infrequent.
Blood sugar changes—possible but do appear clinically significant.

Serious Adverse Effects
Development of heart rhythm disorders, chest pain, and heart attack—case reports.
Increased bleeding risk with low blood platelets—possible.

▷ **Possible Effects on Sexual Function:** None reported.

Possible Effects on Laboratory Tests
Bleeding time: extended.
Complete blood cell counts: rarely lowers red cells.
Blood sugar: variable changes.
Triglycerides: decreased (beneficial effect).
May increase HDL (beneficial effect).

CAUTION
1. May worsen migraines.
2. DO NOT USE IF YOU HAVE CONGESTIVE HEART FAILURE.

Precautions for Use
By Infants and Children: Safety and effectiveness for those less than 18 years of age not established. Use by this age group is not anticipated.
By Those Over 60 Years of Age: You may be more susceptible to effects of this medicine. Observe closely for any adverse effects and report these promptly.

▷ **Advisability of Use During Pregnancy**
    Pregnancy Category: C. See Pregnancy Risk Categories at the back of this book.
    Animal Studies: Increased fetal cardiovascular, kidney, and skeletal problems.
    Human Studies: Adequate studies of pregnant women are not available.
    Talk to your doctor.

Advisability of Use If Breast-Feeding
    Presence of this drug in breast milk: Yes in rats, expected in humans.
    Avoid drug or refrain from nursing.

Habit-Forming Potential: None.

Effects of Overdose: Limited data: severe headache, diarrhea, low blood pressure, fast heart rate, and possible abnormal heartbeats.

Possible Effects of Long-Term Use: None reported.

Suggested Periodic Examinations While Taking This Drug (at physician's discretion)
    Blood pressure measurements.
    Evaluation of heart and blood vessel status. Check of HDL and triglycerides.

▷ **While Taking This Drug, Observe the Following**
    Foods: Best taken on an empty stomach. Some data finds L-arginine to be helpful in intermittent claudication, but head to head trials are needed.
    Herbal Medicines or Minerals: Many herbal medicines may interact with cilostazol because of its potential action on blood clotting. Examples include ginkgo, garlic, ginger, ginseng, white willow bark, and feverfew. DO NOT COMBINE THESE HERBAL MEDICINES WITH CILOSTAZOL. Capsaicin (Zostrix, others) and evening primrose oil may increase bleeding risk.
    Beverages: DO NOT TAKE WITH GRAPEFRUIT JUICE.
▷   *Alcohol:* Alcohol may increase the blood pressure lowering effect of this drug.
    Tobacco Smoking: Smoking decreases cilostazol benefits. Avoid tobacco.
▷   *Other Drugs*
    Cilostazol may *increase* the effects of
- antihypertensive drugs and cause excessive lowering of blood pressure.
- antiplatelet medicines on blood clotting, leading to a benefit to risk decision.
- aspirin on blood clotting, but clinical significance is not known.
- clot busters (thrombolytics) leading to a benefit to risk decision.

    The following drugs may *increase* the effects of cilostazol:
- any medicine that interferes with cytochrome (CYP3A4-major or 2C9-minor) will potentially increase cilostazol blood levels (such as sibutramine [Meridia] that uses CYP3A4). In some cases, I expect that cilostazol dosing will need to be adjusted, and in others, the combination should be avoided.
- cimetidine (Tagamet).
- diltiazem (Cardizem).
- erythromycins (see Drug Classes erythromycin and clarithromycin).
- fluconazole (Diflucan).
- itraconazole (Sporanox).
- ketoconazole (Nizoral).
- metronidazole (Flagyl).
- miconazole (Monistat).
- nefazodone (Serzone).
- nelfinavir (Viracept) and perhaps other protease inhibitors (see Drug Classes), which may increase cilostazol blood levels and effects.
- sertraline (Zoloft).

Cilostazol *taken concurrently* with
- CYP-3A4 (diltiazem-Cardizem, erythromycin). Itraconazole, others or CYP 2C19 inhibitors such as omeprazole (Prilosec) may result in excessively high cilostazol levels and increased risk of cilostazol toxicity unless doses are lowered.
- glipizide (Glucotrol) or other medicines that lower blood sugar may result in excessively low blood sugar.
- omeprazole (Prilosec) may lead to increased adverse effects if the cilostazol dose is not reduced to 50 mg twice daily.
- warfarin (Coumadin, etc.) finds that multiple dosing effects are not known.

The following drugs may *decrease* the effects of cilostazol:
- carbamazepine (Tegretol).
- phenytoin (Dilantin).
- rifabutin (Mycobutin).
- rifampin (Rifadin, Rimactane).

▷ *Driving, Hazardous Activities:* This drug may cause dizziness. Restrict activities as necessary.

Aviation Note: The use of this drug *may be a disqualification* for piloting. Consult a designated Aviation Medical Examiner.

Exposure to Sun: No restrictions.

CIMETIDINE (si MET i deen)

Please see the histamine (H2) blocking drug family profile.

CIPROFLOXACIN (sip roh FLOX a sin)

Please see the fluoroquinolone antibiotic family profile.

CISAPRIDE (SIS a pryde)

Introduced: 1993   **Class:**   Gastrointestinal   drug   **Prescription:** USA: Yes   **Controlled Drug:**   USA: No; Canada: No   **Available as Generic:**   USA: No; Canada: No

Brand Names: ✿Prepulsid, Propulsid

Author's Note: This medicine is only available under severely restricted medication guidelines and as such is no longer covered as a full profile—the information in this profile has been shortened.

CITALOPRAM (SIH tal oh prahm)

Introduced: 1998   **Class:**   Antidepressant   **Prescription:**   USA: Yes   **Controlled Drug:**   USA: No   **Available as Generic:**   USA: No

Brand Name: Celexa

```
┌─────────────────────────────────────────────────────────────────┐
│                     BENEFITS versus RISKS                         │
│      Possible Benefits                    Possible Risks          │
│   EFFECTIVE TREATMENT OF          Headache                        │
│     DEPRESSION                    Dry mouth                        │
│   Rapidly goes to work (reaches steady   Sleepiness               │
│     state)                        Constipation                    │
└─────────────────────────────────────────────────────────────────┘
```

▷ **Principal Uses**

As a Single Drug Product: Uses currently included in FDA-approved labeling: (1) Treats depression.

Other (unlabeled) generally accepted uses: (1) may have a role in alcohol abuse; (2) can ease the frequency and intensity of tension headaches; (3) may have a role in obsessive-compulsive disorder; (4) relieves symptoms of premenstrual dysphoria syndrome (PDS); (5) eases depression that can occur after a stroke; (6) effective in panic disorder—particularly useful where headache is also seen; (7) one small study found improvement in seven 12–18 year old patients with post-traumatic stress disorder (PTSD) which warrants additional research.

How This Drug Works: It restores normal levels of a nerve transmitter (serotonin) by selectively inhibiting the reuptake of serotonin.

▷ **Widely Used Guidelines That Involve This Medicine (representative sample):** Please look at the section at the very beginning of this profile called "Class." Next, turn to Table 22 and you will find guidelines listed by the class involved!

Available Dosage Forms and Strengths

Oral solution — 10 mg per 5 mL

Tablets — 10 mg, 20 mg, 40 mg

▷ **Usual Adult Dosage Ranges:** *Depression:* Starts with 20 mg, if no improvement after a week, dose may be increased by 20 mg/day as needed and tolerated. Most people don't have to take more than 40 mg a day, but the dose can be increased up to a maximum of 60 mg daily.

Alcohol abuse: 40 mg once daily.

Depression or crying after a stroke: 20 mg once daily with lower doses being used in older patients.

Obsessive-compulsive disorder: 20 mg to 60 mg once daily.

Infants and Children: Safety and efficacy not established.

Note: Actual dose and schedule must be determined for each patient individually.

Conditions Requiring Dosing Adjustments

Liver Function: The dose should be decreased to 20 mg daily in treating depression. One drug maker in Germany suggests a limit of 30 mg a day in liver dysfunction.

Kidney Function: Dosing changes do not appear to be needed. Patients with mild to moderate kidney failure should be closely watched for adverse effects as less than 15% of the original (parent) drug and 20% of metabolites are removed by the kidneys. Use of this medicine in people with severe kidney failure has not been studied.

▷ **Dosing Instructions:** The capsule may be opened and the contents mixed with any convenient food. The contents may be mixed with orange juice or apple juice (NOT GRAPEFRUIT JUICE). The liquid form should always be measured with a dosing spoon. Some clinicians have patients take this medicine at night in order to avoid possible drowsiness, while others have patients take this drug in the morning. If you forget a dose: Take the dose right away, unless it is nearly time for your next dose—then simply take the next scheduled dose. DO NOT double doses. Call your doctor if you find yourself forgetting doses.

Usual Duration of Use: Use on a regular schedule for 1 week may reveal start of benefits in depression. Up to 6 weeks may be needed for peak effects in (1) relieving depression and (2) the pattern of both favorable and unfavorable effects. Since there are active metabolites and a long half-life, it may take several weeks before the benefits of a change in dose are seen. Long-term use requires periodic physician evaluation. Some clinical guidelines suggest that 4–9 months of treatment should continue after the symptoms of depression go away. Some clinicians use lower ongoing doses to prevent depression. People who take their medicine regularly are least likely to have a recurrence.

Typical Treatment Goals and Measurements (Outcomes and Markers)
Depression: The general goal: to at least help lessen the degree and severity of depression, letting patients return to their daily lives. Specific measures of depression involve testing or inventories (such as the Hamilton Depression Scale-HAMD) can be valuable in helping check benefits from this medicine.

Possible Advantages of This Drug: Does not cause weight gain, a common side effect of tricyclic antidepressants. Less likely to cause dry mouth, constipation, urinary retention, orthostatic hypotension (see Glossary), and heart rhythm disturbances than tricyclic antidepressants. Since a large National Cancer Institute study found that those who suffer depression for 6 years or more have a generally increased risk of cancer, one benefit of effective treatment of depression with this drug may be a generally reduced risk of cancer.

▷ **This Drug Should Not Be Taken If**
  • you had an allergic reaction to it previously.
  • you take, or took in the last 14 days, a monoamine oxidase (MAO) type A inhibitor (see Drug Classes).

▷ **Inform Your Physician Before Taking This Drug If**
  • you have had any adverse effects from antidepressant drugs.
  • you have impaired liver or kidney function.
  • you have a seizure disorder.
  • you have a history of suicide attempt.
  • you are pregnant or plan pregnancy while taking this drug.

Possible Side Effects (natural, expected, and unavoidable drug actions)
Increased sweating or cough—may be frequent.
Weight loss.
Withdrawal symptoms if this medicine is stopped suddenly (best to slowly decrease or taper the dose over 2–4 weeks or longer).
Excessive lowering of the blood pressure upon standing (orthostatic hypotension; see Glossary)—may be frequent.

▷ **Possible Adverse Effects** (unusual, unexpected, and infrequent reactions)
If any of the following develop, consult your physician promptly for guidance.
Mild Adverse Effects
Allergic reactions: skin rash, itching—may be frequent.

Headache, insomnia, drowsiness, tremor, dizziness—infrequent to frequent (these central nervous system symptoms tend to diminish over time).
Agitation/anxiety syndrome (acathesia-like)—may be frequent.
Altered taste, increased saliva, or nausea—frequent.
Increased appetite or gas (flatulence)—may be frequent.
Nausea, vomiting, constipation—infrequent to frequent.
Increased heart rate—frequent.
Slowing of the heart rate—case reports.
Increased urination—frequent.
Increased liver enzymes—possible.
Blurred vision—infrequent.
Excessive sweating (diaphoresis)—frequent.
Serious Adverse Effects
Allergic reactions: not reported.
Drug-induced seizures—rare and questionable cause and effect.
Changes in sodium levels—possible (SIADH or low sodium).
Suicidal preoccupation—possible.
Serotonin syndrome—case reports.
Activation of mania/hypomania—possible.
This medicine caused some degeneration of the retina in rats. The significance of this for humans is not known.

▷ **Possible Effects on Sexual Function:** Inhibition of ejaculation or inhibited orgasm in men and women—infrequent.
Amenorrhea—frequent.

Natural Diseases or Disorders That May Be Activated by This Drug
Latent epilepsy.

Possible Effects on Laboratory Tests
Blood sodium level: possibly decreased.

CAUTION
1. If dry mouth develops and persists for more than 2 weeks, consult your dentist for help.
2. Ask your doctor or pharmacist before taking any other prescription or over-the-counter drug while taking this medicine
3. A withdrawal syndrome can happen if this medicine is stopped suddenly. Best to slowly decrease this medicine (taper) over 2–4 weeks or more.
4. If you must start any monoamine oxidase (MAO) type A inhibitor (see Drug Classes), allow an interval of 5–6 weeks after stopping this drug before starting the MAO inhibitor.
5. Pediatric and adult patients treated with this medicine should be closely watched for worsening depression or suicidal thinking. The FDA has required makers of antidepressants such as this one to alert healthcare professionals to the fact that children and adults with major depression may develop worsening depression or suicidal thoughts and behavior whether they take medicine for depression or do not take it. Patients should be carefully followed for such clinical worsening (particularly when treatment is started or doses are increased or decreased).

Precautions for Use
By Infants and Children: Safety and effectiveness are not established.
By Those Over 60 Years of Age: Lower or less frequent doses are recommended by the German manufacturer with a maximum dose of 40 mg daily.

▷ **Advisability of Use During Pregnancy**
Pregnancy Category: C. See Pregnancy Risk Categories at the back of this book.
Animal Studies: No birth defects due to this drug found in rat or rabbit studies.
Human Studies: Adequate studies of pregnant women are not available.
  Use this drug in pregnancy is a benefit-to-risk decision that MUST be discussed with your doctor.

Advisability of Use If Breast-Feeding
  Presence of this drug in breast milk: Yes.
  Use is a benefit-to-risk decision. There have been a few reports of weight loss, excessive somnolence and decreased feeding in babies breast-fed while the mother was taking citalopram.

Habit-Forming Potential: Not systematically studied, but a withdrawal syndrome is possible.

Effects of Overdose: Post-marketing reports of drug overdoses that included citalopram include 12 fatalities. Symptoms include agitation, sweating, tremor, nausea, vomiting, seizures, ECG changes, and one possible case of Torsades de Pointes.

Possible Effects of Long-Term Use: None reported.

Suggested Periodic Examinations While Taking This Drug (at physician's discretion)
  Check of electrolytes if symptoms of SIADH begin.

▷ **While Taking This Drug, Observe the Following**
Foods: No specific guidance.
Beverages: Best taken with milk or water.
Herbal Medicines or Minerals: Since citalopram and St. John's wort may act to increase serotonin, the combination is not advised. St. John's wort also increases sun sensitivity. Ginkgo may have some MAO activity—hence this combination cannot be recommended. Ma huang (no longer on the market), yohimbe, Indian snakeroot, and kava kava are also best avoided while taking this medicine.
▷ *Alcohol:* This combination is NOT advisable.
Tobacco Smoking: No interactions expected, but I advise everyone to quit smoking.
Marijuana Smoking or injestion: Mania resulted from combination of a selective serotonin reuptake inhibitor (fluoxetine) and marijuana in one report.

▷ *Other Drugs*
  Citalopram may *increase* the effects of
  • dofetilide (Tikosyn) requiring dosing decreases.
  • imipramine (Tofranil).
  • medicines that change clotting (NSAIDS, anticoagulants such as warfarin-Coumadin, even aspirin)–see Drug Classes) caution and close follow up for any signs of bleeding are needed.
  • metoprolol (Toprol, Lopressor, others) by increasing metoprolol blood levels.
  • sildenafil (Viagra) by competing for CYP3A4. Caution is advised.
  Citalopram *taken concurrently* with
  • azole antifungals (such as fluconazole, itraconazole, and ketoconazole) may lead to higher than expected citalopram blood levels and increased risk of adverse effects.
  • buspirone (Buspar) may lead to serotonin syndrome. Avoid the combination.
  • carbamazepine (Tegretol, others) may blunt benefits of citalopram, however, this combination has been used where the carbamazepine is used as a mood stabolizer.

- cimetidine (Tagamet) may theoretically lead to increased citalopram levels.
- cisapride (Propulsid) may lead to excessive cisapride levels and risk of serotonin syndrome.
- clarithromycin (Biaxin) may lead to citalopram toxicity—avoid the combination.
- delavirdine (Rescriptor) may lead to citalopram toxicity.
- dextromethorphan (a cough suppressant in many "DM"-labeled nonprescription cough medicines) has resulted in visual hallucinations when combined with fluoxetine, a related medicine. Caution is advised if these drugs are combined.
- diltiazem (Cardizem) may lead to excessive citalopram levels and possible serotonin syndrome.
- fenfluramine (Pondimin) may lead to serotonin syndrome—DO NOT combine.
- linezolid (Zyvox) may lead to serotonin syndrome—(an antibiotic that also acts as a MAOI). Combination is not recommended.
- lithium (Lithobid, others) may increase risk of enhanced effects from serotonin. Caution is advised.
- medicines that inhibit CYP3A4 or CYP2C19 may lead to higher than expected citalopram blood levels and increased citalopram toxicity risk.
- monoamine oxidase (MAO) type A inhibitor drugs (see Drug Classes) may cause confusion, agitation, high fever, seizures, and dangerous elevations of blood pressure. Avoid combining these drugs.
- naratriptan (Amerge), rizatriptan (Maxalt), sumatriptan (Imitrex), almotgriptan (Axert), or zolmitriptan (Zomig) or other members of this family may lead to increased risk of incoordination, weakness or excessive reflex responses.
- selegiline (Eldepryl) can result in serotonin toxicity syndrome. Avoid this combination.
- sibutramine (Meridia) may lead to serotonin syndrome—AVOID COMBINING.
- tryptophan will result in central nervous system toxicity. Avoid the combination.
- any tricyclic antidepressant (amitriptyline, nortriptyline, etc) may result in increased antidepressant drug levels and serotonin syndrome. Extreme caution is advised.
- tramadol (Ultram) may increase seizure risk. DO NOT COMBINE.
- verapamil (Calan) may lead to excessive citalopram levels and possible serotonin syndrome.

▷ *Driving, Hazardous Activities:* This drug may cause drowsiness, dizziness, impaired judgment, and delayed reaction time. Restrict activities as necessary.

Aviation Note: The use of this drug *is a disqualification* for piloting. Consult a designated Aviation Medical Examiner.

Exposure to Sun: No restrictions.

Discontinuation: Best to slowly decrease (taper) the medicine over 2–4 weeks or longer. Call your doctor if you plan to stop this drug for any reason.

Controversies in Drug Management: A review of relevant literature on the subject of depression and suicide reveals that the development or intensification of suicidal thoughts during treatment (regardless of the severity of depression) has been documented repeatedly for many patients who were also taking some of the antidepressant drugs in wide use. If you or a loved one are taking this medicine talk to your doctor immediately if suicidal thinking begins.

CLARITHROMYCIN (klar ith roh MY sin)

Please see the macrolide antibiotic family profile.

CLINDAMYCIN (klin da MY sin)

Introduced: 1973 **Class:** Antibiotic **Prescription:** USA: Yes
Controlled Drug: USA: No; Canada: No **Available as Generic:** USA: Yes; Canada: No
Brand Names: Cleocin, Cleocin Pediatric, Cleocin T, Cleocin Vaginal Cream, ✤Dalacin C, ✤Dalacin T

BENEFITS versus RISKS	
Possible Benefits	*Possible Risks*
EFFECTIVE TREATMENT FOR SERIOUS INFECTIONS OF THE LOWER RESPIRATORY TRACT, ABDOMINAL CAVITY, GENITAL TRACT IN WOMEN, BLOODSTREAM (SEPTICEMIA), SKIN, AND RELATED TISSUES CAUSED BY SUSCEPTIBLE ORGANISMS	SEVERE DRUG-INDUCED COLITIS (FATALITIES REPORTED— SYSTEMIC USE)
Combination treatment of *Pneumocystis carinii* pneumonia	Liver injury with jaundice—rare
Effective for local treatment of acne	Reduction in white blood cell and platelet counts—rare

▷ **Principal Uses**
   As a Single Drug Product: Uses currently included in FDA-approved labeling: (1) Treats serious and unusual infections of the lungs and bronchial tubes, organs and tissues within the abdominal cavity, the genital tract, and pelvic organs in women, the skin and soft tissue structures and generalized infections involving the bloodstream; (2) used in topical form to treat acne. Other (unlabeled) generally accepted uses: (1) Treatment of resistant gum disease and malaria; (2) prevention of infection of the heart; (3) combination treatment of *Pneumocystis carinii* pneumonia (PCP), an infection associated with AIDS; (4) may have a role in combination therapy of toxoplasmosis infections of the brain in AIDS patients.
   Author's Note: This profile has been shortened to make room for more widely used medicines.

CLOMIPRAMINE (kloh MI pra meen)

Introduced: 1970 **Class:** Antidepressant **Prescription:** USA: Yes **Controlled Drug:** USA: No; Canada: No **Available as Generic:** Yes
Brand Names: Anafranil, ✤Apo-Clomipramine, ✤Novo-Clopamine, Maronil

```
┌─────────────────────────────────────────────────────────────────────┐
│                      BENEFITS versus RISKS                            │
│        Possible Benefits                    Possible Risks            │
│   EFFECTIVE TREATMENT OF          DRUG-INDUCED SEIZURES               │
│      SEVERE OBSESSIVE-            ADVERSE BEHAVIORAL EFFECTS           │
│      COMPULSIVE NEUROSIS          Conversion of depression to mania in │
│   Effective relief of symptoms of some   manic-depressive (bipolar)   │
│      types of depression            disorders                         │
│   Relief in some pain syndromes   Aggravation of schizophrenia        │
│                                   Liver toxicity                      │
│                                   Bone marrow depression and blood    │
│                                      cell disorders                   │
└─────────────────────────────────────────────────────────────────────┘
```

▷ **Principal Uses**

As a Single Drug Product: Uses currently included in FDA-approved labeling: Relieves severe, disabling obsessive-compulsive disorder.

Other (unlabeled) generally accepted uses: (1) eases depression; (2) relieves symptoms of panic attacks; (3) helps some phobias; (4) may help repetitive symptoms in autistics; (5) could have a role in diabetic neuropathy and some low back pain problems; (6) can help premature ejaculation; (7) may relieve severity of hair-pulling (trichotillomania), nail-biting, or arm-burning in obsessive-compulsive patients; (8) can ease symptoms in severe premenstrual syndrome.

How This Drug Works: By increasing brain nerve transmitters (mostly serotonin), it reduces frequency/intensity of obsessive-compulsive behavior.

▷ **Widely Used Guidelines That Involve This Medicine (representative sample):** Please look at the section at the very beginning of this profile called "Class." Next, turn to Table 22 and you will find guidelines listed by the class involved!

Available Dosage Forms and Strengths

Capsules — 10 mg (Canada only), 25 mg, 50 mg, 75 mg
Tablet, sustained release — 75 mg

▷ **Usual Adult Dosage Ranges:** Starts at 25 mg daily in the evening. If needed, may be increased by 25 mg daily at 3- to 4-day intervals up to 100 mg daily (reached in 2 weeks). The 100 mg should be divided and taken after meals. Usual maintenance dose is 50 mg to 150 mg daily. Maximum daily dose is 250 mg. (Once identified, the daily dose can be given at bedtime as a single dose to help ease sleepiness problems during the day and confer sleep at night.)

Note: Actual dose and schedule must be determined for each patient individually.

Conditions Requiring Dosing Adjustments

Liver Function: The dose should be decreased in patients with liver compromise.

Kidney Function: Changes in dose are not usually needed.

▷ **Dosing Instructions:** May be taken without regard to meals, but when starting this medicine it is smart to take this medicine with meals to lower GI problems. If needed, the capsule may be opened and mixed with soft goods such as applesauce—but the beads of medicine should NOT be chewed. If you forget a dose: Take the missed dose right away, unless it's nearly time for your next dose. If you only take one dose at bedtime, call your doctor. DO NOT double doses.

Usual Duration of Use: Regular use for 4 to 10 weeks often needed to see benefits in controlling obsessive-compulsive behavior. Intravenous dosing gives an initial response in less than 6 days. Long-term use (months to years) requires periodic evaluation.

Typical Treatment Goals and Measurements (Outcomes and Markers) Obsessive-compulsive disorder: The general goal is to ease the severity of the OCD in order to let the patient resume his or her usual activities. There should involve less time spent with prior obsessions or compulsions. Blood levels of 100 to 250 ng/mL plus 230 to 550 ng/mL for desmethylclomipramine (an active chemical that your body changes this medicine into) have been designated as the therapeutic range, but the effective level varies patient to patient.

Possible Advantages of This Drug: Used as first line treatment of obsessive compulsive disorder. May be beneficial in people who also have one kind of movement disorder (akathisia) or problems sleeping.

▷ **This Drug Should Not Be Taken If**
  • you have had an allergic reaction to it previously.
  • you are taking, or have taken within the past 14 days, any monoamine oxidase (MAO) type A inhibitor drug (see Drug Classes).
  • you have active bone marrow depression or a current blood cell disorder.
  • you have had a recent heart attack (myocardial infarction).

▷ **Inform Your Physician Before Taking This Drug If**
  • you have had an adverse reaction to an antidepressant drug, especially one of the tricyclic class.
  • you have a history of bone marrow or blood cell disorder.
  • you have any type of seizure disorder.
  • you have any type of heart disease, especially coronary artery disease or a heart rhythm disorder.
  • you are subject to bronchial asthma.
  • you have impaired liver or kidney function.
  • you have any type of thyroid disorder or are taking thyroid medication.
  • you have a history of suicide attempts.
  • you have an adrenaline-producing tumor.
  • you are pregnant.
  • you have prostatism (see Glossary).
  • you have a history of alcoholism.
  • you will have surgery with general anesthesia.

Possible Side Effects (natural, expected, and unavoidable drug actions)
Drowsiness, increased sweating, light-headedness, blurred vision, dry mouth, constipation, impaired urination.

▷ **Possible Adverse Effects** (unusual, unexpected, and infrequent reactions)
If any of the following develop, consult your physician promptly for guidance.
Mild Adverse Effects
Allergic reactions: skin rash, itching, drug fever (see Glossary)—case reports.
Headache, dizziness, nervousness, impaired memory, weakness, tremors, insomnia, muscle cramps, flushing—infrequent.
Tremor—frequent.
Sweating—infrequent.
Increased appetite, weight gain—infrequent.
Altered taste, indigestion, nausea, vomiting, diarrhea—infrequent.

Serious Adverse Effects

Allergic reactions: drug-induced hepatitis, with or without jaundice—case reports.

Idiosyncratic reactions: hyperthermia, neuroleptic malignant syndrome (see Glossary)—case reports.

Adverse behavioral effects: confusion, delirium, delusions, hallucinations, paranoia—case reports.

Seizures, reduced control of epilepsy—case reports to rare.

Aggravated paranoid psychoses or schizophrenia—case reports.

Heart rhythm disturbances—case report.

Bone marrow depression (see Glossary): fatigue, weakness, fever, sore throat, infections, abnormal bleeding or bruising—case reports.

SIADH and severe lowering of blood sodium—case reports.

Liver toxicity—infrequent.

Serotonin syndrome—case reports.

▷ **Possible Effects on Sexual Function:** Altered libido, impaired (delayed) ejaculation, impotence, inhibited male orgasm, inhibited female orgasm, abnormal sperm formation, female breast enlargement with milk production (galactorrhea), absence of menstruation—case reports. The delay in ejaculation is useful in males who are troubled by premature ejaculation.

Adverse Effects That May Mimic Natural Diseases or Disorders

Liver toxicity may suggest viral hepatitis.

Natural Diseases or Disorders That May Be Activated by This Drug

Latent epilepsy, glaucoma, prostatism, schizophrenia.

Possible Effects on Laboratory Tests

Complete blood cell counts: decreased red cells, hemoglobin, white cells, and platelets.

Liver function tests: increased liver enzymes (ALT/GPT, AST/GOT)—liver damage.

Thyroid function tests: decreased TT3 and FT3.

Blood sodium: severely lowered in cases of drug-induced SIADH.

CAUTION

1. Watch for toxicity: confusion, agitation, rapid heart rate, heart irregularity. Blood levels clarify the situation.
2. Use with caution in schizophrenia. Watch closely for deterioration of thinking or behavior.
3. Use with caution in epilepsy. Watch for any change in the frequency or severity of seizures.
4. Complete blood counts should be obtained in patients who develop sore throat or fever while taking this medicine.

Precautions for Use

By Infants and Children: Safety and effectiveness for those under 10 years of age not established. Dose and management should be supervised by a properly trained pediatrician. Dosing is started at 25 mg daily and is then increased over 2 weeks to 200 mg or 3 mg per kg of body mass, whichever number is smaller.

By Those Over 60 Years of Age: Started with 10 mg at bedtime. Dose is increased as needed and tolerated to 75 mg daily in divided doses. During first 2 weeks, watch for behavioral reactions: restlessness, agitation, forgetfulness, disorientation, hallucinations. Unsteadiness or instability may predispose to falling. Prostate problems may also be aggravated.

▷ **Advisability of Use During Pregnancy**

Pregnancy Category: C. See Pregnancy Risk Categories at the back of this book.

Animal Studies: No drug-induced birth defects seen in mouse or rat studies.

Human Studies: Adequate studies of pregnant women are not available.

Use only if clearly needed. Avoid use during the last 3 months, if possible, to prevent withdrawal symptoms in the newborn infant: irritability, tremors, and seizures.

Advisability of Use If Breast-Feeding

Presence of this drug in breast milk: Yes.

Talk with your doctor about this benefit to risk decision.

Habit-Forming Potential: Withdrawal symptoms have been reported (nausea, vomiting, dizziness, headache, and temperature changes), and the drug should be slowly decreased in dose (tapered) if it is to be stopped.

Effects of Overdose: Confusion, delirium, hallucinations, drowsiness, tremors, unsteadiness, heart irregularity, seizures, stupor, sweating, fever.

Possible Effects of Long-Term Use: Neuroleptic malignant syndrome (see Glossary): Fever, fast or irregular heartbeat, fast breathing, sweating, weakness, muscle stiffness, seizures, loss of bladder control.

Suggested Periodic Examinations While Taking This Drug (at physician's discretion)

Monitoring of blood drug levels as appropriate.

Complete blood cell counts.

Liver and kidney function tests.

Serial blood pressure readings and electrocardiograms.

Visual acuity checks.

▷ **While Taking This Drug, Observe the Following**

Foods: No specific restrictions. May need to limit food intake to avoid excessive weight gain.

Herbal Medicines or Minerals: Since clomipramine and St. John's wort may act to increase serotonin, the combination is not advised. St. John's wort also increases sun sensitivity. Since part of the way ginkgo biloba works may be as a MAO inhibitor, do not combine with this medicine. Ma huang and yohimbe are best avoided while taking clomipramine. Indian snakeroot and kava kava (kava is no longer recommended in Canada) are also best avoided while taking this medicine.

Beverages: No restrictions. May be taken with milk.

▷ *Alcohol:* Avoid completely. This drug can markedly increase the intoxicating effects of alcohol; the combination can depress brain function significantly.

Tobacco Smoking: May delay the elimination of this drug and require dosage adjustment. I advise everyone to quit smoking.

Marijuana Smoking or injestion: Increased drowsiness and mouth dryness; reduced effectiveness and increased cardiovascular problems.

▷ *Other Drugs*

Clomipramine may ***increase*** the effects of

• all drugs with atropine-like effects (see Drug Classes).

• all sedating drugs. Watch for excessive sedation.

Clomipramine may ***decrease*** the effects of

• clonidine (Catapres).

• guanadrel (Hylorel).

• guanethidine (Ismelin, Esimil).

Clomipramine *taken concurrently* with

- anticonvulsants (see Drug Classes) such as carbamazepine (Tegretol) requires careful monitoring for changes in seizure patterns and the need to adjust anticonvulsant dosage.
- bepridil (Vascor) may lead to dangerous heart rhythms.
- cisapride (Propulsid) may lead to dangerous heart rhythms.
- dofetilide (Tikosyn) may lead to dangerous heart rhythms. Do not combine.
- gatifloxacin (Tequin), grepafloxacin (Raxar), moxifloxacin (Avelox), or sparfloxacin (Zagam) may lead to dangerous heart rhythms. Combination is NOT recommended.
- medicines that affect the QTc interval of the heart may worsen the QTc interval changes if combined with clomipramine.
- monoamine oxidase (MAO) type A inhibitor drugs (see Drug Classes) may cause high fever, seizures and hypertension. Avoid combining these drugs—14 days should separate doses of either.
- phenytoin (Dilantin) or fosphenytoin (Cerebyx) may lead to phenytoin or fosphenytoin toxicity.
- salmeterol (Serevent) may lead to excessive heart stimulation. Caution is advised.
- SAMe (S-adenosylmethionine) may lead to serotonin syndrome (mental status changes, muscle movement problems, high temperature, and high blood pressure).
- stimulant drugs (amphetamine, cocaine, epinephrine, methylphenidate, etc) may cause severe high blood pressure and/or high fever.
- thyroid preparations may increase risk of heart rhythm disorders.
- tramadol (Ultram) may increase seizure risk.
- valproic acid (Depakote) may lead to clomipramine toxicity. Clomipramine doses should be lowered if these two medicines must be combined.
- venlafaxine (Effexor) may lead to venlafaxine and clomipramine toxicity.
- warfarin (Coumadin) may cause an increased warfarin effect and bleeding. More frequent INR (prothrombin time) testing is needed.

The following drugs may *increase* the effects of clomipramine:

- ACE inhibitors (see Drug Classes).
- birth control pills (oral contraceptives).
- cimetidine (Tagamet).
- enalapril (Vasotec, Vaseretic).
- estrogens (various).
- fluoxetine (Prozac).
- fluvoxamine (Luvox).
- haloperidol (Haldol).
- medicines that interfere with or inhibit cytochrome P450 2D6, a liver enzyme that is responsible for removing clomipramine from the body.
- methylphenidate (Ritalin).
- modafinil (Provigil).
- paroxetine (Paxil).
- phenothiazines (see Drug Classes).
- propafenone (Rythmol).
- quinidine (Quinaglute).
- ranitidine (Zantac).
- ritonavir (Norvir), amprenavir (Agenerase), atazanavir (Reyataz) and perhaps other protease inhibitors (see Drug Classes).
- sertraline (Zoloft).
- verapamil (Calan, others).

The following drugs may **decrease** the effects of clomipramine:
- barbiturates (see Drug Classes).
- carbamazepine (Tegretol).
- chloral hydrate (Noctec, Somnos, etc).
- lithium (Lithobid, Lithotab, etc).
- reserpine (Serpasil, Ser-Ap-Es, etc).

▷ *Driving, Hazardous Activities:* This drug may cause seizures and impair alertness, judgment, physical coordination and reaction time. Restrict activities as necessary.

Aviation Note: The use of this drug *is a disqualification* for piloting. Consult a designated Aviation Medical Examiner.

Exposure to Sun: No restrictions.

Exposure to Heat: Use caution. This drug may impair the body's adaptation to hot environments, increasing the risk of heatstroke. Avoid saunas.

Exposure to Environmental Chemicals: This drug may mask the symptoms of poisoning due to handling certain insecticides (organophosphorous types). Read their labels carefully.

Discontinuation: It is best to slowly reduce the dose over 3 to 4 weeks. Abrupt withdrawal after prolonged use may cause nausea, vomiting, diarrhea, headache, dizziness, malaise, disturbed sleep, and irritability. Obsessive-compulsive behavior may worsen if drug is stopped. Other drug doses may need to be changed to adjust.

CLONAZEPAM (kloh NA ze pam)

Introduced: 1977   **Class:** Anticonvulsant, benzodiazepines   **Prescription:** USA: Yes   **Controlled Drug:** USA: C-IV*; Canada: No   **Available as Generic:** Yes

Brand Names: ✦Apo-clonazepam, Klonopin, Klonopin Wafers, ✦Med-clonazepam, ✦Novo-clonazepam, ✦Rhoxal-clonazepam, ✦Rivotril

Warning: Klonopin and the generic clonidine have similar names and can be mistaken for each other—a serious error. Make sure you are taking the correct drug.

BENEFITS versus RISKS	
Possible Benefits	*Possible Risks*
EFFECTIVE CONTROL OF SOME TYPES OF PETIT MAL, AKINETIC AND MYOCLONIC SEIZURES	Paradoxical reactions: excitement, agitation, and hallucinations
EFFECTIVE IN MANAGING PANIC DISORDER	Minor impairment of mental functions
ORPHAN DRUG FOR STARTLE DISEASE	Blood cell disorders: anemia, abnormally low white blood cell and platelet counts—rare
Can help restless leg syndrome	Increased salivation (difficult in people with chronic lung disease)
Klonopin Wafers offers the ability to take the drug without water	

*See Schedules of Controlled Drugs at the back of this book.

▷ **Principal Uses**

As a Single Drug Product: Uses currently included in FDA-approved labeling: (1) Treats several types of epilepsy: petit mal variations, akinetic, myoclonic, and absence seizure patterns; (2) effective in panic disorder; (3) an orphan drug for startle disease (hyperekplexia).

Other (unlabeled) generally accepted uses: (1) Eases symptoms of Tourette's syndrome; (2) relieves trigeminal neuralgia; (3) helps resistant depression; (4) can ease drug-induced mania; (5) may be of help in restless leg syndrome (Ekbom syndrome); (6) may help essential tremor symptoms; (7) eases alprazolam withdrawal.

How This Drug Works: Increases the action of a nerve transmitter (gamma-aminobutyric acid or GABA), which blocks seizures.

▷ **Widely Used Guidelines That Involve This Medicine (representative sample):** Please look at the section at the very beginning of this profile called "Class." Next, turn to Table 22 and you will find guidelines listed by the class involved!

Available Dosage Forms and Strengths

Orally disintegrating tablets — 0.125 mg, 0.25 mg, 0.5 mg, 1 mg and 2 mg (Wafers)

Tablets — 0.125 mg, 0.25 mg, 0.5 mg, 1 mg, 2 mg

▷ **Usual Adult Dosage Ranges**

Seizures: Starts with 0.5 mg three times daily. Increased by 0.5 mg to 1.0 mg every 3 days, as needed and tolerated. Maximum daily dose 20 mg.

Panic disorder: Not established for those less than 18 years old.

Note: Actual dose and schedule must be determined for each patient individually.

Conditions Requiring Dosing Adjustments

Liver Function: The dose must be decreased in liver compromise.

Kidney Function: Watch for signs and symptoms of accumulation (see "Effects of Overdose" below).

▷ **Dosing Instructions:** May be taken on empty stomach or with food or milk. Klonopin Wafers are orally disintegrating tablets that dissolve without water. The tablet may be crushed. Do not stop this drug abruptly if taken for seizure control, or if taken for more than 4 weeks to control panic attacks. If your forget a dose: take the dose as soon as you remember it, unless it's nearly time for your next dose—if that is the case, skip the missed dose and simply take the next scheduled dose. DO NOT double doses.

Usual Duration of Use: Regular use for 2 to 3 weeks may be needed to see benefit in reducing frequency or severity of seizures. Peak control requires dose adjustments over several months. Long-term use (months to years) requires evaluation by your doctor.

Typical Treatment Goals and Measurements (Outcomes and Markers)

Seizures: The general goal for this medicine is effective seizure control. Neurologists tend to define effective on a case-by-case basis depending on the seizure type and patient factors. IF goals have not been reached, combination treatment may be needed.

Panic: Goals for panic tend to be more vague and subjective than for hypertension or cholesterol. Frequently, the patient (in conjunction with physician assessment) will largely decide if panic has been successfully controlled. Additional markers include: decreased number of trips to the hospital or

ER visits may be a useful measure. The ability of the patient to return to normal activities is a hallmark of successful treatment.

Possible Advantages of This Drug: The wafer form may be particularly suited to treatment of panic attacks, offering a medicine that goes to work quickly (rapid onset) and does not require water to take it.

▷ **This Drug Should Not Be Taken If**
• you have had an allergic reaction to it previously.
• you have sudden (acute) narrow-angle glaucoma.
• you have active liver disease.

▷ **Inform Your Physician Before Taking This Drug If**
• you are allergic to any benzodiazepine (see Drug Classes).
• you have a history of alcoholism or drug abuse.
• you are pregnant or planning pregnancy.
• you have palpitations, as this drug may worsen palpitations.
• you have impaired liver or kidney function.
• you have a history of serious depression or mental disorder.
• you have asthma, emphysema, chronic bronchitis, or myasthenia gravis.
• you have acute intermittent porphyria or lung disease.

Possible Side Effects (natural, expected, and unavoidable drug actions)
Drowsiness—frequent (may diminish with time).
Increased salivation.

▷ **Possible Adverse Effects** (unusual, unexpected, and infrequent reactions)
If any of the following develop, consult your physician promptly for guidance.
Mild Adverse Effects
Allergic reactions: skin rash, hives, itching.
Ataxia—frequent.
A feeling that the mouth is burning (burning mouth syndrome)—case report.
Weight gain—frequent.
Headache, dizziness, blurred vision, double vision, slurred speech, impaired memory, confusion, depression—possible.
Muscle weakness, uncontrolled body movements—possible.
Palpitations or hair loss—rare.
Nausea, vomiting, constipation, diarrhea, impaired urination, incontinence—case reports in older patients.
Serious Adverse Effects
Idiosyncratic reactions: paradoxical responses of excitement, hyperactivity, agitation, anger, hostility—case reports.
Hallucinations, seizures—case reports.
Blood disorders: abnormally low platelet counts—case reports.
Porphyria—case reports.
Increased secretions and breathing problems, especially in those with chronic lung disease—case reports.

▷ **Possible Effects on Sexual Function:** Increased libido, enlargement of male breasts. May cause abnormally early (precocious) secondary sex characteristics in children—case reports.

Possible Effects on Laboratory Tests
Complete blood cell counts: low red or white cells, hemoglobin, or platelets.
Urine tests for drug abuse: may be positive. (Results depend on amount of drug taken and test method.)
Liver function tests: increased.

CAUTION
1. Drug should not be stopped abruptly if used to control seizures (rebound seizures may occur), and should be slowly decreased (see discontinuation) if it must be stopped.
2. Some over-the-counter products containing antihistamines (allergy and cold preparations, sleep aids) can cause excessive sedation if combined with clonazepam.
3. Adverse behavioral reactions are more common in people with brain damage, mental retardation or psychiatric disorders.
4. Decreased drug response seen in about 30% of users 3 months after therapy starts. Dose increase often needed to restore seizure control.

Precautions for Use
By Infants and Children: This drug has data for use in infants and children of all ages. Careful dosage adjustment based on weight and age is mandatory. Abnormal behavioral responses are more common in children.
By Those Over 60 Years of Age: Smaller doses and longer intervals are suggested. Watch for lethargy, indifference, fatigue, unsteadiness, disturbing dreams, paradoxical excitement, agitation, anger, hostility, or rage.

▷ **Advisability of Use During Pregnancy**
Pregnancy Category: C. See Pregnancy Risk Categories at the back of this book.
Animal Studies: This drug causes cleft palates, open eyelids, fused rib structures, and limb defects in rabbits.
Human Studies: Adequate studies of pregnant women are not available.
Avoid drug during the first 3 months if possible. Frequent use in late pregnancy may cause the "floppy infant" syndrome in newborns: weakness, lethargy, unresponsiveness, low body temperature, depressed breathing.

Advisability of Use If Breast-Feeding
Presence of this drug in breast milk: Yes.
Avoid drug or refrain from nursing.

Habit-Forming Potential: This drug can produce psychological and/or physical dependence (see Glossary), especially with large doses for extended periods.

Effects of Overdose: Marked drowsiness, weakness, confusion, slurred speech, staggering gait, tremor, stupor progressing to deep sleep or coma.

Possible Effects of Long-Term Use: Benefits versus risks must be considered carefully.

Suggested Periodic Examinations While Taking This Drug (at physician's discretion)
During long-term use: Complete blood cell counts; liver function tests.

▷ **While Taking This Drug, Observe the Following**
Foods: No restrictions.
Herbal Medicines or Minerals: Hawthorn may react antagonistically to clonazepam. Valerian and kava kava may interact additively (drowsiness). Avoid these combinations. Kola nut, Siberian ginseng, mate, ephedra, and ma huang may blunt the benefits of this medicine. While St. John's wort is indicated for anxiety, it is also thought to increase (induce) cytochrome P450 enzymes and will tend to blunt clonazepam effectiveness if combined with clonazepam. Evening primrose oil may increase risk of seizures and is not recommended. Some forms of ginkgo are contaminated with 4'-O-methylpyridoxine which can be toxic to nerves. Caution is advised.
Beverages: No restrictions. May be taken with milk.
▷ *Alcohol:* Use with extreme caution. Alcohol may increase the depressant effects of this drug on the brain. It is advisable to avoid alcohol

completely—throughout the day and night—if it is necessary to drive or to engage in any hazardous activity.

Tobacco Smoking: No interactions expected. I advise everyone to quit smoking.

Marijuana Smoking: Increased sedation and significant impairment of intellectual and physical performance.

▷ *Other Drugs*

Clonazepam *taken concurrently* with

- amiodarone (Cordarone) may decrease elimination of clonazepam and also worsen toxicity by causing low thyroid function.
- carbamazepine (Tegretol) may decrease blood levels and hence benefits of both medications.
- desipramine, imipramine and other tricyclic antidepressants (see Drug Classes) can decrease the tricyclic antidepressant blood level and lessen its therapeutic benefit.
- MAO inhibitors (see Drug Classes) may result in very low blood pressure and worsening of sedation and respiratory depression.
- phenytoin (Dilantin) or fosphenytoin (Cerebyx) may result in decreased phenytoin or fosphenytoin levels.
- primidone (Mysoline) may lead to excessive drowsiness.
- ritonavir (Norvir), amprenavir (Agenerase), atazanavir (Reyataz) and perhaps other protease inhibitors (see Drug Classes), may lead to clonazepam toxicity.
- valproic acid (Depakene, etc) may cause continuous absence seizures, and is a benefit to risk decision.

The following drugs may *increase* the effects of clonazepam:

- antifungal medicines such as itraconazole (Sporanox) and ketoconazole (Nizoral).
- cimetidine (Tagamet).
- disulfiram (Antabuse).
- macrolide antibiotics such as azithromycin, clarithromycin, or erythromycin (see Drug Classes).
- omeprazole (Prilosec).
- oral contraceptives (birth control pills).

The following drugs may *decrease* the effects of clonazepam:

- rifampin (Rifater) or rifabutin (Mycobutin).
- theophylline (aminophylline, Theo-Dur, etc).

▷ *Driving, Hazardous Activities:* This drug can impair mental alertness, judgment, physical coordination, and reaction time. Avoid hazardous activities accordingly.

Aviation Note: The use of this drug *is a disqualification* for piloting. Consult a designated Aviation Medical Examiner.

Exposure to Sun: No restrictions.

Discontinuation: Do not stop clonazepam suddenly if it was controlling any type of seizure, or if it was taken for more than 4 weeks. Dosing should be slowly decreased (tapered) to prevent a withdrawal syndrome.

CLONIDINE (KLOH ni deen)

Introduced: 1969 **Class:** Antihypertensive, analgesic **Prescription:** USA: Yes **Controlled Drug:** USA: No; Canada: No **Available as Generic:** USA: Yes; Canada: No

Brand Names: ✤Apo-Clonidine, Catapres, Catapres-TTS, Combipres [CD], Dixarit, Duraclon, ✤Novo-Clonidine, ✤Nu-Clonidine

---

BENEFITS versus RISKS

Possible Benefits	*Possible Risks*
EFFECTIVE ANTIHYPERTENSIVE IN MILD TO MODERATE HIGH BLOOD PRESSURE	ACUTE WITHDRAWAL SYNDROME (rebound hypertension) with abrupt discontinuation
Effective control of menopausal hot flashes (in selected cases)	Raynaud's phenomenon (cold fingers or toes)
Effective help in narcotic withdrawal	
Has an anesthetic sparing effect in some cases	
May have a role as a second-line medicine for people who are trying to quit smoking	

▷ **Principal Uses**

As a Single Drug Product: Uses currently included in FDA-approved labeling: (1) Used in combination with other medicines to treat mild to moderate high blood pressure; (2) helpful in adjunctive treatment of cancer pain (helps narcotics or opioids work better).

Other (unlabeled) generally accepted uses: (1) Helps prevent migraine headache; (2) helps improve outcomes in some head injuries (may be a drug of choice there); (3) can aid menopausal hot flashes and severe menstrual cramps; (4) lessens symptoms of alcohol or narcotic drug withdrawal; (5) helped atrial fibrillation in one study; (6) second-line drug in controlling high blood pressure in congestive heart failure patients; (7) useful in some diabetic nerve damage (peripheral neuropathy) and cancer pain; (8) may have a use protecting the kidneys (renal protective) from cyclosporine or in coronary artery bypass surgery; (9) useful in Tourette's syndrome; (10) given preoperatively, it was shone to lower pain coming from propofol injection in gynecological laparotomy.

As a Combination Drug Product [CD]: Available in combination with chlorthalidone. The different ways in which these drugs work complement each other, making the combination a more effective antihypertensive.

How This Drug Works: Decreases action of the brain (vasomotor center), limiting the sympathetic nervous system's constriction of blood vessels and blood pressure increases. Chlorthalidone combination helps remove excess water from the body ("water pill") that contributes to high blood pressure.

▷ **Widely Used Guidelines That Involve This Medicine (representative sample):** Please look at the section at the very beginning of this profile called "Class." Next, turn to Table 22 and you will find guidelines listed by the class involved!

Available Dosage Forms and Strengths

Patches — 2.5 mg, 5.0 mg, 7.5 mg

Tablets — 0.1 mg, 0.2 mg, 0.3 mg

Tablets, combination — 0.1 mg, 0.2 mg and 0.3 mg of clonidine with 15 mg chlorthalidone

▷ **Usual Adult Dosage Ranges:** *Tablets:* Initially 0.1 mg twice daily. Increased by 0.1 to 0.2 mg daily as needed and tolerated. Usual range is 0.2 to 0.6 mg daily, taken in two doses. Maximum daily dose is 2.4 mg. Some clinicians set maximum of 1.2 mg daily. *Patches:* Applied once a week. Dosing begins with the 0.1mg a day system (Catapres TTS-1) Dosing greater than a 0.6 milligram daily dose does not often result in added therapeutic effects.

Note: Actual dose and schedule must be determined for each patient individually.

Conditions Requiring Dosing Adjustments

Liver Function: This drug is changed into six active forms. The dose must be decreased in liver compromise.

Kidney Function: Some kidney patients may require higher ongoing doses to get the best blood pressure.

▷ **Dosing Instructions:** Tablets may be taken without regard to eating. The tablet may be crushed. Patches should not be altered. If you forget a dose: For the patch form—put the patch on as soon as you remember it. If you are more than 3 days late, call your doctor. If you forget a regular release tablet, take the missed dose right away unless it is nearly time for your next dose, then skip the missed dose and take the regularly scheduled dose. DO NOT double doses. If you have trouble remembering this medicine, talk with your doctor. If a change is being made from oral treatment to the patches, it's important to remember that the blood pressure lowering effect often does not start for 2–3 days. The maker of this medicine recommends placing the patch, then on day one taking 100% of the usual dose, on day two taking 50% of the usual dose and on day three taking 25% of the usual dose. Your doctor will decide which strength patch to give you based on how large your oral dose is.

Usual Duration of Use: Use on a regular schedule for 2 to 3 weeks may be needed to see this drug's full benefit in lowering high blood pressure. If target goals are not met by the expected time frame, changes should be made. Long-term use (months to years) requires physician supervision and guidance.

Typical Treatment Goals and Measurements (Outcomes and Markers)

Blood Pressure: Guidelines (JNC VII) define normal blood pressure (BP) as **less than** 120/80 and **pre-hypertension** as 120/80 to 139/89. This new range is intended to help doctors encourage lifestyle changes (or in the case of people with a risk factor for high blood pressure, start treatment) much earlier—so that damage to blood vessels, your heart, kidneys, sexual potency, or eyes might be minimized or avoided altogether. Stage 1 hypertension is 140/90 to 159/99 and stage 2 hypertension equal to or greater than: 160/100 mm Hg. These guidelines also recommend that clinicians work with their patients to agree on the goals and a plan of treatment. The first-ever guidelines for blood pressure (hypertension) in African Americans recommends that MOST black patients be started on TWO antihypertensive medicines with the goal of lowering blood pressure to 130/80 for those with high risk for heart and blood vessel disease or with diabetes. The American Diabetes Association also recommends 130/80 as the target for diabetics and less than 125/75 for those who spill more than one gram of protein into their urine. Most clinicians try to achieve a BP that confers the best balance of lower cardiovascular risk and avoids the problem of too low a blood pressure. Blood pressure duration is generally increased with beneficial restriction of sodium. If goals are not met, it is not unusual to intensify doses or add on medicines.

▷ **This Drug Should Not Be Taken If**

- you have had an allergic reaction to it previously.
- you have a problem in your heart that impacts the timing of the heartbeat or transmission of electrical impulses through the heart.

▷ **Inform Your Physician Before Taking This Drug If**
- you have a circulatory disorder of the brain.
- you have angina or coronary artery disease.
- you recently had a heart attack (MI).
- you have or have had serious emotional depression.
- you have a very slow heart rate.
- you have kidney failure.
- you have Buerger's disease or Raynaud's phenomenon.
- you are taking a tricyclic antidepressant (see Drug Classes).
- you are taking any sedative or hypnotic drugs or an antidepressant.
- you will have surgery with general anesthesia.

Possible Side Effects (natural, expected, and unavoidable drug actions)
Drowsiness, dry nose and mouth, constipation—common.
Decreased heart rate, mild orthostatic hypotension (see Glossary).
Serious abnormal heartbeats possible if drug is stopped suddenly. Skin irritation (contact dermatitis) with the patch—infrequent to frequent.

▷ **Possible Adverse Effects** (unusual, unexpected, and infrequent reactions)
If any of the following develop, consult your physician promptly for guidance.

Mild Adverse Effects
Allergic reactions: skin rash, hives, localized swellings, itching—rare to infrequent.
Drowsiness—infrequent to frequent.
Headache, dizziness, fatigue, anxiety, sleep disorders (nightmares or vivid dreaming), dry and burning eyes—possible.
Painful parotid (salivary) gland, nausea, vomiting—case reports.
Dry mouth—frequent.
Urination at night—rare.
Increased liver function tests—case reports.

Serious Adverse Effects
Idiosyncratic reaction: Raynaud's phenomenon (see Glossary)—case reports.
Aggravation of congestive heart failure, heart rhythm disorders—case reports.
Depression, hallucinations or psychosis—case reports.

▷ **Possible Effects on Sexual Function:** Decreased libido or impotence—infrequent.
Enlargement of male breasts (gynecomastia)—rare.
Precocious puberty in females—case report.

Possible Effects on Laboratory Tests
Blood cholesterol or triglyceride levels: no consistent or significant effects.
Blood sodium level: increased.
Liver function: rare increases of enzymes (ALT/GPT, AST/GOT, alkaline phosphatase).

CAUTION
1. ***Do not stop this drug suddenly.*** Sudden withdrawal can cause a severe and possibly fatal reaction.
2. Hot weather or fever can reduce blood pressure significantly. Dose adjustments may be necessary.
3. Report any tendency to depression.
4. Lowered response to the beneficial effects on blood pressure may happen over time (tolerance). This may require alternate medicines for blood pressure control.

Precautions for Use

By Infants and Children: Initial doses of 5–10 mcg per kg of body mass per day, divided into two or three doses, have been used. A larger evening dose and smaller morning dose can help minimize sedation during school hours when used for attention deficit hyperactivity disorder (ADHD).

By Those Over 60 Years of Age: ***Proceed cautiously*** with this drug. High blood pressure should be reduced slowly without the risks associated with excessively low blood pressure. Low initial doses and frequent blood pressure checks are needed. Watch for development of light-headedness, dizziness, unsteadiness, fainting, and falling. Sedation and dry mouth occur in 50% of elderly users. Promptly report any changes in mood or behavior: depression, delusions, hallucinations.

▷ **Advisability of Use During Pregnancy**

Pregnancy Category: C. See Pregnancy Risk Categories at the back of this book.
Animal Studies: No birth defects reported. However, this drug is toxic to the embryo in low dosage.
Human Studies: Adequate studies of pregnant women are not available. The manufacturer recommends that women who are or who may become pregnant avoid this drug. Ask your doctor for help.

Advisability of Use If Breast-Feeding

Presence of this drug in breast milk: Yes.
This drug may impair milk production. Monitor nursing infant closely. Stop drug or nursing if adverse effects begin.

Habit-Forming Potential: A small number of reports regarding abuse of this drug have surfaced. It may cause extreme grogginess and lethargy when combined with diazepam (Valium). It may produce (with large doses of 1–3 mg) an altered mental state (nod effect) which may have lead to some abuse of this medicine. A withdrawal syndrome (rebound hypertension) is possible if this medicine is stopped suddenly, but is not withdrawal as it is used relative to opioids.

Effects of Overdose: Marked drowsiness, weakness, dry mouth, slow pulse, low blood pressure, vomiting, stupor progressing to coma.

Possible Effects of Long-Term Use: Development of tolerance (see Glossary) with loss of drug effect; weight gain due to salt and water retention; temporary sexual impotence.

Suggested Periodic Examinations While Taking This Drug (at physician's discretion)

Blood pressure measurements.
Monitoring of body weight.

▷ **While Taking This Drug, Observe the Following**

Foods: Avoid excessive salt and ask your doctor for help with salt restriction.
Herbal Medicines or Minerals: Ginseng, bitter orange, country mallow, guarana, hawthorn, saw palmetto, ma huang (no longer on the market), goldenseal, yohimbe, and licorice may cause increased blood pressure. Calcium and garlic may help lower blood pressure and Indian snakeroot has a German Commission E monograph indication for hypertension—talk to your doctor to see if those combinations may allow some lowering of prescription medicine doses. Eleuthero root and ephedra should be avoided by people living with hypertension.
Beverages: No restrictions. May be taken with milk.

▷   *Alcohol:* Use with extreme caution. Combined effects can cause marked drowsiness and exaggerated reduction of blood pressure.

    Tobacco Smoking: No expected interactions. I advise everyone to quit smoking.

▷   *Other Drugs*

    Clonidine may *decrease* the effects of

- levodopa (Larodopa, Sinemet, etc), causing an increase in Parkinsonism symptoms.

    Clonidine *taken concurrently* with

- beta-adrenergic blocking drugs (Inderal, Lopressor, Coreg, etc) may increase rebound hypertension risk if clonidine is stopped first. It is best to stop the beta-blocker first and then withdraw clonidine gradually.
- cyclosporine (Sandimmune) may lead to cyclosporine toxicity.
- ephedrine (various) may dangerously increase the blood pressure raising effect of ephedrine.
- mirtazapine (Remeron) resulted in a large increase in blood pressure in one case report. Caution is advised.
- naloxone (Narcan, Talwin NX) may blunt the therapeutic effect of clonidine and result in a hypertensive response.
- niacin may decrease the facial-flushing side effect of niacin.
- nonsteroidal anti-inflammatory drugs (NSAIDs—see Drug Classes) may blunt blood pressure lowering benefits of clonidine.
- verapamil (Calan, others) may lead to problems in conduction of the heart.

    The following drugs may *decrease* the effects of clonidine:

- nonsteroidal anti-inflammatory drugs (NSAIDs—see Drug Classes).
- tricyclic antidepressants (Elavil, Sinequan, etc—see Drug Classes), possibly reducing clonidine's effectiveness in lowering blood pressure.

▷   *Driving, Hazardous Activities:* Use caution. Can cause drowsiness and impair alertness, judgment, and coordination.

    Aviation Note: Hypertension (high blood pressure) *is a disqualification* for piloting. Consult a designated Aviation Medical Examiner.

    Exposure to Sun: No restrictions.

    Exposure to Heat: Use caution. Hot environments may reduce blood pressure, making orthostatic hypotension (see Glossary) more likely.

    Exposure to Cold: Use caution. May cause painful blanching and numbness of the hands and feet on exposure to cold air or water (Raynaud's phenomenon).

    Heavy Exercise or Exertion: Use caution. This drug may intensify the hypertensive response to isometric exercise. Ask your doctor for help.

    Occurrence of Unrelated Illness: Fever may lower blood pressure. Repeated vomiting may prevent the regular use of this drug and cause an acute withdrawal reaction. Consult your physician.

    Discontinuation: **Do not stop this drug suddenly.** A severe withdrawal reaction can occur within 12 to 48 hours after the last dose. It is best to gradually decrease the dose over 3 to 4 days, and check blood pressure often.

CLOPIDOGREL (KLOH pi doh grel)

Introduced: 1998   **Class:**   Antiplatelet (platelet aggregation inhibitor)
Prescription: USA: Yes   **Controlled Drug:**   USA: No; Canada: No
Available as Generic: No
Brand Name: Plavix

BENEFITS versus RISKS

Possible Benefits	*Possible Risks*
PREVENTION OF HEART ATTACK (CARDIOVASCULAR EVENTS IN PEOPLE WITH USTABLE ANGINA)	Stomach irritation, bleeding, and/or ulceration (less than aspirin)
	Lowered white blood cells
EFFECTIVE PREVENTION OF ATHEROSCLEROTIC EVENTS	Liver toxicity
	Thrombotic thrombocytopenic purpura
PREVENTION OF BLOOD CLOTS	
PREVENTION OF HEART ATTACK	
PREVENTION OF STROKE	
PREVENTION OF VASCULAR DEATH	
PREVENTION OF CARDIOVASCULAR COMPLICATIONS (SUCH AS STROKE, HEART ATTACK, OR CARDIOVASCULAR DEATH) IN PEOPLE WITH ACUTE CORONARY SYNDROMES UNSTABLE ANGINA AND NON-Q-WAVE MI WHEN COMBINED WITH ASPIRIN	
LONG-TERM BENEFIT (THREE YEARS IN THE CAPRIE STUDY) IN PREVENTING DEATH, HEART ATTACK, OR STROKE	

▷ **Principal Uses**

As a Single Drug Product: Uses currently included in FDA-approved labeling: (1) Reduces atherosclerotic events (vascular death, stroke or heart attack, [MI]) in people who have atherosclerosis (shown by recent MI, peripheral artery disease or stroke); (2) used to lower the number of repeat problems (events) caused by clogging of the arteries (atherosclerosis) such as stroke, heart attack, or vascular death in people who have artery clogging (atherosclerosis) which is documented by a recent stroke, heart attack, or peripheral artery disease; (3) FDA approved this medicine in the first quarter of 2002 to prevent cardiovascular problems (events such as heart attack, cardiovascular death, or stroke) in patients with acute coronary syndrome (unstable angina/non-Q-wave MI) in combination with 75–325 mg of aspirin once daily.

Other (unlabeled) generally accepted uses: (1) Combined use of clopidogrel with dalteparin or when used alone helped heal wounds (refractory venous stasis ulcers); (2) Used for up to one year in the Clopidogrel for the Reduction of Events During Observation (CREDO) study in patients after percutaneous coronary intervention (PCI) showing that long-term use gave a 38% reduction in heart attack, stroke, or death.

How This Drug Works: Permanently (irreversibly) inhibits adenosine diphosphate (ADP)-induced platelet clumping (aggregation). Combination of clopidogrel with aspirin decreases a compound important to platelet function (down regulates P-selectin expression) and also decreases C Reactive Protein (CRP) in stroke (acute ischemic kind).

▷ **Widely Used Guidelines That Involve This Medicine (representative sample):** Please look at the section at the very beginning of this profile called "Class." Next, turn to Table 22 and you will find guidelines listed by the class involved!

Available Dosage Forms and Strengths: Tablets — 75 mg

▷ **Usual Adult Dosage Ranges**

In patients with *Acute Coronary Syndromes or ACS* (unstable angina/non-Q-wave Myocardial Infarction): 300 mg is given as a priming (loading dose) to quickly gain the therapeutic effect, and then 75 mg is given by mouth each day. Aspirin (75-325 mg once a day) should also be started and used together with clopidogrel. In this population, therapy must clearly be individualized. In the CURE trial most patients were also given heparin.

After a heart attack or stroke: 75 mg once a day by mouth. This approach may take 2–3 days to have a full anti-clot effect.

In coronary stenting: A 300 mg clopidogrel dose before the procedure was given, followed by 75 mg.

In percutaneous coronary intervention (PCI): 300 mg given as a loading dose from three to 24 hours before the procedure. After PCI, 75 mg a day was continued for up to one year.

In peripheral artery disease (severe enough to cause symptoms): 75 mg once a day.

Conditions Requiring Dosing Adjustments

Liver Function: No change needed in mild to moderate cirrhosis (Child-Pugh class A or B). Dose lowering may be needed in moderate to severe liver disease and the drug used with caution.

Kidney Function: No changes thought to be needed.

▷ **Dosing Instructions:** May be taken with or without food. Talk to your doctor or pharmacist BEFORE combining this medicine with any other pill, herbal or nutritional medicine. If you forget a dose: take the missed dose as soon as you remember it, unless it is nearly time for your next dose. If this is the case, skip the missed dose and simply take the next scheduled dose. DO NOT double doses.

Usual Duration of Use: Ongoing use for prevention of atherosclerotic events MUST continue until your doctor tells you to stop this medicine. In Acute Coronary Syndrome (this includes unstable angina/Non-Q-wave MI). The latest FDA approval is for COMBINED USE WITH ASPIRIN and includes people who are going to be managed with medicines and those who have percutaneous coronary intervention (with or without a stent) or coronary artery bypass graft (CABG). The ongoing dose (75 mg) of clopidogrel in ACS patients is given WITH aspirin (75–325 mg) once a day for a duration of up to a year (CURE trial). The Caprie trial showed benefits for up to three years. The Clopidogrel for the Reduction of Events During Observation (CREDO) trail showed the benefit (38% decrease in heart attack, stroke or death) with a loading dose followed by 75 mg daily for up to a year. Ongoing physician supervision is required and more recent trends toward longer duration of use.

Typical Treatment Goals and Measurements (Outcomes and Markers)

Atherosclerotic events: Most clinicians view preventing, rather than treating an atherosclerotic event such as stroke or heart attack, as the ultimate goal of this therapy. Measurement then becomes straightforward in that fewer than expected (based on the severity of the atherosclerosis that you face) heart attack or stroke occurrences is the end point of therapy. Electron beam computed tomography (EBCT) may help define the severity of circulatory compromise.

Unstable angina: Avoidance of a cardiovascular problem (event) such as a heart attack, cardiovascular death, or a stroke.

Possible Advantages of This Drug: Combined use of clopidogrel with aspirin showed dramatic results in the CURE (Clopidogrel in Unstable angina to prevent Recurrent Events) trial. One researcher estimated that 50,000 to 100,000 strokes, heart attacks or deaths in patients with acute coronary syndromes could be prevented EACH YEAR with combined aspirin and clopidogrel use. As a result of a New Drug Application (NDA 20-839/S-019) clopidogrel was approved to use in Acute Coronary Syndrome (this includes unstable angina/Non-Q-wave MI). The added approval includes people who are going to be managed with medicines and those who have percutaneous coronary intervention (with or without a stent) or coronary artery bypass graft (CABG). The advantage of this use is that clopidogrel decreased the rate of measures (combined endpoints) of cardiovascular death, MI or stroke as well as cardiovascular death, MI, stroke or resistant lowering of circulation (refractory ischemia). The CREDO (see above) trial showed a 38% reduction in heart attack (MI), stroke and death when a loading dose and up to a year of clopidogrel was used. The CAPRIE trial showed clopidogrel benefits for up to three years. A novel, hospital-based program called STRIVE (Strategies and Therapies for Reducing Ischemic and Vascular Events) was created by the makers of this medicine. This program is a unique advantage in that it gives hospital clinicians the tools needed to most appropriately treat acute coronary syndromes (unstable angina-UA and non-ST-segment elevation myocardial infarction-NSTEMI) in the hospital where they work.

▷ **This Drug Should Not Be Taken If**
  • you have had an allergic reaction to this drug or to any substance in the pill.
  • you have any type of bleeding disorder (such as hemophilia).
  • you are actively bleeding, such as from an ulcer or hemorrhage in the head (intracranial).

▷ **Inform Your Physician Before Taking This Drug If**
  • you are taking any anticoagulant drug or you have an increased risk of bleeding.
  • you are pregnant or planning pregnancy.
  • you have high blood pressure.
  • you plan to have general surgery (drug is usually stopped 5–7 days BEFORE major surgery). The exception to this in PCI where the medicine is given.
  • you have a low white blood cell count.
  • you have a history of liver problems.

Possible Side Effects (natural, expected, and unavoidable drug actions)
  Interference with usual blood clotting.

▷ **Possible Adverse Effects** (unusual, unexpected, and infrequent reactions)
  SAFETY DATA: This drug has been evaluated for safety in more than 17,500 patients at the time of this writing.
  If any of the following develop, consult your physician promptly for guidance
  Mild Adverse Effects
  Allergic reactions: skin rash, itching—infrequent.

Headache, fatigue, depression, or dizziness—infrequent.

Flu-like symptoms—infrequent.

Loss of taste (ageusia)—case reports.

Nose bleeds—infrequent.

Sudden (acute) arthritis—case reports.

Cough—infrequent.

Increased cholesterol—infrequent.

Stomach irritation, nausea, vomiting, or diarrhea—infrequent to frequent.

Increased blood pressure—infrequent.

Serious Adverse Effects

Allergic reactions: possible.

Erosion of stomach lining, with silent bleeding—possible.

Bone marrow depression (see Glossary): fatigue, weakness, fever, sore throat, abnormal bleeding or bruising—possible.

Thrombotic thrombocytopenic purpura (low blood platelets, anemia, fever, nerve and kidney changes)—21 cases reported to date (onset mostly within 2 weeks after treatment was started but one more than 3 weeks after starting).

Hemothorax—rare.

Hemolytic uremic syndrome—case report.

Ischemic necrosis—rare.

Hepatitis with jaundice (see Glossary): yellow skin and eyes, dark-colored urine, light-colored stool—possible.

Intracranial bleeding—possible.

▷ **Possible Effects on Sexual Function:** Excessive menstrual flow (menorrhagia)—case reports.

Adverse Effects That May Mimic Natural Diseases or Disorders

Liver damage may suggest viral hepatitis or reveal (unmask) low-level (subclinical) liver disease.

Possible Effects on Laboratory Tests

Bleeding time: prolonged.

Cholesterol: possibly increased.

Complete blood counts: decreased white blood cells (agranulocytosis, neutropenia, or granulocytopenia)—possible.

Liver function tests: increased ALT/GPT, AST/GOT, alkaline phosphatase.

CAUTION

1. You may take longer than usual to stop bleeding.
2. Since this medicine is indicated for preventing problems in people with atherosclerosis, the atherosclerosis needs to be diagnosed by: recent heart attack or stroke or established peripheral artery disease. Make certain you also understand the goal of the cholesterol-lowering medicine you are taking.
3. If you are planning surgery, talk to your doctor about how soon before surgery they want you to stop this medicine (usually 7 days if zero antiplatelet effect is desired).
4. Call your doctor if you start to develop infections more often than usual.

Precautions for Use

By Infants and Children: Safety and efficacy not evaluated.

By Those Over 60 Years of Age: The blood levels achieved with the standard dose are significantly higher than those in younger patients, but no dosing changes are presently thought to be needed. Watch for gray- to black-colored stools, an indication of stomach bleeding.

▷ **Advisability of Use During Pregnancy**
  Pregnancy Category: B. See Pregnancy Risk Categories at the back of this book.
  Animal Studies: No changes in rats at up to 78 times the human dose.
  Human Studies: Adequate human studies are not available.
  Talk to your doctor to see if benefit outweighs the risk.

Advisability of Use If Breast-Feeding
  Presence of this drug in breast milk: Yes in rats, unknown in humans.
  Avoid drug or refrain from nursing.

Habit-Forming Potential: None.

Effects of Overdose: One overdose (1,050 mg) resulted in no special treatment
  or adverse effects.

Possible Effects of Long-Term Use: Prolonged bleeding time, critical in the
  event of injury or surgery.

Suggested Periodic Examinations While Taking This Drug (at physician's discretion)
  Complete blood cell counts.
  Liver function tests.

▷ **While Taking This Drug, Observe the Following**
  Foods: No effect by food on how much gets into your body.
  Herbal Medicines or Minerals: Many herbal medicines may interact with clopidogrel. Examples include capsaicin, primrose oil (EPO), ginkgo, garlic, ginger, ginseng, guggul, hawthorn, anise, skull cap, white willow bark, and feverfew. Combining those medicines with clopidogrel is not recommended. Talk to your doctor BEFORE adding any herbal medicine.
  Beverages: No restrictions. May be taken with milk.
▷ *Alcohol:* Use of alcohol and clopidogrel at the same time may increase risk of stomach damage and may prolong bleeding time.
  Tobacco Smoking: No interactions expected, but I advise everyone to quit smoking.
▷ *Other Drugs*
  Clopidogrel may ***increase*** the effects of
  • aspirin (various), posing an increased bleeding risk—however the CURE trial showed a dramatic benefit in Acute Coronary Syndrome patients where aspirin was combined with clopidogrel. The indication for clopidogrel is for COMBINED USE WITH ASPIRIN for people with acute coronary syndromes (unstable angina/non Q wave heart attack-MI). See dosing above. The ongoing dose (75 mg) of clopidogrel in those patients is given WITH aspirin (75-325 mg) once a day for a duration of up to a year. Talk to your doctor about this important combination and what he or she wants you to do if any conflicting information arises from a pharmacy computer.
  • eptifibatide (Integrilin), leading to an increased bleeding risk.
  • fluvastatin (Lescol) (blood levels may be increased because of overlapping liver removal-CYP-2C9).
  • heparin, leading to increased bleeding risk (used with caution).
  • medicines removed by cytochrome P450 2C9 may be increased if combined with clopidogrel (an inhibitor of this enzyme).
  • oral anticoagulants (see Drug Classes) such as warfarin (Coumadin), low molecular weight heparins (see Drug Classes) and cause abnormal bleeding.
  • phenytoin (Dilantin) and fosphenytoin (Cerebyx). More frequent blood levels and dosage adjustments are prudent.

- tamoxifen (Nolvadex), leading to tamoxifen toxicity.
- tolbutamide (Orinase), leading to tolbutamide toxicity.

Clopidogrel *taken concurrently* with

- alendronate (Fosamax) may result in increased risk of stomach upset/diarrhea.
- atorvastatin (Lipitor) blunted the benefits of clopidogrel in one study using measures outside the body. Other clinical studies have not revealed any significant difference in clinical results or outcomes when the medicines were combined. This interaction may only be of laboratory versus clinical interest.
- capsaicin (Zostrix, others) may increase bleeding risk because of overlapping effects on platelets.
- cortisonelike drugs (see Drug Classes) increases risk of stomach ulcers.
- high blood pressure medicines (antihypertensives) may lessen lowering of elevated blood pressure.
- thrombolytic agents ("clot busters" such as TPA, streptokinase, TNKase, others) may lead to increased bleeding risk.
- torsemide (Demadex), leading to excessive torsemide effect.
- zafirlukast (Accolate) may cause additive inhibition of the CYP2C9 isoenzyme, possibly increasing blood levels of other medicines removed by CYP2C9.

The following drug may *decrease* the effects of clopidogrel:

- cholestyramine (Questran, others) might decrease the amount of clopidogrel that goes to work—separate doses by 30 minutes.

▷ *Driving, Hazardous Activities:* No restrictions or precautions.

Aviation Note: It is advisable to watch for dizziness and fatigue and restrict activities accordingly.

Exposure to Sun: No reports of problems.

Discontinuation: Talk to your doctor before stopping this medicine for any reason.

CLOTRIMAZOLE (kloh TRIM a zohl)

Introduced: 1976 **Class:** Antifungal **Prescription:**USA:Yes, though some are nonprescription **Controlled Drug:** USA: No; Canada: No **Available as Generic:** USA: Yes; Canada: No

Brand Names: ✤Canesten, Clotrimaderm, ✤Desenex, Desenex AF, Femcare, Femzol-7, Gyne-Lotrimin (1% cream and insert are nonprescription), ✤Lotriderm, Lotrimin, Lotrimin AF (nonprescription), Lotrisone [CD], Mycelex (1% vaginal cream is nonprescription), Mycelex-G, Mycelex-7, ✤Myclo, ✤Myclo-Gyne, ✤Neo-Zol

Warning: The brand names Mycelex and Myoflex sound similar. This can lead to serious errors. Make sure you are using the correct drug.

BENEFITS versus RISKS

Possible Benefits

EFFECTIVE TREATMENT AND
  PREVENTION OF *CANDIDA*
  (YEAST) INFECTIONS OF THE
  MOUTH AND THROAT (THRUSH)
EFFECTIVE TREATMENT OF
  CANDIDA (YEAST) INFECTIONS
  OF THE SKIN
EFFECTIVE TREATMENT OF
  CANDIDA (YEAST) INFECTIONS
  OF THE VULVA AND VAGINA
EFFECTIVE TREATMENT OF TINEA
  (RINGWORM) INFECTIONS OF
  THE SKIN

Possible Risks

Skin and mucous membrane
  irritation due to sensitization (drug-
  induced allergy)
Nausea, vomiting, stomach cramping,
  diarrhea (when swallowed)

▷ **Principal Uses**

As a Single Drug Product: Uses currently included in FDA-approved labeling: (1) Treats *Candida* (yeast) infections of skin, mouth, throat, vulva, and vagina; (2) treats tinea and related infections: ringworm of the body, groin (jock itch), or feet (athlete's foot), due to susceptible fungi; (3) treats pityriasis.

Other (unlabeled) generally accepted uses: (1) Prevention of *Candida* (yeast) infections of the mouth and throat in the management of HIV; an orphan drug for treatment of sickle cell disease.

How This Drug Works: It damages cell walls and blocks critical enzymes, inhibiting fungal growth (with low drug levels) and kills fungus (with high drug concentrations).

▷ **Widely Used Guidelines That Involve This Medicine (representative sample):** Please look at the section at the very beginning of this profile called "Class." Next, turn to Table 22 and you will find guidelines listed by the class involved!

Available Dosage Forms and Strengths

Cream — 1% (10 mg/g)
Lotion — 1% (10 mg/g)
Mouth lozenges — 10 mg
Topical solution — 1% (10 mg/mL)
Vaginal cream — 1% (10 mg/g), 2% (20 mg/g)
Vaginal tablets — 100 mg, 200 mg, 500 mg

▷ **Recommended Dosage Ranges** (Actual dosage and schedule must be determined for each patient individually.)

Infants and Children: Use of lozenges not recommended for children under 5 years of age; for 5 years and older, dissolve one lozenge slowly and completely in mouth five times a day for 14 days, longer if necessary.

12 to 60 Years of Age:

For Candida infections of mouth and throat: Dissolve 1 lozenge slowly and completely in mouth five times a day for 14 days; extended treatment will be necessary for people with AIDS.

For PREVENTING Candida infections of mouth and throat: One lozenge (troche) is dissolved in the mouth three times a day while patients are getting medicines that blunt the immune system (such as in kidney transplants, leukemia, and some tumors). Your doctor will decide when to stop the prophylactic use.

For Candida and tinea infections of skin: Apply cream, lotion, or solution to infected areas twice a day, morning and evening. Make certain that you use this product for the length of time specified by your doctor (if a prescription form) or by the label if you are using a nonprescription form.

For Candida infections of vulva and vagina: One applicatorful (5 g) of cream intravaginally at bedtime for 7 consecutive days; or one 100-mg tablet intravaginally at bedtime for 7 days; or one 200-mg tablet intravaginally at bedtime for 3 days; or as a single-dose treatment, one 500-mg tablet intravaginally at bedtime, one time only.

Over 60 Years of Age: Same as 12 to 60 years of age.

Conditions Requiring Dosing Adjustments

Liver Function: This drug is removed via the bile—dose should be decreased if bile duct is blocked.

Kidney Function: Dosing changes are not needed.

▷ **Dosing Instructions:** Dissolve lozenge in mouth completely, swallowing saliva as it accumulates. Do not chew the lozenge or swallow it whole. Take full course prescribed. Vaginal forms will seep out of the vagina. It's prudent to wear a minipad to protect your clothing. If symptoms persist after or worsen during a course of nonprescription forms, see your doctor. Many clinicians prefer multiple-day regimens for more complicated or severe vulvovaginal yeast infections. If you forget a dose: Take the missed dose right away, unless it is nearly time for your next dose—then skip the missed dose and just take the next scheduled dose. DO NOT double doses.

Usual Duration of Use: Regular use for a weeks usually needed to see benefit in controlling yeast or tinea infection. Some single-, 3- or 7-day courses are appropriate for some creams or tablets. Long-term use (as in AIDS management) requires periodic physician evaluation. Treatment failure may indicate need for new combination HIV therapy in HIV positive patients.

Typical Treatment Goals and Measurements (Outcomes and Markers)

Infections: The most commonly used measures of serious infections are white blood cell counts and differentials (the kind of blood cells that occur most often in your blood) and temperature. For uncomplicated vaginal yeast infections, many clinicians look for positive changes in 48 hours. If this is a multi-day course, NEVER stop an antifungal because you start to feel better. The goals and time frame (see peak benefits above) should be discussed with you when the prescription is written.

Possible Advantages of This Drug

Reasonably effective with minimal toxicity. More palatable than nystatin.

▷ **This Drug Should Not Be Taken If**
- you have had an allergic reaction to it previously.

▷ **Inform Your Physician Before Taking This Drug If**
- you are allergic to related antifungal drugs: fluconazole, itraconazole, ketoconazole, miconazole.
- you have liver problems and take oral clotrimazole troche.
- you think you are pregnant.

Possible Side Effects (natural, expected, and unavoidable drug actions)

None.

▷ **Possible Adverse Effects** (unusual, unexpected, and infrequent reactions)

If any of the following develop, consult your physician promptly for guidance.

Mild Adverse Effects

Allergic reactions: skin rash, hives, itching, burning, swelling, blistering (not present prior to treatment)—possible.

Depression, disorientation, or drowsiness—may be frequent with oral therapy.

Nausea, vomiting, stomach cramping, diarrhea (when swallowed)—frequent.

Serious Adverse Effects

Allergic reactions: sensitization of tissues (where applied locally) that will react allergically with future drug application—possible.

Inverted T waves on the ECG—case report.

Liver toxicity (with oral form)—infrequent.

Author's Note: Side effects with topical forms are rare.

▷ **Possible Effects on Sexual Function:** None.

Possible Delayed Adverse Effects: Local tissue sensitization to this drug.

Possible Effects on Laboratory Tests

Liver function tests: increased liver enzyme AST/GOT in 15% of oral form users.

CAUTION

1. Avoid contact of cream, lotion, and solution with the eyes.
2. Do not cover applied cream or lotion with an occlusive dressing.
3. Failure of treatment may mean resistant fungi.
4. Failure of treatment in AIDS patients may mean resistant HIV.

Precautions for Use

By Infants and Children: Use of lozenges by those under 5 years of age is not recommended.

By Those Over 60 Years of Age: No specific problems reported.

▷ **Advisability of Use During Pregnancy**

Pregnancy Category: B for vaginal or topical use. C for troches. See Pregnancy Risk Categories at the back of this book.

Animal Studies: No drug-induced birth defects were found in mouse, rat, or rabbit studies.

Human Studies: Adequate studies of pregnant women are not available.

Ask your physician for guidance.

Advisability of Use If Breast-Feeding

Presence of this drug in breast milk: Unknown.

Watch infant closely. Stop drug or nursing if adverse effects.

Habit-Forming Potential: None.

Effects of Overdose: Excessive use of lozenges may cause nausea, vomiting, or diarrhea.

Possible Effects of Long-Term Use: None reported.

Suggested Periodic Examinations While Taking This Drug (at physician's discretion)

Ongoing oral use: liver function tests.

▷ **While Taking This Drug, Observe the Following**

Foods: No restrictions.

Herbal Medicines or Minerals: Echinacea: Some patients use echinacea to attempt to boost their immune systems. Unfortunately, use of echinacea is not recommended in people with damaged immune systems. This herb may also actually weaken any immune system if it is used too often or for too long a time. Do NOT take mistletoe herb, oak bark or F.C. of marsh-mallow root, and licorice.

Beverages: No restrictions.

▷ *Alcohol:* No interactions expected.

Tobacco Smoking: No interactions expected. I advise everyone to quit smoking.

▷ *Other Drugs:*

Clotrimazole (oral dosage forms) **taken concurrently** with

- amphotericin B lipid complex (Abelcet) may blunt benefits.
- aspirin (various) may lead to additive stomach and intestinal (GI upset, bleeding) problems.
- betamethasone (Betaderm, Diprolene, others) resulted in enhanced fungal growth (Majocchi's granulomas) in one case report.
- benzodiazepines (see drug classes) may result in benzodiazepine toxicity. Caution required and dosage adjustments may be needed.
- cyclosporine (Sandimmune) may result in cyclosporine toxicity.
- dofetilide (Tikosyn) may result in dofetilide toxicity.
- ergot derivatives (see Drug Classes) should not be combined because of possible toxicity.
- sirolimus (Rapamune) and tacrolimus (Prograf) can result in increased sirolimus or tacrolimus levels and increased risk of kidney toxicity and increased potassium and glucose.
- trimetrexate (Neutrexin) may result in trimexate toxicity.

▷ *Driving, Hazardous Activities:* No restrictions.

Aviation Note: No restrictions.

Exposure to Sun: No restrictions.

Discontinuation: As directed by your doctor.

CLOXACILLIN (klox a SIL in)

Please see the penicillin family profile.

CLOZAPINE (KLOH za peen)

Introduced: 1975 **Class:** Antipsychotic, atypical antipsychotic **Prescription:** USA: Yes **Controlled Drug:** USA: No **Available as Generic:** USA: Yes

Brand Names: ❧Apo-Clozaril, Clozaril

Author's Note: In the United States, this drug is available only by special arrangement through the Clozaril National Registry. Your doctor will call 800-448-5938 to register you and then a form is filled out by the MD and pharmacy, which is faxed to 800-648-6015. The medicine can then be ordered directly from the pharmacy wholesaler. This is to make certain that required blood tests are obtained, and proper follow up undertaken. Ask your doctor for help. The FDA has required manufacturers of all atypical antipsychotics to include warnings about increased risk of diabetes and increased blood sugar (hyperglycemia) in their product labels.

BENEFITS versus RISKS	
Possible Benefits	*Possible Risks*
EFFECTIVE CONTROL OF SEVERE SCHIZOPHRENIA THAT HAS FAILED TO RESPOND ADEQUATELY TO OTHER APPROPRIATE DRUGS	SERIOUS BLOOD CELL DISORDERS: ABNORMALLY LOW WHITE BLOOD CELL AND PLATELET COUNTS
Improvement in many refractory cases	DRUG-INDUCED SEIZURES (DEPENDING ON SIZE OF DOSE)
Useful in patients who have tardive dyskinesia	DIABETES AND/OR INCREASED BLOOD SUGAR
This class of medicines may be drugs of choice in older adults	HEART MUSCLE INFLAMMATION (MYOCARDITIS)

▷ **Principal Uses**

As a Single Drug Product: Uses currently included in FDA-approved labeling: (1) Manages severe schizophrenia that fails to respond to adequate trials of other standard antipsychotic medicines. Because of potential for serious blood cell disorders and seizures, its use is reserved for severely ill schizophrenic patients; (2) helps control suicidal behavior.

Other (unlabeled) generally accepted uses: (1) Severe and refractory bipolar disorder; (2) severe tardive dyskinesia (dystonic subtype)—a syndrome that can happen after some medicines are used to treat psychosis; (3) psychosis occurring after labor with lactation; (4) may help excessive urination (polydipsia) caused by other neuroleptic agents.

How This Drug Works: By blocking the place (receptor) where dopamine works, this drug corrects an imbalance of nerve impulses causing schizophrenic thought disorders.

▷ **Widely Used Guidelines That Involve This Medicine (representative sample):** Please look at the section at the very beginning of this profile called "Class." Next, turn to Table 22 and you will find guidelines listed by the class involved!

Available Dosage Forms and Strengths

Tablets — 25 mg, 100 mg

▷ **Usual Adult Dosage Ranges:** *Resistant schizophrenia:* Starts with 12.5 mg (half of a 25 mg tablet) once or two times a day; the dose is gradually increased by 25 mg to 50 mg daily, as tolerated, to reach a dose of 300 mg to 450 mg daily (divided into three doses) by the end of 2 weeks. Later increases should be limited to 100 mg one or two times a week. For ongoing (maintenance) doses, the lowest effective dose should be used. One researcher commented on dosing ranges from 50 to 900 mg daily.

Note: Actual dose and schedule must be determined for each patient individually.

Conditions Requiring Dosing Adjustments

Liver Function: Eliminated in the liver; however, no specific dosing guidelines are available.

Kidney Function: Patients with kidney failure should be watched closely for adverse effects.

▷ **Dosing Instructions:** White blood cell checks are MANDATORY with this medicine. May be taken without regard to meals or with food if necessary to reduce stomach irritation. The tablet may be crushed. If you forget a dose: Take the missed dose as soon as you remember it, unless it is nearly time for the next scheduled dose—then skip the missed dose and take the scheduled dose on time. DO NOT double doses.

Usual Duration of Use: Benefits may be seen after 2 to 4 weeks of regular use. Peak effect may require 3 to 12 months. If no significant benefit is seen, many clinicians stop the drug. Long-term use requires periodic evaluation for desirable results, laboratory testing and checks to see if lower doses and continued treatment is needed.

Typical Treatment Goals and Measurements (Outcomes and Markers)
Schizophrenia: The general goal: to ease the severity of symptoms in order to let the patient resume his or her usual activities. There should be lessened time spent with prior intrusions of abnormal thinking into more normal life. This improved quality of life (QOL) and the patient perception of QOL may be measured by the Quality of Life Enjoyment and Satisfaction Questionnaire. Numerous clinical ratings such as the Brief Psychiatric Rating Scale (BPRS24) and the Physician Global Rating Scale (PhGRS) as well as dimensions of temperament such as the tridimensional personality questionnaire (TPQ) have been used to check results of therapy. The Minnesota Multiphasic personality Inventory and several subscales are also used.

Possible Advantages of This Drug: Rarely causes significant sexual dysfunction. Low incidence of Parkinson-like reactions (see Glossary). Medicines in this class are probably drugs of choice in older adults. Additional information is available at *www.clozapineregistry.com; www.nimh.nih.gov.*

Currently a Drug of Choice: For treatment of severe schizophrenia in patients who have not responded to other standard antipsychotic drugs.

▷ **This Drug Should Not Be Taken If**
- you have had an allergic reaction to it previously.
- you have had severe bone marrow depression (impaired white blood cell production) with previous use of this drug.
- you have a bone marrow or blood cell disorder.
- you have epilepsy that is not controlled.
- you have severe kidney failure.
- you take any other drug that can cause bone marrow depression (see Glossary).

▷ **Inform Your Physician Before Taking This Drug If**
- you have a history of any type of seizure disorder.
- you have a history of narrow-angle glaucoma.
- you have any type of heart or circulatory disorder, especially heart rhythm abnormalities or hypertension.
- you have diabetes or glucose intolerance.
- your body is very depleted (cachectic).
- you have impaired liver or kidney function.
- you have prostatism (see Glossary).

Possible Side Effects (natural, expected, and unavoidable drug actions)
Drowsiness, sedation—frequent.
Weight gain—frequent.
Dizziness, light-headedness—infrequent to frequent.
Orthostatic hypotension (see Glossary)—possible.
Blurred vision, salivation, dry mouth, impaired urination, constipation—possible.

▷ **Possible Adverse Effects** (unusual, unexpected, and infrequent reactions)
If any of the following develop, consult your physician promptly for guidance.
Mild Adverse Effects
Allergic reactions: skin rash; drug fever (see Glossary), which usually occurs within the first 3 weeks of treatment and is self-limiting—rare.
Headache, tremor, fainting, sleep disorders, restlessness, confusion, depression—rare.
Edema (in the ankles and around the eyes)—rare.
Increased salivation—frequent.
Rapid heartbeat (tachycardia), hypertension, chest pain—rare to infrequent.
Nausea, indigestion, vomiting, diarrhea—rare.

Serious Adverse Effects
Allergic reactions: asthmatic-type respiratory reaction—case reports.
Bone marrow depression: specific impairment of white blood cell production with potential for serious infection—rare.
Increased eosinophils (a type of white blood cell) above 4,000 per cubic millimeter—rare.
Systemic lupus erythematosus like reaction—case reports.
Glucose intolerance—case reports.
Build up of lactic acid (lactic acidosis)—case reports.
Drug-induced seizures, dose-related—rare.
Tardive dyskinesia—case reports.
Heart muscle inflammation (myocarditis-now in a boxed warning in the FDA labeling)—possible.
Lung clot (pulmonary thromboembolism)—case reports.
Anticholinergic syndrome—rare.
Neuroleptic malignant syndrome—case reports.

▷ **Possible Effects on Sexual Function:** Decreased libido and impotence—infrequent and dose-related (over 150 mg).
Abnormal ejaculation or priapism (see Glossary)—rare.

Adverse Effects That May Mimic Natural Diseases or Disorders
Drug-induced fever may suggest systemic infection. Because of the risk of bone marrow depression and secondary infection, any occurrence of fever must be carefully evaluated. Drug-induced seizures may suggest the possibility of epilepsy. Blood sugar changes not completely understood but mimic diabetes.

Natural Diseases or Disorders That May Be Activated by This Drug
Latent glaucoma, prostatism, diabetes.

Possible Effects on Laboratory Tests
White blood cell counts: decreased.
Eosinophils: may be rarely increased significantly.
Blood sugar: possibly increased.

CAUTION
1. Baseline white blood cell counts must be checked before clozapine treatment is started; follow-up counts must be made every week during the entire course of treatment and for 4 weeks after discontinuation of clozapine. Periodic checks of blood sugar are prudent.
2. Promptly report any signs of infection: fever, sore throat, flu-like symptoms, skin infections, painful urination, etc.
3. Report promptly light-headedness or dizziness on rising from a sitting or lying position—this could be orthostatic hypotension (see Glossary).

4. There have been case reports of glucose intolerance and diabetes mellitus with this medicine.
5. Call your doctor before taking any other medication. (ANY prescription or over-the-counter drug.)

Precautions for Use
By Infants and Children: Safety and effectiveness have NOT been established.
By Those Over 60 Years of Age: Starting doses of 6.25 to 12.5 mg are prudent with required increases not exceeding 25 mg a day. There is an increased risk of orthostatic hypotension, confusion, blood problems, and prostatism. Report related symptoms promptly.

▷ **Advisability of Use During Pregnancy**
Pregnancy Category: B. See Pregnancy Risk Categories at the back of this book.
Animal Studies: No birth defects due to this drug reported.
Human Studies: Adequate studies of pregnant women are not available.
   Use this drug only if clearly needed.

Advisability of Use If Breast-Feeding
   Presence of this drug in breast milk: Yes, in animal studies.
   Avoid drug or refrain from nursing.

Habit-Forming Potential: None, but a withdrawal syndrome has been reported after suddenly stopping long-term therapy.

Effects of Overdose: Marked drowsiness, delirium, hallucinations, rapid and irregular heartbeat, irregular breathing, fainting.

Possible Effects of Long-Term Use: Movement disorders, changes in blood sugar.

Suggested Periodic Examinations While Taking This Drug (at physician's discretion)
   White blood and differential counts prior to starting therapy, every week during therapy, and for 4 weeks after stopping therapy.
   Serial blood pressure measurements and electrocardiograms.
   Plasma drug levels (controversial)—350–420 micrograms per liter.

▷ **While Taking This Drug, Observe the Following**
Foods: Because many non-prescription diet aids have large amounts of caffeine, make certain that you carefully read the label and talk to your doctor and pharmacist before combining such a product with clozapine. Dehydroepiandrosterone (DHEA) supplementation may lower benefits from clozapine.
Herbal Medicines or Minerals: Kava and valerian may worsen drowsiness. Since part of the way that ginkgo biloba may work is as a MAO inhibitor, combination with this medicine is not advisable. Evening primrose has some case reports of increasing seizure risk when combined with medicines that are structurally similar to clozapine. St. John's wort may increase the removal of clozapine from the body—combined use is NOT recommended. Because the active ingredient of guarana and mate is caffeine—these products should be avoided.
Beverages: The caffeine in coffee can block the removal of clozapine if 400 to 1000 mg of caffeine a day is taken. For this reason, guarana, and mate should be avoided. May be taken with milk.
▷ *Alcohol:* Avoid completely. Alcohol increases clozapine-induced sedation and can worsen possible undesirable side effects of clozapine on blood pressure and brain function.
Tobacco Smoking: May accelerate the elimination of this drug and require increased dosage. I advise everyone to quit smoking.

Marijuana Smoking: Moderate increase in drowsiness, worsening of orthostatic hypotension, increased risk of aggravating psychosis.

▷ *Other Drugs*

Clozapine may ***increase*** the effects of
- antihypertensive drugs; observe for excessive lowering of blood pressure.
- drugs with atropine-like actions (see Drug Classes).
- drugs with sedative actions (see benzodiazepines, etc); observe for excessive sedation.

Clozapine ***taken concurrently*** with
- other bone marrow depressant drugs, such as carbamazepine (Tegretol), may increase the risk of impaired white blood cell production.
- amprenavir (Agenerase), atazanavir (Reyataz) and perhaps other protease inhibitors may lead to increased clozapine levels. Caution is advised.
- buspirone (Buspar) may excessively elevate blood sugar and also lead to bleeding.
- carbamazepine (Tegretol) may increase risk of low white blood cells.
- cimetidine (Tagamet) can result in a toxic level of clozapine.
- erythromycin (E-Mycin, others) can result in increased clozapine concentrations and potential toxicity. This has been seen in a single case report, but caution is advised.
- fluoxetine (Prozac) can result in clozapine toxicity.
- fluvoxamine (Luvox) can result in clozapine toxicity.
- lithium (Lithobid, Lithotab, etc) may increase the risk of confusional states, seizures and neuroleptic malignant syndrome (see Glossary).
- monoamine oxidase inhibitors (MAO inhibitors; see Drug Class) may cause abnormally low blood pressure and exaggerated central nervous system response.
- nefazodone (Serzone) may lead to clozapine toxicity.
- other medicines that interfere with cytochrome P450 3A4 may increase clozapine levels and increase risk of clozapine side effects or toxicity.
- paroxetine (Paxil) may lead to toxicity from either medicine.
- phenytoin (Dilantin) and fosphenytoin (Cerebyx) can cause a decreased clozapine level and result in breakthrough schizophrenia.
- risperidone (Risperdal) may lead to increased risperidone levels.
- ritonavir (Norvir), and perhaps other protease inhibitors (see Drug Classes). Monitor closely.
- sertraline (Zoloft) can result in clozapine toxicity.
- tramadol (Ultram) may increase seizure risks.
- venlafaxine (Effexor) may lead to clozapine toxicity.
- zotepine (Nipolept) may increase seizure risk.

▷ *Driving, Hazardous Activities:* This drug may cause drowsiness, dizziness, blurred vision, confusion, and seizures. Restrict activities as necessary.

Aviation Note: The use of this drug ***is a disqualification*** for piloting. Consult a designated Aviation Medical Examiner.

Exposure to Sun: No restrictions except for heat adaptation (see below).

Exposure to Heat: Use caution. This drug can cause fever and can impair the body's adaptation to heat.

Occurrence of Unrelated Illness: Infections must be vigorously treated. White blood cell response to infection must be followed closely.

Discontinuation: If possible, this drug should be discontinued gradually over a period of 1 to 2 weeks. If abrupt withdrawal is necessary, observe carefully for recurrence of psychotic symptoms. Headache, diarrhea, nausea, and vomiting are frequent.

CODEINE (KOH deen)

Introduced: 1886   **Class:** Analgesic, narcotic, opioid   **Prescription:** USA: Yes   **Controlled Drug:** USA: C-II*; Canada: No   **Available as Generic:** Yes

Brand Names: A.B.C. Compound w/Codeine [CD], AC&C [CD], Accopain, Actagen-C [CD], Actifed w/Codeine [CD], Afed-C [CD], Alamine-C [CD], Alamine Expectorant [CD], Ambenyl Expectorant [CD], Ambenyl Syrup [CD], Anacin 3 w/Codeine #2–4, Anacin w/Codeine [CD], APC w/Codeine [CD], Atasol-8,-15,-30 [CD], Ban-Tuiss C [CD], Benylin Syrup w/Codeine [CD], Bitex [CD], Bromanyl Cough Syrup [CD], Bromotuss, Bromphen DC [CD], Brontex [CD], Bufferin w/Codeine [CD], Butalbital Compound [CD], Chemdal Expectorant [CD], Chem-Tuss NE [CD], Cheracol [CD], Chlor-Trimeton Expectorant [CD], Coactifed [CD], Codecon-C [CD], Codehist DH, Codehist Elixir, ♣Codeine Contin (timed release), ♣Coricidin w/Codeine [CD], ♣Coryphen-Codeine [CD], ♣C2 Buffered, ♣C2 w/Codeine, Deproist [CD], Dimetane Cough Syrup-DC [CD], Dimetane Expectorant-C [CD], Dimetapp-C [CD], Dimetapp w/Codeine [CD], Empirin w/Codeine No. 2, 4 [CD], ♣Empracet-30,-60 [CD], Empracet w/Codeine No. 3, 4 [CD], ♣Emtec-30 [CD], ♣Exdol-8,-15,-30 [CD], ♣Extra Strength Acetaminophen with Codeine [CD], ♣Fiorinal-C 1/4,-C 1/2 [CD], Fiorinal w/Codeine No. 1, 2, 3 [CD], Gecil [CD], Glydeine, Isoclor Expectorant [CD], ♣Lenoltec w/Codeine No. 1, 2, 3, 4 [CD], ♣Mersyndol, Naldecon-CX [CD], Normatane [CD], Novadyne DH [CD], ♣Novahistex C [CD], ♣Novo-Gesic, Nucochem [CD], Nucofed [CD], ♣Omni-Tuss [CD], Oridol-C [CD], Panadol w/Codeine [CD], ♣Paveral, Pediacof [CD], Penntuss [CD], ♣Phenaphen No. 2, 3, 4 [CD], Phenaphen w/Codeine No. 2, 3, 4 [CD], Phenergan w/Codeine [CD], Poly-Histine [CD], Promethazine CS [CD], Pyra-Phed [CD], ♣Robaxacet-8, Robaxisal-C [CD], ♣Rounox w/Codeine [CD], SK-Apap [CD], Tamine Expectorant DC [CD], ♣Tecnal C [CD], Terpin Hydrate and Codeine [CD], ♣318 AC&C [CD], Triafed w/Codeine [CD], Triaminic Expectorant w/Codeine [CD], ♣Triatec-8, 30 [CD], ♣Tussaminic C Forte [CD], ♣Tussaminic C Ped [CD], ♣Tussi-Organidin [CD], ♣222 [CD], ♣282 [CD], ♣292 [CD], ♣Tylenol w/Codeine [CD], Tylenol w/Codeine No. 1, 2, 3, 4 [CD], Tylenol w/Codeine Elixir [CD], ♣VC Expectorant w/Codeine, ♣Veganin [CD]

BENEFITS versus RISKS	
Possible Benefits	*Possible Risks*
RELIEF OF MILD TO MODERATE PAIN	Potential for habit formation (dependence)
VERY EFFECTIVE CONTROL OF COUGH	Mild allergic reactions—infrequent
	Nausea, constipation

▷ **Principal Uses**

As a Single Drug Product: Uses currently included in FDA-approved labeling: (1) Relieves mild to moderate pain; (2) controls cough—its widest use is as an ingredient in analgesic preparations and cough remedies.

Other (unlabeled) generally accepted uses: (1) Limited role in controlling diarrhea; (2) migraine during pregnancy.

As a Combination Drug Product [CD]: Codeine is combined with other analgesics (aspirin and acetaminophen) on the World Health Organization pain ladder to increase overall pain control. It is also added to cough mixtures containing antihistamines, decongestants, and expectorants.

How This Drug Works: By depressing some brain functions, this drug decreases pain perception, calms emotional responses to pain, and reduces cough reflex sensitivity.

▷ **Widely Used Guidelines That Involve This Medicine (representative sample):** Please look at the section at the very beginning of this profile called "Class." Next, turn to Table 22 and you will find guidelines listed by the class involved!

Available Dosage Forms and Strengths
   Combination form — 15mg codeine, 300 mg acetaminophen (number 2)
                    — 30 mg codeine, 300 mg acetaminophen (number 3)
                    — 60 mg codeine, 300 mg acetaminophen (number 4)
       Injection — 30 mg/mL, 60 mg/mL
       Tablets — 15 mg, 30 mg, 60 mg
   Tablets, soluble — 15 mg, 30 mg, 60 mg

▷ **Usual Adult Dosage Ranges:** *As analgesic:* 15 to 60 mg (dosed as the codeine content) every 4 hours.

   Author's Note: Current pain treatment theory calls for timed or scheduled dosing. This tends to prevent pain, rather than allowing pain to recur and then having to be treated. Some clinicians will use timed dosing immediately after surgery and then revert to as-needed dosing once the most severe period of pain has passed. Pain is now the fifth vital sign.

   For cough (non-combination forms): 10 to 20 mg every 4 to 6 hours as needed. Maximum daily dose 200 mg for pain, 120 mg for cough.

   Note: Actual dose and schedule must be determined for each patient individually.

Conditions Requiring Dosing Adjustments
   Liver Function: The dose must be decreased in liver compromise.
   Kidney Function: Dose decreased by up to 50% in moderate to severe failure.

▷ **Dosing Instructions:** Tablet may be crushed and then taken with or following food to reduce stomach irritation or nausea. If you forget a dose: take it as soon as you remember, unless it's nearly time for your next dose—then omit the dose you forgot and take the next scheduled dose. DO NOT double doses.

Usual Duration of Use: As long as it is needed to control cough (usually the shortest time required). Use for pain should not exceed 5 to 7 days without reassessment of need.

Typical Treatment Goals and Measurements (Outcomes and Markers)
   Pain: Most clinicians treating pain use a device called an algometer to check your pain. This looks like a small ruler. The goals of treatment then relate to where the level of pain started (for example, a rating of 7 on a 0–10 scale) and what the cause of the pain was. Pain medicines may also be used together (in combination) to get the best result or outcome. If your pain control is not acceptable to YOU, be sure to call your doctor as you may need a different medicine or combination.
   Cough: The frequency and severity of cough should decrease as discussed with you by your physician. If coughing persists at its prior level, it is prudent to call your doctor.

▷ **This Drug Should Not Be Taken If**
  • you have had an allergic reaction to any form of it.
  • you are having an acute attack of asthma.
  • your breathing is depressed (respiratory depression).

▷ **Inform Your Physician Before Taking This Drug If**
  • you have a history of drug abuse or alcoholism.
  • you have impaired liver or kidney function.
  • you have gallbladder disease, a seizure disorder, or an underactive thyroid gland.
  • you have chronic obstructive pulmonary disease (COPD) or other lung problems such as asthma.
  • you have low blood calcium (increased sensitivity to this medicine).
  • you have a history of porphyria.
  • you tend to be constipated.
  • you are taking any other drugs that have a sedative effect.
  • you will have surgery with general anesthesia.

Possible Side Effects (natural, expected, and unavoidable drug actions)
  Drowsiness, light-headedness, dry mouth, urinary retention—possible.
  Constipation—frequent and dose-related. (Best to start a stool softener or related medicine before codeine is started if you are prone to constipation.)

▷ **Possible Adverse Effects** (unusual, unexpected, and infrequent reactions)
  If any of the following develop, consult your physician promptly for guidance.
  Mild Adverse Effects
  Allergic reactions: skin rash, hives, itching—case reports.
  Dizziness, impaired concentration, sensation of drunkenness, confusion, depression, blurred or double vision—infrequent.
  Nausea, vomiting—frequent and may be dose-related.
  Serious Adverse Effects
  Allergic reactions: anaphylaxis, severe skin reactions—case reports.
  Idiosyncratic reactions: delirium, hallucinations, excitement, increased pain sensitivity once the medicine wears off.
  Seizures—rare.
  Impaired breathing—dose-related (children and people with low calcium levels may be more sensitive to this medicine).
  Porphyria—case reports.
  Pancreatitis—case reports (all patients had previously had their gallbladders removed).
  Liver or kidney toxicity—case reports.

▷ **Possible Effects on Sexual Function:** Opiates have a variety of effects on sexual response. These may range from blunting of sexual response to increased response if anxiety has been a factor inhibiting response—case reports.

Adverse Effects That May Mimic Natural Diseases or Disorders
  Paradoxical behavioral disturbances may suggest psychotic disorder.

Possible Effects on Laboratory Tests
  Blood platelet counts: decreased.
  Blood amylase and lipase levels: increased (natural side effect).
  Urine screening tests for drug abuse: may be positive. (Test results depend upon amount of drug taken and testing method used.)

CAUTION
1. If you have asthma, chronic bronchitis, or emphysema, use of this drug may cause respiratory difficulty, thickening of secretions, and decrease of needed cough reflex.
2. Combining this drug with atropinelike drugs can increase the risk of urinary retention and reduced intestinal function.
3. Do not take this drug following acute head injury.
4. It is easy to forget about the acetaminophen in combination codeine products and also in many other products. Make sure to add up ALL the acetaminophen you are taking and stay less than the 4,000 mg a day limit.

Precautions for Use
By Infants and Children: Do not use this drug in children under 2 years of age (possible life-threatening respiratory depression). Children 2 to 6 years old can receive 1 mg per kg of body mass per day, divided into four equal doses. Maximum dose is 30 mg per day. Children 6 to 12 years of age can receive 5 to 10 mg per dose every 4 to 6 hours, to a maximum of 60 mg every 24 hours.
By Those Over 60 Years of Age: Small starting doses and short-term use is indicated. Expect increased risk of drowsiness, dizziness, unsteadiness, falling, urinary retention, and constipation (often leading to fecal impaction).

▷ **Advisability of Use During Pregnancy**
Pregnancy Category: C; D if used in high doses or for prolonged periods near the time the baby is about to be born. See Pregnancy Risk Categories at the back of this book.
Animal Studies: Skull defects reported in hamster studies.
Human Studies: Adequate studies of pregnant women are not available. Some studies suggest an increase in significant birth defects when this drug is taken during the first 6 months of pregnancy. Codeine taken during the last few weeks before delivery can cause withdrawal symptoms in the newborn.
Use only if clearly needed and in small, infrequent doses.

▷ **Advisability of Use If Breast-Feeding**
Presence of this drug in breast milk: Yes, in small amounts.
Discuss this benefit to risk decision with your doctor.

▷ **Habit-Forming Potential:** Psychological and/or physical dependence can develop with use of large doses for an extended period of time. True dependence is infrequent, however, and unlikely with prudent use.

Effects of Overdose: Drowsiness, restlessness, agitation, nausea, vomiting, dry mouth, vertigo, weakness, lethargy, stupor, coma, seizures.

Possible Effects of Long-Term Use: Psychological and physical dependence, chronic constipation.

Suggested Periodic Examinations While Taking This Drug (at physician's discretion)
Periodic check for constipation, especially in older patients.

▷ **While Taking This Drug, Observe the Following**
Foods: No restrictions.
Herbal Medicines or Minerals: Valerian and kava kava may interact additively (drowsiness). Avoid these combinations. St. John's wort can change (inducing or increasing) P450 3A4 enzymes, blunting the effects of this

medicine. Talk to your doctor BEFORE you combine any herbals with codeine.

Beverages: No restrictions. May be taken with milk.

▷ *Alcohol:* DO NOT COMBINE. Codeine intensifies alcohol, and alcohol intensifies codeine depressant effects on brain function, breathing, and circulation.

Tobacco Smoking: Tobacco smoking may cause decreased pain tolerance and require an increased or more frequent dose of codeine. I advise everyone to quit smoking.

Marijuana Smoking: Increases drowsiness and pain relief. Mental and physical performance will be impaired.

▷ *Other Drugs*

Codeine may ***increase*** the effects of

- atropinelike drugs and increase the risk of constipation and urinary retention.
- monoamine oxidase (MAO) inhibitors and also increase central nervous system symptoms and depression.
- other drugs with sedative effects.
- tramadol (Ultram).

Codeine ***taken concurrently*** with

- acetaminophen (Tylenol, others) may lead to overlap of acetaminophen dose if you are taking a codeine and acetaminophen form (exceeding the 4 gram daily limit). This can increase risk of liver toxicity. Read the label, total the acetaminophen and keep it at 4,000 mg or less.
- naltrexone (ReVia, others) may lead to withdrawal symptoms.
- quinidine may decrease codeine pain control.
- rifabutin (Mycobutin) may decrease codeine effectiveness.
- ritonavir (Norvir) may blunt codeine benefits.

▷ *Driving, Hazardous Activities:* This drug can impair mental alertness, judgment, reaction time, and physical coordination. Avoid hazardous activities accordingly.

Aviation Note: The use of this drug ***is a disqualification*** for piloting. Consult a designated Aviation Medical Examiner.

Exposure to Sun: No restrictions.

Discontinuation: Best to limit use to short-term. If extended use occurs, gradual decreases in dose are prudent to minimize possible withdrawal (usually mild with codeine).

COLCHICINE (KOL chi seen)

Introduced: 1763   **Class:** Antigout   **Prescription:** USA: Yes
Controlled Drug: USA: No; Canada: No   **Available as Generic:** Yes
Brand Names: Colbenemid [CD], Col-Probenecid [CD], Colsalide, Proben-C [CD]

BENEFITS versus RISKS

Possible Benefits	*Possible Risks*
EFFECTIVE RELIEF OF ACUTE GOUT SYMPTOMS	Loss of hair
Prevention of recurrent gout attacks	Rare bone marrow depression (see Glossary)
Prevention of attacks of Mediterranean fever	Rare peripheral neuritis (see Glossary)
	Rare liver damage

▷ **Principal Uses**

As a Single Drug Product: Uses currently included in FDA-approved labeling: (1) Reduces pain, swelling, and inflammation seen in acute gout attacks (many clinicians prefer NSAIDs [see Drug Classes] as drugs of first choice in acute gout); (2) also used in smaller doses to prevent recurrent gout attacks.

Other (unlabeled) generally accepted uses: (1) Prevention and control of attacks of familial Mediterranean fever; (2) may have a role in easing symptoms of Behçet's disease; (3) some use in biliary cirrhosis of the liver and in hepatitis B patients who can't tolerate usual interferon treatment; (4) may have a role in recurrent pericarditis; (5) can be of help in pseudo-gout; (6) treats some cases of refractory immune thrombocytopenic purpura.

As a Combination Drug Product [CD]: Colchicine combined with probenecid enhances its ability to prevent recurrent attacks of gout. Colchicine is most effective in relieving acute gout; it has some effect in preventing recurrent and chronic discomfort. Probenecid increases removal of uric acid by the kidneys and reduces risk of acute gout. This dual action is more effective than either drug used alone in long-term management of gout.

How This Drug Works: Decreasing joint tissue acid, lowering painful uric acid deposits and acute inflammation and pain. (Colchicine does not lower uric acid in the blood or increase urine removal.)

▷ **Widely Used Guidelines That Involve This Medicine (representative sample):** Please look at the section at the very beginning of this profile called "Class." Next, turn to Table 22 and you will find guidelines listed by the class involved!

Available Dosage Forms and Strengths

Granules — 0.5 mg
Injection — 1 mg/2 mL
Tablets — 0.5 mg, 0.6 mg, 0.65 mg (also 1 mg in Canada)

▷ **Usual Adult Dosage Ranges:** *For acute attack:* 1.0 to 1.2 mg, followed by 0.5 to 0.65 mg every 2 hours until pain eases or nausea, vomiting, or diarrhea occurs. Maximum total dose is 8 mg per attack. *For preventing recurrent attacks:* If you have had less than one attack a year, 0.5 to 0.65 mg per day, taken three or four times a week. If you have more than one attack a year, 0.5 to 0.65 mg per day. The maximum dose in preventing gout is 0.5 to 0.65 taken two or three times a day. *Pericarditis:* 3 mg daily to start, followed by 0.5 mg up to one mg daily.

Note: Actual dose and schedule must be determined for each patient individually.

Conditions Requiring Dosing Adjustments

Liver Function: Caution must be used, and the dose decreased, if there is a bile obstruction. This drug should NOT be used in people with both liver and kidney compromise.

Kidney Function: For creatinine clearance of 10 to 50 mL/min (see Glossary), up to 0.6 mg every other day is given. Ongoing preventive use NOT prudent in moderate (creatinine clearance less than 50 mL/min) kidney problems. In severe kidney failure, the medicine should not be given.

▷ **Dosing Instructions:** The tablet may be crushed and then either taken on an empty stomach or with food to reduce nausea or stomach irritation. Talk to your doctor about how much water you should drink. Some clinicians recommend 8–10 full glasses a day. Start this medicine at the first sign of an acute attack. Take the exact dose prescribed. While dosing should be individualized, once the dose needed to abort a sudden (acute) attack is identified, the patient should keep that supply on hand in order to stop an acute attack. Remember that if diarrhea or stomach and intestine (gastrointestinal) side effects happen, the drug needs to be stopped. If you forget a dose: take the dose you forgot as soon as you remember it, unless it's nearly time for your next dose. If it's nearly time for your next dose, skip the dose you missed and simply take the next scheduled dose. DO NOT double doses.

Usual Duration of Use: For acute attack, stop the drug when pain is relieved or when nausea, vomiting, or diarrhea occurs; do not restart this drug for 3 days without asking your doctor. Total doses of 8 mg should not be exceeded. For prevention, use the smallest dose that works. Ask your doctor about dosing.

Typical Treatment Goals and Measurements (Outcomes and Markers)

Gout: Blood uric acid levels are not changed by this medicine (tissue deposits are), but gout pain decreases (lowered by ongoing use of this drug as in dosing section) or limiting nausea defines response or highest tolerable dose of colchicine. Call your doctor if an acute attack of gout is not stopped or if you have reached dose-limiting nausea or vomiting.

▷ **This Drug Should Not Be Taken If**
- you have had an allergic reaction to it previously.
- you have an active stomach or duodenal ulcer.
- you have active ulcerative colitis.
- you have a severe kidney or liver disorder.
- you have a serious heart disorder.
- you are pregnant.
- you have a history of blood cell disorders.

▷ **Inform Your Physician Before Taking This Drug If**
- you have peptic ulcer disease or ulcerative colitis.
- you develop diarrhea and vomiting while taking this drug.
- you have any type of heart disease.
- you have impaired liver or kidney function.
- you plan to have surgery in the near future.

Possible Side Effects (natural, expected, and unavoidable drug actions)

Nausea, vomiting, abdominal cramping, diarrhea—frequent, especially with maximum doses.

▷ **Possible Adverse Effects** (unusual, unexpected, and infrequent reactions)

If any of the following develop, consult your physician promptly for guidance.

Mild Adverse Effects

Allergic reactions: skin rash, hives, fever—rare.

Hair loss—reported after overdoses.

Serious Adverse Effects

Allergic reaction: anaphylactic reaction (see Glossary)—case reports.

Bone marrow depression (see Glossary): fatigue, weakness, fever, sore throat, abnormal bleeding, or bruising—case reports.

Peripheral neuritis (see Glossary): numbness, tingling, pain, weakness in hands and/or feet or myopathy with nerve symptoms (facial palsy and weakness, especially with long-term use in patients with declines in kidney function)—case reports.

Rhabdomyolysis—case reports.

Porphyria—case reports.

Drooping of the eyes (ptosis)—case reports.

Inflammation of colon with bloody diarrhea—case reports.

Thrombophlebitis with intravenous use—case reports.

▷ **Possible Effects on Sexual Function:** Reversible absence of sperm (azoospermia).

Possible Delayed Adverse Effects: Impaired production of sperm, possibly resulting in birth defects.

A rare combined muscle and nerve damage syndrome.

Natural Diseases or Disorders That May Be Activated by This Drug

Peptic ulcer disease, ulcerative colitis.

Possible Effects on Laboratory Tests

Complete blood cell counts: decreased red cells, hemoglobin, white cells, and platelets; increased white cells (follows initial decrease).

Prothrombin time: decreased (with concurrent use of warfarin).

Blood vitamin B12 level: decreased.

Liver function tests: increased liver enzymes (ALT/GPT, AST/GOT, and alkaline phosphatase), increased bilirubin.

Fecal occult blood test: positive.

Sperm counts: decreased (may be marked).

CAUTION

1. If this drug causes vomiting and/or diarrhea before relief of joint pain, stop it and call your doctor.
2. Try to limit each course of treatment for acute gout to 4 to 8 mg. Do not exceed 3 mg every 24 hours or a total of 8 mg per course.
3. Omit drug for 3 days between courses to avoid toxicity.
4. Carry this drug with you while traveling if you are subject to attacks of acute gout.
5. Surgical stress can cause a gout attack. Ask your doctor how much colchicine should be taken before and after surgery to prevent gout.
6. This medicine may inhibit healing of the cornea. Talk to your doctor about this if you will have eye surgery.

Precautions for Use

By Infants and Children: Use for preventing (prophylaxis) familial Mediterranean fever in children 5 years old or older: 0.5 mg twice per day and increased by 0.5 mg per day, to symptom control or a maximum of 2 mg per day. Safety and efficacy have not been established for conditions other than familial Mediterranean fever.

By Those Over 60 Years of Age: Because the dosage needed to relieve acute gout often causes vomiting and/or diarrhea, extreme caution is advised if you have heart or circulatory disorders, reduced liver or kidney function, or general debility.

▷ **Advisability of Use During Pregnancy**

Pregnancy Category: C by one manufacturer, and D by another source. See Pregnancy Risk Categories at the back of this book.

Animal Studies: This drug causes significant birth defects in hamsters and rabbits.

Human Studies: Adequate studies of pregnant women are not available. However, it is reported that colchicine can cause harm to the fetus.

Avoid during entire pregnancy if possible. Ask your physician for guidance.

Advisability of Use If Breast-Feeding

Presence of this drug in breast milk: Yes.

Ask your doctor for help. The American Academy of Pediatrics considers this medicine compatible with breast-feeding.

Habit-Forming Potential: None.

Effects of Overdose: Nausea, vomiting, abdominal cramping, diarrhea (may be bloody), burning sensation in throat and skin, weak and rapid pulse, progressive paralysis, inability to breathe.

Possible Effects of Long-Term Use: Hair loss, aplastic anemia (see Glossary), peripheral neuritis (see Glossary).

Suggested Periodic Examinations While Taking This Drug (at physician's discretion)

Complete blood cell counts.

Uric acid blood levels to monitor status of gout.

Sperm analysis for quantity and condition.

Liver function tests.

▷ **While Taking This Drug, Observe the Following**

Foods: Follow your doctor's advice about a low-purine diet.

Herbal Medicines or Minerals: Acerola is high in vitamin C. Inosine, like acerola, may increase uric acid levels. Aspen should be avoided in gout. Lipase may worsen gout. Goutweed (*Aegopodium podagraria*) does not have enough data to assess effectiveness. Some "herbal teas" (promoted as being beneficial for arthritis) contain phenylbutazone and other potentially toxic ingredients. Avoid herbal teas if you are not certain of their source, content, and medicinal effects. This drug is derived from a plant called Colchicum autumnale. Carefully read the labels of any herbal products you take to make sure autumn crocus or meadow saffron are not in the product. If they are, you may be unknowingly adding extra doses of this medicine.

Beverages: Drink at least 3 quarts of liquids every 24 hours. This drug may be taken with milk.

▷   *Alcohol:* No interactions expected. Combination may increase the risk of gastrointestinal irritation or bleeding and raise uric acid blood levels.

Tobacco Smoking: No interactions expected. I advise everyone to quit smoking.

▷   *Other Drugs*

Colchicine ***taken concurrently*** with

- allopurinol (Zyloprim), probenecid (Benemid), or sulfinpyrazone (Anturane) can prevent attacks of acute gout that often occur when treatment with these drugs is first started.
- cyanocobalamin will decrease absorption of the vitamin B_{12}. Higher doses of oral cyanocobalamin may be required by patients on colchicine.

- cyclosporine (Sandimmune) may increase cyclosporine levels and result in toxicity.
- erythromycins (E.E.S., clarithromycin) can result in toxic colchicine blood levels.
- insulin may inhibit the response (biphasic) of the body to sugar.
- interferon alfa-2A may blunt the antiviral benefits of the interferon.

▷ *Driving, Hazardous Activities:* Usually no restrictions when taken continually in small (preventive) doses.

May cause nausea, vomiting, and/or diarrhea when taken in larger (treatment) doses.

Aviation Note: The use of this drug **may be a disqualification** for piloting. Consult a designated Aviation Medical Examiner.

Exposure to Sun: No restrictions.

Exposure to Cold: This drug can lower body temperature. Use caution to prevent excessive lowering (hypothermia), especially in those over 60 years of age.

Occurrence of Unrelated Illness: Acute attacks of gout may result from injury or illness. Call your doctor for dosing adjustment if injury or new illness occurs.

COLD SORE AND GENITAL HERPES TREATMENT FAMILY

Acyclovir   (ay SI kloh veer)   **Famciclovir**   (fam SEYE klo veer)
Penciclovir   (PEN SI kloh veer)   **Valacyclovir**   (val a SY klo veer)
Docosanol cream (Abreva)   (a BREE vah):
Author's Note: Once head-to-head trials have been conducted with prescription antivirals and this relatively new non-prescription medicine for cold sores, a decision will be made as to inclusion in this profile. (Docosanol needs to be applied 12 hours after itching or redness and appears to work by inhibiting fusion between the skin membrane and the herpes virus envelope.)

Other Names: *Acyclovir*: Acycloguanosine, *penciclovir*: BRL-39123, *valacyclovir*: BW256U87   **Introduced:**   1979, 1994, 1997, 1996   **Class:** Antiviral, cold sore medicines, antiherpes virus   **Prescription:**   USA: Yes   **Controlled Drug:**   USA: No; Canada: No   **Available as Generic:**   Yes acyclovir (capsule, suspension, and tablets). No for famciclovir, penciclovir, valacyclovir

Brand Names: *Ayclovir*: ✿Apo-Acyclovir, ✿Gen-Acyclovir, Zovirax; *Famciclovir*: Famvir; *Penciclovir*: Denavir; *Valacyclovir*: Valtrex

---

BENEFITS versus RISKS

Possible Benefits	*Possible Risks*

Acyclovir:
TREATMENT OF ENCEPHALITIS
CAUSED BY HERPES SIMPLEX
TREATMENT OF CHICKENPOX

Acyclovir, famciclovir, and valacyclovir:
FASTER RECOVERY FROM INITIAL
EPISODE OF GENITAL HERPES
TREATMENT OF SUDDEN (ACUTE)
SHINGLES (HERPES ZOSTER)
PREVENTION OF RECURRENCE
OF GENITAL HERPES

Valacyclovir:
ORAL (BY MOUTH) DOSING
ACHIEVES BLOOD LEVELS
SIMILAR TO THOSE OBTAINED
FROM INTRAVENOUS DOSING
3-DAY DOSING OF VALACYCLOVIR
IN RECURRENT GENITAL
HERPES WILL HELP PEOPLE
TAKE IT (ADHERENCE)

Acyclovir, famciclovir, and penciclovir:
TREATMENT OF HERPES SIMPLEX
OF THE LIPS (COLD SORES OR
MUCOCUTANEOUS HERPES)

Acyclovir systemic use:
Nausea, vomiting, diarrhea
Joint and muscle pain
Seizures or coma with IV use—rare

Famciclovir:
Purpura
Paresthesias

Valacyclovir:
Rare reports of thrombotic
thrombocytopenic purpura (TTP) in
HIV and bone marrow or kidney
transplant patients

Valacyclovir, acyclovir, and penciclovir topical use:
Skin redness or irritation

Author's Note: Acyclovir has been rejected by the FDA for a change to nonprescription "over-the-counter" (OTC) status. This was based on fear of development of viral resistance—NOT on safety issues.

▷ **Principal Uses**

As a Single Drug Product: Uses currently included in FDA-approved labeling:

Acyclovir only: (1) Used to treat varicella (chickenpox) in children over a year old who have a chronic lung disease or skin condition, who take aspirin regularly, who are receiving short courses of corticosteroids via the lungs, or who are over 13 years old and are otherwise healthy (must be started within 24 hours of signs and symptoms); (2) used to treat brain infections caused by herpes simplex (encephalitis); (3) used to prevent herpes simplex virus infections in bone marrow transplant patients.

Acyclovir, famciclovir, and valacyclovir: (1) Treats or helps prevent (suppress) genital herpes; (2) treats shingles (herpes zoster).

Acyclovir and famciclovir: (1) Treats skin and mucous membrane infections (mucocutaneous) caused by herpes simplex in patients with immune problems (immunocompromised); (2) treatment of cold sores (mucocutaneous herpes) of the lips and face.

Penciclovir: (1) Treatment of cold sores (mucocutaneous herpes) of the lips and face.

Famciclovir only: Used in severe damage to the retina (retinal necrosis syndrome) in cases where acyclovir has failed to work.

Other (unlabeled) generally accepted uses: (1) Acyclovir helps treat herpes simplex infections of the eye and rectum (proctitis), and pneumonia caused by the chickenpox (varicella) virus; (2) some data support acyclovir use in nonmalignant skin growths in the throat (laryngeal papillomatosis); (3) prevention of repeat episodes of herpes eye infections; (4) penciclovir may have a role in herpes infections of the genitals—phase three trials have started in treating herpes simplex skin infections in immunocompromised patients; (5) famciclovir may help treat hepatitis B; (6) some combination data with interferon alpha and famciclovir in treating polyarteritis nodosa are promising; (7) valacyclovir may have a role in erythema multiforme and in decreasing risk of cytomegalovirus disease in kidney and heart transplant patients.

Author's Note: A study of 455 patients reported in JAMA found that when famciclovir was correctly taken for 1 year to suppress herpes simplex virus (HSV), nearly 75% of those patients did NOT have any HSV outbreaks during that year.

How These Drugs Work: By blocking genetic material formation of the herpes simplex virus, these drugs stop viral multiplication and spread, reducing severity and duration of the herpes infection. Use at the first sign of infection (such as the "itch" of a cold sore) can prevent a full blown lesion. Famciclovir is changed in the body to penciclovir. Valacyclovir is rapidly changed into acyclovir in the body and enters the body to a much greater extent than acyclovir. Docosanol prevents fusion between the skin and the virus.

▷ **Widely Used Guidelines That Involve This Medicine (representative sample):** Please look at the section at the very beginning of this profile called "Class." Next, turn to Table 22 and you will find guidelines listed by the class involved!

Available Dosage Forms and Strengths
Acyclovir:
Capsules — 200 mg, 400 mg, 800 mg
Intravenous — 500 mg, 1 g
Oral suspension — 200 mg/5 mL
Tablets — 200 mg, 400 mg, 500 mg, 800 mg
Ointment — 5%, 50 mg/g (Canada)
Famciclovir:
Tablets — 125 mg, 250 mg, 500 mg
Penciclovir:
Ointment — 1%
Valacyclovir:
Caplets — 500 mg, 1,000 mg
Coated tablets — 500 mg (Canada)

▷ **Recommended Dosage Ranges** (Actual dose and schedule must be determined for each patient individually.)
Infants and Children:
Acyclovir: In children less than 12 who have deficient immune systems (immunocompromised), intravenous acyclovir has been used (250 mg per square meter given over 1 hour) every 8 hours in a week-long treatment for skin and mouth herpes simplex infections. Safety and efficacy of oral use in children younger than 6 weeks of age have NOT been established.
Famciclovir, penciclovir, and valacyclovir: Safety and efficacy in infants and children not established.
18 to 65 Years of Age:
Acyclovir: For first episode of genital herpes: 200 mg every 4 hours for a total of five capsules daily for 7 to 10 days (or until what your doctor describes

as "clinical resolution" happens). Some clinicians use 400 mg three times a day for 7 to 10 days. Initial cases of herpes proctitis may require 400–800 mg five times daily by mouth (orally) for 10 days or until clinical resolution or 800 mg three times daily for 7–10 days until clinical resolution.

For intermittent recurrence: 200 mg every 4 hours for a total of five capsules daily for 5 consecutive days (total dose of 25 capsules) or 400 mg three times a day for 5 days. Start treatment at the earliest sign of recurrence.

For prevention of frequent recurrence: 400 mg taken twice daily for up to 12 months and then evaluation of ongoing need for this medicine.

For the ointment form: Cover all infected areas every 3 hours for a total of six times daily for 7 consecutive days. Start treatment at the earliest sign of infection (this can avoid a full-blown lesion).

In attempting to decrease the pain of herpes zoster: 800 mg five times daily (every 4 hours) for 7–10 days. Ointment use six times a day for 10 days helps the crusts form sooner.

Treatment of chickenpox: For those over 12 months old with a long-standing skin or lung condition, those being given aerosolized steroids, those taking long-term salicylates, or those 13 years old (otherwise healthy as outlined by the American Academy of Pediatrics): In those 2 or older: 20 mg per kg of body mass (do not exceed 800 mg) orally, four times a day for 5 days. If over 40 kg: 800 mg four times daily for 5 days. Start treatment at the first symptom or sign.

Treatment of herpes infections of the eye: 400 mg by mouth five times a day for at least 5 days.

Prevention of repeat herpes eye infections: One study used 400 mg twice a day (decreased recurrence by 45%).

Famciclovir: Shingles (herpes zoster): 500 mg is given every 8 hours for 7 days. It is important to start this medicine promptly after the diagnosis is made (within 48 hours of rash is best).

Recurrent genital herpes: 125 mg twice a day for 5 days. Once the initial infection is controlled, 250 mg twice a day has been given for up to a year (for suppression).

Hepatitis B: 500 mg three times daily.

Penciclovir: For the cream form: Cover all infected areas every 2 hours for a total of six times daily (during waking hours) for 4 consecutive days. Start treatment at the earliest sign of infection.

Valacyclovir: Herpes zoster (shingles): Best started within 48 hours of the zoster rash; 1 g (1,000 mg) three times a day for 7 days. Genital herpes simplex: This medicine is best started within 48 hours of the onset of symptoms and is taken as 1,000 mg twice daily for 7–10 days. It has not been shown to work if started more than 72 hours after symptoms start.

Recurrent genital herpes simplex: 500 mg twice a day for 3–5 days.

Suppression of genital herpes: 1 gram taken once a day. Some clinicians use 500 mg once a day in patients who have nine *or fewer recurrences a year. Safety and result (efficacy) have not been established for use more than a year.*

Over 65 Years of Age (all four medicines): The dose must be adjusted if the kidneys are impaired.

Conditions Requiring Dosing Adjustments

Liver Function: All medicines: Specific adjustment in liver dysfunction is not defined. Valacyclovir is NOT recommended in people with cirrhosis.

Kidney Function:

Acyclovir: The dose MUST be adjusted in people with compromised kidney function. For example: Creatinine clearance of 25–50 mL/min gets usual dose every 12 hours; 10–25 mL/min gets usual dose once daily.

Famciclovir: In people with mild kidney compromise (creatinine clearance greater than 60 mL/min), 500 mg is given every 8 hours. Mild to moderate compromise (creatinine clearance 40 to 59 mL/min) receives 500 mg every 12 hours. Moderate to severe (creatinine clearance 20 to 39 mL/min) receives 500 mg every 24 hours.

Penciclovir: Dosing may need to be lowered in ongoing dosing cases of oral dosing. Topical use generally results in no detectable drug in the blood.

Valacyclovir: Dosing changes MUST be made in patients with compromised kidneys (500 mg once a day for creatinine clearance less than 30 mL/min).

Obesity: Acyclovir: Dosing (intravenous form) should be made on ideal body weight and given as 10 mg per kg of body mass. Maximum dose is 500 mg per square meter every 8 hours.

▷ **Dosing Instructions:**

Acyclovir, famciclovir, and valacyclovir: May be taken without regard to food. Acyclovir only: Capsule may be opened. The maker of acyclovir recommends drinking 1 liter of water for each gram (1,000 mg) taken.

All medicines: Take or apply the full course of the exact dose prescribed—interrupted therapy can make the virus smarter (lead to resistant viruses). Apply ointment forms to the lesions every 2 hours while you are awake. Start treatment at the earliest sign of infection. Use a finger cot or rubber glove to apply the ointment forms. If you forget a dose: Take or apply the missed dose as soon as you remember it, unless it is nearly time for your next dose—if that is the case, simply take the next dose right on schedule. DO NOT double doses.

Usual Duration of Use:

Acyclovir: Use on a regular schedule for 10 days is usually needed to see this drug's effect in reducing the severity and duration of the initial infection. Continual use for 6 months may be needed to prevent frequent recurrence of herpes eruptions.

Famciclovir: For herpes zoster: Regular use for 2 days determines effectiveness. Then the medicine is typically continued for 7 days. Your doctor should decide when to stop the medicine.

For recurrent genital herpes: Start at first sign of recurrence and dosing is continued for 5 days.

Penciclovir: Use on a regular schedule for 4 days usually needed to see this drug's effect in reducing the severity and duration of the infection.

Valacyclovir: Best started within 48 hours of onset of the zoster rash. Use on a regular schedule for 7 days for herpes zoster has been effective. Start therapy within 24 hours of signs of genital herpes; regular use for 10 days is appropriate for initial cases. Take the full course as prescribed. Missing doses may lead to resistance. For recurrent genital herpes, 500 mg twice a day for 3–5 days.

If you forget a dose: Apply the cream or ointment form as soon as you remember, but skip the missed dose if it is nearly time for your next dose. If you are taking the "pill" forms, take the missed dose as soon as you remember it, unless it is nearly time for your next dose—then skip the missed dose and continue with your next scheduled dose. DO NOT double doses.

Typical Treatment Goals and Measurements (Outcomes and Markers)

Infections: The most commonly used measures of serious infections are white blood cell counts and differentials (the kind of blood cells that occur most often in your blood) and temperature. With herpes infections, clinicians look for positive changes in the appearance of the infection (shortened time to crusting, etc.) as well as shortened time for postherpetic neuralgia. Suppressive use finds decreased frequency of outbreaks (for example, with genital herpes) and shorter duration of any recurrences as a goal.

Possible Advantages of These Drugs: Valacyclovir: Achieves blood levels similar to INTRAVENOUS acyclovir with a medicine taken by mouth (the oral route). Patients do not have to take it as many times a day as acyclovir (should help people stay on the medicine-adherence). Newer dosing for valacyclovir in recurrent genital herpes should also help adherence. Famciclovir also offers less frequent dosing (three times a day) in shingles versus acyclovir. Penciclovir may give results even if started later in a "cold sore" case.

▷ **These Drugs Should Not Be Taken If**
  • you have had an allergic reaction to them previously.

▷ **Inform Your Physician Before Taking These Drugs If**
Valacyclovir:
  • your immune system is compromised (immunocompromised patients) or you have shingles (herpes zoster) that has spread (disseminated). Valacyclovir benefits not established in this population.
  • you have advanced HIV disease or have had a bone marrow or kidney transplant (increased risk of thrombotic thrombocytopenic purpura).
Acyclovir and valacyclovir:
  • you take other medicines that may cause kidney damage.
  • you think you are dehydrated and can't or will not drink water.
Famciclovir:
  • you have a first episode of genital herpes or your immune system is compromised (immunocompromised) and you have shingles (herpes zoster).
All medicines:
  • your liver (hepatic), kidney (renal), or nerve (neurologic) function is impaired.
  • you are unsure of how much or how often to take them.

Possible Side Effects (natural, expected, and unavoidable drug actions)
Acyclovir and valacyclovir:
Possible increased sensitivity to light (photophobia).
With IV acyclovir—possible irritation of the vein (thrombophlebitis) up to 9%. Tissue death (necrosis) can occur if this acyclovir form is given in a vein and the vein "blows" letting the drug into the tissue around the IV site. A special IV line (peripherally inserted central catheter) is prudent.
All medicines with ointment forms:
With use of ointment—mild pain or stinging at site of application.

▷ **Possible Adverse Effects** (unusual, unexpected, and infrequent reactions)
  If any of the following develop, consult your physician promptly for guidance.
Mild Adverse Effects: Allergic reaction: skin rash, itching.
  Acyclovir: Headache (valacyclovir, penciclovir, famciclovir as well and may be frequent), dizziness, nervousness, confusion, insomnia, depression, fatigue—rare. Nausea, vomiting, diarrhea—infrequent with IV form. Joint pains, muscle cramps—rare. Acne, hair loss—rare.
  Famciclovir: Nausea or diarrhea—infrequent to frequent.
  Valacyclovir: fast heart rate—case reports.
Serious Adverse Effects
  Acyclovir: Superficial thrombophlebitis—infrequent with IV form. Seizures, hallucinations or coma with IV use—rare. Kidney problems—rare

(especially if adequate water is taken). Low platelets or red or white blood cells—case reports—rare. Colitis—case reports.

Famciclovir: Purpura or paresthesias—case reports. Rigors or movement disorders—case reports to rare. Increased breast cancer in male rats given extremely high doses. Does not appear to increase risk in humans.

Valacyclovir: Thrombotic thrombocytopenic purpura—rare and in immunocompromised patients.

Aseptic meningitis (stiff neck, disorientation, sleepiness, and incontinence)—case report. Erythema multiforme—case report.

▷ **Possible Effects on Sexual Function:** None reported for these medicines.

Possible Effects on Laboratory Tests

Acyclovir and valacyclovir: Complete blood cell counts: decreased red or white cells or hemoglobin—rare.

Blood urea nitrogen (BUN)/creatinine: increased—rare.

Liver function tests: increased—rare.

CAUTION

1. These drugs do not eliminate all herpes virus and are not a cure. The infection often returns. Restart treatment at the earliest sign of infection.
2. Avoid intercourse if herpes blisters and swelling are present.
3. Do not exceed the prescribed dose.
4. If severity/frequency of infections don't improve, call your doctor.
5. The manufacturer recommends drinking 1 liter (1,000 mL) of fluid for each gram (1,000 mg) of oral or intravenous form taken of acyclovir.
6. Other medicines that can form damaging crystals in the urine may lead to added kidney problem risk if combined with acyclovir.
7. Some managed care organizations suggest pill splitting (valacyclovir is an example). If you are required to split pills, get a pill splitter to help ensure accuracy.

Precautions for Use

By Infants and Children: Acyclovir: Specific dosing required. Fluid intake must be adequate.

Famciclovir, penciclovir, and valacyclovir: Safety and efficacy not established.

By Those Over 60 Years of Age: Acyclovir and valacyclovir:

Avoid dehydration. Talk to your doctor about how much water you should take or can tolerate. Make sure dosing is adjusted for age-related decline in kidney function.

Famciclovir and penciclovir: Age-related declines in kidney function may require dosing adjustment.

▷ **Advisability of Use During Pregnancy**

Pregnancy Category:

Acyclovir: B for the oral and intravenous forms. C for the topical form. See Pregnancy Risk Categories at the back of this book.

Famciclovir, penciclovir, and valacyclovir: B. See Pregnancy Risk Categories at the back of this book.

Animal Studies:

Acyclovir: No birth defects found in mouse, rat, or rabbit studies.

Famciclovir and penciclovir: No birth defects found in animals.

Valacyclovir: NOT teratogenic in rabbits or rats (up to 10 times the human dose).

Human Studies:

Acyclovir: The pregnancy registry has followed more than 600 cases to date. Sixteen birth defects occurred, with no pattern. Widespread (disseminated) or life-threatening herpes virus infections may warrant use of this medicine during pregnancy. Talk with your doctor about use.

Famciclovir and penciclovir: Studies not available.

Valacyclovir: Adequate studies of pregnant women are not available. A valacyclovir pregnancy registry can be accessed by physicians at 1-800-722-9292, extension 39437.

Advisability of Use If Breast-Feeding

Presence of this drug in breast milk: Acyclovir: Yes. *Famciclovir:* Yes in lab animals, unknown in humans. *Penciclovir:* Unknown. *Valacyclovir:* Yes (documented in two women; 0.6 to 4.1 times the plasma levels).

Ask your physician for guidance: Acyclovir: Often okay to breast-feed. While the drug is in the milk, it is in small amounts. *Famciclovir:* Stop nursing or discontinue drug. *Valacyclovir:* Discuss discontinuing the medicine or stopping nursing with your doctor. Discuss benefits and risk factors with your doctor for other medicines in this profile also.

Habit-Forming Potential: None.

Effects of Overdose: Possible impairment of kidney function with acyclovir and valacyclovir, not defined or symptomatic management for famciclovir or penciclovir.

Possible Effects of Long-Term Use: Resistant strains of herpes virus may emerge. See your doctor.

Suggested Periodic Examinations While Taking This Drug (at physician's discretion)

Kidney function tests for acyclovir and valacyclovir, not defined for famciclovir or penciclovir.

▷ **While Taking This Drug, Observe the Following**

Foods: No restrictions. Some claims have been made for lysine (an amino acid) in cold sores, but specific scientifically rigorous studies have not been made.

Herbal Medicines or Minerals: Some patients use echinacea to attempt to boost their immune systems. Unfortunately, use of echinacea is not recommended in people with damaged immune systems. This herb may also actually weaken any immune system if it is used too often or for too long a time. Since St. John's wort and valacyclovir can increase sensitivity to the sun—caution is advised.

Beverages: No restrictions. Acyclovir may be taken with milk. Drink 2 to 3 quarts of liquids daily (if not contraindicated for you) when you take acyclovir or valacyclovir.

▷ *Alcohol:* Acyclovir and valacyclovir: Use caution; dizziness or fatigue may be accentuated. Penciclovir and famciclovir: No restrictions.

Tobacco Smoking: No interactions expected. I advise everyone to quit smoking.

▷ *Other Drugs*

Penciclovir: No significant interactions for the cream as it results in undetectable blood levels.

The following drugs may ***increase*** the effects of acyclovir and valacyclovir:
- cyclosporine (Sandimmune)—use may result in increased risk of kidney toxicity.
- probenecid (Benemid)—may delay acyclovir or valacyclovir elimination.

Acyclovir or valacyclovir ***taken concurrently*** with or by
- a patient with an allopurinol (Zyloprim) allergy may result in cross-allergenicity and allergic reaction.
- cimetidine (Tagamet) increases risk of antiviral toxicity.

- fosphenytoin (Cerebyx) or phenytoin (Dilantin) may cause loss of seizure control (lower blood levels of this seizure medicine).
- meperidine (Demerol) may result in neurologic problems.
- valproic acid (Depakote) may cause loss of seizure control (lower valproic blood levels).
- varicella vaccine (Varivax) will blunt the vaccine effectiveness.
- zidovudine (AZT) may result in severe fatigue and lethargy.

Famciclovir *taken concurrently* with
- digoxin (Lanoxin) may increase peak digoxin blood level slightly.
- probenecid (Benemid) may increase famciclovir blood levels as both medicines are removed from the body by active tubular secretion in the kidney.

▷ *Driving, Hazardous Activities:* Use caution if dizziness or fatigue occurs from acyclovir or famciclovir. Caution is advised if significant headache results from these medicines.

Aviation Note: The use of acyclovir, famciclovir, or valacyclovir *may be a disqualification* for piloting. Penciclovir is probably not a disqualification. Consult a designated Aviation Medical Examiner.

Exposure to Sun: No restrictions; however, some data indicate that sun exposure may trigger release of herpes simplex from its dormant state (from the optic nerve).

COLESEVELAM (koh lee SEV eh lamb)

Introduced: 2000 **Class:** Anticholesterol **Prescription:** USA: Yes **Controlled Drug:** USA: No; Canada: No **Available as Generic:** USA: No; Canada: No
Brand Name: Welchol

BENEFITS versus RISKS	
Possible Benefits	*Possible Risks*
EFFECTIVE REDUCTION OF TOTAL CHOLESTEROL AND LOW-DENSITY CHOLESTEROL IN TYPE IIA CHOLESTEROL DISORDERS	Constipation
	Reduced absorption of fat, fat-soluble vitamins (A, D, E, K, etc.)
ADDITIVE EFFECTS WHEN COMBINED WITH HMG-CoA REDUCTASE INHIBITORS	

▷ **Principal Uses**

As a Single Drug Product: Uses currently included in FDA-approved labeling: (1) Used in combination with diet and exercise to decrease blood cholesterol and low-density (LDL) cholesterol in Type IIa cholesterol disorders; (2) used in combination with "statin" type (see Drug Classes) medicines to achieve cholesterol lowering goals.

Other (unlabeled) generally accepted uses: None at present.

How This Drug Works: This medicine (a cross-linked hydrogel polymer) holds onto (binds) bile acids in the intestine, which prevents them from being absorbed. Because bile acids are not absorbed, more cholesterol is converted to bile acids. This effect works to lower cholesterol (upregulate the LDL receptor) by removing cholesterol from the blood (plasma).

▷ **Widely Used Guidelines That Involve This Medicine (representative sample):**
Please look at the section at the very beginning of this profile called "Class."
Next, turn to Table 22 and you will find guidelines listed by the class involved!

Available Dosage Forms and Strengths
Tablets—625 mg

▷ **Usual Adult Dosage Ranges:** *When used alone:* This medicine is started with 3
tablets twice a day (with meals) or 6 tablets once a day with a meal. The
dose can then be increased if goals are not met to 7 tablets a day (4,375 mg
a day maximum).
Combination therapy (with an HMG-CoA inhibitor—see Drug Classes): Four to
six tablets per day has worked. To gain maximum effect, 3 colesevelam
tablets twice a day with meals or 6 tablets a day with a meal combined
with a statin has been used.
**Note: Actual dose and schedule must be determined for each patient
individually.**

Conditions Requiring Dosing Adjustments
Liver Function: No changes needed (zero to minimal absorption).
Kidney Function: No changes needed (zero to minimal absorption).

▷ **Dosing Instructions:** Always take just before or with a meal and with liquids. If
you forget a dose: Take the missed dose as soon as you remember it, unless
it is nearly time for the next dose. DO NOT DOUBLE DOSES. Call your
doctor if you find yourself forgetting doses. While not included in official
FDA labeling, the recent National Cholesterol Education Program (NCEP)
ATP 3 guidelines call for use of TLC or therapeutic lifestyle changes (see
Glossary) in order to augment results in achieving cholesterol goals.

Usual Duration of Use: Initial response often occurs in 2 weeks. Regular use for
up to a month may be needed to see peak benefits in lowering cholesterol.
If no acceptable response in 3 months with peak doses, combination therapy with an HMG-CoA is advisable. Long-term use (months to years)
requires periodic follow-up with your doctor. Treat cholesterol for life!

Typical Treatment Goals and Measurements (Outcomes and Markers)
Cholesterol: Current guidelines (National Cholesterol Education Program, or
NCEP) acknowledge diabetes as one of the conditions that increases risk
of heart disease, modifying risk factors, therapeutic lifestyle changes
(TLC), and recommending routine testing for all of the cholesterol fractions (lipoprotein profile) versus total cholesterol alone. Goals are: a total
cholesterol of 200 mg/dL, and optimal bad cholesterol (LDL) of less than
100 mg/dL. Less than 70 mg/dL (see Grundy, S.M. in Sources) is a reasonable optional goal for very high risk patients (such as diabetics with acute
coronary syndromes, etc.). 130–159 mg/dL as borderline high, 160 mg/dL
as high and 190 mg/dL as very high. Did you know that there are at least
five different kinds of "good cholesterol" or HDL? The "too low" measure
for HDL is still 40mg/dL, but in order to learn more about cholesterol
types some doctors are starting to order lipid panels. There are at least
seven different kinds of "bad cholesterol." The new panels tell doctors
about the kinds of cholesterol that your body makes. This is important
because some kinds (small dense particles) tend to stick to blood vessels
(are highly atherogenic). Take your medicine to reach your goals! Two
additional tests you will hear about will be electron beam computed
tomography (EBCT) and CRP. EBCT is an important tool used in conjunction with laboratory studies. Findings show that even patients who meet

cholesterol goals (particularly females over 55) can still be at significant cardiovascular risk. EBCT then defines risk by giving a calcium score and a "virtual tour" of the coronary arteries. C Reactive Protein or CRP is a relatively new and apparently independent predictor of heart disease risk. A large study (see Ridker, P.M. in Sources) found that CRP predicted heart disease risk independently of bad cholesterol (low density lipoprotein). Talk to your doctor about this laboratory test and ask about current guidelines for who should be tested (see Pearson, T.A. in Sources).

▷ **This Drug Should Not Be Taken If**
- you have had an allergic reaction to it previously.
- you have a bowel block (obstruction).

▷ **Inform Your Physician Before Taking This Drug If**
- you are prone to constipation.
- you have low thyroid function (hypothyroidism).
- you have stomach or intestinal problems (gastrointestinal disorders).
- you have a bleeding disorder of any kind.
- you have a fat-soluble vitamin (especially vitamin K) deficiency.

Possible Side Effects (natural, expected, and unavoidable drug actions)
Constipation; interference with normal fat digestion and absorption; reduced absorption of vitamins A, D, E, and K and folic acid. Binds to vitamin B_{12}-intrinsic factor complex.

▷ **Possible Adverse Effects** (unusual, unexpected, and infrequent reactions)
If any of the following develop, consult your physician promptly for guidance.
Mild Adverse Effects
Allergic reactions: not reported as yet.
Joint pains or muscle aches (myalgia)—possible.
Constipation or indigestion (dyspepsia)—most frequent.
Loss of appetite, indigestion, heartburn, abdominal discomfort, excessive gas, nausea, vomiting, diarrhea—case reports.
Serious Adverse Effects
Fat-soluble vitamin deficiency—possible.

▷ **Possible Effects on Sexual Function:** None reported.

Natural Diseases or Disorders That May Be Activated by This Drug
Fat-soluble vitamin deficiency.

Possible Effects on Laboratory Tests
Blood cholesterol and triglyceride levels: decreased (therapeutic effect).

CAUTION
1. Watch carefully for constipation; use stool softeners and laxatives as needed.

Precautions for Use
By Infants and Children: Safety and effectiveness for those under 12 years of age not established.
By Those Over 60 Years of Age: Increased risk of severe constipation.

▷ **Advisability of Use During Pregnancy**
Pregnancy Category: B. See Pregnancy Risk Categories at the back of this book.
Animal Studies: No information available.
Human Studies: Adequate studies of pregnant women are not available.
Use this drug only if clearly needed. Ensure adequate intake of vitamins and minerals to satisfy needs of mother and fetus.

Advisability of Use If Breast-Feeding
Presence of this drug in breast milk: None.
Breast-feeding is permitted.

Habit-Forming Potential: None.

Effects of Overdose: Progressive constipation.

Possible Effects of Long-Term Use: Deficiencies of vitamins A, D, E, and K and folic acid. Binding of the B12-intrinsic factor complex may lead to blood cell problems.

Suggested Periodic Examinations While Taking This Drug (at physician's discretion)
Measurements of blood levels of total cholesterol, low-density (LDL) cholesterol and high-density (HDL) cholesterol. HDL and LDL patterns, CRP.

▷ **While Taking This Drug, Observe the Following**
Foods: Avoid foods that tend to constipate (cheeses, etc.). Talk to your doctor if you are considering adding soy milk or other soy products to your diet. Follow a standard low-cholesterol diet. Your doctor may also recommend some specific foods such as increased vegetables or functional foods such as Benecol (see TLC in Glossary). Three well-designed studies were published in April 2002 found that both in women and men and before and after a heart attack, people who ate more fish (2–4 servings a week) appeared to avoid heart disease. Additionally, putting supplements containing Omega 3 polyunsaturated fatty acids (PUFA) into the diet also appeared to protect against abnormal heart rhythms and sudden death from heart attack. Your doctor may also recommend increasing B vitamins. See Tables 19 and 20 about lifestyle changes and risk factors you can fix.
Herbal Medicines or Minerals: Some studies show garlic to reduce cholesterol. Since it probably works by a different mechanism than colesevelam, the combination use may be reasonable if dosing is separated. Discuss this with your doctor. Policosanol may also work by a different mechanism. Soy milk offers some lowering of cholesterol. Current cholesterol therapy sets a goal for treatment, and these herbs may help reach that goal when combined with this prescription medicine. Talk to your doctor before combining any herbals with colesevelam.
Nutritional Support: Ask your doctor if you need supplements of vitamins A, D, E, K, folic acid, and calcium.
Beverages: Ensure adequate liquid intake (up to 2 quarts daily). This drug may be taken with milk.
▷ *Alcohol:* No interactions expected.
Tobacco Smoking: No interactions expected. I advise everyone to quit smoking.
▷ *Other Drugs*
Colesevelam may ***decrease*** the effects of
- alendronate (Fosamax); take 2 hours before colesevelam.
- fibrates (Tricor, others); take 2 hours before colestipol or 4 to 6 hours after colestipol.
- verapamil (Calan, others). Caution and careful patient follow up is prudent.
- vitamin B_{12} and fat-soluble vitamins.
Colesevelam may ***increase*** the effects of
- atorvastatin (Lipitor), lovastatin (Mevacor), simvastatin (Zocor), and other statins (see Drug Classes) as well as ezetimibe (Zetia) [desirable and beneficial effect].

▷ *Driving, Hazardous Activities:* No restrictions.
Aviation Note: The use of this drug is usually not a disqualification for piloting. Consult a designated Aviation Medical Examiner.
Exposure to Sun: No restrictions.
Discontinuation: Once colesevelam is stopped, cholesterol levels usually return to pretreatment levels in 1 month.

COLESTIPOL (koh LES ti pohl)

Introduced: 1974 **Class:** Anticholesterol **Prescription:** USA: Yes **Controlled Drug:** USA: No; Canada: No **Available as Generic:** USA: No; Canada: No
Brand Names: Colestid, Lestid

BENEFITS versus RISKS	
Possible Benefits	*Possible Risks*
EFFECTIVE REDUCTION OF TOTAL CHOLESTEROL AND LOW-DENSITY CHOLESTEROL IN TYPE IIA CHOLESTEROL DISORDERS	Constipation (may be severe) Reduced absorption of fat, fat-soluble vitamins (A, D, E, and K) and folic acid
EFFECTIVE RELIEF OF ITCHING associated with biliary obstruction	Reduced formation of prothrombin with possible bleeding
Treatment of some pseudomembranous colitis cases	

▷ **Principal Uses**
As a Single Drug Product: Uses currently included in FDA-approved labeling: (1) Used in combination with diet changes to decrease blood cholesterol and low-density (LDL) cholesterol in Type IIa cholesterol disorders; (2) eases itching due to deposit of bile acids in skin.
Other (unlabeled) generally accepted uses: (1) Data from one study showed that colestipol in combination with lovastatin actually caused regression of plaque buildup (atherosclerosis) inside blood vessels; (2) some data show that colestipol is useful in pseudomembranous colitis.

How This Drug Works: Binds bile acids and is removed in feces. Removal of bile acids stimulates conversion of cholesterol to bile acids, which then reduces cholesterol. By reducing levels of bile acids, this drug hastens removal of bile acids in the skin and relieves itching.

▷ **Widely Used Guidelines That Involve This Medicine (representative sample):** Please look at the section at the very beginning of this profile called "Class." Next, turn to Table 22 and you will find guidelines listed by the class involved!

Available Dosage Forms and Strengths
Bottles — 250 g, 500 g
Flavored Colestid
granules for oral
suspension — 5 g per dose (7.5 grams in Canada)
Packets — 5 g
Tablet, coated — 1 g

▷ **Usual Adult Dosage Ranges:** Starts with 5 g of powder mixed in an approved liquid (such as orange juice, apple juice, water, or grape juice) and taken three times daily. May be increased slowly as needed and tolerated to 30 g daily in two to four divided doses. The tablet form is taken as 2 to 16 grams a day as a single dose or divided into several equal doses. Dose is increased as needed and tolerated every 30–60 days.

> **Note: Actual dose and schedule must be determined for each patient individually.**

Conditions Requiring Dosing Adjustments
Liver Function: No changes needed.
Kidney Function: No changes needed.

▷ **Dosing Instructions:** Always take just before or with a meal; drug does not work if taken without food. Mix the powder thoroughly in 4 to 6 ounces of water, fruit juice, tomato juice, milk, thin soup or a soft food such as applesauce. **Do not take the powder in its dry form.** If you forget a dose, take the missed dose as soon as you remember it, unless it is nearly time for the next dose. DO NOT DOUBLE DOSES. Call your doctor if you find yourself forgetting doses. The tablet form should be swallowed whole and taken with a liquid such as water.

Usual Duration of Use: Regular use for up to a month may be needed to see peak benefits in lowering cholesterol. If no acceptable response in 3 months, combination treatment with an HMG-CoA inhibitor should be considered. Long-term use (months to years) requires periodic follow-up with your doctor as cholesterol tends to increase as we age.

Typical Treatment Goals and Measurements (Outcomes and Markers)
Cholesterol: Current guidelines (National Cholesterol Education Program, or NCEP) acknowledge diabetes as one of the conditions that increases risk of heart disease, modifying risk factors, therapeutic lifestyle changes (TLC), and recommending routine testing for all of the cholesterol fractions (lipoprotein profile) versus total cholesterol alone. Goals are: a total cholesterol of 200 mg/dL, and optimal bad cholesterol (LDL) of less than 100 mg/dL. Less than 70 mg/dL (see Grundy, S.M. in Sources) is a reasonable optional goal for very high risk patients (such as diabetics with acute coronary syndromes, etc.). 130–159 mg/dL as borderline high, 160 mg/dL as high and 190 mg/dL as very high. Did you know that there are at least five different kinds of "good cholesterol" or HDL? The "too low" measure for HDL is still 40mg/dL, but in order to learn more about cholesterol types some doctors are starting to order lipid panels. There are at least seven different kinds of "bad cholesterol." The new panels tell doctors about the kinds of cholesterol that your body makes. This is important because some kinds (small dense particles) tend to stick to blood vessels (are highly atherogenic). Take your medicine to reach your goals! Two additional tests you will hear about will be electron beam computed tomography (EBCT) and CRP. EBCT is an important tool used in conjunction with laboratory studies. Findings show that even patients who meet cholesterol goals (particularly females over 55) can still be at significant cardiovascular risk. EBCT then defines risk by giving a calcium score and a "virtual tour" of the coronary arteries. C Reactive Protein, or CRP, is a relatively new and apparently independent predictor of heart disease risk. A large study (see Ridker, P.M. in Sources) found that CRP predicted heart disease risk independently of bad cholesterol (low density lipoprotein).

Talk to your doctor about this laboratory test and ask about current guidelines for who should be tested (see Pearson, T.A. in Sources).

▷ **This Drug Should Not Be Taken If**
- you have had an allergic reaction to it previously.
- you have complete biliary obstruction.

▷ **Inform Your Physician Before Taking This Drug If**
- you are prone to constipation.
- you have low thyroid function (hypothyroidism).
- you have peptic ulcer disease.
- you have a bleeding disorder of any kind.
- you have impaired kidney function.

Possible Side Effects (natural, expected, and unavoidable drug actions)
Constipation; interference with normal fat digestion and absorption; reduced absorption of vitamins A, D, E, and K, and folic acid. Binds to vitamin B_{12}-intrinsic factor complex.

▷ **Possible Adverse Effects** (unusual, unexpected, and infrequent reactions)
If any of the following develop, consult your physician promptly for guidance.

Mild Adverse Effects
Allergic reactions: skin rash—rare; hives, tongue irritation, anal itching—case reports.
Headache, dizziness, weakness, muscle and joint pains—possible.
Constipation—most frequent.
Loss of appetite, indigestion, heartburn, abdominal discomfort, excessive gas, nausea, vomiting, diarrhea—case reports.

Serious Adverse Effects
Vitamin K deficiency and increased bleeding tendency—possible.
Impaired absorption of calcium; predisposition to osteoporosis—possible.
Hypothyroidism—possible.
Disruption of normal acid-base balance of the body (metabolic acidosis)—possible with long-term use.

▷ **Possible Effects on Sexual Function:** None reported.

Natural Diseases or Disorders That May Be Activated by This Drug
Peptic ulcer disease; steatorrhea (excessive fat in stools) with large doses.

Possible Effects on Laboratory Tests
Blood cholesterol and triglyceride levels: decreased (therapeutic effect).
Blood thyroxine (T4) level: decreased when colestipol and niacin are taken concurrently (in presence of normal thyroid function).

CAUTION
1. Never take the dry powder; always mix thoroughly with a suitable liquid before swallowing.
2. Watch carefully for constipation; use stool softeners and laxatives as needed.
3. This drug may bind other drugs taken concurrently and impair their absorption. It is advisable to take all other drugs 1 to 2 hours before or 4 to 6 hours after taking this drug.
4. If triglycerides rise significantly, the dose may need to be decreased (talk to your doctor).

Precautions for Use
By Infants and Children: Safety and effectiveness for those under 12 years of age not established. Watch carefully for the possible development of

acidosis and vitamin A or folic acid deficiency. (Ask your physician for guidance.)

By Those Over 60 Years of Age: Increased risk of severe constipation. Impaired kidney function may predispose to the development of acidosis.

▷ **Advisability of Use During Pregnancy**

Pregnancy Category: Not established, B2 in Australia. See Pregnancy Risk Categories at the back of this book.

Animal Studies: No information available.

Human Studies: Adequate studies of pregnant women are not available.

Use this drug only if clearly needed. Ensure adequate intake of vitamins and minerals to satisfy needs of mother and fetus.

Advisability of Use If Breast-Feeding

Presence of this drug in breast milk: Not known.

Talk to your doctor about breast-feeding.

Habit-Forming Potential: None.

Effects of Overdose: Progressive constipation, skin changes (skin drying).

Possible Effects of Long-Term Use: Deficiencies of vitamins A, D, E, and K and folic acid. Calcium deficiency, osteoporosis. Acidosis due to excessive retention of chloride. Binding of the B_{12}-intrinsic factor complex may lead to blood cell problems such as macrocytic anemia.

Suggested Periodic Examinations While Taking This Drug (at physician's discretion)

Appropriate testing to rule out low thyroid, diabetes, or other causes (secondary) of hypercholesterolemia before the medicine is started.

Measurements of blood levels of total cholesterol, low-density (LDL) cholesterol and high-density (HDL) cholesterol, HDL and LDL fraction testing, and CRP.

Hemoglobin and red blood cell studies for possible anemia.

Thyroid function tests.

▷ **While Taking This Drug, Observe the Following**

Foods: Avoid foods that tend to constipate (cheeses, etc.). Follow the diet that your doctor recommends (plus some specific foods such as increased vegetables or functional foods such as Benecol). Three well-designed studies found that both in women and men and before and after a heart attack, people who ate more fish (2–4 servings a week) appeared to avoid heart disease. Additionally putting supplements containing Omega 3 polyunsaturated fatty acids (PUFA) into the diet also appeared to protect against abnormal heart rhythms and sudden death from heart attack. Your doctor may also recommend increasing B vitamins. See Tables 19 and 20 about lifestyle changes and risk factors you can fix.

Herbal Medicines or Minerals: Some studies show garlic to reduce cholesterol. Since it probably works by a different mechanism than colestipol, the combination use may be reasonable if dosing is separated. Discuss this with your doctor. Policosanol and soy milk may also offer some lowering of cholesterol. Current cholesterol therapy sets a goal for treatment, and these herbs may help reach that goal when combined with this prescription medicine. Talk to your doctor before combining any herbals with colestipol.

Nutritional Support: Ask your doctor if you need supplements of vitamins A, D, E, K, folic acid, and calcium.

Beverages: Ensure adequate liquid intake (up to 2 quarts daily). This drug may be taken with milk.

▷ *Alcohol:* No interactions expected.

Tobacco Smoking: No interactions expected. I advise everyone to quit smoking.

▷ *Other Drugs*

Colestipol may ***decrease*** the effects of

- acetaminophen (Tylenol); take 2 hours before colestipol.
- alendronate (Fosamax); take 2 hours before colestipol.
- aspirin; take 2 hours before colestipol.
- atorvastatin (Lipitor); take 2 hours before colestipol.
- cephalexin (Keflex); take 2 hours before colestipol.
- diclofenac (various); take 2 hours before colestipol.
- digitoxin and digoxin (Lanoxin); take 2 hours before colestipol.
- fibrates (Tricor, others); take 2 hours before colestipol or 4 to 6 hours after colestipol.
- folic acid; take 2 hours before colestipol.
- furosemide (Lasix); take 2 hours before colestipol or 4 to 6 hours after colestipol.
- hydrocortisone; take 2 hours before colestipol.
- iron preparations; take 2 to 3 hours before colestipol.
- leflunomide (Arava); take 2 hours before colestipol.
- penicillin G (Pentids); take 2 hours before colestipol.
- phenobarbital; take 2 hours before colestipol.
- pravastatin (Pravachol); take 2 hours before colestipol.
- oral antidiabetic drugs (see Drug Classes).
- raloxifene (Evista); take 2 hours before colestipol.
- tetracycline (various); take 2 hours before or 3 hours after colestipol.
- thiazide diuretics (see Drug Classes); take 2 hours before colestipol.
- thyroxine (see Thyroid Hormones Drug Class); take 5 hours before colestipol.
- vancomycin (various oral forms); take 2 hours before colestipol or 4 to 6 hours after colestipol.
- vitamin B12.

▷ *Driving, Hazardous Activities:* No restrictions.

Aviation Note: The use of this drug is usually ***not a disqualification*** for piloting. Consult a designated Aviation Medical Examiner.

Exposure to Sun: No restrictions.

Discontinuation: The dose of any toxic drug combined with colestipol must be reduced when this drug is stopped. Once colestipol is stopped, cholesterol levels usually return to pretreatment levels in 1 month.

COX II INHIBITOR FAMILY (KOX too)

Celecoxib   (SELL ah kox ib)   **Rofecoxib**   (ROW fah kox ib)

Introduced: 1999, 1999 **Class:** COX II Inhibitor, selective NSAID
Prescription: USA: Yes **Controlled Drug:** USA: No; Canada: No
Available as Generic: No

Brand Names: *Celecoxib:* Celebrex; *Rofecoxib:* Vioxx, *Valdecoxib:* Bextra, *Etoricoxib:* Arcoxia (investigational)

Author's Note: Some sound-alike errors have been made with Celexa and Celebrex. One drug is an antidepressant, while the other is a COX II inhibitor. Caution is advised. Information on Bextra will be included in subsequent editions if clinical data and use warrant inclusion.

BENEFITS versus RISKS

Possible Benefits	*Possible Risks*
EFFECTIVE TREATMENT OF OSTEOARTHRITIS	INCREASED BLOOD PRESSURE
EFFECTIVE RELIEF OF INFLAMMATION	ROFECOXIB USED WITH CAUTION IN PEOPLE WITH ISHEMIC HEART DISEASE
EFFECTIVE SHORT-TERM RELIEF OF SUDDEN (ACUTE) NONARTHRITIC PAIN	Stomach irritation, bleeding, and/or ulceration—possible but less likely than earlier NSAIDS
TREATMENT OF PRIMARY DYSMENORRHEA	Anemia—rare
REDUCTION OF ADENOMATOUS COLON POLYPS IN FAMILIAL ADENOMATOUS POLYPOSIS (FAP) (CELECOXIB ONLY)	Bronchospasm in asthmatics—possible
TREATMENT OF RHEUMATOID ARTHRITIS PAIN	CELECOXIB only—allergic reactions in people allergic to sulfa drugs
ROFECOXIB NOW HAS LABELING THAT SAYS IT HAS A BETTER STOMACH AND INTESTINAL SIDE EFFECT PROFILE THAN NAPROXEN	
ROFECOXIB NEWLY APPROVED FOR TREATING MIGRAINE HEADACHE (ACUTE)	
May have a role in treating a kind of bladder cancer (carcinoma *in situ*)	
Both medicines reduce fevers	
Rofecoxib may have a role in acute migraines	
Both may have a role in Alzheimer's	

▷ **Principal Uses**

As a Single Drug Product: Uses currently included in FDA-approved labeling: (1) Both medicines relieve sudden (acute) nonarthritic pain in adults (orthopedic and dental pain); (2) relieves signs and symptoms of osteoarthritis (both medicines); (3) treats primary dysmenorrhea; (4) relieves signs and symptoms of rheumatoid arthritis; (5) celecoxib reduces the number of adenomatous colorectal polyps in familial adenomatous polyposis (FAP); (6) rofecoxib now approved to treat migraine headaches.

Other (unlabeled) generally accepted uses: (1) Based on the way that they work, both could have a role in Alzheimer's disease; (2) may have a role in treating carcinoma *in situ* of the bladder; (3) could be useful in ankylosing spondylitis; (4) rofecoxib may have a role in sudden (acute) migraines.

How These Drugs Work: Inhibit cyclooxygenase (COX) II. Since COX II is the COX type (isoform) that is mostly responsible for inflammation and pain, this results in relief of pain and inflammation. COX II also causes fever in humans (along with other compounds), so these medicines work to lower fevers if they occur. Because COX I works to maintain kidney function and has a protective role in the stomach, lack of inhibition of this isoform by both medicines should result in a much more favorable gastrointestinal side effect profile than nonselective NSAIDs for most patients.

▷ **Widely Used Guidelines That Involve This Medicine (representative sample):** Please look at the section at the very beginning of this profile called "Class." Next, turn to Table 22 and you will find guidelines listed by the class involved!

Available Dosage Forms and Strengths
Celecoxib:
Capsules — 100 mg, 200 mg
Rofecoxib:
Oral suspension — 12.5 mg/5 mL, 25 mg/5 mL
Tablets — 12.5 mg, 25 mg, 50 mg

▷ **Usual Adult Dosage Ranges**
Celecoxib:
Osteoarthritis: 100 mg twice daily or 200 mg once a day.
Rheumatoid arthritis: 100 mg twice a day, increased as needed and tolerated to 200 mg twice daily.
Sudden pain or primary dysmenorrhea: Acute pain treatment is started with 400 mg right away (stat) an option for an additional 200 mg on the first day. Dosing is continued at 200 mg twice a day if needed.
FAP: 400 mg twice a day (taken with food).
Rofecoxib:
Osteoarthritis: Dosing is started at 12.5 mg once daily. The dose may be increased as needed and tolerated to 25 mg daily. The lowest effective dose should be used.
Migraine headache (acute): 25 mg once a day. Some people may benefit from up to 50 mg a day. Data for treating more than 5 headaches a month are not available.
Rheumatoid arthritis: 25 mg once a day is appropriate and is also the maximum dose.
Sudden pain or primary dysmenorrhea: 50 mg once daily is used (use for more than 5 days). May have an opioid sparing effect in patients taking opioids (medicines such as morphine).
Note: Actual dosage and schedule must be determined for each patient individually.

Conditions Requiring Dosing Adjustments
Liver Function: Celecoxib: Lower doses recommended for celecoxib in moderate liver compromise. Lowering usual doses by half (50%) is appropriate. Not recommended for use in severe liver (hepatic) problems. Rofecoxib: Use in mild (Child-Pugh score of less than 6) liver problems (dysfunction) showed that rofecoxib achieves similar blood levels as in healthy patients. A small amount of data in moderate (Child-Pugh 7–9) liver disease shows that blood levels are roughly 53% increased. Dose decreases by half (50%) appear prudent, and the lowest possible dose should be used. This medicine has NOT been studied in severe liver failure.
Kidney Function: Rofecoxib and celecoxib have not been studied in advanced kidney (renal) disease and are NOT recommended for use in those situations.

▷ **Dosing Instructions:** Celecoxib and rofecoxib: May be taken with or without food. Higher doses of celecoxib are best taken with food to increase how much gets into the body. Taking these medicines with a full glass of water is a good idea. Use of rofecoxib in treating pain or in primary dysmenorrhea has only been studied for up to 5 days. An oral rofecoxib suspension is available if you have trouble swallowing pills. The suspension should be shaken well before a dose is taken. The pill and suspension form give the benefit of equal dosing (are bioequivalent). For both medicines: If you forget a dose: take the missed dose as soon as you remember it, unless it's nearly time for your next scheduled dose—if this is the case, skip the missed dose and simply take the regularly scheduled dose. DO NOT double doses.

Usual Duration of Use: Celecoxib may generally take 1–2 weeks of regular use to work in osteoarthritis and 2 weeks in rheumatoid arthritis. Onset for the treatment of more complicated Familial Adenomatous Polyposis (FAP) may require 6 months. In any case, use on a regular basis delivers the best results.

Short-term use of rofecoxib is recommended (up to 5 days) for nonarthritic pain or dysmenorrhea. The medicine usually goes to work in 30 minutes but may take up to an hour. Use on a regular schedule for 1 week usually needed to see benefit in relieving osteoarthritis symptoms. Use of the 50 mg rofecoxib dose on an ongoing (chronic) basis is not recommended. Both medicines are best used in the smallest possible dose and for the shortest possible length of time (minimizes the possibility of GI adverse effects). Treatment of osteo or rheumatoid arthritis duration will be decided by your doctor. Follow up with your doctor on a regular basis is needed.

Typical Treatment Goals and Measurements (Outcomes and Markers)

Pain: Most clinicians treating pain use a device called an algometer to check your pain. This looks like a small ruler, but lets the clinician better understand your pain. The goals of treatment then relate to where the level of pain started (for example, a rating of 7 on a 0–10 scale) and what the cause of the pain was. Pain medicines may also be used together (in combination) in order to get the best result or outcome. For example, many clinicians use acetaminophen (Tylenol, others) rescue doses (NOT NSAID rescue) to help breakthrough pain previously controlled by a COX II inhibitor. If your pain control is not acceptable to YOU (remember, in hospitals and outpatient settings, etc., pain control is a patient right and the fifth vital sign) and if after a week of arthritis pain treatment, results are not what you expect, be sure to call your doctor. It is not unusual to combine medicines or change them to get the best results.

Arthritis: Control of arthritis symptoms (pain, loss of mobility, decreased ability to accomplish activities of daily living, range of motion, etc.) is paramount in returning patient quality of life and to checking the results (beneficial outcomes) from these medicines. Clinicians use the WOMAC osteoarthritis index (see Glossary) to globally assess the health status of people living with osteoarthritis. Many arthritis management or pain centers use interdisciplinary teams (physicians from several specialties, nurses, physician's assistants, physical and occupational therapists, pharmacotherapists, psychotherapists, social workers, and others) to get the best results. Laboratory measures of results for rheumatoid arthritis include decreases in chemicals released by the body (acute phase reactants) such as C-reactive protein. A more general test to roughly measure inflammation is a sed rate (erythrocyte sedimentation rate). In rheumatoid arthritis (RA), the American College of Rheumatologists (ACR) has a scoring system ACR 20, etc. that gives a measure of the degree of response. The higher the ACR number, the better the response.

Migraine headache: Control of headache pain, relief of nausea and sensitivity to sound and light and decreased use of rescue medicines.

Possible Advantages of These Drugs: Both compounds: Do NOT inhibit the COX I isoenzyme. Rofecoxib is now the only COX II inhibitor that can claim better gastrointestinal safety based on approved FDA labeling. Rofecoxib: Is NOT a sulfonamide compound and avoids possible allergic sulfonamide reactions of celecoxib. Metabolic differences are present between the medicines in this profile. Rofecoxib is mainly removed by cycotosolic enzymes, versus CYP 450 2C9 removal of celecoxib. Because of the mechanism of both medicines, combined use of low-dose (81 mg) aspirin may be advisable for patients who have already suffered a heart attack. The GI effects of this combination are not fully defined, but are expected to increase the risk of ulcers versus the medicines taken alone, therefore this issue should be discussed with your doctor. In a head-to-head study of 382 arthritis patients, rofecoxib was reported to relieve pain at night more effectively than celecoxib. In a head-to-head trial of 800 patients with osteoarthritis and high blood pressure, only 6% of celecoxib versus 12% of rofecoxib patients developed higher blood pressure. Rofecoxib offers dosing flexibility with a suspension form (offers an easy way to take the medicine for those who have trouble swallowing).

▷ **These Drugs Should Not Be Taken If**
- you have had an allergic reaction to any COX II inhibitor or NSAID.
- you have active peptic ulcer disease.
- you are in the last 3 months of pregnancy.
- you have severe liver disease (not studied).
- you have a history of urticaria/angioedema or spasm of the bronchi with rhinoconjunctivitis with aspirin or other NSAID (adults who developed nasal polyps, asthma, chronic rhinitis, or ongoing angioedema or urticaria make these reactions more likely).

▷ **Inform Your Physician Before Taking These Drugs If**
- you smoke, have ulcerative colitis, take corticosteroids or abuse alcohol.
- you have a bleeding disorder.
- you have a history of peptic ulcer disease.
- you have a history of heart disease or high blood pressure.
- you have ischemic heart disease (rofecoxib only).
- you are pregnant or planning pregnancy.
- you have asthma, carditis, or nasal polyps.
- you have a history of liver or kidney problems.
- you drink three or more alcoholic drinks a day (see Caution).

Possible Side Effects (natural, expected, and unavoidable drug actions)
Not defined at present.

▷ **Possible Adverse Effects** (unusual, unexpected, and infrequent reactions)
If any of the following develop, consult your physician promptly for guidance.
Mild Adverse Effects
Allergic reactions: skin rash, itching.
Dizziness—infrequent.
Auditory hallucinations (celecoxib)—case report.
Stomach irritation, heartburn—infrequent.
Increased liver enzymes—up to 15% of people who take NSAIDs. (This was a rare effect for rofecoxib in clinical trials, and 6% of people had this effect.)
Diarrhea—infrequent.
Edema/fluid accumulation (call your doctor if you develop swelling in your legs or ankles)—infrequent.

Serious Adverse Effects

Allergic reactions: acute anaphylactic reaction (see Glossary)—not reported, but possible based on NSAID experience.

Erosion of stomach lining, with silent bleeding—possible (rofecoxib has labeling minimizing this risk).

Gastrointestinal (GI) bleeding, ulceration or perforation (call your doctor if you have a black, tarry stool, unexplained stomach pain, or vomit that has a coffee ground look)—possible to infrequent.

Anemia—rare.

Kidney function decline—possible similar to other NSAIDs.

Liver function changes with possible severe reactions—rare.

Lowered white blood cells, platelets, or bone marrow suppression—rare (rofecoxib).

Bronchospasm when used in patients with nasal polyps, asthma—possible.

May worsen angina attacks and increase their frequency—possible (because of fluid retention and increased heart work).

Clot-related (thrombotic) cardiovascular problems (events)—rofecoxib (from the VIGOR study) appeared to have increased risk and the label was changed. Celecoxib has had four cases of blood clots (thrombosis) when used in patients with connective tissue diseases.

▷ **Possible Effects on Sexual Function:** None reported.

Adverse Effects That May Mimic Natural Diseases or Disorders

Increased liver enzymes may suggest viral hepatitis. Other NSAIDs have led to decline in kidney function in people with borderline kidney disease. Accumulation of fluid may mimic worsening of congestive heart failure.

Possible Effects on Laboratory Tests

Complete blood counts: decreased red cells or hemoglobin.

Liver function tests: increased ALT/GPT, AST/GOT, alkaline phosphatase.

Fecal occult blood test: may be positive.

CAUTION

1. The FDA requires a warning noting that people who have three or more alcoholic drinks a day may have increased risk of stomach bleeding if they also use NSAIDs (problems may also occur with lower alcohol use).

2. NSAIDs should be used with extreme caution in people with a previous history of gastrointestinal bleeding or ulcer disease.

3. People with asthma may have aspirin-sensitive asthma. Cross-reactivity between aspirin and these medicines may be possible.

4. When NSAIDs are taken long term, kidney damage is possible. Caution is needed if these medicines are to be used in a patient with kidney damage or in one who is dehydrated (should be rehydrated BEFORE these medicines are started).

5. Rofecoxib and celecoxib may lead to anemia. Patients should be evaluated if they are taking rofecoxib and start to show signs or symptoms of anemia.

6. Part of the removal of rofecoxib from the body happens in a way that can become full or saturated. This means a small change in dose could result in a larger than expected increase in blood level. Take this medicine exactly as prescribed.

7. People who take NSAIDS such as these medicines can develop serious stomach or intestinal (gastrointestinal) problems. Elderly people or patients with debilitating diseases or conditions may be at increased risk for gastrointestinal problems from these medicines. The FDA recently

ruled that data on rofecoxib (VIGOR) supported favorable modification (but not removal) of the gastrointestinal side effect labeling. To lower risk of possible GI problems, the lowest effective dose should be used for rofecoxib or celecoxib for the shortest amount of time.

8. These medicines may cause fluid retention, complicating high blood pressure or heart failure treatment—this effect may generally be managed by an inexpensive and well-tolerated water pill (diuretic) such as low-dose hydrochlorothiazide.

9. Rofecoxib has FDA labeling saying that it should be used with caution in people with ischemic heart disease. Higher doses may warrant risk.

10. It is important to realize that while the lack of effect on platelets is a benefit, it is also a challenge. In patients who require prevention of cardiovascular problems (prophylaxis), rofecoxib is NOT a substitute for a cardioprotective drug.

11. Celecoxib is primarily removed by a liver enzyme called P450 2C9. Caution is advised if consideration is being given to medicines that effect this enzyme. Celecoxib also acts as an inhibitor of a liver enzyme called P450 2D6. Caution should be used in considering prescribing celecoxib for patients already receiving a medicine removed by 2D6.

Precautions for Use

By Infants and Children: Safety and efficacy in those less than 18 years old have NOT been established.

By Those Over 60 Years of Age: Clinical studies included many patients who were more than 75 years old. These patients showed no difference in drug levels from younger patients. For people less than 50 kg, the lowest dose of celecoxib should be used to start treatment. Rofecoxib labeling says that doctors should use caution in prescribing it for patients with ischemic heart disease.

▷ ### Advisability of Use During Pregnancy

Pregnancy Category: C for both medicines. See Pregnancy Risk Categories at the back of this book.

Animal Studies: Slight increase in vertebral malformations in rabbits for rofecoxib. Celecoxib caused skeletal defects at two times the usual human dose.

Human Studies: Adequate studies of pregnant women have NOT been performed.

These medicines should be avoided in pregnancy because of possible premature closure of the ductus arteriosus.

Advisability of Use If Breast-Feeding

Presence of this drug in breast milk: Yes for both medicines in rats, unknown in humans.

Avoid drug or refrain from nursing.

Habit-Forming Potential: None.

Effects of Overdose:
No overdose data were reported in clinical trials. Supportive measures consistent with patient symptoms as well as removal of unabsorbed drug from the stomach is reasonable.

Possible Effects of Long-Term Use:
Anemia due to chronic blood loss from erosion of stomach lining.

Suggested Periodic Examinations While Taking These Drugs (at physician's discretion)

Check for signs or symptoms of serious GI toxicity.

Complete blood cell counts.

Liver function tests if signs or symptoms of liver problems begin.

Increased range of motion and decreased pain in arthritis.

▷ **While Taking These Drugs, Observe the Following**

Foods: May be taken with or without food (take it with food if the medicine upsets your stomach).

Herbal Medicines or Minerals: Ginseng, ginkgo, alfalfa, clove oil, feverfew, cinchona bark, white willow bark, and garlic may change clotting, so combining those herbals with these medicines is not recommended. NSAIDs may decrease feverfew effects. Hay flower, mistletoe herb, and white mustard seed carry German Commission E monograph indications for arthritis and may be complementary. White willow bark contains salicylate (aspirin) and may increase GI toxicity risk. Talk to your doctor BEFORE combining any herbal medicines or prescription medicines.

Beverages: No restrictions. May be taken with milk.

▷ *Alcohol:* Use of alcohol and these medicines at the same time may increase risk of stomach irritation. See alcohol/NSAIDs warning in Cautions.

Tobacco Smoking: May increase risk of stomach irritation. I advise everyone to quit smoking.

▷ *Other Drugs*

These medicines may ***increase*** the effects of

- adrenocortical steroids (see Drug Classes), which may lead to additive stomach irritation and bleeding.
- methotrexate—not by increasing blood levels, but by possible increased GI effects.
- oral anticoagulants (see Drug Classes) such as warfarin (Coumadin) and require more frequent INR testing.

The following drugs may ***decrease*** the effects of these medicines:

- cholestyramine (Questran, others) may decrease the amount of drug that goes to work (not reported, but possible in theory). Separate doses by 30 minutes.

These medicines ***taken concurrently*** with

- ACE inhibitors—since vein-opening or vasodilator prostaglandins may account for some of the ACE beneficial effects and since data from combined use with benazepril (Lotensin) showed blunting of beneficial effects from benazepril, caution with all ACE inhibitors is prudent.
- alendronate (Fosamax) may blunt alendronate absorption and may also result in increased risk of stomach upset/diarrhea (not reported, but theoretically possible).
- cortisonelike drugs (see Drug Classes) increase risk of stomach ulcers.
- high blood pressure (antihypertensive) medicines may blunt their therapeutic benefit, especially those that are diuretics such as furosemide (Lasix) or other loop diuretics, spironolactone, or thiazides (see Drug Classes).
- lithium (Lithobid) may increase lithium blood levels.
- other NSAIDs (see Drug Classes) (such as aspirin) may increase risk of stomach or intestine (GI) toxicity. The benefit-to-risk decision of combined use of aspirin with these medicines in patients who have had a heart attack (secondary prevention) may be desirable because of the lack of a needed effect on platelets or to overcome a possible effect of these medicines on clotting. Further study is needed.

The following drugs may ***increase*** the effects of celecoxib:

- any medicine that inhibits the liver enzyme that removes celecoxib from the body (CYP 2C9).

- fluconazole (Diflucan) by inhibiting liver enzymes that remove celecoxib from the body. Celecoxib dose decreases are prudent if these medicines are to be combined.
- fluoxetine (Prozac) by inhibiting liver enzymes that remove celecoxib from the body. Celecoxib dose decreases may be prudent if these medicines are to be combined.
- propafenone (Rythmol) by inhibiting liver enzymes that remove celecoxib from the body. Celecoxib dose decreases may be prudent if these medicines are to be combined.
- ritonavir (Norvir) and perhaps other protease inhibitors by inhibiting liver enzymes that remove celecoxib from the body. Celecoxib dose decreases may be prudent if these medicines are to be combined.
- sertraline (Zoloft) by inhibiting liver enzymes that remove celecoxib from the body. Celecoxib dose decreases may be prudent if these medicines are to be combined.

The following drugs may *decrease* the effects of celecoxib:
- carbamazepine (Tegretol), phenytoin (Dilantin), and rifampin (Rifater, others) by increasing the liver enzyme that removes it from the body (not yet reported, but these medicines are known CYP 2C9 inducers).

The following drugs *taken concurrently with* celecoxib:
- diltiazem (Cardizem, others) may lead to increased blood pressure. Careful monitoring of blood pressure is prudent.

▷ *Driving, Hazardous Activities:* May cause dizziness. Use caution until full effects are known.

Aviation Note: The use of these drugs *may be a disqualification* for piloting. Consult a designated Aviation Medical Examiner.

Exposure to Sun: No reported problems.

Discontinuation: May be stopped abruptly, but talk to your doctor before making any changes in your medicines.

CROMOLYN (KROH moh lin)

Other Names: Cromolyn sodium, sodium cromoglycate

Introduced: 1968   **Class:**   Antiasthmatic drug, mast cell stabilizing agent, asthma attack preventive   **Prescription:**   USA: Yes   **Controlled Drug:**   USA: No; Canada: No   **Available as Generic:**   USA: Yes; Canada: Yes

Brand Names: Children's Nasalcrom, Crolom, Fisoneb [CD], Gastrocrom, Intal, ♣Gen-cromolyn, ♣Intal Spincaps, ♣Intal Syncroner, ♣Nalcrom, Nasalcrom, ♣Novo-cromolyn, Opticrom, ♣Rynacrom, Vistacrom

Author's Note: Cromolyn sodium (4%) as Nasalcrom is available without a prescription.

```
┌─────────────────────────────────────────────────────────────────────┐
│                        BENEFITS versus RISKS                          │
│         Possible Benefits                    Possible Risks           │
│    LONG-TERM PREVENTION OF          Anaphylactic reaction (see Glossary)│
│      RECURRENT ASTHMA ATTACKS       Spasm of bronchial tubes, increased│
│    Prevention of acute asthma due to   wheezing                       │
│      allergens or exercise          Allergic pneumonitis (allergic reaction│
│    Prevention and treatment of allergic   in lung tissue)             │
│      rhinitis                                                         │
│    Prevention of bronchospasm                                         │
│    RELIEF OF ALLERGIC EYE                                             │
│      INFLAMMATION                                                     │
│      (CONJUNCTIVITIS)                                                 │
│    Treatment of giant papillary                                       │
│      conjunctivitis                                                   │
└─────────────────────────────────────────────────────────────────────┘
```

▷ **Principal Uses**

> *As a Single Drug Product:* Uses currently included in FDA-approved labeling: (1) Prevents allergic reactions in the nose (allergic rhinitis, hay fever) and the bronchial tubes (bronchial asthma); (2) used to treat eye inflammation (allergic conjunctivitis); (3) helps prevent exercise- or environmental-induced asthma; (4) treats mastocytosis and manages several allergy-related skin disorders.

> Other (unlabeled) generally accepted uses: (1) Can be used to help stop cough from ACE inhibitors (see Drug Classes); (2) helps modify the reactions in food allergies.

How This Drug Works: Blocks the release of histamine (and other chemicals) from mast cells that worsens allergic reactions. Prevents sequence of events leading to swelling, itching and constriction of bronchial tubes (asthma).

▷ **Widely Used Guidelines That Involve This Medicine (representative sample):** Please look at the section at the very beginning of this profile called "Class." Next, turn to Table 22 and you will find guidelines listed by the class involved!

Available Dosage Forms and Strengths

> Capsules, oral — 20 mg, 100 mg
> Eyedrops — 2% (such as Vistacrom) and 4%
> Inhalation aerosol — 0.8 mg per metered spray
> Inhalation capsules (powder) — 20 mg
> Inhalation solution — 20 mg per ampule
> Nasal insufflation (powder) — 10 mg per cartridge
> Nasal solution — 40 mg/mL
> Nasal spray — 5.2 mg per spray in a 26 mL bottle

▷ **Usual Adult Dosage Ranges**

> *Eyedrops:* One to two drops of the 4% solution in each eye four to six times daily at regular intervals.

> *Inhalation aerosol:* 1.6 mg (two inhalations) four times daily at regular intervals for prevention of asthma, or two inhalations 10 to 15 minutes before exposure to prevent allergen- or exercise-induced asthma.

> *Inhalation powder:* 20 mg (one capsule) four times daily at regular intervals for long-term prevention of asthma; 20 mg (one capsule) as a single dose 10 to 15 minutes before exposure to prevent acute allergen- or exercise-induced asthma. Total daily maximum dosage is 160 mg (eight capsules).

Inhalation solution: Same as inhalation powder.

Nasal insufflation: Initially 10 mg in each nostril every 4 to 6 hours as needed; reduce to every 8 to 12 hours for maintenance.

Nasal solution: 5.2 mg in each nostril three to six times daily as needed.

Oral powder: ALL of the contents of capsules for oral use are poured into a half glass of hot water. This is stirred, and a half glass of cold water is added while mixing. Drink all the liquid and add more water to be sure you drink any leftover medicine. Mix cromolyn with water only, not with fruit juice, milk, or foods.

Note: Actual dose and schedule must be determined for each patient individually.

Conditions Requiring Dosing Adjustments

Liver Function: If the bile duct is damaged by liver disease, the dose must be decreased.

Kidney Function: The dose should be decreased in kidney failure.

▷ **Dosing Instructions:** Follow instructions provided with all of the dosage forms, especially inhalers and eyedrops. Do not swallow capsules intended for inhalation. (If the capsule is accidentally swallowed, drug will cause no beneficial or adverse effects.) Capsules for mouth (oral) use can be poured into 4 ounces (one half glass) of hot water as above. If you forget a dose, take it right away unless it's nearly time for your next regular dose. If it IS nearly time, just take the scheduled dose. DO NOT double doses. The Nasalcrom form if best used 1–2 weeks BEFORE you are going to be exposed to something that you are allergic to (allergen).

Usual Duration of Use: Regular use for 6 weeks or more is often needed for benefits in preventing asthma attacks. Onset in perennial allergic rhinitis can be 1 to 2 weeks. Eye use (ophthalmic) may work in a few days up to 6 weeks. Long-term use (months to years) requires periodic evaluation.

Typical Treatment Goals and Measurements (Outcomes and Markers)

Asthma: The frequency of asthma attacks as well as the severity of asthma attacks that occur (such as those requiring an emergency department visit) are a benchmark of effectiveness. Some clinicians also use the number of times a rescue inhaler must be used as a clinical fine point. Pulmonary function tests such as FEV1 may also be used. Goals should be communicated and checked.

Possible Advantages of This Drug

May be quite effective in young asthmatics. Well tolerated. Serious adverse effects are very rare. Works against immediate responses to allergens as well as late nasal responses and isolated late nasal responses. Usually regarded as the drug of choice in adding medicines to step one of current asthma treatments for children under five years old.

▷ **This Drug Should Not Be Taken If**
- you have had an allergic reaction to any dosage form of it previously.

▷ **Inform Your Physician Before Taking This Drug If**
- you are allergic to milk, milk products, or lactose. (The inhalation powder contains lactose.)
- you have impaired liver or kidney function.
- you have soft contact lenses (these should not be worn while using the eyedrops).
- you have angina or a heart rhythm disorder. (Some inhalation aerosol forms have propellants that could be hazardous.)

Possible Side Effects (natural, expected, and unavoidable drug actions)

    Unpleasant taste with use of inhalation aerosol. Mild throat irritation, hoarseness, cough (minimized by a few swallows of water after each powder inhalation). Painful or difficult urination (dysuria)—rare. For the eye (ocular) form—the most common problem (adverse reaction) is stinging or burning.

▷ **Possible Adverse Effects** (unusual, unexpected, and infrequent reactions)

    If any of the following develop, consult your physician promptly for guidance. (Frequency and probable severity of adverse effects is greatly reduced or not applicable for the eye [ophthalmic] form.)

Mild Adverse Effects

    Allergic reactions: skin rash, hives, itching—possible.

    Headache, dizziness, drowsiness—rare.

    Nausea, vomiting, urinary urgency and pain (dysuria), joint pain—infrequent.

    Muscle pain (myositis)—rare.

    Stinging or burning of the eyes with ophthalmic use—possible.

    Cough and bronchial irritation—rare.

    Nosebleed or itching with nasal solution use—rare.

Serious Adverse Effects

    Allergic reactions: rare anaphylactic reaction (see Glossary).

    Allergic pneumonitis (allergic reaction in lung tissue)—case reports.

    Propellants in the metered dose inhaler may cause problems in patients with disease of the heart arteries or a history of abnormal heart rhythms—possible.

    Pericarditis—case report.

    Inflammation of the arteries—case reports.

▷ **Possible Effects on Sexual Function:** None reported.

Possible Effects on Laboratory Tests

    None reported.

CAUTION

1. This drug only helps **prevent** bronchial asthma—use **before** the start of acute bronchial constriction (asthmatic wheezing).
2. **Do not** use during an acute asthma attack—may worsen and prolong asthmatic wheezing.
3. This drug does not block the benefits of drugs that relieve acute asthma attacks after they start. Cromolyn is used *before and between* acute attacks to help keep them from starting; bronchodilators are used during acute attacks.
4. If you are using a bronchodilator drug by inhalation, it is best to take it about 5 minutes before inhaling cromolyn.
5. If this drug has allowed you to decrease or eliminate steroids and you are unable to tolerate cromolyn, ask your doctor about the need to start steroids once again.

Precautions for Use

    By Infants and Children: Safety and effectiveness for those under 5 years of age not established for the metered dose inhaler. Inhalation capsules: For children 2 years and older—20 mg (contents of one capsule) inhaled four times a day. Young children may find a nebulized solution easier than the powder.

    By Those Over 60 Years of Age: This drug does not work in the management of chronic bronchitis or emphysema.

▷ **Advisability of Use During Pregnancy**
  Pregnancy Category: B. See Pregnancy Risk Categories at the back of this book.
  Animal Studies: Mouse, rat, and rabbit studies revealed no birth defects due to this drug.
  Human Studies: Adequate studies of pregnant women are not available.
  Use this drug only if clearly needed.

Advisability of Use If Breast-Feeding
  Presence of this drug in breast milk: Unknown.
  Avoid drug or refrain from nursing.

Habit-Forming Potential: None.

Effects of Overdose: No significant effects reported.

Possible Effects of Long-Term Use: Allergic reaction of lung tissue (allergic pneumonitis)—very rare.

Suggested Periodic Examinations While Taking This Drug (at physician's discretion) sputum analysis and X-ray if symptoms suggest allergic pneumonitis. FEV1.

▷ **While Taking This Drug, Observe the Following**
  Foods: Follow physician-prescribed diet. Avoid all foods to which you are allergic.
  Herbal Medicines or Minerals: If you are allergic to plants in the Asteraceae family (aster, chrysanthemum, daisy, or ragweed), you may also be allergic to echinacea, chamomile, feverfew, and St. John's wort. Fir or pine needle oil should NOT be used by asthmatics. Ephedra alone does carry a German Commission E monograph indication for asthma treatment. Talk to your doctor before using any herbal medicine.
  Beverages: Avoid all beverages to which you may be allergic.
▷ *Alcohol:* No interactions expected.
  Tobacco Smoking: No interactions with the medicine, but smoking can irritate your airways. I advise everyone to quit smoking.
▷ *Other Drugs:* Cromolyn may allow reduced dosage of cortisonelike drugs in the management of chronic asthma. Ask your doctor about dosage adjustment.
▷ *Driving, Hazardous Activities:* This drug may cause dizziness. Restrict activities as necessary.
  Aviation Note: The use of this drug *may be a disqualification* for piloting. Consult a designated Aviation Medical Examiner.
  Exposure to Sun: No restrictions.
  Heavy Exercise or Exertion: This drug may prevent exercise-induced asthma if taken 10 to 15 minutes before exertion. It is most effective in young people.
  Discontinuation: If cromolyn has made it possible to reduce or stop maintenance doses of cortisonelike drugs and you find it necessary to discontinue cromolyn, watch closely for a sudden return of asthma. A slow withdrawal (over a week) is advisable. You may have to start a cortisonelike drug as well as take other measures to control asthma and prevent a recurrence if this medicine is stopped.
  Special Storage Instructions: Keep the powder cartridges in a dry, tightly closed container. Store in a cool place, but not in the refrigerator. Do not handle the cartridges or the inhaler when hands are wet.

CYCLOPHOSPHAMIDE (si kloh FOSS fa mide)

Introduced: 1959 **Class:** Anticancer, immunosuppressive **Prescription:** USA: Yes **Controlled Drug:** USA: No; Canada: No **Available as Generic:** Yes
Brand Names: Cycloblastin, Cytoxan, Neosar, ✤Procytox

```
┌─────────────────────────────────────────────────────────────────────────┐
│                         BENEFITS versus RISKS                             │
│        Possible Benefits                    Possible Risks                │
│  CURE OR CONTROL OF CERTAIN        REDUCED WHITE BLOOD CELL                │
│    TYPES OF CANCER                   COUNT                                 │
│  PREVENTION OF REJECTION IN        SECONDARY INFECTION                     │
│    ORGAN TRANSPLANTATION           URINARY BLADDER                         │
│  Possibly beneficial in rheumatoid BLEEDING HEART                         │
│    arthritis or lupus erythematosus LUNG, LIVER OR KIDNEY DAMAGE          │
│  May help selected cases of childhood Loss of hair                        │
│    nephrotic syndrome                                                     │
└─────────────────────────────────────────────────────────────────────────┘
```

▷ **Principal Uses**
   As a Single Drug Product: Uses currently included in FDA-approved labeling: (1) Combination treatment of various cancers: malignant lymphomas, multiple myeloma, sarcomas, retinoblastomas, leukemias, as well as breast and ovarian cancer; (2) also used to prevent rejection in organ transplantation and in some autoimmune disorders; (3) treats some resistant forms of nephrotic syndrome.
   Other (unlabeled) generally accepted uses: (1) Used to prepare patients for autologous bone marrow transplants; (2) part of several combination chemotherapy regimens; (3) helps overall survival in combination therapy of lung or fallopian tube cancer; (4) can be part of combination therapy for Ewing's sarcoma; (5) may be of help in patients with lupus erythematosus who have interstitial lung disease or nephritis; (6) secondary role in prostate cancer; (7) high-dose therapy of anemia (aplastic anemia); (8) helps in resistant rheumatoid arthritis or RA (and in pachymeningitis associated with RA); (9) may have a role in drug-induced serious skin reactions (such as Stevens-Johnson syndrome or toxic epidermal necrolysis, etc.).

How This Drug Works: Kills cancer cells during all phases of development. Suppresses primary growth and secondary spread (metastasis) of some types of cancer.

▷ **Widely Used Guidelines That Involve This Medicine (representative sample):** Please look at the section at the very beginning of this profile called "Class." Next, turn to Table 22 and you will find guidelines listed by the class involved!

Available Dosage Forms and Strengths
   Injection — vials of 100 mg, 200 mg, 500 mg, 1 g, 2 g
   Tablets — 25 mg, 50 mg

▷ **Usual Adult Dosage Ranges:** *Oral form:* Many different ways of using and dosing this medicine have been reported. In general, doses range from one to five mg/kg of body weight per day through starting (induction) phases and ongoing (maintenance) dosing. Doses are adjusted to the response of the tumor as well as to development of toxicity such as low white blood cell count (leukopenia). Some clinicians use 60 to 120 mg per square meter of body surface area daily or 400 mg per square meter of body surface area on days 1 to 5, every 3 to 4 weeks. Once again as therapy continues, the dose is adjusted according to how the tumor responds or unacceptable low white blood cell counts develop. *Intravenous:* 1,000 to 1,500 mg per square meter every 3 to 4 weeks, adjusted the same as the oral form. Current experimental approaches for combination therapy can be found at *www.cancer.org* and *www.clinicaltrials.gov*.

Note: Actual dose and schedule must be determined for each patient individually.

Conditions Requiring Dosing Adjustments
Liver Function: Dose changes are not required in liver compromise. Toxicity may be more likely in people with liver failure.
Kidney Function: In moderate to severe kidney problems, the dose is decreased by 25–50%.

▷ **Dosing Instructions:** Tablets may be crushed and are best taken on an empty stomach. If nausea or indigestion occurs, may be taken with or following food. Liquid intake should be no less than 3 quarts every 24 hours to reduce risk of bladder irritation and help keep your kidneys flushed. If you forget a dose, take it right away unless it's nearly time for your next regular dose. If it IS nearly time, just take the scheduled dose. DO NOT double doses.

Usual Duration of Use: Use on a regular schedule is required to achieve and maintain a significant cancer remission. Initial response often happens in 1 to 3 weeks. Duration depends on response of the cancer and patient tolerance of the drug. Your doctor will help decide.

Typical Treatment Goals and Measurements (Outcomes and Markers)
Cancer chemotherapy: The balance here is a difficult one of killing cancer cells versus toxic effects of the medicine itself (bone marrow suppression, heart, and others). Complete blood cell counts, assessment of the cancer (as in disappearance of soft tissue bumps or masses in multiple myeloma), and resolution of increased calcium are typical markers.

▷ **This Drug Should Not Be Taken If**
- you have had an allergic reaction to it previously.
- you have an active infection of any kind, or your bone marrow is severely suppressed.
- you have bloody urine for any reason.
- you are pregnant (exposure through a sexual partner may also cause fetal damage) or are breast-feeding your infant.

▷ **Inform Your Physician Before Taking This Drug If**
- you have impaired liver, heart, or kidney function.
- you have a blood cell or bone marrow disorder.
- you have had previous chemotherapy or X-ray therapy for any type of cancer.
- you take, or have taken within the past year, any cortisonelike drug (adrenal corticosteroids).
- you have diabetes.
- you will have surgery with general anesthesia.

Possible Side Effects (natural, expected, and unavoidable drug actions)
Bone marrow depression (see Glossary)—low production of white blood cells and, to a lesser degree, red blood cells, and blood platelets (see Glossary). Fever, chills, sore throat, fatigue, weakness, abnormal bleeding, or

bruising. Leukemia has been reported following cyclophosphamide therapy. Impairment of natural resistance (immunity) to infection. Weakening of the heart muscle (cardiomyopathy). Excessive urination (SIADH). Cystitis or hemorrhagic cystitis. Up to ninefold increase in bladder cancer risk. Some combination regimens (such as cyclophosphamide, methotrexate, and fluorouracil-CMF) have been associated with changes in thinking (mental status change).

▷ **Possible Adverse Effects** (unusual, unexpected, and infrequent reactions)
   If any of the following develop, consult your physician promptly for guidance.
   Mild Adverse Effects
   Allergic reaction: skin rash—rare.
   Headache, dizziness, blurred vision—possible.
   Loss of scalp hair (50% of users), darkening of skin and fingernails, transverse ridging of nails.
   Nausea, vomiting (dose-related)—frequent.
   Ulceration of mouth, diarrhea (may be bloody)—possible.
   Serious Adverse Effects
   Idiosyncratic reaction: hemolytic anemia—case reports.
   Allergic reaction: anaphylaxis—possible.
   Heart damage (cardiomyopathy)—possible and associated with higher doses (18-270 mg/kg).
   Liver damage with jaundice: yellow eyes and skin, dark-colored urine, light-colored stools—rare.
   Kidney damage: impaired kidney function, reduced urine volume, bloody urine—case reports.
   Lowered white blood cell (granulocyte) colony formation—possible even with rheumatoid arthritis use.
   Leukemia—reported.
   Severe inflammation of bladder: painful urination, bloody urine—infrequent to frequent.
   Syndrome of inappropriate antidiuretic hormone secretion (SIADH)—rare.
   Increased potassium (hyperkalemia)—possible.
   Intestinal or stomach bleeding (hemorrhagic colitis or GI bleed)—possible.
   Drug-induced damage of heart and lung (interstitial pneumonitis) tissue—case reports.
   Pancreatitis—case reports.

▷ **Possible Effects on Sexual Function:** Suppression of ovaries (ovarian function)—irregular menstrual pattern or cessation of menstruation (amenorrhea): 18 to 57%, depending upon dose and duration of use.
   Testicular suppression—reduced or no sperm production (100% of users).

Possible Delayed Adverse Effects: Development of other types of cancer (secondary malignancies). Development of severe cystitis with bleeding from the bladder wall (may occur many months after the last dose).

Possible Effects on Laboratory Tests
   Complete blood cell counts: decreased red cells, hemoglobin, white cells, and platelets.
   Blood sodium levels: decreased in SIADH (rare).
   Blood potassium: may be increased.
   INR (prothrombin time): increased.
   Liver function tests: increased liver enzymes (ALT/GPT, AST/GOT, and alkaline phosphatase), increased bilirubin.

CAUTION

1. This drug may interfere with the normal healing of wounds.
2. This drug can cause significant changes in genetic material in both men and women (sperm and eggs or ova). Patients taking this drug must understand the potential for serious defects in children who are conceived during or following the course of medication.
3. This drug can suppress natural resistance (immunity) to infection, resulting in life-threatening illness.
4. Avoid live-virus vaccines while taking this drug (talk with your doctor about this and other vaccines prior to starting therapy).

Precautions for Use

By Infants and Children: This drug should not be given if the child is dehydrated. Adequate fluid intake to ensure a copious urine volume for 4 hours following each dose is needed. Prevent exposure of child to anyone with active chickenpox or shingles. This drug may cause ovarian or testicular sterility.

By Those Over 60 Years of Age: Increased risk of serious bladder problems (chemical cystitis). Patients MUST drink large amounts of water in order to keep the bladder flushed. This may increase the risk of urinary retention in men with prostatism (see Glossary).

▷ **Advisability of Use During Pregnancy**

Pregnancy Category: D. See Pregnancy Risk Categories at the back of this book.

Animal Studies: Significant birth defects reported in mice, rat, and rabbit studies.

Human Studies: Information from studies of pregnant women indicates that this drug can cause serious birth defects or fetal death.

Avoid completely during the first 3 months. Use of this drug during the last 6 months must be carefully individualized.

Advisability of Use If Breast-Feeding

Presence of this drug in breast milk: Yes.

Avoid drug or refrain from nursing.

Habit-Forming Potential: None.

Effects of Overdose: Nausea, vomiting, diarrhea, bloody urine, water retention, weight gain, severe bone marrow depression, severe infections.

Possible Effects of Long-Term Use: Development of fibrous tissue in lungs; secondary malignancies.

Suggested Periodic Examinations While Taking This Drug (at physician's discretion)

Complete blood cell counts, every 2 to 4 days during initial treatment and then every 3 to 4 weeks during maintenance treatment. Signs and symptoms of bleeding.

Liver and kidney function tests, potassium.

Thyroid function tests (if symptoms warrant).

▷ **While Taking This Drug, Observe the Following**

Foods: No restrictions.

Herbal Medicines or Minerals: Echinacea: Some patients use echinacea to attempt to boost their immune systems. Unfortunately, use of echinacea is not recommended in people with damaged immune systems. This herb may also actually weaken any immune system if it is used too often or for too long a time. Talk to your doctor before taking any herbal medicine with cyclophosphamide.

Beverages: No restrictions. May be taken with milk.

▷   *Alcohol:* No interactions expected.

Tobacco Smoking: No interactions expected. I advise everyone to quit smoking.

▷   *Other Drugs*

Cyclophosphamide *taken concurrently* with

- allopurinol (Zyloprim) may increase the extent of bone marrow depression.
- amphotericin (Abelcet and others) may increase risk of kidney toxicity.
- chloramphenicol can decrease cyclophosphamide effectiveness.
- ciprofloxacin (Cipro) can result in lowered ciprofloxacin levels and the need for a larger than usual dose.
- digoxin (Lanoxin) may decrease digoxin absorption and impair digoxin's effectiveness.
- flu (influenza) vaccine, and perhaps other vaccines, may decrease the vaccine's ability to confer immunity.
- hydrochlorothiazide and other thiazide diuretics (see Drug Classes) may worsen the lowering of white blood cells (myelosuppression) caused by cyclophosphamide. Watch for combination blood pressure pills that may contain "hidden thiazides."
- indomethacin (Indocin) can cause fluid retention.
- live-virus vaccines should be avoided.
- ondansetron (Zofran) may blunt benefits of cyclophosphamide.
- pentostatin may cause fatal heart damage.
- ritonavir (Norvir) may lead to cyclophosphamide toxicity.
- succinylcholine can result in succinylcholine toxicity.
- tamoxifen (Nolvadex) can increase blood clot risk.
- traztuzumab (Herceptin) may increase the risk of heart problems (congestive heart failure or ventricular dysfunction).

▷   *Driving, Hazardous Activities:* Use caution if dizziness occurs.

Aviation Note: The use of this drug *may be a disqualification* for piloting. Consult a designated Aviation Medical Examiner.

Exposure to Sun: No restrictions.

Occurrence of Unrelated Illness: Any signs of infection—fever, chills, sore throat, cough, or flu-like symptoms—must be promptly reported. This drug may have to be stopped until the infection is controlled. Consult your physician.

CYCLOSPORINE (SI kloh spor een)

Other Names: Ciclosporin, cyclosporin A

Introduced: 1983   **Class:**   Immunosuppressant   **Prescription:**
USA: Yes   **Controlled Drug:**   USA: No; Canada: No   **Available as**
Generic: USA: Yes; Canada: No

Brand Names: Neoral, Sandimmune, SangCya, Sangstat

336   Cyclosporine

<table>
<tr><td colspan="2" align="center">**BENEFITS versus RISKS**</td></tr>
<tr><td align="center">*Possible Benefits*</td><td align="center">*Possible Risks*</td></tr>
<tr><td>EFFECTIVE PREVENTION AND TREATMENT OF REJECTION IN ORGAN TRANSPLANTATION
Some use treating severe rheumatoid arthritis, psoriasis, and other inflammatory (autoimmune) conditions</td><td>MARKED KIDNEY TOXICITY
DEVELOPMENT OF HYPERTENSION
HIGH BLOOD PRESSURE
Liver toxicity
Low white blood cell count
Development of lymphoma
Excessive hair growth
Blunted response to vaccines (best given 3–4 weeks BEFORE cyclosporine is started)</td></tr>
</table>

▷ **Principal Uses**

As a Single Drug Product: Uses included in FDA-approved labeling: (1) Helps prevent (in conjunction with cortisonelike drugs) organ rejection in kidney, liver and heart transplantation; (2) helps treat rejection crisis; (3) the Neoral microemulsion form and Sandimmune treats severe active rheumatoid arthritis; (4) treats refractory psoriasis.

Other (unlabeled) generally accepted uses: (1) Used in transplantation of the bone marrow; (2) used investigationally in a variety of diseases involving the immune system such as: Sjögren's, Crohn's, and Grave's diseases; ulcerative colitis; psoriasis; myasthenia gravis; bullous pemphigoid; pulmonary fibrosis associated with rheumatoid arthritis; Sweet's syndrome; insulin-dependent diabetes; systemic lupus erythematosus (SLE); large granular lymphocytic leukemia; and some anemias; (3) severe, steroid-dependent asthma; (4) treats severe skin reactions (toxic epidermal necrolysis) to phenytoin (Dilantin).

How This Drug Works: By inhibiting some lymphocytes (white blood cells) and their growth factors, this drug suppresses the rejection of transplanted organs.

▷ **Widely Used Guidelines That Involve This Medicine (representative sample):** Please look at the section at the very beginning of this profile called "Class." Next, turn to Table 22 and you will find guidelines listed by the class involved!

Available Dosage Forms and Strengths
Capsules, soft gelatin — 25 mg, 100 mg
Injection, intravenous — 50 mg/mL
Oral solution — 100 mg/mL (Note: The microemulsion Neoral is NOT the same as Sandimmune.)

▷ **Usual Adult Dosage Ranges:** *Transplantation:* Initially 15 mg per kg of body mass intravenously (some clinicians use higher doses, but this is not common), the chosen dose is given 4–12 hours prior to transplantation surgery. The drug is then continued after surgery at the same dose for up to 14 days. Clinicians use the lowest blood levels (trough) to adjust dosing. After this, the dose is usually lowered (tapered) by 5% per week to an ongoing dose taken by mouth that is equal to 5–10 mg per kg of body weight each day. Sandimmune should be given with corticosteroids.

If a conversion is made from oral Sandimmune to Neoral, Neoral dose is usually started at the same daily dose as Sandimmune, given at the same time each day in two equally divided doses. Cyclosporine trough levels should be measured twice weekly in people who were taking more than 10 mg per kg of body mass per day of Sandimmune. Dosing of SangCya and Neoral is always given in two divided doses.

Crohn's disease or severe/refractory ulcerative colitis: Therapy is started with 8–10 mg/kg/day with the medicine adjusted to response and a maximum treatment length of 6 months.

Note: Actual dose and schedule must be determined for each patient individually.

Conditions Requiring Dosing Adjustments

Liver Function: The dose must be adjusted (based on blood levels) in liver compromise. Much of the drug is eliminated in the bile.

Kidney Function: This drug is capable of causing marked kidney toxicity. Caution is critical. One set of guidelines for rheumatoid arthritis suggested that cyclosporine dosing should be adjusted to serum creatinine. For example, if serum creatinine increases more than 30% above the starting level (baseline) in two tests taken a week apart, then the cyclosporine dose is lowered by 0.5 to 0.75 mg/kg/day. If the creatinine returns to less than 30% of the starting level—cyclosporine can be continued. If the serum creatinine stays up, cyclosporine is stopped for 30 days and is restarted if creatinine decreases to 15% of the starting level. As in other cases of increasing creatinine, the medicines being taken at the same time should be evaluated for possible adverse impact on kidney function.

Diabetes: People who are diabetic and subsequently have kidney or pancreatic transplants will need larger than usual doses.

Hypercholesterolemia: If the blood cholesterol is 50% above normal, the dose must be decreased by 50% in order to avoid toxicity.

Obesity: Dosing **must** be based on ideal (a calculation that helps eliminate the weight that is fat) body weight.

Cystic Fibrosis: It is very difficult to appropriately dose this medication in patients who have this disease. Some patients will require as much as two times the usual dose. The dose should be adjusted to drug levels.

Multiple Organ Transplants: Patients with multiple transplants (such as pancreas and kidney) often need an increased dose of cyclosporine in order to achieve the desired effect. The dose should be determined based on blood levels.

▷ **Dosing Instructions:** Preferably taken with or immediately following food to reduce stomach irritation. The capsule should be swallowed whole; do not open, crush, or chew. The oral solution should be carefully measured and can be mixed with milk, chocolate milk, or orange juice (at room temperature) in a glass or ceramic cup; do not use a wax-lined or plastic cup or container. Stir well and drink immediately. Use the same liquid to dilute the dose, because different liquids may change the amount that gets into your body. Blood levels are important. DO NOT take this medicine with grapefruit juice. It is also best to take this drug at the same time each day to maintain steady blood levels.

Usual Duration of Use: Use on a regular schedule for several weeks is usually needed to prevent organ rejection or stop rejection already underway. Benefits in psoriasis or rheumatoid arthritis may take 4 to 8 weeks. Long-term use (months to years) requires follow-up by your doctor. If you forget a dose: Take the dose you missed as soon as possible, unless it's nearly time for your next dose. If that is the case, skip the missed dose and take the next scheduled dose. DO NOT double doses. If you find yourself missing doses, talk to your doctor.

▷ **This Drug Should Not Be Taken If**
   • you have had an allergic reaction to it previously. Attention should be paid to the ingredients also present in many forms of this medicine (such as castor oil).
   • you are getting radiation treatment.
   • you have uncontrolled high blood pressure and are taking this medicine to treat rheumatoid arthritis.
   • you have an active lymphoma or a malignancy of any type.
   • you are taking this medicine to control psoriasis and are getting PUVA treatment.
   • you have an active, uncontrolled infection, especially chickenpox or shingles.

▷ **Inform Your Physician Before Taking This Drug If**
   • you are taking any immunosuppressant drug other than cortisonelike preparations.
   • you are pregnant or breast-feeding.
   • you have a history of liver or kidney disease or impaired liver or kidney function.
   • you have a history of hypertension or gout.
   • you have a chronic gastrointestinal disorder.
   • you are taking a potassium supplement or drugs that can raise the blood level of potassium.
   • you have a seizure disorder.
   • you have a history of a blood cell disorder.
   • you take other medicines toxic to the kidney.

Possible Side Effects (natural, expected, and unavoidable drug actions)
   Predisposition to infections (such as pneumocystis). Drug fever—possible.

▷ **Possible Adverse Effects** (unusual, unexpected, and infrequent reactions)
   If any of the following develop, consult your physician promptly for guidance.
   Mild Adverse Effects
   Allergic reactions: skin rash, itching—case reports.
   Excessive hair growth—frequent in transplant patients.
   Acne—rare.
   Headache, confusion, anxiety, or mood alterations—infrequent.
   Tremors (dose dependent)—frequent.
   Mouth sores—rare.
   Gum overgrowth—frequent in some reports.
   Nausea/vomiting, diarrhea—infrequent.
   Changes in facial features (dysmorphosis)—possible with longer-term therapy.
   Serious Adverse Effects
   Allergic reactions: anaphylactic reaction (see Glossary) to intravenous solution—case reports.
   Kidney injury (25% kidney transplant, 37% liver, and 38% heart)—frequent.
   Hypertension, mild to severe (up to half of patients getting this drug)—frequent.
   Blood total cholesterol: increased (while HDL decreased).
   Seizures—rare to frequent (kidney, 1.8%; bone marrow, 5.5%; up to 25% of liver transplant patients).
   Cortical blindness—case reports.

Hearing loss (ototoxicity)—rare.

Hallucinations, movement problems (catatonia), dementia, or coma (may all derive from encephalopathy)—case reports.

Nerve damage (neurotoxicity)—possible and usually reversible when the medicine is stopped, but may be permanent.

Liver injury—infrequent and dose dependent.

Pancreatitis—rare.

Low white blood cell count (leukopenia)—infrequent.

Low blood platelets (thrombocytopenia)—rare.

Abnormal blood clots (thromboembolic complications)—case reports (usually in the first week, but up to 30 days after the medicine was started).

High blood potassium levels, blood sugar (glucose) increases, uric acid levels (and gout), increased blood cholesterol, or low blood magnesium—all possible.

Lymphoma, possibly drug-induced—rare to infrequent.

Relapse of lupus erythematosus—case reports.

Increased risk of skin cancers (risk increased by sun or UV light exposure).

▷ **Possible Effects on Sexual Function:** Enlargement and tenderness of male breast (gynecomastia—1 to 4%)—rare to infrequent.

Adverse Effects That May Mimic Natural Diseases or Disorders

Liver toxicity may suggest viral hepatitis.

Natural Diseases or Disorders That May Be Activated by This Drug

Latent infections, hypertension, gout.

Possible Effects on Laboratory Tests

Complete blood cell counts: decreased red cells, hemoglobin, and white cells.

Blood potassium level or uric acid level: increased.

Blood platelets, white cells, magnesium: decreased.

Liver function tests: increased liver enzymes (ALT/GPT, AST/GOT, and alkaline phosphatase), increased bilirubin.

Kidney function tests: blood creatinine and urea nitrogen levels (BUN) increased; urine casts present.

Total cholesterol: increased. HDL: decreased.

CAUTION

1. Report promptly any indications of infection of any kind.
2. Promptly report swollen glands, sores or lumps in the skin, abnormal bleeding or bruising.
3. Call your doctor immediately if you become pregnant.
4. Periodic laboratory tests are mandatory.
5. It is best to avoid live-virus vaccines, and contact with people who have recently taken them (such as oral poliovirus vaccine). Other shots (vaccines) should be given 3–4 weeks BEFORE cyclosporine is started in order to get the best results from them.

Precautions for Use

By Infants and Children: This drug has been used successfully and safely in children of all ages. Dosing is made on the adult schedule in some cases, while others require increased dosing.

By Those Over 60 Years of Age: The dose must be adjusted to any decline in kidney function.

▷ **Advisability of Use During Pregnancy**

Pregnancy Category: C. See Pregnancy Risk Categories at the back of this book.

Animal Studies: Rat and rabbit studies reveal that this drug is toxic to the embryo and fetus. No drug-induced birth defects were found.

Human Studies: Adequate studies of pregnant women are not available.

Avoid this drug during entire pregnancy unless it is clearly needed.

Advisability of Use If Breast-Feeding

Presence of this drug in breast milk: Yes.

Avoid drug or refrain from nursing.

Habit-Forming Potential: None.

Effects of Overdose: Headache, pain, facial flushing, gum soreness and bleeding, high blood pressure, atrial fibrillation, respiratory distress, seizures, coma, hallucinations, neurotoxicity, electrolyte disturbances, liver toxicity.

Possible Effects of Long-Term Use: Irreversible kidney damage, severe hypertension, abnormal growth of gums.

Suggested Periodic Examinations While Taking This Drug (at physician's discretion)

Cyclosporine blood levels.

Complete blood counts.

Liver and kidney function tests.

Magnesium, potassium, and uric acid blood levels.

Cholesterol with fractions (including LDL fractions).

Blood pressure checks.

▷ **While Taking This Drug, Observe the Following**

Foods: Food may increase the peak blood level of cyclosporine.

Herbal Medicines or Minerals: Some patients use echinacea to attempt to boost their immune systems when they are ill. Use of echinacea is not recommended in people taking medicines to suppress their immune systems. Do NOT take mistletoe herb, oak bark, F.C. of marshmallow root, and licorice. There have been case reports of heart transplant rejection with combined use of cyclosporine and St. John's wort. DO NOT COMBINE THESE. Cyclosporine may deplete magnesium from the body. Ask your doctor if supplementation with magnesium makes sense for you. Potassium levels may be increased by cyclosporine. Avoid excessive intake of high-potassium foods. See Table 13.

Beverages: Grapefruit juice and other fruit juices increase blood levels. Milk may increase blood levels.

▷ *Alcohol:* Large amounts of alcohol may increase cyclosporine levels.

Tobacco Smoking: This interaction has not been well studied. I advise everyone to quit smoking.

▷ *Other Drugs*

Cyclosporine *taken concurrently* with

- ACE inhibitors (see Drug Classes) may increase the risk of kidney problems.
- acyclovir (Zovirax) may lead to increased cyclosporine levels. CAREFUL check of cyclosporine blood levels is recommended.
- aminoglycoside antibiotics (see Drug Classes) may increase kidney toxicity.
- amphotericin B (Abelcet, others) can cause serious kidney toxicity.
- amprenavir (Agenerase) may increase blood levels, resulting in cyclosporine toxicity. More frequent cyclosporine blood levels are prudent.
- aspirin substitutes (nonsteroidal anti-inflammatory drugs or NSAIDs) may increase kidney toxicity.

- atorvastatin (Lipitor), fluvastatin (Lescol), lovastatin (Mevacor, Advicor), pravastatin (Pravachol), rosuvastatin (Crestor), and simvastatin (Zocor) may result in increased risk of muscle damage or rhabdomyolysis. If a patient requires combination therapy, very close patient follow-up and education regarding immediately reporting unexplained muscle pain, weakness, or tenderness should be given along with instructions as to who to call.
- azathioprine (Imuran) may increase immunosuppression.
- calcium channel blockers (see Drug Classes) may result in cyclosporine toxicity.
- clonidine (Catapres) can increase risk of kidney problems.
- ciprofloxacin (Cipro) and other fluoroquinolones—(see Drug Classes) may increase risk of kidney toxicity.
- cotrimoxazole (Bactrim, others) may result in decreased cyclosporine effectiveness as well as kidney toxicity.
- cyclophosphamide (Cytoxan) may increase immunosuppression.
- digoxin (Lanoxin) may result in serious digoxin toxicity.
- furosemide (Lasix) may result in increased risk of gout.
- ganciclovir (Cytovene) may result in increased kidney toxicity.
- histamine (H2) inhibitors (see Drug Classes) and ketoconazole may experience decreased cyclosporine blood levels.
- imipenem/cilastatin (Primaxin) may result in neurotoxicity.
- methylprednisolone (Medrol) may cause seizures.
- metronidazole (Flagyl) may result in increased cyclosporine levels and toxicity.
- nifedipine (Adalat) may worsen abnormal gum growth (gingival hyperplasia) and also cause nifedipine toxicity (low blood pressure and abnormal heartbeats).
- propafenone (Rythmol) may increase risk of cyclosporine toxicity.
- saquinavir (Fortovase, Invirase) may increase risk of cyclosporine toxicity.
- sirolimus (Rapamune) can cause sirolimus toxicity. Separate dosing by four hours.
- spironolactone (various) may increase risk of excessive potassium levels.
- sulfamethoxazole and/or trimethoprim (Septra) may increase kidney toxicity.
- tacrolimus (Prograf) can cause kidney toxicity.
- thiazide diuretics (see Drug Classes) may increase adverse effects on the blood (myelosuppression).
- triamterine (various) may increase risk of excessive potassium levels.
- vaccines may blunt the benefit of the vaccine. Vaccines are best given 3–4 weeks BEFORE cyclosporine is started.
- valproic acid (Depakene, others) lead to liver toxicity in one patient.
- verapamil (Calan) may increase immunosuppression.
- warfarin (Coumadin) may lower anticoagulant benefits of warfarin.

The following drugs may **increase** the effects of cyclosporine:
- acetazolamide.
- allopurinol (Zyloprim).
- amiodarone (Cordarone).
- ceftriaxone (Rocephin).
- cimetidine (Tagamet).
- cisapride (Propulsid).
- clarithromycin (Biaxin).
- clotrimazole (Mycelex, Gyne-Lotrimin, others).
- colchicine (Colbenemid).
- dalfopristin (Synercid or quinupristin/dalfopristin).

- danazol or other anabolic steroids.
- diltiazem (Cardizem).
- econazole (Spectazole).
- erythromycin (E.E.S., others).
- fluconazole (Diflucan).
- fluvoxamine (Luvox).
- glipizide (Glucotrol) or glyburide (Diabeta).
- grepafloxacin (Raxar).
- imatinib (Gleevec).
- itraconazole (Sporanox).
- ketoconazole (Nizoral).
- medicines that inhibit cytochrome P-450 3A4 liver enzymes. Caution is advised.
- methotrexate (Rheumatrex).
- methyltestosterone (various).
- metoclopramide (Reglan).
- miconazole (Lotrimin, Micatin).
- nonsteroidal anti-inflammatory agents (see Drug Classes).
- oral contraceptives (birth control pills).
- ritonavir (Norvir), amprenavir (Agenerase), and atazanavir (Reyataz).
- tamoxifen (Nolvadex).
- terconazole (Terazol).
- ticarcillin/clavulanic acid (Timentin).

The following drugs may **decrease** the effects of cyclosporine:
- carbamazepine (Tegretol).
- carvedilol (Coreg).
- clindamycin (various).
- isoniazid (INH).
- nafcillin.
- octreotide (Sandostatin).
- orlistat (Xenical).
- omeprazole (Prilosec).
- phenobarbital.
- phenytoin (Dilantin) or fosphenytoin (Cerebyx).
- quinine.
- rifabutin (Mycobutin).
- rifampin (Rifadin).
- sulfadimidine, sulfadiazine, and/or trimethoprim.
- ticlopidine (Ticlid).
- warfarin (Coumadin).

▷ *Driving, Hazardous Activities:* This drug may cause confusion or seizures. Restrict activities as necessary.

Aviation Note: The use of this drug **may be a disqualification** for piloting. Consult a designated Aviation Medical Examiner.

Exposure to Sun: Exposure to sunlight or other ultraviolet (UV) radiation may increase the risk of skin cancer.

Discontinuation: Do not stop this drug without your physician's guidance.

Special Storage Instructions: Keep the gelatin capsules in the blister packets until ready for use. Store below 77 degrees F. (25 degrees C.). Keep the oral solution in a tightly closed container. Store below 86 degrees F. (30 degrees C.). Do not refrigerate or freeze it.

Observe the Following Expiration Times: The oral solution must be used within 2 months after opening.

DESIPRAMINE (des IP ra meen)

Introduced: 1964 **Class:** Antidepressant **Prescription:** USA: Yes **Controlled Drug:** USA: No; Canada: No **Available as Generic:** USA: Yes; Canada: Yes

Brand Names: ✤Apo-desipramine, Deprexan, Norpramin, Pertofrane

Author's Note: Information in this profile has been shortened to make room for more widely used medicines.

DEXAMETHASONE (dex a METH a sohn)

Introduced: 1958 **Class:** Cortisonelike drugs **Prescription:** USA: Yes **Controlled Drug:** USA: No; Canada: No **Available as Generic:** USA: Yes; Canada: Yes

Brand Names: Aeroseb-Dex, ✤Ak-Dex, Ak-Trol [CD], Baldex, Dalalone, Dalalone DP, Dalalone LA, Decaderm, Decadron, Decadron Nasal Spray, Decadron-LA, Decadron Phosphate Ophthalmic, Decadron Phosphate Respihaler, Decadron Phosphate Turbinaire, Decadron w/Xylocaine [CD], Decadron dose pack, Decaject, Decaject LA, Decaspray, Deenar [CD], Deone-LA, ✤Deronil, Dex-4, Dexacen-4, Dexacen LA-8, Dexacidin [CD], Dexacort, Dexameth, Dexasone, Dexasone-LA, Dexo-LA, Dexon, Dexone-E, Dexone-4, Dexone-LA, Dexsone, Dexsone-E, Dexsone-LA, Dezone, Duo-dezone, Gammacorten, Hexadrol, Maxidex, Mymethasone, ✤Neodecadron Eye-Ear, Neodexair, Neomycin-Dex, Ocu-Trol [CD], ✤Oradexon, ✤PMS-Dexamethasone, ✤SK-Dexamethasone, ✤Sofracort, Solurex, Solurex-LA, ✤Spersadex, Tobradex [CD], Turbinaire

---

BENEFITS versus RISKS

Possible Benefits	*Possible Risks*
EFFECTIVE RELIEF OF SYMPTOMS IN A WIDE VARIETY OF INFLAMMATORY AND ALLERGIC DISORDERS EFFECTIVE IMMUNOSUPPRESSION IN SELECTED BENIGN AND MALIGNANT DISORDERS COMBINED WITH TOBRAMYCIN TO FIGHT BOTH INFECTION AND INFLAMMATION IN THE EYE	Ongoing systemic use (variable onset) can be associated with increased possible emergence of effects such as: ALTERED OR CHANGED MOOD AND PERSONALITY, CATARACTS, GLAUCOMA, HYPERTENSION, ARRHYTHMIAS, PEPTIC ULCERS, PANCREATITIS, OSTEOPOROSIS, INCREASED SUSCEPTIBILITY TO INFECTIONS, AND OTHERS ASCEPTIC BONE NECROSIS (OSTEONECROSIS) IS AN AREA OF CONTROVERSY, UNCLEAR ONSET, PATIENT RISK FACTORS, AND CORRELATION VERSUS CAUSATION (SEE CONTROVERSIES IN MEDICINE)

▷ **Principal Uses**

As a Single Drug Product: Uses currently included in FDA-approved labeling: (1) Used to manage serious skin disorders (such as Stevens-Johnson syndrome, exfoliative dermatitis, etc.), asthma, allergic rhinitis, lymphoma, brain edema, shock, systemic lupus erythematosus, and all types of major rheumatic disorders including bursitis, tendonitis, and most forms of arthritis; (2) ulcerative disease of the colon; (3) topical cream is used to treat eczema, psoriasis, dermatitis, and lichen planus; (4) used in conjunction with antibiotics in meningitis; (5) helps ease swelling in otitis media.

Other (unlabeled) generally accepted uses: (1) Adrenal insufficiency; (2) acute airway obstruction; (3) mountain sickness; (4) vomiting caused by chemotherapy; (5) cardiopulmonary bypass; (6) refractory depression; (7) relief of brain cancer symptoms; (8) combination with other drugs in multiple myeloma; (9) cases of *Pneumocystis carinii* pneumonia; (10) can help suppress male hormones (androgens) in women with acne, hirsutism, or hair loss (androgenic alopecia) caused by androgens; (11) eases vomiting after cancer treatment (chemotherapy); (12) single doses may have a role in croup.

How This Drug Works: Inhibits defensive functions of certain white blood cells. It reduces the production of lymphocytes and some antibodies and acts as an immunosuppressant. When combined with tobramycin or other antibiotics in the eye, it helps relieve inflammation and pain while the antibiotic kills the infection.

▷ **Widely Used Guidelines That Involve This Medicine (representative sample):** Please look at the section at the very beginning of this profile called "Class." Next, turn to Table 22 and you will find guidelines listed by the class involved!

Available Dosage Forms and Strengths

Aerosol — 0.01% and 0.04%

Aerosol inhaler — 84 mcg per spray

Cream — 0.1%

Elixir — 0.5 mg/5 mL

Eye ointment — 0.05%

Eye solution — 0.1%

Eye suspension — 0.1% dexamethasone, 0.3% tobramycin

Gel — 0.1%

Injection — 4 mg/mL, 8 mg/mL, 10 mg/mL, 16 mg/mL, 20 mg/mL, 24 mg/mL

Oral solution — 0.5 mg/0.5 mL, 0.5 mg/5 mL

Solution — 0.1%

Spray, topical — 10 mg/25 g

Suspension — 0.1%

Tablets — 0.25 mg, 0.5 mg, 0.75 mg, 1 mg, 1.5 mg, 2 mg, 4 mg, 6 mg

▷ **Usual Adult Dosage Ranges**

Respihaler: For asthma, three inhalations taken three to four times a day in asthmatics whose asthma is unresponsive to other medicines.

Turbinaire form: Two sprays in each nostril two or three times daily. Twelve sprays is the daily maximum.

Decadron dose pack form: On the first day, 1 or 2 mL is given as an intramuscular injection (IM). On the second day, four tablets are taken—divided into two equal doses (such as two in the morning at 9 A.M. and two at 9 P.M.). The third day, the same tablet dose is given, the fourth day two tablets are given in two equal doses, the fifth and sixth day one tablet a day is given, and treatment is stopped on the seventh day (tapering schedule).

Ophthalmic: Tobradex form is often started as one to two drops into the eye sac or sacs (conjunctival) every 2 hours during the first day or two of treatment. The dosing frequency is then gradually decreased to one or two drops every 4–6 hours depending on the severity and response of the infection to treatment.

Oral: 0.75 to 9 mg daily divided into two to four doses—depending on the condition.

Topical (0.1% cream): Apply thin film of medicine on the affected area three or four times a day.

Oral dose for children: 0.03 to 0.15 mg per kg of body mass per day, divided into equal doses given every 6 to 12 hours, or 1–5 mg per square meter divided into equal doses and given every 6 to 12 hours.

Note: Actual dose and schedule must be determined for each patient individually.

Conditions Requiring Dosing Adjustments

Liver Function: This drug is eliminated via the liver; however, no specific guidelines for dosing adjustments are available.

Kidney Function: Use with caution as it can cause alkalosis (a change toward a more basic condition in the body's chemistry).

Obesity: Deciding how much medicine (dosing) on a mg-per-kg-of-body-mass-per-day basis is recommended. It is best to measure free urinary cortisol as well.

▷ **Dosing Instructions:** Tablet may be crushed (if required) and taken with or following food to prevent stomach irritation, preferably in the morning. If you forget a dose: (suspension, solution): take the missed dose right after you remember it. If it is nearly time for your next scheduled dose, skip the missed dose and continue with the scheduled dose. DO NOT double doses. If you only take this medicine every other day, take the dose you forgot right away, unless it's late in the day. If you only remember late in the day, wait until the next morning to take the missed dose and then continue on your every other day schedule. If you forget a dose of the shot (IM injection), call your doctor for instructions.

Usual Duration of Use: Varies with the problem: 4 to 10 days, generally. Dose, patient reaction to tapering, disease flare, and other factors must be considered and individualized to the condition being treated.

For chronic disorders: varies. Length of therapy should not exceed time needed for adequate symptomatic relief in sudden (acute) self-limiting conditions or time required to stabilize a chronic condition and permit gradual and appropriate, individualized withdrawal. Disease flares may indicate need for reassessment of dosing and/or tapering.

Typical Treatment Goals and Measurements (Outcomes and Markers)

Inflammation: The general goal is to relieve the swelling and the inflammatory response. Use in asthma should help decrease the frequency and severity of acute attacks. Some clinicians use decreased frequency of rescue inhaler use as a measure of success. Lung (pulmonary function) testing and improvement in those tests also helps define results in asthma. Lastly, clinical signs and symptoms such as wheezing, tightness in the chest, and exercise tolerance should all move in favorable directions.

▷ **This Drug Should Not Be Taken If**
- you have had an allergic reaction to it previously.
- you have active peptic ulcer disease.

- you have an active herpes simplex, fungal or mycobacterial infection of the eye, or fungal ear infection.
- you have a systemic fungal infection (talk with your doctor).
- your sputum consistently grows *Candida albicans* (a yeast that may grow very quickly if steroids suppress your immune system).
- you have a psychoneurosis or psychosis.
- you have active tuberculosis.

▷ **Inform Your Physician Before Taking This Drug If**
- you have had unfavorable reactions to cortisonelike drugs.
- you have a history of peptic ulcer disease, thrombophlebitis, low blood platelets, or tuberculosis.
- you have diabetes, glaucoma, high blood pressure, deficient thyroid function, or myasthenia gravis.
- you start to have restricted motion, unexplained or increased pain (as in knees, hips, or shoulders), fever, or joint swelling while taking or after taking this medicine—may be early signs of aseptic necrosis (osteonecrosis). Call your doctor immediately.
- you have osteoporosis.
- you are taking an "in the nose form" (intranasal) and you have ongoing irritation of the nose.
- you have recently had a heart attack (may have a serious effect on the wall of the left ventricle).
- you plan to have surgery of any kind in the near future.

▷ **Possible Side Effects** (natural, expected, and unavoidable drug actions)
Increased appetite, weight gain, retention of salt and water, benign increase in head (intracranial) pressure—rare, but more likely with long-term use, excretion of potassium, increased susceptibility to infection (yeast infections can be frequent in cancer patients treated with a corticosteroid)—superinfection due to immune system suppression. Increased facial hair. Increased white blood cell count (release from the bone marrow versus a sign of infection). Nose irritation with nasal forms. **All of the possible and mild or serious adverse effects may happen with inhaled or even ophthalmic steroid use, but generally to a much reduced extent and/or severity.**

▷ **Possible Adverse Effects** (unusual, unexpected, and infrequent reactions)
If any of the following develop, consult your physician promptly for guidance.
Mild Adverse Effects
Allergic reaction: skin rash—case reports.
Headache, dizziness, insomnia—possible.
Mild depression or euphoria—most common possible central nervous system (CNS) effects.
High blood pressure (may be lessened by alternate-day therapy): more likely in older patients and those who already have high blood pressure—possible.
Acid indigestion, abdominal distention—possible.
Muscle cramping and weakness—case reports.
Slowing of growth in infants—possible and minimized by use of lowest effective dose and or alternate day treatment if possible.
Easy bruising (ecchymosis) or acne lesions—common after long-term high dose use.
Vaginal itching—may be frequent with intravenous dosing.
Serious Adverse Effects
Allergic reaction: anaphylaxis—case reports.

Mental and emotional disturbances of serious magnitude—infrequent.

Reactivation of latent tuberculosis—possible.

Pneumocystis carinii pneumonia—possible with immunosuppression and chronic use.

Development of peptic ulcer—rare, but risk increases with higher doses and preexisting ulcers.

Inflammation of the pancreas (pancreatitis)—rare.

Thrombophlebitis (inflammation of a vein with the formation of blood clot): pain or tenderness in thigh or leg or swelling of the foot, ankle, or leg—possible with intravenous use.

Abnormal lipids (cholesterol-mean increase 88mg/dL, triglyceride-mean increase 30 mg/mL, LDLs)—possible (may need to be addressed by lowest possible dose, diet, exercise, and even added medicines).

Abnormal heart rhythm—case reports.

Cushing's syndrome—possible with chronic use and high doses (supraphysiologic).

Suppression of the adrenal gland—possible with chronic use and more common with larger doses.

High blood sugar—risk increases with use in pre-diabetes, patients with family history of diabetes, with higher doses, and longer treatment duration.

Excessively low blood potassium—case reports.

Abnormally slow heartbeat in infants—case reports.

Increased pressure in the eye or cataracts or glaucoma—rare to frequent.

Precipitation of porphyria—case reports.

Excessive thyroid function (questionable causality)—case reports.

Fluid buildup in the lungs (pulmonary edema)—possible (more likely with combined ritodrine and dexamethasone treatment in threatened premature labor).

Muscle changes (myopathy)—infrequent, but more likely with higher doses and some steroids.

Bone death (aseptic necrosis, osteonecrosis, or avascular necrosis)—questions remain as to correlation versus causation, but may be more likely with high initial doses, long-term treatment, and cumulative doses of 4.32 grams—although cumulative dose is NOT an absolute. May also happen with short-term modest doses. Individual patient risk factors appear to be important. See controversies in medicine below.

Osteoporosis—more likely with long-term and higher-dose use.

▷ **Possible Effects on Sexual Function:** Altered timing and pattern of menstruation—case reports.

Adverse Effects That May Mimic Natural Diseases or Disorders

Pattern of symptoms and signs resembling Cushing's syndrome.

Natural Diseases or Disorders That May Be Activated by This Drug

Latent diabetes, glaucoma, peptic ulcer disease, tuberculosis.

Possible Effects on Laboratory Tests

Blood amylase level: increased (possible pancreatitis).

Blood glucose level: increased.

DEXA: possible decreased BMD.

Digoxin testing: may falsely increase digoxin results.

Glucose tolerance test (GTT): increased.

Blood potassium level: decreased.

Thyroid function tests: may be increased (questionable causation).

Cholesterol, LDL, triglycerides: increased.

CAUTION

1. It is best to carry a card noting that you are taking this drug, if your course of treatment is to exceed 1 week.
2. Do not stop this drug abruptly if it is used for long-term treatment.
3. If vaccination against measles, rabies, smallpox, or yellow fever is required, stop this drug 72 hours before vaccination and do not resume it for at least 14 days after vaccination.
4. Children may be more sensitive to topical application because there is a larger skin surface area to body weight ratio.
5. A variety of patient risk factors appear to be important in possible development of osteonecrosis. Talk to your doctor about the current list.

Controversies in Medicine: Medicines in this class have had conflicting reports regarding correlation with or causation of aseptic bone necrosis (osteonecrosis[ON]). There appear to be patient risk factors, possible delayed onset, occurrence even after the medicine is stopped, and some diseases or conditions where corticosteroids are often used and ON is more frequent than the general population. It is unclear if this is because of the disease/condition, patient risk factors, or the use of corticosteroids. Previous data regarding cumulative dosing (4.32 grams) appears controversial, with more recent case reports of 6 days of treatment with some doses being associated with ON. Some existing/emerging patient risk factors include alcohol use versus abuse, initial high doses, HIV positive patients who weight trained, Systemic Lupus Erythematosus, some clotting disorders, and high homocysteine levels amongst others appear to increase risk. Early research regarding use of alendronate (Fosamax) to treat ON appears to show that it is important for patients to quickly return to their doctors if unexplained joint pain (such as in the hip or knee) happens. Some centers note that ON has been poorly studied, and while the weight of data is growing, it is yet too early to say more than ON is correlated with corticosteroid use.

Precautions for Use

By Infants and Children: Avoid prolonged use if possible. During long-term use, watch for suppression of normal growth and the possibility of increased intracranial pressure. Following long-term use, the child may be at risk for adrenal gland deficiency during stress for as long as 18 months after cessation.

By Those Over 60 Years of Age: Avoid prolonged use of this drug if possible. Continual use (even in small doses) can increase the severity of diabetes, enhance fluid retention, raise blood pressure, weaken resistance to infection, induce stomach ulcer, and accelerate the development of cataracts and osteoporosis.

▷ Advisability of Use During Pregnancy

Pregnancy Category: C. See Pregnancy Risk Categories at the back of this book.
Animal Studies: Birth defects reported in mice, rats, and rabbits.
Human Studies: Adequate studies of pregnant women are not available.

Avoid completely during the first 3 months. Limit use during the last 6 months as much as possible. If used, examine infant for possible deficiency of adrenal gland function.

Advisability of Use If Breast-Feeding

Presence of this drug in breast milk: Yes.
Avoid drug or refrain from nursing.

Habit-Forming Potential: Use to suppress symptoms over an extended period of time may produce a state of functional dependence (see Glossary). In treating asthma and rheumatoid arthritis, it is best to keep the dose as small as possible and to attempt drug withdrawal after periods of reasonable improvement. Such procedures may reduce the degree of "steroid rebound"—the return of symptoms as the drug is withdrawn.

Effects of Overdose: Fatigue, muscle weakness, stomach irritation, acid indigestion, excessive sweating, facial flushing, fluid retention, swelling of extremities, increased blood pressure.

Possible Effects of Long-Term Use: Increased blood sugar (possible diabetes), increased fat deposits on the trunk of the body ("buffalo hump"), rounding of the face ("moon face"), thinning and fragility of skin, loss of texture and strength of bones (osteoporosis, aseptic necrosis—questionable correlation versus causation), cataracts, glaucoma, increased body hair (hirsutism), retarded growth and development in children.

Suggested Periodic Examinations While Taking This Drug (at physician's discretion)

Measurements of blood pressure, blood sugar, and potassium levels.

Complete eye examinations at regular intervals.

Chest X-ray if history of tuberculosis.

Determination of the rate of development of the growing child to detect retardation of normal growth.

Bone mineral density testing to assess risk of osteoporosis or thinning of bones.

Check on patient visit for unexplained joint pain (such as in the knee, hip, or shoulder). Further evaluation of any such development by MRI is prudent.

Homocysteine level (increased Homocysteine levels appear to be a risk factor for osteonecrosis).

▷ **While Taking This Drug, Observe the Following**

Foods: No interactions expected. Ask your physician about salt restriction or need for potassium-rich foods. During long-term use of this drug, it is advisable to eat a high-protein diet.

Herbal Medicines or Minerals: Hawthorn, ginger, garlic, ma huang, ginseng, and nettle may change blood sugar. Since dexamethasone may also change blood sugar control, caution is advised. Licorice may interfere with removal of this medicine—dexamethasone doses may need to be decreased and the combination is not recommended.

Fir or pine needle oil should NOT be used by asthmatics. Ephedra alone does carry a German Commission E monograph indication for asthma treatment. If you are allergic to plants in the Asteraceae family (aster, chrysanthemum, daisy, or ragweed), you may also be allergic to echinacea, chamomile, feverfew, and St. John's wort. Echinacea and ginseng may reverse some of the desired immunosuppression from this medicine. Combination is not advised.

During long-term use, take a vitamin D supplement and increase calcium. During wound repair, take a zinc supplement. Talk to your doctor BEFORE adding any herbal to any other medicines that you already take.

Beverages: No restrictions. Drink all forms of milk liberally.

▷ *Alcohol:* Alcohol use is a risk factor seen in osteonecrosis cases. Talk to your doctor about how he or she would like you to approach any alcohol use. Caution needed as well if you are prone to peptic ulcer disease.

Tobacco Smoking: Nicotine increases the blood levels of naturally produced cortisone and related hormones. Heavy smoking may add to the expected actions of this drug and requires close observation for excessive effects. I advise everyone to quit smoking.

Marijuana Smoking: May cause additional impairment of immunity and also is a risk factor for toxoplasmosis.

▷ *Other Drugs*

Dexamethasone may ***decrease*** the effects of

- amprenavir (Agenerase) and indinavir (Crixivan).
- caspofungin (Cancidas), requiring dosing increases in caspofungin.
- donepezil (Aricept). A different steroid should be used in patients on donepezil.
- imatinib (Gleevec), requiring dosing changes of imatinib (may need up to twice the usual dose).
- isoniazid (INH, Niconyl, etc.).
- quetiapine (Seroquel).
- salicylates (aspirin, sodium salicylate, etc.), increasing ulcer risk.
- vaccines (such as flu vaccine), by blunting the immune response to them.

Dexamethasone ***taken concurrently*** with

- aprepitant (Emend) may increase how much dexamethasone stays in your body. Dexamethasone doses should be decreased—some sources recommend half the usual dose.
- aspirin (various) and other NSAIDS (see Drug Classes) increases the risk of stomach and intestinal (gastrointestinal) ulceration.
- birth control pills (oral contraceptives) may increase dexamethasone's therapeutic effects.
- carbamazepine (Tegretol) will reduce the effectiveness of dexamethasone.
- irinotecan (Camptosar) may increase risk of low white blood cells (lymphocytopenia) and increase hyperglycemia risk. Caution and close patient monitoring advisable.
- loop diuretics such as furosemide (Lasix) or bumetanide (Bumex) can result in additive potassium loss.
- oral anticoagulants may either increase or decrease their effectiveness; ask your doctor about increased INR testing and dose adjustment.
- oral antidiabetic drugs (see Drug Classes) will decrease their effectiveness.
- neuromuscular blocking agents (such as pancuronium [Pavulon] or vecuronium [Norcuron]) may antagonize the neuromuscular blockade, increasing risk or severity of flaccid paralysis. Dose adjustments or unparalyzed periods may be advisable.
- ritodrine (Yutopar) increases the risk of pulmonary edema. Extreme caution and close patient monitoring are needed if this combination must be used.
- ritonavir (Norvir), saquinavir (Fortovase), and possibly other protease inhibitors (PI—see Drug Classes) may decrease PI blood levels and increase dexamethasone blood levels.
- thalidomide (various) increases risk of a serious skin problem (TEN). Combination not advisable except in closely followed clinical trials.
- thiazide diuretics (see Drug Classes) will decrease their blood-pressure-lowering ability.

The following drugs may ***decrease*** the effects of dexamethasone:

- antacids—may reduce its absorption.
- barbiturates (Amytal, Butisol, phenobarbital, etc.).
- fosphenytoin (Cerebyx).
- phenytoin (Dilantin, etc.).
- primidone (Mysoline).

- rifabutin (Mycobutin).
- rifampin (Rifadin, Rimactane, etc.).

▷ *Driving, Hazardous Activities:* Usually no restrictions. Be alert to the rare occurrence of dizziness.

Aviation Note: The use of this drug **may be a disqualification** for piloting. Consult a designated Aviation Medical Examiner.

Exposure to Sun: No restrictions.

Occurrence of Unrelated Illness: This drug may decrease natural resistance to infection. Call your doctor if you develop an infection of any kind. It may also reduce your body's ability to respond to the stress of acute illness, injury, or surgery. Keep your physician fully informed of any significant health changes.

Discontinuation: Do not stop this drug abruptly after chronic use. Ask your doctor for help about gradual, individualized withdrawal. Some clinicians change from daily to every other day therapy for four weeks BEFORE starting to lower the dose in a stepwise fashion. Many patients tolerate dose reductions of 2.5 mg of prednisone (other steroids are calculated on the basis of prednisone equivalents) with those decreases made every 3–7 days. If a disease flare occurs (worsening of symptoms), the dose should be increased to the last dose before the disease flare and should be tapered more slowly down to 5–10 mg or lower. Some clinicians use 8 AM predose plasma cortisol to guide tapering. If this lab test is less than 10 mcg/deciliter, tapering is continued until the daily prednisone equivalent is 2–5 mg. In general, if long-term treatment or high doses were used, prednisone equivalents should be tapered over 9–12 months. For up to 2 years after stopping this drug, you may require it again if you have an injury, surgery, or an illness.

DEXMETHYLPHENIDATE (DEX meth il FEN i dayt)

Introduced: 2001 **Class:** Amphetaminelike drug, anti-attention-deficit-disorder drug **Prescription:** USA: Yes **Controlled Drug:** USA: C-II*; Canada: Yes **Available as Generic:** USA: Yes; Canada: Yes

Brand Names: Focalin

Author's Note: Focalin is a recent addition for treatment of ADHD. This medicine is NOT the same as methylphenidate. This drug is dexmethylphenidate. The usual dose is only half of the methylphenidate dose. Information on Focalin will be broadened if ongoing studies and results warrant this.

DIAZEPAM (di AZ e pam)

Introduced: 1963 **Class:** Antianxiety drug, benzodiazepines, mild tranquilizer **Prescription:** USA: Yes **Controlled Drug:** USA: C-IV*; Canada: No **Available as Generic:** Yes

Brand Names: ✤Apo-Diazepam, Diastat, ✤Diazemuls, Diazepam Intensol Oral Solution, Dizac, E-Pam, ✤Meval, ✤Novo-Dipam, Q-pam, ✤Rival, T-Quil, Valcaps, Valium, Valrelease, Vazepam, ✤Vivol, Zetran

*See Schedules of Controlled Drugs at the back of this book.

BENEFITS versus RISKS

Possible Benefits	*Possible Risks*
RELIEF OF ANXIETY AND NERVOUS TENSION	Habit-forming potential with prolonged use
Wide margin of safety with therapeutic doses	Minor impairment of mental functions
	Respiratory depression
	Jaundice—very rare

▷ **Principal Uses**

As a *Single Drug Product:* Uses included in FDA-approved labeling: (1) Provides short-term relief of mild to moderate anxiety; (2) relieves the symptoms of acute alcohol withdrawal: agitation, tremors, hallucinations, incipient delirium tremens; (3) eases skeletal muscle spasm; (4) provides short-term control of certain types of seizures (epilepsy, fever-induced and status epilepticus); (5) short-term relief of insomnia; (6) adjunctive use in endoscopic procedures; (7) decreases anxiety prior to electrical defibrillation of the heart (cardioversion); (8) eases severe muscle spasms; (9) rectal gel is approved as an orphan drug for intermittent sudden (acute) seizure control in some patients who fail to respond to other treatments.

Other (unlabeled) generally accepted uses: (1) Helps prevent LSD flashbacks; (2) short-term treatment of sleepwalking; (3) treatment of persistent hiccups; (4) adjunctive treatment of catatonia; (5) helpful in easing chest pain in patients who have taken cocaine and have acute heart (coronary) syndromes; (6) further study is needed to define use in movement disorder caused by antipsychotic medicines (akathisia).

How This Drug Works: This drug calms higher brain centers by enhancing a nerve transmitter (gamma-aminobutyric acid, or GABA).

▷ **Widely Used Guidelines That Involve This Medicine (representative sample):** Please look at the section at the very beginning of this profile called "Class." Next, turn to Table 22 and you will find guidelines listed by the class involved!

Available Dosage Forms and Strengths

Capsules, prolonged action (sustained release) — 15 mg

Concentrate — 5 mg/mL

Injection — 5 mg/mL

Oral solution — 1 mg/ mL, 5 mg/5 mL, 10 mg/10 mL

Rectal gel — 2.5 mg, 5 mg, 10 mg, 15 mg, 20 mg

Tablets — 2 mg, 5 mg, 10 mg

▷ **Usual Adult Dosage Ranges:** *For anxiety:* 2 to 10 mg, two to four times daily. Dose may be increased cautiously as needed and tolerated. After 1 week of continual use, the total daily dose may be taken at bedtime. Maximum daily dose is 60 mg. Sustained-release form can be given once daily (15 mg) if it is replacing use of the immediate-release form that has been taken as a total daily dose of 15 mg divided into 5-mg doses three times a day.

Seizures: 2–10 mg two to four times daily.

Alcohol withdrawal: 10 mg given every 8 hours up to every 6 hours during the first day. This is then lowered to 5 mg three or four times daily as needed and tolerated.

Note: Actual dose and schedule must be determined for each patient individually.

Conditions Requiring Dosing Adjustments

Liver Function: The dose must be decreased by 50% in patients with liver compromise.

Kidney Function: Caution—if 15 mg or more is given daily, diazepam metabolites may accumulate.

Obesity: Obese patients may take longer than nonobese patients to accumulate this medicine. The time that it takes to remove diazepam (elimination half-life) is prolonged in obese people. This means that obese people may take a much longer time to get the peak effect of diazepam and will also take a longer time to remove the drug from their bodies.

▷ **Dosing Instructions:** The tablet may be crushed and taken on empty stomach or with food or milk. The prolonged-action capsule should not be opened, broken, or chewed. Always use a measuring spoon for oral liquid forms to get the correct dose. Do not stop this drug abruptly if taken for more than 4 weeks (medicine should be slowly withdrawn or tapered). If you forget a dose, take the dose as soon as you remember it, unless it's nearly time for your next dose. If you remember when it's nearly time for your next dose, skip the missed dose and take the next dose right on schedule. DO NOT double doses.

Usual Duration of Use: Regular use for 3 to 5 days is usually needed to see benefits in relieving moderate anxiety. Severity and probability of addiction (physical dependence) is associated with increasing dose and ongoing nature of use. Best to limit continual use to 1 to 3 weeks. Avoid uninterrupted and prolonged use if possible. Use for seizures may be ongoing, and appropriate cautions should be taken.

Author's Note: The National Institute of Mental Health has an information page on anxiety. It can be found on the World Wide Web (*www.nimh.nih.gov/anxiety*).

Typical Treatment Goals and Measurements (Outcomes and Markers)

Goals for anxiety tend to be more vague and subjective than hypertension or cholesterol. Frequently, the patient (in conjunction with physician assessment) will largely decide if anxiety has been modified to a successful extent. The ability of the patient to return to normal activities is a hallmark of successful treatment. The Hamilton Anxiety Scale is a useful measurement tool.

▷ **This Drug Should Not Be Taken If**
- you have had an allergic reaction to any dosage form of it previously.
- you have acute narrow-angle glaucoma.
- it is prescribed for a child under 6 months of age.

▷ **Inform Your Physician Before Taking This Drug If**
- you are allergic to any benzodiazepine (see Drug Classes).
- you have a history of alcoholism or drug abuse.
- you are pregnant or planning pregnancy.
- you have impaired liver or kidney function.
- you have a history of serious depression or a mental disorder.
- you have asthma, emphysema, or other lung problems that limit appropriate breathing (limited pulmonary reserve), epilepsy, or myasthenia gravis.

Possible Side Effects (natural, expected, and unavoidable drug actions)
Drowsiness—frequent.

Irritation of the vein with the intravenous form—possible.

Lethargy, unsteadiness—rare.

"Hangover" effects on the day following bedtime use.

▷ **Possible Adverse Effects** (unusual, unexpected, and infrequent reactions)

If any of the following develop, consult your physician promptly for guidance.

Mild Adverse Effects

Allergic reactions: rashes, hives—rare.

Dizziness, fainting, blurred or double vision, slurred speech, sweating, nausea—possible.

Increased liver enzymes—case report.

Ringing in the ears—case reports.

Impaired motor skills (dose-related to some extent)—frequency varies.

Serious Adverse Effects

Allergic reactions: liver damage with jaundice (see Glossary), kidney damage, abnormally low blood platelet count, anaphylaxis—case reports.

Respiratory depression—dose-related.

Bone marrow depression: low white blood cells, fever, sore throat—case reports.

Severe lowering of blood pressure, slow heart rate, and cardiac arrest have been reported after rapid intravenous dosing—case reports.

Hip fracture—possible indirect effect of the medicine arising from unsteadiness.

Amnesia—dose-related.

Vein irritation and or blood clots—possible with intravenous (IV) form.

Heart arrhythmia (intravenous form)—possible.

Obsessive-compulsive disorder following extended use and abrupt withdrawal—possible.

Paradoxical responses of excitement, agitation, anger, rage—case reports.

▷ **Possible Effects on Sexual Function:**

Altered timing and pattern of menstruation.

Small doses (2 to 5 mg/day) may help the anxiety seen in many cases of impotence in men and inhibited sexual responsiveness in women. Larger doses (10 mg/day or more) can decrease libido, impair potency in men, and inhibit orgasm in women.

Swelling and tenderness of male breast tissue (gynecomastia).

Abnormally prolonged erections (priapism)—case reports.

Adverse Effects That May Mimic Natural Diseases or Disorders

Liver reaction with jaundice may suggest viral hepatitis.

Possible Effects on Laboratory Tests

White blood cell counts: decreased.

Blood thyroxine (T4) level: decreased.

Liver function tests: increased liver enzymes (ALT/GPT, AST/GOT, and alkaline phosphatase), increased bilirubin—all rare.

Urine sugar tests: no drug effect with Tes-Tape; low test results with Clinistix and Diastix.

Urine screening tests for drug abuse may be positive. (Test results depend upon amount of drug taken and testing method used.)

CAUTION

1. This drug should not be stopped abruptly if it has been taken continually for more than 4 weeks.

2. Some nonprescription (over-the-counter, or OTC) drug products that

contain antihistamines (allergy and cold preparations, sleep aids) can cause excessive sedation if combined with diazepam.

Precautions for Use

By Infants and Children: This drug should not be used in hyperactive or psychotic children. Watch for excessive sedation and incoordination. Usual dose in children for muscle relaxation or sedation is 0.1 to 0.8 mg per kg of body mass per day, divided into equal doses and given every 8 hours or as often as every 6 hours. The drug has been used intravenously to help seizures in neonates.

By Those Over 60 Years of Age: Small doses are indicated (two to 2.5 mg once or twice a day). Watch for lethargy, indifference, fatigue, weakness, unsteadiness, disturbing dreams, nightmares, and paradoxical reactions of excitement, agitation, anger, hostility, and rage.

▷ **Advisability of Use During Pregnancy**

Pregnancy Category: D. See Pregnancy Risk Categories at the back of this book.

Animal Studies: Cleft palate reported in mice; skeletal defects in rats.

Human Studies: Available information is conflicting and inconclusive. Some findings of increased serious birth defects. Other studies have found no significant increase in birth defects.

Frequent use in late pregnancy can cause the "floppy infant" syndrome in the newborn: weakness, lethargy, unresponsiveness, depressed breathing, low body temperature. Avoid use during entire pregnancy.

Advisability of Use If Breast-Feeding

Presence of this drug in breast milk: Yes.

Avoid drug or refrain from nursing.

Habit-Forming Potential: This drug can produce psychological and/or physical dependence (see Glossary), especially if used in large doses for an extended period of time.

Effects of Overdose: Marked drowsiness, weakness, feeling of drunkenness, staggering gait, tremor, stupor progressing to deep sleep or coma.

Possible Effects of Long-Term Use: Psychological and/or physical dependence, rare blood cell disorders.

Suggested Periodic Examinations While Taking This Drug (at physician's discretion)

Complete blood cell counts during long-term use.

▷ **While Taking This Drug, Observe the Following**

Foods: Grapefruit and grapefruit juice can increase diazepam concentrations. Caution and moderation advised.

Herbal Medicines or Minerals: Kava, skull cap, and valerian may increase central nervous system depression (avoid this combination). Kola nut, Siberian ginseng, guarana, mate, ephedra (no longer on the market), and hawthorn may blunt the benefits of this medicine. While St. John's wort is indicated for anxiety, it is also thought to increase (induce) cytochrome P450 enzymes and will tend to blunt diazepam effectiveness if combined with diazepam. Dong quai inhibits removal of diazepam in some animal models. Evening primrose oil increased seizure risk in some patients. If diazepam is being used to treat a seizure disorder, this combination is not recommended. Ginkgo is also not recommended in seizure patients as some extracts have a contaminant (4'-O-methylpyridoxine) that may blunt anticonvulsant benefits. Do not combine any herbal medicines without talking to your doctor first.

Beverages: Avoid excessive intake of caffeine-containing beverages: coffee, tea, cola. May be taken with milk. Caffeine use may be recommended by your doctor to ease some cases of excessive diazepam-caused drowsiness. Grapefruit juice will concentrate substances in grapefruit that can inhibit removal of diazepam from the body. Better to take this medicine with water.

▷ *Alcohol:* Avoid this combination. Alcohol increases the absorption of this drug and adds to its depressant effects on the brain. It is advisable to avoid alcohol completely—throughout the day and night—if it is necessary to drive or to engage in any hazardous activity.

Tobacco Smoking: Heavy smoking may reduce the calming action of this drug. I advise everyone to quit smoking.

Marijuana Smoking: Increased sedation and impairment of intellectual and physical performance.

▷ *Other Drugs*

Diazepam may ***increase*** the effects of
• digoxin (Lanoxin) and cause digoxin toxicity.
• phenytoin (Dilantin) or fosphenytoin (Cerebyx) and cause toxicity.

Diazepam may ***decrease*** the effects of
• levodopa (Sinemet, etc.) and reduce its effectiveness in treating Parkinson's disease.

Diazepam ***taken concurrently*** with
• fluoxetine (Prozac) may lead to diazepam toxicity.
• fluvoxamine (Luvox) can result in serious accumulation of diazepam and toxicity.
• macrolide antibiotics (see Drug Classes) may lead to toxicity. Lowering doses by half to 75% may be prudent.
• MAO inhibitors (see Drug Classes) may exaggerate breathing depression.
• mirtazapine (Remeron) may worsen motor skills. Avoid operating dangerous machinery or tasks requiring coordination.
• narcotics or other centrally active medicines may cause additive respiratory depression or decreased levels of consciousness.
• olanzapine (Zyprexa) may cause blood pressure lowering when you stand (orthostatic hypotension).
• propoxyphene (various) may lead to benzodiazepine (diazepam) intoxication.
• quinupristin/dalfopristin (Synercid) may lead to diazepam toxicity.

The following drugs may ***increase*** the effects of diazepam:
• amprenavir (Agenerase), atazanavir (Reyataz), ritonavir (Norvir), and perhaps other protease inhibitors.
• birth control pills (oral contraceptives).
• cimetidine (Tagamet).
• cisapride (Propulsid).
• disulfiram (Antabuse).
• isoniazid (INH, Rifamate, etc.).
• itraconazole (Sporanox), ketoconazole (Nizoral), or other azole antifungals.
• macrolide antibiotics such as erythromycin or clarithromycin.
• omeprazole (Prilosec).
• sertraline (Zoloft).
• valproic acid (Depakene, Depakote).

The following drugs may ***decrease*** the effects of diazepam:
• ranitidine (Zantac).

- rifampin (Rimactane, etc.).
- rifabutin (Mycobutin).
- theophylline (aminophylline, Theo-Dur, etc.).

▷ *Driving, Hazardous Activities:* This drug can impair mental alertness, judgment, physical coordination, and reaction time. Avoid hazardous activities accordingly.

Aviation Note: The use of this drug **is a disqualification** for piloting. Consult a designated Aviation Medical Examiner.

Exposure to Sun: No restrictions.

Exposure to Heat: Because of reduced urine volume, this drug may accumulate in the body and produce effects of overdose.

Discontinuation: Avoid stopping this drug suddenly if taken for over 4 weeks. Prudent to taper gradually to prevent a withdrawal syndrome (sweating, tremor, depression, hallucinations, seizures, and vomiting).

DICLOFENAC (di KLOH fen ak)

Please see the acetic acid (nonsteroidal anti-inflammatory drug) family profile.

DIDANOSINE (di DAN oh seen)

Other Names: DDI, dideoxyinosine

Introduced: 1991 **Class:** Antiviral **Prescription:** USA: Yes **Controlled Drug:** USA: No; Canada: No **Available as Generic:** USA: No; Canada: No

Brand Names: Videx, Videx EC

BENEFITS versus RISKS	
Possible Benefits	*Possible Risks*
DELAYED PROGRESSION OF DISEASE IN HIV-POSITIVE PATIENTS	DRUG-INDUCED PANCREATITIS DRUG-INDUCED PERIPHERAL NEURITIS
USE IN COMBINATION THERAPY OF AIDS	Drug-induced seizures
ONCE- OR TWICE-DAILY DOSING	Liver damage—rare

▷ **Principal Uses**

As a Single Drug Product: Uses currently included in FDA-approved labeling: (1) Combination treatment of human immunodeficiency virus (HIV) infections in adults and children (6 months of age or older).

Author's Note: Adherence or taking medicines for HIV exactly on time and in the right amount is ABSOLUTELY critical to getting the best possible results or outcomes (see STI note).

Antiretroviral therapy guidelines from NIAID take into account how easily the medicine treating HIV can fit into a patient's life.

Other (unlabeled) generally accepted uses: None at present.

How This Drug Works: By interfering with essential HIV enzyme systems, this drug prevents growth and reproduction of HIV particles in infected cells, limiting the severity and extent of HIV infection.

▷ **Widely Used Guidelines That Involve This Medicine (representative sample):** Please look at the section at the very beginning of this profile called "Class." Next, turn to Table 22 and you will find guidelines listed by the class involved!

Available Dosage Forms and Strengths
> Capsules, extended release — 125 mg, 200 mg, 250 mg, 400 mg
Powder for oral solution (bottle) — 2 g, 4 g
Powder for oral solution (packet) — 100 mg, 167 mg, 250 mg, 375 mg
> Tablets, chewable/dispersible — 25 mg, 50 mg, 100 mg, 150 mg, 200 mg

▷ **Recommended Dosage Ranges** (Actual dose and schedule must be determined for each patient individually.)
Infants and Children: For those 2 weeks to 8 months is 100 mg per square meter. Eight months of age or older, dose is based on drug form and body surface area with 120 mg per square meter twice daily used. Once-daily dosing HAS NOT been studied as yet in children.
12 to 60 Years of Age: (Twice daily dosing is preferred for all forms.) Chewable/dispersible tablets: 400 mg once a day or 200 mg every 12 hours for those weighing more than 60 kg; 250 mg once daily or 125 mg every 12 hours for those weighing less than 60 kg.
EC form: 200-mg EC tablets are only part of a 400-mg once-daily regimen and dosing is based on a mg per kg of body weight basis. For example—if a patient weighs more than 60 kg, 400 mg of Videx EC should be taken daily.
Over 60 Years of Age: Same as 12 to 60 group, but the dose should be reduced if there is an age-related decline in kidney function.

Conditions Requiring Dosing Adjustments
Liver Function: Increased risk of liver toxicity if used in people with compromised liver. Doses must be decreased in liver failure.
Kidney Function: Dose must be decreased in mild to moderate kidney failure. For example: those with creatinine clearance of 30–59 mL/min who weigh 60 kg or more would receive 100 mg twice daily or 200 mg each day of the oral tablets, 100 mg twice daily of the buffered powder and 200 mg each day of Videx EC. Care must also be taken as there is an increased risk of magnesium toxicity (chewable dispersible tablets have 8.6 MEQ of magnesium each). Risk of drug-induced pancreatitis also increases in patients with kidney problems.

▷ **Dosing Instructions:** Best taken on an empty stomach, 30 minutes before or 2 hours after eating. Patients MUST take at least two of the needed chewable/dispersible tablets at each dose in order to make sure that there is adequate buffer present. This actually protects the drug itself from being destroyed by stomach acid. The Videx EC should be swallowed whole (not crushed or altered).
Pediatric oral solution first reconstituted with water and then combined with equal amounts of antacid (such as Mylanta or Maalox). Shake this mixture thoroughly BEFORE you measure each dose.
Adult oral solution is made by stirring one packet into 120 mL (4 ounces) of water until the powder is dissolved; this may take up to 3 minutes. Do not mix powder with fruit juice or other acidic liquid. Swallow all of the 4-ounce solution immediately.
The chewable/dispersible buffered tablets should be thoroughly chewed, crushed, or dispersed in water before swallowing. To disperse the tablet(s), stir in at least 30 mL (1 ounce) of water until all the medicine is in the water.

Swallow all of preparation immediately. The mandarin orange flavor formulation of Videx disperses in water in as little as 2 minutes. These tablets are dropped whole into a glass of water and are stirred to speed dispersion in the water. If you forget a dose: take the missed dose as soon as you remember it, unless it's nearly time for your next dose—then skip the missed dose and take the next scheduled dose right on time. DO NOT double doses. Talk openly with your doctor if you are having trouble remembering doses. Some patients benefit greatly from beeper-based reminder systems.

Author's Note: Current HIV therapy involves combination use of agents from different drug classes to attack the AIDS virus from different points and delay resistance. Clinicians use viral load (see Glossary) to indicate success or failure of therapy.

Usual Duration of Use: Regular use for several months with repeat viral load and CD4 tests are needed check benefits in slowing HIV progression. Long-term use requires follow-up with your doctor.

Typical Treatment Goals and Measurements (Outcomes and Markers)

HIV: Goals for HIV treatment presently are maximum suppression of viral replication, maximum lowering of the amount of virus in your body (viral load or burden), and maximum patient survival. Markers of successful therapy include undetectable viral load, increased CD4 cells, absence of indicator or opportunistic infections (OIs), and in the case of the HIV-positive patient, delay of the infection to progress to AIDS.

Possible Advantages of This Drug

Does not cause serious bone marrow depression (production of blood cells). Less frequent liver toxicity than some other antiretrovirals. Once-daily dosing can be a great advantage in adherence.

This Drug Should Not Be Taken If

- you have had an allergic reaction to it previously.
- you have active liver disease.
- you have had pancreatitis recently.

▷ **Inform Your Physician Before Taking This Drug If**

- you have had allergic reactions to any drugs in the past.
- you are taking any other drugs currently.
- you have a history of pancreatitis or peripheral neuritis.
- you have a history of gout or high blood uric acid level.
- you have a history of alcoholism.
- you have a history of eye problems.
- you have a history of diarrhea.
- you have had nerve damage (peripheral neuropathy) from other medicines.
- you have a history of phenylketonuria (PKU).
- you have a history of low blood platelets or blood disorder.
- you are pregnant—increased chance of metabolic problems (lactic acidosis risk).
- you have a history of low blood potassium.
- you have a history of heart failure.
- you have a seizure disorder.
- you have impaired liver or kidney function.

Possible Side Effects (natural, expected, and unavoidable drug actions)

Mild decreases in red blood cell, white blood cell, and platelet counts in adults.

Mild increases in blood uric acid levels. Increased sodium load (each buffered powder packet has 1,380 mg of sodium).

Increased magnesium levels in patients with kidney problems.

▷ **Possible Adverse Effects** (unusual, unexpected, and infrequent reactions)
If any of the following develop, consult your physician promptly for guidance.

Mild Adverse Effects

Allergic reactions: skin rash and itching—occasional in adults and common in pediatric patients.

Headache, dizziness, insomnia, nervousness, confusion—infrequent.

Visual disturbances—rare.

Nausea, vomiting—may be frequent in pediatrics.

Stomach pain and diarrhea (25% of adults and frequent in pediatric patients), dry mouth and altered taste, yeast infection of mouth—rare to infrequent.

Lowered blood pressure—rare to infrequent.

Loss of color in the retina (retinal depigmentation)—case reports.

Nose bleeds—frequent in clinical trials in children.

Increased urination—infrequent in pediatric patients.

Cough—infrequent.

Loss of hair, muscle and joint pains—rare to infrequent.

Serious Adverse Effects

Skin reaction: Stevens-Johnson syndrome—case report.

Drug-induced pancreatitis, usually seen in the first 6 months—infrequent.

Drug-induced peripheral neuritis (see Glossary), usually occurring after 2 to 6 months of treatment (this effect also appears to be dose-related)—infrequent to frequent.

Muscle damage (myalgia and/or rhabdomyolysis including sudden kidney failure)—case reports.

Electrolyte imbalance (low potassium or calcium)—variable.

Increased triglycerides—frequent.

Asthma—frequent in children.

Abnormal heart rhythm, heart failure—rare.

High blood sugar—possible.

Excessive lowering of blood pressure and passing out (syncope)—case reports to infrequent.

Serious skin rash (Stevens-Johnson syndrome)—case report.

Seizures (may be due to electrolyte problems)—rare.

Lowered white blood cell counts, lowered granulocyte (a specific white blood cell) counts and lowered blood platelets (69%) in pediatric patients—infrequent to frequent.

Lactic acidosis—case reports.

Optic neuritis and blindness—case reports.

Liver damage—rare to infrequent.

Kidney damage—rare.

▷ **Possible Effects on Sexual Function:** Gynecomastia—case report.

Adverse Effects That May Mimic Natural Diseases or Disorders

Drug-induced liver reaction—rare at less than 0.2%—may suggest viral hepatitis.

Possible Effects on Laboratory Tests

Complete blood cell counts: decreased red cells and white cells—variable; decreased platelets—infrequent.

Blood amylase or uric acid level: increased—infrequent.

Blood electrolytes: low calcium, potassium and magnesium.

Liver function tests: increased liver enzymes (ALT/GPT, AST/GOT, and alkaline phosphatase), increased bilirubin—infrequent in adults, higher in pediatric patients.

CAUTION

1. This drug **does not cure HIV infection.** Ongoing CD4 and viral load tests are prudent. The AIDS virus may still be passed to other people while you are taking this medicine.
2. Report stomach pain with nausea and vomiting to your doctor; this could indicate pancreatitis.
3. Report pain, numbness, tingling, or burning in the hands or feet—could be peripheral neuritis. Drug may need to be stopped.
4. If your kidneys are damaged or your creatinine elevated, ask your doctor if accumulating magnesium will be a problem for you.
5. One current therapy approach uses STI or structured therapy interruptions also called structured interruptions in therapy (SIT) by one group to carefully attempt to evoke an immune response to HIV. This approach is presently controversial and should NOT be attempted without the supervision of your doctor.

Precautions for Use

By Infants and Children: Safety and effectiveness for those under 6 months of age not established. Children are also at risk for developing pancreatitis and peripheral neuritis. It is recommended that detailed eye examinations be performed every 6 months and at any time that visual disturbance occurs.

By Those Over 60 Years of Age: Reduced kidney function may require dose reduction.

▷ Advisability of Use During Pregnancy

Pregnancy Category: B. See Pregnancy Risk Categories at the back of this book.

Animal Studies: Rat and rabbit studies show no birth defects.

Human Studies: Adequate studies of pregnant women not available.

Consult your physician for specific guidance.

Advisability of Use If Breast-Feeding

Presence of this drug in breast milk: Yes in rats, unknown in humans.

Avoid drug or refrain from nursing.

Note: HIV has been found in human breast milk. Breast-feeding may result in transmission of HIV infection to the nursing infant.

Habit-Forming Potential: None.

Effects of Overdose: Nausea, vomiting, stomach pain, diarrhea, pain in hands and feet, irritability, confusion.

Possible Effects of Long-Term Use: Peripheral neuritis (see Glossary).

Suggested Periodic Examinations While Taking This Drug (at physician's discretion)

Complete blood cell counts before starting treatment and weekly thereafter until tolerance is established.

Electrolytes.

Blood amylase levels, fractionated for salivary gland and pancreatic origin.

Liver and kidney function tests.

Viral load or viral burden in order to assess success of treatment.

CD4 counts.

▷ **While Taking This Drug, Observe the Following**

Foods: Best taken on an empty stomach.

Herbal Medicines or Minerals: Echinacea: Some patients use echinacea to attempt to boost their immune systems. Unfortunately, use of echinacea is not recommended in people with damaged immune systems. This herb may also actually weaken any immune system if it is used too often or for too long a time. Some cancer patients are looking to mistletoe (Iscador) to boost their immune systems. This **HAS NOT** been studied in HIV-positive patients.

Beverages: Do not take with acidic fruit juices.

▷ *Alcohol:* No interactions expected.

Tobacco Smoking: No interactions expected. I advise everyone to quit smoking.

▷ *Other Drugs*

Didanosine may *increase* the effects of
- zidovudine (Retrovir) and enhance its antiviral effect against HIV.

Didanosine may *decrease* the effects of
- amprenavir (Agenerase), atazanavir (Reyataz), and indinavir (Crixivan) and blunt therapeutic benefits; separate dosing by 2 hours.
- ciprofloxacin (Cipro) and other fluoroquinolones (gatifloxacin [Tequin] and grepafloxacin [Raxar], levofloxacin [Levaquin]; see Drug Classes), if taken at the same time; take fluoroquinolones at least 4 hours before taking didanosine buffered solution, tablets, or the oral powder.
- dapsone and render it ineffective; avoid concurrent use.
- itraconazole (Sporanox). Separate dosing by at least 2 hours.
- ketoconazole (Nizoral), if taken at the same time; take ketoconazole at least 2 hours before taking didanosine.
- tetracyclines (see Drug Classes), if taken at the same time; take tetracyclines at least 2 hours before taking didanosine.

Didanosine *taken concurrently* with
- allopurinol (various) increased didanosine absorption in two patients with damaged kidneys. Caution and blood levels are prudent if this medicine is used in patients with kidney failure.
- amprenavir (Agenerase) will probably decrease amprenavir absorption. Separate doses by at least 1 hour.
- antacids will decrease didanosine absorption and lower its therapeutic benefit.
- delavirdine (Rescriptor) may lower both drug levels. Separate doses by an hour.
- fluconazole (Diflucan) and other azole antifungals may decrease fluconazole benefits.
- histamine (H2) blocking drugs (see Drug Classes)—cimetidine, etc.—may increase didanosine toxicity.
- hydroxyurea (Droxia) and increase risk of pancreatitis or liver toxicity. Careful patient monitoring is critical.
- pentamidine or sulfamethoxazole may increase the risk of drug-induced pancreatitis; watch for significant symptoms.
- ritonavir (Norvir) will inactivate both medicines. Separate doses by 2 to 3 hours.
- tenofovir (Viread) increases didanosine levels by up to 60% (particularly if taken with a light meal)—possibly leading to didanosine toxicity. If the medicines must be combined, dosing changes appear prudent. Talk to your doctor.
- zalcitabine (Hivid) may cause increased neurotoxicity.

▷ *Driving, Hazardous Activities:* This drug may cause dizziness and impaired vision. Restrict activities as necessary.

Aviation Note: The use of this drug *is a disqualification* for piloting. Consult a designated Aviation Medical Examiner.

Exposure to Sun: No restrictions.

Discontinuation: Do not stop this drug without your physician's knowledge and guidance.

DIFLUNISAL (di FLU ni sal)

Please see the acetic acid (nonsteroidal anti-inflammatory drug) family profile.

DIGITOXIN (di ji TOX in)

See the digoxin profile for further information.

DIGOXIN (di JOX in)

Introduced: 1934 **Class:** Digitalis preparations **Prescription:** USA: Yes **Controlled Drug:** USA: No; Canada: No **Available as Generic:** Yes

Brand Names: ✤Digitaline Nativelle, Digitek, Lanoxicaps, Lanoxin, Novodigoxin, SK-Digoxin

---

BENEFITS versus RISKS

Possible Benefits	*Possible Risks*
EFFECTIVE HEART STIMULANT IN CONGESTIVE HEART FAILURE	NARROW TREATMENT RANGE
EFFECTIVE PREVENTION AND TREATMENT OF CERTAIN HEART RHYTHM DISORDERS	Frequent and sometimes serious disturbances of heart rhythm Controversial in heart failure in women (may relate to levels)

▷ **Principal Uses**

As a Single Drug Product: Uses in current FDA-approved labeling: (1) Treats congestive heart failure; (2) restores and helps keep normal heart rate and rhythm in cases of atrial fibrillation and flutter; (2) is a second-line agent behind verapamil (drug of choice in Paroxysmal Atrial Tachycardia).

Controversies in Medicine: Some clinicians found that lower than previously advocated levels of digoxin (0.5–0.8 ng/mL) reduced death (mortality) in heart failure patients. One research group found 0.5–0.8 mg/mL to be ideal (optimal) for men in stable heart failure who have normal heart rhythm (see Rosenberg, J. in Sources). A group at Yale questioned the safety of digoxin in treating heart failure in women. Further research on blood levels is required (see Ratthore, S.S. in Sources). A most recent study in JAMA found the lower levels of digoxin (0.5–0.8 ng/mL) to reduce death in heart failure patients.

Other (unlabeled) generally accepted uses: (1) Postoperative arrhythmias; (2) helps to increase left ventricular function in patients with pacemakers; (3) may have a role in treating Wolff-Parkinson-White syndrome.

How This Drug Works: Increases force of heart muscle contraction. Delays electrical transmission through the heart, helping restore normal rate and rhythm.

▷ **Widely Used Guidelines That Involve This Medicine (representative sample):** Please look at the section at the very beginning of this profile called "Class." Next, turn to Table 22 and you will find guidelines listed by the class involved!

Available Dosage Forms and Strengths

    Capsules — 0.05 mg, 0.1 mg, 0.2 mg
     Elixir — 0.25 mg/5 mL, 0.125 mg/5 mL
  Elixir, pediatric — 0.05 mg/mL
     Injection — 0.1 mg/mL, 0.25 mg/mL
    Tablets — 0.0625 mg (Canada), 0.125 mg, 0.25 mg, 0.5 mg

Author's Note: Dosing and timing of doses are critical for this medicine. The difference between toxic blood levels and therapeutic blood levels is small. Be CERTAIN you understand how and when to take this medicine.

▷ **Usual Adult Dosage Ranges:** For loading dose, 10 mcg per kilogram of lean body mass (some clinicians use ideal body weight as the math is less complicated); 8–12 mcg per kg of body mass may be needed if digoxin is being used to control abnormal heart rhythms (such as atrial fibrillation); 8–12 mcg per kg is typical if this medicine is being used for heart failure (0.75 to 1.25 mg by mouth). Loading dose can be given orally or intravenously. Once decided, it is often given as 50% in the first dose with remainder divided into smaller doses and given at 6- to 8-hour intervals until the desired response is achieved. Usual ongoing dose after loading is 0.125 to 0.5 mg per day, and is calculated by a specific formula. Divided versus once daily dosing is recommended for patients who are likely to have toxic levels, in those who require 300 mcg a day or more and in people who have had digoxin toxicity previously. Newer guidance on lower ongoing blood levels may lead to lower loading and ongoing doses. Further research is needed. In neonatal and pediatric patients, a similar loading and ongoing strategy is used, but the amount on a mg-per-kg-of-body-mass basis is very different.

 Note: Actual dose and schedule must be determined for each patient individually.

Conditions Requiring Dosing Adjustments

 Liver Function: Use with caution; blood levels should be obtained more frequently.

 Kidney Function: Dose must be adjusted in kidney compromise. Smaller doses and some cases of dosing every other day may be needed.

▷ **Dosing Instructions:** Tablet may be crushed and is best taken at the same time each day (to help keep blood levels about the same) on an empty stomach. The elixir form can be useful if swallowing is a problem, and should be measured using a dosing spoon or measured medicine cup. Can be taken with or following food; milk and dairy products may delay absorption but do not reduce the amount of drug absorbed. The capsule should be swallowed whole. If you forget a dose: Take the dose you missed as soon as you remember it, unless you are more than 12 hours late. If that is the case, skip the missed dose and simply take the next scheduled dose. DO NOT double doses. If you forget your medicine for 2 days, call your doctor for directions.

Usual Duration of Use: Regular use for 7 to 10 days needed to see benefits in relieving heart failure or controlling heart rhythm disorders. Long-term use requires physician supervision and checks of blood levels. Treatment of heart rhythm disorders and congestive heart failure will usually be ongoing.

Typical Treatment Goals and Measurements (Outcomes and Markers)

Heart failure: The level of this medicine in the blood must be kept in a certain range. When this medicine is in the correct range, it helps the heart beat more strongly, increasing the amount of work that it can do (see Controversies in Medicines above). Your doctor may use terms like cardiac output (the amount of work that your heart can do in a given amount of time), contractile force (the strength of your heart action), and edematous decrease (lower ankle swelling) to describe how much better your heart is working. Surrogate end points (a marker that offers vital information about how well a patient is responding to a treatment) is useful to clinicians. Two possible surrogate markers for CHF are left ventricular end diastolic volume (LVEDV) and b-type natriuretic peptide (BNP). These will be updated as more information becomes available. The goals and time frame should be discussed with you when the prescription is written.

▷ **This Drug Should Not Be Taken If**
- you have had an allergic reaction to any form of it.
- you are in ventricular fibrillation (a life-threatening heart rhythm).

▷ **Inform Your Physician Before Taking This Drug If**
- you have had an unfavorable reaction to digitalis.
- you have taken digitalis in the past 2 weeks.
- you take (or have recently taken) any diuretic drug.
- you have a history of severe lung disease.
- you have abnormal heart rhythms (such as severe slowing or bradycardia), sick sinus syndrome, rapid rate arising in the ventricles (ventricular tachycardia), or certain aortic problems.
- you have had damage to the heart muscle (myocardium), such as in a heart attack or myocarditis.
- you have ongoing (chronic) inflammation of part of the heart (constrictive pericarditis).
- you have a history of low blood potassium or magnesium.
- you have impaired liver or kidney function or develop impaired function while taking this medicine.
- you have a history of thyroid function disorder.

Possible Side Effects (natural, expected, and unavoidable drug actions)

Slow heart rate.

May cause blackening of feces.

Enlargement or sensitivity of the male breast—rare.

▷ **Possible Adverse Effects** (unusual, unexpected, and infrequent reactions)

If any of the following develop, consult your physician promptly for guidance.

Mild Adverse Effects

Allergic reactions: skin rash, hives—rare.

Headache, drowsiness, lethargy, confusion, changes in vision: "halo" effect, blurring, spots, double vision, yellow-green vision—infrequent.

Changes in vaginal tissue (vaginal cornification)—case reports.

Nightmares—case reports.

Loss of appetite, nausea, vomiting, diarrhea (can be early signs of adult toxicity)—frequent.

Serious Adverse Effects

Idiosyncratic reactions: hallucinations, facial neuralgias, peripheral neuralgias, blindness—case reports.

Low blood platelets (thrombocytopenia)—case reports and probably an immune reaction.

Psychosis and hallucinations—associated with toxic levels.

Seizures—rare.

Serious skin rash (Stevens-Johnson syndrome)—rare.

Disorientation—most common in the elderly.

Trigeminal neuralgia—case report.

Heart rhythm disturbances—possible and dose-related.

▷ **Possible Effects on Sexual Function:**

Decreased libido and impotence in 35% of male users. Enlargement and tenderness of male breasts (gynecomastia)—case reports. Both effects are attributed to digoxin's estrogenlike action. May cause cornification of the vagina in women after menopause. Caution is advised, as this has been mistaken for cancer (endometrial).

Adverse Effects That May Mimic Natural Diseases or Disorders

Drug-induced mental changes may be mistaken for senile dementia or psychosis. May cause cornification of the vagina in women after menopause. Caution is advised as this has been mistaken for cancer (endometrial).

Possible Effects on Laboratory Tests

Blood platelet counts: rarely decreased.

Blood testosterone level: may be decreased with long-term use.

CAUTION

1. Take this medicine EXACTLY as prescribed.
2. If you take calcium supplements, ask your doctor. May be best to avoid large doses.
3. Prudent to carry a card that says you are taking this drug.
4. Avoid over-the-counter antacids and cold, cough, or allergy remedies without first asking your doctor or pharmacist.
5. Because blood levels are so important, make sure you stay on the same brand or generic form that you are started on. If you are changed from one form or one generic to the other, blood level checks are usually prudent. If your blood potassium is lowered you can have signs and symptoms of toxicity with a "therapeutic level and a normal dose."
6. May cause changes (cornification) in the vagina in women after menopause. Caution is advised, as this has been mistaken for cancer (endometrial).

Precautions for Use

By Infants and Children: Watch for indications of toxicity: slow heart rate (below 60 beats/min), irregular heart rhythms.

By Those Over 60 Years of Age: Reduced drug tolerance; smaller doses are prudent. Watch for toxicity: headache, dizziness, fatigue, weakness, lethargy, depression, confusion, nervousness, agitation, delusions, difficulty with reading. Call your doctor if these happen.

▷ **Advisability of Use During Pregnancy**

Pregnancy Category: C. See Pregnancy Risk Categories at the back of this book.

Animal Studies: No birth defects reported.

Human Studies: Adequate studies of pregnant women not available. However, no birth defects from the therapeutic use of this drug have been reported. Use this drug only if clearly needed. Overdose can be harmful to the fetus.

Advisability of Use If Breast-Feeding
Presence of this drug in breast milk: Yes.
Monitor nursing infant closely and discontinue drug or nursing if adverse effects develop.

Habit-Forming Potential: None.

Effects of Overdose: Loss of appetite, excessive saliva, nausea, vomiting, diarrhea, serious disturbances of heart rate and rhythm, intestinal bleeding, drowsiness, headache, confusion, delirium, hallucinations, convulsions.

Possible Effects of Long-Term Use: May cause cornification of the vagina in women after menopause. Caution is advised, as this has been mistaken for cancer (endometrial).

Suggested Periodic Examinations While Taking This Drug (at physician's discretion)
Measurements of blood levels of digoxin, calcium, magnesium, and potassium. (Time to sample blood for digoxin level: 6–8 hours after last dose or just before next dose.) Recommended broad therapeutic range: 0.5–2.0 ng/mL, but 5–0.8 ng/mL has been recommended for heart failure patients—see above Controversies in Medicine note.
Electrocardiograms.

▷ **While Taking This Drug, Observe the Following**
Foods: Talk to your doctor about high-potassium foods. The peak level and rate that digoxin enters your body will decrease if taken with food.
Herbal Medicines or Minerals: Hawthorn and co-enzyme Q10 (co-Q10) can affect the way the heart works. Issues remain regarding optimum doses, monitoring strategies, and possible interactions. One objective review recognized co-Q10 as adjunctive therapy for congestive heart failure. BE CERTAIN to tell your doctor that you are taking or are considering taking these herbs if you are taking digoxin or if a digoxin prescription is being considered for you or a loved one. Co-Q10 may also interact badly with aspirin. Soy (milk, tofu, etc.) contains phytoestrogens that have led to an FDA-approved health claim for reducing risk of heart disease (if they have at least 6.25 grams of soy protein per serving). It is important that potassium and magnesium levels be kept in the normal range while you are taking digoxin. Aloe can work as a laxative and can cause excess potassium loss—caution is advised as low potassium or magnesium can lead to digoxin toxicity with "normal" dosing and blood levels.
St. John's wort appears to lower digoxin levels by about 25%. This decrease may lead to loss of digoxin benefits and can be a very serious drug interaction. Couch grass or nettle should NOT be taken by patients who have increased fluid (edema) caused by heart weakness. Patients taking digoxin should NOT take lily of the valley herb, pheasant's eye, or squill. Hawthorn (Crataegus variety) has been used to help heart failure, but should not be combined with heart medicines as combination use has not been studied. Use of intravenous calcium may cause a fatal interaction with digoxin. A case report of ginseng falsely elevating digoxin test levels has been made.
Beverages: Avoid excessive amounts of caffeine-containing beverages or herbs: coffee, tea, cola. May be taken with milk.

▷   *Alcohol:* No interactions expected.

Tobacco Smoking: Nicotine can cause heart muscle irritability and predispose to serious rhythm disturbances. I advise everyone to quit smoking.

Marijuana Smoking: Possible accentuation of heart failure; reduced digoxin effect; possible changes in electrocardiogram, confusing interpretation.

▷   *Other Drugs*

Digoxin **taken concurrently** with

- acarbose (Precose) may result in decreased digoxin blood levels and loss of digoxin's benefits.
- calcium (intravenously) may cause a fatal interaction.
- digoxin immune Fab (Digibind) will result in decreased blood levels. This is used to therapeutic advantage in digoxin toxicity.
- diuretics (except spironolactone or triamterene) can cause serious heart rhythm problems due to loss of potassium.
- dofetilide (Tikosyn) has been found to result in increased occurrence of an abnormal heart effect (Torsades de pointes). Presently, it is unclear if this is an interaction or is a result of medicines used in sicker patients. Caution is advised.
- metformin (Glucophage) may increase metformin levels and lead to excessively low blood sugar.
- pancuronium (Pavulon) or vecuronium (Norcuron) may cause abnormal heartbeats (arrhythmia).
- propranolol or other beta-blocking medicines (see Drug Classes) may cause very slow heart rate.
- quinidine may result in decreased digoxin effectiveness and increased digoxin toxicity; careful dose adjustments are needed.
- succinylcholine may lead to abnormal heart rhythms.

The following drugs may **increase** the effects of digoxin:

- alprazolam (Xanax).
- amiloride (Midamor).
- amiodarone (Cordarone).
- amphotericin B (Abelcet, Fungizone).
- atorvastatin (Lipitor), simvastatin (Zocor); blood levels should be checked more frequently and digoxin dosing adjusted as needed.
- benzodiazepines (Librium, Valium, etc.; see Drug Classes).
- captopril (Capoten, Capozide).
- carvedilol (Coreg) may lead to abnormal heart conduction and increased blood digoxin levels. Caution is prudent. A small study in children from 14 days to 8 years old found that this combination slowed the removal of digoxin by 50%. Lower doses and more frequent blood levels are prudent if this combination must be used—particularly in children.
- cotrimoxazole (various).
- cyclosporine (Sandimmune).
- diltiazem (Cardizem) and other calcium channel blockers (see Drug Classes).
- disopyramide (Norpace).
- erythromycin (E.E.S., Erythrocin, etc.). May also occur with clarithromycin and azithromycin.
- ethacrynic acid.
- esomeprazole (Nexium), omeprazole (Prilosec).
- flecainide (Tambocor).
- fluoxetine (Prozac, Sarafem) and fluvoxamine (Luvox).
- gatifloxacin (Tequin).

- hydroxychloroquine.
- ibuprofen (Advil, Medipren, Motrin, Nuprin, etc.).
- indomethacin (Indocin) and other NSAIDs.
- itraconazole (Sporanox).
- methimazole (Tapazole).
- mibefradil (Posicor).
- nefazodone (Serzone).
- nifedipine (Adalat, Procardia).
- omeprazole (Prilosec), rabeprazole (Aciphex).
- phenytoin (Dilantin).
- propafenone (Rythmol) (30–100% increased blood level).
- propylthiouracil (Propacil).
- quinine.
- quinupristin/dalfopristin (Synercid).
- ritonavir (Norvir).
- spironolactone (Aldactone).
- telmisartan (Micardis).
- tetracyclines (see Drug Classes).
- tolbutamide (Orinase).
- tramadol (Ultram).
- trazodone (Desyrel).
- trimethoprim (Septra, others).
- verapamil (Calan, Verelan, others).

The following drugs may **decrease** the effects of digoxin:
- activated charcoal (various).
- aluminum, magnesium hydroxide, and magnesium trisilicate-containing antacids (Amphojel, Maalox, Mylanta, etc.).
- bleomycin (Blenoxane).
- carmustine (BiCNU).
- cholestyramine (Questran).
- colestipol (Colestid).
- cyclophosphamide (Cytoxan).
- cytarabine (Cytosar).
- doxorubicin (Adriamycin).
- fluvoxamine (Luvox).
- kaolin/pectin (Donnagel, others).
- methotrexate (Mexate).
- metoclopramide (Reglan).
- miglitol (Glyset).
- neomycin.
- penicillamine (Cuprimine, Depen).
- procarbazine (Matulane).
- rifampin or rifabutin.
- St. John's wort (hypericum).
- sucralfate (Carafate).
- sulfa antibiotics or sulfasalazine.
- thyroid hormones.
- vincristine (Oncovin).

▷ *Driving, Hazardous Activities:* Usually no restrictions. This drug may cause drowsiness, vision changes, and nausea. Restrict activities as necessary.

Aviation Note: Heart function disorders **are a disqualification** for piloting. Consult a designated Aviation Medical Examiner.

Exposure to Sun: No restrictions.

Occurrence of Unrelated Illness: Vomiting or diarrhea can seriously alter this drug's effectiveness. Notify your physician promptly.

Discontinuation: This drug may be continued indefinitely. Do not stop it without consulting your physician.

DILTIAZEM (dil TI a zem)

Introduced: 1977   **Class:** Anti-anginal, antihypertensive, calcium channel blocker   **Prescription:** USA: Yes   **Controlled Drug:** USA: No; Canada: No   **Available as Generic:** Yes

Brand Names: ✤Abert Diltiazem CD, ✤Apo-Diltiaz, ✤Alti-Diltiazem, Cardizem, Cardizem CD, Cardizem LA, Cardizem SR, Cartia XT, Dilacor XR, Diltia XT, Diltiazem, Diltiazem ER, Med Diltiazem SR, ✤Novo-Diltiazem, ✤Nu-Diltiaz, Pharma-Diltiaz, ✤Syn-Diltiazem, Teczem [CD], Tiamate, Tiazac

Controversies in Medicine: Medicines in this class have had many conflicting reports. The FDA has held hearings on the calcium channel blocker (CCB) class. Research at New York University found that nifedipine is a cause of reversible male infertility. CCBs are currently second-line agents for high blood pressure according to the JNC VII (see Glossary).

BENEFITS versus RISKS

Possible Benefits	*Possible Risks*
EFFECTIVE PREVENTION OF BOTH MAJOR TYPES OF ANGINA	Depression, confusion
	Low blood pressure
EFFECTIVE CONTROL OF MILD TO MODERATE HYPERTENSION	Heart rhythm disturbance
	Fluid retention—possible worsening of CHF
HELPS CONTROL ATRIAL FIBRILLATION	
	Liver damage—case reports
May help prevent repeat blockage of coronary arteries in heart transplant patients	Muscle damage—case reports
May inhibit the inflammatory response of the body in heart bypass patients	
Reduces frequency of slowed heart circulation in patients with end-stage kidney disease	
CARDIZEM LA FORM MAY GIVE ENHANCED ANGINA CONTROL WHEN TAKEN AT BEDTIME	

▷ **Principal Uses**

As a Single Drug Product: Uses currently included in FDA-approved labeling: Treats (1) angina pectoris (coronary artery spasm or spontaneous Prinzmetal's variant angina) or associated with exertion; (2) classical angina-of-effort (due to atherosclerotic disease); (3) mild to moderate hypertension; (4) atrial fibrillation.

Other (unlabeled) generally accepted uses: (1) Unstable angina; (2) congestive heart failure; (3) migraine prophylaxis; (4) prevention of abnormal protein excretion in the urine; (5) abnormal heart rhythms; (6) treats abnormal plaques inside blood vessels (atherosclerosis); (7) may help prevent abnormal growth of the left side of the heart (left ventricular hypertrophy) after a heart attack; (8) treats some esophageal disorders; (9) eases symptoms of an overactive thyroid gland (hyperthyroidism); (10) can ease symptoms of Raynaud's phenomenon; (11) can have a role in preserving function in kidney and heart transplant patients; (12) may protect against heart attacks or variant or unstable angina that can occur after (postoperatively) coronary artery bypass grafting; (13) could have a role in slowing the advance of low tension glaucoma; (14) may help prevent repeat blockage (restenosis) in heart transplant patients; (15) appears to reduce the frequency of heart blood flow decreases in patients with end-stage kidney disease.

How This Drug Works: This drug blocks normal passage of calcium through cell walls, inhibiting coronary artery and peripheral arteriole narrowing. As a result, this drug
- prevents spontaneous coronary artery spasm (Prinzmetal's angina).
- decreases heart rate and contraction force in exertion, making effort-induced angina less likely.
- opens contracted peripheral arterial walls, lowering blood pressure (also lessens heart work and helps prevent angina).

Appears to work as an anti-inflammatory drug (inhibits IL-6) in people getting a heart bypass.

▷ **Widely Used Guidelines That Involve This Medicine (representative sample):** Please look at the section at the very beginning of this profile called "Class." Next, turn to Table 22 and you will find guidelines listed by the class involved!

Available Dosage Forms and Strengths

Capsules, extended release — 120 mg, 180 mg, 240 mg, 300 mg
Capsules, extended release (Tiazac only) — 120 mg, 180 mg, 240 mg, 300 mg, 360 mg, 420 mg
Capsules, sustained release — 60 mg, 90 mg, 120 mg
Tablets, immediate release — 30 mg, 60 mg, 90 mg, 120 mg

▷ **Usual Adult Dosage Ranges:** High blood pressure: Sustained-release capsules are started at 60 to 120 mg twice daily or 180 to 240 mg daily (for example, Cardizem LA is started at 180–240 mg when used alone). Effective dose for many patients is 120 to 180 mg twice a day. Daily maximum is 360 mg a day for Cardizem SR. Extended release capsules (Dilacor XR) are started at 120 to 240 mg once a day. Many patients benefit from 240–360 mg daily. Maximum dose is 540 mg once a day. *Angina:* Extended release (such as Cardizem CD, Dilacor XR, or Tiazac) forms may be started at 120 to 180 mg daily. The dose can then be increased as needed and tolerated to 480 mg over 1 to 2 weeks. Maximum dose is 540 mg.

Note: Actual dose and schedule must be determined for each patient individually.

Conditions Requiring Dosing Adjustments

Liver Function: Maximum daily dose in patients with liver compromise should be 90 mg. Rarely causes hepatoxicity, and a benefit-to-risk decision must be made.

Kidney Function: May be one of the best calcium channel blockers to use in kidney compromise (large liver and fecal removal). Caution must still be used. Drug can be a rare cause of kidney compromise.

▷ **Dosing Instructions:** Immediate-release form may be crushed and is best taken before meals and at bedtime. Extended-release forms should NEVER be crushed or altered. Tiazac form may be taken with or without food. Tiazac capsules have been cautiously opened and the contents sprinkled on applesauce. This mixture is then swallowed without chewing. Dilacor XR form is best taken on an empty stomach in the morning. Cardizem LA form has data finding more than a 200% improvement in angina control when taken at bedtime (see Glasser, S.P. in Sources, and talk to your doctor). If you forget a dose, take it as soon as you remember it, unless it is nearly time for your next dose—then skip the missed dose and take the next dose right on schedule. DO NOT double doses. If you find yourself forgetting doses, please talk to your doctor about possible reminder systems to help.

Usual Duration of Use: Use for 2 to 4 weeks is required to see effectiveness in decreasing angina frequency and severity and in lowering blood pressure. Smallest effective dose should be used in long-term therapy (months to years). Take control of your blood pressure for life!

Typical Treatment Goals and Measurements (Outcomes and Markers)

Blood Pressure: Guidelines (JNC VII) define normal blood pressure (BP) as **less than** 120/80 and **pre-hypertension** as 120/80 to 139/89. This new range is intended to help doctors encourage lifestyle changes (or in the case of people with a risk factor for high blood pressure, start treatment) much earlier—so that damage to blood vessels, heart, kidneys, sexual potency, or eyes might be minimized or avoided altogether. Stage 1 hypertension is 140/90 to 159/99 and stage 2 hypertension equal to or greater than: 160/100 mm Hg. These guidelines also recommend that clinicians work with their patients to agree on the goals and a plan of treatment. The first-ever guidelines for blood pressure (hypertension) in African Americans recommends that MOST black patients be started on TWO antihypertensive medicines with the goal of lowering blood pressure to 130/80 for those with high risk for heart and blood vessel disease or with diabetes. The American Diabetes Association also recommends 130/80 as the target for diabetics and less than 125/75 for those who spill more than one gram of protein into their urine. Most clinicians try to achieve a BP that confers the best balance of lower cardiovascular risk and avoids the problem of too low a blood pressure. Blood pressure duration is generally increased with beneficial restriction of sodium. If goals are not met, it is not unusual to intensify doses or add on medicines.

Possible Advantages of This Drug

Minimal kidney removal may make this a drug of choice in people with kidney damage who require a calcium channel blocker. Works in ongoing suppressive treatment in patients who will not tolerate beta blockers. Cardizem LA form offered a 200% improvement in angina control when taken at bedtime.

▷ **This Drug Should Not Be Taken If**
- you have had an allergic reaction to it previously.
- you have "sick sinus" syndrome, second or third degree heart block (and do not have an artificial pacemaker).
- you've recently had a heart attack and your lungs are not working well (acute MI with pulmonary congestion).
- you have atrial fibrillation or flutter and an IV form is being considered.
- you have a particular kind of fast heart rate (ventricular tachycardia with a

wide [QRS more than 0.12 sec] complex and an IV form is being considered).
- you have low blood pressure—systolic pressure below 90.

▷ **Inform Your Physician Before Taking This Drug If**
- you had an unfavorable response to any calcium blocker drug.
- you take digitalis or a beta-blocker (see Drug Classes).
- you have a history of or have congestive heart failure.
- you have a narrowing or stenosis of the aorta.
- you have atrial fibrillation (talk with your doctor).
- you have impaired liver or kidney function.
- your blood pressure is excessively low.
- you have a blockage in your stomach or intestines or they are moving excessively (gastrointestinal obstruction or hypermotility).
- you develop a skin rash.
- you have a history of drug-induced liver damage.

Possible Side Effects (natural, expected, and unavoidable drug actions)
Fatigue—rare.
Light-headedness, heart rate and rhythm changes in some people—rare.
Excessive growth of gum tissue (gingival hyperplasia)—possible.
Difficulty breathing or cough—possible.
Drug fever—one case report—possible.

▷ **Possible Adverse Effects** (unusual, unexpected, and infrequent reactions)
If any of the following develop, consult your physician promptly for guidance.
Mild Adverse Effects
Allergic reactions: skin rash, hives, itching—rare.
Headache—may be self-limiting but frequent.
Drowsiness, dizziness—occasional and dose-related.
Nervousness, sleep problems, depression, confusion, hallucinations—case reports.
Overgrowth of the gums (gingival hyperplasia)—may be frequent.
Impaired sense of smell or taste—possible.
Increased urination—rare.
Flushing, palpitations, fainting, slow heart rate, low blood pressure—rare.
Edema—infrequent (up to 8% with Diltiazem LA form).
Nausea, indigestion, heartburn, vomiting, diarrhea, constipation—rare to infrequent.
Serious Adverse Effects
Serious skin rashes (Stevens-Johnson syndrome, others).
Movement disorder (akathisia)—case report.
Serious disturbances of heart rate and/or rhythm, fluid retention (edema), congestive heart failure—rare.
Drug-induced myopathy or liver damage—rare.
Lowering of a specific kind of white blood cell (granulocytes)—case reports with this and other calcium channel blockers.
Lowering of blood platelets or function—case reports.
Sudden kidney failure—case reports to rare.
Systemic lupus erythematosus—rare.

▷ **Possible Effects on Sexual Function:** Impotence—rare.
Swelling or tenderness of the male breast tissue (gynecomastia)—case reports.
One reported case of heavy vaginal bleeding. Male sexual dysfunction—1–2% reported with other calcium antagonists.

Possible Effects on Laboratory Tests
Blood total cholesterol and triglyceride levels; no effects.
Blood HDL cholesterol level: increased (beneficial).
Blood LDL and VLDL cholesterol levels: no effects.

CAUTION
1. Tell health care providers that you take this drug. Carry a card in your purse or wallet saying you take diltiazem.
2. Nitroglycerin and other nitrate drugs as needed may still be used to relieve acute angina pain. If your angina attacks become more frequent or intense, call your doctor promptly.

Precautions for Use
By Infants and Children: Safety and effectiveness for those under 12 years of age not established.
By Those Over 60 Years of Age: May be more likely to have weakness, dizziness, fainting, and falling. Take necessary precautions to prevent injury. Report promptly any changes in your pattern of thirst and urination.

▷ **Advisability of Use During Pregnancy**
Pregnancy Category: C. See Pregnancy Risk Categories at the back of this book.
Animal Studies: Embryo and fetal deaths and skeletal birth defects reported in mice, rats, and rabbits.
Human Studies: Adequate studies of pregnant women not available.
Avoid this drug during the first 3 months. Use during the last 6 months only if clearly needed. Ask your physician for help.

Advisability of Use If Breast-Feeding
Presence of this drug in breast milk: Yes.
Avoid drug or refrain from nursing.

Habit-Forming Potential: None.

Effects of Overdose: Weakness, light-headedness, fainting, slow pulse, low blood pressure, shortness of breath, congestive heart failure.

Possible Effects of Long-Term Use: None reported.

Suggested Periodic Examinations While Taking This Drug (at physician's discretion)
Evaluations of heart function, including electrocardiograms.
Liver and kidney function tests, with long-term use.

▷ **While Taking This Drug, Observe the Following**
Foods: May increase absorption and cause a 30% increase in blood levels. Avoid excessive salt intake.
Herbal Medicines or Minerals: Ginseng, bitter orange, country mallow, guarana, hawthorn, saw palmetto, ma huang (no longer on the market as a weight loss form but available in traditional Chinese medicine), goldenseal, yohimbe, and licorice may cause increased blood pressure. Garlic and calcium may work to lower blood pressure. The combination may work to require lower diltiazem doses. St. John's wort may work to lower calcium channel blocker levels (because it increases P-glycoprotein in the gut). This combination may also increase sun sensitivity. Guggul and gugulipid will reduce effectiveness of diltiazem—do not combine. Eleuthero root and ephedra should be avoided by people living with hypertension.
Indian snakeroot has a German Commission E monograph indication for hypertension—talk to your doctor. Discuss any plans for herbal medicines or minerals with your doctor.
Beverages: No restrictions. May be taken with milk.

▷   *Alcohol:* Use with caution. Alcohol may exaggerate the drop in blood pressure.

Tobacco Smoking: Nicotine reduces benefits. I advise everyone to quit smoking.

Marijuana Smoking: Possible reduced effectiveness of this drug; mild to moderate increase in angina; possible changes in electrocardiogram, confusing interpretation.

▷   *Other Drugs*

Diltiazem ***taken concurrently*** with

- alfentanil (various) may lead to accumulation of alfentanil. Caution and lower doses of alfentanil are prudent.
- amiodarone (Cordarone) may lead to abnormal heart rhythm.
- anticoagulants (see Drug Classes) may lead to stomach or intestinal bleeding.
- aprepitant (Emend) can result in increased levels and toxicity from BOTH medicines. Cautions and possible dosage decrease are needed.
- aspirin can result in prolonged bleeding time or hemorrhage. This is a benefit to risk decision.
- beta-blocker drugs or digitalis preparations (see Drug Classes) may affect heart rate and rhythm. Careful patient monitoring is necessary if these drugs are combined.
- carbamazepine (Tegretol) may result in toxicity and seizures.
- celecoxib (Celebrex) or rofecoxib (Vioxx) may increase blood pressure secondary to fluid retention.
- cilostazol (Pletal) may result in cilostazol toxicity. Lower cilostazol doses are prudent.
- cisapride (Propulsid) may lead to heart toxicity.
- cyclosporine (Sandimmune) may result in cyclosporine toxicity and kidney failure.
- digoxin (Lanoxin) can result in digoxin toxicity.
- dofetilide (Tikosyn) may result in dofetilide toxicity. Checks of dofetilide levels and dosing adjustments to levels are prudent.
- lithium (Lithobid, others) can result in psychosis and neurotoxicity.
- lovastatin (Mevacor) and simvastatin (Zocor) may increase these (and perhaps other) HMG CoA reductase inhibitor levels that rely on CYP 450 3A4 for removal, and increase risk of muscle damage. Lower HMG CoA doses and careful patient monitoring are prudent.
- midazolam (Versed) may result in midazolam toxicity. Lower doses (by 50%) and careful patient monitoring are critical.
- nifedipine (various) may result in nifedipine toxicity. Alternative medicines or nifedipine dosing adjusted to blood levels is prudent.
- nonsteroidal anti-inflammatory drugs (NSAIDs—see Drug Classes) may lead to stomach or intestinal bleeding.
- oral anticoagulants (warfarin—Coumadin, others) may result in higher than expected anticoagulation. Increased INRs and careful patient following are prudent.
- oral antidiabetic drugs (see Drug Classes) such as glipizide (Glucotrol) may result in greater than expected lowering of blood sugar and hypoglycemia.
- phenytoin (Dilantin) and fosphenytoin (Cerebyx) decrease phenytoin and fosphenytoin metabolism and may cause toxicity. Lower doses and blood level checks are prudent.
- quinidine (Quinaglute, others) may lead to quinidine toxicity.
- rifabutin (Mycobutin) may decrease diltiazem blood levels.
- rifampin (Rifadin) may result in decreased diltiazem effectiveness.

- ritonavir (Norvir), amprenavir (Agenerase), atazanavir (Reyataz), and other protease inhibitors (see Drug Profiles) may lead to diltiazem toxicity.
- Sirolimus (Rapamune) or tacrolimus (Prograf) may result in sirolimus or tacrolimus accumulation and toxicity. Blood levels and dosing adjustments as needed are prudent.
- theophylline (Theo-Dur, others) may lead to theophylline toxicity.
- tretinoin (Vesanoid, others) may lead to tretinoin toxicity.
- triazolam (Halcion) may lead to triazolam toxicity.

The following drugs may *increase* the effects of diltiazem:
- cimetidine (Tagamet).
- fluoxetine (Prozac).
- fluvoxamine (Luvox).
- quinupristin/dalfopristin (Synercid).
- ranitidine (Zantac).
- sertraline (Zoloft).
- voriconazole (Vfend).

▷ *Driving, Hazardous Activities:* Usually no restrictions. This drug may cause drowsiness or dizziness. Limit activities as necessary.

Aviation Note: Coronary artery disease *is a disqualification* for piloting. Consult a designated Aviation Medical Examiner.

Exposure to Sun: This drug may cause photosensitivity (see Glossary).

Exposure to Heat: Caution is advised. Hot environments can exaggerate the blood-pressure-lowering effects of this drug. Observe for light-headedness or weakness.

Heavy Exercise or Exertion: May improve ability to be more active without angina pain. Use caution, and avoid exercise that might be excessive and yet not result in warning pain.

Discontinuation: **Do not stop this drug abruptly.** Ask your doctor about gradual withdrawal.

DIPHENHYDRAMINE (di fen HI dra meen)

Introduced: 1946   **Class:** Antihistamine (ethanolamine type), hypnotic   **Prescription:**   USA: Varies with dose (50 mg is prescription form)   **Controlled Drug:**   USA: No*; Canada: No   **Available as Generic:**   Yes

Author's Note: This medicine is available without a prescription in lower doses and is found in many products.

Brand Names: Acetaminophen-PM, AID to Sleep, Allerdryl, Allergy Capsules, Allergy Formula, Allermax, ✤Ambenyl Expectorant [CD], Ambenyl Syrup [CD], Anacin P.M. Aspirin-Free, Banophen, Bayer Select, Beldin Syrup, Bena-D, Benadryl, Benadryl 25, Benadryl Allergy, Benahist, Benylin, ✤Benylin Decongestant [CD], ✤Benylin Pediatric Syrup, ✤Benylin Syrup w/Codeine [CD], ✤Caladryl [CD], Caldyphen Lotion, Children's Complete Allergy, Complete Allergy Medication, Compoz, Dermarest, Di-Delamine, Dihydrex, Diphendryl, Diphenhist, Dormarex 2, ✤Ergodryl [CD], Excedrin P.M. [CD], Extra Strength Tylenol PM, Gecil, Genahist, Gen-D-Phen, Hydramine, ✤Insomnal, Kolex, ✤Mandrax [CD], Maximum Strength Nytol, Medi-Phedryl, Midol-PM, Nervine Nighttime

---

*See Schedules of Controlled Drugs at the back of this book.

Sleep, Nidryl Elixir, Nighttime Cold Medicine [CD], Nite-Time, Noradryl [CD], Noradryl 25, Nytol, Pain Relief PM [CD], Pathadryl, ❧PMS-Diphenhydramine, Sinutab Maximum Strength, SK-Diphenhydramine, Sleep, ❧Sleep-Eze D, Sleep-Eze 3, Sominex, Sominex 2, Theraflu Cold Medicine (Nighttime Strength), Twilite, Tylenol PM Extra Strength, Unisom Sleepgels, Valdrene, Valu-Dryl Allergy Medicine [CD], Wal-Ben, Wal-Dryl, Wehydryl

---

BENEFITS versus RISKS

Possible Benefits	*Possible Risks*
EFFECTIVE RELIEF OF ALLERGIC RHINITIS AND ALLERGIC SKIN DISORDERS	Marked sedation
	Atropinelike effects
	Accentuation of prostatism (see Glossary)
EFFECTIVE, NONADDICTIVE SEDATIVE AND HYPNOTIC	Difficulty driving or operating hazardous machinery
Treatment of anaphylaxis	
Prevention and relief of motion sickness	
Partial relief of symptoms of Parkinson's disease	

▷ **Principal Uses**

As a *Single Drug Product:* Uses currently included in FDA-approved labeling: (1) Prevention or treatment of motion sickness (control of dizziness, nausea, and vomiting); (2) treatment of drug-induced Parkinsonian reactions, especially in children or the elderly; (3) treatment of conditions caused by histamine release (such as allergic drug reactions and allergic rhinitis (hay fever); (4) used as a short-term sleep aid; (5) helps hives (urticaria) that have an unknown cause (idiopathic); (6) approved to help treat symptoms of the common cold.

Other (unlabeled) generally accepted uses: (1) Cough suppression; (2) can have a role in easing the discomfort of mucositis caused by radiation therapy; (3) used in combination with metoclopramide (Reglan) to help stop vomiting caused by chemotherapy (moderately emetogenic); (4) intravenous or intramuscular use can help serious eye spasm (oculogyric crisis).

As a *Combination Drug Product [CD]:* This drug has a mild suppressant effect on coughing. It is combined with expectorants and codeine or dextromethorphan in some cough products.

How This Drug Works: Blocks the action of histamine. Its natural side effects are used to advantage: sedative action used to help people fall asleep; atropinelike action used in motion sickness and Parkinson-related disorders.

▷ **Widely Used Guidelines That Involve This Medicine (representative sample):** Please look at the section at the very beginning of this profile called "Class." Next, turn to Table 22 and you will find guidelines listed by the class involved!

Available Dosage Forms and Strengths
Capsules, nonprescription — 5 mg
Capsules, prescription — 50 mg
Cream — 1%
Elixir — 12.5 mg/5 mL (14% alcohol)

Spray — 1%
Syrup — 12.5 mg/5 mL, 13.3 mg/5 mL
Tablets, nonprescription — 25 mg
Tablets, prescription — 50 mg

▷ **Usual Adult Dosage Ranges:** *Antihistamine, to prevent motion sickness, or in Parkinsonism:* 25 to 50 mg every 6 to 8 hours. Maximum daily dose is 300 mg. Cough control (antitussive): 25 mg every 4 to 6 hours. Maximum daily dose is 150 mg. *As a sleep aid (hypnotic):* 50 mg at bedtime is often used. To prevent vomiting from chemotherapy: 50 mg of diphenhydramine combined with 50 mg of metoclopramide every 6 hours for 2 to 4 days.
Note: Actual dose and schedule must be determined for each patient individually.

Conditions Requiring Dosing Adjustments
Liver Function: Caution—single doses are not expected to be a problem; however, the use of multiple doses in patients with liver compromise has not been studied.
Kidney Function: In mild kidney failure (creatinine clearance more than 50 mL/min), usual dose is given every 6 hours; every 6–12 hours in mild-moderate failure; and every 12–18 hours in severe kidney failure.

▷ **Dosing Instructions:** Tablet may be crushed and capsule may be opened and is best taken with or following food. Elixirs are available if swallowing is a difficulty, and should be measured with a dosing spoon or medicine cup. If you forget a dose, take the missed dose as soon as you remember unless it is almost time for your next dose—if that is the case, simply skip the missed dose and take the next dose right on schedule. DO NOT double doses.

Usual Duration of Use: Regular use for 2 to 3 days is needed to see effectiveness in easing allergic rhinitis and dermatosis symptoms. If it doesn't work after 5 days, this drug should be stopped. As a bedtime sedative (hypnotic), use only as needed. Avoid long-term use.

▷ **This Drug Should Not Be Taken If**
• you have had an allergic reaction to it previously.
• you are nursing your infant.
• you are taking, or took during the past 2 weeks, any monoamine oxidase (MAO) type A inhibitor (see Drug Classes).
• cream (topical 1%) should NOT be used on the eye lids or in the eyes.

▷ **Inform Your Physician Before Taking This Drug If**
• you have had an unfavorable response to any antihistamine.
• you have narrow-angle glaucoma.
• you have peptic ulcer disease, with any degree of pyloric obstruction.
• you have chickenpox and are considering the topical form of this medicine.
• you have prostatism (see Glossary).
• you are subject to bronchial asthma or seizures (epilepsy).
• you have difficulty urinating.
• you have glucose-6-phosphate dehydrogenase (G6PD) deficiency.

Possible Side Effects (natural, expected, and unavoidable drug actions)
Drowsiness (diphenhydramine is the most sedating antihistamine); weakness; dryness of nose, mouth, and throat; constipation; thickening of bronchial secretions.

▷ **Possible Adverse Effects** (unusual, unexpected, and infrequent reactions)
If any of the following develop, consult your physician promptly for guidance.

Mild Adverse Effects

Allergic reactions: skin rash, hives—rare.

Headache, dizziness, inability to concentrate, blurred or double vision, difficult urination—infrequent.

Reduced tolerance for contact lenses—possible.

Nausea, vomiting, diarrhea—possible.

Serious Adverse Effects

Allergic reaction: anaphylactic reaction (see Glossary)—case reports.

Idiosyncratic reactions: insomnia, excitement, hallucinations, confusion—case reports.

Severe constriction of blood vessels (vasoconstriction)—possible with injection use as a local anesthetic.

Hemolytic anemia (see Glossary) or porphyria—case reports.

Reduced white blood cell count: fever, sore throat, infections, or blood platelet destruction (abnormal bleeding or bruising; see Glossary)—case reports.

Movement disorders (dyskinesias, dystonias)—case reports.

Impaired reaction time—dose related and greater impairment than 0.1% blood alcohol in some people.

Hip fractures—case reports resulting in older patients from unsteadiness from the drug versus the drug itself.

▷ **Possible Effects on Sexual Function:** Shortened menstrual cycle (early arrival of expected menstrual onset).

Natural Diseases or Disorders That May Be Activated by This Drug

Latent epilepsy, glaucoma, prostatism.

Possible Effects on Laboratory Tests

Red blood cell counts and hemoglobin: decreased—possible.

Urine screening tests for drug abuse: initial test result may be falsely **positive;** confirmatory test result will be **negative.** (Test results depend upon amount of drug taken and testing method used.)

CAUTION

1. Stop this drug 5 days before diagnostic skin testing procedures in order to prevent false-negative test results.
2. Do not use if you have active bronchial asthma, bronchitis, or pneumonia.
3. May lead to unsteadiness in older patients (generally more sensitive to this drug), resulting in falls. Caution is advised.
4. Benylin Elixir has 19 mg (0.8 MEQ) of sodium in each 5 mL.

Precautions for Use

By Infants and Children: This drug should not be used in premature or full-term newborn infants. Doses for children should be small, as the young child is especially sensitive to the effects of antihistamines on the brain and nervous system. For use to decrease coughing (antitussive) in children 6 to 12 years old: 12.5 mg every 4 to 6 hours. The maximum daily dose here is 75 mg/day. Avoid the use of this drug in the child with chickenpox or a flu-like infection—may lead to altered mental status and loss of coordination.

By Those Over 60 Years of Age: Increased risk of drowsiness, dizziness, un-steadiness, and impairment of thinking, judgment, and memory. Can

380   Diphenhydramine

increase the degree of impaired urination associated with prostate enlargement (prostatism). Sedative effects may be misinterpreted as senility or emotional depression.

▷ **Advisability of Use During Pregnancy**

Pregnancy Category: B by the manufacturer. See Pregnancy Risk Categories at the back of this book.

Animal Studies: No birth defects reported in rats or rabbits.

Human Studies: Some case reports of fetal toxicity have been made. Information from studies of pregnant women is not available. A withdrawal syndrome of tremor and diarrhea was reported in a 5-day-old infant whose mother used this drug (150 mg daily) during pregnancy.

Use is a benefit-to-risk decision. Ask your doctor for help.

Advisability of Use If Breast-Feeding

Presence of this drug in breast milk: Yes.

Avoid drug or refrain from nursing.

Habit-Forming Potential: Combination use of pentazocine and diphenhydramine has become an abused intravenous drug combination. There have been rare reports of a withdrawal syndrome after use of high doses. Intravenous use has led to some rare cases of drug abuse.

Effects of Overdose: Marked drowsiness, confusion, incoordination, muscle tremors, fever, dilated pupils, stupor, coma, seizures.

Possible Effects of Long-Term Use: The development of tolerance (see Glossary) and reduced effectiveness of drug.

Suggested Periodic Examinations While Taking This Drug (at physician's discretion)

Complete blood cell counts.

▷ **While Taking This Drug, Observe the Following**

Foods: No restrictions.

Herbal Medicines or Minerals: Valerian and kava kava (kava no longer recommended in Canada) may interact additively (drowsiness). Avoid these combinations. Ginkgo biloba leaf extract has a German Commission E indication for vertigo, but has not been studied in combination with antihistamines and cannot presently be recommended. Talk to your doctor BEFORE adding any herbal medicines.

Beverages: No restrictions. May be taken with milk.

▷ *Alcohol:* Use extreme caution. The combination of alcohol and antihistamines can cause rapid and marked sedation.

Tobacco Smoking: No interactions expected. I advise everyone to quit smoking.

Marijuana Smoking: Increased drowsiness and mouth dryness; accentuation of impaired thinking.

▷ *Other Drugs*

Diphenhydramine may ***increase*** the effects of

- all drugs with a sedative effect such as benzodiazepines, tricyclic antidepressants, and narcotics (see Drug Classes) and cause oversedation.
- amitriptyline (Elavil) and cause increased urinary retention.
- atropine and atropinelike drugs (see Drug Classes).
- metaproterenol (Alupent, others) leading to increased risk of metaproterenol toxicity.
- tramadol (Ultram), leading to increased sedation risk.

The following drugs may *increase* the effects of diphenhydramine:

- monoamine oxidase (MAO) type A inhibitor drugs (see Drug Classes); can delay elimination, exaggerating and prolonging its action.

Diphenhydramine *taken concurrently* with

- metoprolol (see Drug Profiles) may result in increased risk of metoprolol toxicity. Careful patient follow-up and dose changes are prudent.
- phenothiazines (see Drug Classes) may result in increased difficulty urinating, intestinal obstruction, or glaucoma, especially in those over 70 years old.
- temazepam (Restoril) in pregnancy may increase risk of death of the fetus.
- tricyclic antidepressants (see Drug Classes) may cause increased risk of urinary retention.

▷ *Driving, Hazardous Activities:* This drug may impair alertness, judgment, coordination, and reaction time. Restrict activities as necessary.

Aviation Note: The use of this drug *is a disqualification* for piloting. Consult a designated Aviation Medical Examiner.

Exposure to Sun: Caution—this drug may cause phototoxicity (eczematous eruptions) if the lotion is applied and you go in the sun (see Glossary).

Exposure to Environmental Chemicals: The insecticides Aldrin, Dieldrin, and Chlordane may decrease the effectiveness of this drug. Sevin may increase the sedative effects of this drug.

DISOPYRAMIDE (di so PEER a mide)

Introduced: 1969   **Class**: Antiarrhythmic (group or class 1A)   **Prescription:**   USA: Yes   **Controlled Drug:**   USA: No; Canada: No
Available as Generic: USA: Yes; Canada: No

Brand Names: Norpace, Norpace CR, Pisopyramide, Rythmical, ❦Rythmodan, ❦Rythmodan-LA

BENEFITS versus RISKS	
Possible Benefits	*Possible Risks*
EFFECTIVE TREATMENT OF SELECTED HEART RHYTHM DISORDERS	NARROW TREATMENT RANGE LOW BLOOD PRESSURE LOW BLOOD SUGAR (INFREQUENT) AGRANULOCYTOSIS—RARE Peripheral neuropathy Liver toxicity Heart conduction and rhythm abnormalities Frequent atropinelike side effects

▷ **Principal Uses**

As a Single Drug Product: Uses currently included in FDA-approved labeling: Treats abnormal rhythms in the heart ventricles (ventricular arrhythmias). It is classified as a Type 1A antiarrhythmic agent.

Author's Note: Information in this profile has been shortened to make room for more widely used medicines.

DISULFIRAM (di SULF i ram)

Introduced: 1948   **Class:**   Antialcoholism   **Prescription:**   USA:
Yes   **Controlled Drug:**   USA: No; Canada: No   **Available as Generic:**
USA: Yes; Canada: No
Brand Name: Antabuse

BENEFITS versus RISKS

Possible Benefits	*Possible Risks*
EFFECTIVE ADJUNCT IN THE TREATMENT OF CHRONIC ALCOHOLISM	DANGEROUS REACTIONS WITH ALCOHOL INGESTION Acute psychotic reactions Drug-induced liver damage Drug-induced optic and/or peripheral neuritis Low blood platelets

---

▷ **Principal Uses**
  As a Single Drug Product: Uses currently included in FDA-approved labeling:
    Deters abusive drinking of alcoholic beverages. It does not abolish the
    craving or impulse to drink.
  Other (unlabeled) generally accepted uses: (1) Limited use in helping skin
    problems (dermatitis) caused by nickel exposure; (2) some data showing
    benefit in people addicted to narcotics who subsequently abused cocaine.

How This Drug Works: This drug blocks normal liver enzyme activity after alcohol is changed to acetaldehyde. This causes accumulation of acetaldehyde
  and causes the disulfiram (Antabuse) reaction (see Glossary).

▷ **Widely Used Guidelines That Involve This Medicine (representative sample):** Please look at the section at the very beginning of this profile called
  "Class." Next, turn to Table 22 and you will find guidelines listed by the
  class involved!

Available Dosage Forms and Strengths
  Tablets — 250 mg, 500 mg

▷ **Usual Adult Dosage Ranges:** Once all signs of intoxication are gone and no less
    than 12 hours after the last alcohol drink, therapy begins with 500 mg/day
    for 1 to 2 weeks, followed by an ongoing dose of 250 mg/day. Range is 125
    mg to 500 mg daily and is individually determined. Maximum daily dose is
    500 mg.
  **Note: Actual dose and schedule must be determined for each patient
  individually.**

Conditions Requiring Dosing Adjustments
  Liver Function: This drug is a benefit-to-risk decision in mild liver compromise.
    Disulfiram is clearly contraindicated in portal hypertension and active
    hepatitis.
  Kidney Function: Dosing adjustments are not indicated.
  Diabetes: People with diabetes who take disulfiram can be at increased risk for
    diabetic blood vessel (micro- and macrovascular) problems. The risk is
    worsened by potential adverse drug effects such as increased cholesterol
    levels and peripheral neuropathy.

Lung Disease: Accumulation of a metabolite may occur in severe lung problems. Drug levels or dose reduction will be needed.

▷ **Dosing Instructions:** The tablet may be crushed and taken with or following food to decrease stomach irritation. The dose can be given in the evening if sleepiness from the drug is a problem. If you forget a dose: take the missed dose right away, unless it is 12 hours after you should have taken the dose—if that is the case, simply take the next scheduled dose. DO NOT double doses.

Usual Duration of Use: Use on a regular schedule for several months required to see effectiveness in deterring alcohol use. If tolerated well, use should continue until self-control and sobriety are ongoing (use is highly individualized, but may be required for years).

Typical Treatment Goals and Measurements (Outcomes and Markers)

Alcoholism: This medicine does NOT cure alcoholism, but reduces the desire to drink. The goal is to stop drinking and return self-control and sobriety. Combination of this medicine with psychological help (psychotherapy) gets the best results.

▷ **This Drug Should Not Be Taken If**
- you have had a severe allergic reaction to disulfiram. (Note: The interaction of disulfiram and alcohol is not an allergic reaction.)
- you have taken any form of alcohol within the past 12 hours.
- you are pregnant.
- you have a history of psychosis.
- you are taking paraldehyde.
- you have significant exposure to ethylene dibromide where you live or work. Disulfiram inhibits the removal of this chemical and enhances the ability of ethylene dibromide to cause cancer.
- you are taking (or have taken recently) metronidazole (Flagyl).
- you have coronary blood vessel occlusion (block in a coronary artery) or a serious heart rhythm disorder.

▷ **Inform Your Physician Before Taking This Drug If**
- you are allergic to rubber (contact dermatitis from it).
- you have used disulfiram in the past.
- you do not intend to avoid alcohol completely while taking this drug.
- you do not understand what will happen if you drink alcohol while taking this drug.
- you are planning pregnancy in the near future.
- you have a history of diabetes, epilepsy, or kidney or liver disease.
- you take oral anticoagulants, digitalis, isoniazid, paraldehyde, or phenytoin (Dilantin).
- you have a history of low thyroid function (hypothyroidism).
- you have a history of lung disease.
- you plan to have surgery under general anesthesia while taking this drug.

Possible Side Effects (natural, expected, and unavoidable drug actions)

Drowsiness, lethargy during early use.
Offensive breath and body odor.

▷ **Possible Adverse Effects** (unusual, unexpected, and infrequent reactions)
If any of the following develop, consult your physician promptly for guidance.

Mild Adverse Effects

Allergic reactions: skin rash, hives—case reports.
Headache, dizziness, restlessness, tremor—infrequent.

Metallic or garlic-like taste, indigestion (usually subsides in 2 weeks).

Increased cholesterol after 3–6 weeks of treatment—possible (taking 50 mg per day of pyridoxine appears to stop this).

Decreased or increased blood pressure—possible.

Serious Adverse Effects

Allergic reactions: severe skin rashes, drug-induced hepatitis—rare.

Idiosyncratic reaction: acute toxic effect on brain, including abnormal movements and psychotic behavior—case reports.

Optic or peripheral neuritis (see Glossary)—case reports.

Seizures or catatonia—case reports.

Movement changes (akinesia)—case report.

Decreased thyroid gland function—possible.

May increase risk for blood vessel problems in people with diabetes or cause low blood platelets—case reports.

Carpal tunnel syndrome, peripheral neuropathy—case reports.

▷ **Possible Effects on Sexual Function:** Decreased libido and/or impaired erection in users taking recommended doses of 125 to 500 mg daily—case reports.

Adverse Effects That May Mimic Natural Diseases or Disorders

Liver reaction may suggest viral hepatitis.

Brain toxicity may suggest spontaneous psychosis.

Possible Effects on Laboratory Tests

Blood cholesterol level: increased.

INR (prothrombin time): increased (taken concurrently with warfarin).

Liver function tests: liver enzymes increased (ALT/GPT, AST/GOT, and alkaline phosphatase), increased bilirubin.

CAUTION

1. No one intoxicated with alcohol should take this drug.
2. Patients must be fully informed about purpose drug action **before** treatment is started.
3. Long-term use requires exam for reduced thyroid function.
4. Carry a personal identification card noting you are taking this drug.
5. Many liquid herbal medicines contain alcohol—do not combine.

Precautions for Use

By Infants and Children: Safety and effectiveness for those under 12 years of age not established.

By Those Over 60 Years of Age: Watch for excessive sedation when the drug is started. **Do not** perform an "alcohol trial" to see the effects of this drug.

▷ **Advisability of Use During Pregnancy**

Pregnancy Category: C. See Pregnancy Risk Categories at the back of this book.

Animal Studies: No defects reported in rats and hamsters.

Human Studies: Two reports indicate that four of eight fetuses exposed had serious birth defects. Adequate studies of pregnant women are not available.

Avoid this drug completely if possible.

Advisability of Use If Breast-Feeding

Presence of this drug in breast milk: Unknown.

Talk with your doctor, as this is a question of benefit of the drug versus the risk of adverse effects to the fetus.

Habit-Forming Potential: None.

Effects of Overdose: Marked lethargy, impaired memory, altered behavior, confusion, unsteadiness, weakness, stomach pain, nausea, vomiting, diarrhea.

Possible Effects of Long-Term Use: Decreased function of thyroid gland.

Suggested Periodic Examinations While Taking This Drug (at physician's discretion)
Visual acuity.
Liver function tests.
Thyroid function tests.

▷ **While Taking This Drug, Observe the Following**
Foods: Avoid all foods prepared with alcohol, including sauces, marinades, vinegars, desserts, etc. Ask when dining out about use of alcohol in cooking food. Increased cholesterol after 3–6 weeks of treatment is possible. Taking 50 mg per day of pyridoxine seems to stop this side effect. Talk to your doctor.
Herbal Medicines or Minerals: Many liquid herbal medicines such as ginseng and echinacea contain alcohol. DO NOT combine them with disulfiram. Using St. John's wort, guarana, ma huang (no longer on the market), bitter orange, country mallow, ephedrine-like compounds, or kola while trying to stop drinking may worsen jitteriness and anxiety.
Beverages: Avoid all punches, fruit drinks, etc. that may contain alcohol. This drug may be taken with milk.
▷ *Alcohol:* **Avoid completely in all forms** while taking this drug and for 14 days after the last dose. Disulfiram and alcohol—even in small amounts—produces the disulfiram (Antabuse) reaction. This starts 5 to 10 minutes after alcohol: intense flushing, severe headache, shortness of breath, chest pains, nausea, repeated vomiting, sweating, and weakness. If large amounts of alcohol: reaction may progress to blurred vision, vertigo, confusion, severely low blood pressure, and loss of consciousness. May go on to convulsions and death. Reaction may last 30 minutes to hours, depending upon amount of alcohol and disulfiram.
Tobacco Smoking: No interactions expected. I advise everyone to quit smoking.
Marijuana Smoking: Possible increase in drowsiness or lethargy and one case report of hypomania.
▷ *Other Drugs*
Disulfiram may ***increase*** the effects of
- chlordiazepoxide (Librium) and diazepam (Valium) and cause oversedation. Other benzodiazepines such as alprazolam, clonazepam, clorazepate, flurazepam, halazepam, prazepam, or triazolam may also be subject to this interaction.
- oral anticoagulants (warfarin, etc.) and increase the risk of bleeding; dose adjustments may be necessary.
- paraldehyde and cause excessive depression of brain function.
- phenytoin (Dilantin) or fosphenytoin (Cerebyx) and cause toxicity; dose must be decreased.
Disulfiram may ***decrease*** the effects of
- perphenazine (Trilafon, etc.).
Disulfiram ***taken concurrently*** with
- amprenavir (Agenerase) has propylene glycol in the oral solution. Combined use with disulfiram can lead to toxicity. Do not combine.
- bacampicillin (Spectrobid) can theoretically cause a disulfiram reaction, but no cases have been reported.

- cisplatin (Platinol) can increase risk of toxicity of cisplatin.
- cyclosporine (Sandimmune) may result in a disulfiram reaction, as there is alcohol in the intravenous and oral forms of cyclosporine.
- isoniazid (INH, etc.) may cause acute mental problems and incoordination.
- metronidazole (Flagyl) may cause acute mental and behavioral disturbances, making it necessary to stop treatment.
- omeprazole (Prilosec) and possibly esomeprazole (Nexium) may result in increased disulfiram levels and toxicity.
- over-the-counter (OTC) cough syrups, tonics, etc. containing alcohol may cause a disulfiram (Antabuse) reaction; avoid concurrent use (see Over-the-Counter Drugs in Glossary).
- paraldehyde may result in a disulfiram reaction.
- theophylline (Theo-Dur, others) can lead to theophylline toxicity because the metabolism of theophylline is decreased.
- tranylcypromine (Parnate) can increase risk of hallucinations, disorientation, and agitation. Monitor the patient closely if these two medicines must be used together.
- warfarin will result in an increased risk of bleeding. More frequent INR testing is recommended.

The following drugs may *increase* the effects of disulfiram:
- amitriptyline (Elavil) and perhaps other tricyclic antidepressants may enhance the disulfiram-alcohol interaction; avoid concurrent use of these drugs.

▷ *Driving, Hazardous Activities:* This drug may cause drowsiness or dizziness. Limit activities as necessary.

Aviation Note: Alcoholism *is a disqualification* for piloting. Consult a designated Aviation Medical Examiner.

Exposure to Sun: No restrictions.

Exposure to Environmental Chemicals: Thiram, a pesticide, and carbon disulfide, a pesticide and industrial solvent, can have additive toxic effects. Watch for toxic effects on the brain and nervous system.

Discontinuation: This medicine is only part of your program. Do not stop it unless you have talked with your doctor. Even if it is stopped, no alcohol should be ingested for 14 days.

DOFETILIDE (Doh FET ill eyed)

Introduced: 1999   **Class:** Antiarrhythmic   **Prescription:** USA: Yes   **Controlled Drug:** USA: No; Canada: No   **Available as Generic:** USA: No; Canada: No

Brand Name: Tikosyn

Author's Note: Information on this medicine will be broadened in subsequent editions as clinical use and medication benefits warrant.

DORNASE ALPHA (Door nase AL fa)

Introduced: 1994 **Class:** Anti-cystic-fibrosis agent **Prescription:**
USA: Yes **Controlled Drug:** USA: No; Canada: No **Available as**
Generic: USA: No; Canada: No
Brand Name: Pulmozyme

BENEFITS versus RISKS	
Possible Benefits	*Possible Risks*
DECREASED MUCUS VISCOSITY	Hoarseness
IMPROVED LUNG FUNCTION	Antibodies to DNA
DECREASED OCCURRENCE OF	Facial swelling (edema)
RESPIRATORY INFECTIONS	
DECREASED NUMBER OF	
HOSPITALIZATIONS	

▷ **Principal Uses**
As a Single Drug Product: Uses currently included in FDA-approved labeling:
Eases symptoms of cystic fibrosis (used with standard therapies).
Other (unlabeled) generally accepted uses: None at present.

How This Drug Works: Large amounts of DNA are found in sputum of people
with cystic fibrosis, making it thicker than normal. Dornase breaks the
DNA down, making the sputum easier to remove. Other undiscovered
mechanisms may also account for its benefits.

▷ **Widely Used Guidelines That Involve This Medicine (representative sample):**
Please look at the section at the very beginning of this profile called "Class."
Next, turn to Table 22 and you will find guidelines listed by the class involved!

Available Dosage Forms and Strengths
Solution — 2.5-mL ampules of 1.0 mg/mL dornase alpha (2.5 mg)

▷ **Recommended Dosage Ranges** (Actual dose and schedule must be determined
for each patient individually.)
Infants and Children: Patients 3 months to less than 5 years of age. Rashes,
cough, and runny nose (rhinitis) may happen at a higher rate in this population than in older patients.
5 to 60 Years of Age: One 2.5-mg dose administered by one of the tested nebulizers each day. Some selected patients (FVC greater than 85%) may benefit from twice-daily dosing.
Over 60 Years of Age: Same as 5 to 60 years of age.

Conditions Requiring Dosing Adjustments
Liver Function: Not defined.
Kidney Function: Not defined.

▷ **Dosing Instructions:** Solution must be refrigerated and protected from strong light.
The drug should not be used if it is cloudy or discolored. DO NOT mix dornase with other medicines. Clinical trials have only been conducted with the
Hudson T Up-Draft 2, Marquest Acorn II, and Pulmo-Aide compressor. The
reusable PARI LC and PARI BABY Jet nebulizers and PARI PRONEB compressor were also tested. The Durable Sidestream nebulizer with the Moilaire
or Porta-Neb compressors have been tested as well. DO NOT use with other
equipment. If you forget a dose, administer the missed dose as soon as you
remember it, unless it is almost time for your next dose—if that is the case,
simply administer the next scheduled dose. DO NOT double doses.

Usual Duration of Use: Regular use for up to 8 days may be needed in cystic fibrosis. Long-term use (up to 12 months has been studied) requires periodic physician evaluation.

Typical Treatment Goals and Measurements (Outcomes and Markers)
Cystic fibrosis: Lung (pulmonary) function tests (FEV1 or FEC) are used to measure the success of treatment. Improvements in these tests may be seen in as little as 3 days. Patient clinical signs and symptoms of cystic fibrosis (such as easing of breathing difficulty or dyspnea and clearing of sputum) may also be a measure of treatment results. If the usual benefit is not realized, call your doctor.

Possible Advantages of This Drug
Reduction in number of infections, use of antibiotics and hospitalizations with minimal side effects.

▷ **This Drug Should Not Be Taken If**
  • you have had an allergic reaction to it.
  • you have an allergy to Chinese hamster ovary cells.

▷ **Inform Your Physician Before Taking This Drug If**
  • you had a rash after the last dose was taken.
  • you are uncertain how to use the nebulizer or compressor.
  • you are uncertain how much to take or how often to take it.

Possible Side Effects (natural, expected, and unavoidable drug actions)
Hoarseness—may be frequent.

▷ **Possible Adverse Effects** (unusual, unexpected, and infrequent reactions)
  If any of the following develop, consult your physician promptly for guidance.
  Mild Adverse Effects
  Allergic reactions: rash or itching—infrequent to frequent (may be more likely in those 3 months to less than 5 years old).
  Cough or runny nose—infrequent (may be more likely in those 3 months to less than 5 years old).
  Mild pharyngitis or laryngitis—frequent.
  Conjunctivitis—infrequent.
  Chest pain—has been reported.
  Facial swelling—rare.
  Serious Adverse Effects
  Allergic reactions: none defined at present.
  Antibodies to DNA (2–4%).

▷ **Possible Effects on Sexual Function:** None reported.

Possible Delayed Adverse Effects: None reported.

Possible Effects on Laboratory Tests
Antibodies to DNA.

CAUTION
  1. This drug should only be used with one of the studied nebulizers and compressors.
  2. Do not use the drug if it is cloudy or discolored.

Precautions for Use
By Infants and Children: Rash, cough, and runny nose may be more likely in those 3 months to 5 years old.
By Those Over 60 Years of Age: No changes or precautions.

▷ **Advisability of Use During Pregnancy**
  Pregnancy Category: B. See Pregnancy Risk Categories at the back of this book.
  Animal Studies: Studies in rats and rabbits at up to 600 times the usual human dose have not revealed any harm to the fetus.
  Human Studies: Adequate studies of pregnant women are not available.
  Ask your doctor for guidance.

Advisability of Use If Breast-Feeding
  Presence of this drug in breast milk: Unknown.
  Avoid drug or refrain from nursing.

Habit-Forming Potential: None.

Effects of Overdose: Single doses of up to 180 times the usual human dose in rats and monkeys have been well tolerated.

Possible Effects of Long-Term Use: Not defined.

Suggested Periodic Examinations While Taking This Drug (at physician's discretion)

Periodic pulmonary function tests. Improved clearing of sputum.

▷ **While Taking This Drug, Observe the Following**
  Foods: No restrictions.
  Herbal Medicines or Minerals: Some herbals such as anise seed and fennel oil have German commission E monograph indications for catarrh or upper respiratory tract difficulties, but since no studies have been performed in combination with this medicine, they cannot be recommended.
  Nutritional Support: Continued enzyme and nutritional support is still needed.
  Beverages: No specific restrictions.
▷ *Alcohol:* Follow your doctor's advice relative to alcohol use.
  Tobacco Smoking: No interaction, but smoking irritates airways. I advise everyone to quit smoking.
▷ *Other Drugs*
  Clinical studies have revealed that dornase is compatible with medicines typically used to manage cystic fibrosis. Specific drug interactions are not documented at present.
▷ *Driving, Hazardous Activities:* Specific limitations because of drug effects are not defined at present.
  Aviation Note: The use of this drug ***may be a disqualification*** for piloting. Consult a designated Aviation Medical Examiner.
  Exposure to Sun: No restrictions.
  Discontinuation: This drug's benefits stop soon after its regular use is stopped. It must be continued indefinitely to maintain benefit.
  Special Storage Instructions: This drug should be stored at 36–46 degrees F. and should be protected from light. Unused ampules should be stored in their protective pouch in the refrigerator.

DOXAZOSIN (dox AY zoh sin)

Introduced: 1986   **Class:**   Antihypertensive   **Prescription:** USA: Yes   **Controlled Drug:**   USA: No   **Available as Generic:**   Yes
Brand Names: ♣Apo-Doxazosin, Cardura, Cardura-1, Doxaloc, ♣Gen-Doxazosin, ♣Med-Doxazosin

Author's Note: Data from the ALLHAT trial found that alpha blockers are not drugs of first choice in high blood pressure. A recent FDA panel decided not to change the product label. Information in this profile has been truncated to make room for more widely used medicines. Combination use with Proscar (finasteride) to treat benign prostatic hyperplasia (BPH) will be addressed in the finasteride profile.

DOXEPIN (DOX e pin)

Introduced: 1969   **Class:** Antidepressant   **Prescription:** USA: Yes   **Controlled Drug:** USA: No; Canada: No   **Available as Generic:** USA: Yes; Canada: No

Brand Names: Adapin, Sinequan, ✦Triadapin, Zonalon

BENEFITS versus RISKS

Possible Benefits	*Possible Risks*
EFFECTIVE RELIEF OF ENDOGENOUS DEPRESSION	ADVERSE BEHAVIORAL EFFECTS: Confusion, disorientation, hallucinations, delusions
EFFECTIVE RELIEF OF ANXIETY AND NERVOUS TENSION	CONVERSION OF DEPRESSION TO MANIA in manic-depressive (bipolar) disorders
EFFECTIVE RELIEF OF SOME KINDS OF ITCHING (TOPICAL FORM)	Aggravation of schizophrenia and paranoia
Possibly beneficial in other depressive disorders	Rare blood cell disorders
	Rare liver toxicity
	Low blood pressure on standing

Author's Note: Information in this profile has been truncated to make room for more widely used medicines.

EFAVIRENZ (e FAV i rinz)

Introduced: 1998   **Class:** Non-nucleoside reverse transcriptase inhibitor, antiretroviral, antiviral   **Prescription:** USA: Yes   **Controlled Drug:** USA: No; Canada: No   **Available as Generic:** USA: No; Canada: No

Brand Name: Sustiva

```
┌─────────────────────────────────────────────────────────────────┐
│                     BENEFITS versus RISKS                          │
│      Possible Benefits              Possible Risks                 │
│ EFFECTIVE COMBINATION        SIGNIFICANT CENTRAL NERVOUS           │
│   TREATMENT OF HIV             SYSTEM EFFECTS                       │
│ IS PART OF THE STRONGLY      Rash                                  │
│   RECOMMENDED MEDICINES IN                                         │
│   THE CURRENT NIAID                                                │
│   GUIDELINES                                                       │
│ May be the most effective non-                                    │
│   nucleoside reverse transcriptase                                │
│   inhibitor currently available when                              │
│   used in combination with other                                  │
│   antiretrovirals. Convenient once-                               │
│   daily dosing schedule decreases pill                            │
│   burden and will improve adherence.                              │
└─────────────────────────────────────────────────────────────────┘
```

Author's Note: Information in this profile will be broadened or shortened as more information and outcomes become available.

ENALAPRIL (e NAL a pril)

Class: Antihypertensive, ACE inhibitor

Please see the angiotensin converting enzyme (ACE) inhibitor family profile.

ENFUVIRTIDE (En FOO vur tyde)

Introduced: 2003   **Class:**   Fusion inhibitor, antiretroviral, antiviral
Prescription: USA: Yes   **Controlled Drug:**   USA: No; Canada: No
Available as Generic: USA: No; Canada: No

Brand Name: Fuzeon

▷ **Usual Adult Dosage Ranges**

Subqutaneous: Ninety micrograms (MCG) are injected under the skin (subqutaneously) twice daily into the upper arm, thigh (anterior part), or belly (abdomen). Sites should be changed (rotated) from day to day.

Author's Note: Information on this drug will be broadened further in subsequent editions if present promise holds up.

EPINEPHRINE (ep ih NEF rin)

Other Name: Adrenaline   **Introduced:**   1900   **Class:**   Antiasthmatic, antiglaucoma, decongestant   **Prescription:**   USA: Varies   **Controlled Drug:**   USA: No; Canada: No   **Available as Generic:**   USA: Yes; Canada: No

Brand Names: Adrenalin, Adreno-Mist, Ana-Kit, Asthmahaler, Asthmanephrine, Bronkaid Mist, ❧Bronkaid Mistometer, ❧Citanest Forte,

Duranest [CD], ♣Dysne-Inhal, Epifrin, E-Pilo Preparations [CD], Epinal Ophthalmic, EpiPen, Epitrate, Marcaine, Medihaler-Epi Preparations, Micronephrine, Norocaine, Octocaine, P1E1, P2E1, P3E1, P4E1, P6E1, Primatene Mist, Propine Ophthalmic, Sensorcaine, Sus-Phrine, Thalfed [CD], Therex [CD], ♣Ultracaine, Vaponefrin, Xylocaine

---

BENEFITS versus RISKS

Possible Benefits	*Possible Risks*
EFFECTIVE RELIEF OF SEVERE ALLERGIC (ANAPHYLACTIC) REACTIONS	Significant increase in blood pressure (in sensitive people)
TEMPORARY RELIEF OF ACUTE BRONCHIAL ASTHMA	Idiosyncratic reaction: pulmonary edema (fluid formation in lungs)
Reduction of internal eye pressure (treatment of glaucoma)	Heart rhythm disorders (in sensitive people)
Relief of allergic congestion of the nose and sinuses	

▷ **Principal Uses**

As a Single Drug Product: Uses currently included in FDA-approved labeling: (1) Inhalation to relieve acute attacks of bronchial asthma; (2) as a decongestant for symptomatic relief of allergic nasal congestion and as eyedrops in the management of glaucoma; (3) treats anaphylactic shock; (4) emergency treatment of abnormal heart rhythms (such as ventricular fibrillation) and in cardiopulmonary resuscitation; (5) increases beneficial effects of topical anesthetics.

Other (unlabeled) generally accepted uses: (1) Septic shock; (2) wheezing in infants; (3) croup; (4) can have a role in easing painful erections (priapism); (5) may be used in cataract surgery.

How This Drug Works: By stimulating some nerve (sympathetic) terminals, this drug:
- contracts blood vessel walls, raising blood pressure.
- inhibits histamine release into skin and internal organs.
- dilates constricted bronchial tubes, increasing the size of the airways and improving the ability to breathe.
- decreases fluid formation in the eye, increases its outflow, and reduces internal eye pressure.
- decreases blood flow in the nose, shrinking swelling (decongestion) and expanding nasal airways.

▷ **Widely Used Guidelines That Involve This Medicine (representative sample):** Please look at the section at the very beginning of this profile called "Class." Next, turn to Table 22 and you will find guidelines listed by the class involved!

Available Dosage Forms and Strengths

Aerosol — 0.2, 0.27, 0.3 mg per spray
Eyedrops — 0.1%, 0.25%, 0.5%, 1%, 2%
Injection — 0.01, 0.1, 1, 5 mg/mL
Nose drops — 0.1%
Solution for nebulizer — 1%, 1.25%, 2.25%

▷ **Usual Adult Dosage Ranges**

Aerosols: One inhalation, repeated in 1 to 2 minutes if needed; wait 4 hours before next inhalation.

Eyedrops: One drop every 12 hours. Dose may vary with product; follow printed instructions and label directions.

Note: Actual dose and schedule must be determined for each patient individually.

Conditions Requiring Dosing Adjustments

Liver Function: Dose reduction is not needed in liver compromise.

Kidney Function: Dose adjustment is not defined in kidney compromise.

Diabetes: People with diabetes benefit more from standard-dose epinephrine when they are undergoing cardiopulmonary resuscitation (CPR) than they do from high dose.

▷ **Dosing Instructions:** Aerosols and inhalation solutions: Do not use Adrenalin solutions if the are colored (possibly pink to brown) or if they contain particles (precipitates). For inhalers: After first inhalation, wait 1 to 2 minutes to see if a second inhalation is needed. If relief does not occur within 20 minutes of use, stop this drug and seek medical attention **promptly. Avoid prolonged and excessive use.** Eyedrops: Place one drop of the 0.25% to 2.0% solution in the eye. During instillation of drops and for 2 minutes after, press finger against the tear sac (inner corner of eye) to prevent rapid absorption of drug into body. If you forget a dose: take (instill) the missed dose as soon as you remember it, unless it is nearly time for your next dose—then simply skip the missed dose and instill the next dose right on schedule.

Usual Duration of Use: According to individual needs. Long-term use requires physician supervision.

Typical Treatment Goals and Measurements (Outcomes and Markers)

Asthma: Short-acting sympathomimetics like epinephrine are used to prevent or treat reversible spasms of the bronchial tubes. The peak effect happens 1 to 2 hours after dosing. Goals are to return bronchial status to more acceptable status (relief of respiratory distress) FEV1 is useful. If the usual benefit to your breathing is not realized, call your doctor right away.

▷ **This Drug Should Not Be Taken If**
- you have had an allergic reaction to it previously.
- you have narrow-angle glaucoma.
- you are in shock.
- you have organic brain damage.
- you are in labor—it may delay the second stage of labor.
- you are to undergo general anesthesia with cyclopropane or halogenated hydrocarbons.
- your heart is dilated and you have a coronary deficiency.
- you have experienced a recent stroke or heart attack.

▷ **Inform Your Physician Before Taking This Drug If**
- you have any degree of high blood pressure.
- you have any form of heart disease, especially coronary heart disease (with or without angina) or a heart rhythm disorder.
- you have diabetes or overactive thyroid function (hyperthyroidism).
- you have a history of stroke.
- you have ongoing (chronic) lung disease.

- you take monoamine oxidase (MAO) type A inhibitors, phenothiazines (see Drug Classes), digitalis preparations, or quinidine.

Possible Side Effects (natural, expected, and unavoidable drug actions)
In some people—restlessness, anxiety, headache, tremor, palpitation, cold hands and feet, dryness of mouth and throat (with use of aerosol). Temporary increase in blood platelets. Discoloration of soft contact lenses—possible.

▷ **Possible Adverse Effects** (unusual, unexpected, and infrequent reactions)
If any of the following develop, consult your physician promptly for guidance.
Mild Adverse Effects
Allergic reactions: skin rash; eyedrops may cause redness, swelling, and itching of the eyelids.
Weakness, dizziness, pallor.
Serious Adverse Effects
Idiosyncratic reaction: sudden development of excessive fluid in the lungs (pulmonary edema).
Gas gangrene after injection into a muscle (intramuscular)—possible.
In predisposed people—excessive rise in blood pressure with risk of stroke (cerebral hemorrhage).
Rapid heart rate and arrhythmias and heart attack—case reports.
Passing out (syncope)—possible.
Seizures or porphyria—rare.
Pulmonary edema—case reports.
Constriction of the bowel (mesenteric) blood vessels leading to necrosis—possible.
Pigmentation of the eye—case reports.
Kidney toxicity—rare.

▷ **Possible Effects on Sexual Function:** May ease painful and abnormally prolonged erections (priapism).

Possible Effects on Laboratory Tests
Complete blood counts: red cells and white cells increased; eosinophils decreased.
Blood glucose level: increased.
Urine sugar tests: false low or negative results with Clinistix; true positive with Benedict's or Fehling's solution.
Acidosis—possible.
Blood platelets: temporarily increased.

CAUTION
1. Medication failure can result from frequent repeat use at short intervals. If this develops, avoid use for 12 hours, and a normal response should return.
2. Excessive use of aerosol preparations in asthmatics has been associated with sudden death.
3. May cause significant irritability of nerve pathways (conduction system) and heart muscle, predisposing to serious heart rhythm disorders. Talk with your doctor about this.
4. This drug can increase blood sugar level. If you have diabetes, test for sugar often to detect significant changes.
5. If this drug no longer works for you and you substitute isoproterenol (Isuprel), allow 4 hours between drugs.

6. Promptly throw this drug away if a pinkish-red to brown coloration or cloudiness (precipitation) occurs.

Precautions for Use
By *Infants and Children:* Use cautiously in small doses until tolerance is determined. Watch for weakness, light-headedness, or fainting.
By *Those Over 60 Years of Age:* Small doses are prudent. Watch for nervousness, headache, tremor, rapid heart rate. If you have hardening of the arteries (arteriosclerosis), heart disease, high blood pressure, Parkinson's disease, or prostatism (see Glossary), this drug may aggravate your disorder. Ask your doctor for help.

▷ **Advisability of Use During Pregnancy**
Pregnancy Category: C. See Pregnancy Risk Categories at the back of this book.
Animal Studies: Birth defects reported in rats.
Human Studies: Adequate studies of pregnant women are not available.
This drug can cause significant reduction of oxygen supply to the fetus. Use it only if clearly needed and in small, infrequent doses. Avoid during the first 3 months and during labor and delivery.

Advisability of Use If Breast-Feeding
Presence of this drug in breast milk: Yes.
Avoid drug or refrain from nursing.

Habit-Forming Potential: Tolerance to this drug (see Glossary) can develop with frequent use, but dependence does not occur.

Effects of Overdose: Nervousness, throbbing headache, dizziness, tremor, palpitation, disturbance of heart rhythm, difficult breathing, abdominal pain, vomiting of blood.

Possible Effects of Long-Term Use: "Epinephrine fastness": loss of ability to respond to this drug's bronchodilator effect. With long-term treatment of glaucoma: pigment deposits on eyeballs and eyelids, possible damage to retina, impaired vision, blockage of tear ducts.

Suggested Periodic Examinations While Taking This Drug (at physician's discretion)
Blood pressure measurements.
Blood or urine sugar measurements in diabetics.
Vision testing and measurement of internal eye pressure in glaucoma.

▷ **While Taking This Drug, Observe the Following**
Foods: No restrictions, except those that cause you to have an asthma attack.
Herbal Medicines or Minerals: Using St. John's wort, bitter orange, country mallow, ma huang (no longer on the market), guarana, paullinia, ephedrine-like compounds, or kola while taking this medicine may result in unacceptable central nervous system stimulation. Fir or pine needle oil should NOT be used by asthmatics. Ephedra alone does carry a German Commission E monograph indication for asthma treatment, but combining it with this medicine would be like using two medicines from the same family and does not make sense. If you are allergic to plants in the Asteraceae family (aster, chrysanthemum, daisy, or ragweed), you may also be allergic to echinacea, chamomile, feverfew, and St. John's wort. Talk to your doctor BEFORE combining herbal meds with epinephrine.

Beverages: No restrictions.

▷ *Alcohol:* Alcoholic beverages can increase the urinary excretion of this drug.

Tobacco Smoking: No interactions expected. I advise everyone to quit smoking.

▷ *Other Drugs*

Epinephrine *taken concurrently* with

- some beta-blockers (carvedilol, carteolol, nadolol, propranolol) may cause increased blood pressure response to epinephrine and decreased heart rate and resistance to epinephrine if it is used in anaphylaxis.
- chlorpromazine (Thorazine) or other phenothiazines (see Drug Classes) may cause decreased blood pressure and increased heart rate.
- dihydroergotamine (D.H.E.) may cause extreme increases in blood pressure.
- furazolidone (Furoxone) may cause increased blood pressure.
- guanethidine (Esimil, Ismelin) may cause increased blood pressure.
- halothane may cause abnormal heartbeats (ventricular arrhythmia).
- monoamine oxidase (MAO) inhibitors (see Drug Classes) may lead to large and undesirable increases in blood pressure.
- pilocarpine (Ocusert) may cause increased myopia.
- tricyclic antidepressants (amitriptyline, etc.) may cause increased blood pressure and heart rhythm disturbances.
- zotepine (Nipolept) may lead to low blood pressure and reversal of epinephrine benefits.

▷ *Driving, Hazardous Activities:* This drug may cause dizziness or nervousness. Limit activities as necessary.

Aviation Note: The use of this drug *may be a disqualification* for piloting. Consult a designated Aviation Medical Examiner.

Exposure to Sun: No restrictions.

Heavy Exercise or Exertion: No interactions expected, but exercise can induce asthma in sensitive individuals.

Occurrence of Unrelated Illness: Use caution in severe burns. This drug can increase drainage from burned tissue and cause serious loss of tissue fluids and blood proteins.

Special Storage Instructions: Protect drug from exposure to air, light, and heat. Keep in a cool place, preferably in the refrigerator.

Discontinuation: If this drug fails after an adequate trial, stop using it and call your doctor. It is dangerous to increase the dose or frequency.

EPLERENONE (EH plair ih noan)

Introduced: 2002   **Class:** aldosterone receptor antagonist (selective), antihypertensive   **Prescription:** USA: Yes   **Controlled Drug:** USA: No; Canada: No   **Available as Generic:** USA: No

Brand Names: Inspra

Author's Note: A study called Eplerenone Post-AMI Heart Failure Efficacy and Survival Trial (EPHESUS) showed that this medicine in combination with optimal use of other medicines decreased overall death (mortality) in people with left ventricular dysfunction (LVD) and heart failure by 15%. This profile will be broadened in future editions if clinical research warrants.

ERGOTAMINE (er GOT a meen)

Introduced: 1926   **Class:** Antimigraine, ergot derivative   **Prescription:** USA: Yes   **Controlled Drug:** USA: No; Canada: No   **Available as Generic:** Yes

Brand Names: Bellamine [CD], Bellaspas [CD], ✤Bellergal [CD], Bellergal-S [CD], ✤Bellergal Spacetabs [CD], Cafergot [CD], Cafergot P-B [CD], Cafetrate [CD], Drummergal [CD], Duragal-S [CD], Ercaf [CD], Ergobel [CD], Ergocaf [CD], ✤Ergodryl [CD], Ergomar, Ergostat, Genergen, ✤Gravergol [CD], ✤Gynergen, Medihaler Ergotamine, ✤Megral [CD], Oxoid, Phenerbrel-S [CD], Spastrin [CD], Wigraine [CD], ✤Wigraine [CD], Wigrettes

---

BENEFITS versus RISKS	
Possible Benefits	*Possible Risks*
PREVENTION AND RELIEF OF CLUSTER HEADACHES	GANGRENE OF THE FINGERS, TOES, OR INTESTINE
RELIEF OF MIGRAINE HEADACHE	AGGRAVATION OF CORONARY ARTERY DISEASE (ANGINA)
	INCREASED RISK OF ABORTION (if used during pregnancy)

▷ **Principal Uses**

As a Single Drug Product: Uses currently included in FDA-approved labeling: Treats vascular headaches, especially migraine and "cluster" headaches. Often effective in stopping headache if taken in the first hour following start of pain. Short-term basis use is a valid attempt to prevent or abort "cluster" headaches. The inhalation form provides rapid onset of action.

Other (unlabeled) generally accepted uses: None at present.

As a Combination Drug Product [CD]: Combined with caffeine to enhance its absorption. This makes a smaller dose of ergotamine effective and reduces risk of adverse effects with repeated use. This drug is also combined with belladonna (atropine) and barbiturates to help premenstrual tension and the menopausal syndrome—nervousness, nausea, hot flushes, and sweating.

How This Drug Works: It constricts blood vessel walls in the head, preventing or relieving dilation that causes pain of migrainelike headaches.

▷ **Widely Used Guidelines That Involve This Medicine (representative sample):** Please look at the section at the very beginning of this profile called "Class." Next, turn to Table 22 and you will find guidelines listed by the class involved!

Available Dosage Forms and Strengths

Aerosol — 9 mg/mL (0.36 mg/inhalation)

Nasal inhaler (Canada) — 9 mg/mL (360 mcg/dose)

Suppositories — 2 mg (in combination with 100 mg of caffeine)

Tablets, sublingual — 2 mg

▷ **Usual Adult Dosage Ranges:** *Inhalation:* One spray (0.36 mg) when headache starts; repeat 1 spray after 30 to 60 minutes as needed for relief, up to a maximum of 6 sprays every 24 hours. Do not exceed 15 sprays (5.4 mg) per week.

Oral dose: 1–2 mg immediately, then 1–2 mg every 30–60 minutes. Dosing up **to 6 mg in 24 hours or 10 mg per week**. *Sublingual tablets:* Dissolve 2 mg under tongue at the start of headache; repeat 2 mg in 30 minutes as needed, up to a maximum of 6 mg per day. Do not exceed 6 mg every 24 hours or 10 mg/week.

Note: Actual dose and schedule must be determined for each patient individually.

Conditions Requiring Dosing Adjustments

Liver Function: Should be used with caution by patients with liver compromise.
Kidney Function: This drug is a rare cause of acute renal failure and should be used with caution by patients with compromised kidneys.

▷ **Dosing Instructions:** Follow written instructions and doses **carefully.** The regular tablets (combination drug) may be crushed; sustained-release tablets should be taken whole (not crushed). Sublingual tablets should be dissolved under the tongue, not swallowed. If you forget a dose: Call your doctor as this medicine gets the best results if you take it at the first sign of migraine.

Usual Duration of Use: Regular use for several headache episodes often needed to see effectiveness in aborting or relieving vascular headache. Do not exceed recommended schedules. If headaches are not controlled after several trials of maximal doses, ask your doctor about other treatments. There are also a variety of medicines to prevent (prophylactic use) for migraines.

Typical Treatment Goals and Measurements (Outcomes and Markers)

Pain: Most clinicians treating pain use a device called an algometer to check your pain. This looks like a small ruler, but lets the clinician better understand your pain. The goals of treatment then relate to where the level of pain started (for example, a rating of 7 on a 0 to 10 scale) and what the cause of the pain was. Pain medicines may also be used together (in combination) in order to get the best result or outcome. Specific results to migraine relate to stopping (aborting) an attack or easing the severity of an attack. Once again, the role of prophylactic medicines is clear in helping some patients avoid attacks altogether.

▷ **This Drug Should Not Be Taken If**
- you have had an allergic reaction to any dose form.
- you are pregnant or are breast-feeding.
- you have a severe infection (sepsis).
- you have any of the following conditions:
  angina pectoris (coronary artery disease)
  Buerger's disease
  hardening of the arteries (arteriosclerosis)
  high blood pressure (severe hypertension)
  ischemic heart disease or angina
  stroke
  peptic ulcer
  malnutrition
  kidney disease or impaired kidney function
  liver disease or impaired liver function
  Raynaud's phenomenon
  thrombophlebitis
  glaucoma

▷ **Inform Your Physician Before Taking This Drug If**
- you are allergic or overly sensitive to any ergot preparation.
- you have a prolonged aura and migraines (aura may be further prolonged).
- you are planning to have a face-lift (rhytidectomy) or other plastic surgery. This drug may cause serious skin flap problems.

Possible Side Effects (natural, expected, and unavoidable drug actions)
Usually infrequent and mild with recommended doses.
Some people may have cold hands and feet, with mild numbness and tingling.

▷ **Possible Adverse Effects** (unusual, unexpected, and infrequent reactions)
If any of the following develop, consult your physician promptly for guidance.
Mild Adverse Effects
Allergic reactions: localized swellings (angioedema), itching—case reports.
Headache, drowsiness, dizziness, confusion—possible.
Chest pain, abdominal pain, numbness and tingling of fingers and toes, muscle pains in arms or legs—infrequent.
Nausea, vomiting, diarrhea—possible.
Serious Adverse Effects
Gangrene of the extremities: coldness; numbness; pain; dark discoloration; eventual loss of fingers, toes, or feet—possible.
Gangrene of the intestine: severe abdominal pain and swelling; emergency surgery required—case reports.
Retroperitoneal fibrosis—case reports.
Fibrous changes in the lung (pleuropulmonary fibrosis)—case reports.
Pain syndromes (reflex sympathetic dystrophy)—possible.
Insufficient blood flow to the heart (myocardial ischemia) or arrhythmias—case reports.
Clots in a large artery (superior mesenteric)—case reports.
Decreased heart circulation (myocardial ischemia)—case reports and dangerous in ischemic or occult/hidden heart disease.
Fibrous changes in the heart (myocardial fibrosis) or porphyria—case reports.
Lesions of the rectum or anus (anorectal lesions)—case reports.
Kidney failure—case reports.

▷ **Possible Effects on Sexual Function:** None reported.

Natural Diseases or Disorders That May Be Activated by This Drug
Angina pectoris (coronary artery insufficiency), Buerger's disease, Pheochromocytoma (hypertensive crisis), Raynaud's phenomenon.

Possible Effects on Laboratory Tests: None reported.

CAUTION
1. Excessive use of this drug can actually provoke migraines and increase their frequency.
2. Do not exceed a total dose of 6 mg daily or 10 mg/week of the oral form.
3. Individual drug sensitivity varies greatly. Some may have early toxic effects while taking recommended doses. Promptly report numbness in fingers or toes, muscle cramping, or chest pain.

Precautions for Use
By Infants and Children: Safety and effectiveness for those under 12 years of age are not established.

By Those Over 60 Years of Age: Natural circulation changes may make you more susceptible to adverse effects of this drug. See the preceding list of disorders that are contraindications for the use of this drug.

▷ **Advisability of Use During Pregnancy**
Pregnancy Category: X. See Pregnancy Risk Categories at the back of this book.
Animal Studies: Fetal deaths reported due to this drug.
Human Studies: Information from studies of pregnant women indicates that this drug can cause abortion.
This drug should be avoided during the entire pregnancy.

Advisability of Use If Breast-Feeding
Presence of this drug in breast milk: Yes.
Avoid drug or refrain from nursing. May also suppress prolactin secretion.

Habit-Forming Potential: Functional dependence is possible with a withdrawal syndrome (nausea, vomiting, and headache) reported. This has been treated with naproxen (500 mg twice a day).

Effects of Overdose: "Ergotism": cold skin, severe muscle pain, tingling or burning pain in hands and feet, loss of blood supply to extremities resulting in tissue death (gangrene) in fingers and toes. Acute ergot poisoning: nausea, vomiting, diarrhea, cold skin, numbness of extremities, confusion, seizures, coma.

Possible Effects of Long-Term Use: A form of functional dependence (see Glossary) may develop, resulting in withdrawal headaches if the drug is stopped. Tolerance to beneficial effects.

Suggested Periodic Examinations While Taking This Drug (at physician's discretion)
Evaluation of circulation (blood flow) to the extremities.
Observation for emergence of tolerance. Headache diaries can be very helpful in identifying triggers.

▷ **While Taking This Drug, Observe the Following**
Foods: No interactions expected. Avoid all foods to which you are allergic; some migraine headaches are due to food allergies. There are also often "trigger" foods. Keep a diary and try to identify, then avoid these.
Herbal Medicines or Minerals: Using ma huang or ephedrine-like compounds (ephedra) may result in additive and undesirable vasoconstriction. If you are allergic to plants in the Asteraceae family (aster, chrysanthemum, daisy, or ragweed), you may also be allergic to echinacea, chamomile, feverfew, and St. John's wort. St. John's wort can cause changes in the liver enzymes that help remove this medicine—talk to your doctor before combining any herbal medicine or mineral with ergotamine.
Beverages: No restrictions.
▷ *Alcohol:* Best avoided; alcohol can intensify vascular headache.
Tobacco Smoking: Best avoided; nicotine can further reduce the restricted blood flow produced by this drug.
Marijuana Smoking: Best avoided; additive effects can increase the coldness of hands and feet.
▷ *Other Drugs*
Ergotamine may ***decrease*** the effects of
• nitroglycerin and reduce its effectiveness in preventing or relieving angina pain.

The following drugs may *increase* the effects of ergotamine:
- amprenavir (Agenerase), atazanavir (Reyataz), indinavir (Crixivan), nelfinavir (Viracept), ritonavir (Norvir), saquinavir (Fortovase), and efavirenz (Sustiva) are removed by the same enzymes that remove ergotamine. Ritonavir actually has had reports of sudden (acute) ergotism. These combinations are to be avoided.
- beta-blockers (see Drug Classes).
- delavirdine (Rescriptor).
- dopamine (Intropin).
- erythromycins: clarithromycin (Biaxin), dirithromycin (Dynabac), or E-Mycin, ERYC, etc. Azithromycin (Zithromax) has not been reported to cause this effect.
- medicines that inhibit cytochrome P450 3A4 or compete for elimination by it will lead to increased ergotamine levels (such as fluconazole [Diflucan] or voriconazole [Vfend])—do not combine, increasing toxicity risk, and those that induce P450 3A4 (such as St. John's wort) will blunt therapeutic effects.
- troleandomycin (TAO).

Ergotamine *taken concurrently* with
- triptans (naratriptan [Amerge], rizatriptan [Maxalt], sumatriptan [Imitrex], or zolmitriptan [Zomig]) may lead to prolonged vasospastic reaction. One day should pass between an ergotamine dose and triptan use.
- zileuton (Zyflo) increases risk of ergotism—do not combine.

▷ *Driving, Hazardous Activities:* This drug may cause drowsiness or dizziness. Restrict activities as necessary.

Aviation Note: Vascular headache *is a disqualification* for piloting. Consult a designated Aviation Medical Examiner.

Exposure to Sun: No restrictions.

Exposure to Cold: Avoid as much as possible. Cold further reduces restricted blood flow to the extremities.

Discontinuation: Following long-term use, it may be necessary to withdraw this drug gradually to prevent withdrawal headache. Ask your doctor for help.

ERYTHROMYCIN (er ith roh MY sin)

Please see the macrolide antibiotic family profile.

ESCITALOPRAM (EH sih tal oh pram)

Introduced: 2002 **Class:** Antidepressant, SSRI **Prescription:** USA: Yes **Controlled Drug:** USA: No **Available as Generic:** USA: No

Brand Name: Lexapro

Author's Note: This medicine is a different chemical form (isomer) of citalopram (Celexa). Additional clinical study is needed to define the role of this medicine versus other SSRIs, but it appears to offer decreased side effects and increased beneficial results. Information in this profile will be broadened in the next edition if clinical studies warrant.

ESTROGENS (ES troh jenz)

Other Names: Chlorotrianisene, conjugated estrogens, esterified estrogens, estradiol, estriol, estrone, estropipate, quinestrol

Introduced: 1933, 2000, 2003 (low dose Prempro form)   **Class:** Female sex hormone, hormone replacement therapy   **Prescription:**   USA: Yes   **Controlled Drug:**   USA: No; Canada: No   **Available as Generic:** USA: Yes; Canada: No

Brand Names: Activella, Alora, ✤C.E.S., ✤Climacteron, Climara, ✤Clime- strone, ✤Congest, Delestrogen, Depo-Estradiol, DV, Esclim, Estinyl, Estrace, Estraderm, Estraguard, Estratab, Estrovis, Feminone, ✤Femogen, ✤Femogex, Femhrt, Gynetone, Gynodiol, Gynogen LA, Men- est, Menotab, Menotab-M, Menrium [CD], Milprem [CD], ✤Minestrin, ✤Neo-Pause, ✤Oesclim, ✤Oestrilin, Ogen, PMB [CD], Ortho-Prefest, PMS-Estradiol, Premarin, Premphase [CD], Prempro [CD] (a lower dose Prempro was approved March 2003), Progynon Pellet, TACE, Valergen-10, Vivelle, Vivelle-Dot, White Premarin

Author's Note: The estrogen alone part of the Women's Health Initiative (WHI) was stopped in February 2004 because there was no lowering of risk of coronary heart disease and there was found to be an increased risk of stroke. (Visit *www.nhlbi.nih.gov* for more information. At the time of this writing, there is a press release at *www.nhlbi.nih.gov/new/press/04-04- 13.htm.*) Controversy about estrogen therapy (ERT) and use of combi- nation hormone replacement therapy (HRT) started with the HERS (Heart and Estrogen/progestin Replacement Study). HERS negated the role of estrogen/progestin in preventing a second heart attack. The Women's Health Initiative (WHI) combination arm was stopped early (see *www. whi.org;* July 17, 2002 JAMA article, especially Table 4; *www.acog.org;* and *www.menopause.org.*) Importantly, the WHI data showed that if 10,000 women took the 0.626 mg conjugated estrogens and 2.5 mg medrox- yprogesterone daily (as in Prempro), versus not taking it: 8 more women would develop invasive breast cancer, 7 more would have a heart attack or other coronary, and 8 more would have blood clots in the lungs or a stroke. Five fewer would have hip fracture and 6 fewer would have col- orectal cancers. The WHIMS group (Women's Health Initiative Memory Study) of the WHI (May 27, 2003—see FDA talk paper T03-39 in Sources) found that this medicine should NOT be used to help prevent dementia or Alzheimer's, and for the data analyzed, showed an increased risk of unde- sirable mental status change (dementia) in women over 65 who used the combination for longer periods. A two month time frame of use was rec- ommended by the WHI panel (shortest period and in the lowest dose to meet treatment goals).

A continued analysis of the 16,608 women from the Women's Health Ini- tiative (WHI), published in the July 25, 2003 issue of JAMA reported that in women who used the combination of estrogen plus progesterone who developed breast cancer, the tumors tended to be larger than those of women who did not take the combination. Additionally, 25.4% of the com- bined product users who developed breast cancer had tumors that had begun to spread. In general, women who took the combination formulation had a 24% increased breast cancer risk. Increased risk did not become apparent in the first two years of those studied. Some question regarding difficulty of discovering tumors because of increased breast density caused by the hormone progestin has been postulated.

The low-dose Prempro form contains 0.45 mg of conjugated estrogens and 1.5 mg of medroxyprogesterone acetate. This combination form is indicated for use by women who have a uterus and is used to treat moderate to severe vasomotor symptoms (night sweats and hot flashes) as well as moderate to severe vulvar and vaginal changes (atrophy) that may show as vaginal dryness. Topical forms should be considered if the combination is only being used for vulvar and vaginal atrophy. Alternatives for patients who can't take estrogen currently include: clonidine, fluoxetine (Prozac), gabapentin (Neurontin), and venlafaxine (Effexor).

BENEFITS versus RISKS	
Possible Benefits	*Possible Risks*
COMBINATION WITH SIMVASTATIN MAY REDUCE UNDESIRABLE CLOTTING FACTORS AND INFLAMMATION	INCREASED RISK OF INVASIVE BREAST CANCER (combo form with time frame of use uncertain, yet showing after 2 years)
RELIEF OF MENOPAUSAL HOT FLASHES AND NIGHT SWEATS	INCREASED RISK OF HEART ATTACK
PREVENTION OR RELIEF OF ATROPHIC VAGINITIS, ATROPHY OF THE VULVA AND URETHRA	INCREASED RISK OF STROKE INCREASED RISK OF LONG OR DEEP VEIN CLOTS (THROMBOSIS)
PREVENTION OF POSTMENOPAUSAL OSTEOPOROSIS	INCREASED RISK OF CANCER OF THE UTERUS (endometrium— possible and risk increases with
PATCH FORM MAY GIVE UP TO A WEEK OF ESTROGEN	longer use)
DECREASED RISK OF HIP FRACTURE	Accelerated growth of preexisting fibroid tumors of the uterus
DECREASED RISK OF COLORECTAL CANCER	Fluid retention Postmenopausal bleeding
Prevention of thinning of the skin	Increased gall stone risk Increased blood pressure risk Decreased sugar tolerance (glucose)

▷ **Principal Uses**

As a Single Drug Product: Uses currently included in FDA-approved labeling: "Replacement" therapy in (1) ovarian failure or surgical removal; (2) the menopausal syndrome; (3) postmenopausal atrophy of genital tissues; (4) postmenopausal osteoporosis; (5) selected cases of breast cancer and prostate cancer; (6) treats difficulty having sexual intercourse (dyspurunia) caused by vaginal secretion drying (topical forms may be most desirable).

Other (unlabeled) generally accepted uses: (1) Used in combination with simvastatin (Zocor) (in one study of women averaging 57 years old) lowered LDL, increased HDL, reduced undesirable blood clotting factors and inflammation; (2) may have a role in some selected cases of Turner's syndrome (beneficial changes in blood vessels and sensitivity to insulin).

As a Combination Drug Product [CD]: Estrogen is available in combination with chlordiazepoxide (Librium) and with meprobamate (Equanil, Miltown). These drugs provide a calming effect and ease symptoms in selected cases of menopause. See oral contraceptives profile for a discussion of estrogens and progestins.

In the Pipeline: Prempro product with 0.3 mg of conjugated estrogens and 1.5 mg of MPA is being studied and has been submitted to the FDA.

How This Drug Works: When used to correct hormonal deficiency states, estrogens restore normal cellular activity by increasing nuclear material and protein synthesis. Frequency and intensity of menopausal symptoms are reduced when normal levels of estrogen are restored. Blood vessel effects appear to work through both nongenetic and genetic ways.

▷ **Widely Used Guidelines That Involve This Medicine (representative sample):** Please look at the section at the very beginning of this profile called "Class." Next, turn to Table 22 and you will find guidelines listed by the class involved!

Available Dosage Forms and Strengths
Capsules — 12 mg, 25 mg
Capsules (TACE) — 72 mg
Combination form — 0.45 conjugated estrogens/1.5 mg medroxyprogesterone acetate (new)
Combination form — 0.625 mg conjugated estrogens/1.5 mg medroxyprogesterone acetate
Tablets — 0.02 mg, 0.05 mg, 0.1 mg, 0.3 mg, 0.5 mg, 0.625 mg, 0.9 mg, 1.25 mg, 2.5 mg
Transdermal patch — 0.01 mg per day, 0.05 mg per day, 0.025 mg per day, 0.075 mg per day, 0.0375 mg per day, 1.5 mg, 2.3 mg, 3 mg
Transdermal patch — 10, 20, 30 mg (Canada only)
Vaginal cream — 0.1, 0.625, 1.5 mg/g

▷ **Usual Adult Dosage Ranges:** *For conjugated and esterified estrogens:* lowest doses that will control moderate to severe vasomotor symptoms that happen in menopause should be used for the shortest amount of time: Starting doses of 0.45 mg with increases up to 1.25 mg daily are used. Cenestin product notes attempts to lower doses or taper the medicine should be made. Premarin product notes use of 1.25 mg daily for treatment of moderate to severe vasomotor symptoms. Dosing is undertaken for 21 days with 1 week off. Addition of a progestin for the last 10–14 days of the cycle is recommended to lower the occurrence of effects (endometrial hyperplasia or carcinoma) caused by estrogen alone (unopposed). Some studies suggested that combined estrogen and progestin use actually increases breast cancer risk. For other forms of estrogen: Ask your doctor. Patch forms give a week of estrogen replacement in a small patch.
Note: Actual dose and schedule must be determined for each patient individually.

Conditions Requiring Dosing Adjustments
Liver Function: The dose should probably be decreased in mild liver disease as they are poorly removed (metabolized). Estrogens should not be used in acute or severe liver compromise. This drug can be lithogenic (capable of causing stones) in bile.
Kidney Function: In severe kidney compromise requiring dialysis, blood levels are higher than in those with normal kidneys. Lower doses appear prudent.

▷ **Dosing Instructions:** The tablets may be crushed and taken without regard to food. The capsules should be taken whole. If you forget a dose, take the dose you forgot as soon as you remember it, unless it is nearly time for your next dose—if that is the case, simply skip the missed dose and take the next dose right on schedule. DO NOT double doses. Talk to your doctor if you find yourself forgetting doses.

Usual Duration of Use: Transdermal products such as Climara, Estroderm, and Vivelle increase estradiol levels above the starting point (baseline) in about 4 hours. Regular use for 10 to 20 days needed to see effectiveness in easing menopausal symptoms. These medicines should be used in the lowest possible dose for the shortest amount of time in order to reach the goals and avoid the risks of treatment. Use requires periodic evaluation by your doctor (individualized) to see if the benefits of this medicine are being realized (depending on the use) and if it is still needed.

Typical Treatment Goals and Measurements (Outcomes and Markers)
Menopause: Most clinicians treating menopause seek goals of reduction or cessation of hot flashes, and avoidance of rapid bone loss (which can also be measured by some laboratory tests and DEXA testing).

▷ **This Drug Should Not Be Taken If**
- you have had an allergic reaction to the medicine or the substances in the pills previously.
- you have a history of thrombophlebitis, embolism, heart attack, or stroke.
- you have seriously impaired liver function or recent onset of liver disease.
- you are trying to prevent heart and blood vessel (cardiovascular) disease.
- you have abnormal and unexplained genital/vaginal bleeding.
- you are pregnant.
- you have sickle cell disease.
- you have or are suspected to have breast cancer (may be used to treat some kinds of breast cancer) or cancer of the uterus.
- you have known or suspected estrogen-dependent cancer (your doctor will determine this)—except in selected patients being treated for cancer.

▷ **Inform Your Physician Before Taking This Drug If**
- you have had an unfavorable reaction to estrogen therapy previously or if you have an allergy to horses.
- you have a history of breast or reproductive organ cancer.
- you have fibrocystic breast changes, fibroid tumors or bleeding of the uterus, endometriosis, migraine headaches, epilepsy, asthma, vision disturbances, high blood pressure, gallbladder disease, diabetes, or porphyria.
- you tend to retain fluid.
- you have low calcium or kidney disease.
- you smoke tobacco on a regular basis.
- you have a history of blood-clotting (increased likelihood of forming blood clots-hypercoagulability) disorders.
- you plan to have surgery in the near future.
- you are depressed or have a history of depression.

Possible Side Effects (natural, expected, and unavoidable drug actions)
Fluid retention, weight gain, "breakthrough" bleeding (spotting in middle of menstrual cycle), altered menstrual pattern, resumption of menstrual flow ("periods") after natural cessation (postmenopausal bleeding), increased yeast infection susceptibility of the genitals.

▷ **Possible Adverse Effects** (unusual, unexpected, and infrequent reactions)
If any of the following develop, consult your physician promptly for guidance.

Mild Adverse Effects

Allergic reactions: skin rash, hives, itching—rare.

Headache, nervous tension/anxiety, irritability, depression, accentuation of migraine headaches—infrequent.

Nausea, vomiting, bloating, diarrhea—infrequent to frequent.

Tannish pigmentation of the face—possible.

Serious Adverse Effects

Allergic reactions: anaphylaxis—case reports.

Idiosyncratic reaction: cutaneous porphyria—fragility and scarring of the skin.

Erythema multiforme or nodosum—reported.

Can produce or worsen high blood pressure—more likely with higher doses.

Gallbladder disease, pancreatitis, benign liver tumors, jaundice, rise in blood sugar—case reports.

Erosion of uterine cervix, enlargement of uterine fibroid tumors—possible.

Thrombophlebitis (inflammation of a vein with formation of blood clot): pain or tenderness in thigh or leg, with or without swelling of foot or leg—low dose has minimal increased risk; higher doses may carry more risk.

Thromboembolism—increased risk of stroke and blood clots in the veins or lung in women after menopause who have a uterus (risk was greater than benefits for estrogen plus progestin) (see WHI note above).

Pulmonary embolism (movement of blood clot to lung): sudden shortness of breath, pain in chest, coughing, bloody sputum—increased risk (see WHI note above).

Benign liver tumors (adenomas)—possible.

Systemic lupus erythematosus or porphyria—rare.

Stroke (blood clot in brain): headaches, blackout, sudden weakness or paralysis of any part of the body, severe dizziness, altered vision, slurred speech, inability to speak—increased risk (see WHI note above).

Endometrial cancer—increased risk (risk from using estrogen alone [unopposed estrogen]) may be 2 to 12 times greater than for people who do not use estrogen. Many studies do not show an increased endometrial cancer risk if estrogens are used for less than a year. Risk with longer term use may persist for 8–15 years after estrogen treatment is stopped.

Ovarian cancer—Short-term, combined estrogen-progestin use didn't appear to increase risk, but increased risk based on years of use was found once age, oral contraceptive use, and menopause type was considered with a 7% increase in rate ratio per year that estrogen alone was used (found in patients in the Breast Cancer Detection Demonstration Project).

Retinal thrombosis (blood clot in eye vessels): sudden impairment or loss of vision—case reports.

Heart attack (blood clot in coronary artery)—sudden pain in chest, neck, jaw, or arm; weakness; sweating; nausea—increased risk (see WHI note above).

Severe hypercalcaemia—reported in patients with breast cancer that spread to the bone.

Breast cancer—increased risk with combination form use. The Women's Health Initiative (WHI) found a 26% increase in invasive breast cancer in women with a uterus who took estrogen plus progestin treatment (see WHI note above). A re-analysis of the WHI data found that increased tumor risk did not appear in the first two years that the combination form was used (see Chlepowski, R.T. in Sources). A subset analysis of 975 women from 65–79 found that the greatest risk of breast cancer was seen in women who used the combination for at least five years (see Li, C.I. in Sources). Patients using estrogen alone (data women who have had a hysterectomy and for use as long as 25 years) did not show any appreciable increased risk of breast cancer.

▷ **Possible Effects on Sexual Function:** Swelling and tenderness of breasts, milk production.

Increased vaginal secretions. Gynecomastia in males exposed to custom compounded cream used by a parent—case report.

Possible Delayed Adverse Effects: Estrogens taken during pregnancy may predispose a female child to the later development of cancer of the vagina or cervix following puberty.

▷ **Adverse Effects That May Mimic Natural Diseases or Disorders**

Liver reactions may suggest viral hepatitis.

Natural Diseases or Disorders That May Be Activated by This Drug

Latent hypertension, diabetes mellitus, acute intermittent porphyria.

Possible Effects on Laboratory Tests

Arginine test of the pituitary (human growth hormone increase)—falsely increased.

Red blood cells, hemoglobin, and platelets: decreased.

Blood calcium level: increased.

Blood total cholesterol level: decreased (treatment effect); increased in postmenopausal women.

Blood LDL cholesterol level: decreased in postmenopausal women.

Blood triglyceride level: increased.

HDL: increased.

Blood glucose level: increased.

Glucose tolerance test (GTT): decreased.

Blood thyroid hormone (T3 and T4) levels: increased.

Blood uric acid level: decreased.

Liver function tests: increased liver enzymes (ALT/GPT, AST/GOT, and alkaline phosphatase), increased bilirubin.

CAUTION

1. To avoid prolonged (uninterrupted) stimulation of breast and uterine tissues, estrogen should be taken in cycles of 3 weeks on and 1 week off of medication.
2. The estrogen in estrogen vaginal creams is absorbed systemically. It may also be absorbed through the penis during sexual intercourse and can cause enlargement and tenderness of male breast tissue.
3. Some patients may benefit from lower or may require higher than usual doses to prevent osteoporosis. Bone mineral density tests (DEXA or PDEXA) are prudent to see whether a selected dose is working.
4. See WHI note above regarding breast cancer, heart disease, blood clots, etc. Best to take this medicine as a benefit to risk decision in its present dosing for the shortest possible time consistent with treatment goals. Results and continued need should be quickly assessed.
5. Patch forms should not be stored above 86 degrees—be careful when traveling in the summer.

6. The active ingredient of many forms of estrogen replacement comes from pregnant horse urine. Talk to your doctor if you are allergic to horses.

Precautions for Use

By Those Over 60 Years of Age: In this age group, it is advisable to attempt relief of hot flashes with nonestrogenic medicines, yet benefits have been shown in osteoporosis. During use, report promptly any indications of impaired circulation: speech disturbances, altered vision, sudden hearing loss, vertigo, sudden weakness or paralysis, angina, leg pains.

▷ **Advisability of Use During Pregnancy**

Pregnancy Category: X. See Pregnancy Risk Categories at the back of this book.

Animal Studies: Genital defects reported in mice and guinea pigs; cleft palate reported in rodents.

Human Studies: Information from studies of pregnant women indicates that estrogens can masculinize the female fetus. In addition, limb defects and heart malformations have been reported.

It is now known that estrogens taken during pregnancy can predispose the female child to the development of cancer of the vagina or cervix following puberty. **Avoid estrogens completely during entire pregnancy.**

Advisability of Use If Breast-Feeding

Presence of this drug in breast milk: Yes, in minute amounts.

Estrogens in large doses can suppress milk formation. Breast-feeding is considered to be safe during the use of estrogens. Malnourished mothers may have unacceptable decreases in protein and nitrogen in their breast milk if this drug is used while breast-feeding. Discuss benefits and risks with your doctor. The infant should be closely followed and growth checked.

Habit-Forming Potential: There has been some suggestion of estrogens having potential for psychological dependence and tolerance because of their mood-elevating properties, but clinical reports have not been presented.

Effects of Overdose: Headache, drowsiness, nausea, vomiting, fluid retention, abnormal vaginal bleeding, breast enlargement, and discomfort.

Possible Effects of Long-Term Use: Long-term use of combination form is no longer recommended. Ongoing study of the WHI is for estrogens alone. Prudence dictates that women with intact uteri should use estrogens only when symptoms justify it and with proper supervision and attempts every 3–6 months to assess continued need and possible discontinuation.

Suggested Periodic Examinations While Taking This Drug (at physician's discretion)

Checks every few months for benefits and continued need. Regular evaluation of the breasts (self exam) and annual mammography. Check of pelvic organs including Pap smears, and check for urinary tract infection. Periodic lipid panels and blood pressure checks are prudent. Liver function tests as indicated.

▷ **While Taking This Drug, Observe the Following**

Foods: Avoid excessive use of salt if fluid retention occurs. Combining DHEA with estrogen can lead to signs and symptoms (such as nausea, colitis, or breakthrough bleeding) of excess estrogen.

Herbal Medicines or Minerals: Black cohosh appears to work by: (1) suppressing lutenizing hormone; (2) binding to estrogen receptors in the pituitary; and (3) inhibiting lutenizing hormone release. The net effect is that this herb eases symptoms of menopause, but little is known about long-term use or heart and bone protective effects. This herb may interfere with the benefits of estrogen replacement therapy. Talk to your doctor before starting black cohosh if you are currently taking estrogen. Other herbal or integrative approaches to women's health are always best discussed with your doctor to develop an evidence-based approach to overall therapy and avoid possible undesirable additive or side effects.

Use of St. John's wort, echinacea, or ginkgo completely blocked or lowered the ability of sperm to penetrate eggs in one study. DO NOT use these herbs if you are using a conjugated estrogen product to augment mucus quality and help infertility. Combined use of calcium and vitamin D can be a further step to help avoid osteoporosis. St. John's wort may lead to additive sun sensitivity. Talk to your doctor BEFORE adding any herbal medicines.

Beverages: Caffeine levels will be increased—limited consumption of caffeine is prudent. May be taken with milk.

▷ *Alcohol:* No interactions expected.

Tobacco Smoking: Some studies show that heavy smoking (15 or more cigarettes daily) in association with use of estrogen-containing oral contraceptives significantly increases risk of heart attack (coronary thrombosis). I advise everyone to stop smoking.

▷ *Other Drugs*

Estrogens ***taken concurrently*** with

- alendronate (Fosamax) have not been well studied. One small clinical study suggested the combination was beneficial in preventing postmenopausal osteoporosis. The combination of alendronate and hormone replacement therapy (HRT) is now approved in Canada because of excellent combination results.
- amprenavir (Agenerase) may blunt benefits of amprenavir in fighting HIV, and may also result in loss of contraceptive benefits (efficacy). Other protease inhibitors such as nelfinavir (Viracept) may lead to contraceptive failure also.
- atazanavir (Reyataz) may lead to increased birth control pill medicine (estrogen) levels.
- atorvastatin (Lipitor) may lead to increased birth control pill medicine levels.
- fluconazole (Diflucan) may increase contraceptive medicine blood levels (ethinyl estradiol).
- lamotrigene (Lamictal) may increase or decrease lamotrigene levels. More frequent blood level checks are needed with doses adjusted accordingly.
- naratriptan (Amerge) may increase naratriptan as well as zolmitriptan (Zomig) blood levels. Patients should be closely followed for increased naratriptan or zolmitriptan adverse effects.
- oral antidiabetic drugs (see Drug Classes) or oral blood-sugar-lowering medicines may cause loss of glucose control and high blood sugars.
- progestins (various) may increase risk of breast cancer versus estrogen use by itself.
- tacrine (Cognex) increases the risk of tacrine adverse effects.
- thyroid hormones may increase the bound (inactive) drug and require an increase in thyroid dose.
- tricyclic antidepressants (Elavil, Sinequan, etc.) may enhance their adverse effects and reduce their antidepressant effectiveness.
- vitamin C (ascorbic acid, various brands) in higher doses may result in increased estrogen effects. A lower dose of estrogens may be indicated if higher-dose vitamin C will be taken on an ongoing basis.

- warfarin (Coumadin) may cause alterations of prothrombin activity. Increased doses may be needed.

The following drugs may *decrease* the effects of estrogens:

- carbamazepine (Tegretol).
- penicillin (various) may blunt contraceptive benefits.
- phenobarbital (Belladonna, others).
- phenytoin (Dilantin), fosphenytoin (Cerebyx).
- primidone (Mysoline).
- rifampin (Rifadin, Rimactane).

▷ *Driving, Hazardous Activities:* Usually no restrictions. Consult your physician for assessment of individual risk and for guidance regarding specific restrictions.

Aviation Note: Usually no restrictions, but watch for the rare occurrence of disturbed vision and restrict activities accordingly. Consult a designated Aviation Medical Examiner.

Exposure to Sun: Caution—may cause photosensitivity (see Glossary).

Discontinuation: Best to use estrogens in the smallest effective dose, for the shortest amount of time consistent with the benefit to risk profile of the patient and the goals of treatment. If used to control menopausal symptoms, the dose is reduced gradually to prevent acute withdrawal hot flashes. Avoid continual, uninterrupted use of large doses. Ask your doctor for help.

ETANERCEPT (ee TAN err sept)

Other Names: TNFR: Fc (Tumor necrosis factor receptor p75 Fc fusion protein)

Introduced: 1998 **Class:** Disease-modifying antirheumatic drug (DMARD), biologic response modifier **Prescription:** USA: Yes **Controlled Drug:** USA: No; Canada: No **Available as Generic:** No

Brand Name: Enbrel

BENEFITS versus RISKS

Possible Benefits	*Possible Risks*
USEFUL IN RHEUMATOID ARTHRITIS	INFECTIONS CAUSED BY IMMUNOSUPPRESSION FROM THE MEDICINE ITSELF
HAS A ROLE IN MANY CASES OF JUVENILE RHEUMATOID ARTHRITIS	Injection site reactions
	Possible development of antibodies
CAN BE USED IN COMBINATION WITH METHOTREXATE	Questionable cause of heart failure or worsening of existing failure
MAY GIVE A RESPONSE WHERE OTHER AGENTS HAVE FAILED	
THE FIRST PRODUCT TO BE APPROVED FOR PSORIATIC ARTHRITIS (either alone or in combination with methotrexate)	
APPROVED FOR ANKYLOSING SPONDYLITIS	
APPROVED ON APRIL 30, 2004 TO TREAT MODERATE TO SEVERE PLAQUE PSORIASIS	
Emerging data may evolve into a role for this drug in immune thrombocytopenic purpura	

▷ **Principal Uses**

As a Single Drug Product: Uses currently included in FDA-approved labeling: (1) Approved for INITIAL treatment of rheumatoid arthritis (RA) where previously it was used in treatment of moderate to severe rheumatoid arthritis (RA) in patients who have not responded to one or more disease-modifying antirheumatic drugs (DMARD); (2) approved for use in RA in children over 4 years old (juvenile rheumatoid arthritis); (3) treats psoriatic arthritis (either alone or in combination with methotrexate); (4) treats ankylosing spondylitis; (5) approved to treat moderate to severe plaque psoriasis.

Other (unlabeled) generally accepted uses: (1) May have a role in some kinds of wasting (cachexia) where tumor necrosis factor (TNF) is involved; (2) data from the cholesterol and recurrent events (CARE) trial found that decreasing tumor necrosis factor (TNF) (see how this drug works, below) reduces risk of repeat heart attacks; (3) appears to have a role in ongoing (chronic) nerve problems (demyelinating polyneuropathy); (4) early data showed a complete recovery from resistant (refractory) platelet problems (immune thrombocytopenic purpura).

How This Drug Works: Binds with tumor necrosis factor alpha (TNF-alpha) in the body, as well as to lymphotoxin alpha (TNF-beta), and stops their biologic actions. This drug also works to change the body's responses that are caused or regulated by TNF, such as increased levels of matrix metalloproteinase-3, serum levels of cytokines, and release of substances that control white blood cell migration.

▷ **Widely Used Guidelines That Involve This Medicine (representative sample):** Please look at the section at the very beginning of this profile called "Class." Next, turn to Table 22 and you will find guidelines listed by the class involved!

Available Dosage Forms and Strengths
    Injection—25 mg with a syringe containing 1 mL of bacteriostatic water.

▷ **Recommended Dosage Ranges** (Actual dose and schedule must be determined for each patient individually.)
    Infants and Children: Not studied in children less than 4 years old.
        Children 4–17 years old who have moderate to severely active juvenile rheumatoid arthritis (JRA) and who did not respond to or tolerate methotrexate were given 0.4 mg/kg up to a maximum of 25 mg twice a week (subcutaneously). Twice-weekly dosing is best, given 72 to 96 hours apart.
    Usual Adult Dosage Ranges: For rheumatoid arthritis (adults): 25 mg injected under the skin (subcutaneously), twice a week. (Remember to change or rotate where you inject.)
        Author's Note: A medicine also used in rheumatoid arthritis (infliximab or Remicade) has added a black box (more stringent) warning about increased risk of infections in patients who use that medicine. Etanercept now has a bold warning about infections in post-marketing reports. Enbrel should be stopped if the patient develops a serious infection while taking this medicine. Members of an FDA advisory panel found that more data was required for the three existing TNF blockers (adalimumab-Humira, etanercept-Enbrel, and infliximab-Remicade) relative to their possible role in causing lymphoma in patients that use them.

Conditions Requiring Dosing Adjustments
    Liver Function: No changes needed, as the drug is removed by the reticuloendothelial system.
    Kidney Function: Dosing changes are not known to be needed in people with kidney problems.

▷ **Dosing Instructions:** It is very important that you understand how to inject this drug under the skin (subcutaneously) and NOT in a vein (intravenously). Please ask your doctor or pharmacist if you do not understand the patient information on injecting. Please also remember to change (rotate) where you inject (the injection site). Do not use places where the skin is tender, red, or puffy. Talk to your doctor before injecting etanercept if you have an infection. If you forget a dose, take the missed dose right away, unless it is nearly time for your next dose—if that is the case, skip the missed dose and take the next dose right on schedule. Call your doctor if you find yourself missing doses.

Usual Duration of Use: Use on a regular schedule determines benefit. In rheumatoid arthritis this drug usually goes to work in 1 to 4 weeks. Long-term use (months to years) requires physician supervision. Data for use as long as five years has accumulated for this medicine.

Typical Treatment Goals and Measurements (Outcomes and Markers)
    Arthritis: Control of arthritis symptoms (pain, loss of mobility, decreased ability to accomplish activities of daily living, range of motion, etc.) is paramount in returning patient quality of life and to checking the results (beneficial outcomes) from this medicine. The American College of Rheumatology uses scales that define the degree of benefit from a medicine treating rheumatoid arthritis. You will hear these mentioned as ACR 20, 50, and 70. Many arthritis management or pain centers use interdisciplinary teams (physicians from several specialties, nurses, physician's assistants, physical and occupational therapists, pharmacotherapists, psychotherapists, social workers, and others) to get the best results. Specific mobility goals are often set by the

doctor and administered by a physical/occupational therapist. Laboratory tests include C Reactive Protein (CRP), rheumatoid factor or "sed" rate (erythrocyte sedimentation rate, or ESR). The arthritis foundation has additional information at *www.arthritis.org*.

Possible Advantages of This Drug Uses: A novel mechanism (against TNF) to fight arthritis. Works to prevent joint damage better than methotrexate and also eases symptoms faster than methotrexate. Convenient dosing schedule. A patient enrollment program has been started and can be entered by patients by calling 1-888-4EN-BREL. The only agent FDA approved to treat psoriatic arthritis.

▷ **This Drug Should Not Be Taken If**
- you have had an allergic reaction to it previously.
- you currently have an active infection (including chronic or localized infections).

▷ **Inform Your Physician Before Taking This Drug If**
- you have poorly controlled diabetes or a suppression of the immune system or any other disease or condition that predisposes you to infections.
- you develop a serious infection or sepsis while taking this medicine (the drug should be stopped).
- you have recently received a live-virus vaccine.
- you have a history of malignancy.
- you are pregnant or planning pregnancy in the near future.
- you are breast-feeding your infant.
- you have an allergy to latex.
- you develop signs and symptoms of heart failure while taking this medicine or have a history of heart failure.
- you have impaired kidney function.
- you have a history of asthma or allergies to other medicines.

Possible Side Effects (natural, expected, and unavoidable drug actions)

Report any of the following developments to your physician promptly.
Discomfort at the injection site. Immune system suppression. Emergence of latent or quiescent tuberculosis in patients previously exposed.

▷ **Possible Adverse Effects** (unusual, unexpected, and infrequent reactions)
If any of the following develop, consult your physician promptly for guidance.
Mild Adverse Effects
Allergic reactions: skin rash at the injection site—possible.
Development of antinuclear antibodies—infrequent to frequent.
Cough—frequent.
Sinusitis—possible.
Upper respiratory infections—up to 29%.
Vomiting—may be frequent in some children.
Serious Adverse Effects
Allergic reactions: anaphylaxis, injection site reactions—possible.
Central nervous system damage (demyelination)—case reports with unclear causality.
Suppression of the immune system/cells (pancytopenia/aplastic anemia)—possible.
Emergence of tuberculosis in patients previously exposed.
Systemic lupus erythematosus—case reports.
Lymphoma—questionable correlation or causation for all three TNF blockers.

Skin cancer (squamous cell carcinoma)—case reports.

Development of or worsening of heart failure—47 patient case reports receiving etanercept or infliximab.

Excessive activity of the thyroid (hyperthyroidism)—case report.

▷ **Possible Effects on Sexual Function:** None reported.

Possible Delayed Adverse Effects: Possible development of antinuclear antibodies. Long-term effects on infections and malignancies is not fully understood.

Possible Effects on Laboratory Tests

Antinuclear antibodies (ANA): positive.

CAUTION

1. This drug must be monitored carefully by a qualified physician.
2. Make certain you understand how to inject this medicine under the skin.
3. Live-virus vaccines should be avoided during use of this drug. Live-virus vaccines could actually produce infection rather than stimulate an immune response.
4. Positive antinuclear antibodies (ANA) have been reported, but the clinical importance is not yet known.
5. The manufacturer advises against using this medicine if you have an active infection.
6. Patients should be followed closely if they develop an infection while taking etanercept, and treatment should be STOPPED in patients with serious infections or sepsis.
7. All three TNF blockers have come into question relative to correlation or causative agents in lymphoma.

Precautions for Use

By Those Over 60 Years of Age: Specific changes are not indicated at present.

▷ **Advisability of Use During Pregnancy**

Pregnancy Category: B. See Pregnancy Risk Categories at the back of this book.
Human Studies: Adequate studies are NOT available.
Talk to your doctor about benefits versus risks of use.

Advisability of Use If Breast-Feeding

Presence of this drug in breast milk: Unknown.
Avoid drug or refrain from nursing.

Habit-Forming Potential: None.

Effects of Overdose: One patient injected 62 mg twice a week for 3 weeks without any significant adverse effects.

Possible Effects of Long-Term Use: Positive antinuclear antibodies—significance not presently known. One case of diabetes mellitus.

Suggested Periodic Examinations While Taking This Drug (at physician's discretion)

Beneficial response to the medicine (ACR category).
Sedimentation rate (ESR) and rheumatoid factor or C-reactive protein.
CBC with differential (see lymphoma note above).
ANA and fasting glucose tests.
If used in congestive heart failure, tests of heart function and symptom-free walking time.

▷ **While Taking This Drug, Observe the Following**

Foods: No specific recommendations.

Herbal Medicines or Minerals: There are NO DATA on combined use of etanercept with glucosamine. There are also no data on use of etanercept with hay flower, mistletoe herb, or white mustard seed. Echinacea may actually blunt the immune response if used on an ongoing basis, and therefore combination with etanercept is not advisable. Talk to your doctor before combining any herbal medicine with etanercept.

Beverages: No restrictions.

▷ *Alcohol:* No specific recommendations.

Tobacco Smoking: No interactions expected. I advise everyone to quit smoking.

Marijuana Smoking: May cause impairment of immunity.

▷ *Other Drugs*

Etanercept **taken concurrently** with

- anakinra (Kineret) may pose an increased risk of infections, and combined use had NOT been decided.
- medicines that blunt the immune system may lead to additive immune system depression if combined with etanercept.
- yellow fever, pneumococcal, smallpox, or any other live vaccine may result in decreased immune response to the vaccine as well as possible transmission of the infection BY the vaccine.

▷ *Driving, Hazardous Activities:* No restrictions.

Aviation Note: The use of this drug is **probably not a disqualification** for piloting, but the condition being treated may be. Consult a designated Aviation Medical Examiner.

Exposure to Sun: No restrictions.

ETHAMBUTOL (eth AM byu tohl)

Introduced: 1971 Class: Anti-infective, antituberculosis drug **Prescription:** USA: Yes **Controlled Drug:** USA: No; Canada: No **Available as Generic:** USA: No; Canada: No

Brand Names: ✤Etibi, Myambutol

BENEFITS versus RISKS	
Possible Benefits	*Possible Risks*
EFFECTIVE ADJUNCTIVE TREATMENT OF PULMONARY TUBERCULOSIS	RARE OPTIC NEURITIS WITH IMPAIRMENT OR LOSS OF VISION
EFFECTIVE ADJUNCTIVE TREATMENT OF AIDS-RELATED *MYCOBACTERIUM AVIUM-INTRACELLULARE* COMPLEX INFECTIONS	Rare peripheral neuritis (see Glossary)
Possibly effective treatment of tuberculous meningitis	Activation of gout

▷ **Principal Uses**

As a Single Drug Product: Uses currently included in FDA-approved labeling: Treats lung (pulmonary) tuberculosis. Used with other antitubercular drugs (currently three other medicines are added to ethambutol).

416 Ethanol

Other (unlabeled) generally accepted uses: (1) Treatment of tuberculous meningitis; (2) treatment of AIDS-related *Mycobacterium avium-intracellulare* (MAI) complex infections, in combination with other antimycobacterial drugs.

▷ **Widely Used Guidelines That Involve This Medicine (representative sample):** Please look at the section at the very beginning of this profile called "Class." Next, turn to Table 22 and you will find guidelines listed by the class involved!

Available Dosage Forms and Strengths
Tablets — 100 mg, 400 mg

▷ **Recommended Dosage Ranges** (Actual dose and schedule must be determined for each patient individually.)

Infants and Children: Dose not established. Some authorities recommend that children under 13 years of age not be given this drug.

13 to 60 Years of Age: To start—15 mg per kg of body mass, once daily. Daily maximum is 500–1,500 mg.

For retreatment of tuberculosis—25 mg per kg of body mass, once daily for 60 days; then 15 mg per kg of body mass. Total daily dose should not exceed 900–2,500 mg. A variety of dosing schedules have been used, but all of them depend on clinical judgment and a balance of the organism being treated and the ability of the patient to keep taking the medicine.

For tuberculous meningitis or AIDS-related MAI infections—15 mg per kg of body mass, once daily in combination with other medicines.

Over 60 Years of Age: Same as 13 to 60 years of age.

▷ **This Drug Should Not Be Taken If**
• you have had an allergic reaction to it previously.
• you currently have optic neuritis or peripheral neuritis.
• you currently have active gout.
• you are not able to have visual acuity testing.

Author's Note: The information in this profile has been shortened to make room for more widely used medicines.

ETHANOL (ETH an all)

Other Names: **Prescription:** None

Nonprescription: Moonshine, alcohol, jack, white lightning, wine, beer, whiskey, vodka, others

Introduced: 1980 (prescription); 6,000 years ago (nonprescription) **Class:** Antianxiety drug (nonprescription form) **Prescription:** USA: Yes (IV) **Controlled Drug:** USA: No; Canada: Yes (IV) **Available as Generic:** USA: Yes; Canada: Yes

Brand Names: **Prescription:** ❦Dilusol (38.7%), Eskaphen B, Novahistine DMX Liquid, Nyquil Nighttime Cold Medicine, Temaril (5.7%), Tuss-Ornade (5%), Vicks Formula 44D (often used as part of liquid combination medicines) **Nonprescription:** Robert Alison Chardonnay (12% by volume), Bud Dry, Glenlivet, Smirnoff (40% by volume), Cabernet, others

Warning: Clinical use is limited to intravenous treatment of methanol and antifreeze (ethylene glycol) poisoning and as a preservative. Many products contain alcohol. Ask your pharmacist for help if you must avoid alcohol. Widely used in nonprescription form as an antianxiety agent. Some data

show heart (cardiac) benefit of moderate use—however, other data show increased cancer risks. Data from the UK show that heavy drinking may actually **DOUBLE** the risk of strokes. Some people may not have any mental or physical changes even though a breath or blood alcohol test shows they are "legally drunk."

BENEFITS versus RISKS	
Possible Benefits	*Possible Risks*
EFFECTIVE TREATMENT OF METHANOL OR ETHYLENE GLYCOL POISONING	WITHDRAWAL SYMPTOMS SEIZURES
MODERATE USE MAY DECREASE HEART DISEASE/HEART ATTACK RISK	LIVER DAMAGE (with prolonged use)
LIGHT TO MODERATE USE (AS LITTLE AS ONE DRINK PER WEEK) MAY DECREASE RISK OF STROKE AND ISCHEMIC STROKE IN MEN	Possible increased cancer risk Heavy drinking may increase the risk of type 2 diabetes Pancreatitis Encephalopathy Low white blood cell counts and anemia
Moderate drinking may lower the risk of type 2 diabetes	Myopathy

▷ **Principal Uses**

As a Single Drug Product: Uses currently included in FDA-approved labeling: (1) Intravenously (as 10% ethanol and 5% dextrose) in very specific depletion cases as a calorie source.

Other (unlabeled) generally accepted uses: (1) Treatment of methanol or antifreeze (ethylene glycol) poisoning; (2) adjunctive treatment of cancer pain; (3) intravenous treatment of DTs (delirium tremens); (4) used to sclerose esophageal varices and stop bleeding; (5) treatment of hepatocellular cancer where severe liver problems preclude surgery; (6) used to sclerose thyroid cysts; (7) used to destroy nerve tissue (neurolytic block) in chronic pain therapy; (8) widely used in nonprescription form as an antianxiety agent; (9) one large study appears to show that use ranging up to moderate (and NO GREATER than 0.7 mg per kg of body mass for 3 days in a row) may actually help prevent coronary heart disease and heart attacks; (10) a large study of more than 22,000 men showed that light to moderate use (as little as one drink per week) appears to decrease risk of stroke and ischemic stroke in men; (11) moderate drinking (one to two drinks per day) appears to lower the risk of type 2 diabetes; (12) ethanol injection may have a role in managing benign prostatic hypertrophy (BPH); (13) injected (Percutaneous Ethanol Injection, or PEI) therapy of liver carcinoid tumors that had spread (metastasized) and use of PEI combined with transcatheter arterial chemoembolization therapy (TAE) has been helpful in cases of unresectable cancer (hepatocellular carcinoma) of the liver.

As a Combination Drug Product [CD]: Uses currently included in FDA-approved labeling: Widely present in elixirs and other liquid vehicles for drugs as a preservative and partial drug action enhancer.

How This Drug Works: In antifreeze (ethylene glycol) or methanol poisoning, ethanol prevents ethylene glycol or methanol from being changed (metabolized) into toxic chemicals, letting the body remove antifreeze or methanol harmlessly. If used in nonprescription form in excess, it depresses nerve function, leading to emotional changes and disturbances of perception, coordination, and intoxication. Nonprescription use of up to moderate amounts appears to decrease risk of heart and blood vessel disease, but how it works is unknown. Theories include increased HDL, decreased ADP, antioxidant levels in red wine, fibrinolytic system (anticoagulant) effects, and increased levels of prostacyclin have all been presented. Some researchers found that red wine—particularly Cabernet has the greatest protective value. Antioxidant substances are postulated to be active in some reports of cardioprotective effects. One report found that beer containing vitamin B6 helps protect against heart disease by lowering homocysteine—a risk factor for heart disease.

▷ **Widely Used Guidelines That Involve This Medicine (representative sample):** Please look at the section at the very beginning of this profile called "Class." Next, turn to Table 22 and you will find guidelines listed by the class involved!

Available Dosage Forms and Strengths
Intravenous — 5%, 10%, 95%
Nonprescription — Each ounce of 100-proof whiskey has 15 mL of ethanol
— 6 ounces (12%) wine has 22 mL of ethanol
— 12 ounces of beer (4.9%) has 18 mL of ethanol

▷ **Recommended Dosage Ranges** (Actual dose and schedule must be determined for each patient individually.)

Infants and Children: Methanol or ethylene glycol poisoning: 40 mL per kg of body mass per day.

18 to 60 Years of Age: Ethylene glycol poisoning: A loading dose of 0.6 to 0.7 grams per kg of body mass is given (by mouth, NG tube, or intravenously) and followed by 66 to 154 mg per kg of body mass per hour intravenously to maintain a blood level of 100 to 200 mg/dL (milligrams per deciliter) until ethylene glycol levels are undetectable. Methanol poisoning: 0.80 to 1 mL per kg by mouth of 95% ethanol in 6 ounces of orange juice over 30 minutes. Some centers use 1.5 to 2 milliliters per kilogram by mouth of 40% v/v ethanol given in 6 ounces of orange juice over 30 minutes. Dosing is continued to keep a blood level as above until methylene glycol levels are less than 10 mg/dL and/or metabolic changes (such as acidosis, amylase, bicarb, and clinical findings) have resolved.

Coronary heart disease or heart attack prevention: It appears that use of moderate amounts (up to 0.8 mg per kg of body mass per day or no more than 0.7 mg per kg of body mass per day for 3 days in a row) of alcohol may help in preventing risk of this kind of blood vessel disease and myocardial infarctions.

Ischemic stroke or stroke prevention: It appears that as little as one drink per week decreases risk.

Over 60 Years of Age: Same as 18 to 60 years of age for poisonings. Older people may be less able to tolerate the same amount as a younger person for the nonprescription forms. A smaller dose will generally cause an equal or greater loss of coordination or mental ability. Hypothermia risk is also increased.

Conditions Requiring Dosing Adjustments
Liver Function: Ethanol is extensively metabolized in the liver to acetaldehyde and acetyl CoA. The drug is also a clear cause of liver toxicity. The dose must be decreased in liver compromise.

Kidney Function: Kidneys are minimally involved. No changes needed.

▷ **Dosing Instructions:** If methanol or ethylene glycol poisoning is suspected: The nearest poison control center should be contacted (national number is 800-222-1222). Oral dosing (use vodka mixed in orange juice) may be of benefit, depending on distance from a hospital or free-standing emergency center.

For nonprescription antianxiety use: Dose of this drug and the blood alcohol level varies with many factors. Critical ones are weight, metabolic activity of the liver, how much food is in the stomach, strength of alcohol in the beverage, number of "drinks" consumed over a given period of time, and how well hydrated (whether there has been extreme exercise and fluid loss) you are. In general, most of the ethanol consumed is absorbed in the small intestine in fasting patients and the remaining 20% of ethanol is absorbed in the stomach. Food does not change absorption from the small intestine, but delays absorption in the stomach by 2–6 hours.

A blood or breath alcohol test is a marker for mental or physical changes; some people may not have physical or mental changes and will actually have a blood or breath alcohol level in the state-defined range of "legally drunk." Specific levels of blood or breath alcohol do not absolutely predict impairment. Each 10 mL of ethanol increases blood ethanol of an average 150-lb (70-kg) person by 16.6 mg percent (3.6 mmol/L).

The legal definition of intoxication varies state to state, but generally, the legal definition of intoxication is a blood alcohol level of 0.10% or 100 mg/dL. "Under the influence" in Maryland is 0.07% or 70 mg/dL. Driving impairment may occur at blood levels of 0.05% (50 mg/dL) or lower.

Usual Duration of Use: Use on a regular schedule for 48 hours determines effectiveness in methanol overdose. Long-term excessive use as an antianxiety agent is NOT recommended. If you forget a dose: not applicable. Small daily doses appear to have heart protective effects.

Typical Treatment Goals and Measurements (Outcomes and Markers)

Prevention of coronary heart disease: Information from big and small studies shows that taking two or fewer (see dosing above) drinks per day can help decrease the risk of coronary heart disease. Red wine appears to have the most data, but some recent information appears to show a benefit from vitamin B_6–containing beer. Goals then relate to probability of a coronary problem, and time gained without experiencing a coronary problem.

▷ **This Drug Should Not Be Taken If**
- you have had an allergic reaction to any dose form of it previously.
- you have epilepsy.
- you have a history of alcohol addiction.
- you have a urinary tract infection.
- you are pregnant.
- you are in diabetic coma.

▷ **Inform Your Physician Before Taking This Drug If**
- you are in shock or have had surgery on the head (cranium).
- you have liver or kidney compromise.
- you have gout.
- you are prone to low blood sugars.
- you are a diabetic.
- you have congestive heart failure.

Possible Side Effects (natural, expected, and unavoidable drug actions)
Intoxication, perception, coordination, and mood changes.

▷ **Possible Adverse Effects** (unusual, unexpected, and infrequent reactions)
  If any of the following develop, consult your physician promptly for guidance.
  Mild Adverse Effects
  Allergic reactions: itching, rash, hives, and flushing.
  Headache "hangover": nausea, headache, and malaise—dose-related.
  Sedation—dose-dependent.
  Disorientation, memory loss—dose-dependent.
  Color blindness or neuropathy (tingling, burning, or numbness)—with chronic use.
  Vitamin deficiency or muscle changes (myopathy)—with chronic use.
  Stomach irritation—frequent.
  Serious Adverse Effects
  Allergic reactions: anaphylaxis (rash, swelling of tongue, breathing problems, flushing)—case reports.
  Bronchospasm (asthmatics at increased risk)—case reports.
  Respiratory depression—dose-related.
  Elevated or decreased white blood cell count—possible.
  Increased or decreased platelets—case reports.
  Anemia with large red blood cells (megaloblastic)—possible and dose-related.
  Heart dysfunction (myopathy) or anemia (megaloblastic)—possible with chronic, particularly high dose use.
  High blood pressure—possible to frequent.
  Abnormal heart rhythms (atrial and ventricular) or chest pain (angina)—increased risk.
  Liver toxicity—cirrhosis possible with chronic use.
  Liver cancer—may be a relationship to heavy drinking.
  Osteoporosis—increased risk with chronic use.
  Pancreatitis—increased risk with chronic higher-dose use.
  Encephalopathy or cerebrovascular bleeding—increased risk with higher-dose chronic use.
  Nerve damage (peripheral neuropathy)—commonly seen in alcoholism.
  Low blood sugar or ketoacidosis—especially if meals are missed or with chronic or high dose "binge" use.
  Vitamin deficiency (folic acid, vitamins B_1 and B_6) or low magnesium—with chronic use.
  Low potassium (especially with acute intoxication in children)—possible.
  Gout (precipitated by alcohol use in those with gout)—possible.
  Tolerance (with chronic use)—possible.
  Withdrawal: nausea, fever, rapid heart rate, hallucinations. May progress to delirium tremens (5%): profound confusion, hallucinations, etc.—possible.
  Breast cancer—controversial (some case studies found an association while others did not, some data for more dose-related effect in women).
  Gastroesophageal (tongue, mouth, oral pharynx, hypopharynx, and esophagus) and/or liver cancer—increased associated with heavy drinking.

▷ **Possible Effects on Sexual Function:** Decreased libido, impotence (with excessive chronic use). Difficulty achieving an erection in males and decreased vaginal dilation in females. Chronic alcohol use may lead to tenderness and swelling of male and female breast tissue, testicular atrophy, low sperm counts, decreased menstrual blood flow, and diminished capability for orgasm in females. Patients with carcinomas, Hodgkin's disease, lymphoma, and some non-malignant conditions have described intense pain associated with drinking alcohol.

Possible Delayed Adverse Effects: Liver toxicity, anemia, low or high platelets, vitamin deficiency.

▷ **Adverse Effects That May Mimic Natural Diseases or Disorders**
Alcoholic cirrhosis may mimic hepatitis.

Natural Diseases or Disorders That May Be Activated by This Drug
Peptic ulcer disease.

Possible Effects on Laboratory Tests
Liver function tests: elevated ALT.
Complete blood count: decreased white blood cells, decreased hemoglobin, increased or decreased platelets, large (macrocytic) red blood cells, macrocytic anemia.
Amylase: elevated.
Acidosis: possible.
Sperm count: decreased with chronic use.
Sodium and phosphorous: decreased.
Magnesium: decreased with chronic use.
Iron: increased serum iron levels.
Uric acid: increased.

CAUTION
1. The FDA now requires a warning label on all nonprescription pain (analgesic) and fever (antipyretic) products that have aspirin or other salicylates, ibuprofen, naproxen sodium, ketoprofen, or acetaminophen in them (NSAIDs) that says:
Alcohol Warning: If you consume 3 or more alcoholic drinks every day, ask your doctor whether you should take [the medicine in question] or other pain relievers/fever reducers. [The ingredient] may cause stomach bleeding.
This is a warning intended to help protect patients from possible stomach or liver damage.
2. Nonprescription form may cause FATAL increases in blood pressure if combined with cocaine.
3. With high doses (nearly pure "grain" alcohol) or many drinks (frequent dosing) over a short period of time, FATAL blood alcohol levels may be reached with the nonprescription form.
4. Some alcoholic beverages have tyramine in them. Combination of these beverages with MAO inhibitors (see Drug Classes) may lead to extreme increases in blood pressure (hypertensive crisis).
5. Data from a study of 5,766 men over more than 21 years showed that heavy drinking may DOUBLE the risk of strokes.
6. Data from a study of more than 22,000 men showed that light to moderate use (from one drink per week up to one drink per day) of alcohol decreased the risk of stroke or ischemic stroke. Having more than one drink per day DID NOT further decrease risk.
7. Some data says that drinking alcohol (dose-related or heavy use according to different researchers) while taking a corticosteroid (see Drug Classes) type medicine increases risk of bone death (osteonecrosis or avascular necrosis). Talk to your doctor to see how he or she wants to advise you on this. If you do drink alcohol while taking corticosteroids, promptly report any unexplained joint (such as hip, knee, or shoulder) pain.

Precautions for Use

By Infants and Children: Safety and effectiveness for those under 12 years of age not established. Accidental and unsupervised drinking of the nonprescription form may result in severe consequences in children. Seriously low blood sugar may happen and be delayed up to 6 hours after drinking. Low potassium may also occur with high ethanol levels. Therapy is guided by blood sugar, potassium, and blood alcohol (ethanol) levels. Fatality caused by low blood sugar was reported in a 4-year-old child who drank 12 ounces of a mouthwash that contained 10% ethanol.

By Those Over 60 Years of Age: Poisoning with methanol or ethylene glycol is an emergency situation, and while there may be an increased sensitivity to effects, dosing is adjusted to blood levels. The nonprescription form dosing (number of drinks) tolerated would be expected to decrease with increasing age.

▷ **Advisability of Use During Pregnancy**

Pregnancy Category: D, X if used for long periods. See Pregnancy Risk Categories at the back of this book.

Human Studies: Fetal alcohol syndrome—a collection of limb, neurological, and behavioral defects—occurs with excessive alcohol use.

Avoid use of this drug during your **entire** pregnancy.

Advisability of Use If Breast-Feeding

Presence of this drug in breast milk: Yes.

Avoid drug or refrain from nursing.

Habit-Forming Potential: Clearly defined alcoholism exists and occurs. Tolerance also occurs. Severe withdrawal (delirium tremens, or DTs) is well documented.

Effects of Overdose: Toxic levels result in ataxia, loss of consciousness progressing to coma, anesthesia, respiratory failure, and death. Levels of 150 to 300 mg/dL may result in exaggerated emotional states, confusion, and incoordination. Fatalities most often result with blood concentrations greater than 400 mg/dL. Fatal blood levels vary greatly, however, and death has been reported following levels as low as 260 mg/dL. Once again, some people will not have any mental or physical changes with an alcohol level that is in the "legally drunk" range and even with higher levels.

Possible Effects of Long-Term Use: Liver toxicity, anemia, esophageal varices, low white blood cell counts, compromised heart function, high blood pressure, depression, peripheral neuropathy, seizures, cerebrovascular accident (with acute high levels), water intoxication, vitamin and electrolyte disturbances, gastritis or ulcers, pancreatitis, some cancers (see above) muscle pain, osteoporosis, tolerance, and withdrawal.

Suggested Periodic Examinations While Taking This Drug (at physician's discretion)

Blood alcohol levels and methanol or ethylene glycol levels guide therapy in poisonings.

Chronic alcohol abuse: Complete blood counts, liver function tests, amylase, lipase, bone mineral density test such as DEXA, electrocardiograms.

▷ **While Taking This Drug, Observe the Following**

Foods: Food may decrease the absorption of ethanol from the stomach and reduce chances of intoxication.

Nutritional Support: Vitamin support, particularly thiamin (B_1), folic acid, B_6, and vitamin A are needed with chronic use. Vitamin C may help eliminate ethanol.

Herbal Medicines or Minerals: Valerian and kava kava (kava is now not recommended in Canada because of possible liver damage) may interact additively (drowsiness). Avoid these combinations. Magnesium replacement may be needed.

Tobacco Smoking: No interactions expected. I advise everyone to quit smoking.

Marijuana Smoking: Additive central nervous system depression and possible increases in ethanol blood levels.

▷ *Other Drugs*

Ethanol may ***increase*** the effects of
- some antibiotics (such as doxycycline, others).
- central nervous system depressants, such as benzodiazepines, barbiturates, opioids (codeine, oxycodone, morphine, others), and anesthetic agents.
- chlorpromazine (Thorazine) and will result in increased sedation.
- cocaine and result in dangerous increases in blood pressure.
- cyclosporine (Sandimmune)—with large amounts of ethanol.
- diphenhydramine (Benadryl, others) and will increase sedation.
- paroxetine (Paxil), venlafaxine (Effexor), and other antidepressants may increase CNS effects of both drugs.
- warfarin (Coumadin) and require more frequent INR testing and possible dose changes.

Ethanol may ***decrease*** the effects of
- phenytoin (Dilantin) or fosphenytoin (Cerebyx) by reducing blood levels.
- propranolol (Inderal) by increasing propranolol elimination.

Ethanol ***taken concurrently*** with
- abacavir (Ziagen) may result in increased blood levels of abacavir and possibly an increased risk of toxicity.
- acetaminophen (Tylenol) poses an increased risk of liver damage.
- some antihistamines may increase sedation.
- amprenavir (Agenerase) solution may carry a risk of propylene glycol toxicity. Combination is NOT recommended.
- aspirin may result in increased blood loss from the stomach.
- bupropion (Wellbutrin) lowers the seizure threshold in chronic alcohol users. This combination should at least be minimized and better avoided.
- cefamandole (Mandol), cefotetan (Cefotan), metronidazole (Flagyl), cotrimoxazole, sulfamethoxazole, and cefoperazone (Cefobid) may result in disulfiramlike reaction (see Glossary).
- cimetidine (Zantac) may decrease the amount of alcohol that it takes to make you drunk (intoxicated).
- cisapride (Propulsid) may increase ethanol blood levels.
- corticosteroids (various) may increase risk of bone death (aseptic necrosis, avascular necrosis, or osteonecrosis). Talk to your doctor about drinking BEFORE you take any alcoholic beverage.
- disulfiram (Antabuse) will result in severe vomiting and intolerance.
- dronabinol (Marinol) may increase ethanol levels.
- escitalopram (Lexapro) is NOT recommended by the manufacturer.
- fexofenadine (Allegra) showed NO driving performance decrease in one study of 24 healthy men.
- griseofulvin (Fulvicin) can increase the effects of alcohol.

- insulin (various, see insulin profile) may result in potential severe hypoglycemia.
- isoniazid may result in elevated isoniazid levels.
- ketoconazole (Nizoral) may result in disulfiramlike reactions.
- lithium (Lithobid) may result in worsened impairment of coordination and intoxication.
- metformin (Glucophage) may increase risk of lactic acidosis with ongoing or excessive ethanol use.
- methotrexate (Rheumatrex, others) may increase risk of liver damage (especially with long-term ethanol use).
- metronidazole (Flagyl) may result in a disulfiramlike reaction.
- mirtazapine (Remeron) may lead to increased risk of psychomotor impairment.
- nitroglycerin (Nitrostat, others) may result in excessive decreases in blood pressure.
- nonsteroidal anti-inflammatory drugs (NSAIDs; see Drug Classes) may lead to increased risk of stomach bleeding or liver damage.
- olanzapine (Zyprexa) may lead to excessive depression of the central nervous system.
- oral hypoglycemic agents (see Drug Classes) poses an increased risk of seriously low glucose levels.
- quetiapine (Seroquel) may worsen thinking and motor skill depression caused by ethanol.
- ranitidine (Zantac) lead to increased ethanol levels in one study. Ethanol intake is best minimized in patients taking ranitidine.
- sibutramine (Meridia) is not recommended by the manufacturer.
- sulfonylurea oral hypoglycemic agents (such as glipizide, glyburide, others; see Drug Classes) poses an increased risk of seriously low glucose levels and disulfiram-like reactions.
- tramadol (Ultram) may lead to excessive depression of the central nervous system.
- tricyclic antidepressants (see Drug Classes) may result in increased antidepressant levels and toxicity.
- trimethoprim/sulfamethoxazole (Cotrimoxazole, Septra, Bactrim, others) may lead to a disulfiram-like reaction.
- valproic acid (Depakene, Depakote, others) may enhance central nervous depression from ethanol.
- venlafaxine (Effexor) is not advised by the manufacturer.
- verapamil (Calan, others) may increase the amount of time ethanol stays in the body and may pose an increased risk of intoxication.
- zaleplon (Sonata) may result in increased additive central nervous depression (impairing psychomotor functions). Combination should be avoided.
- zolpidem (Ambien) may result in increased additive central nervous depression (impairing psychomotor functions). Combination should be avoided.

▷ *Driving, Hazardous Activities:* This drug may cause drowsiness, mental impairment, and coordination problems. Driving skill may be impaired at very low blood levels with the perception that capabilities are *not* reduced. Drinking and driving is not recommended. Restrict activities as necessary.

Aviation Note: The use of this drug ***is a disqualification*** for piloting. Consult a designated Aviation Medical Examiner.

Exposure to Sun: May result in additive dehydration.

Heavy Exercise or Exertion: May worsen the adverse effects of this drug.

Discontinuation: Abrupt discontinuation after chronic use may result in a serious withdrawal syndrome known as DT, or delirium tremens.

ETHOSUXIMIDE (eth oh SUX i myde)

Introduced: 1960   **Class:** Anticonvulsant   **Prescription:** USA: Yes
Controlled Drug: USA: No; Canada: No   **Available as Generic:** Yes
Brand Name: Zarontin

BENEFITS versus RISKS

Possible Benefits	*Possible Risks*
EFFECTIVE CONTROL OF ABSENCE SEIZURES (PETIT MAL EPILEPSY)	RARE APLASTIC ANEMIA (see Aplastic Anemia and Bone Marrow Depression in Glossary)
EFFECTIVE CONTROL OF MYOCLONIC AND AKINETIC EPILEPSY IN SOME PATIENTS	Rare decrease in white blood cells and blood platelets

---

▷ **Principal Uses**

As a Single Drug Product: Uses currently included in FDA-approved labeling: Used to treat petit mal epilepsy and is a drug of choice in absence seizures. Other (unlabeled) generally accepted uses: None at present.

How This Drug Works: Alters some nerve impulses, suppressing abnormal electrical activity that causes absence seizures (petit mal epilepsy). In general succinimides inhibit (suppress) paroxysmal three-cycle per second wave activity that is seen (associated) with lapses of consciousness in absence seizures. Ethosuximide action is possible related to inhibition at the synapse, which is caused by GABA (GABA mediated chloride conductants).

▷ **Widely Used Guidelines That Involve This Medicine (representative sample):** Please look at the section at the very beginning of this profile called "Class." Next, turn to Table 22 and you will find guidelines listed by the class involved!

Available Dosage Forms and Strengths

Capsules or
　　Gelcaps — 250 mg
　　Solution — 250 mg/5 mL
　　Syrup — 250 mg/5 mL

▷ **Usual Adult Dosage Ranges:** Dosing starts with 500 mg daily and can be increased by 250 mg every 4 to 7 days until acceptable seizure control is achieved. Ending dose may be 20 to 30 mg per kg daily. Daily maximum is 1,500 mg. IMPORTANT: Blood levels increase more quickly in females than males. *For children 3 to 6 years old:* Usual starting dose is 250 mg per day. May increase by 250-mg doses every 4 to 7 days as needed. Usually 20–30 mg per kg is the once-daily dose. *More than 6 years old with absence seizures:* Same as adults.

Note: Actual dose and schedule must be determined for each patient individually.

Conditions Requiring Dosing Adjustments

Liver Function: Blood levels are recommended if the liver is damaged.
Kidney Function: No specific changes needed, but a more frequent check of blood levels may be prudent.

▷ **Dosing Instructions:** Capsule may be opened and taken with food to reduce stomach irritation. If you forget a dose: take the dose you missed as soon as you remember it, unless it is nearly time for your next dose—if that is the case, simply skip the missed dose and take the next scheduled dose right on schedule. DO NOT double doses.

Usual Duration of Use: Regular use for 1 to 2 weeks may be needed to identify the best dose and reduce frequency of absence seizures. Long-term use requires physician supervision and use is ongoing.

Typical Treatment Goals and Measurements (Outcomes and Markers)

Seizures: The general goal for this medicine is effective seizure control. Neurologists tend to define effective on a case-by-case basis depending on the seizure type and patient factors. Blood levels can help guide dosing. If this medicine is being used to treat absence seizures, EEG can be used to check clinical progress.

Currently a Drug of Choice

For ongoing (maintenance) therapy of **absence** seizures.

▷ **This Drug Should Not Be Taken If**
  • you are allergic to any succinimide anticonvulsant (see Drug Classes).
  • you currently have a blood cell or bone marrow disorder.

▷ **Inform Your Physician Before Taking This Drug If**
  • you have a history of or active liver or kidney disease.
  • you have any type of blood disorder, especially one caused by drugs.
  • you have serious depression or mental illness.

Possible Side Effects (natural, expected, and unavoidable drug actions)

Drowsiness, lethargy, fatigue.

▷ **Possible Adverse Effects** (unusual, unexpected, and infrequent reactions)

If any of the following develop, consult your physician promptly for guidance.

Mild Adverse Effects

Allergic reactions: skin rash, hives—case reports.

Headache, unsteadiness, euphoria, impaired vision, numbness and tingling in extremities—infrequent.

Loss of appetite, nausea, vomiting, dizziness, hiccups, stomach pain, diarrhea—infrequent to frequent.

Thickening and overgrowth of gums—possible.

Serious Adverse Effects

Allergic Reaction: Swelling of tongue—case reports.

Severe skin eruptions (Stevens-Johnson syndrome, erythema multiforme)—occasional.

Aggravation of emotional depression and paranoid mental disorders—case reports.

Severe bone marrow depression: fatigue, fever, sore throat, abnormal bleeding or bruising—case reports.

Porphyria, myasthenia gravis, or systemic lupus erythematosus—rare.

▷ **Possible Effects on Sexual Function:** Increased libido (questionable); nonmenstrual vaginal bleeding—case reports.

Natural Diseases or Disorders That May Be Activated by This Drug

Latent psychosis, systemic lupus erythematosus.

Possible Effects on Laboratory Tests

Complete blood cell counts: decreased red cells, hemoglobin, white cells, and platelets; increased eosinophils.

Blood aspartate aminotransferase (AST) level: increased in 33% of users.

Blood bilirubin level: increased (rare liver damage).

Blood lupus erythematosus (LE) cells: positive—rare.
Kidney function tests: increased blood urea nitrogen (BUN) level, increased urine protein content.

CAUTION
1. May increase the frequency of grand mal seizures in people with mixed seizure disorders.
2. Periodic blood counts and other tests are mandatory.
3. Plasma levels increase faster in women than men.

Precautions for Use
By Infants and Children: If a single daily dose causes nausea or vomiting, give in two or three divided doses 8 to 12 hours apart. Large differences in response occur and require blood levels. Watch for a lupuslike reaction: fever, rash, arthritis.
By Those Over 60 Years of Age: Rarely used in this age group.

▷ **Advisability of Use During Pregnancy**
Pregnancy Category: C. See Pregnancy Risk Categories at the back of this book.
Animal Studies: Bone defects reported in rodents.
Human Studies: Three instances of birth defects have been reported. Adequate studies of pregnant women are not available.
Avoid during first 3 months. Use only if clearly needed during the final 6 months.

Advisability of Use If Breast-Feeding
Presence of this drug in breast milk: Yes, but not usually a significant level.
Watch nursing infant closely and discontinue drug or nursing if adverse effects develop. If mother requires high doses, refrain from nursing. Ask your doctor for help.

Habit-Forming Potential: None, but sudden withdrawal may lead to seizures.

Effects of Overdose: Drowsiness, lethargy, dizziness, nausea, vomiting, stupor progressing to coma.

Possible Effects of Long-Term Use: Systemic lupus erythematosus.

Suggested Periodic Examinations While Taking This Drug (at physician's discretion)
Complete blood counts every 2 weeks during the first months of use and then monthly thereafter.
Liver and kidney function tests.

▷ **While Taking This Drug, Observe the Following**
Foods: No restrictions.
Herbal Medicines or Minerals: Valerian and kava kava may interact additively (drowsiness). Avoid these combinations. Kava is no longer recommended in Canada due to liver problems. Evening primrose oil should not be used in people with seizures. A contaminant (4'-o-methylpyridoxine) in some ginkgo preparations can increase seizure risk. Talk to your doctor about this benefit to risk decision. Evening primrose oil can lower the point where seizures happen (seizure threshold). Do not use.
Beverages: No restrictions. May be taken with milk.
▷ *Alcohol:* Use caution—this drug may increase the sedative effects of alcohol. Excessive alcohol may precipitate seizures.
Tobacco Smoking: No interactions expected. I advise everyone to quit smoking.
▷ *Other Drugs*
Ethosuximide may **increase** the effects of
• phenytoin (Dilantin) and fosphenytoin (Cerebyx), by slowing elimination.

Ethosuximide *taken concurrently* with
- carbamazepine (Tegretol) may change ethosuximide blood levels.
- phenobarbital may decrease seizure control success.
- ritonavir (Norvir) and perhaps other protease inhibitors (see Drug Classes) may lead to toxicity.
- tramadol (Ultram) may increase seizure risk.
- valproic acid (Depakene, Depakote) may unpredictably alter ethosuximide effects.

The following drug may *increase* the effects of ethosuximide:
- isoniazid (INH, Niconyl, etc.).

▷ *Driving, Hazardous Activities:* This drug may cause drowsiness, dizziness, unsteadiness, and impaired vision. Restrict activities as necessary.

Aviation Note: Seizure disorders and the use of this drug *are disqualifications* for piloting. Consult a designated Aviation Medical Examiner.

Exposure to Sun: No restrictions.

Discontinuation: Do not stop taking this drug abruptly as sudden withdrawal may lead to seizures. Slow and stepwise lowering is prudent (over at least three months). Some clinicians have obtained superb results by lowering the dose in increments of three months and discontinuing the medicine over 9 months. Ask your physician for help with gradual dose reduction.

ETIDRONATE (e ti DROH nate)

Introduced: 1976 **Class:** Anti-osteoporotic **Prescription:**
USA: Yes **Controlled Drug:** USA: No; Canada: No **Available as**
Generic: USA: No; Canada: No
Brand Name: Didronel

BENEFITS versus RISKS	
Possible Benefits	*Possible Risks*
PARTIAL RELIEF OF SYMPTOMS OF PAGET'S DISEASE OF BONE	Increased bone pain
	Bone fractures
EFFECTIVE PREVENTION AND TREATMENT OF ABNORMAL CALCIFICATION	Kidney failure
	Focal osteomalacia
Effective adjunctive treatment of abnormally high blood calcium levels (associated with malignant disease)	
Treatment of postmenopausal osteoporosis	

▷ **Principal Uses**

As a Single Drug Product: Uses currently included in FDA-approved labeling: (1) Treatment of symptomatic Paget's disease of bone (excessive bone growth of skull, spine, and long bones); (2) prevention and treatment of abnormal bone formation (ossification) following total hip replacement or spinal cord injury; (3) adjunctive treatment of excessively high blood calcium levels due to malignant bone disease.

Other (unlabeled) generally accepted uses: (1) treatment of Paget's disease of bone that is not yet causing symptoms; (2) treatment of abnormal calcium levels that may result from prolonged immobilization; (3) helps hyperparathyroidism; (4) helps pulmonary alveolar microlithiasis (PAM); (5) treatment (with cyclic dosing) of postmenopausal osteoporosis.

How This Drug Works: This drug attaches to the surface of bone and slows the abnormally accelerated processes of "bone turnover" that occur in Paget's disease. In malignant bone disease, this drug slows bone destruction and reduces excessive transfer of calcium from bone to blood.

Available Dosage Forms and Strengths
Injection — 50 mg/mL
Tablets — 200 mg, 400 mg

▷ **Recommended Dosage Ranges** (Actual dose and schedule must be determined for each patient individually.)

Infants and Children: Dose not established.

12 to 60 Years of Age:

For Paget's disease: Initially 5 mg per kg of body mass daily, as a single dose, for up to 6 months. Discontinue for a drug-free period of 6 months. As needed, repeat, alternating 6-month courses of drug treatment and abstention. Doses above 10 mg per kg of body mass per day are only used if there is a critical need to decrease increased work output of the heart or to quickly slow down increased bone turnover.

For ossification associated with hip replacement: 20 mg per kg of body mass daily for 1 month before and 3 months after surgery.

For ossification associated with spinal cord injury: Initially 20 mg per kg of body mass daily for 2 weeks after injury; then decrease dose to 10 mg per kg of body mass daily for an additional 10 weeks.

For high blood calcium associated with malignant bone disease: 20 mg per kg of body mass daily for 30 days; if needed and tolerated, continue for a maximum of 90 days. The total daily dose should not exceed 20 mg per kg of body mass.

Over 60 Years of Age: Same as 12 to 60 years of age.

Author's Note: The information in this profile has been shortened to allow room for more widely used medicines.

ETODOLAC (e TOE do lak)

Please see the acetic acids (nonsteroidal anti-inflammatory drug) family profile.

ETRETINATE (e TRET i nayt)

Introduced: 1976   **Class:**   Antipsoriasis
Brand Name: Tegison
Author's Note: The manufacturer has stopped marketing this medicine.

EXTENDED RELEASE NIACIN/LOVASTATIN
(NIGH a sin/loh VAH sta tin)

Introduced: 2002   **Class:**   Anticholesterol, cholesterol lowering medicine, vasodilator   **Prescription:**   USA: Yes   **Controlled Drug:**   USA: No   **Available as Generic:**   USA: No; Canada: No
Brand Name: Advicor

BENEFITS versus RISKS

Possible Benefits	*Possible Risks*
EFFECTIVE REDUCTION OF TOTAL BLOOD CHOLESTEROL, LOW DENSITY LIPOPROTEINS (LDL), AND TRIGLYCERIDES IN TYPES II, III, IV, AND FIVE CHOLESTEROL DISORDERS	FLUSHING (minimized by taking aspirin 30 minutes before this product and also by taking at bedtime)
PREVENTS CORONARY HEART DISEASE IN PATIENTS WHO DO NOT HAVE SYMPTOMS, BUT HAVE INCREASED TOTAL CHOLESTEROL, LDL-C, AND LOW HDL-C	Drug-induced hepatitis (without jaundice) Drug-induced myositis (muscle inflammation) Decreased co-enzyme Q10 (possible effect of the lovastatin component)
INCREASES HIGH DENSITY LIPOPROTEINS (HDL)	Possible aggravation of diabetes or gout
DECREASES Lp (a)	
SLOWS PROGRESSION OF HEART (CORONARY) ATHEROSCLEROSIS	
May reduce risk of stroke, like other medicines in this class	
May lower the risk of some cancers	

▷ **Principal Uses**

As a Single Drug Product: Uses currently included in FDA-approved labeling: (1) Reduces abnormally high total blood cholesterol levels in people with primary hypercholesterolemia (heterozygous familial and nonfamilial increased cholesterol) as well as mixed dyslipidemia (otherwise known as Frederickson Types IIa and IIb) where the patients have (1) attempted a low cholesterol diet and other nonpharmacologic measures and have: (2) been treated with lovastatin, but need to have their triglycerides lowered more or their HDL raised, or (3) who would benefit from taking niacin. Additionally, this combination drug should be used in people who have been taking niacin—yet require to have their LDL lowered more and who would benefit from taking lovastatin.

Other (unlabeled) generally accepted uses: (1) None at present.

How This Drug Works: The combination of these two distinct medicines offers the benefit of niacin actions and while not completely understood, it is thought that: (1) the niacin part of this combination increases lipoprotein lipase activity that then quickens removal of triglyceride (via chylomicrons) from the plasma; (2) decreases the speed that the liver makes LDL and VLDL; (3) may inhibit release of free fatty acids from fat (adipose tissue). Via the lovastatin component, this medicine blocks a liver enzyme that starts making cholesterol. It decreases low-density lipoproteins (LDL), the fraction of total blood cholesterol that increases risk of coronary heart disease. Since the amount of cholesterol is reduced in the liver, the VLDL fraction may also be decreased. There is a growing body of evidence that "statins" also have beneficial effects on undesirable compounds in the blood, on blood flow and even on the blood vessel walls themselves. Specific compounds or effects on platelet derived growth factor (PDGF), undesirable clotting via thrombin-antithrombin III, thrombomodulin, and other chemicals are probably changed in desirable ways by statins. The original (prodrug) form of this medicine increases CDKI P21 and P27 and may account for the ability of lovastatin to lower the risk of cancer.

▷ **Widely Used Guidelines That Involve This Medicine (representative sample):** Please look at the section at the very beginning of this profile called "Class." Next, turn to Table 22 and you will find guidelines listed by the class involved!

Available Dosage Forms and Strengths
> Tablets, extended action niacin/lovastatin — 500 mg niacin/20 mg lovastatin
> 750 mg niacin/20 mg lovastatin
> 1,000 mg niacin/20 mg lovastatin.

▷ **Usual Adult Dosage Ranges:** *For cholesterol disorders:* Usual Niaspan starting dose is 500 mg taken at bedtime. People who already take Niaspan can be switched directly to the appropriate (niacin equivalent) dose of Advicor. The typical lovastatin starting dose is 20 mg daily. Increases are made at 4 week intervals as needed to reach goals and tolerated. One 500/20 mg tablet at bedtime, which is increased as needed and tolerated at four-week intervals to 750 and 1,000 mg daily. Taking more than 2,000 mg/40 mg daily is NOT recommended. If Advicor is stopped for more than 7 days, it should be restarted at the lowest dose and increased as above all over again (re-titrated).

Note: Actual dose and dosing schedule must be determined for each patient individually.

Conditions Requiring Dosing Adjustments
> *Liver Function:* Both medicines in this combination are removed via the liver and have not been studied in liver compromised populations. Advicor is contraindicated in liver disease/dysfunction.
> *Kidney Function:* Specific dosing adjustments for the combination medicine are not available, but great caution should be used in considering doses above 20 mg per day of the lovastatin component for patients with severe kidney problems (creatinine clearance less than 30 mL/min).

▷ **Dosing Instructions:** Other (secondary causes) of hypercholesterolemia (such as low thyroid function, poorly controlled diabetes, alcoholism, or certain kidney problems) should be ruled out before a cholesterol lowering medicine is started. Take at night with a low fat snack to help prevent stomach irritation and avoid the problem of flushing (a common side effect). Taking aspirin half an hour before taking this medicine can help prevent facial flushing and itching. Taking hot drinks close to the time this medicine is taken may worsen the feeling of flushing. This medicine should not be crushed or altered. If you forget a dose, take the missed dose as soon as you remember it, unless it's nearly time for your next dose—if that is the case, skip the missed dose and take the next dose right on schedule. Talk with your doctor if you find yourself missing doses.

Usual Duration of Use: Use on a regular schedule for 3 to 5 weeks determines benefit in reducing levels of cholesterol and triglycerides. Long-term use (months to years) requires periodic physician evaluation. Treatment of high cholesterol is an ongoing therapy in order to help avoid heart disease and stroke.

Typical Treatment Goals and Measurements (Outcomes and Markers)

Cholesterol: Current guidelines (National Cholesterol Education Program, or NCEP) acknowledge diabetes as one of the conditions that increases risk of heart disease, modifying risk factors, therapeutic lifestyle changes (TLC), and recommending routine testing for all of the cholesterol fractions (lipoprotein profile) versus total cholesterol alone. Goals are: a total cholesterol of 200 mg/dL, and optimal bad cholesterol (LDL) of less than 100 mg/dL. Less than 70 mg/dL (see Grundy, S.M. in Sources) is a reasonable optional goal for very high risk patients (such as diabetics with acute coronary syndromes, etc.). 130–159 mg/dL as borderline high, 160 mg/dL as high and 190 mg/dL as very high. Did you know that there are at least five different kinds of "good cholesterol" or HDL? The "too low" measure for HDL is still 40 mg/dL, but in order to learn more about cholesterol types some doctors are starting to order lipid panels. There are at least seven different kinds of "bad cholesterol." The new panels tell doctors about the kinds of cholesterol that your body makes. This is important because some kinds (small dense particles) tend to stick to blood vessels (are highly atherogenic). Take your medicine to reach your goals! Two additional tests you will hear about will be electron beam computed tomography (EBCT) and CRP. EBCT is an important tool used in conjunction with laboratory studies. Findings show that even patients who meet cholesterol goals (particularly females over 55) can still be at significant cardiovascular risk. EBCT then defines risk by giving a calcium score and a "virtual tour" of the coronary arteries. C Reactive Protein or CRP is a relatively new and apparently independent predictor of heart disease risk. A large study (see Ridker, P.M. in Sources) found that CRP predicted heart disease risk independently of bad cholesterol (low density lipoprotein). Talk to your doctor about this laboratory test and ask about current guidelines for who should be tested (see Pearson, T.A. in Sources).

Author's Note: The Advicor Versus Other Cholesterol-modifying Agents Trial Evaluation (ADVOCATE) study showed significant advantage of this medicine over 16 weeks versus atorvastatin (Lipitor) and simvastatin (Zocor). Comparison was made with checks of LDL, HDL, triglycerides, and Lp(a) and the Advicor 1000/40 versus Lipitor and Zocor (20 mg).

Possible Advantages of This Drug Combination

Provides benefits of two proven medicines, which work both to lower cholesterol and increase reverse cholesterol transport via an increase in HDL. May have specific benefits in women who are having trouble meeting their cholesterol lowering goals. Advicor benefits lipid profiles in both sexes, but has a significantly larger beneficial effect in women than in men. Lovastatin portion of this medicine increases some substances that may reduce the risk of cancer.

▷ **This Drug Should Not Be Taken If**
- you have had an allergic reaction to any component of it previously.
- you have active peptic ulcer disease.
- you have active liver disease or unexplained increases in liver enzymes.
- you are bleeding from an artery.

▷ **Inform Your Physician Before Taking This Drug If**
- you are prone to low blood pressure.
- you regularly drink substantial amounts of alcohol.
- you have cataracts or impaired vision.
- you have a heart rhythm disorder of any kind.
- you have a history of peptic ulcer disease, inflammatory bowel disease, liver disease, jaundice, or gallbladder disease.
- you have any type of chronic muscular disorder.
- you are not using any method of birth control or you are planning pregnancy.
- you have diabetes or gout.

Possible Side Effects (natural, expected, and unavoidable drug actions)
Flushing, itching, tingling, and feeling of warmth, usually in the face and neck. Sensitive people may experience orthostatic hypotension (see Glossary). Development of abnormal liver function tests without associated symptoms. Increases CDKI P21 and P27 and may decrease cancer risk.

▷ **Possible Adverse Effects** (unusual, unexpected, and infrequent reactions)
If any of the following develop, consult your physician promptly for guidance.
Mild Adverse Effects
Allergic reactions: skin rash, itching, hives.
Headache, dizziness, faintness, impaired vision—infrequent to frequent.
Indigestion, nausea, altered taste, impaired sense of smell, excessive gas, vomiting, and diarrhea—rare to infrequent.
Flushing and tingling—infrequent to frequent (modified by this form of niacin and can be further modified by taking aspirin 30 minutes before Advicor).
Dryness of skin, grayish-black pigmentation of skin folds—infrequent.
Prolonged protime (prothrombin time)—possible.
Gum pain—case reports with one component.
Serious Adverse Effects
Drug-induced hepatitis with jaundice (see Glossary): yellow eyes and skin, dark-colored urine, light-colored stools—case reports with lovastatin. Hypersensitivity syndrome (positive ANA, anaphylaxis, angioedema, arthritis, fever, toxic epidermal necrolysis, or other features) has been reported.
Worsening of diabetes (hyperglycemia) and gout—possible.
Neuropathy or systemic lupus erythematosuslike syndrome—case reports with the single ingredient lovastatin.
Blood clotting problem (increased prothrombin time) and/or low blood platelets (thrombocytopenia)—case reports.
Development of heart rhythm disorders—case reports to infrequent.
Sudden unexplained muscle pain and tenderness (myopathy) or rhabdomyolysis—case reports with lovastatin, no reports in clinical trials at doses up to 2,000/40 mg Advicor for two years.
Peptic ulcers—case reports.
Vision changes (macular edema)—case reports with lovastatin.

▷ **Possible Effects on Sexual Function:** None reported.

▷ **Adverse Effects That May Mimic Natural Diseases or Disorders**
Liver reactions may suggest viral hepatitis.

Possible Delayed Adverse Effects: Myopathy.

Natural Diseases or Disorders That May Be Activated by This Drug
Latent diabetes, gout, inflammatory bowel disease, or peptic ulcer.

Possible Effects on Laboratory Tests

Complete blood cell counts: decreased eosinophils and lymphocytes.

Platelet counts: may be decreased (more likely in men).

Blood total cholesterol, LDL cholesterol, triglyceride, and Lp(a) levels: decreased.

Blood phosphorous levels: may be decreased.

Blood HDL cholesterol level: increased.

Blood glucose level: increased.

Glucose tolerance test (GTT): decreased.

Blood uric acid level: increased.

Liver function tests: increased enzymes (ALT/GPT, AST/GOT, alkaline phosphatase) or bilirubin.

Urine sugar tests: inaccurate test results with Benedict's solution.

INR (PT) or protime may be increased.

CAUTION

1. Periodic measurements of blood cholesterol and triglyceride levels are essential for monitoring response and determining the need for changes in dose or medication. Talk to your doctor if goals are not reached.
2. Stop the drug immediately and call your doctor if you become pregnant.
3. Muscle problems and rhabdomyolysis have been seen when niacin (some release forms not used in the Advicor combination) has been used in combination with lovastatin. Risk of these problems is increased with high levels of lovastatin in the body. Because of this, careful attention should be paid to taking medicines (see Drug Interactions) that can block a liver enzyme called P450 3A4.
4. Call your doctor if you have unexplained muscle tenderness, weakness, or pain—especially during the first month of treatment. It is prudent to check a lab test called creatine kinase during the first month of treatment and if the dose of this medicine is increased. While checking this test periodically is prudent, no assurance is present that such testing will prevent muscle problems (myopathy).
5. In people who have just had a heart attack (acute MI phase) and in patients with unstable angina, this combination of medicines should be used with caution—especially if they are already being given medicines that work to dilate blood vessels (such as adrenergic blockers, calcium channel blockers, or nitrates).
6. The Advicor combination product should NOT be exchanged (substituted) for immediate release (crystalline) niacin. This switch can be made, but treatment in those cases should be started with the 500/20 mg Advicor dose.

Precautions for Use

By Infants and Children: Safety and effectiveness for use by those less than 18 years of age have not been established.

By Those Over 60 Years of Age: Watch for possible development of low blood pressure (light-headedness, dizziness, faintness) and heart rhythm changes.

▷ Advisability of Use During Pregnancy

Pregnancy Category: X. See Pregnancy Risk Categories at the back of this book.

Animal Studies: Significant birth defects due to one component of this drug were found in chicks. Mouse and rat studies reveal skeletal birth defects due to the lovastatin part of this medicine.

Human Studies: Adequate studies of pregnant women are not available.

Should NOT be used in pregnancy. Given to women of childbearing potential only after careful instruction about contraception and where they are highly unlikely to get pregnant. If a pregnancy occurs, the drug should be stopped immediately and your doctor notified.

Advisability of Use If Breast-Feeding

Presence of this drug in breast milk: Yes for one component, probably for another.

Avoid drug or refrain from nursing.

Habit-Forming Potential: None.

Effects of Overdose: Generalized flushing, nausea, vomiting, stomach cramps, diarrhea, weakness, fainting, low blood pressure (reported for the niacin component).

Possible Effects of Long-Term Use: Increased blood levels of sugar and uric acid; increased liver enzymes. Studies in rats with three to four times the human lovastatin dose resulted in increases in hepatocellular carcinoma (cancer). Clinical significance in human is not known. Research published in July 2002 in the *National Academy of Sciences Proceedings* shows that the lovastatin component of this medicine increases cyclin-dependent kinase inhibitors P21 and P27. This effect may reduce cancer risk in general in humans.

Suggested Periodic Examinations While Taking This Drug (at physician's discretion)

Measurements of blood levels of total cholesterol, HDL and LDL cholesterol fractions, triglycerides, sugar, and uric acid.

Liver function tests and creatine kinase (CK). CK testing is prudent particularly during the first month of treatment.

▷ **While Taking This Drug, Observe the Following**

Foods: Follow the low-cholesterol diet prescribed by your doctor. Your doctor may also recommend some specific foods such as increased vegetables or functional foods such as Benecol. Three well-designed studies found that both in women and men and before and after a heart attack, people who ate more fish (2–4 servings a week) appeared to help avoid heart disease. Additionally using Omega 3 polyunsaturated fatty acids (PUFA) appeared to protect against abnormal heart rhythms and sudden death from heart attack. The studies appeared in *JAMA, Circulation,* and the *New England Journal of Medicine.* Vitamins that have a large amount of niacin or niacin-like compounds may increase the effects of this medicine.

Herbal Medicines or Minerals: The FDA has allowed one dietary supplement called Cholestin to continue to be sold. This preparation actually contains lovastatin, or lovastatin-like compounds, and since increasing the amount of HMG-CoA inhibitor may increase risk of muscle problems, the combination is NOT advised. Be on the look out for red rice yeast products as they are similar. No data exist from well-designed clinical studies about garlic and this product, but the combination is probably complementary in lowering cholesterol. One other consideration is that garlic may inhibit blood-clotting (platelet) aggregation—something to consider if you are already taking a platelet inhibitor.

Soy products (milk, tofu, etc.) contain phytoestrogens that have led to an FDA-approved health claim for reducing risk of heart disease (if they have at least 6.25 g of soy protein per serving). Use of soy products have been proven to lower cholesterol. Policosanol also has this effect. Talk to your doctor to see if this makes sense for you. Because the lovastatin part of this medicine may lower co-enzyme Q10, supplementation may be needed.

Beverages: Grapefruit juice may increase the lovastatin portion of this medicine. Prudent NOT to combine. May be taken with milk or water.

▷ *Alcohol:* Use with caution. Alcohol used with large doses of this drug may cause excessive lowering of blood pressure and may also increase flushing or itching. There has been one case report of delirium.

Tobacco Smoking: May increase risk of flushing and dizziness. I advise everyone to quit smoking.

▷ *Other Drugs*

Niacin may ***increase*** the effects of
• some antihypertensive drugs and cause excessive lowering of blood pressure.

Niacin may ***decrease*** the effects of
• antidiabetic drugs (insulin and oral antidiabetic drugs; see Drug Classes), by raising the level of blood sugar.
• aspirin (various), which may decrease flushing but may also increase niacin blood levels; talk to your doctor.
• probenecid (Benemid) and sulfinpyrazone (Anturane), by raising the level of blood uric acid.

Niacin ***taken concurrently*** with
• isoniazid (INH) may result in decreased niacin levels and require increased niacin dosing.
• cholestyramine (Cholybar, Questran) or colestipol (Colestid) may result in decreased niacin levels and require increased niacin dosing. Separate dosing by 4–6 hours.
• lovastatin and other HMG-CoA type medicines does increase the chance of muscle problems (myositis or even rhabdomyolysis). Your doctor will make this a benefit-to-risk decision.
• nicotine (particularly transdermal) may result in increased risk of flushing and dizziness

▷ *Other Drugs*

Lovastatin ***taken concurrently*** with
• amprenavir (Agenerase), atazanavir (Reyataz), ritonavir (Norvir), and perhaps other protease inhibitors may lead to lovastatin toxicity (damaged muscles [rhabdomyolysis]).
• clofibrate (Atromid-S, others) may damage muscles (rhabdomyolysis).
• colesevelam (Welchol) can help further lower cholesterol.
• cyclosporine (Sandimmune) can cause a severe myopathy.
• diltiazem (Cardizem) may increase risk of myopathy.
• erythromycin (E.E.S.) and other macrolide antibiotics clarithromycin (Biaxin) or dirithromycin may result in severe rhabdomyolysis.
• fluconazole (Diflucan), itraconazole (Sporanox), ketoconazole (Nizoral), and voriconazole (Vfend) may increase risk of muscle damage (rhabdomyolysis).
• gemfibrozil (Lopid) and other fibrates may cause myopathy and the combination is not recommended.
• levothyroxine (various) may decrease thyroxine benefits.
• medicines that change the liver enzyme cytochrome P450 3A4 will change the levels of lovastatin and could lead to a subtherapeutic effect or toxicity. Talk to your doctor and pharmacist before adding other medicines.
• nefazodone (Serzone) may lead to myopathy.
• quinupristin/dalfopristin (Synercid) may increase risk of muscle damage (rhabdomyolysis).
• warfarin (Coumadin, others) may result in bleeding; increased frequency of INR (prothrombin time or protime) testing is suggested.

▷ *Driving, Hazardous Activities:* This drug may cause dizziness or impaired vision. Restrict activities as necessary.

Aviation Note: The use of this drug *may be a disqualification* for piloting. Consult a designated Aviation Medical Examiner.

Exposure to Sun: No restrictions.

Discontinuation: Do not stop this drug without your physician's knowledge and guidance. Patients who have acute coronary syndromes, or ACS (such as unstable angina, heart attack [non-p; Q-wave myocardial infarction], and Q-wave myocardial infarction) were reviewed as part of the Platelet Receptor Inhibitor in Ischemic Syndrome Management (PRISM) study. It was found that pretreatment with statin type medicines (HMG-CoA reductase inhibitors such as the medicine in this profile) significantly lowered risk during the first 30 days after ACS symptoms started. Most importantly, it was found that if a statin type medicine is stopped in ACS patients, there was a three-fold increased risk of nonfatal heart attack or death (see Heeschen, C. in Sources). Talk with your doctor BEFORE stopping any statin type medicine.

EZETIMIBE (Ee ZET ih mybe)

Introduced: 2003, 2004   **Class:** Anticholesterol, selective cholesterol absorption inhibitor **Prescription:** USA: Yes **Controlled Drug:** USA: No **Available as Generic:** No

Brand Names: Zetia, Vytorin (ezetimibe/simvastatin)

Author's Note: This medicine is presently approved for add-on therapy (for example, in people who do not reach their cholesterol lowering or cholesterol goals with their present medicine). Growing data appears to show a well-tolerated medicine with excellent combined (as with a statin-type medicine) results in lowering cholesterol. While present strategy is for add-on treatment, conjecture remains as to possible benefits in earlier add-on in order to avoid HMG-CoA reductase (statin) dosing increases and possible adverse effects. It is crucial to understand that this medicine works on the cholesterol that comes from your diet (one of the two sources of cholesterol), while medicines such as statins (HMG-CoA reductase inhibitors) work on cholesterol that YOU make in your liver, which is the second source of cholesterol. The new combination offers the benefits of blocking cholesterol from the diet AND the cholesterol that you make in your liver with a single pill. Information in this profile will be broadened in subsequent editions if ongoing research and comparative trials warrant.

FAMOTIDINE (fa MOH te deen)

Please see the histamine (H2) drug family profile.

FELODIPINE (feh LOH di peen)

Introduced: 1986 **Class:** Antihypertensive, dihydropyridine derivative calcium channel blocker **Prescription:** USA: Yes **Controlled Drug:** USA: No **Available as Generic:** No

Brand Names: Plendil, Altace plus felodipine [CD], Lexxel [CD], ✤Logimax [CD], ✤Renedil

Controversies in Medicine: Medicines in this class have had many conflicting reports. The FDA has held hearings on the calcium channel blocker (CCB) class. Amlodipine got the first FDA approval to treat high blood pressure or angina in people with congestive heart failure. Early research at NYU found that nifedipine is a cause of reversible male infertility. CCBs are currently second-line agents for high blood pressure according to the JNC VII (see Glossary).

BENEFITS versus RISKS

Possible Benefits	*Possible Risks*
EFFECTIVE TREATMENT OF MILD TO MODERATE HYPERTENSION	Peripheral edema (fluid retention in feet and ankles)

▷ **Principal Uses**

As a Single Drug Product: Uses currently included in FDA-approved labeling: Treats mild to moderate hypertension.

Other (unlabeled) generally accepted uses: (1) Treats angina; (2) arrhythmias; (3) may inhibit progression of atherosclerosis; (4) can be used in some cases of premature labor; (5) may have a role in kidney disease in diabetes (diabetic nephropathy); (6) helps kidney toxicity caused by cyclosporine (nephropathy).

As a Combination Drug Product [CD]: Available combined with enalapril (an ACE inhibitor) as the brand name Lexxel. The combination puts two different actions to work to lower blood pressure. Logimax combines felodipine with metoprolol, and Altace plus felodipine combines ramipril (an ACE inhibitor) with felodipine.

How This Drug Works: Blocks normal passage of calcium through some cell walls. This slows spread of electrical activity and reduces contraction of peripheral arterial walls, lowering blood pressure. Combination form adds the benefits of an ACE inhibitor to this calcium blocker.

▷ **Widely Used Guidelines That Involve This Medicine (representative sample):** Please look at the section at the very beginning of this profile called "Class." Next, turn to Table 22 and you will find guidelines listed by the class involved!

Available Dosage Forms and Strengths

Tablets, sustained release — 5 mg, 10 mg

Coated tablet (Lexxel) — 5 mg enalapril and 2.5 mg or 5 mg felodipine

Extended-release tablet (Plendil) — 2.5 mg, 5 mg, 10 mg felodipine

Sustained-release tablet (Logimax) — 5 mg felodipine and 47.5 mg metoprolol

Author's Note: Information in this profile has been truncated pending a combination family profile based on utilization and clinical data for the next edition.

FENAMATE (NONSTEROIDAL ANTI-INFLAMMATORY DRUG) FAMILY

Meclofenamate   (MEK low fen a mate)   **Mefenamic Acid**   (MEF en amik a sid)

Introduced: 1977, 1966   **Class:**   Analgesic, mild; NSAIDs   **Prescription:**   USA: Yes   **Controlled Drug:**   USA: No; Canada: No   **Available as Generic:**   Yes

Brand Names: *Meclofenamate:* Meclodium, Meclofenaf, Meclomen; *Mefenamic Acid:* ♣Apo-Mefanamic, ♣Novo-Mefanamic, Ponstel, ♣Ponstan

BENEFITS versus RISKS	
Possible Benefits	*Possible Risks*
EFFECTIVE RELIEF OF MILD TO MODERATE PAIN AND INFLAMMATION	Diarrhea (frequent for meclofenamate)
	Gastrointestinal pain, ulceration, bleeding
	Kidney damage
	Fluid retention
	Bone marrow depression (mefenamic acid)
	Hemolytic anemia (mefenamic acid)
	Systemic lupus erythematosus (mefenamic acid)
	Pancreatitis (mefenamic acid)

Author's Note: Information in this profile has been truncated to make room for more widely used medicines.

FENOPROFEN (fen oh PROH fen)

Please see the propionic acid (nonsteroidal anti-inflammatory drug) family profile.

FENTANYL (FEN ta nil)

Introduced: 1991   **Class:**   Analgesic, strong   **Prescription:** USA: Yes   **Controlled Drug:**   USA: C-II*; Canada: Yes   **Available as Generic:**   USA: No; Canada: No

Brand Names: Actiq, Duragesic, ♣Innovar, Oralet, Sublimaze

Author's Note: An investigational form of fentanyl is being studied and is sprayed into the mouth (buccal dosing see *www.medicineinfo.com*). The company that makes Duragesic has an excellent personal pain diary available from their Web site at *www.duragesic.com/files/pain_diary_other.pdf*

```
┌─────────────────────────────────────────────────────────────────────┐
│                        BENEFITS versus RISKS                          │
│         Possible Benefits                    Possible Risks           │
│  EFFECTIVE PAIN RELIEF              Habit-forming potential with       │
│  SKIN PATCH APPLICATION                prolonged use                  │
│    NEEDED ONLY ONCE EVERY 3         Impairment of mental function     │
│    DAYS                             Methemoglobinemia                 │
│  EFFECTIVE RELIEF OF                Respiratory depression            │
│    BREAKTHROUGH CANCER PAIN                                           │
│    WITH A MEDICINE TAKEN BY                                           │
│    MOUTH (Actiq)                                                      │
└─────────────────────────────────────────────────────────────────────┘
```

▷ **Principal Uses**

As a Single Drug Product: Uses currently included in FDA-approved labeling: (1) Treatment of chronic pain; (2) Actiq approved for treatment of break-through cancer pain (contains the same medicine as Oralet) for people ALREADY taking or who are tolerant to opioid therapy for cancer pain; (3) balanced anesthesia and cardiac and neurosurgery anesthesia (injection form); (4) anesthesia induction (injection form); (5) premedication (Oralet); (6) transdermal or epidural form is approved for chronic pain.

Other (unlabeled) generally accepted uses: None at present.

How This Drug Works: Acts at specific pain receptors (Mu agonist) to block pain.

▷ **Widely Used Guidelines That Involve This Medicine (representative sample):** Please look at the section at the very beginning of this profile called "Class." Next, turn to Table 22 and you will find guidelines listed by the class involved!

Available Dosage Forms and Strengths

Buccal lozenge (Actiq) — 400 mcg, 600 mcg, 800 mcg, 1,200 mcg, 1,600 mcg

Transdermal patch — 2.5 mg (25 mcg/hour), 5 mg (50 mcg/hour), 7.5 mg (75 mcg/hour), 10 mg (100 mcg/hour)

Lozenge on a handle — 100 mcg, 200 mcg, 300 mcg, 400 mcg

Author's Note: Injectable forms are not presented in this profile.

▷ **Recommended Dosage Ranges** (Actual dose and schedule *must* be determined for each patient individually.)

Children: Lozenge on a handle form: Based on weight. For those more than 40 kg may need 5–15 mcg/kg and those less than 40 kg may need 10–15 mcg/kg range as a premedication to lower anxiety and give pain relief before surgery.

18 to 60 Years of Age:

Patch (transdermal): Not generally indicated for patients less than 12 or those 18 years old who weigh less than 50 kg (110 lb). In patients who are not opioid tolerant, the 25 mcg/hour (10 cm) patch has been used. In people who used opioids previously, the amount needed to control pain on a 24-hour basis is calculated, converted to an equal amount of morphine (morphine equianalgesic dose), and then converted to fentanyl. It is important for patients to have the benefit of a judicious amount of short acting opioid during the first 24 hours after the patch is applied. After this, a "rescue dose" of short acting opioids is used. A circumspect review of rescue dose use should be made, and subsequently used to decide if any increases in the fentanyl patch is needed. Some centers use intravenous fentanyl and make a transition to a patch that is equal to the final ongoing fentanyl infusion rate. In that case, the continuous infusion fentanyl was lowered by half (50%) 6 hours after the patch was applied, and was stopped 12 hours after the patch was first applied. Patches are generally replaced every 72 hours, but some patients require replacement every 48 hours.

Oralet form: Used to treat pain/anxiety before surgery; 400 mcg for those with a body mass of 50 kg or more.

Buccal lozenge (Actiq)—used for patients with breakthrough cancer pain: 200 mcg (in cancer patients already receiving and who are tolerant to opioid [such as morphine] treatment—as defined by taking at least 50 mcg of transdermal fentanyl per hour, 60 mg of morphine a day, or an equianalgesic dose of a different opioid for 7 days or longer). They can subsequently be given another of the same dose (IF NEEDED) in 30 minutes. No more than 2 units should be taken for each breakthrough cancer pain episode. When the medicine is being added to the baseline opioid and a dose that works is found, patients should take no more than 4 units in a single day. Current pain treatment dictates that if more than 4 units are needed, the dose of the ongoing long-acting opioid should be evaluated, the cause of increasing assessed, and then dose increased as appropriate.

Over 60 Years of Age: Should receive 25 mcg per hour (2.5 mg) patch, unless already receiving equivalent of 135 mg of oral morphine or an equivalent opioid dose daily. Intravenous fentanyl clears more slowly in those over 60 than in younger patients. Watch carefully for overdose. If a decision is made to use the Actiq form, 200 mcg is used as a starting dose, and those over 75 generally require lower total doses than younger patients.

Conditions Requiring Dosing Adjustments
Liver Function: The dose must be decreased in liver compromise.

Kidney Function: In moderate to severe kidney failure, 75% of the usual dose. Dose reduced by 50% in severe kidney failure. People in end-stage kidney disease may be more sensitive to this medicine.

Dosing Instructions
Patch: Take the patch from pouch. Remove stiff protective liner from sticky side of patch. Do not cut the system. Place sticky side on a hair-free, dry area (back, chest, side, or upper arm). Avoid burned, irritated, or oily areas. Hold the patch in place for 30 seconds, paying close attention to the edges of the patch. Wash hands after patch is applied. Apply a new patch to a different area after 3 days. Fold the old patch onto itself and flush it down the toilet. Avoid heat such as electric blankets or heating pads.

Lozenge or sucker: Slowly dissolve in the mouth. Do not bite or chew it. For Actiq, place medicine between cheek and lower gum, and rotate occasionally using the handle.

If the patient feels sleepy or otherwise has signs of excessive fentanyl effects, the medicine should be removed. Subsequent doses MUST be decreased if the above effects occur.

Usual Duration of Use: Regular use for 1 to 3 days determines benefits in pain control. Immediate-release morphine or similar drug should be available while this drug reaches peak effect (patch form). Long-term use requires evaluation by your doctor. If you forget a dose: apply the missed patch as soon as you remember it, and then continue on the same three-day schedule or on the schedule that your doctor has prescribed. Make sure you tell your doctor as your use of rescue medication may increase. DO NOT double doses or apply two patches at the same time unless your doctor has told you to do so.

Typical Treatment Goals and Measurements (Outcomes and Markers)

Pain: Most clinicians treating pain use a device called an algometer to check your pain. This looks like a small ruler, but lets the clinician better understand your pain. The goals of treatment then relate to where the level of pain started (for example, a rating of 7 on a zero to ten scale) and what the cause of the pain was. I use the PQRSTG system. Pain medicines may also be used together (in combination) in order to get the best result or outcome. If your pain control is not acceptable to YOU (remember, in hospitals and outpatient settings, etc., pain control is a patient right and the fifth vital sign) or if after applying the patch or using the sucker form, and if there is no other pain contingency, ask your doctor about a different rescue medicine. If pain treatment results are not what you expect, be sure to call your doctor as you may need a different medicine or combination. Cancer pain can vary, and it is not unusual to need different doses.

Possible Advantages of This Drug

Effective pain relief with patch placement once every 3 days and no injections. Effective pain relief with a medicine used by mouth. Effective rescue pain relief.

▷ ## This Drug Should Not Be Taken If

- you had an allergic reaction to any form of it previously.
- you have had an allergic reaction to the adhesive in the patch.
- you are less than 12 years old. Oralet should NOT be used in children weighing less than 22 pounds (10 kg).
- you are at home and a Fentanyl Oralet is prescribed—these are only to be used in hospital settings.
- you weigh less than 50 kg and are less than 18 years old.
- you have mild pain.
- you have acute or postoperative pain without opportunity for proper dose adjustment.

▷ ## Inform Your Physician Before Taking This Drug If

- you have liver or kidney compromise.
- you have chronic lung disease (such as COPD).
- you have an abnormally slow heartbeat or other heart disease.
- you develop or have a fever.
- you have not taken narcotic pain medicines before and you are given a dose more than 25 mcg per hour.
- you take, or took in the last two weeks, an MAO inhibitor (see Drug Classes).
- you have a brain tumor or seizure disorder.
- you are elderly or debilitated.
- a benzodiazepine (such as diazepam or Valium—see Drug Classes) has been prescribed for you.
- you are anemic or have heart disease.
- you have a history of alcoholism or drug abuse.
- you take prescription or nonprescription drugs not discussed with your doctor when fentanyl was prescribed.

Possible Side Effects (natural, expected, and unavoidable drug actions)

Constipation, dry mouth. Dose-related respiratory depression.
Sleepiness (somnolence) or euphoria—infrequent to frequent.

▷ ## Possible Adverse Effects (unusual, unexpected, and infrequent reactions)

If any of the following develop, consult your physician promptly for guidance.

Mild Adverse Effects
Allergic reactions: skin rash and itching.
Blurred vision or amblyopia—rare to infrequent.
Nausea or vomiting—infrequent.
Urinary retention—infrequent.
Tremor or muscular rigidity—possible.
Sweating or itching (transdermal)—infrequent to frequent.

Serious Adverse Effects
Allergic reactions: exfoliative dermatitis and/or anaphylactic reactions—case reports.
Arrhythmias—rare.
Paranoid reaction, depersonalization, speech problems (aphasia)—rare, dose-related.
Increased or decreased blood pressure—possible.
Benign increases in pressure in the head (pseudotumor cerebri)—possible.
Seizures or hallucinations—case reports.
Methemoglobinemia or porphyrias—rare.
Paresthesias—rare.
Respiratory depression (this effect may last longer than the pain-relieving effect)—dose-related and possible.

▷ **Possible Effects on Sexual Function:** Impotence and blunted orgasm sensation in men. Irregular menstrual periods and blunted orgasm sensation in women.

Possible Delayed Adverse Effects: Dependence and tolerance.

Possible Effects on Laboratory Tests
Screening tests for opioids: positive.

CAUTION
1. Extreme caution should be used if this drug is combined with other opioids, narcotic drugs, benzodiazepines, or alcohol.
2. May cause serious constipation in older patients. Many clinicians use an appropriate drug to PREVENT constipation in older patients or those prone to constipation by starting a medicine to keep the bowels open (such as Senokot) when the medicine is started.
3. Do not expose the patch site to external sources of heat such as heating pads or electric blankets, as an increased rate of drug release may occur.
4. If there are children living in the same house as someone using Actiq or any form of fentanyl, great care must be taken to avoid accidentally having a child take one of the lozenges, or other dosage form as the dose would be fatal. A child-resistant container is provided in case a lozenge is not fully taken.
5. If this medicine is to be stopped, gradual withdrawal is required.
6. Dosing is individualized based on numerous factors such as: underlying conditions or diseases, age and weight, physical status, other ongoing medicines, liver function, any anesthesia that may be used and others.

Precautions for Use
By Infants and Children: Safety and effectiveness for those less than 12 years of age are not established.
By Those Over 60 Years of Age: The 2.5-mg patch should NOT be used as a starting dose unless you are already taking more than 135 mg of morphine daily. Those with cardiac, respiratory, kidney, or liver compromise or dehydration should be given low doses and carefully monitored.

▷ **Advisability of Use During Pregnancy**

Pregnancy Category: C, D if used in high doses when the baby is born or for prolonged periods. See Pregnancy Risk Categories at the back of this book.

Animal Studies: Some fetal death data with intravenous use in rats.

Human Studies: Adequate studies of pregnant women are not available.

Ask your doctor for guidance.

Advisability of Use If Breast-Feeding

Presence of this drug in breast milk: Yes.

Avoid drug or refrain from nursing.

Habit-Forming Potential: Fentanyl is a Schedule II narcotic and can cause dependence similar to morphine dependence. Physical and psychological dependence and tolerance can occur with repeated use.

Effects of Overdose: Dizziness, amnesia, and stupor. Respiratory depression and apnea may occur.

Possible Effects of Long-Term Use: Tolerance and physical or psychological dependence.

Suggested Periodic Examinations While Taking This Drug (at physician's discretion)

PQRSTG assessment of pain (see Glossary). Liver function tests.

Check for constipation.

▷ **While Taking This Drug, Observe the Following**

Foods: No restrictions.

Herbal Medicines or Minerals: Valerian and kava kava may interact additively (drowsiness). Avoid these combinations. Kava is no longer recommended in Canada at the time of this writing because of liver damage reports. St. John's wort can change (inducing or increasing) P450 3A4 or 2D6 enzymes, blunting the effects of fentanyl. Talk to your doctor BEFORE you combine any herbal medicines with fentanyl.

Beverages: No restrictions.

▷ *Alcohol:* **DO NOT DRINK ALCOHOL** while you are taking this drug—leads to additive loss of mental status, respiratory depression, and confusion.

Tobacco Smoking: No interactions expected. I advise everyone to quit smoking.

Marijuana Smoking: Additive adverse effects; however, marijuana may block the vomiting effect of fentanyl.

▷ *Other Drugs*

Fentanyl may *increase* the effects of

- benzodiazepines such as diazepam (Valium) and alprazolam (Xanax).
- central nervous system depressants such as opiates, barbiturates, tranquilizers, anesthetics, and tricyclic antidepressants.

Fentanyl *taken concurrently* with

- amiodarone (Cordarone) may result in heart (cardiac) toxicity.
- clonidine (Catapres, others) may result in greater than expected fentanyl effects. The fentanyl dose may need to be decreased if these medicines are to be combined.
- MAO inhibitors (see Drug Classes) may worsen the lowering of blood pressure and depression of breathing seen with fentanyl.
- rifabutin (Mycobutin) and rifampin may decrease pain control by fentanyl.
- medicines that block (inhibit) or use cytochrome P-450 3A4 to get out of the body (such as ketoconazole or voriconazole or macrolide antibiotics such as erythromycin) will increase effects of fentanyl and medicines that

induce cytochrome P-450 3A4 in the liver (such as fosphenytoin-Cerebyx or phenytoin-Dilantin) will blunt the benefits of fentanyl.

- ritonavir (Norvir) and perhaps other protease inhibitors (see Drug Classes) can lead to major fentanyl toxicity by inhibiting removal of this medicine from the body.
- sibutramine (Meridia) may increase risk of serotonin syndrome. DO NOT COMBINE.
- sildenafil (Viagra) may lead to changes in sildenafil or in fentanyl levels. Caution is advised (both drugs are removed by CYP450 3A4).

▷ *Driving, Hazardous Activities:* This drug may cause drowsiness, sedation, and respiratory depression. Restrict activities as necessary.

Aviation Note: The use of this drug *is a disqualification* for piloting. Consult a designated Aviation Medical Examiner.

Exposure to Sun: No restrictions.

Discontinuation: Once the patch is removed, fentanyl will still be released from the site for 17 hours or more. If pain medicine is still needed, the alternative should be substituted once the fentanyl level is low enough. The level from the lozenge declines more rapidly, and replacement medicine is required sooner if the fentanyl lozenge is stopped. If the lozenge has been used routinely, the drug should be slowly tapered, NOT stopped abruptly.

FILGRASTIM (fil GRA stim)

Other Name: Recombinant G-CSF

Introduced: 1991 **Class:** Hematopoietic agent **Prescription:** USA: Yes **Controlled Drug:** USA: No; Canada: No **Available as Generic:** USA: No; Canada: No

Brand Name: Neupogen

Author's Note: Pegfilgrastim (Neulasta) is NOT the same as filgrastim. Pegfilgrastim is given in a dose of 6 mg under the skin per each cycle of chemotherapy.

BENEFITS versus RISKS	
Possible Benefits	*Possible Risks*
PREVENTION OF INFECTIONS DUE TO LOWERED WHITE BLOOD CELL COUNTS FOLLOWING CHEMOTHERAPY, FOLLOWING BONE MARROW TRANSPLANT IN PATIENTS WITH CHRONIC OR CYCLIC NEUTROPENIA	Bone pain Changes in heart waves
INCREASED BLOOD CELLS IN AIDS PATIENTS	
CORRECTION OF DRUG-INDUCED LOWERING OF WHITE BLOOD CELLS	

▷ **Principal Uses**

   As a Single Drug Product: Uses currently included in FDA-approved labeling:
   (1) Used to help white blood cell counts recover after bone marrow transplants; (2) used subcutaneously or intravenously to reduce or prevent low
   white blood cell counts that occur after cancer chemotherapy; (3) treats
   patients who have an absence of white blood cells at birth; (4) used to help
   patients with Kostmann syndrome have improved white blood cell counts;
   (5) used to help patients who have low white blood cell counts (neutropenia) of unknown cause (idiopathic); (6) helps cyclic low white blood cells
   (cyclic neutropenia); (7) used in adults to move blood-forming cells
   (hematopoietic progenitors) into the blood stream (peripheral blood) so
   that they can be collected by leukopharesis.

   Other (unlabeled) generally accepted uses: (1) Helps patients recover from a
   particular kind of lack of white blood cells (agranulocytosis) that has been
   caused by medicines (drug-induced); (2) used in AIDS (orphan drug status) patients (taking ganciclovir) to help restore white blood cell counts;
   (3) used to treat patients with severe long-term (chronic) low white blood
   cell counts; (4) used to treat patients with abnormally low white blood cell
   and neutrophil counts (myelodysplastic syndrome).

In the Pipeline: A phase three study comparing 5 or 10 mcg/kg per day for mobilization with chemotherapy, followed by autologous transplantation in
   patients with nonmyeloid malignancies is underway (see Andre, M. in
   Sources). One case report was made for patients resistant to other antipsychotics who developed white blood cell problems with clozapine, who
   were successfully managed with filgrastim so that they could take clozapine (see Hagg, S., et al. in Sources). In leukemia patients treated with imatinib (Gleevec), filgrastim was successfully used to mobilize peripheral
   blood stem cells (PBSC) in people who achieved complete cytogenetic
   response (CCR). The yield of CD 34+ cells was improved when imatinib
   was withheld temporarily (see Hui, C.H. in Sources).

How This Drug Works: Regulates proliferation and release of early (progenitor)
   forms of white blood cells. In effect, this medicine can tell bone marrow
   (where important blood cells are actually made) to increase the rate at
   which it makes white blood cells. Filgrastim may also work with other factors to increase the production of blood platelets.

▷ **Widely Used Guidelines That Involve This Medicine (representative sample):** Please look at the section at the very beginning of this profile called
   "Class." Next, turn to Table 22 and you will find guidelines listed by the
   class involved!

Available Dosage Forms and Strengths

   Solution for injection — 300 mcg/mL (supplied as a 300- or 480-mcg vial),
                 600 mcg/mL

How to Store

   The prepared solution should be stored at 36 to 46 degrees F. (2 to 8 degrees
   C.). This medicine should not be frozen. Some centers draw up a 7-day
   supply of syringes that are then stored in a refrigerator.

▷ **Recommended Dosage Ranges** (Actual dose and schedule must be determined
   for each patient individually.)

   Infants and Children: Studied doses of 0.6 to 120 mcg per kg of body mass per
   day for up to 3 years have been well tolerated in children 3 months to 18
   years of age. In low blood cells (neutropenia) that occur after chemotherapy,
   a starting dose of 5 mcg/kg per day has been used by giving 15–30-minute

intravenous infusions or via ongoing infusions. Doses are subsequently increased in steps of 5 mcg/kg/day while the patient is getting a cycle of chemotherapy. Dosing is adjusted in response to the severity and length of time that the lowest point (nadir) of the neutrophil count. In the studies leading to approval (phase III), 4–8 mcg/day were typically successful. In chronic low white blood cell counts (chronic neutropenia), doses of 5 to 10 mcg per kg of body mass per day have been used. Safety and efficacy in pediatric patients with neutropenia that is a result of one's own immune system working against oneself (autoimmune) have not been established.

18 to 60 Years of Age: Patients having bone marrow destroyed (myeloablative treatment) and getting a bone marrow transplant: Wait 24 hours after chemo was given and 24 hours after bone marrow transplant. Then 10 mcg per kg of body mass per day to start. The dose is given over 4 to 24 hours. Ongoing daily dosing is adjusted to increase of white blood cells (absolute neutrophil count).

Patients receiving bone marrow suppression should wait until 24 hours after or before the chemotherapy is given. Filgrastim is started with 5 mcg per kg of body mass per day, increased by 5 mcg per kg per day for each cycle of chemotherapy. Dosing is based on severity of white blood cell count decrease (nadir) and how long lowered white cell (absolute neutrophil) count lasts. Drug can be given daily for up to 14 days.

Guidelines released by the Infectious Disease Society of America talk about using this medicine (on a non-routine basis) to reverse low white blood cell counts (neutropenia) associated with HIV infection. The dose noted there was 5–10 mcg/kg per day subcutaneously or 250 mcg/square meter intravenously infused over 2 hours each day. The use period listed was 2 to 4 weeks.

Peripheral blood progenitor cell mobilization: Conflicting data about once versus twice a day dosing in this unique donor situation. One group received 6 mcg per kg intravenously every 12 hours and another received 12 mcg/kg intravenously once daily for 3 days before leukopharesis. In this study, each patient then received 6 mcg/kg on the fourth day within 2 hours before the first leukopharesis. The results in harvesting the needed donor cells were roughly (statistically) the same.

Over 60 Years of Age: Same as 18 to 60 years of age.

Conditions Requiring Dosing Adjustments

Liver Function: Not significantly involved in the elimination of this drug.

Kidney Function: Roughly 90% of a given filgrastim dose is eliminated by the kidneys. Changes in dosing are not defined.

▷ **Dosing Instructions:** The solution in the reconstituted vial should be colorless and clear. Once your doctor or nurse has taught you how to inject the medicine:

- Make certain the solution has not expired (check the expiration date).
- Make certain that albumin (human) has been added to the 2 mg per mL Neupogen to protect it from attaching (adsorbing) to the plastic material of the container.
- Make certain you have the correct kind of syringe (talk this over with your doctor, nurse, or nurse practitioner).
- Follow the provided patient instructions carefully, not using saline to dilute, and not diluting to a final concentration of less than 5 mcg/mL.
- If you are using a syringe, make certain you inject the medicine under the skin (subcutaneously or Sub Q), not into a vein.
- This medicine can also be given intravenously over a period of 15 to 30 minutes.

- If you forget a dose: call your doctor and ask what he or she would like you to do.

Usual Duration of Use: Ten to 14 days of regular use may be needed to see benefits in correcting low white blood cell (absolute neutrophil) counts after chemotherapy. Bone marrow transplant patients may take still longer to respond. Long-term problems with white blood cells (such as chronic neutropenia) may require years of therapy. Long-term use requires periodic evaluation of response and dose adjustment. See your doctor on a regular basis.

Typical Treatment Goals and Measurements (Outcomes and Markers)
Neutropenia: Most clinicians will check laboratory tests (white blood cell counts with differentials) two to three times per week and adjust dosing to results. Additionally, bone marrow tests (aspiration) will be done periodically to check granulocyte-macrophage counts, morphology, myeloid/erythroid ratios, and even colony-forming unit counts.

Possible Advantages of This Drug
Effective recombinant product with few side effects.

▷ **This Drug Should Not Be Taken If**
- you had an allergic reaction to it previously.
- you have a known allergy to products derived from *E. coli* (a bacteria).

▷ **Inform Your Physician Before Taking This Drug If**
- you have a history of gout or psoriasis.
- you have received chemotherapy within the last 24 hours.
- you have a history of heart problems (heart rhythm should be closely monitored).
- you have a history of leukemia (myeloid type). The safety and efficacy of this medicine are not established in that condition.
- you have a history of cancer (with myeloid characteristics). There is a possibility that this drug may act as a growth factor for these tumors. Use, however, in a small number of leukemia patients has not resulted in worsening of their leukemia.
- you have an excessive increase in white blood cells (leukocytosis).

Possible Side Effects (natural, expected, and unavoidable drug actions)
Pain on injection.
Bone pain (up to 33%).
Extreme sensitivity to light (photophobia) possible and dose limiting with 30–100,000 mcg/square meter daily.

▷ **Possible Adverse Effects** (unusual, unexpected, and infrequent reactions)
If any of the following develop, consult your physician promptly for guidance.
Mild Adverse Effects
Allergic reactions: skin rash or itching—infrequent.
Mild decreases in blood pressure or increases in uric acid—case reports.
Drug-induced fever—infrequent to frequent.
Headache—infrequent.
Nausea and anorexia—rare.
Irritation of the eye (iridocyclitis, conjunctival erythema)—case reports.
Enlargement of the spleen: reported in patients with chronic lowering of the white blood cells (chronic neutropenia)—frequent, though asymptomatic in these patients.
Taste disorders—case reports.

Serious Adverse Effects
   Allergic reactions: anaphylaxis—case report.
   Sweet syndrome (acute neutrophilic dermatosis)—possible.
   Worsening of psoriasis—case report.
   Low oxygen in the blood (hypoxemia)—very rare.
   Anemia—possible (happened in peripheral blood progenitor donations).
   Low blood platelets (thrombocytopenia)—infrequent to frequent.
   Depression of part of the heart action (ST depression)—rare to infrequent.
   Myocardial infarction (heart attack)—happened in 11 of 375 cancer patients
      in one study, but the relationship to filgrastim is unclear.
   Liver or kidney toxicity—case reports and of unclear relationship.
   Potential for this medicine to act as a growth factor for certain cancers:
      breast, colon, lung, and lymphoma—possible (use in preleukemia is an
      area of controversy).
   Myelodysplastic syndrome (MDS) or acute myeloid leukemia—annual rate
      of 2% and cumulative rate of 16.5% when patients with congenital neu-
      tropenia are treated.
   Capillary leak syndrome—possible, case reports.
   Respiratory distress syndrome in patients with serious (septic) infections,
      because white blood cells may travel to the infected area—possible.
   Hypothyroidism—case report.

▷ **Possible Effects on Sexual Function:** None reported.

Possible Delayed Adverse Effects: Increased uric acid. Formation of neutraliz-
      ing antibodies.

▷ **Adverse Effects That May Mimic Natural Diseases or Disorders**
   None reported.

Natural Diseases or Disorders That May Be Activated by This Drug
   Gout.

Possible Effects on Laboratory Tests
   Absolute neutrophil count: increased.
   Alkaline phosphatase: increased markedly.
   Uric acid: increased mildly.
   Lactate dehydrogenase (LDH): increased.
   Formation of neutralizing antibodies—possible.

CAUTION
   1. Bone pain may be prevented by taking acetaminophen (Tylenol, others)
      BEFORE this medicine is injected.
   2. Call your doctor if you have chills, fever, or any other sign of infection.
   3. Be certain to follow up with your laboratory testing as scheduled.
   4. The solution in the vial should be clear. Do not inject any discolored or
      cloudy solution.
   5. Make sure you have the correct kind of syringe before you inject this
      medicine.
   6. This medicine can be given intravenously when it is appropriately pre-
      pared. If your doctor has instructed you on how to give yourself an injec-
      tion using a syringe, the medicine should be given under the skin. Be
      certain you understand the technique.
   7. Always change the site in which you inject this medicine, as your doctor
      instructed.

Precautions for Use

By Infants and Children: This medicine has been used in children with long-term lowering of white blood cell counts (chronic neutropenia) in doses of 5 to 10 mcg per kg of body mass per day.

By Those Over 60 Years of Age: No specific precautions.

▷ **Advisability of Use During Pregnancy**

Pregnancy Category: C. See Pregnancy Risk Categories at the back of this book.

Animal Studies: In rabbits given 80 mcg per kg of body mass per day (very high doses), increased abortion and death of embryos were observed.

Human Studies: Information from adequate studies of pregnant women is not available.

Ask your doctor for help with this benefit-to-risk decision.

Advisability of Use If Breast-Feeding

Presence of this drug in breast milk: Unknown.

Ask your doctor for guidance.

Habit-Forming Potential: None.

Effects of Overdose: No maximum tolerated dose has been identified.

Possible Effects of Long-Term Use: Enlarged spleens may occur in up to 25% of patients (splenomegaly) with severe chronic neutropenia. Skin rashes may occur in up to 6% of patients.

Suggested Periodic Examinations While Taking This Drug (at physician's discretion)

Complete blood cell counts and platelet counts should be obtained prior to chemotherapy and twice weekly during filgrastim therapy.

▷ **While Taking This Drug, Observe the Following**

Foods: No restrictions.

Herbal Medicines or Minerals: Echinacea: Some patients use echinacea to attempt to boost their immune systems. Unfortunately, use of echinacea is not recommended in people with damaged immune systems. This herb may also actually weaken any immune system if it is used too often or for too long a time. **Caution:** St. John's wort may also cause extreme reactions to the sun. Additive photosensitivity may be possible—combination is not advised.

Beverages: No restrictions.

▷ *Alcohol:* No restrictions.

Tobacco Smoking: No interactions expected. I advise everyone to quit smoking.

▷ *Other Drugs*

Filgrastim *taken concurrently* with

• lithium (Lithobid, others) may (in theory) result in additive release of white blood cells.

• topotecan (Hycamtin) may cause extended low white blood cells.

• vincristine (Oncovin) has led to nerve problems (peripheral neuropathy).

▷ *Driving, Hazardous Activities:* No restrictions presently attributed to this medicine.

Aviation Note: The use of this drug is ***probably not a disqualification*** for piloting. Consult a designated Aviation Medical Examiner.

Exposure to Sun: SEVERE intolerance of sunlight (photophobia) has been a treatment-limiting factor. **Caution:** See the Herbal Medicines note on St. John's wort above.

Occurrence of Unrelated Illness: Report development of chills, fever, or other signs or symptoms of infection immediately to your doctor.

Discontinuation: In people taking bone marrow suppressing drugs: Filgrastim is usually stopped when white blood cell (absolute neutrophil count) reaches 10,000 per cubic mm (once the lowest white blood cell count was reached for the chemotherapy given).

In people taking bone marrow destroying medicine who then have a bone marrow transplant: The drug is started as described above. If white blood cell count reaches 1,000 per cubic mm, dose is decreased to 5 mcg per kg of body mass per day. Once white cell count reaches 1,000 per cubic mm for 6 consecutive days, filgrastim can be stopped.

Special Storage Instructions: This drug should be stored at 36 to 46 degrees F. (2 to 8 degrees C.) in the refrigerator once it has been mixed with the diluent (reconstituted). Care should be taken **not to shake** the prepared drug, as it may lose activity. Care should also be taken **not to freeze** the prepared medicine, as it will clump and lose therapeutic activity.

Observe the Following Expiration Times: Once the medicine is prepared, it is stable for 1 day (24 hours) if it is refrigerated. If the drug is stored at room temperature, it is stable for 6 hours. Medicine left at room temperature for more than 6 hours should be returned.

FINASTERIDE (fin ASS tur ide)

Introduced: 1992 **Class:** 5-alpha reductase inhibitor **Prescription:** USA: Yes **Controlled Drug:** USA: No; Canada: No **Available as Generic:** USA: No; Canada: No

Brand Names: Propecia, Proscar

Author's Note: A study called the Prostate Cancer Prevention Trial (see Thompson, I.M. in Sources) looked at 18,882 men. From the study results, it appeared that finasteride offers a 25% reduction of prostate cancer, which must be balanced against the risk of higher grade (more aggressive or advanced) cancers if a cancer does occur. The FDA approved changes to product labeling for use of finasteride (Proscar) combined WITH doxazosin (Hytrin) to treat benign prostatic hyperplasia (and keep it from progressing over time).

BENEFITS versus RISKS	
Possible Benefits	*Possible Risks*
NONSURGICAL TREATMENT OF SYMPTOMATIC BENIGN PROSTATIC HYPERPLASIA	Impotence (small percentage)
	Decreased libido (small percentage)
	Gynecomastia (rare)
Shrinkage of prostatic tissue and increase in urine flow	HIGHER GRADE CANCER IF IT HAPPENS
RETENTION OF HAIR OR INCREASED HAIR GROWTH IN MEN	
25% DECREASE IN PROSTATE CANCER	
COMBINED USE WITH DOXAZOSIN LOWERS THE RISK OF PROSTATE SYMPTOMS GETTING WORSE OVER TIME	

▷ **Principal Uses**

As a Single Drug Product: Uses currently included in FDA-approved labeling: (1) Treats symptomatic benign prostatic hyperplasia (BPH)—peak decrease in prostate size has occurred after 6 months of therapy; (2) approved to decrease risk of urine retention and need for prostate surgery in BPH; (3) used as Propecia brand (1 mg) to retain or regrow hair; (4) combined use WITH doxazosin to prevent benign prostatic hypertrophy from getting worse over time (see McConnell, J.D. in Sources).

Other (unlabeled) generally accepted uses: Reduces excessive hair in women (hirsutism).

How This Drug Works: Blocks an enzyme (5-alpha reductase) that decreases change of testosterone to dihydrotestosterone (in liver); this causes the prostate to shrink. Symptoms such as urgency and trouble urinating improve. Inhibiting 5-alpha reductase also leads to hair growth.

▷ **Widely Used Guidelines That Involve This Medicine (representative sample):** Please look at the section at the very beginning of this profile called "Class." Next, turn to Table 22 and you will find guidelines listed by the class involved!

Available Dosage Forms and Strengths

Proscar tablets — 5 mg
Propecia tablets — 1 mg

▷ **Recommended Dosage Ranges** (Actual dose and schedule must be determined for each patient individually.)

Infants and Children: Not indicated.

12 to 60 Years of Age: Symptomatic benign prostatic hyperplasia often does not occur in the younger end of this adult dosing range; however, the dose for this age range is 5 mg each day, taken by mouth. Note combination treatment in McConnell, J.D., above.

Hair-restoring agent: 1 mg daily dose.

Over 60 Years of Age: Same as 12 to 60 years of age, unless liver function has decreased.

Conditions Requiring Dosing Adjustments

Liver Function: People with abnormal liver tests should be closely followed by their doctors.

Kidney Function: No changes thought to be needed.

▷ **Dosing Instructions:** May be taken without regard to food. Food changes time to peak blood concentration only. If you forget a dose: Take the missed dose as soon as you remember it, unless it is nearly time for your next dose—if that is the case, omit the missed dose and take the next scheduled dose right on schedule. DO NOT double doses.

Usual Duration of Use: Use on a regular schedule for at least 6 months is needed to see this drug's peak benefit in shrinking the prostate and decreasing symptoms. Use for 5 years has been documented. Use for 1 year may be required to demonstrate hair regrowth.

Typical Treatment Goals and Measurements (Outcomes and Markers)

Hair loss: Most clinicians use hair counts, or lack of further hair loss, to define results. Use for that indication will be ongoing.

BPH: Urologists use improvement in urinary flow as well as subjective measures such as relief of difficulty urinating and lowered feeling of urgency.

Digital rectal examination for prostate cancer should be done prior to therapy and periodically.

Possible Advantages of This Drug: May give you symptomatic relief of benign prostatic hyperplasia (BPH) without surgery. May be more effective than other available agents in helping hair regrowth. Few clinically significant drug interactions. Twenty-five percent decrease in prostate cancer in one study and improved outcomes over time with combination therapy in the most recent study (McConnell).

▷ **This Drug Should Not Be Taken If**
- you had an allergic reaction to it previously and you are a woman or child.
- you are pregnant.

▷ **Inform Your Physician Before Taking This Drug If**
- you have impaired liver function or liver disease.
- you are a woman or a child.
- you have kidney problems of any nature.
- your sexual partner is pregnant.

Possible Side Effects (natural, expected, and unavoidable drug actions)
May or may not increase testosterone levels; however, the significance of this effect is not known.

▷ **Possible Adverse Effects** (unusual, unexpected, and infrequent reactions)
If any of the following develop, consult your physician promptly for guidance.
Mild Adverse Effects
Allergic reactions: skin rash, hives—rare.
Plasma testosterone—decreased.
Headaches—infrequent.
Serious Adverse Effects
Allergic reactions: hypersensitivity reactions—case reports.
Handling Propecia or Proscar tablets by pregnant females may harm male fetuses.
Muscle changes (myopathy—progressive leg or arm weakness)—case report.
Low blood platelets (thrombocytopenia)—case report.
Higher grade prostate cancer—possible associated higher grade cancers if a cancer does happen.
Possible increase in more aggressive tumors if cancer (neoplasm) does happen—possible.

▷ **Possible Effects on Sexual Function:** Impotence, decreased libido, or decreased volume of ejaculate—infrequent. Adverse sexual effects may resolve in more than 60% of patients who continue this medication.

Possible Delayed Adverse Effects: Possible enlargement of male breast tissue (gynecomastia), decreased libido, impotence, and decreased volume of ejaculate—infrequent.

Possible Effects on Laboratory Tests
Decreased PSA (prostate specific antigen).

CAUTION
1. A digital rectal exam and other prostate cancer exams are prudent before this medicine is started and periodically thereafter. PSA will be falsely decreased by this medicine. More frequent checks may be prudent given the Thompson data.
2. If you have a change in liver function, inform your doctor.

3. If your sexual partner is pregnant, avoid exposing your partner to your semen. Exposure to finasteride-containing semen may cause genital abnormalities in male offspring.
4. If cancer of the prostate does happen, it may be more aggressive.

Precautions for Use
By Infants and Children: Safety and effectiveness for infants and children are not established.

By Those Over 60 Years of Age: No specific precautions other than changes related to decreased liver function.

▷ **Advisability of Use During Pregnancy**
Pregnancy Category: X. See Pregnancy Risk Categories at the back of this book.

Animal Studies: When administered to pregnant rats, the male offspring developed hypospadias. The offspring experienced decreased prostatic and seminal vesicular weight, slow preputial separation, and transient nipple problems.

Human Studies: Contraindicated in women who are pregnant or who plan to become pregnant. Women who are pregnant must avoid exposure to crushed tablets and semen of a sexual partner who is on finasteride.

Ask your physician for guidance.

Advisability of Use If Breast-Feeding
Refrain from nursing if you have been exposed to finasteride or finasteride-containing semen.

Habit-Forming Potential: None.

Effects of Overdose: Multiple doses of up to 80 mg per day have been taken without adverse effect.

Possible Effects of Long-Term Use: Adverse effects of long-term use are similar to short-term use effects.

Suggested Periodic Examinations While Taking This Drug (at physician's discretion)
Patients should be monitored for signs and symptoms of hypersensitivity.

Periodic digital rectal exam and PSA.

Patients should be monitored for improvement in symptoms of BPH.

▷ **While Taking This Drug, Observe the Following**
Foods: This medicine is best taken on an empty stomach.

Herbal Medicines or Minerals: Saw palmetto works by anti-androgenic and anti-inflammatory actions. The combination of this herb and finasteride has not been studied, but both drugs appear to work by different mechanisms. Talk to your doctor before combining. Autumn crocus should be avoided in alopecia.

Beverages: No restrictions.

▷   *Alcohol:* No restrictions.

Tobacco Smoking: No interactions expected. I advise everyone to quit smoking.

Marijuana Smoking: No interactions expected.

▷   *Other Drugs*
Finasteride *taken concurrently* with
• tirilazad (Freedox) will be increased by up to 29% if combined with finasteride. Caution is advised.

▷   *Driving, Hazardous Activities:* No restrictions.

Aviation Note: No restrictions.

Exposure to Sun: No restrictions.

Special Storage Instructions: Keep at room temperature. Avoid exposure to extreme humidity.

FLUCONAZOLE (flu KOHN a zohl)

Introduced: 1985 **Class:** Antifungal (triazole) **Prescription:**
USA: Yes **Controlled Drug:** USA: No; Canada: No **Available as**
Generic: USA: No; Canada: No
Brand Names: ✸Apo-Fluconazole, Diflucan, ✸Dom-Fluconazole, ✸Gen-Fluconazole, ✸Nu-Flucon

BENEFITS versus RISKS	
Possible Benefits	*Possible Risks*
EFFECTIVE PREVENTION OF YEAST (CANDIDIASIS) INFECTIONS	Severe skin reactions
	Possible liver damage
	Many possible drug interactions
EFFECTIVE TREATMENT AND SUPPRESSION OF CRYPTOCOCCAL MENINGITIS	
EFFECTIVE TREATMENT OF *CANDIDA* INFECTIONS OF THE MOUTH, THROAT, AND ESOPHAGUS	
EFFECTIVE TREATMENT OF SYSTEMIC *CANDIDA* INFECTIONS	
EFFECTIVE SINGLE-DOSE TREATMENT OF VAGINAL YEAST INFECTIONS	

▷ **Principal Uses**

As a Single Drug Product: Uses currently included in FDA-approved labeling: (1) *Candida* (yeast) infections of the mouth, throat, esophagus (may be AIDS related); (2) systemic *Candida* infections: lungs, peritonitis, urinary tract infections (may be AIDS related); (3) treats vaginal yeast infections (approved for single use); (4) treatment of cryptococcal meningitis in HIV-positive patients.

Other (unlabeled) generally accepted uses: (1) Prevention of yeast infections in patients with low white blood cell counts or cancer or those taking steroids; (2) treatment of some fungal eye infections (endophthalmitis); (3) treatment of Aspergillus pneumonia; (4) treatment of candidal urinary tract infections; (5) used to treat some fungal infections that may occur in people who have received transplanted organs; (6) may be a drug of choice for Sporothrix schenckii infections or for prevention of relapse of some Histoplasma infections; (7) some use as an alternative to amphotericin B in presumptive (empiric) treatment of cancer patients with prolonged fever and low white blood cell counts.

How This Drug Works: By damaging cell walls and blocking essential cell enzymes, this drug inhibits cell growth and reproduction (with low drug concentrations) and destroys fungal cells (with high drug concentrations).

▷ **Widely Used Guidelines That Involve This Medicine (representative sample):** Please look at the section at the very beginning of this profile called "Class." Next, turn to Table 22 and you will find guidelines listed by the class involved!

Available Dosage Forms and Strengths
> Injection — 2 mg in 1 mL
> Tablets — 50 mg, 100 mg, 150 mg, 200 mg
> Oral suspension — 10 mg in 5 mL,
> 40 mg in 5 mL

▷ **Recommended Dosage Ranges** (Actual dose and schedule must be determined for each patient individually.)

Infants and Children: From 3 to 13 years of age: 3–6 mg per kg of body mass daily, depending on the kind and site of infection. Intravenous use should be infused over 2 hours in this population.

Cryptococcal meningitis: 12 mg per kg on the first day and then 6 mg per kg daily for 10 to 12 weeks after cerebrospinal fluid culture becomes negative.

13 to 60 Years of Age: Cryptococcal meningitis: 400 mg once daily until improvement occurs; then 200 to 400 mg once daily for 10 to 12 weeks after cerebrospinal fluid culture becomes negative.

Suppression of cryptococcal meningitis: 50–200 mg once daily for up to 21 months have been used.

Candida infections of mouth and throat: 200 mg first day and then 100 mg once daily for 2 weeks.

Candida infection of the esophagus: 200 mg first day and then 100 mg once daily for at least 3 weeks; treat for 2 weeks after all signs of infection are gone. Doses up to 400 mg daily may be used. Some patients with chronic mucocutaneous *Candida* infections have benefited from 50 mg/day of this medicine.

Systemic *Candida* infections: 400 mg daily for at least 4 weeks; treating for 2 weeks after all symptoms of infection are gone.

Vaginal yeast infections (*Candida*): One 150-mg tablet by mouth.

Over 60 Years of Age: Same as 13 to 60, adjusted if kidneys are impaired (ask your doctor about creatinine clearance).

Conditions Requiring Dosing Adjustments

Liver Function: Caution: Rare cause of hepatitis.

Kidney Function: Mild to moderate failure—usual dose every 48 hours. In severe kidney failure—half (50%) of usual dose every 48 hours.

▷ **Dosing Instructions:** The tablet may be crushed; may be taken with or after food to reduce stomach upset. Suspension forms are available if swallowing is a problem. Shake them well before dosing and use a measuring spoon for suspension forms. If you forget a dose, take the missed dose as soon as you remember it—unless it is nearly time for your next dose. If that is the case, skip the missed dose and take the next pill right on schedule. DO NOT double doses. Fungal infections will return if you do not take this medicine as long as you are supposed to.

Usual Duration of Use: Use on a regular schedule for 2 to 4 weeks is usually needed to see this drug's benefit in controlling candidal or cryptococcal infections. Actual cures or long-term suppression often require continual treatment for many months. May be continuous therapy in AIDS patients.

Typical Treatment Goals and Measurements (Outcomes and Markers)

Candida *infections:* Goals for treatment of infections include resolution of signs and symptoms (such as sore throat and white coloration in candidal throat infections), return of white blood cell count and differential to normal (for systemic infections), negative growth of fungus in appropriate cultures and failure of the infection to return in prophylactic use.

Currently a "Drug of Choice"
For maintenance therapy to prevent relapse following control of AIDS-related candidal esophagitis. Because oral absorption is so complete, oral and intravenous dosing are the same.

▷ **This Drug Should Not Be Taken If**
- you have had an allergic reaction to it previously.
- you have active liver disease.

▷ **Inform Your Physician Before Taking This Drug If**
- you are allergic to clotrimazole, itraconazole, ketoconazole, or miconazole.
- you have impaired liver or kidney function.
- you develop light stools, unexplained abdominal pain, dark urine, nausea, or yellow eyes (signs of liver problems).
- you tend to have low blood potassium.
- you get a skin rash while taking this medicine.

Mild Adverse Effects
Allergic reactions: skin rash—rare.
Hair loss—very rare with usual doses. Reversible hair loss (alopecia) may be more common with high doses of fluconazole given for 2 months or longer.
Headache—rare.
Nausea, vomiting, stomach pain, diarrhea—frequent.

Serious Adverse Effects
Allergic reactions: severe dermatitis (Stevens-Johnson syndrome)—very rare.
Anaphylactic reactions—case reports.
Liver toxicity—rare.
Abnormally low platelet counts: abnormal bruising/bleeding or low white blood cell counts—rare.
Seizures or adrenal suppression—case reports, rare.
Low blood potassium (hypokalemia)—case reports in 3 acute myeloid leukemia patients.
Abnormal heart rhythm (Torsades de Pointes)—case report.

▷ **Possible Effects on Sexual Function:** Amenorrhea—one case report.

Possible Delayed Adverse Effects: Liver toxicity.

▷ **Adverse Effects That May Mimic Natural Diseases or Disorders**
Possible liver reaction may suggest viral hepatitis.

Possible Effects on Laboratory Tests
Blood platelet counts: decreased.
Liver function tests: increased liver enzymes (ALT/GPT, AST/GOT, and alkaline phosphatase), increased bilirubin.
Blood potassium: lowered—case reports.

Precautions for Use
By Infants and Children: Safety and effectiveness for those under 13 years of age are not established, but any infusions for age-appropriate patients should be given over 2 hours.
By Those Over 60 Years of Age: Age-related decrease in kidney function may require adjustment of dose.

▷ **Advisability of Use During Pregnancy**
Pregnancy Category: C. See Pregnancy Risk Categories at the back of this book.
Animal Studies: Rat studies revealed significant abnormalities in bone growth and development.
Human Studies: Adequate studies of pregnant women are not available.
Use this drug only if clearly needed. Ask your doctor for help.

Advisability of Use If Breast-Feeding
Presence of this drug in breast milk: Yes.
Avoid drug or refrain from nursing.

Habit-Forming Potential: None.

Effects of Overdose: Possible nausea, vomiting, diarrhea.

Possible Effects of Long-Term Use: None reported.

Suggested Periodic Examinations While Taking This Drug (at physician's discretion)
Liver function tests (medicine should be stopped in patients who have signs and symptoms of liver disease while taking this medicine). Kidney function tests, potassium levels in patients with one kind of leukemia (acute myeloid). Check for skin rashes.

▷ **While Taking This Drug, Observe the Following**
Foods: Caution is advised regarding grapefruit or grapefruit juice. Avoid eating grapefruit.
Herbal Medicines or Minerals: Echinacea: Some patients use echinacea to attempt to boost their immune systems. Unfortunately, use of echinacea is not recommended in people with damaged immune systems. This herb may also actually weaken any immune system if it is used too often or for too long a time. Eucalyptus may increase risk of liver toxicity. Kava is no longer recommended in Canada because of liver toxicity.
Beverages: Grapefruit juice should be avoided. May be taken with milk or water.
▷ *Alcohol:* No interactions expected.
Tobacco Smoking: No interactions expected. I advise everyone to quit smoking.
▷ *Other Drugs*
Fluconazole may ***increase*** the effects of
- benzodiazepines (see Drug Classes).
- birth control pills (oral contraceptives with ethinyl estradiol and levonorgestrel) may lead to adverse effects.
- celecoxib (Celebrex).
- cyclosporine (Sandimmune).
- dofetilide (Tikosyn) and other medicines for abnormal heart beats (see Drug Classes) or those which prolong the QTc interval increase risk of heart toxicity.
- felodipine (Plendil).
- nicardipine (Cardene) and nifedipine (Adalat, others) leading to excessively low blood pressure. Lower doses of one or both drugs are prudent with careful patient follow up.
- oral antidiabetic drugs (chlorpropamide, glipizide, glyburide, tolbutamide, others) and cause hypoglycemia; check sugar levels carefully.
- phenytoin (Dilantin, etc.) or fosphenytoin (Cerebyx) and cause toxicity, monitor blood levels.
- sirolimus (Rapamune), and tacrolimus (Prograf). Sirolimus and tacrolimus levels should be used to guide dosing.
- triazolam (Halcion), leading to toxicity.
- tricyclic antidepressants (see Drug Classes).

- trimetrexate (Neutrexin).
- warfarin (Coumadin) and cause unwanted bleeding. Dosing changes and more frequent INRs are prudent.
- zidovudine (AZT) and result in toxicity. The zidovudine dose may need to be decreased if this combination is to be continued.
- zolpidem (Ambien) and result in toxicity. The zolpidem dose may need to be decreased if this combination is to be continued.

The following drugs may *decrease* the effects of fluconazole:

- cimetidine (Tagamet).
- rifampin (Rifadin, Rimactane, etc.).

Fluconazole *taken concurrently* with

- amphotericin B (Amphotec, others) may decrease amphotericin benefits.
- astemizole (Hismanal—now removed from the U.S. market) may result in fatal toxicity to the heart.
- atorvastatin (Lipitor), and other HMG-CoA inhibitors, may increase risk of muscle toxicity.
- cisapride (Propulsid) may lead to adverse effects on the heart. DO NOT COMBINE.
- cotrimoxazole (various) may lead to adverse effects on the heart. DO NOT COMBINE.
- ergot-type medicines (Cafergot, others) may lead to increased ergotism risk. DO NOT COMBINE.
- hydrochlorothiazide (Esidrix, others) may increase potassium loss.
- loratadine (Claritin) may result in increased blood levels of loratadine, but to date, toxicity to the heart has not been reported. Since blood levels may be increased if combined use is undertaken, it is prudent to decrease the dose of loratadine.
- losartan (Cozaar) may blunt blood pressure control.
- oral contraceptives (birth control pills) may blunt contraception and result in pregnancy.
- prednisone (various) may lead to increased removal (metabolism) of prednisone if the two medicines are taken at the same time, then the fluconazole is stopped and the prednisone dose is left the same.
- quetiapine (Seroquel) may lead to quetiapine toxicity.
- ritonavir (Norvir) may increase ritonavir blood levels.
- terfenadine (Seldane—now removed from the U.S. market) may result in toxicity to the heart.
- ziprasidone (Geodon) may result in toxicity to the heart (QT prolongation—see Glossary). DO NOT combine.

▷ *Driving, Hazardous Activities:* No restrictions.

Aviation Note: The use of this drug *is probably not a disqualification* for piloting. Consult a designated Aviation Medical Examiner.

Exposure to Sun: No restrictions.

Discontinuation: Take all of the medicine. Ongoing therapy for months may be needed. Ask your doctor when it is okay to stop this medicine.

FLUCYTOSINE (flu SI toh seen)

Other Names: 5-fluorocytosine, 5-FC **Introduced:** 1977 **Class:** Antifungal **Prescription:** USA: Yes **Controlled Drug:** USA: No; Canada: No **Available as Generic:** USA: No; Canada: No

Brand Names: Ancobon, ✤Ancotil, ✤Novo-triphyl

```
┌─────────────────────────────────────────────────────────────────────┐
│                      BENEFITS versus RISKS                            │
│     Possible Benefits                    Possible Risks               │
│  EFFECTIVE ADJUNCTIVE            BONE MARROW DEPRESSION                │
│   TREATMENT OF CERTAIN           DRUG-INDUCED LIVER DAMAGE             │
│   INFECTIONS CAUSED BY           Peripheral neuritis                  │
│   CANDIDA, CRYPTOCOCCUS                                                │
│   FUNGI, AND ASPERGILLUS                                              │
│  Effective adjunctive treatment of                                    │
│   chromomycosis infection                                             │
└─────────────────────────────────────────────────────────────────────┘
```

▷ **Principal Uses**

As a Single Drug Product: Uses currently included in FDA-approved labeling: (1) Treats endocarditis, osteomyelitis, arthritis, meningitis, pneumonia, septicemia, and urinary tract infections caused by *Candida*; (2) treats meningitis, pneumonia, septicemia, endocarditis, and urinary tract infections caused by *Cryptococcus*.

Other (unlabeled) generally accepted uses: (1) Treatment of disseminated candidiasis, chromoblastomycosis, and cryptococcosis (these infections may be AIDS related); (2) treatment of general fungal infections.

Author's Note: Flucytosine is usually used together with amphotericin B to treat widely distributed (disseminated) fungal infections.

How This Drug Works: This drug goes into fungal cells and blocks production of RNA and DNA, inhibiting fungal development and reproduction.

▷ **Widely Used Guidelines That Involve This Medicine (representative sample):** Please look at the section at the very beginning of this profile called "Class." Next, turn to Table 22 and you will find guidelines listed by the class involved!

Available Dosage Forms and Strengths

Capsules — 200 mg, 250 mg, 500 mg

Injection — 2.5 grams/250 mL

▷ **Recommended Dosage Ranges** (Actual dose and schedule must be determined for each patient individually.)

Infants and Children: Safety and efficacy in children have not been established.

12 to 60 Years of Age: 50 to 150 mg per kg of body mass, divided into equal doses and given every 6 hours. Some severe infections have required 250 mg per kg of body mass per day. Capsules are often taken a few at a time and the total dose taken over 15 minutes.

Over 60 Years of Age: Same as 12 to 60 years of age. If kidney function is impaired, dose reduction is mandatory.

Conditions Requiring Dosing Adjustments

Liver Function: No changes needed in mild to moderate liver compromise. This drug may cause liver toxicity (with blood levels greater than 100 mcg/mL). Used with caution in liver compromise.

Kidney Function: In mild to moderate kidney failure, the usual dose can be given every 12–24 hours (GFR 10–50 mL/min). In severe kidney failure the usual dose can be given every 24–48 hours.

▷ **Dosing Instructions:** If a single dose requires more than one capsule, space doses over a period of 15 minutes to reduce stomach upset and nausea. The capsule may be opened and taken with or after food. If you forget a dose: Take the omitted dose as soon as you remember it, unless it is nearly time for your next dose—if that is the case, skip the missed dose and take the next scheduled dose right on time. DO NOT double doses.

Usual Duration of Use: Use on a regular schedule for 4 to 6 weeks is needed to see effectiveness in controlling *Candida* or cryptococcal infection. Long-term use requires physician evaluation.

Typical Treatment Goals and Measurements (Outcomes and Markers)
Fungal infections: Goals for treatment of infections include resolution of signs and symptoms, return of white blood cell count and differential to normal (for systemic infections), and checks of blood levels of flucytosine (levels more than 100–125 mcg/mL increase toxicity risk) are prudent.

Currently a "Drug of Choice"
For the treatment of Chromomycosis with or without amphotericin B.

▷ **This Drug Should Not Be Taken If**
  • you have had an allergic reaction to it previously.
  • you have an active blood cell or bone marrow disorder.
  • you have active liver disease.

▷ **Inform Your Physician Before Taking This Drug If**
  • you have a history of drug-induced bone marrow depression.
  • you have a history of peripheral neuritis.
  • you have impaired liver or kidney function.

Possible Side Effects (natural, expected, and unavoidable drug actions)
Dose-related nausea and vomiting.

▷ **Possible Adverse Effects** (unusual, unexpected, and infrequent reactions)
If any of the following develop, consult your physician promptly for guidance.
Mild Adverse Effects
Allergic reactions: skin rash, itching.
Headache, dizziness, drowsiness, confusion, hallucinations—infrequent.
Loss of appetite, nausea, vomiting, stomach pain, diarrhea—possible and dose-related.
Serious Adverse Effects
Allergic reactions: anaphylactic reactions, toxic epidermal necrolysis (TEN)—case reports.
Bone marrow depression (see Glossary): fatigue, weakness, fever, sore throat, abnormal bleeding, or bruising—rare.
Liver toxicity, with or without jaundice (see Glossary)—may be frequent.
Peripheral neuritis (see Glossary)—possible.
Hallucinations—case reports.
Bowel perforation or kidney damage—rare.
Heart toxicity (ventricular dysfunction, toxicity, or cardiac arrest)—infrequent.

▷ **Possible Effects on Sexual Function:** None reported.

▷ **Adverse Effects That May Mimic Natural Diseases or Disorders**
Drug-induced hepatitis may suggest viral hepatitis.

Natural Diseases or Disorders That May Be Activated by This Drug
Crohn's disease, ulcerative colitis.

Possible Effects on Laboratory Tests
Complete blood counts: decreased red cells, hemoglobin, white cells, and platelets.
Liver function tests: increased liver enzymes (ALT/GPT, AST/GOT, and alkaline phosphatase), increased bilirubin.

Kidney function tests: increased blood urea nitrogen (BUN) and creatinine.
Serum creatinine: may be falsely increased if tested by some methods.

CAUTION
1. When this drug is used alone, resistance can occur rapidly. It is usually used concurrently with amphotericin B (Abelcet) (given intravenously).
2. This drug may cause false increases in creatinine laboratory values tested by the Ektachem method. DuPont ACA does not appear to have this problem.

Precautions for Use
By Infants and Children: No information available.
By Those Over 60 Years of Age: If necessary, adjust dose for age-related decrease in kidney function.

▷ ### Advisability of Use During Pregnancy
Pregnancy Category: C. See Pregnancy Risk Categories at the back of this book.
Animal Studies: Rat studies reveal drug-induced birth defects.
Human Studies: Adequate studies of pregnant women are not available.
Use this drug only if clearly needed. Ask your physician for guidance.

Advisability of Use If Breast-Feeding
Presence of this drug in breast milk: Yes.
Avoid drug or refrain from nursing.

Habit-Forming Potential: None.

Effects of Overdose: Nausea, vomiting, stomach pain, diarrhea, confusion.

Possible Effects of Long-Term Use: Bone marrow depression, liver or kidney damage.

Suggested Periodic Examinations While Taking This Drug (at physician's discretion)
Measurement of blood levels of flucytosine.
Complete blood cell counts.
Liver and kidney function tests.

▷ ### While Taking This Drug, Observe the Following
Foods: No restrictions.
Herbal Medicines or Minerals: Echinacea: Some patients use echinacea to attempt to boost their immune systems. Unfortunately, use of echinacea is not recommended in people with damaged immune systems. This herb may also actually weaken any immune system if it is used too often or for too long a time. **Caution:** St. John's wort may also cause extreme reactions to the sun. Additive photosensitivity may be possible. Eucalyptus may increase risk of liver toxicity. Kava is no longer recommended in Canada because of liver toxicity.
Beverages: No restrictions. May be taken with milk.
▷ *Alcohol:* No interactions expected.
Tobacco Smoking: No interactions expected. I advise everyone to quit smoking.
▷ *Other Drugs*
The following drugs may ***decrease*** the effects of flucytosine:
- antacids.
- cytarabine (Cytosar).

Flucytosine ***taken concurrently*** with
- amphotericin B may result in increased risk of kidney toxicity; lipid-associated form (Abelcet) may help avoid this.
- zidovudine (AZT) may result in additive and serious blood (hematological) toxicity.

▷ *Driving, Hazardous Activities:* This drug may cause dizziness, drowsiness, or confusion. Limit activities as necessary.

Aviation Note: The use of this drug *may be a disqualification* for piloting. Consult a designated Aviation Medical Examiner.

Exposure to Sun: Use caution—may cause photosensitivity (see Glossary). See Herbal Medicines note above.

Discontinuation: This drug may be needed for an extended period. Your doctor must decide when to stop it.

FLUNISOLIDE (flu NIS oh lide)

Introduced: 1980   **Class:**   Antiasthmatic, cortisonelike drugs   **Prescription:**   USA: Yes   **Controlled Drug:**   USA: No; Canada: No   **Available as Generic:**   No

Brand Names: AeroBid, AeroBid-M, ✦Bronalide, Nasalide, Nasarel, ✦Nu-Flunisolide, ✦Ratio-Flunisolide, ✦Rhinalar

---

BENEFITS versus RISKS

Possible Benefits	*Possible Risks*
EFFECTIVE CONTROL OF SEVERE,CHRONIC BRONCHIAL ASTHMA	Yeast infections of mouth and throat (inhaler form)
FIRST-LINE TREATMENT OF ALLERGIC RHINITIS WITH INTRANASAL FORM	Increased susceptibility to respiratory tract infections (inhaler form)
	Localized areas of "allergic" pneumonia (inhaler form)
	Possible osteoporosis with long-term use

Principal Uses

As a Single Drug Product: Uses currently included in FDA-approved labeling: (1) Treats chronic bronchial asthma in people requiring cortisonelike drugs for asthma control; (2) treats various kinds of "hay fever" (seasonal or perennial allergic rhinitis).

Other (unlabeled) generally accepted uses: (1) Treatment of nasal polyps; (2) treats bronchopulmonary dysplasia; (3) may have a role in acute or chronic sinusitis in combination with an antibiotic (amoxicillin/clavulanate in one study).

How This Drug Works: Increases cyclic AMP, which may increase epinephrine, an effective bronchodilator and antiasthmatic. Also reduces local allergic reaction and inflammation.

▷ **Widely Used Guidelines That Involve This Medicine (representative sample):** Please look at the section at the very beginning of this profile called "Class." Next, turn to Table 22 and you will find guidelines listed by the class involved!

Available Dosage Forms and Strengths

Inhalation aerosol — 0.25 mg (250 mcg) per metered spray

Nasal solution — 25 mcg per actuation

▷ **Recommended Dosage Ranges** (Actual dose and schedule must be determined for each patient individually.)

Infants and Children:
   Oral inhalation: Less than 6 years old—not recommended. Six to 15 years old—two inhalations that are 500 mcg twice a day. Maximum daily dose is 1 mg.
   Nasal inhalation: Up to 6 years old—not recommended. Six to 15 years old—0.25 mcg (one spray in each nostril) three times a day. Once the peak effect is seen, the dose should be reduced to the smallest dose and frequency that works. Maximum is four sprays in each nostril (200 mcg/day).
   Aqueous nasal form: Up to 6 years old—not recommended. Six to 14 years old—two sprays in each nostril twice daily or one spray in each nostril three times a day. Once the peak effect is seen, the dose should be reduced to the smallest dose and frequency that works.
15 to 60 Years of Age:
   Oral inhalation: 0.5 to 1 mg (2 to 4 metered sprays) twice a day, morning and evening. Limit total daily dose to 2 mg (four inhalations twice daily). Once the peak effect is seen, the dose should be reduced to the smallest dose and frequency that works.
   Nasal inhalation: Two sprays (50 mcg) per nostril twice a day. The dose may be increased to two sprays in each nostril three times a day (300 mcg/day) if required. Maximum dose with this route is eight sprays (400 mcg) in each nostril daily. Once the peak effect is seen, the dose should be reduced to the smallest dose and frequency that works.
   Aqueous nasal form: Two sprays in each nostril twice daily to start. Maintenance dosing is continued with the lowest dose that is effective. This may be as low as one spray in each nostril daily.
Over 60 Years of Age: Same as 15 to 60 years of age.

Conditions Requiring Dosing Adjustments
   Liver Function: Specific guidelines are not available.
   Kidney Function: No specific changes needed—dual kidney and fecal elimination (Nasalide).

▷ **Dosing Instructions:** May be used as needed without regard to eating. Shake the container well before using. Carefully follow the printed patient instructions provided with the inhaler; rinse the mouth and throat (gargle) with water thoroughly after each inhalation. A decongestant is prudent BEFORE flunisolide is used in people with blocked nose (nasal) passages. If you forget a dose: take the next dose as soon as you remember it, unless it is nearly time for your next dose—if that is the case, skip the dose you forgot, and take the next dose right on schedule. DO NOT double doses. Once the peak benefit is seen, the dose should be lowered to the smallest dose that works.

Usual Duration of Use: Use on a regular schedule for 1 to 3 weeks is necessary to see effectiveness in controlling allergic rhinitis. It may take 4 weeks to see the greatest benefit in severe, chronic asthma. In patients who are dependent on systemic steroids, changing to oral flunisolide inhalations may be more difficult since recovering from suppressed adrenal gland function can be slow. When therapy is started, the inhaler form is typically used at the same time as the prior systemic steroid and continued for 7–14 days. After this, gradual reductions of the daily dose of the previous steroid are undertaken. As with other steroids, if severe asthma attacks or stress, systemic steroids may need to be restarted. Ongoing use requires physician supervision and guidance.

Typical Treatment Goals and Measurements (Outcomes and Markers)

Asthma: Frequency and severity of asthma attacks should ease. Some clinicians also use decreased frequency of rescue inhaler use as a further clinical indicator. It is critical that this medicine is used regularly to get the best results. An additional goal of therapy is to use the lowest effective dose. Some people keep their improvements when doses are lowered, while others relapse. Specific testing goals include improvement in PEFR and other lung (pulmonary) function tests. Wheezing and difficulty breathing (Dyspnea) should ease as well as asthma caused (induced) by exercise. If the usual benefit is not realized, call your doctor.

Allergic rhinitis: Signs and symptoms of allergic rhinitis such as runny or stuffy nose, postnasal drip, and sneezing should ease. Scratch testing for a specific immune substance (IgE) can also be done to check progress at a cellular level.

Possible Advantages of These Dosage Forms and Medicines: Intranasal or inhaled flunisolide has not been reported to be related to suppression of the adrenal gland. The localized nature of the dosing appears, the dose amount and/or the medicine to offer systemic exposure or medicine action different than other approaches to corticosteroids use.

▷ **This Drug Should Not Be Taken If**
  • you have had an allergic reaction to it previously.
  • you are having severe acute asthma or status asthmaticus that requires more intense treatment for prompt relief.
  • you have been taking this medicine and have repeat nosebleeds.
  • you have a form of nonallergic bronchitis with asthmatic features.

▷ **Inform Your Physician Before Taking This Drug If**
  • you are now taking or have recently taken any cortisone-related drug (including ACTH by injection; see Drug Classes) for any reason.
  • you have a history of tuberculosis (inhalation form).
  • you have herpes simplex infection of the eye.
  • you have chicken pox or measles or have been exposed to them.
  • you have had recent surgery of the nose or have ulcers of the nose or nosebleeds—this medicine should be used cautiously until the site has healed.
  • you are a child and your growth has slowed.
  • you have chronic bronchitis or bronchiectasis.
  • you think you may have an active infection of any kind, especially a respiratory infection (such as tuberculosis).

Possible Side Effects (natural, expected, and unavoidable drug actions)

Yeast infections (thrush) of the mouth and throat. Suppression of the adrenal gland (possible and more likely with higher doses).

Unpleasant taste. Orally inhaled flunisolide can cause flu-like symptoms occasionally in people taking the drug by oral inhalation. Difficulty in making usual voice sounds (dysphonia)—may be frequent with the inhaled form. The most frequent adverse effect of the nasal form is irritation of the nose (nasal mucosa).

▷ **Possible Adverse Effects** (unusual, unexpected, and infrequent reactions)

If any of the following develop, consult your physician promptly for guidance.

Mild Adverse Effects

Allergic reactions: skin rash, hives, itching.

Headache, dizziness, nervousness, moodiness, insomnia, loss of smell or taste—rare to infrequent.

Aftertaste (nasal form)—frequent.

Upper respiratory infections, cough—possible.

Heart palpitation, increased blood pressure, swelling of feet and ankles (inhalation form)—possible to infrequent.

Loss of appetite, indigestion, nausea, vomiting, stomach pain, diarrhea—infrequent.

Sore throat, stinging of the nose—infrequent to frequent.

Nasal irritation—infrequent to frequent (less common with the aqueous form).

Slowing of growth rate in children—possible.

Impaired sense of smell—possible.

Serious Adverse Effects

Allergic reaction: localized areas of "allergic" pneumonitis (lung inflammation).

Bronchospasm, asthmatic wheezing—rare with the inhalation form.

Tachycardia or hypertension—rare with the inhalation form.

Osteoporosis—possible with long-term use, even in people who do not usually get osteoporosis, such as men, blacks, and women before menopause. Cumulative dose and how long the corticosteroids have been used impacts this problem, but exact cumulative doses (cut point) are not known (often greatest in the first 6 months of treatment and in the spine and ribs—alendronate or raloxifene plus calcium replacement may prevent this). The British Royal College of Physicians recommends that patients at high risk for osteoporosis should also start bone protective treatment at the same time.

Increased risk of cataracts (posterior subcapsular)—possible, though less likely than with other corticosteroid dosing strategies.

▷ **Possible Effects on Sexual Function:** None reported.

Natural Diseases or Disorders That May Be Activated by This Drug

Cortisone-related drugs (used by inhalation) that produce systemic effects can impair immunity and lead to reactivation of "healed" or quiescent tuberculosis. People with a history of tuberculosis should be watched closely during use of cortisonelike drugs by inhalation.

Possible Effects on Laboratory Tests

None reported.

CAUTION

1. Does NOT act primarily as a bronchodilator. **Should not be used for immediate relief of acute asthma**.

2. If you were using any cortisone-related drugs for treatment of your asthma before changing to this inhaler, the cortisone-related drug may be required if you are injured, have an infection, or require surgery. Tell your doctor about prior use of cortisone-related drugs. Slow downward adjustment of the prior steroid is typical. For example, if prednisone was being taken, 2.5 mg per week decreases in prednisone (as outlined above) would be a usual occurrence.

3. If severe asthma returns while using this drug, call your doctor immediately.

4. If you have used cortisone-related drugs in the past year, carry a card that says so.

5. Five to ten minutes should separate the inhalation of bronchodilators, such as albuterol, epinephrine, pirbuterol, etc. (which should be used first), and the inhalation of this drug. This lets more flunisolide reach the bronchial tubes and reduces risk of adverse effects from the propellants used in the two inhalers.

6. A decongestant may be a good idea in people with blocked nasal passages. Talk with your doctor or pharmacist.

7. Osteoporosis risk is increased with long-term use of this medicine. Bone mineral density (BMD) tests are prudent as well as the use of alendronate (Fosamax) as a preventive (prophylactic) medicine in some high-risk patients (based on BMD results).

8. Unlike other corticosteroids, reports of osteonecrosis (avascular necrosis or aseptic necrosis) have not been made for this medicine. Caution is prudent, and patients should report any unexplained joint (such as knee, hip, or shoulder) pain to their doctor.

9. Up to 50% of an intranasal dose may reach the rest of the body (systemic circulation).

Precautions for Use

By Infants and Children: Safety and effectiveness for those under 4 years of age are not established. To obtain maximal benefit, the use of a spacer device is recommended for inhalation therapy in children.

By Those Over 60 Years of Age: People with chronic bronchitis or bronchiectasis should be watched closely for the development of lung infections.

▷ **Advisability of Use During Pregnancy**

Pregnancy Category: C. See Pregnancy Risk Categories at the back of this book.

Animal Studies: Rat and rabbit studies reveal significant birth defects due to this drug.

Human Studies: Adequate studies of pregnant women are not available.

Avoid drug during the first 3 months. Use infrequently and only as clearly needed during the final 6 months.

Advisability of Use If Breast-Feeding

Presence of this drug in breast milk: Unknown.

Avoid drug or refrain from nursing.

Habit-Forming Potential: With recommended dose, a state of functional dependence (see Glossary) is not likely to develop.

Effects of Overdose: Indications of cortisone excess (due to systemic absorption)—fluid retention, flushing of the face, stomach irritation, nervousness.

Possible Effects of Long-Term Use: Development of acne, cataracts, altered menstrual pattern. Osteoporosis (periodic bone mineral density tests are prudent).

Suggested Periodic Examinations While Taking This Drug (at physician's discretion)

Inspection of mouth and throat for evidence of yeast infection.

Check of adrenal function in people who have used cortisone-related drugs for an extended period of time before using this drug.

X-ray of the lungs of people with a prior history of tuberculosis.

Bone mineral density testing (osteoporosis test DEXA or PDEXA) with long-term use.

▷ **While Taking This Drug, Observe the Following**

Foods: No specific restrictions beyond those advised by your physician.

Herbal Medicines or Minerals: Fir or pine needle oil should NOT be used by asthmatics. Ephedra alone does carry a German Commission E monograph indication for asthma treatment. If you are allergic to plants in the Asteraceae family (aster, chrysanthemum, daisy, or ragweed), you may also be allergic to echinacea, chamomile, feverfew, and St. John's wort.

Increased calcium and vitamin D are prudent while taking this medicine. Talk to your doctor BEFORE adding any herbals to this medicine.

Beverages: No specific restrictions.

▷ *Alcohol:* No direct interactions expected, but excessive alcohol use may be a risk factor for osteoporosis. Since long-term use of this medicine may lead to osteoporosis, excessive use of alcohol must be avoided.

Tobacco Smoking: No direct drug interactions expected; however, smoking can worsen asthma and reduce benefits of flunisolide. I advise everyone to quit smoking.

▷ *Other Drugs*

The following drugs may ***increase*** the effects of flunisolide:

• inhalant bronchodilators—albuterol, bitolterol, epinephrine, etc.
• oral bronchodilators—aminophylline, ephedrine, terbutaline, theophylline, etc.

Flunisolide ***taken concurrently*** with

• bupropion (Wellbutrin and Zyban) may result in increased risk of seizures (more possible with systemic forms of this medicine).
• stanozolol (Winstrol) may result in increased risk of acne or edema.
• some antiepileptic medicines such as phenytoin (Dilantin) may increase risk of osteoporosis.
• inhalant bronchodilators—epinephrine, isoetharine, isoproterenol—may offer improved results in asthma treatment.

▷ *Driving, Hazardous Activities:* No restrictions.

Aviation Note: The use of this drug and the disorder for which this drug is prescribed ***may be disqualifications*** for piloting. Consult a designated Aviation Medical Examiner.

Exposure to Sun: No restrictions.

Occurrence of Unrelated Illness: Acute infections, serious injuries, or surgical procedures can create an urgent need for cortisone-related drugs given by mouth and/or injection. Call your doctor immediately in the event of new illness or injury.

Special Storage Instructions: Store at room temperature. Avoid exposure to temperatures above 120 degrees F. (49 degrees C.). Do not store or use this inhaler near heat or open flame.

Discontinuation: If this drug has made it possible to reduce or discontinue cortisonelike drugs by mouth, do not stop this drug abruptly. If you must stop this drug, call your doctor promptly. Cortisone preparations and other measures may be necessary.

FLUOROQUINOLONE ANTIBIOTIC FAMILY

Ciprofloxacin   (sip roh FLOX a sin)   **Gatifloxacin**   (GAT ih flox a sin)
Grepafloxacin   (GREP ah flox a sin)   **Levofloxacin**   (leev oh FLOX a sin)   **Lomefloxacin**   (loh me FLOX a sin)   **Norfloxacin**   (nor FLOX a sin)   **Ofloxacin**   (oh FLOX a sin)   **Sparfloxacin**   (SPAR flox a sin)
Trovafloxacin   (TROV ah flox a sin)

Introduced: 1984, 2000, 1997, 1996, 1992, 1986, 1984, 1996, 1997, respectively **Class:** Anti-infective, fluoroquinolone **Prescription:** USA: Yes **Controlled Drug:** USA: No **Available as Generic:** USA: Yes, ciprofloxacin, no, others; Canada: Yes (IV)

Brand Names: *Ciprofloxacin*: Ciloxan, Cipro, Cipro Cystitis pack, Cipro HC [CD], Cipro-XR; *Gatifloxacin*: Tequin; *Grepafloxacin* (removed from the market); *Levofloxacin:* Levaquin, Maxaquin, Quixin; *Moxifloxacin:* Avelox; *Norfloxacin:* Chibroxin, Noroxin, Noroxin Ophthalmic; *Ofloxacin:* ✦Apo-Oflox, Floxin, Floxin Otic, Floxin Uropak, Ocuflox, ✦Ofloxacine; *Sparfloxacin:* Zagam; *Trovafloxacin:* Trovan, Trovan/Zithromax Compliance Pak

Author's Note: Information in this profile will be broadened to include data on gatifloxacin and moxifloxacin once more data are available. It does carry a precautionary note regarding QTc interval prolongation and avoidance in people with QTc prolongation and in those taking other medicines that can cause QTc prolongation.

Warning: Some prescribers use "Norflox" to identify norfloxacin. This is not an accepted name in any setting for any reason. Using this name has resulted in serious medication errors—that is, the dispensing of Norflex, the generic drug orphenadrine, a skeletal muscle relaxant. Check to be sure you get the right drug.

Warning: There have been reports for some drugs in this class that find tendon rupture as a rare adverse effect. Ask your doctor about limits on strenuous exercise while you are taking this medicine. A rare idiosyncratic reaction has also been reported that presents as mental confusion and disorientation. Use of these medicines after head trauma may be a risk factor. If you have suffered a fall, ask your doctor if a medicine in a different antibiotic class should be substituted. If you are taking this drug and notice a change in your thinking, call your doctor. **THE FDA HAS RESTRICTED TROVAFLOXACIN USE TO EMERGENCIES.** The CDC has stopped recommending quinolones to treat gonorrhea in Hawaii and California due to resistant gonorrhea.

BENEFITS versus RISKS

Possible Benefits	*Possible Risks*
HIGHLY EFFECTIVE TREATMENT FOR INFECTIONS OF THE LOWER RESPIRATORY TRACT (ciprofloxacin and ofloxacin), URINARY TRACT, BONES, JOINTS, AND SKIN TISSUES due to susceptible organisms	TROVAFLOXACIN PATIENTS WERE WARNED (IN EUROPE) TO STOP TROVAFLOXACIN IF THEY DEVELOP SKIN RASH OR HIVES, YELLOWING OF THE SKIN OR EYES, DARK URINE, OR NAUSEA AND VOMITING WITH STOMACH PAIN; THE DRUG IS NO LONGER SOLD IN DRUG STORES
EFFECTIVE TREATMENT OF BACTERIAL (EYE) INFECTIONS	
CIPRO XR FORM OFFERS THREE-DAY TREATMENT FOR URINARY TRACT INFECTIONS	SOME OF THESE MEDICINES CAN CAUSE SEVERE SUN SENSITIVITY
Effective treatment for some forms of bacterial gastroenteritis (diarrhea)	PROLONGATION OF THE QT INTERVAL with some
Effective treatment for some infections of the prostate gland	Nausea, Indigestion
	Drug-induced colitis
	Hallucination or seizure
	Tendon rupture

▷ **Principal Uses**

As a Single Drug Product: Uses currently included in FDA-approved labeling: Treats responsive infections (in adults) of (1) the lower respiratory tract (lungs and bronchial tubes); (2) the urinary tract (kidneys, bladder, urethra [CDC recommends against using these medicines where resistant gonorrhea may be more likely such as in men who have sex with men], and prostate gland); (3) the digestive tract (small intestine and colon); (4) bones and joints (ciprofloxacin; ofloxacin—unlabeled); (5) skin and related tissues; (6) used in ophthalmic preparations to treat bacterial conjunctivitis caused by susceptible organisms; (7) ciprofloxacin has been approved to treat mild to moderate acute sinusitis caused by *Streptococcus pneumoniae, Haemophilus influenzae,* or *Moraxella catarrhalis;* (8) sparfloxacin is very active against Streptococcus; (9) ciprofloxacin/hydrocortisone is used for sudden infections of the outside of the ear *(acute otitis externa)*; (10) ciprofloxacin is used in post-exposure anthrax cases; (11) gatifloxacin is approved for a short course (5-day regimen) for acute exacerbation of chronic bacterial bronchitis; Cipro XR form is approved for uncomplicated bladder (cystitis) as once-a-day treatment for three days.

Other (unlabeled) generally accepted uses: (1) Can have a role in treating cholera where the organisms are resistant to doxycycline (ciprofloxacin); (2) lessens symptoms or prevents traveler's diarrhea; (3) ciprofloxacin can be of use in treating some unusual organisms such as Aeromonas, cat-scratch fever, or chancroid; (4) ofloxacin and sparfloxacin may help in combination therapy of leprosy; (5) levofloxacin is listed as an alternative medicine for treating chlamydia or gonorrhea (where the gonorrhea did NOT come from the Pacific or Asia or in cases where men have had sex with men leading to this infection—resistance problem).

Author's Note: Given the restricted use of trovafloxacin, information on that medicine will be truncated.

As a Combination Drug Product [CD]: Combined with hydrocortisone in the Cipro HC form to give the benefit of a corticosteroid in reducing inflammation and the antibiotic ciprofloxacin to kill the causative bacteria.

How These Drugs Work: These medicines block the bacterial enzyme DNA gyrase (required for DNA synthesis and cell reproduction), arrest bacterial growth (in low concentrations), and kill bacteria (in high concentrations).

▷ **Widely Used Guidelines That Involve This Medicine (representative sample):** Please look at the section at the very beginning of this profile called "Class." Next, turn to Table 22 and you will find guidelines listed by the class involved!

Available Dosage Forms and Strengths

Ciprofloxacin:

　　Ophthalmic solution — 0.3%

　　　　Otic suspension — 2 mg/mL ciprofloxacin and 10 mg/mL hydrocortisone

　　　Suspension — 250 mg, 500 mg per 5 mL

　　　　Tablets — 250 mg, 500 mg, 750 mg

　　　Tablets, XR — 500 mg

　Tablets Ciprocystitis pack — 100 mg

Levofloxacin:

　　Ophthalmic solution — 0.5%

　　Solution for injection — 5 mg per mL, 25 mg per mL

　　　　Tablets — 250 mg, 500 mg, 750 mg

Lomefloxacin:

　　　Tablets — 400 mg

Norfloxacin:

　　Ophthalmic solution — 3 mg/mL

　　　　Tablets — 400 mg

Ofloxacin:
> Ophthalmic solution — 3 mg/mL
> Otic solution — 0.3%
> Tablets — 200 mg, 300 mg, 400 mg

Sparfloxacin:
> Tablet — 200 mg

▷ **Recommended Dosage Ranges** (Actual dose and schedule for all these medicines must be determined for each patient individually.)

Infants and Children: None of these medicines is recommended.

18 to 60 Years of Age:

Ciprofloxacin: 250 mg to 750 mg every 12 hours (depends on nature and severity of infection). Daily maximum is 1,500 mg. Mild to moderate sinusitis (caused by organisms outlined above) treated with 500 mg every 12 hours for 10 days in adults. Cipro XR form is used for uncomplicated bladder (cystitis) infections with 500 mg once a day for 3 days.

Anthrax (after exposure): 500 mg by mouth every 12 hours (started as soon as possible after exposure) and continued **for 60 days. Please note, the 60-day time frame is critical. Amazingly, many patients who thought they were exposed did NOT continue the medicine as directed according to some sources.**

Ophthalmic—one or two drops instilled in the eye every 2 hours while awake for 2 days and then one or two drops for 5 more days (given every 4 hours while awake). *Otic:* After shaking the bottle well and warming it in your hand, children one year and older and adults should be given 3 drops of the suspension into the affected ear twice a day for seven days.

Levofloxacin: 500 mg orally every 24 hours for 7–14 days for community-acquired pneumonia, 500 mg a day for 7 days for chlamydia in people who can't take azithromycin or doxycycline.

Ophthalmic: On the first and second day—one to two drops in the affected eye every 2 hours (up to 8 times a day) while you are awake. On the 3rd through 7th day—1–2 drops every 4 hours (up to 4 times a day) while you are awake.

Lomefloxacin: For bronchitis—400 mg daily for 10 days. For bladder infections (cystitis)—400 mg daily for 10 days. For complicated urinary tract infections—400 mg daily for 14 days. For preoperative prevention of urinary tract infection—400 mg (single dose) taken 2 to 6 hours before surgery.

Norfloxacin: Uncomplicated urinary tract infections—400 mg every 12 hours for 3 days. Complicated urinary tract infections—400 mg every 12 hours for 10 to 21 days. Total daily dose should not exceed 800 mg. Ophthalmic dosing—1 to 2 drops to the affected eye 4 times daily.

Ofloxacin: 200 mg to 400 mg every 12 hours (for 10 days for lower respiratory infections), depending on nature and severity of infection. Daily maximum is 800 mg. Ophthalmic dosing (conjunctivitis)—1 to 2 drops every 2 to 4 hours for 2 days and then four times a day for 7 to 10 days. *Otic:* For patients 12 or older, the Floxin Otic form is used to treat otitis externa and 10 drops are placed into the affected ear twice a day for 10 days (in otitis media that is ongoing and suppurative, the same dose is used for 14 days).

Sparfloxacin: 400 mg now; then 200 mg a day for 10 days for pneumonia.

Over 60 Years of Age: Same as 18 to 60 years of age unless kidney function is an issue.

Conditions Requiring Dosing Adjustments

Liver Function: Use ciprofloxacin, norfloxacin used with caution in severe liver failure. No changes for levofloxacin, ofloxacin, or sparfloxacin. Because of possible liver toxicity trovafloxacin use not prudent in liver compromise.

Kidney Function: Ciprofloxacin, levofloxacin, lomefloxacin, norfloxacin, ofloxacin, and sparfloxacin **must** be decreased (or time between doses increased) in kidney compromise. For moderate to severe kidney compromise, ofloxacin dose is decreased to 400 mg daily. For patients with moderate kidney failure, the usual ofloxacin dose can be taken every 24 hours. For patients with severe failure, one-half the usual dose should be taken every 24 hours. Since some of these medicines can form crystals in urine, drink adequate quantities of water.

Cystic Fibrosis: A loading dose for ciprofloxacin, as well as ongoing doses of 750 mg every 8 hours, is taken by cystic fibrosis patients. This dosing gives blood levels that are more aggressive versus the bacteria that usually cause infections in these patients. No changes for the other drugs are presented.

▷ **Dosing Instructions:** Ciprofloxacin, levofloxacin, lomefloxacin, norfloxacin, or sparfloxacin may be taken with or without food (NOT dairy products), and all immediate release forms may be crushed. Extended release forms should NOT be crushed, chewed, or changed and should be taken whole. Ofloxacin is best taken 2 hours after eating. Drink large amounts of fluids while taking any of these drugs. For suspension forms, shake them well BEFORE taking them to resuspend the medicine and measure the dose with a dosing spoon or calibrated medicine measuring cup. Avoid aluminum or magnesium antacids, iron, zinc, or calcium for 2 hours before and after drug doses. If you forget a dose: take the missed dose as soon as you remember it, unless it is nearly time for your next dose—then skip the missed dose and take the next dose right on schedule. Then return to your usual schedule. If you are taking one of the every-12-hour quinolones, take any remaining doses for the day at an evenly spaced time period. If you miss more than one dose, please call your doctor. The otic ciprofloxacin suspension should be warmed by rolling the container in your hand for several minutes.

Usual Duration of Use: Regular use for 7 to 14 days is needed to see benefits in eradicating infection. Dosing should be continued for at least 2 days after all indications of infection have disappeared. Bone and joint infections (ciprofloxacin or ofloxacin) or prostate gland infections may be treated for 6 weeks or longer. Anthrax treatment using ciprofloxacin REQUIRES 60 days of treatment. Long-term use requires periodic evaluation of response by a physician. Cipro XR form is used once a day for three days for uncomplicated bladder infections (cystitis).

Typical Treatment Goals and Measurements (Outcomes and Markers)

Infections: The most commonly used measures of serious infections are white blood cell counts and differentials (the kind of blood cells that occur most often in your blood), and temperature. Many clinicians look for positive changes in 24–48 hours. NEVER stop an antibiotic because you start to feel better. For many infections, a full 14 days is REQUIRED to kill the bacteria. The goals and time frame (see Benefits) should be discussed with you when the prescription is written. Response to eye (ophthalmic) and ear (otic) forms can be assessed by reduced redness and itching of the eye and reduced swelling of the ear (auditory) canal and lessened severity and subsequent disappearance of earache.

Possible Advantages of These Drugs: Ciprofloxacin and ofloxacin have very broad spectrums of antibacterial activity of all currently available oral antimicrobial drugs. Highly effective in treating numerous types of infection caused by a wide spectrum of bacteria. Provide effective drug levels in the prostate gland (a difficult place to penetrate). Lomefloxacin has not had significant effects on kidney function. Sparfloxacin has better gram positive (Strep and Staph) activity than other medicines in this family. Cipro XR form treats uncomplicated bladder infections (cystitis) with only *a once-a-day dose taken for three days*. Ciprofloxacin and levofloxacin offer the opportunity to change (streamline) from intravenous to pill forms taken by mouth once clinically appropriate. This can offer treatment with a very potent antibiotic without the use of an intravenous line, and also allow treatment at home, shortening hospital stay.

▷ **These Drugs Should Not Be Taken If**
- you take an antiarrhythmic drug (see Drug Classes) or have a prolonged QTc (heartbeat interval) or take medicines known to cause Torsades de Pointes. Talk with your doctor (gatifloxacin, levofloxacin, moxifloxacin, sparfloxacin—perhaps others).
- you had an allergic reaction to any quinolone antibiotic.
- you have swelling (inflammation), pain, or bursting (rupture) of a tendon.
- you are pregnant or breast-feeding.
- you have a poorly controlled seizure disorder.
- you are less than 18 years of age.

▷ **Inform Your Physician Before Taking These Drugs If**
- you are allergic to cinoxacin (Cinobac), naladixic acid (NegGram), or other quinolone drugs.
- you have a seizure disorder or a brain circulatory disorder.
- you have increased lipids (dyslipidemia) as this may increase risk of tendonitis.
- you have impaired liver or kidney function.
- you have a history of mental disorders (psychosis).
- you are taking any form of probenecid, theophylline, or steroids.
- your work requires you to be in the sun. Sparfloxacin can cause severe phototoxicity, ciprofloxacin increases sensitivity as well.
- your urine is alkaline (talk to your doctor) as this may increase risk of crystals in the urine from some members of this medicine family.
- your work requires heavy manual labor. (Several cases of tendon rupture have been reported with fluoroquinolone use.) Heavy exercise or work may be contraindicated. Call your doctor immediately if you develop inflammation or pain in a tendon.

Possible Side Effects (natural, expected, and unavoidable drug actions)
Superinfections (see Glossary). Permanent greenish tooth discoloration if used in infants (ciprofloxacin). Photosensitivity.

▷ **Possible Adverse Effects** (unusual, unexpected, and infrequent reactions)
If any of the following develop, consult your physician promptly for guidance.
Mild Adverse Effects
Allergic reaction: rash, itching, localized swelling—rare.
Dizziness, headache (frequent with lomefloxacin), weakness, migraine, anxiety, abnormal vision—rare.
Nausea, diarrhea, vomiting, indigestion—rare to frequent.
Muscle aches—case reports.

Burning feeling in the eye when the ophthalmic solutions are used—possible.

Decreased vision (with ophthalmic use)—case reports.

Serious Adverse Effects

Allergic reaction: anaphylaxis—case reports.

Serious skin rashes—case reports for some (for example, ciprofloxacin has a case report of bullous pemphigoid, ofloxacin has a report as a probable cause of toxic epidermal necrolysis [TEN], and levofloxacin has a case report for TEN also). Call your doctor immediately if you develop a rash.

Idiosyncratic reactions—central nervous system stimulation (restlessness, tremor, confusion), hallucinations, seizures (lowers seizure threshold). One medication of this class has had reports of severe neurological compromise. Stop the drug immediately and call your doctor if you become confused or have trouble speaking while taking this drug—case reports. An idiosyncratic reaction between levofloxacin and warfarin leading to increased INR has been reported. Careful consideration of alternative antibiotics is advisable, more frequent INR checks and patient instruction on self-monitoring of possible bleeding is prudent if those medicines must be combined.

Kidney disease (interstitial nephritis)—case reports.

Tendon rupture—case reports for some family members (talk to your doctor about how much if at all to exercise or undertake strenuous work). Risk may be increased for people with high cholesterol or triglycerides, those who have kidney (renal) failure, those taking corticosteroids, and in people over 60 years old.

Abnormal heartbeats (even Torsades de Pointes) or palpitations—rare, but may be additive or worse if these medicines are taken with other medicines that change QT interval.

Liver toxicity—rare (trovafloxacin availability changed because of this).

Blood sugar disturbances—possible (more likely in diabetics taking insulin or an oral hypoglycemic medicine).

Bone marrow depression—case reports with ciprofloxacin, norfloxacin, and levofloxacin.

Intracranial hypertension (ciprofloxacin or ofloxacin)—case reports.

Worsening of myasthenia gravis—case reports.

▷ **Possible Effects on Sexual Function:** Vaginitis with discharge has been reported. Painful menstruation, excessive menstrual bleeding (ofloxacin only), urethral bleeding (ciprofloxacin)—case reports. Intermenstrual bleeding—case reports (lomefloxacin).

Natural Diseases or Disorders That May Be Activated by These Drugs

Latent epilepsy, latent gout.

Possible Effects on Laboratory Tests

Kidney function: increased blood creatinine and urea nitrogen (BUN)—rare.

Liver function tests: increased as a sign of liver toxicity—rare.

Red and white blood cell counts: rarely decreased (norfloxacin and ciprofloxacin)—case reports.

Blood glucose levels: rare fluctuations.

CAUTION

1. If you develop skin rash, hives, fatigue, or skin yellowing with nausea and vomiting while taking these medicines (especially trovafloxacin), call your doctor immediately.

2. With high doses or prolonged use, crystal formation in the kidneys may occur. This can be prevented by drinking large amounts of water, up to 2 quarts daily.

3. These drugs may decrease saliva formation, making dental cavities or gum disease more likely. Consult your dentist if dry mouth persists.
4. Changes in heart rhythm have been reported (QT interval). Sparfloxacin, gatifloxacin, and moxifloxacin appear to cause this problem more often than ciprofloxacin. Only polymorphic ventricular tachycardia reported for levofloxacin.
5. Strenuous exercise is NOT recommended while these medicines are being taken.
6. If a sudden change in mental status is noticed, call your doctor immediately.
7. The ciprofloxacin suspension must be reconstituted with the special diluent that comes with the powder. DO NOT reconstitute with water.
8. Case reports of bone marrow depression have been made in patients taking some of the medicines in this family. The drug should be suspect if white blood cell counts and platelets fall while taking this medicine.
9. Sun sensitivity that may be severe (phototoxicity) is possible with sparfloxacin (Zagam), lomefloxacin (Maxaquin), levofloxacin (Levaquin), and ciprofloxacin (Cipro). Sun should be avoided while sparfloxacin is being taken and for 5 days after the medicine is stopped. Sun sensitivity may be minimized by taking lomefloxacin in the evening.

Precautions for Use

By Infants and Children: Avoid the use of these drugs completely. Impairs normal bone growth and development.

By Those Over 60 Years of Age: Impaired kidney function may require dose reduction.

▷ Advisability of Use During Pregnancy

Pregnancy Category: C. See Pregnancy Risk Categories at the back of this book.

Animal Studies: Rabbit studies showed maternal weight loss and increased abortions (ciprofloxacin). Mild skeletal defects due to ofloxacin were found in rat studies; toxic effects on the fetus were shown in rat and rabbit studies. These drugs can impair normal bone development in immature dogs.

Human Studies: Adequate studies of pregnant women are not available.

The potential for adverse effects on fetal bone development contraindicates the use of these drugs during entire pregnancy.

Advisability of Use If Breast-Feeding

Presence of these drugs in breast milk: yes for levofloxacin, ofloxacin, and ciprofloxacin—probably for the rest.

Avoid drug or refrain from nursing.

Habit-Forming Potential: None.

Effects of Overdose: Confusion, headache, abdominal pain, diarrhea, liver toxicity, seizures, kidney toxicity, hallucinations.

Possible Effects of Long-Term Use: Superinfections (see Glossary); crystal formation in kidneys.

Suggested Periodic Examinations While Taking These Drugs (at physician's discretion)

Liver function tests. (Specific baseline and follow-up liver function tests prudent for trovafloxacin and perhaps others in this class.)

Urine analysis.

While Taking These Drugs, Observe the Following

Foods: Caffeine may remain in your system longer than usual. Use care in the amount of caffeine consumed. Dairy foods (such as milk and cheese) will decrease the effectiveness of these drugs by decreasing the amount absorbed. Separate 2 hours before or 6 hours after a dose.

Herbal Medicines or Minerals: Calcium supplements, iron pills, or zinc will decrease the amount of these medicines that go to work fighting infection. Separate doses by 2 hours before or 6 hours after the antibiotic. Some dandelion preparations may have a high enough concentration of metal ions to bind these medicines and blunt their benefits. Fennel seeds may have enough cations to also blunt benefits of these antibiotics. Separation by 2 hours before or 4–6 hours after is recommended. Use of St. John's wort may lead to additive sensitivity to the sun. Some patients use echinacea to attempt to boost their immune systems. Unfortunately, use of echinacea is not recommended in people with damaged immune systems. This herb may also actually weaken any immune system if it is used too often or for too long a time. Do NOT take mistletoe herb, oak bark, or F.C. of marshmallow root, and licorice.

Beverages: No restrictions (see Foods note on caffeine, above).

▷ *Alcohol:* No interactions expected, but since heavy alcohol intake can blunt the immune system, limit alcohol if you are ill enough to require an antibiotic.

Tobacco Smoking: No interactions expected. I advise everyone to quit smoking.

▷ *Other Drugs*

The following drug may ***increase*** the effects of fluoroquinolones:
- probenecid (Benemid).

Fluoroquinolones ***taken concurrently*** with
- amiodarone (Cordarone) may lead to heart toxicity.
- azlocillin may result in toxicity.
- caffeine will result in increased caffeine levels.
- corticosteroids (such as methylprednisolone, prednisone, and others) may result in increased risk of tendon rupture.
- cyclosporine (Sandimmune) may result in increased risk of kidney toxicity.
- dofetilide (Tikosyn) may lead to prolonged QT intervals and even possible Torsades de Pointes.
- foscarnet (Foscavir) may result in an increased risk of seizures.
- ibutilide (Corvert) may lead to prolonged QT intervals and even possible Torsades de Pointes.
- lithium led to lithium toxicity in one patient who took it with levofloxacin.
- live typhoid vaccine (Vivotif Bernia) may lead to blunted immunological response.
- olanzapine (Zyprexa) may lead to increased olanzapine levels (reported for ciprofloxacin, but caution advised for all quinolones acting on CYP1A2).
- phenytoin (Dilantin) or fosphenytoin (Cerebyx) may result in increased or decreased phenytoin levels.
- riluzole (Rilutek) combined with ofloxacin (because of P450 1A2 inhibition) may lead to riluzole toxicity. Riluzole doses may need to be lowered.
- theophylline (Theo-Dur, others) may lead to theophylline toxicity over time (norfloxacin or ciprofloxacin).
- warfarin (Coumadin) can result in increased risk of bleeding or blunted warfarin response. More frequent INR testing is needed and prudent.

The following drugs may ***decrease*** the effects of fluoroquinolones:
- antacids containing aluminum or magnesium, reducing absorption and lessening effectiveness.
- calcium supplements.
- didanosine (ciprofloxacin only).
- iron salts.

- magnesium, decreasing therapeutic benefits.
- morphine (only reported for trovafloxacin).
- nitrofurantoin (Macrodantin, etc.), which may antagonize the antibacterial action in the urinary tract. Avoid this combination.
- sucralfate (Carafate).
- zinc salts.

Sparfloxacin *taken concurrently* with the following drugs may cause abnormal heartbeats (also to be used with extreme caution with any new medicines that can prolong the QTc interval):

- amiodarone (Cordarone).
- astemizole (Hismanal).
- bepridil (Vascor).
- beta-blockers (see Drug Classes).
- chlorpromazine (Thorazine).
- cisapride (Propulsid).
- disopyramide (Norpace).
- macrolide antibiotics (erythromycin, dirithromycin, others).
- phenothiazines (see Drug Classes).
- procainamide (Pronestyl) (see Drug Classes).
- quinidine (Quinaglute, various).
- tricyclic antidepressants (see Drug Classes).

Moxifloxacin *taken concurrently* with

- class 1A or class III antiarrhythmic agents (see Drug Classes) may lead to abnormal heart changes (QT prolongation or even Torsades de Pointes). DO NOT combine.

Norfloxacin *taken concurrently* with

- dofetilide (Tikosyn) may lead to dofetilide toxicity via inhibition of CYP 3A4.

▷ *Driving, Hazardous Activities:* May cause dizziness or impair vision. Restrict activities as necessary.

Aviation Note: The use of these drugs *may be a disqualification* for piloting. Consult a designated Aviation Medical Examiner.

Exposure to Sun: Some members of this class have caused photosensitivity (see Glossary) and have limiting sun warnings. Sunglasses are advised if eyes are overly sensitive to bright light. A strong sun block is advised for your skin. Sparfloxacin users should avoid the sun while taking that medicine and for 5 days after the medicine is stopped. Lomefloxacin sun sensitivity may be reduced by taking the medicine at night. Excessive sun exposure should be avoided by levofloxacin users.

Heavy Exercise or Exertion: Several reports have surfaced regarding tendon rupture in patients with some of the medicines in this class. It is prudent to avoid heavy exercise or exertion while you are taking a fluoroquinolone.

Discontinuation: If you experience no adverse effects from these drugs, take the full course prescribed for best results. Ask your doctor when to stop treatment.

FLUOXETINE (flu OX e teen)

Introduced: 1978, 2001 **Class:** Antidepressant **Prescription:** USA: Yes **Controlled Drug:** USA: No **Available as Generic:** USA: Yes

Brand Names: ✦Alti-Fluoxetine, ✦Apo-Fluoxetine, ✦Gen-Fluoxetine, ✦Med-Fluoxetine, Prozac, Prozac Weekly, Sarafem, Symbyax [CD]

BENEFITS versus RISKS

Possible Benefits	*Possible Risks*
EFFECTIVE TREATMENT OF MAJOR DEPRESSIVE DISORDERS	Serious allergic reactions
	Conversion of depression to mania in manic-depressive (bipolar) disorders
EFFECTIVE PREVENTION OF RECURRENCE OF DEPRESSION	
EFFECTIVE IN SEVERE PMS (premenstrual dysphoric syndrome or PMDS)	
TREATS BULIMIA NERVOSA	
TREATS OBSESSIVE-COMPULSIVE DISORDER	
ONCE-WEEKLY FORMULATION FOR DEPRESSION WILL HELP ADHERENCE	
APPROVED FOR PREMENSTRUAL DYSPHORIC THERAPY WHEN USED 14 DAYS BEFORE THE PERIOD WILL START	
May reduce hot flashes in some cancer survivors	

▷ **Principal Uses**

As a Single Drug Product: Uses currently included in FDA-approved labeling: Treats (1) major forms of depression (including depression in HIV-positive patients and in geriatric depression); (2) obsessive-compulsive disorder; (3) bulimia; (4) approved for use in severe PMS (PMDS either every day or for the 14 days before menstruation is expected to start).

Other (unlabeled) generally accepted uses: (1) Refractory diabetic neuropathy; (2) may help control kleptomania; (3) can be of help in treating obesity, especially when obesity is accompanied by depression; (4) eases symptoms of panic attacks; (5) used to treat seasonal affective disorder (such as depression limited to winter months); (6) treats some forms of sexual problems; (7) some data for use of childhood anxiety disorder; (8) may ease ringing in the ears (tinnitus) that has not responded to other medicines; (9) may reduce the severity and frequency of hot flashes (by about half) in cancer survivors; (10) could have a role after a stroke in decreasing emotionalism and improving motor performance; (11) may have a role in anorexia nervosa when weight is returned to prior levels in order to help prevent relapse; (12) improved some measures of thinking in a small trial of patients with traumatic brain injury.

As a Combination Drug Product [CD]: Combined with olanzapine in treating depression that happens with bipolar disorder.

How This Drug Works: It restores normal levels of a nerve transmitter (serotonin). May work to stimulate Brain Derived Neurotrophic Factor (BDNF) and a specific receptor (tyrosine kinase receptor) resulting in remodeling of nerves. While this mechanism is derived from rat data, early clinical trials show improved performance in some small studies where fluoxetine gained improvements in thinking in adults who had suffered traumatic injuries.

▷ **Widely Used Guidelines That Involve This Medicine (representative sample):** Please look at the section at the very beginning of this profile called "Class." Next, turn to Table 22 and you will find guidelines listed by the class involved!

Available Dosage Forms and Strengths

Capsules — 10 mg, 20 mg, 40 mg
Capsules — 90 mg (Prozac Weekly form)
Capsules — 10 mg, 20 mg (28-pill blister packs Sarafem form)
Combination Capsules — 6 mg olanzapine and 25 mg fluoxetine
Oral solution — 20 mg/5 mL
Tablet — 10 mg

▷ **Usual Adult Dosage Ranges:**

Depression: Starts with 20 mg in the morning; if no improvement after several weeks, dose may be increased by 20 mg/day. Doses over 20 mg/day should be divided into two equal doses and taken twice daily. Maximum daily dose is 80 mg. Prozac Weekly form is intended for people who are already stabilized on the daily 20 mg form. The once weekly form is started seven days after the last 20 mg dose was given and is continued at 90 mg per week.

Depression with bipolar disorder: Dosing is started with one of the 6 mg olanzapine/25 mg fluoxetine capsules.

Bulimia: 60 mg once daily in the morning.

PMDS (severe PMS): A 28-pill blister pack is available (Sarafem form). In clinical studies, some patients used 20–60 mg during the entire month to check sign and symptom decreases (this is the recommended dose in current labeling). One part of the clinical study group obtained an 86% symptom reduction using 20 mg a day on days 14–28 of each menstrual cycle. Your doctor may adjust dosing strategies to the severity of your symptoms. This drug is now approved in PMDS for use only in the 14 days (luteal phase) BEFORE menstruation is expected to start.

Hot flashes in cancer survivors: 20 mg per day.

Obsessive-compulsive disorder: 20 to 80 mg daily.

Note: Actual dose and schedule must be determined for each patient individually.

Conditions Requiring Dosing Adjustments

Liver Function: The dose should be decreased or the dosing interval lengthened for patients with liver compromise. Some clinicians decrease the dose by 50% in compensated cirrhosis. This drug is also a rare cause of liver toxicity and should be used with caution by this patient population.

Kidney Function: Dosing changes are needed for severely impaired kidney function. Patients should be closely watched for adverse effects.

▷ **Dosing Instructions:** The capsule may be opened and the contents mixed with any convenient food. To make smaller doses, the contents may be mixed with orange juice or apple juice (NOT GRAPEFRUIT JUICE) and refrigerated; doses of 5–10 mg may prove effective and better tolerated. If you forget a dose: take the dose you missed as soon as you remember it, unless it is nearly time for your next dose—if that is the case, skip the missed dose and take the next dose right on schedule. DO NOT DOUBLE DOSES. If you find yourself missing doses, talk to your doctor.

Usual Duration of Use: Use on a regular schedule for 1 to 2 weeks may reveal start of benefits in depression. Up to 4 weeks may be needed for peak effects in (1) relieving depression and (2) the pattern of both favorable and unfavorable effects. An article in the *American Journal of Psychiatry* (see Quitkin, F.M. in Sources) advocated that 8 weeks of treatment should be undertaken BEFORE this medicine in treatment of depression is assessed and declared unsuccessful. Since there is an active metabolite and a long half-life, it may take several weeks before the benefits of a change in dose are seen. Benefits in obsessive-compulsive disorder may take 5 weeks or even longer in some cases. Long-term use (months to years) requires periodic physician evaluation. Some clinical guidelines suggest that 4 to 9 months of treatment should continue after the symptoms of depression go away. Some clinicians use lower doses to prevent or use as prophylaxis of depression. People who take their medicine regularly are least likely to have a recurrence. Will often take several weeks to work in reducing hot flashes in cancer survivors. PMDS use is recommended as 20 mg per day in the package insert, but acknowledges the need for reassessment of ongoing patient need. Bulimia treatment is often ongoing; however, there should be periodic checks to see if the medicine is still needed.

Typical Treatment Goals and Measurements (Outcomes and Markers)

Depression: The general goal is to lessen the degree and severity of depression, letting patients return to their daily lives. Specific measures of depression involve testing or inventories and can be valuable in helping check benefits from this medicine. The Hamilton Depression Scale (HAM-D) is widely used to assess depression. In the case of PMDS, control of irritability and decreased number and/or severity of symptoms and the ability of the patient to return to normal activities or not have them interrupted is a hallmark of successful treatment.

PMDS: The goal is to lessen the degree and severity of menstrual difficulties (such as pain, irritability, etc.) or to prevent menstruation-associated problems altogether.

Possible Advantages of This Drug

Does not cause weight gain, a common side effect of tricyclic antidepressants. May actually cause weight loss. Less likely to cause dry mouth, constipation, urinary retention, or orthostatic hypotension (see Glossary) than tricyclic antidepressants. Since a large National Cancer Institute study found that those who suffer depression for 6 years or more have a generally increased risk of cancer, one benefit of effective treatment of depression with this drug may be a generally reduced risk of cancer.

▷ **This Drug Should Not Be Taken If**
- you had an allergic reaction to it previously.
- you take, or took in the last 14 days, a monoamine oxidase (MAO) type A inhibitor (see Drug Classes).

▷ **Inform Your Physician Before Taking This Drug If**
- you have had any adverse effects from antidepressant drugs.
- you have impaired liver or kidney function.
- you have Parkinson's disease.
- you have a seizure disorder.
- you have a history of psychosis.
- you have a history of SIADH (talk with your doctor).
- you are pregnant or plan pregnancy while taking this drug.

Possible Side Effects (natural, expected, and unavoidable drug actions)
Decreased appetite, weight loss.
Case reports of orthostatic hypotension (see Glossary).

▷ **Possible Adverse Effects** (unusual, unexpected, and infrequent reactions)
If any of the following develop, consult your physician promptly for guidance.

Mild Adverse Effects
Allergic reactions: skin rash, hives, itching—rare.
Headache, nervousness, insomnia, drowsiness, tremor, dizziness, tingling of extremities—rare.
Vivid nightmares—case reports.
Altered taste, nausea—frequent.
Vomiting, diarrhea—possible to rare.
Bruising or nosebleeds—rare.
Hair loss—case reports.
Fast heart rate (tachycardia) or palpitations—rare.
Blurred vision—infrequent.
Excessive sweating—frequent.

Serious Adverse Effects
Allergic reactions: serum-sickness-like syndrome (fever, weakness, joint pain and swelling, swollen lymph glands, fluid retention, skin rash, and/or hives).
Drug-induced seizures—rare.
Worsening of Parkinson's disease—possible.
Parkinson-like reactions (extrapyramidal effects)—rare.
Neuroleptic malignant syndrome—case reports.
Intense suicidal preoccupation in severe depression that does not respond to this drug—case reports.
Mania or hypomania and psychosis or hallucinations—rare.
Aplastic anemia—case report.
Abnormal and excessive urination (SIADH)—case reports.
Abnormal heartbeats (even Torsades de Pointes) or palpitations—rare, but may be additive or worse with other medicines that change QT interval.
Liver toxicity—rare.

▷ **Possible Effects on Sexual Function:** Impaired erection (1.9%), inhibition of ejaculation, or inhibited orgasm in men and women—case reports. Worsening of fibrocystic breast disease in a female—case report. Spontaneous and persistent milk production (galactorrhea)—case reports during post-marketing period.

Natural Diseases or Disorders That May Be Activated by This Drug
Latent epilepsy.

Possible Effects on Laboratory Tests
Blood glucose level: decreased.
Blood sodium level: decreased.

CAUTION
1. If any skin reaction develops (rash, hives, etc.), stop this drug and inform your physician promptly.
2. If dry mouth develops and persists for more than 2 weeks, consult your dentist for help.
3. Ask your doctor or pharmacist before taking any other prescription or over-the-counter drug while taking fluoxetine.

4. If you must start any monoamine oxidase (MAO) type A inhibitor (see Drug Classes), allow an interval of 5–6 weeks after stopping this drug before starting the MAO inhibitor.

5. This drug should be withheld if electroconvulsive therapy (ECT, "shock" treatment) is to be used.

6. Be honest with your doctor about how well this medicine is helping you. There are many antidepressants available, and the first one that is tried may or may not work. Call your doctor immediately if you have thoughts of suicide.

7. A study (see above and Quitkin, F.M. in Sources) advocated that 8 weeks of treatment be undertaken before assessing this medicine to be unsuccessful.

8. Pediatric and adult patients treated with this medicine should be closely watched for worsening depression or suicidal thinking. The FDA has required makers of antidepressants such as this one to alert healthcare professionals to the fact that children and adults with major depression may develop worsening depression or suicidal thoughts and behavior whether they take medicine for depression or do not take it. Patients should be carefully followed for such clinical worsening (particularly when treatment is started or doses are increased or decreased).

9. Please see the olanzapine profile for added possible adverse effects of the combination fluoxetine/olanzapine form.

Precautions for Use
By Infants and Children: Safety and effectiveness for those under 7 years of age are not established.

For those 7 to 18 years old, some clinicians have used 5–10 mg per day or 10 mg three times a week. The dose is subsequently increased as needed and tolerated to a maximum of 20 mg per day.

By Those Over 60 Years of Age: Lower or less frequent doses are recommended by the manufacturer.

▷ Advisability of Use During Pregnancy
Pregnancy Category: C (for Symbyax form also). See Pregnancy Risk Categories at the back of this book.

Animal Studies: No birth defects due to this drug found in rat or rabbit studies.

Human Studies: Adequate studies of pregnant women are not available. Of the SSRIs, this medicine probably has the largest amount of data on women who have taken fluoxetine during pregnancy without adverse effects. One study of 228 women appeared to show that it was safer to take fluoxetine in the first two trimesters of pregnancy and discontinue it during the last trimester.

Use of this drug during pregnancy is a benefit-to-risk decision that must be discussed with your doctor.

Advisability of Use If Breast-Feeding
Presence of this drug in breast milk: Yes.

Avoid drug or refrain from nursing.

Habit-Forming Potential: Reports of patients using excess doses of fluoxetine or combining the drug with alcohol have surfaced. It appears possible that a euphoric effect and abuse potential exists.

Effects of Overdose: Agitation, restlessness, excitement, nausea, vomiting, seizures.

Possible Effects of Long-Term Use: None reported.

Suggested Periodic Examinations While Taking This Drug (at physician's discretion)

None.

▷ **While Taking This Drug, Observe the Following**

Foods: No restrictions (see Beverages below).

Beverages: Grapefruit juice may lead to increased blood levels. AVOID IT. May be taken with milk.

Herbal Medicines or Minerals: Since fluoxetine and St. John's wort may act to increase serotonin, the combination is not advised. Since part of the way ginseng works may be as an MAO inhibitor, do not combine with fluoxetine. Ma huang, yohimbe, Indian snakeroot, and kava kava (kava no longer recommended in Canada) are also best avoided while taking this medicine. Calcium has excellent data (1,200–1,600 mg per day unless contraindicated) in helping prevent premenstrual dysphoric syndrome (PMS). This may be an intelligent first-line therapy or valuable adjunctive use. Talk to your doctor to see if this makes sense for you.

▷ *Alcohol:* Does not appear to increase the central nervous system effects of fluoxetine or change the metabolism of alcohol.

Tobacco Smoking: No interactions expected, but I advise everyone to quit smoking.

Marijuana Smoking: Led to one case of mania in a patient who combined the two drugs.

▷ *Other Drugs*

Fluoxetine may ***increase*** the effects of

- atomoxetine (Strattera).
- beta blockers (see Drug Classes).
- diazepam (Valium) and other benzodiazepines (see Drug Classes).
- digitalis preparations (digitoxin, digoxin).
- diltiazem (Cardizem).
- dofetilide (Tikosyn), requiring dosing decreases.
- ergot derivatives (Cafergot, various) may increase risk of ergotism and is NOT advisable.
- flecainide (Tambocor).
- phenytoin (Dilantin), or fosphenytoin (Cerebyx) by increasing the phenytoin or fosphenytoin levels.
- propafenone (Rythmol).
- propranolol (Inderal).
- quinidine (Quinaglute).
- sildenafil (Viagra), by inhibiting CYP3A4.
- valproic acid (Depakote, others).
- warfarin (Coumadin) and related oral anticoagulants. Test INR more often.

Fluoxetine ***taken concurrently*** with

- antidiabetic drugs (insulin, oral hypoglycemics) may increase the risk of hypoglycemic reactions; monitor blood sugar levels carefully.
- aspirin (various) caused hives to reappear in a patient allergic to fluoxetine.
- astemizole (Hismanal), terfenadine (Seldane) (no longer on the U.S. market), or similar drugs may result in increased antihistamine levels and risk of heart arrhythmias. **Avoid** combining.
- azole antifungals (such as fluconazole, itraconazole, and ketoconazole) may lead to higher than expected fluoxetine blood levels and increased risk of adverse effects.

- buspirone (Buspar) may increase underlying anxiety. Combination is best avoided, but if deemed clinically necessary, patients should be closely watched for worsening of symptoms.
- carbamazepine (Tegretol) will increase the carbamazepine level. Drug levels are critical if the drugs are combined.
- cimetidine (Tagamet) may theoretically lead to increased fluoxetine levels.
- clarithromycin (Biaxin) may lead to fluoxetine toxicity—avoid the combination.
- clozapine (Clozaril) may result in increased levels of clozapine. The clozapine dose may need to be decreased if both medicines are to be used at the same time.
- cotrimoxazole (Bactrim) or cyclobenzaprine (Flexaril) may lead to changes in the heart pattern (QTc interval) and are NOT recommended.
- delavirdine (Rescriptor) may lead to delavirdine toxicity.
- dextromethorphan (a cough suppressant in many "DM"-labeled nonprescription cough medicines) may result in visual hallucinations if these drugs are combined. DO NOT COMBINE.
- fenfluramine (Pondimin) may lead to serotonin syndrome—DO NOT COMBINE.
- haloperidol (Haldol) will increase haloperidol levels. Dose decrease and blood levels are needed.
- ketorolac (Toradol) may result in hallucinations. DO NOT COMBINE.
- lithium (Lithobid, etc.) will result in increased lithium levels and increased risk of neurotoxicity. AVOID COMBINING.
- loratadine (Claritin) may result in increased loratadine levels. It may be prudent to decrease the loratadine dose if these medicines are to be combined. Unlike some of the other nonsedating antihistamines (see Drug Classes), loratadine has not (to date) resulted in abnormal heart rhythms.
- medicines that inhibit liver metabolism (removal) of this medicine may lead to higher than expected fluoxetine blood levels and increased toxicity risk.
- monoamine oxidase (MAO) type A inhibitor drugs (see Drug Classes) may cause confusion, agitation, high fever, seizures, and dangerous elevations of blood pressure. AVOID COMBINING.
- morphine (various) blunted pain management benefits of morphine in one case report.
- naratriptan (Amerge), rizatriptan (Maxalt), sumatriptan (Imitrex), zolmitriptan, almotriptan (Axert), or other triptans may lead to incoordination and abnormal reflexes. Caution is advised.
- olanzapine (Zyprexa) may lead to worsening of depression. Extreme caution is advised.
- ondansetron (Zofran) may have undesirable effects on the heart (QT prolongation, as well as other medicines that have a QT prolongation effect). DO NOT COMBINE.
- ritonavir (Norvir) has lead to case reports of heart or nerve adverse effects. Caution is advised.
- selegiline (Eldepryl) can result in serotonin toxicity syndrome. AVOID COMBINING.
- sibutramine (Meridia) may lead to serotonin syndrome. AVOID COMBINING.
- sulfamethoxazole (various) may increase abnormal heartbeat risk (QTc interval changes). DO NOT COMBINE.
- thioridazine (Mellaril) may increase abnormal heartbeat risk. DO NOT COMBINE.

- tramadol (Ultram) may increase seizure risk. DO NOT COMBINE.
- any tricyclic antidepressant (amitriptyline, nortriptyline, etc.) will result in increased antidepressant drug levels that will persist for weeks. Avoid the combination.
- trimethoprim (Septra, others) may increase abnormal heartbeat risk (QTc interval changes). DO NOT COMBINE.
- tryptophan will result in central nervous system toxicity. AVOID COMBINING.
- ziprasidone (Geodon) may increase abnormal heartbeat risk (QTc interval changes). DO NOT COMBINE.
- zolpidem (Ambien) may increase risk of hallucinations.

▷ *Driving, Hazardous Activities:* This drug may cause drowsiness, dizziness, impaired judgment, and delayed reaction time. Restrict activities as necessary.

Aviation Note: The use of this drug *is a disqualification* for piloting. Consult a designated Aviation Medical Examiner.

Exposure to Sun: No restrictions.

Discontinuation: Slow drug elimination makes withdrawal effects unlikely, but call your doctor if you plan to stop this drug for any reason.

FLUPHENAZINE (flu FEN a zeen)

Introduced: 1959 **Class:** Strong tranquilizer, phenothiazines **Prescription:** USA: Yes **Controlled Drug:** USA: No; Canada: No **Available as Generic:** USA: Yes; Canada: Yes

Brand Names: ✤Apo-Fluphenazine, ✤Modecate, ✤Moditan, Permitil, PMS-Fluphenazine, Prolixin

BENEFITS versus RISKS	
Possible Benefits	*Possible Risks*
EFFECTIVE CONTROL OF ACUTE MENTAL DISORDERS	SERIOUS TOXIC EFFECTS ON BRAIN with long-term use
Beneficial effects on thinking, mood, and behavior	Liver damage with jaundice
Decanoate injection gives long-lasting benefit with one shot	Blood cell disorders: abnormally low white blood cell counts

Author's Note: The information in this profile has been shortened to make room for more widely used medicines.

FLURAZEPAM (flur AZ e pam)

Introduced: 1970 **Class:** Hypnotic, benzodiazepines **Prescription:** USA: Yes **Controlled Drug:** USA: C-IV*; Canada: No **Available as Generic:** USA: Yes; Canada: Yes

Brand Names: ✤Apo-Flurazepam, Dalmane, Durapam, ✤Novo-Flupam, Somnol

BENEFITS versus RISKS	
Possible Benefits	*Possible Risks*
EFFECTIVE HYPNOTIC	Habit-forming potential with long-
NO SUPPRESSION OF REM (RAPID	term use
EYE MOVEMENT) SLEEP	Minor impairment of mental
NO REM SLEEP REBOUND after	functions ("hangover" effect)
discontinuation	Jaundice
Wide margin of safety with	Blood cell disorder–Suppression of
therapeutic doses	stage 4 sleep with reduced "quality"
	of sleep

▷ **Principal Uses**

As a Single Drug Product: Uses currently included in FDA-approved labeling: Short-term treatment of insomnia consisting of difficulty in falling asleep, frequent nighttime awakenings, and/or early morning awakenings.

Other (unlabeled) generally accepted uses: None at present.

Author's Note: Information in this profile has been shortened to make room for more widely used medicines.

Author's Note: The National Institute of Mental Health has an information Web page on anxiety. It can be found at *www.nimh.nih.gov/anxiety.*

FLURBIPROFEN (flur BI proh fen)

Please see the propionic acids (nonsteroidal anti-inflammatory drug) family profile.

FLUTAMIDE (FLUTE a myde)

Introduced: 1983   **Class:** Anticancer (antineoplastic), nonsteroidal nonhormonal antiandrogenic   **Prescription:** USA: Yes   **Controlled Drug:** USA: No; Canada: No   **Available as Generic:** USA: Yes; Canada: Yes

Brand Names: ✱Apo-flutamide, ✱Euflex, Eulexin, Flutamex (Germany)

BENEFITS versus RISKS	
Possible Benefits	*Possible Risks*
EFFECTIVE ADJUNCTIVE	Rare drug-induced hepatitis
TREATMENT OF PROSTATE	Breast enlargement and tenderness
CANCER	(gynecomastia)
	Hot flashes

▷ **Principal Uses**

As a Single Drug Product: Uses currently included in FDA-approved labeling: Treatment of metastatic prostate cancer, used concurrently with leuprolide (given by injection), goserelin, or with removal of the testicles (orchiectomy).

Other (unlabeled) generally accepted uses: (1) Some early data on use in bulimia; (2) can help excessive hair growth in women (hirsutism); (3) combination use (with fludrocortisone, reduced hydrocortisone and testolactone helped a group of children with adrenal gland problems present at birth (congenital adrenal hyperplasia); (4) may have a place in improving flow to the uterus in polycystic ovary syndrome (PCOS).

How This Drug Works: Flutamide suppresses effects of dihydrotestosterone (a male sex hormone also called DHT) and testosterone by blocking uptake and binding target tissues (such as the prostate gland). Used in conjunction with leuprolide (a drug that suppresses testosterone from testicles by damping the pituitary gland's testicular stimulation). The combination of these two drug actions—chemical castration by leuprolide and testosterone blockage by flutamide—significantly reduces hormonal stimulation of cancerous prostate tissue.

▷ **Widely Used Guidelines That Involve This Medicine (representative sample):** Please look at the section at the very beginning of this profile called "Class." Next, turn to Table 22 and you will find guidelines listed by the class involved!

Available Dosage Forms and Strengths
Capsules — 125 mg (U.S.)
Tablets — 250 mg (Canada, Germany)

▷ **Recommended Dosage Ranges** (Actual dose and schedule must be determined for each patient individually.)
Infants and Children: Not used in this age group.
12 to 60 Years of Age: In stage B2-C prostate cancer (a measure of the cancer severity): 250 mg by mouth every 8 hours. Flutamide is to be taken at the same time as an LHRH agonist such as leuprolide; the usual dose of leuprolide is 7.5 mg given by injection once a month, starting 8 weeks before radiation treatment. The medicine is also continued during radiation treatment.
Stage D2 prostate cancer: 250 mg by mouth every 8 hours in conjunction with an LHRH agonist. It is continued until there is evidence of progression.
Over 60 Years of Age: Same as 12 to 60 years of age.

Conditions Requiring Dosing Adjustments
Liver Function: Use with caution by patients with liver compromise. It is also a rare cause of cholestatic jaundice.
Kidney Function: Primarily eliminated by the kidneys. Use with caution in kidney compromise.

▷ **Dosing Instructions:** May be taken without regard to food. The capsule may be opened, and the tablet may be crushed. If you forget a dose: take the missed dose as soon as you remember it, unless it is nearly time for your next dose—if that is the case, skip the missed dose and take the next dose right on schedule. DO NOT double doses. Use a condom to keep your semen from contacting your sexual partner.

Warning: Since this medicine is a kind of cancer-killing medicine (antineoplastic agent), proper disposal of urine or vomit MUST be undertaken (ask your doctor).

Usual Duration of Use: Regular use for 2 to 4 months usually needed to see drug's benefits in controlling prostate cancer (tumor response) although symptom relief may happen in 12–28 days. Long-term use (months to years and up to 2.5 years has been reported) requires periodic physician evaluation and check for relapse.

Typical Treatment Goals and Measurements (Outcomes and Markers)

Prostate Cancer: The goal is to decrease bone pain, increase urine outflow, and increase survival time in D2 prostate cancer. Remissions have been gained from this medicine. Monthly bone and liver scans, chest X-ray, excretory urograms, and liver tests are typically obtained for the 4 months of treatment and periodically after that. PSA may also serve as a marker of success. Physical examination and follow-up on bone pain are important. Appropriate therapy and pain medicines to manage pain are critical.

Possible Advantages of This Drug

Ease of use. Less toxicity than other chemotherapeutic drugs.

Currently a "Drug of Choice"

For the management of prostate cancer (in combination with leuprolide) and coupled with castration.

▷ **This Drug Should Not Be Taken If**
   • you have had an allergic reaction to it previously.
   • your liver transaminases levels (ALT) are twice the upper laboratory normal limit.

▷ **Inform Your Physician Before Taking This Drug If**
   • you have a history of liver disease or impaired liver function.
   • you have high blood pressure (hypertension).
   • you have a history of anemia, low white blood cells, or low blood platelets.
   • you have not had a PSA or one has not been checked on a regular basis since starting this medicine.
   • you have a history of lupus erythematosus.

Possible Side Effects (natural, expected, and unavoidable drug actions)

Hot flashes (61%), loss of libido (with combination LHRH therapy), impotence, breast enlargement and tenderness. Bright yellow urine color. Sun sensitivity.

▷ **Possible Adverse Effects** (unusual, unexpected, and infrequent reactions)
   If any of the following develop, consult your physician promptly for guidance.

Mild Adverse Effects
   Allergic reaction: skin rash.
   Drowsiness, confusion, nervousness, depression—rare.
   Indigestion, nausea/vomiting, diarrhea—infrequent.
   Blurred vision—rare.
   Fluid retention (edema) of legs—possible.

Serious Adverse Effects
   Drug-induced hepatitis with jaundice (see Glossary)—rare to infrequent.
   Manic-like mental changes (syndrome)—case reports.
   Low blood platelets, white blood cells, or anemia—rare.
   Lupus erythematosus–like skin rash—case reports.
   Hypertension—rare.
   Heart attack—rare.
   Methemoglobinemia—case report.

▷ **Possible Effects on Sexual Function:** See Possible Side Effects. Flutamide itself does not presently appear to change libido, sexual performance, or the ability to have an erection. Combination therapy does appear to carry the risks of these adverse effects (medicines such as Cialis, Viagra, and Levitra may be of some help here). Swelling and tenderness of male breast tissue (gynecomastia) may be frequent.

▷ **Adverse Effects That May Mimic Natural Diseases or Disorders**
   Drug-induced hepatitis may suggest viral hepatitis.

Possible Effects on Laboratory Tests
   Complete blood counts: decreased red and white cells, hemoglobin, and platelets.
   Liver function tests: increased liver enzymes (ALT/GPT, AST/GOT, and alkaline phosphatase), increased bilirubin.
   PSA: reduced (a marker for cancer treatment results).
   Sperm counts and testosterone levels: decreased.

CAUTION
   1. For best results, flutamide and leuprolide should be started together and continued for the duration of therapy.
   2. During combination therapy with flutamide and leuprolide, symptoms of prostate cancer (difficult urination, bone pain, etc.) may worsen temporarily; these are transient and not significant.
   3. This medicine is not used in women.
   4. Call your doctor immediately if you have light-colored stools, dark urine, yellowing of the eyes or skin, or unexplained weakness or abdominal pain while taking this medicine (may be early signs of liver problems and can be reversible if caught early).
   5. Liver enzyme testing (ALT) should be checked BEFORE starting therapy. Therapy should NOT be started if ALT is twice the upper normal limit.

Precautions for Use
   By Those Over 60 Years of Age: Drug is more slowly excreted. If digestive symptoms or edema are troublesome, ask your doctor about adjusting dose.

▷ **Advisability of Use During Pregnancy**
   Pregnancy Category: D. See Pregnancy Risk Categories at the back of this book.
   Animal Studies: Rat studies reveal malformation of bone structures and feminization of male fetuses.
   Human Studies: Adequate studies of pregnant women are not available.
   Discuss this benefit-to-risk decision with your doctor.

Advisability of Use If Breast-Feeding
   Presence of this drug in breast milk: Unknown, but not intended for women. Stop nursing.

Habit-Forming Potential: None.

Effects of Overdose: Possible drowsiness, unsteadiness, nausea, vomiting.

Possible Effects of Long-Term Use: None reported.

Suggested Periodic Examinations While Taking This Drug (at physician's discretion)
   Prostate-specific antigen (PSA) assays.
   Complete blood cell counts.
   Liver function tests (see Caution note). Digital rectal exam and check for any metastasis (such as bone and liver scans).

▷ **While Taking This Drug, Observe the Following**
   Foods: No restrictions.
   Herbal Medicines: Since St. John's wort may also lead to increased sensitivity to the sun, DO NOT COMBINE. There are no data about use of echinacea with this medicine and the combination cannot be recommended. Herbal products that may be relatively toxic to the liver could increase liver toxicity risk if combined (such as eucalyptus, kava, or valerian).
   Beverages: No restrictions. May be taken with milk.

▷ *Alcohol:* No interactions expected.

Tobacco Smoking: No interactions expected, but I advise everyone to quit smoking.

Marijuana Smoking: Animal studies have shown this combination to result in additive suppression of the immune system. The combination therefore is not advisable.

▷ *Other Drugs*

Flutamide **taken concurrently** with

- influenza, pneumococcal, or yellow fever vaccine may result in blunting of immune response to the vaccine.
- warfarin (Coumadin, others) may cause an increased bleeding risk. More frequent INRs are prudent.

▷ *Driving, Hazardous Activities:* This drug may cause drowsiness. Restrict activities as necessary.

Aviation Note: The use of this drug **may be a disqualification** for piloting. Consult a designated Aviation Medical Examiner.

Exposure to Sun: This drug may cause photosensitivity (see Glossary).

Discontinuation: To be determined by your physician.

FLUTICASONE (flu TIC a zone)

Introduced: 1994   **Class:** Adrenocortical steroids   **Prescription:** USA: Yes   **Controlled Drug:** USA: No; Canada: No   **Available as Generic:** USA: No; Canada: No

Brand Names: ✤Advair [CD], Advair Diskus [CD], Cutivate, Flonase, Flovent, Flovent Diskus, Flovent Rotadisc

Author's Note: Some of the side effects are specific to or more likely with a particular dosing form (product).

BENEFITS versus RISKS

Possible Benefits	*Possible Risks*
EFFECTIVE, ONCE-DAILY RELIEF OF SEASONAL ALLERGIC RHINITIS	Reversible adrenal gland suppression
	Yeast infections of the mouth and throat
EFFECTIVE ONCE-DAILY ECZEMA TREATMENT	Possible osteoporosis with long-term use
EFFECTIVE ASTHMA TREATMENT	Irritation of the nose (nasal form)

▷ **Principal Uses**

As a Single Drug Product: Uses currently included in FDA-approved labeling: (1) Helps perennial and seasonal (hay fever) allergic or nonallergic rhinitis in adults or children who are 12 years of age or older; (2) the topical form is used for a variety of skin conditions from sunburn to eczema or psoriasis; (3) asthma (inhaler form); (4) cream approved for once-daily treatment of eczema.

Other (unlabeled) generally accepted uses: (1) Oral form may have a role in Chronic Obstructive Pulmonary disease (COPD); (2) may have a role in combination treatment of vitiligo using the fluticasone cream plus UV light.

As a Combination Drug Product [CD]: Combined with salmeterol (see drug profile of salmeterol later in this book). These drugs complement each other, making the combination a more effective antiasthmatic.

How This Drug Works: Corticosteroid-type medicines work to ease inflammation, suppress reaction of certain cells, and slow the inflammatory process. Halomethyl carbothionates have very potent anti-inflammatory and blood vessel–contracting (vasoconstrictive) activity.

▷ **Widely Used Guidelines That Involve This Medicine (representative sample):** Please look at the section at the very beginning of this profile called "Class." Next, turn to Table 22 and you will find guidelines listed by the class involved!

Available Dosage Forms and Strengths
Amber glass bottle — 16 g (120 actuations), 9 g (60 actuations)
    Cream — 0.05 mg/g
    Inhalation — 44 mcg, 110 mcg, 220 mcg
Inhalation powder — 50 mcg of salmeterol and 100, 250, or 500 mcg
    (U.S., Canada)   fluticasone per actuation
    ointment — 0.005%
    Nasal spray — 50 mcg per 100 mg

▷ **Recommended Dosage Ranges** (Actual dose and schedule must be determined for each patient individually.)
Infants and Children: Safety and efficacy for those less than 4 have not yet been defined. Nasal dosing for those 4 to 12—start with one spray (50 mcg in each spray) in each nostril (total 100 mcg) once a day. If symptoms are severe, the dose can be increased to two sprays in each nostril (50 mcg each spray) or 200 micrograms a day (for Flovent Rotadisc and Fluticasone Rotadisc). After a few days, the dose should be reduced to 50 micrograms in each nostril once daily.
4 to 11 Years of Age: The combination form of fluticasone 100 micrograms and salmeterol 50 micrograms has been approved for use in those 4–11 who still have symptoms when taking inhaled corticosteroid treatment alone.
12 to 60 Years of Age:
  Nasal dosing: Started with two sprays (50 mcg in each spray) in each nostril once a day when allergic or nonallergic rhinitis is being treated. The same dose can also be given as 100 mcg twice daily (8 A.M. and 8 P.M.). After a few days, the dose can often be decreased to 100 mcg (one spray in each nostril) daily.
  Inhalation for asthma: For those 12 and older: Starting dose is 88 mcg twice a day for patients who were previously treated with bronchodilators alone. Maximum daily dose is 440 mcg. Patients who required an inhaled corticosteroid previously are given 88 to 220 mcg a day. This dose is increased up to 440 mcg twice a day as needed and tolerated. Those taking a corticosteroid by mouth are given 880 mcg twice daily. Once the asthma is under control, the dose is reduced to the lowest effective dose.
  Fluticasone/salmeterol combination: The starting dose is 100 mcg fluticasone and 50 mcg of salmeterol in people who are not presently taking an inhaled steroid (corticosteroid). If they are taking an inhaled corticosteroid such as budesonide and the steroid dose is less than or equal to 400 mcg a day, then the combination inhaler containing 100 mcg of fluticasone

and 50 mcg of salmeterol is substituted and is taken twice a day. Other doses of budesonide or other corticosteroids require different combinations of fluticasone/salmeterol to get the best results.

Over 60 Years of Age: Same as 12 to 60 years of age.

Conditions Requiring Dosing Adjustments

Liver Function: This drug is extensively changed in the liver; however, no specific dosing changes are defined for patients with compromised livers.

Kidney Function: No changes in dosing are needed.

▷ **Dosing Instructions:** Follow the instructions on the patient instruction sheet closely as a limited amount of medicine reaches the lungs with the best inhaler technique. Your doctor should be called if the condition being treated worsens or does not improve. Once an inhalation treatment is completed, rinse your mouth with water. If you forget a dose: use the spray or inhaler as soon as you remember it, unless it's nearly time for your next dose—if this is the case, skip the missed dose and just take the next scheduled dose right on time. DO NOT double doses. This medicine is not used for sudden asthma episodes or status asthmaticus.

Usual Duration of Use: Continual use on a regular schedule for several days is usually necessary to determine this drug's effectiveness in treating seasonal and perennial allergic rhinitis. For the inhaled form, a beneficial response may happen in a day, but it may take two weeks to realize the maximum benefits. Long-term use (months to years) requires periodic evaluation of response and dose adjustment (to the minimum effective dose). Keep appointments with your doctor.

Typical Treatment Goals and Measurements (Outcomes and Markers)

Asthma: Frequency and severity of asthma attacks should ease. Some clinicians also use decreased frequency of rescue inhaler use as a further clinical indicator. It is critical that this medicine is used regularly to get the best results. An additional goal of therapy is to use the lowest effective dose. Some people keep their improvements when doses are lowered, while others relapse. Specific testing goals include improvement in PEFR, FEV1, and other lung (pulmonary) function tests. Wheezing and difficulty breathing (dyspnea) should ease as well as asthma caused (induced) by exercise. If the usual benefit is not realized, call your doctor.

Allergic rhinitis: Signs and symptoms of allergic rhinitis such as runny or stuffy nose, postnasal drip, and sneezing should ease. Scratch testing for a specific immune substance (IgE) can also be done to check progress at a cellular level.

Possible Advantages of This Drug

Once-a-day dosing for the nasal form, and small (roughly 2%) systemic absorption.

▷ **This Drug Should Not Be Taken If**

- you have had an allergic reaction to any dose form of it previously.
- you have sudden onset asthma or status asthmaticus. (Fluticasone or fluticasone/salmeterol WON'T WORK.)

▷ **Inform Your Physician Before Taking This Drug If**

- you are already taking systemic prednisone.
- you are exposed to measles or chicken pox.
- you are unsure how much to take or how often to take it.
- you take prescription or nonprescription medicines not discussed when fluticasone was prescribed.

- you have diabetes.
- you have signs or symptoms of an infection in your nose.
- your skin is shrunken (atrophied) or you have acne, warts, or other skin problems (topical form).
- you've had fungal infections, herpes simplex of the eye, tuberculosis, or other infections.
- you have damage from an accident or surgery to your nose while you are taking this medicine.
- your allergic rhinitis does not improve or worsens.
- you have unexplained joint pain such as knee, hip, or shoulder pain. While not reported for this particular corticosteroid, other medicines in the same family have caused osteonecrosis (aseptic necrosis or avascular necrosis) and caution is prudent.

Possible Side Effects (natural, expected, and unavoidable drug actions)
Irritation of the nose, nosebleeds. Systemic steroid effects—possible. Development of yeast infections of the mouth or throat.

▷ **Possible Adverse Effects** (unusual, unexpected, and infrequent reactions)
If any of the following develop, consult your physician promptly for guidance.
Mild Adverse Effects
Allergic reactions: contact dermatitis.
Nosebleeds or nasal burning—case reports to infrequent.
Dizziness or headache—rare to infrequent.
Unpleasant taste, nausea, or vomiting—rare.
Increased heart rate—case reports.
Serious Adverse Effects
Allergic reactions: anaphylaxis—case report.
Suppression of the hypothalamic pituitary adrenal (HPA) axis—rare (more likely with use in children).
Increased risk from viral infections—possible.
Increased pressure in the head (more likely in children)—possible.
Yeast infections of the nose—rare.
Blood vessel inflammation (vasculitis) including Churg-Strauss-like syndrome—case reports, but of questionable cause.
Loss of control of blood sugar—possible in diabetics and others.
Glaucoma or cataracts—case reports (inhaled form)—increased risk.
Cushing's syndrome (with excessive doses or very sensitive patients)—possible.
Growth suppression in children—possible.
Osteoporosis—increased risk with long-term use.

▷ **Possible Effects on Sexual Function:** None defined.

Possible Delayed Adverse Effects: Yeast infections of the nose—rare. Osteoporosis—increased risk.

▷ **Adverse Effects That May Mimic Natural Diseases or Disorders**
None defined.

Natural Diseases or Disorders That May Be Activated by This Drug
If systemic effects occur, the patient may be more susceptible to infections, or dormant infections may become active. This drug increases osteoporosis risk even in those not predisposed to developing osteoporosis.

Possible Effects on Laboratory Tests
Cortisol levels: decreased.
Eosinophils: increased in rare case reports.

CAUTION

1. Call your doctor if you are exposed to measles or chicken pox.
2. Long-term use requires periodic evaluation for yeast infection of the nose.
3. Call your doctor if your condition does not improve or worsens.
4. Children are in general at greater risk for adrenal gland suppression (HPA axis suppression) and are at greater risk for inadequate levels once therapy is withdrawn. Careful patient follow-up by a qualified specialist is needed.

Precautions for Use

By Infants and Children: Safety and effectiveness for use by those under 12 years of age have not been established for the intranasal form. Many adolescents can be started successfully with one spray in each nostril per day (100 mcg). Maximum total daily dose should not exceed 200 mcg. Children in general are at greater risk for suppression of the HPA axis and glucocorticosteroid insufficiency than adults.

By Those Over 60 Years of Age: No specific precautions.

▷ **Advisability of Use During Pregnancy**

Pregnancy Category: C. See Pregnancy Risk Categories at the back of this book.

Animal Studies: High-dose studies in rats revealed fetal toxicity consistent with changes caused by other steroids.

Human Studies: Information from adequate studies of pregnant women is not available.

Ask your doctor for guidance.

Advisability of Use If Breast-Feeding

Presence of this drug in breast milk: Unknown.

Monitor nursing infant closely and discontinue drug or nursing if adverse effects develop.

Habit-Forming Potential: Not defined.

Effects of Overdose: Not defined.

Possible Effects of Long-Term Use: Rare nasal yeast infections.

Suggested Periodic Examinations While Taking This Drug (at physician's discretion)

Nasal exams, check for osteoporosis (DEXA, PDEXA) with long-term use, periodic CBCs.

▷ **While Taking This Drug, Observe the Following**

Foods: No restrictions.

Herbal Medicines or Minerals: Fir or pine needle oil should NOT be used by asthmatics. Ephedra alone does carry a German Commission E monograph indication for asthma treatment. If you are allergic to plants in the Asteraceae family (aster, chrysanthemum, daisy, or ragweed), you may also be allergic to echinacea, chamomile, feverfew, and St. John's wort. Increased calcium and vitamin D are prudent while taking this medicine. Talk to your doctor BEFORE adding any herbals to this medicine.

Beverages: No restrictions.

▷ *Alcohol:* No interactions expected.

Tobacco Smoking: No interactions expected. I advise everyone to quit smoking.

▷ *Other Drugs*

Fluticasone *taken concurrently* with

- ketoconazole (Nizoral) and perhaps other azole antifungals may increase fluticasone blood levels.

- medicines that inhibit CYP 3A4 (such as ketoconazole) will lead to increased fluticasone effects and those that induce 3A4 will decrease fluticasone benefits.
- ritonavir (Norvir) may increase fluticasone blood levels and lead to Cushing's syndrome. A check of cortisol levels may help make the diagnosis.
- systemic steroids (such as prednisone) may increase the likelihood of suppression of the hypothalamic pituitary adrenal (HPA) axis.

▷ *Driving, Hazardous Activities:* This drug may cause dizziness. Restrict activities as necessary.

Aviation Note: The use of this drug ***may be a disqualification*** for piloting. Consult a designated Aviation Medical Examiner.

Exposure to Sun: No restrictions.

Discontinuation: This medicine should not be stopped abruptly. Talk with your doctor before stopping this drug.

FLUVASTATIN (flu va STAT in)

Introduced: 1994 **Class:** Cholesterol-reducing drug, HMG-CoA reductase inhibitor **Prescription:** USA: Yes **Controlled Drug:** USA: No; Canada: No **Available as Generic:** USA: No; Canada: No
Brand Names: Lescol, Lescol XL

BENEFITS versus RISKS	
Possible Benefits	*Possible Risks*
EFFECTIVE REDUCTION OF TOTAL BLOOD CHOLESTEROL	Increased liver enzymes
REDUCES TRIGLYCERIDES AND APOLIPOPROTEIN B	Muscle pain or weakness
SLOWS PROGRESSION OF CORONARY ATHEROSCLEROSIS	Decreased co-enzyme Q10
REDUCES THE RATE OF HEART ATTACK AND REVASCULARIZATION PROCEDURES IN PATIENTS WHO HAVE PERCUTANEOUS CORONARY INTERVENTION (PCI)	
Short presence in the body (systemic exposure)	
May decrease osteoporosis risk	
May decrease risk of Alzheimer's	
May decrease cancer risk	

▷ **Principal Uses**

As a Single Drug Product: Uses currently included in FDA-approved labeling: (1) Manages abnormally high cholesterol and triglycerides and apolipoprotein B in people with type 2 hypercholesterolemia; (2) slows progression of atherosclerosis in patients with coronary heart disease; (3) decreases risk of heart attack and/or repeat opening of blood vessels (revascularization procedures) in people who have PCI.

Other (unlabeled) generally accepted uses: (1) One case of blue toe syndrome was successfully reversed; (2) worked to lower LDL cholesterol in one study of Type II hyperlipoproteinemia; (3) may have a role in stroke prevention, or deep vein clot (thrombosis) prevention but further studies are needed; (4) like other HMG-CoA reductase inhibitors, may have a role in reducing risk of bone fractures; (5) decreases the number of coronary events in patients with coronary heart disease; (6) could have a role in decreasing risk of dementia; (7) may help decrease fracture risk/osteoporosis; (8) one case-controlled study found a 20% reduction in cancer risk by "statin-type" medicines. Further research is needed.

How This Drug Works: This medicine is changed (hydrolyzed) to a beta-hydroxy-acid form. The beta-hydroxy-acid inhibits HMG-CoA reductase. This enzyme is critical for cholesterol formation. Once inhibited, cholesterol formation slows. Since the amount of cholesterol is reduced in the liver, the VLDL fraction may also be decreased. There is a growing body of evidence that "statins" also have beneficial changes on what is in the blood, blood flow and even the blood vessel walls themselves. Specific compounds or effects of platelet-derived growth factor (PDGF), undesirable blood clotting via thrombin-antithrombin III, thrombomodulin, and other chemicals may be beneficially lowered or effects mitigated by statins.

▷ **Widely Used Guidelines That Involve This Medicine (representative sample):** Please look at the section at the very beginning of this profile called "Class." Next, turn to Table 22 and you will find guidelines listed by the class involved!

Available Dosage Forms and Strengths
Tablets — 10 mg, 20 mg, 40 mg
Tablets extended release — 80 mg

▷ **Recommended Dosage Ranges** (Actual dose and schedule must be determined for each patient individually.)
Infants and Children: Safety and efficacy for those less than 18 years of age have not been established.
18 to 60 Years of Age: **Hypercholesterolemia:** Dosing is started with 20 mg a day, taken with the evening meal or simply in the evening. This dose is increased as needed and tolerated to 80 mg with each evening (24 hours apart) meal. Any needed increases are made at intervals of 4 weeks. Patients who take immunosuppressant medicines are started on 10 mg of lovastatin daily and should not receive more than 20 mg daily with the evening meal. If 80 mg is required to achieve cholesterol and HDL goals, a single evening dose of 80 mg of the Lescol XL form can be taken.
Atherosclerosis: Dosing of 20 mg twice a day was used in a study called the Lipoprotein and Coronary Atherosclerosis Study (LCAS), and 40 mg twice a day in the Lescol Intervention Prevention Study (LIPS).
Over 60 Years of Age: Same as 18 to 60 years of age.

Conditions Requiring Dosing Adjustments
Liver Function: This drug is extensively changed in the liver. Lower doses appear prudent in liver disease.
Kidney Function: Patients with severe failure (creatinine clearance less than 30 mL/min) should be closely followed if given over 20 mg daily.

▷ **Dosing Instructions:** This medicine is best taken in the EVENING (such as with the evening MEAL), as it produces the best cholesterol-lowering results or outcomes. If you forget a dose: Take the next dose as soon as you remember it, unless it is nearly time for your next dose—then skip the dose you missed and just take the next scheduled dose. DO NOT double doses. If you find yourself omitting doses, call your doctor for some added ways to help remember your medicine.

Usual Duration of Use: Continual use on a regular schedule for 3 to 4 weeks may be needed to determine this drug's effectiveness in helping lower low-density lipoprotein (LDL) level. Long-term use may be needed to lead to beneficial effects on the pattern of HDL and LDL. Ongoing (months to years) use requires evaluation of response by your doctor. Know your cholesterol numbers and try to achieve NCEP goals. Take control of cholesterol for life!

Typical Treatment Goals and Measurements (Outcomes and Markers)

Cholesterol: Current guidelines (National Cholesterol Education Program or NCEP) acknowledge diabetes as one of the conditions that increases risk of heart disease, modifying risk factors, therapeutic lifestyle changes (TLC), and recommending routine testing for all of the cholesterol fractions (lipoprotein profile) versus total cholesterol alone. Goals are: a total cholesterol of 200 mg/dL, and optimal bad cholesterol (LDL) of less than 100 mg/dL. Less than 70 mg/dL (see Grundy, S.M. in Sources) is a reasonable optional goal for very high risk patients (such as diabetics with acute coronary syndromes, etc.). 130–159 mg/dL as borderline high, 160 mg/dL as high and 190 mg/dL as very high. Did you know that there are at least five different kinds of "good cholesterol" or HDL? The "too low" measure for HDL is still 40 mg/dL, but in order to learn more about cholesterol types some doctors are starting to order lipid panels. There are at least seven different kinds of "bad cholesterol." The new panels tell doctors about the kinds of cholesterol that your body makes. This is important because some kinds (small dense particles) tend to stick to blood vessels (are highly atherogenic). Take your medicine to reach your goals! Two additional tests you will hear about will be electron beam computed tomography (EBCT) and CRP. EBCT is an important tool used in conjunction with laboratory studies. Findings show that even patients who meet cholesterol goals (particularly females over 55) can still be at significant cardiovascular risk. EBCT then defines risk by giving a calcium score and a "virtual tour" of the coronary arteries. C Reactive Protein, or CRP, is a relatively new and apparently independent predictor of heart disease risk. A large study (see Ridker, P.M. in Sources) found that CRP predicted heart disease risk independently of bad cholesterol (low density lipoprotein). Talk to your doctor about this laboratory test and ask about current guidelines for who should be tested (see Pearson, T.A. in Sources).

Possible Advantages of This Drug

May give a more favorable time of medicine exposure than other medicines of the same family (clinical data are needed to show that this gives a decreased side effect profile). Clinical significance of the inability to cross the blood brain barrier and not being changed into active compounds (active metabolites) have not been clinically demonstrated.

▷ **This Drug Should Not Be Taken If**
- you had an allergic reaction to it previously.
- you have active liver disease or your liver enzymes become elevated (talk to your doctor).
- you are pregnant or breast-feeding your infant.

▷ **Inform Your Physician Before Taking This Drug If**
- you have previously taken any other drugs in this class: lovastatin (Mevacor), pravastatin (Pravachol).
- another doctor prescribes niacin, cyclosporine, erythromycin, or fibrate-type medicines.

- you have a history of liver disease or impaired liver function.
- you are not using birth control or you are planning pregnancy.
- you regularly consume substantial amounts of alcohol.
- you have cataracts or impaired vision.
- you have any type of chronic muscular disorder.
- you develop muscle pain, weakness, or soreness that is unexplained while taking this medicine.
- you plan to have major surgery in the near future.

Possible Side Effects (natural, expected, and unavoidable drug actions)
Development of abnormal liver function tests without associated symptoms. Decreased ubiquinone (co-Q10).

▷ **Possible Adverse Effects** (unusual, unexpected, and infrequent reactions)
If any of the following develop, consult your physician promptly for guidance.
Mild Adverse Effects
Allergic reactions: rash.
Headache, insomnia or dizziness—infrequent.
Indigestion, nausea, excessive gas, constipation, diarrhea—infrequent.
Lowering of the blood pressure—possible.
Serious Adverse Effects
Marked and persistent abnormal liver function tests with focal hepatitis (without jaundice)—case reports.
Acute myositis (muscle pain and tenderness)—occurred rarely during long-term use.
Rhabdomyolysis (simvastatin, atorvastatin, pravastatin, lovastatin, and fluvastatin from highest to lowest probability)—rare.
Sudden kidney failure—rare.
Vision changes—possible, case report.
Lichen planus skin rash—rare.
Neuropathy—case reports.
Systemic lupus erythematosus–like syndrome—case reports.

▷ **Possible Effects on Sexual Function:** None reported.

Possible Delayed Adverse Effects: Doses of 15 to 33 times the human dose of another drug in this class given to rats caused an increase in liver cancers.

Natural Diseases or Disorders That May Be Activated by This Drug
Latent liver disease.

Possible Effects on Laboratory Tests
Blood alanine aminotransferase (ALT) enzyme level: increased (with higher doses of drug).
Blood total cholesterol, LDL cholesterol and triglyceride levels: decreased.
Blood HDL cholesterol level: increased. Beneficial changes in pattern of HDL and LDL.

CAUTION
1. If pregnancy occurs while taking this drug, stop taking the drug immediately and call your doctor.
2. Promptly report any development of muscle pain or tenderness, especially if accompanied by fever or weakness (malaise).
3. Promptly report altered or impaired vision so that appropriate evaluation can be made.

Precautions for Use
By Infants and Children: Safety and effectiveness for those under 20 years of age are not established.

By Those Over 60 Years of Age: Tell your doctor about any personal or family history of vision problems. If periodic eye examinations are recommended, get them. Promptly report any vision changes.

▷ **Advisability of Use During Pregnancy**
Pregnancy Category: X. See Pregnancy Risk Categories at the back of this book.
Animal Studies: Mouse and rat studies reveal skeletal birth defects due to a closely related drug of this class.
Human Studies: Adequate studies of pregnant women are not available.
This drug should be avoided during entire pregnancy.

Advisability of Use If Breast-Feeding
Presence of this drug in breast milk: Unknown, but not thought to be safe. Avoid drug or refrain from nursing.

Habit-Forming Potential: None.

Effects of Overdose: Increased indigestion, stomach distress, nausea, diarrhea.

Possible Effects of Long-Term Use: Abnormal liver function with focal hepatitis. Abnormal liver function tests. Decreased co-enzyme Q10 (co-Q10 or ubiquinone). Loss of beneficial effects—reported with some statin-type medicines.

Suggested Periodic Examinations While Taking This Drug (at physician's discretion)
Blood cholesterol studies: total cholesterol, HDL and LDL fractions (usually every 4 weeks with dose changes). SLE test.
Liver function tests before treatment, 12 weeks after the medicine is started and 12 weeks after any increase in dose.
Complete eye examination at beginning of treatment and at any time that significant change in vision occurs. Ask your physician for guidance.
Electron beam computed tomography (EBCT) can help predict silent ischemia and other problems with blood vessels that supply the heart itself. This also may help define the results (outcomes) you are getting from this medicine.
Ubiquinone levels.

▷ **While Taking This Drug, Observe the Following**
Foods: Follow a standard low-cholesterol diet. Your doctor may also recommend some specific foods such as increased vegetables or functional foods such as Benecol. Three well-designed studies published in early April 2002 found that both in women and men and before and after a heart attack, people who ate more fish (2–4 servings a week) appeared to avoid heart disease. Additionally, putting supplements containing Omega 3 polyunsaturated fatty acids (PUFA) into the diet also appeared to protect against abnormal heart rhythms and sudden death from heart attack. The studies appeared in *JAMA, Circulation*, and the *New England Journal of Medicine*.
Herbal Medicines or Minerals: No data exist from well-designed clinical studies about garlic and fluvastatin combinations and cannot presently be recommended. Additionally, garlic may inhibit blood clotting (platelet) aggregation—something to consider if you are already taking a platelet inhibitor. Herbal medicines that can be toxic to the liver such as kava and valerian should be avoided. The FDA will allow one dietary supplement called Cholestin to be sold. Because this product actually contains lovastatin, and the use of two HMG-CoA inhibitors may increase risk of rhabdomyolysis or myopathy, the combination is NOT advised. Some products containing plant sterols (Benecol) may be useful as complementary care to

lower total and LDL cholesterol. Substituting soy for some of the meat in your diet can help avoid cardiovascular problems. Policosanol has data for lowering cholesterol. Talk to your doctor before starting any herbal medicine. Lastly, because this medicine can deplete co-Q10, supplementation may be needed.

Beverages: No restrictions. May be taken with milk.

▷ *Alcohol:* No interactions expected. Use sparingly.

Tobacco Smoking: No interactions expected. I advise everyone to quit smoking.

▷ *Other Drugs*

Fluvastatin may ***increase*** the effects of
- digoxin (Lanoxin).
- warfarin (Coumadin); more frequent testing of INR (prothrombin time) will be needed.

Fluvastatin ***taken concurrently*** with
- amprenavir (Agenerase) and ritonavir (Norvir) and perhaps other protease inhibitors may increase fluvastatin levels and the risk of muscle damage (myopathy).
- clofibrate (Atromid-S) or other fibrate compounds may result in increased risk of serious muscle toxicity.
- clopidogrel (Plavix) may result in increased fluvastatin levels (because of possible CYP 450 2C9 inhibition). Careful patient follow-up is prudent.
- cyclosporine (Sandimmune) can result in kidney failure and myopathy.
- erythromycin and perhaps other macrolide antibiotics (see Drug Classes) may increase risk of muscle damage (myopathy or rhabdomyolysis).
- fluconazole (Diflucan), itraconazole (Sporanox), or ketoconazole (Nizoral) increases myopathy or rhabdomyolysis risk.
- gemfibrozil (Lopid) may alter the absorption and excretion of fluvastatin; these drugs should not be taken concurrently.
- levothyroxine (various) may blunt the effects of levothyroxine.
- medicines that change cytochrome P450 3A4 (inhibitors will increase fluvastatin levels and inducers will blunt fluvastatin therapeutic effects).
- niacin may cause an increased frequency of muscle problems (myopathy) when combined with a related medicine (lovastatin). Caution is advised. Niacin may also increase homocysteine levels—a risk factor for heart disease.
- omeprazole (Prilosec) and possible esomeprazole (Nexium) may increase fluvastatin levels and lead to toxicity.
- quinupristin/dalfopristin (Synercid) may increase the risk for myopathy by increasing cerivastatin blood levels.
- ranitidine (Zantac) may increase peak blood levels of fluvastatin.
- ritonavir (Norvir) may lead to fluvastatin toxicity.
- sildenafil (Viagra) may change levels of either drug as they both use CYP3A4 to be removed from the body.

The following drug may ***decrease*** the effects of fluvastatin:
- cholestyramine (Questran), by possibly reducing absorption of fluvastatin; take fluvastatin 1 hour before or 4 hours after cholestyramine.

▷ *Driving, Hazardous Activities:* No restrictions.

Aviation Note: No restrictions.

Exposure to Sun: No restrictions.

Discontinuation: Do not stop this drug without your doctor's knowledge and help. There may be a significant increase in blood cholesterol levels if this medicine is stopped. Patients who have acute coronary syndromes, or ACS (such as unstable angina, heart attack [non-p, Q-wave myocardial infarction], and Q-wave myocardial infarction), were reviewed as part of the Platelet Receptor Inhibitor in Ischemic Syndrome Management (PRISM) study. It was found that pretreatment with statin-type medicines (HMG-CoA reductase inhibitors such as the medicine in this profile) significantly lowered risk during the first 30 days after ACS symptoms started. Talk with your doctor BEFORE stopping any statin-type medicine.

FLUVOXAMINE (FLU vox a meen)

Introduced: 1995 **Class:** Antidepressant, selective serotonin reuptake inhibitor **Prescription:** USA: Yes **Controlled Drug:** USA: No; Canada: No **Available as Generic:** USA: Yes; Canada: Yes

Brand Names: ✤Apo-Fluvoxamine, ✤Gen-Fluvoxamine, Luvox, ✤Novo-Fluvoxamine, ✤PMS-Fluvoxamine, ✤Riva-Fluvoxamine

Warning: Do not combine this medicine with terfenadine (Seldane) or astemizole (Hismanal). No longer on the U.S. market, but may still be in some foreign countries.

BENEFITS versus RISKS

Possible Benefits	*Possible Risks*
TREATMENT OF OBSESSIVE-COMPULSIVE DISORDER IN ADULTS	Nausea and vomiting (often resolve with time)
TREATMENT OF OBSESSIVE-COMPULSIVE DISORDER IN CHILDREN (over 8)	
Treatment of depression	
Treatment of panic disorder	
May have a role in helping to control binge eating	
May have a role in helping to treat social anxiety disorder	

▷ **Principal Uses**

As a Single Drug Product: Uses currently included in FDA-approved labeling: Treatment of obsessive-compulsive disorder in adults and children.

Other (unlabeled) generally accepted uses: (1) May have a role in helping compulsive exhibitionism; (2) treats depression; (3) may be useful in eating problems where binge behaviors are a key factor; (4) can help panic attacks; (5) helps prevent long-standing (chronic) tension headaches; (6) eases social anxiety disorder; (7) may help pathological gambling.

How This Drug Works: Inhibits reuptake of the neurotransmitter 5-HT, easing symptoms of treated behaviors or conditions.

▷ **Widely Used Guidelines That Involve This Medicine (representative sample):** Please look at the section at the very beginning of this profile called "Class." Next, turn to Table 22 and you will find guidelines listed by the class involved!

Available Dosage Forms and Strengths

Tablets—25 mg, 50 mg, 100 mg

▷ **Recommended Dosage Ranges** (Actual dose and schedule must be determined for each patient individually.)

Infants and Children: For children 8 years old or older with obsessive-compulsive disorder: Dosing is started with 25 mg at bedtime for 3 days. The dose is then increased by 25-mg steps every 3 to 4 days as needed and tolerated until a maximum of 200 mg is reached. If the required dose is larger than 75 mg, the total daily dose is divided into two equal doses and given twice daily.

18 to 60 Years of Age: Therapy is started with 50 mg taken at bedtime. The dose may then be increased as needed and tolerated by 50-mg intervals every 4 to 7 days to a maximum dose of 300 mg daily. The prescriber should remember that the drug may take from 4 to 14 days to begin to work. If patient needs a daily dose greater than 100 mg, dose is divided in half and taken twice daily.

Over 60 Years of Age: This medicine is removed half as slowly as in younger patients. Plasma concentrations are also roughly 40% higher than in younger patients. Slower time frames for any increases beyond the starting dose and lower maintenance doses are prudent.

Conditions Requiring Dosing Adjustments

Liver Function: This drug is extensively changed by the liver. If it is used by patients with liver disease, lower starting doses, slow dose increases, and careful patient monitoring are indicated.

Kidney Function: A lower starting dose and careful patient monitoring are needed.

▷ **Dosing Instructions:** Take this medicine exactly as prescribed and at the same time each time you take it. This medicine may be taken with or without food. Call your doctor if vomiting (a possible side effect) continues for more than 2 days after you start treatment. If you forget a dose: take the missed dose as soon as you remember it, unless it's nearly time for your next dose—if that is the case, skip the missed dose and take the next dose right on time. DO NOT double doses.

Usual Duration of Use: Continual use on a regular schedule for 4 to 14 days is usually necessary to determine effectiveness in helping obsessive-compulsive disorder. Long-term use (months to years) requires evaluation by your doctor.

Typical Treatment Goals and Measurements (Outcomes and Markers)

Obsessive-compulsive disorder: The general goal: to lessen the degree and severity of obsessions or compulsive behavior, letting patients return to their daily lives. Specific measures of this condition involve testing or inventories (such as the Yale-Brown Obsessive-Compulsive Scale, or Y-BOCS) and can be valuable in checking benefits from this medicine.

Possible Advantages of This Drug

Offers once-daily dosing and has a good side-effect profile.

▷ **This Drug Should Not Be Taken If**
- you had an allergic reaction to it previously.
- you are taking cisapride (Propulsid).

▷ **Inform Your Physician Before Taking This Drug If**
- you continue to have a problem with vomiting 2 days after starting this medicine.
- you feel light-headed when you get up from a sitting position.
- you have a history of seizures.

- you are unsure how much to take or how often to take it.
- you have taken an MAO inhibitor (see Drug Classes) within the last 14 days.
- you have a history of heart problems.
- you take prescription or nonprescription medicines not discussed when fluvoxamine was prescribed.

Possible Side Effects (natural, expected, and unavoidable drug actions)

Nausea and vomiting (usually stops after a few days of treatment). This may be avoided by slowly increasing the dose of this medicine. Dose-related orthostatic hypotension.

▷ **Possible Adverse Effects** (unusual, unexpected, and infrequent reactions)

If any of the following develop, consult your physician promptly for guidance.

Mild Adverse Effects

Allergic reaction: skin rash.

Somnolence, headache, agitation, sleep disorders—infrequent to frequent.

Change in heart waves (R-R, QT, and QTc intervals).

Bruising or nosebleeds—possible (may be stopped by 500 mg of vitamin C daily), usually resolves over time.

Liver toxicity—rare.

Patchy baldness (alopecia)—case report.

Dry mouth, anorexia, or constipation—possible to frequent.

Serious Adverse Effects

Allergic reactions: anaphylactic reaction—case reports.

Serious skin rash (toxic epidermal necrolysis [TEN] or Stevens-Johnson syndrome)—case reports.

Liver toxicity—rare.

Prolonged bleeding time, rectal bleeding, or nose bleeds—stopped by 500 mg of vitamin C daily in one case and usually resolves over time, but the medicine should be stopped if bleeding is significant and does not stop.

Seizures or mania—rare.

Parkinson-like reactions—case reports with SSRI-type medicines.

Tourette's syndrome—case reports.

Serotonin syndrome—case report.

Excessive urination (SIADH)—case reports.

▷ **Possible Effects on Sexual Function:** Delayed or absent orgasm, failure to ejaculate—case reports.

Impotence 2–8%. Galactorrhea—case reports with SSRIs.

Possible Delayed Adverse Effects: Not reported.

▷ **Adverse Effects That May Mimic Natural Diseases or Disorders**

Increased liver enzymes may mimic hepatitis.

Natural Diseases or Disorders That May Be Activated by This Drug

None defined.

Possible Effects on Laboratory Tests

Liver function tests: increased.

Melatonin level: increased.

CAUTION

1. This medicine has several important drug-drug interactions. Be certain to tell all health care professionals that you take this medicine.
2. If nausea and vomiting continue for more than 2 days after you start this medicine, call your doctor.

3. Pediatric and adult patients treated with this medicine should be closely watched for worsening depression or suicidal thinking. The FDA has required makers of antidepressants such as this one to alert health care professionals to the fact that children and adults with major depression may develop worsening depression or suicidal thoughts and behavior whether they take medicine for depression or do not take it. Patients should be carefully followed for such clinical worsening (particularly when treatment is started or doses are increased or decreased).

Precautions for Use
By Infants and Children: Safety and effectiveness for use by those under 18 years of age have not been established.

By Those Over 60 Years of Age: Lowering starting and maintenance doses is indicated.

▷ Advisability of Use During Pregnancy
Pregnancy Category: C. See Pregnancy Risk Categories at the back of this book.

Animal studies: Consistent with category C.

Human studies: Information from adequate studies of pregnant women is not available.

Ask your doctor for help.

Advisability of Use If Breast-Feeding
Presence of this drug in breast milk: Yes, in small amounts.

Monitor nursing infant closely and discontinue drug or nursing if adverse effects develop.

Habit-Forming Potential: None, but a withdrawal syndrome has been reported if the medicine is stopped abruptly (moderate to high occurrence rate).

Effects of Overdose: Nausea, vomiting, seizures.

Possible Effects of Long-Term Use: Not defined.

Suggested Periodic Examinations While Taking This Drug (at physician's discretion)

Liver function tests.

▷ While Taking This Drug, Observe the Following
Foods: No restrictions. Vitamin C (500 mg daily) may stop bruising that is possible with this medicine.

Herbal Medicines or Minerals: Since fluvoxamine and St. John's wort may both act to increase serotonin, the combination is not advised. Since part of the way ginseng and ginkgo work may be as MAO inhibitors, do not combine with fluvoxamine. Ma huang (no longer on the market as a weight loss agent) and yohimbe are also best avoided while taking this medicine. Valerian and kava kava (kava is no longer recommended in Canada) may interact additively (drowsiness). Avoid these combinations. Indian snake-root and dehydroepiandrosterone (DHEA) are also best avoided while taking this medicine. Since fluvoxamine can inhibit a compound that helps remove caffeine from your system, caution with caffeine-containing products such as guarana or mate is advised. Fluvoxamine may also inhibit melatonin removal. Talk to your doctor BEFORE combining any herbal medicine with this medicine.

Beverages: May inhibit an enzyme that removes caffeine—use caution.

▷ *Alcohol:* May worsen drowsiness. Ask your doctor for guidance.

Tobacco Smoking: Fluvoxamine stays in the body of smokers up to one-quarter less time than in nonsmokers, and fluvoxamine benefits may be blunted. I advise everyone to quit smoking.

Marijuana Smoking: Additive sleepiness and one case of mania with an SSRI.
▷ *Other Drugs*
Fluvoxamine ***taken concurrently*** with
- amitriptyline (Elavil, others) can result in amitriptyline toxicity.
- astemizole (Hismanal) may cause ***serious heart arrhythmias.*** DO NOT COMBINE.
- benzodiazepines (see Drug Classes) may result in benzodiazepine toxicity.
- beta blockers (see Drug Classes) may result in decreased drug clearance and toxicity.
- buspirone (Buspar) may lead to very slow heart rates in some patients. One later study found doubling of buspirone levels but no clinical effects. The combination is best avoided, but if deemed clinically necessary, clinical effects on the patient should be closely followed.
- carbamazepine (Tegretol) may cause toxicity. More frequent checks of drug levels needed.
- cimetidine (Tagamet) may lead to toxicity.
- cisapride (Propulsid) may cause heart toxicity. DO NOT COMBINE.
- clomipramine (Anafranil) may cause toxicity.
- clozapine (Clozaril) can result in higher clozapine levels and toxicity.
- cyclosporine (Sandimmune, others) may increase cyclosporine levels.
- dextromethorphan may cause hallucinations (reported with similar medicines).
- diltiazem (Cardizem) may cause diltiazem toxicity.
- dofetilide (Tikosyn) may lead to dofetilide toxicity via inhibition of CYP 3A4 inhibition.
- ergot derivative (such as Cafergot) may lead to toxicity. DO NOT COMBINE.
- imipramine (Tofranil, others) may result in imipramine toxicity.
- lithium (Lithobid) can cause serotonin syndrome.
- MAO inhibitors (see Drug Classes) can cause toxicity. DO NOT COMBINE.
- maprotiline can cause maprotiline toxicity.
- methadone may result in increased opioid effects.
- monoamine oxidase inhibitors (see Drug Classes) may lead to central nervous system toxicity or frank serotonin syndrome.
- olanzapine (Zyprexa) may lead to olanzapine toxicity via inhibition of CYP 1A2.
- oral antidiabetic drugs (see Drug Classes) may remain in the body longer than expected, requiring a dose decrease. This has not been reported with fluvoxamine, but has been reported with sertraline, a medicine in the same pharmacological family.
- phenytoin (Dilantin) or fosphenytoin (Cerebyx) may lead to toxicity. Patients should be watched closely for problems walking (ataxia) or drowsiness (early toxicity signs), and their doctor notified at once if these occur.
- ritonavir (Norvir) and perhaps other protease inhibitors may lead to toxicity.
- sibutramine (Meridia) may lead to serotonin syndrome.
- sumatriptan (Imitrex), naratriptan, almotriptan, zolmitriptan, and any other triptan-type medicines may lead to weakness and confusion—caution is required.
- tacrine (Cognex) may lead to tacrine toxicity.
- terfenadine (Seldane) may cause ***serious heart arrhythmias***. DO NOT COMBINE.

- theophylline may result in theophylline toxicity.
- tramadol (Ultram) may increase seizure risk. DO NOT COMBINE.
- tricyclic antidepressants (imipramine, others) may lead to tricyclic toxicity.
- triptans, such as naratriptan (Amerge), rizatriptan (Maxalt), sumatriptan (Imitrex), or zolmitriptan (Zomig), may lead to weakness and incoordination.
- tryptophan may increase serotonin effects of fluvoxamine and cause severe vomiting.
- warfarin (Coumadin) can result in increased warfarin concentrations and may lead to bleeding; more frequent INR testing is needed.

▷ *Driving, Hazardous Activities:* This drug may cause drowsiness. Restrict activities as necessary.

Aviation Note: The use of this drug *is probably a disqualification* for piloting. Consult a designated Aviation Medical Examiner.

Exposure to Sun: No restrictions.

Discontinuation: A withdrawal syndrome has been reported if this medicine is abruptly stopped. The doses should be slowly tapered.

FORMOTEROL (for MOT er all)

Introduced: 2001   **Class:** Bronchodilator   **Prescription:** USA: Yes   **Controlled Drug:** USA: No; Canada: Not available in Canada   **Available as Generic:** USA: No

Brand Name: Foradil Aerolizer

Author's Note: Information in this profile will be broadened in subsequent editions if evolving patient benefit and research data warrant.

FOSINOPRIL (FOH sin oh pril)

Introduced: 1986   **Class:** Antihypertensive, ACE inhibitor
Please see the angiotensin converting enzyme (ACE) inhibitor family profile.

FUROSEMIDE (fur OH se mide)

Introduced: 1964   **Class:** Antihypertensive, diuretic   **Prescription:** USA: Yes   **Controlled Drug:** USA: No; Canada: No   **Available as Generic:** USA: Yes; Canada: Yes

Brand Names: ✽Albert Furosemide, ✽Apo-Furosemide, Fumide MD, Furocot, Furomide MD, Furose, Furosemide-10, ✽Furoside, Lasaject, Lasimide, Lasix, ✽Lasix Special, Lo-Aqua, Luramide, Myrosemide, Novo-Semide, Ro-Semide, SK-Furosemide, ✽Uritol

```
┌─────────────────────────────────────────────────────────────────┐
│                      BENEFITS versus RISKS                        │
│        Possible Benefits                  Possible Risks          │
│  PROMPT, EFFECTIVE, RELIABLE       WATER AND ELECTROLYTE          │
│    DIURETIC                          DEPLETION with excessive use  │
│  MODEST ANTIHYPERTENSIVE IN        Excessive potassium and magnesium│
│    MILD TO MODERATE                  loss                         │
│    HYPERTENSION                    Increased blood sugar level     │
│  ENHANCES EFFECTIVENESS OF         Decreased blood calcium level   │
│    OTHER ANTIHYPERTENSIVES         Liver damage                   │
│                                    Blood cell disorder            │
└─────────────────────────────────────────────────────────────────┘
```

▷ **Principal Uses**

   As a Single Drug Product: Uses currently included in FDA-approved labeling: (1) Increases urine and removes excessive water (edema), as in congestive heart failure or some forms of liver, lung, and kidney disease; (2) lowers high blood pressure, usually with other drugs.

   Other (unlabeled) generally accepted uses: (1) Inhaled furosemide may help protect the lungs in people with asthma; (2) can have a role in helping infants with lung problems (chronic bronchopulmonary dysplasia); (3) one study found furosemide beneficial in helping lung mechanics of infants after heart surgery; (4) aborted migraine aura in a small number of case reports.

In the Pipeline: The Health and Human Services secretary has identified a group of medicines to be tested for use in children. Furosemide was on that list of the 12 highest priority medicines to be studied in children.

How This Drug Works: By increasing the elimination of salt and water through increased urine production, this drug reduces fluid in the blood and body tissues. These changes also contribute to lowering blood pressure.

▷ **Widely Used Guidelines That Involve This Medicine (representative sample):** Please look at the section at the very beginning of this profile called "Class." Next, turn to Table 22 and you will find guidelines listed by the class involved!

Available Dosage Forms and Strengths
   Injection — 10 mg/mL
   Solution — 10 mg/mL
   Tablets — 20 mg, 40 mg, 80 mg

▷ **Usual Adult Dosage Ranges:** *As antihypertensive:* 40 mg every 12 hours initially. Doses have historically been increased as needed and tolerated. If the response does not meet therapeutic goals, other blood pressure medicines should be added, rather than going above 80 mg a day. *As "water pill" (diuretic):* 20 to 80 mg in a single dose initially; if necessary, increase the dose by 20 to 40 mg every 6 to 8 hours. The smallest effective dose should be used. Daily maximum is 600 mg in treating severe edematous states—but the usual ongoing dose is 40–120 mg a day. Edema removal is often effectively accomplished using intermittent dosing schedules, such as use of furosemide 2 to 4 days in a row each week.

   Note: Actual dose and schedule must be determined for each patient individually.

Conditions Requiring Dosing Adjustments
  Liver Function: Larger doses may be needed for patients with liver compromise, and extreme care must be used to maintain critical electrolytes.
  Kidney Function: Larger initial doses may be needed before any benefit is seen. Drug may cause kidney stones and protein in urine.
  Cystic Fibrosis: Patients with this disease may be more sensitive to the drug, and smaller starting doses are indicated.

▷ **Dosing Instructions:** The tablet may be crushed and taken with or following meals to reduce stomach irritation. Best taken in the morning to avoid nighttime urination. Be certain to measure the oral liquid with a measuring spoon. If you forget a dose: take the missed dose as soon as you remember it, unless it's nearly time for your next dose—if that is the case, skip the missed dose and take the next dose right on time. DO NOT double doses. Call your doctor if you find yourself having problems remembering to use this medicine.

Usual Duration of Use: Use on a regular schedule for 2 to 3 weeks may be required to see effectiveness in lowering high blood pressure. Long-term use (months to years) requires periodic physician evaluation of response. Some cases of mild hypertension may remain normal after therapy with furosemide, lowering blood pressure to goals and allowing gradual furosemide withdrawal.

Typical Treatment Goals and Measurements (Outcomes and Markers)
  Blood Pressure: Guidelines (JNC VII) define normal blood pressure (BP) as **less than** 120/80 and **pre-hypertension** as 120/80 to 139/89. This new range is intended to help doctors encourage lifestyle changes (or in the case of people with a risk factor for high blood pressure, start treatment) much earlier—so that damage to blood vessels, your heart, kidneys, sexual potency, or eyes might be minimized or avoided altogether. Stage 1 hypertension is 140/90 to 159/99 and stage 2 hypertension equal to or greater than: 160/100 mm Hg. These guidelines also recommend that clinicians work with their patients to agree on the goals and a plan of treatment. The first-ever guidelines for blood pressure (hypertension) in African Americans recommends that MOST black patients be started on TWO antihypertensive medicines with the goal of lowering blood pressure to 130/80 for those with high risk for heart and blood vessel disease or with diabetes. The American Diabetes Association also recommends 130/80 as the target for diabetics and less than 125/75 for those who spill more than one gram of protein into their urine. Most clinicians try to achieve a BP that confers the best balance of lower cardiovascular risk and avoids the problem of too low a blood pressure. Blood pressure duration is generally increased with beneficial restriction of sodium. If goals are not met, it is not unusual to intensify doses or add on medicines.
  Congestive heart failure: Used to remove excessive fluid that builds up in the body. Typical treatment markers include resolution of ankle swelling and increased output of fluid (diuresis) as well as improved ease of breathing. Successful withdrawal of furosemide is possible in many elderly heart failure patients.

▷ **This Drug Should Not Be Taken If**
  • you had an allergic reaction to it previously.
  • you have extremely low potassium or sodium.
  • your kidneys are not making urine.

- you have severe fluid depletion (hypovolemia) with or without excessively low blood pressure.
- you are in a coma caused by liver failure.

▷ **Inform Your Physician Before Taking This Drug If**
  - you are allergic to any form of sulfa drug.
  - you are pregnant or planning pregnancy.
  - you have a history of kidney or liver disease.
  - you have diabetes, gout, or lupus erythematosus.
  - you have impaired hearing.
  - you have low blood potassium or other electrolytes (talk with your doctor).
  - you take cortisone, digitalis, oral antidiabetic drugs, or insulin.
  - you will have surgery with general anesthesia.

Possible Side Effects (natural, expected, and unavoidable drug actions)
  Light-headedness on rising from sitting or lying position (see orthostatic hypotension in Glossary).
  Increase in blood sugar level, affecting control of diabetes.
  Increase in blood uric acid level, affecting control of gout.
  Increased cholesterol (may be related to intravascular volume).
  Decrease in blood potassium level, causing muscle weakness and cramping.
  Decreased magnesium level.

▷ **Possible Adverse Effects** (unusual, unexpected, and infrequent reactions)
  If any of the following develop, consult your physician promptly for guidance.
  Mild Adverse Effects
  Allergic reactions: skin rashes, hives, drug fever—case reports.
  Headache, dizziness, blurred or yellow vision, ringing in ears, numbness, and tingling—rare to infrequent.
  Reduced appetite, indigestion, nausea, vomiting, diarrhea—possible.
  Metabolic alkalosis—possible.
  Serious Adverse Effects
  Allergic reactions: hepatitis with jaundice (see Glossary), anaphylactic reaction (see Glossary), severe skin reactions—case reports.
  Idiosyncratic reaction: fluid in lungs—case reports.
  Temporary hearing loss—case reports.
  Inflammation of the pancreas (severe abdominal pain)—rare.
  Bone marrow depression (see Glossary): fatigue, weakness, fever, sore throat, abnormal bleeding or bruising—case reports.
  Low blood pressure on standing or abnormal heartbeats (arrhythmias)—rare.
  Drug-induced porphyria or excessive parathyroid gland action (hyperparathyroidism)—case reports.
  Low blood potassium or magnesium—possible.
  Vitamin deficiency (thiamine)—possible.
  Kidney stones (calcium-containing)—case reports.
  Liver toxicity (cholestatic jaundice)—rare.
  Fever in infants—case reports.
  Skin lesions (erythema multiforme or Stevens-Johnson syndrome)—case reports.
  Hip fractures (may increase risk).

▷ **Possible Effects on Sexual Function:** Impotence—infrequent.

▷ **Adverse Effects That May Mimic Natural Diseases or Disorders**
Liver reaction may suggest viral hepatitis.

Natural Diseases or Disorders That May Be Activated by This Drug
Diabetes, gout, systemic lupus erythematosus.

Possible Effects on Laboratory Tests
Complete blood counts: reduced red cells, hemoglobin, white cells, and platelets.
Blood amylase and lipase levels: increased (possible pancreatitis).
Blood sodium and chloride levels: decreased.
Blood levels of total cholesterol, LDL and VLDL cholesterol, and triglycerides: increased.
Blood glucose level: increased.
Glucose tolerance test (GTT): decreased tolerance.
Blood potassium or magnesium level: decreased.
Blood thyroid hormone (T3 and T4) levels: decreased.
Blood uric acid level or blood urea nitrogen (BUN): increased.
Urine sugar tests: no drug effect (Tes-Tape); false low (Clinistix, Diastix).

CAUTION
1. Take exactly the prescribed dose. Increased doses can cause serious loss of sodium and potassium, with resultant loss of appetite, nausea, fatigue, weakness, confusion, and tingling in the extremities.
2. If you take a digitalis preparation (digitoxin, digoxin), ensure an adequate intake of high potassium foods to prevent potassium deficiency. (See Table 13, High Potassium Foods, Section Six.) Magnesium is also important.
3. Intravenous furosemide should be replaced with oral dosing as soon as possible.

Precautions for Use
By Infants and Children: Significant potassium loss can occur within the first 2 weeks of drug use.
By Those Over 60 Years of Age: Small starting doses are critical. Increased risk of impaired thinking, orthostatic hypotension, potassium loss, and blood sugar increase. Overdose and extended use of this drug can cause excessive loss of body water, thickening (increased viscosity) of the blood, and an increased tendency for the blood to clot, predisposing to stroke, heart attack, or thrombophlebitis (vein inflammation with blood clot).

▷ **Advisability of Use During Pregnancy**
Pregnancy Category: C. See Pregnancy Risk Categories at the back of this book.
Animal Studies: Significant birth defects have been reported.
Human Studies: Adequate studies of pregnant women are not available.
It should not be used during pregnancy unless a very serious complication occurs for which this drug is significantly beneficial. Avoid completely during the first 3 months. Ask your physician for guidance.

Advisability of Use If Breast-Feeding
Presence of this drug in breast milk: Yes.
Avoid drug or refrain from nursing.

Habit-Forming Potential: None.

Effects of Overdose: Dry mouth, thirst, lethargy, weakness, muscle cramping, nausea, vomiting, drowsiness progressing to stupor or coma.

Possible Effects of Long-Term Use: Impaired water, salt, magnesium, and potassium balance; dehydration and increased blood coagulability, with risk of blood clots.

Development of glucose intolerance or hyperglycemia in predisposed individuals.

Suggested Periodic Examinations While Taking This Drug (at physician's discretion)

Complete blood counts.

Measurements of blood levels of sodium, potassium, magnesium, chloride, sugar, and uric acid.

Kidney and liver function tests.

▷ **While Taking This Drug, Observe the Following**

Foods: Ask your doctor if it would benefit you to eat foods rich in potassium. If so advised, see Table 13, High Potassium Foods, Section Six. Follow your physician's advice regarding the use of salt. Food decreases absorption of furosemide by up to 30%. Take this medicine 1 hour before or 2 hours after a meal.

Herbal Medicines or Minerals: Ginseng, guarana, bitter orange (avoid), country mallow (avoid), eleuthero root (avoid), hawthorn, saw palmetto, ma huang (avoid), goldenseal, and licorice may also cause increased blood pressure. Couch grass may worsen edema due to heart or kidney problems. Indian snakeroot, calcium, and garlic may help lower blood pressure. CAUTION: St. John's wort may also lead to photosensitivity. Yohimbe may blunt the blood pressure–lowering benefits of this medicine. Magnesium levels should be checked and magnesium replaced if needed. Talk to your doctor BEFORE adding any herbal medicines or minerals.

Beverages: No restrictions. This drug may be taken with milk.

▷ *Alcohol:* Use with caution—alcohol may exaggerate the blood pressure–lowering effects of this drug and cause orthostatic hypotension.

Tobacco Smoking: No interactions expected. I advise everyone to quit smoking.

▷ *Other Drugs*

Furosemide may **increase** the effects of

- other antihypertensive drugs; dose adjustments may be necessary to prevent excessive lowering of blood pressure.
- digoxin (Lanoxin) and result in digoxin toxicity.
- lithium (Lithobid, others) and cause lithium toxicity.

Furosemide may ***decrease*** the effects of

- oral antidiabetic drugs (sulfonylureas); dose adjustments may be necessary for proper control of blood sugar.

Furosemide ***taken concurrently with***

- activated charcoal (various) will blunt absorption of oral furosemide.
- adrenocortical steroids (see Drug Classes) may cause additive loss of potassium.
- amikacin, gentamicin, tobramycin, or other aminoglycosides may increase risk of hearing toxicity (ototoxicity).
- bepridil (Vascor) may lead to abnormal heart effects if potassium is low.
- cephalosporin antibiotics (see Drug Classes) may increase risk of kidney problems (nephrotoxicity).
- cholestyramine (Questran) may cause loss of furosemide effectiveness.
- clofibrate (Atromid-S) may lead to muscle stiffness and increased diuretic effects.

- colestipol (Colestid) may cause loss of furosemide effectiveness.
- cortisone (various corticosteroids) may lead to excessive potassium loss.
- cyclosporine (Sandimmune) may cause elevated uric acid levels (hyperuricemia) and gout.
- digitalis preparations (digitoxin, digoxin) require blood tests or dose changes to maintain potassium levels and avoid heart rhythm problems.
- lomefloxacin (Maxaquin) may increase lomefloxacin levels and lead to toxicity.
- metformin (Glucophage) may increase metformin and decrease furosemide effects.
- NSAIDs (see Drug Classes) may cause loss of diuretic effectiveness.
- phenytoin (Dilantin) or fosphenytoin (Cerebyx) may decrease furosemide diuretic effects.

▷ *Driving, Hazardous Activities:* Use caution until the possible occurrence of orthostatic hypotension, dizziness, or impaired vision has been determined.

Aviation Note: The use of this drug *may be a disqualification* for piloting. Consult a designated Aviation Medical Examiner.

Exposure to Sun: Use caution—this drug may cause photosensitivity (see Glossary). See Herbal Medicines warning on St. John's wort above.

Exposure to Heat: Avoid excessive perspiring, which could cause additional loss of salt and water from the body.

Heavy Exercise or Exertion: Avoid exertion that produces light-headedness, excessive fatigue, or muscle cramping. Ask your doctor for help about participation in exercise.

Occurrence of Unrelated Illness: Vomiting or diarrhea can produce a serious imbalance of important body chemistry. Ask your doctor for guidance.

Discontinuation: It may be best to discontinue this drug 5 to 7 days before major surgery. Ask your physician, surgeon, and/or anesthesiologist for guidance regarding dose adjustment or drug withdrawal.

GABAPENTIN (GAB ah pen tin)

Introduced: 1981 **Class:** Anticonvulsant, pain syndrome modifier, mood stabilizer **Prescription:** USA: Yes **Controlled Drug:** USA: No; Canada: No **Available as Generic:** USA: No; Canada: No

Brand Name: Neurontin

BENEFITS versus RISKS	
Possible Benefits	*Possible Risks*
ADJUNCTIVE THERAPY OF PARTIAL SEIZURES	Sleepiness
EFFECTIVE TREATMENT OF A VARIETY OF PAIN SYNDROMES	Movement problems
PREVENTION OF MIGRAINES	
MAY HAVE A ROLE AS A MOOD STABILIZER/ANXIOLYTIC	
May have a role in reducing symptoms of social phobia	

▷ **Principal Uses**
  As a Single Drug Product: Uses currently included in FDA-approved labeling:
    (1) As an antiepileptic drug adjunctive to other medicines to control partial
    seizures; (2) treats postherpetic neuralgia pain in adults.
  Other (unlabeled) generally accepted uses: (1) widely used in chronic pain
    syndromes, such as diabetic nerve damage (diabetic neuropathy); (2) may
    have a role in spasticity; (3) possible role in combination treatment of
    resistant bipolar disorder; (4) low-dose gabapentin eased spasms seen in
    multiple sclerosis in one study; (5) a small study found that gabapentin
    reduced symptoms of social phobia; (6) may be of help in essential tremor;
    (7) helps prevent migraines; (8) case reports of gabapentin easing difficult-
    to-treat hot flashes in prostate cancer cases; (9) one report of gabapentin
    easing nicotine addiction.
  How This Drug Works: Similar in chemistry to an inhibitory substance called
    gamma-aminobutyric acid (GABA). Gabapentin appears to increase GABA
    levels in the brain. Works in preventing migraines by stabilizing actions of
    the nerves.
▷ **Widely Used Guidelines That Involve This Medicine (representative sam-
    ple):** Please look at the section at the very beginning of this profile called
    "Class." Next, turn to Table 22 and you will find guidelines listed by the
    class involved!
  Available Dosage Forms and Strengths
        Capsules — 100 mg, 300 mg, 400 mg
        Oral solution — 250 mg/5 mL
        Tablets — 100 mg, 300 mg, 400 mg, 600 mg; 800 mg
▷ **Usual Adult Dosage Ranges**
  Seizures: Initially 300 mg 3 times a day. Dose may be increased to 900 mg a day
    by the third day. Doses up to 2,400 mg have been well tolerated and 3,600
    mg used in some patients.
  Pain syndromes: 100 mg a day, increased as needed and tolerated. Maximum
    doses are as those seen in seizure patients.
  Postherpetic neuralgia: 300 mg on the first day followed by 300 mg twice a day
    on the second day and 300 mg 3 times daily on the third day. Further dos-
    ing is adjusted as needed and tolerated up to 600 mg 3 times a day.
  **Note: Actual dose and schedule must be determined for each patient
    individually.**
  Conditions Requiring Dosing Adjustments
  Liver Function: Not changed by the liver. No dosing changes needed.
  Kidney Function: 300 mg twice daily is given to those with a creatinine clear-
    ance of 30–60 mL/min. For creatinine clearance of 15–30 mL/min, 300 mg
    is given daily.
▷ **Dosing Instructions:** May be taken with or after food to reduce stomach irrita-
    tion. Capsule may be opened, and the tablet may be crushed. The liquid
    should be measured with a measuring spoon or measuring dose cup. If
    you forget a dose: take the missed dose as soon as you remember it, unless
    it's nearly time for your next dose—if that is the case, skip the missed dose
    and take the next dose right on time. DO NOT double doses. Call your doc-
    tor if you find yourself having problems remembering this medicine or if
    you miss two doses.
  Usual Duration of Use: Use on a regular schedule for 2 to 3 weeks usually deter-
    mines benefit in reducing frequency and severity of seizures. Optimal

control will require careful dose adjustments. Use in pain syndromes may take a similar time. Long-term use requires ongoing physician supervision.

Typical Treatment Goals and Measurements (Outcomes and Markers)

Pain: Most clinicians treating pain use a device called an algometer, which looks like a small ruler, but lets the clinician better understand your pain. The goals of treatment then relate to where the level of pain started (for example, a rating of 7 on a 0 to 10 scale) and what the cause of the pain was. Pain medicines may also be used together (in combination) in order to get the best result or outcome. I use the PQRSTG method. If your pain control is not acceptable to YOU, be sure to call your doctor as you may need a different medicine or combination.

▷ **This Drug Should Not Be Taken If**
- you have pancreatitis.
- you have had an allergic reaction to this drug.

▷ **Inform Your Physician Before Taking This Drug If**
- you are taking any other drugs at this time.
- you have a history of kidney disease or impaired kidney function.
- you are less than 12 years old (not studied).
- you have low blood pressure.

Possible Side Effects (natural, expected, and unavoidable drug actions)

Mild fatigue, sluggishness, drowsiness, dizziness—may be frequent.

▷ **Possible Adverse Effects** (unusual, unexpected, and infrequent reactions)

If any of the following develop, consult your physician promptly for guidance.

Mild Adverse Effects

Allergic reactions: skin rashes, hives—possible.

Acne—occasional.

Weight gain or loss—infrequent.

Accumulation of fluid in the ankles (edema)—infrequent.

Nausea, vomiting, constipation—infrequent.

Vision changes—infrequent.

Slurred speech—possible and more likely during the first three days after the medicine is started.

Purpura—may be frequent.

Lowering or increasing of blood pressure—infrequent.

Bed-wetting—case reports, mild and resolved with ongoing therapy.

Serious Adverse Effects

Allergic reactions: severe skin rash (Stevens-Johnson syndrome)—case reports.

Idiosyncratic reactions: none reported.

Seizures or paresthesia—case reports.

Disturbed mood (hostility, mania, labile emotions, and/or depression)—reported (case report for mania).

Amnesia—case reports.

Movement disorders (ataxia)—possible (case reports) and more likely in the first three days after starting therapy—careful follow-up for cogging is important.

Lowered white blood cell counts—rare.

Pancreatitis—case report.

▷ **Possible Effects on Sexual Function:** Impotence—rare. Swelling and tenderness of male breast tissue (gynecomastia) reported.

▷ **Adverse Effects That May Mimic Natural Diseases or Disorders**
Drug-induced hepatitis may suggest viral hepatitis.
Skin reactions may resemble lupus erythematosus.

Natural Diseases or Disorders That May Be Activated by This Drug
Partial seizures.

Possible Effects on Laboratory Tests
Complete blood cell counts: decreased white cells—rare.

CAUTION
1. When used for the treatment of epilepsy, **this drug must not be stopped abruptly.**
2. Taking this medicine exactly as prescribed is essential. Take this drug at the same time each day to help keep the blood level about the same.
3. Carry a personal identification card noting that you are taking this drug.

Precautions for Use
By Infants and Children: Not indicated unless 3 or older. Patients 3–12 for adjunctive partial seizure treatment are given 10–15 mg/kg of body weight per day. The total dose is divided into 3 equal doses and given 3 times a day.
By Those Over 60 Years of Age: You may be more sensitive to all of the actions of this drug and require smaller doses. Some clinicians start with 100 mg at bedtime and slowly increase the dose as needed and tolerated. Watch closely for any adverse effects: drowsiness, fatigue, confusion, "cogging" of arms, vision changes.

▷ **Advisability of Use During Pregnancy**
Pregnancy Category: C. See Pregnancy Risk Categories at the back of this book.
Human Studies: Information from adequate studies of pregnant women is not available. Discuss use of this drug during pregnancy with your doctor.

Advisability of Use If Breast-Feeding
Presence of this drug in breast milk: Unknown.
Monitor nursing infant closely and discontinue drug or nursing if adverse effects develop.

Habit-Forming Potential: None.

Effects of Overdose: Drowsiness, slurred speech, double vision, and diarrhea.

Possible Effects of Long-Term Use: None defined.

Suggested Periodic Examinations While Taking This Drug (at physician's discretion)
Checks of seizure control. Check for "cogging" of arms. For pain assessment, I use the PQRSTG method.

▷ **While Taking This Drug, Observe the Following**
Foods: No restrictions.
Herbal Medicines or Minerals: Ma huang and guarana may cause increased blood pressure and excessive sympathetic stimulation. Ginseng, eleuthero root, hawthorn, saw palmetto, goldenseal, and licorice may also cause increased blood pressure. Evening primrose oil may increase risk of seizures and should be avoided. Some forms of ginkgo have been found to contain a contaminant that is actually a neurotoxin (4'-O-methylpyridoxine). Prudent to avoid ginkgo unless each lot of the product can be checked for this contaminant.
Nutritional Support: None required.
Beverages: No restrictions. May be taken with milk.

▷ *Alcohol:* Use extreme caution. Alcohol (in large quantities or with continual use) may reduce effectiveness in preventing seizures.

Tobacco Smoking: No interactions expected. I advise everyone to quit smoking.

▷ *Other Drugs*

Gabapentin *taken concurrently* with
- antacids (various) may lower beneficial effects.
- cimetidine (Tagamet) may increase blood levels of gabapentin.
- morphine (various) may increase CNS side effects and increase gabapentin concentrations. Doses of either or both medicines should be lowered.
- naproxen (Anaprox, others) may increase gabapentin levels slightly.
- phenytoin (Dilantin) or fosphenytoin (Cerebyx) may lead to phenytoin or fosphenytoin toxicity.
- tramadol (Ultram) may increase seizure risk if gabapentin is being used to treat seizures.

▷ *Driving, Hazardous Activities:* This drug may impair mental alertness, vision, and coordination. Restrict activities as necessary.

Aviation Note: The use of this drug *is a disqualification* for piloting. Consult a designated Aviation Medical Examiner.

Exposure to Sun: No restrictions at present.

Discontinuation: **This drug must not be discontinued abruptly.** Sudden withdrawal can precipitate severe and repeated seizures. If this drug is to be discontinued, gradual reduction in dose should be made. Discuss this with your doctor.

GALANTAMINE (ga LAN tah meen)

Author's Note: please see the Anti-Alzheimer's Drug Family combination profile for further information.

GANCICLOVIR (gan SIGH klo veer)

Introduced: 1995 (tablet)   **Class:**   Antiviral   **Prescription:**
USA: Yes   **Controlled Drug:**   USA: No; Canada: No   **Available as**
Generic: USA: No; Canada: No
Brand Names: Cytovene, Vitrasert

Warning: The oral form of this medicine should be used only by patients who are not candidates for intravenous dosing and for whom the risk of more rapid cytomegalovirus (CMV) retinitis progression is outweighed by the benefit of avoiding the intravenous route.

BENEFITS versus RISKS	
Possible Benefits	*Possible Risks*
Oral, intravenous, or implanted treatment of cytomegalovirus (CMV) retinitis	More rapid progression of CMV disease (capsules)
	Bone marrow suppression
Decreased side effects with the oral form	Reproductive toxicity (see "Infants and Children" section)
Transition to an oral form following intravenous induction	Possible increased cancer risk (see "Infants and Children" section)

▷ **Principal Uses**

As a Single Drug Product: Uses currently included in FDA-approved labeling: (1) Treatment of cytomegalovirus (CMV) retinitis; (2) prevention of CMV retinitis in a variety of patients such as liver, kidney, lung, bone marrow, and heart transplant patients; (3) implantation of the ocular implant into the diseased area—this form may work for 5 months or more; (4) prevention of CMV disease in patients with advanced HIV infection.

Other (unlabeled) generally accepted uses: (1) Treatment of pediatric CMV; (2) may have a role in treating Epstein-Barr virus infection; (3) can have a role in treating leukoplakia; (4) may help outer retinal necrosis; (5) could have a role in some acyclovir-resistant herpes simplex and varicella zoster virus.

How This Drug Works: Changed to an active (triphosphate) form in infected cells. The active form interferes with DNA and the survival of the virus. May be synergistic with some other antiviral medicines (such as foscarnet).

▷ **Widely Used Guidelines That Involve This Medicine (representative sample):** Please look at the section at the very beginning of this profile called "Class." Next, turn to Table 22 and you will find guidelines listed by the class involved!

Available Dosage Forms and Strengths

Capsules — 250 mg, 500 mg
Intravenous — 500 mg/10 mL
Intravitreal insert — 4.5 mg

▷ **Recommended Dosage Ranges** (Actual dose and schedule must be determined for each patient individually.)

Infants and Children: **Author's Note: This drug has potential for reproductive toxicity and the risk of causing cancer. It is used in children only after careful evaluation of benefit to risk and with extreme caution.**

Induction: 2.5 mg per kg of body mass given intravenously three times daily.

Maintenance dose: 6.5 mg per kg of body mass given intravenously once daily 5 to 7 times a week.

12 to 60 Years of Age:

Induction: 5 mg per kg of body mass intravenously (infused over 1 hour) every 12 hours for 14 to 21 days.

Maintenance dose: 2.1 to 6 mg per kg of body mass infused into a vein over 1 hour each day. Some centers have used 6 mg per kg of body mass given once daily 5 days per week. If retinitis progresses, the patient can be restarted on the twice-daily-dosing approach. Maximum dose is 6 mg per kg of body mass infused over 1 hour.

Oral: Once the intravenous induction dosing has been accomplished, oral ganciclovir is given at 1,000 mg 3 times daily. Some centers have opted for 500 mg 6 times per day, given every 3 hours while the patient is awake. If retinitis progresses, intravenous induction therapy should be given.

Intravitreous: This device is surgically implanted and has been effective for 5–8 months. The CDC suggests combination use WITH oral ganciclovir (1–1.5 grams taken three times daily) in order to prevent a repeat CMV retinitis. Use not established in patients younger than 9.

Over 60 Years of Age: Kidney function must be checked, and the dose appropriately adjusted.

Conditions Requiring Dosing Adjustments

Liver Function: The liver is only minimally involved in the elimination of this drug, and dosing changes in liver compromise are not needed.

Kidney Function: The dose must be decreased in kidney compromise. This adjustment is accomplished based on creatinine clearance (see Glossary).

Induction: 5 mg per kg of body mass every 12 hours (70 mL/min or higher); 2.5 mg per kg of body mass every 12 hours (50–69); 2.5 mg per kg of body mass every 24 hours (25–49); 1.25 mg per kg of body mass every 24 hours (10–24); 1.25 mg per kg of body mass 3 times per week (less than 10).

Maintenance: 5 mg per kg of body mass every 24 hours (70 mL/min or higher); 2.5 mg per kg of body mass every 24 hours (50–69); 1.25 mg per kg of body mass every 24 hours (25–49); 0.625 mg per kg of body mass every 24 hours (10–24); 0.625 mg per kg of body mass 3 times per week (less than 10).

▷ **Dosing Instructions:** This medicine should be taken with food if taken by mouth (orally). It is best to take the medicine at the same time each day. Capsule form should not be opened or crushed, because you may have adverse reactions from the toxic powder. If you are taking the capsule form and your vision declines, call your doctor immediately. If you miss a dose: take it as soon as you remember it, unless it's nearly time for your next dose—if that is the case, skip the missed dose and return to taking the medicine on your usual schedule. DO NOT double doses. Call your doctor if you miss more than one dose.

Usual Duration of Use: Continual use on a regular schedule for up to 16 days is usually needed to determine this drug's effectiveness in treating retinitis. Because of a very high frequency of relapse, most centers recommend ongoing maintenance therapy for life. If patients have an ongoing (durable) response to combination antiretroviral therapy (HAART) and CD4 cells improve to more than 100–150 per microliter for more than 6 months, some centers have stopped this medicine. Long-term use (months to years) requires periodic evaluation of response and dose adjustment. The ocular implant form may work for 5 months or more. Keep your follow-up appointments with your doctor.

Typical Treatment Goals and Measurements (Outcomes and Markers)

CMV infections: Goals for treatment of CMV include response to the treatment and avoidance of bone marrow depression and kidney problems. Markers for the infection itself include eyesight improvement, eye exam for retinopathy, slit lamp tests, and eye pressure. Additionally, many patients have been found to gain weight and improve albumin levels.

Possible Advantages of This Drug

Transition from the intravenous form to the oral form (if successful in treatment) offers a clear quality-of-life advantage.

Currently a "Drug of Choice"

For patients with liver failure and CMV.

▷ **This Drug Should Not Be Taken If**
- you had an allergic reaction to it previously.
- your absolute neutrophil count (a specific kind of white blood cell) is less than 500 per cubic mm.
- your platelet count is less than 25,000 per cubic mm.

▷ **Inform Your Physician Before Taking This Drug If**
- you think you are dehydrated (this drug is primarily removed by the kidneys).
- you have a sore throat or fever.
- you have a history of blood cell disorders.
- you are planning pregnancy.

- you are male and are planning pregnancy (attempted conception should be avoided for at least 3 months after ganciclovir therapy).
- you are uncertain of how much ganciclovir to take, how often to take it, how to handle the intravenous solution or if you have the insert form and your vision has not cleared in 14 days.
- you take other prescription or nonprescription medicines that were not discussed with your doctor when ganciclovir was prescribed. This includes natural extracts or herbal remedies and "underground" therapies for AIDS.

Possible Side Effects (natural, expected, and unavoidable drug actions)
Pain at the injection site with the intravenous (IV) form. Possible phlebitis. Visual acuity loss for the first 60 days after the insert form is put in (up to 20% of people lose 3 lines or more).

▷ **Possible Adverse Effects** (unusual, unexpected, and infrequent reactions)
If any of the following develop, consult your physician promptly for guidance.
Mild Adverse Effects
Allergic reactions: skin rash and itching.
Confusion, headache, nervousness, tremor, somnolence, abnormal dreams, ataxia, "pins-and-needles" sensations of the hands (paresthesias)—infrequent.
Muscle aches—rare.
Fever—may be frequent with oral therapy.
Decreased blood glucose or potassium—rare.
Nausea, vomiting, or diarrhea—infrequent to frequent.
Serious Adverse Effects
Allergic reactions: anaphylactic reaction—case reports.
Bone marrow suppression—rare.
Lowered white blood cell (neutropenia) counts—frequent.
Lowered blood platelets—infrequent.
Arrhythmias—rare.
Coma, psychosis, or seizures—case reports.
Neuropathy—infrequent to frequent.
Liver toxicity—rare to infrequent.
Retinal detachment—infrequent.
Visual decline—infrequent to frequent with intravitreal implant.
This drug is a potential cancer-causing (carcinogenic) agent—no percentage defined.

▷ **Possible Effects on Sexual Function:** Reversible infertility in men.

Possible Delayed Adverse Effects: Lowered white blood cell counts or platelets.

▷ **Adverse Effects That May Mimic Natural Diseases or Disorders**
Increased liver enzymes may mimic hepatitis.

Natural Diseases or Disorders That May Be Activated by This Drug
None defined.

Possible Effects on Laboratory Tests
Liver enzymes: increased.
Serum bilirubin or creatinine: increased.
Blood glucose, platelets, or white blood cells: decreased.

CAUTION
1. The oral form may be less effective than the intravenous form. Call your doctor immediately if your vision declines.

2. May cause bone marrow suppression. Call your doctor if you get a sore throat, start to bruise easily, or develop fever.

Precautions for Use

By Infants and Children: Safety and effectiveness for use by those under 18 years of age have not been established. The drug has been used selectively in patients as young as 36 weeks.

By Those Over 60 Years of Age: Because of the age-related decline in kidney function, a creatinine clearance should be obtained and dosing adjusted appropriately.

▷ Advisability of Use During Pregnancy

Pregnancy Category: C. See Pregnancy Risk Categories at the back of this book.

Animal Studies: Rabbits have developed cleft palate, exhibited poorly developed organs, and have experienced fetal death.

Human Studies: Information from adequate studies of pregnant women is not available.

Use of this drug during pregnancy is not recommended.

Advisability of Use If Breast-Feeding

Presence of this drug in breast milk: Unknown.

HIV may be present in breast milk. Avoid drug or refrain from nursing.

Habit-Forming Potential: None.

Effects of Overdose: Nausea and vomiting, excessive salivation, increased liver function tests, bone marrow suppression, kidney failure.

Possible Effects of Long-Term Use: Not defined.

Suggested Periodic Examinations While Taking This Drug (at physician's discretion)

Platelet counts and complete blood counts: every 2 days during induction and weekly thereafter.

Liver function tests: monthly.

Kidney function tests: every 2 weeks.

Eye (ophthalmologic) exams: weekly during induction and every 2 weeks thereafter. These exams may be needed more frequently if the optic nerve or macula of the eye is involved.

▷ While Taking This Drug, Observe the Following

Foods: No restrictions—the oral form should be taken with food.

Herbal Medicines or Minerals: Some patients use echinacea to attempt to boost their immune systems. Unfortunately, use of echinacea is not recommended in people with damaged immune systems. This herb may also actually weaken any immune system if it is used too often or for too long a time. **Caution:** St. John's wort may also cause extreme reactions to the sun. Additive photosensitivity may be possible.

Beverages: No restrictions.

▷ *Alcohol:* No restrictions; however, alcohol may blunt the immune system.

Tobacco Smoking: No interactions expected. I advise everyone to quit smoking.

Marijuana Smoking: May increase somnolence.

▷ *Other Drugs*

Ganciclovir *taken concurrently* with

- amphotericin B (Fungizone, Abelcet) may result in increased bone marrow suppression.
- cancer chemotherapy may result in additive bone marrow suppression.
- cotrimoxazole (Septra) may result in added bone marrow suppression problems.

- cyclosporine (Sandimmune) can result in increased kidney toxicity.
- dapsone is a benefit-to-risk decision, as additive bone marrow suppression may occur.
- didanosine (Videx) can result in increased risk of didanosine toxicity (pancreatitis, nerve damage (neuropathy), or diarrhea.
- flucytosine (Ancobon) can cause additive bone marrow toxicity.
- imipenem/cilastatin (Primaxin) can cause seizures.
- pentamidine may result in additive bone marrow suppression.
- tacrolimus (Prograf) can result in increased risk of kidney toxicity.
- zidovudine (AZT) will often cause a serious increase in bone marrow suppression.

The following drug may *increase* the effects of ganciclovir:
- probenecid (Benemid)—by interfering with elimination by the kidney.

▷ *Driving, Hazardous Activities:* This drug may cause somnolence. Restrict activities as necessary.

Aviation Note: The use of this drug *may be a disqualification* for piloting. Consult a designated Aviation Medical Examiner.

Exposure to Sun: Caution is advised. Photosensitivity has been reported (with IV or oral use). See Herbal Medicines caution on St. John's wort above.

Discontinuation: Talk with your doctor before stopping this medicine.

Special Storage Instructions: Store the intravenous form at 39 degrees F. (4 degrees C.) and use within 12 hours after it has been reconstituted.

Observe the Following Expiration Times: The intravenous form will be stamped or labeled with a specific expiration time if this has been provided by a home infusion company; it should be used within 12 hours after it has been reconstituted.

GEMFIBROZIL (jem FI broh zil)

Introduced: 1976   **Class:**   Anticholesterol   **Prescription:**   USA: Yes   **Controlled Drug:**   USA: No; Canada: No   **Available as Generic:** USA: Yes; Canada: Yes

Brand Names: ✸Apo-Gemfibrozil, Gemcor, ✸Gem-Gemfibrozil, Lopid, ✸Med-Gemfibrozil, ✸Novo-Gemfibrozil, ✸PMS-Gemfibrozil, ✸Riva-Gemfibrozil

BENEFITS versus RISKS	
Possible Benefits	*Possible Risks*
EFFECTIVE REDUCTION OF TRIGLYCERIDE BLOOD LEVELS	Possible myopathy or rhabdomyolysis
INCREASE IN HIGH-DENSITY LIPOPROTEIN (HDL) BLOOD LEVELS	
REDUCES RISK OF CORONARY HEART DISEASE	

▷ **Principal Uses**

As a Single Drug Product: Uses currently included in FDA-approved labeling: (1) Reduces abnormally high blood levels of triglycerides in Types IV and V blood lipid (fat) disorders or Type IIb patients who do not have symptoms or history of existing heart disease (coronary); (2) decreases risk for developing coronary artery heart disease.

Other (unlabeled) generally accepted uses: Could lower the risk of stroke in people with decreased HDL.

How This Drug Works: Reduces triglycerides by inhibiting the liver from making them. Reduces secretion of VLDL and LDL and inhibits VLDL carrier apoproteins. Decreases triglycerides by interfering with liver (hepatic) extraction of free fatty acids and also inhibits peripheral lipolysis. Increases HDL production and does so more than clofibrate. Also appears to increase liver production of more desirable kinds of HDL (small HDL particles).

▷ **Widely Used Guidelines That Involve This Medicine (representative sample):** Please look at the section at the very beginning of this profile called "Class." Next, turn to Table 22 and you will find guidelines listed by the class involved!

Available Dosage Forms and Strengths
Capsules — 300 mg
Tablets — 600 mg

▷ **Usual Adult Dosage Ranges:** 1,200 to 1,600 mg daily in two divided doses (30 minutes before the morning and evening meals). The average dose is 1,200 mg daily. Dose increases should be made gradually over a period of 2 to 3 months. These doses improve lipids and appear to offer a 34% decrease in coronary heart disease after the second year of treatment. **Note: Actual dose and schedule must be determined for each patient individually.**

Conditions Requiring Dosing Adjustments
Liver Function: This drug should not be taken (is contraindicated) in primary biliary cirrhosis and severe liver failure.
Kidney Function: For patients with moderate kidney failure (GFR 10–50 mL/min), 50% of the usual dose should be taken at the usual interval. Patients with severe kidney failure should take 25% of the usual dose at the usual dosing interval.

▷ **Dosing Instructions:** The capsule may be opened and taken 30 minutes before the morning and evening meals. If you forget a dose: take it as soon as you remember it, unless it's nearly time for your next dose—if that is the case, skip the missed dose and return to taking the medicine on your usual schedule. DO NOT double doses. Call your doctor if you find yourself missing doses.

Usual Duration of Use: Regular use for 4 to 8 weeks determines effectiveness in reducing triglycerides. Results in reducing coronary heart disease showed up during the second year of treatment in one study. Long-term use (months to years) requires periodic evaluation by your doctor.

Typical Treatment Goals and Measurements (Outcomes and Markers)
Cholesterol: Current guidelines (National Cholesterol Education Program or NCEP) acknowledge diabetes as one of the conditions that increases risk of heart disease, modifying risk factors, therapeutic lifestyle changes (TLC), and recommending routine testing for all of the cholesterol fractions (lipoprotein profile) versus total cholesterol alone. Goals are: a total cholesterol of 200 mg/dL, and optimal bad cholesterol (LDL) less than 100 mg/dL. Less than 70 mg/dL (see Grundy, S.M. in Sources) is a reasonable optional goal for very high risk patients (such as diabetics with acute coronary syndromes, etc.). 130–159 mg/dL as borderline high, 160 mg/dL as high and

190 mg/dL as very high. Did you know that there are at least five different kinds of "good cholesterol" or HDL? The "too low" measure for HDL is still 40 mg/dL, but in order to learn more about cholesterol types some doctors are starting to order lipid panels. There are at least seven different kinds of "bad cholesterol." The new panels tell doctors about the kinds of cholesterol that your body makes. This is important because some kinds (small dense particles) tend to stick to blood vessels (are highly atherogenic). Take your medicine to reach your goals! Two additional tests you will hear about will be electron beam computed tomography (EBCT) and CRP. EBCT is an important tool used in conjunction with laboratory studies. Findings show that even patients who meet cholesterol goals (particularly females over 55) can still be at significant cardiovascular risk. EBCT then defines risk by giving a calcium score and a "virtual tour" of the coronary arteries. C Reactive Protein, or CRP, is a relatively new and apparently independent predictor of heart disease risk. A large study (see Ridker, P.M. in Sources) found that CRP predicted heart disease risk independently of bad cholesterol (low density lipoprotein). Talk to your doctor about this laboratory test and ask about current guidelines for who should be tested (see Pearson, T.A. in Sources).

Possible Advantages of This Drug
Stronger effect than other fibrates in increasing HDL, decreased risk of death (mortality) from non-heart (noncardiac) causes than other fibric acids. Does not appear to increase homocysteine levels like fenofibrate.

▷ **This Drug Should Not Be Taken If**
  • you have had an allergic reaction to it previously.
  • you have biliary cirrhosis of the liver or liver disease.
  • you have gallbladder disease.
  • you have severe kidney compromise.

▷ **Inform Your Physician Before Taking This Drug If**
  • you have impaired liver or kidney function.
  • you have gallbladder disease or gallstones.
  • you are a diabetic.
  • you are obese and increased exercise and diet have not been attempted.
  • you have a Type IIa cholesterol problem and only have high LDL.
  • you are taking an anticoagulant medicine.
  • you have an underactive thyroid (hypothyroidism).

Possible Side Effects (natural, expected, and unavoidable drug actions)
Moderate increase in blood sugar levels.

▷ **Possible Adverse Effects** (unusual, unexpected, and infrequent reactions)
  If any of the following develop, consult your physician promptly for guidance.
  Mild Adverse Effects
  Allergic reactions: skin rash, hives, itching.
  Headache, dizziness, blurred vision, fatigue, muscle aches and cramps—infrequent.
  Indigestion, excessive gas, stomach discomfort, nausea, vomiting, diarrhea—rare to infrequent.
  Paresthesias—very rare.
  Serious Adverse Effects
  Abnormally low white blood cell count: fever, chills, sore throat—rare.
  Formation of gallstones with long-term use—possible.
  Low blood potassium—possible.

Raynaud's phenomenon—case report.

Liver toxicity—possible.

Myopathy (muscle weakness) or rhabdomyolysis (inability to walk)—case reports to rare.

Kidney failure with muscle damage (rhabdomyolysis with renal failure)—case reports.

▷ **Possible Effects on Sexual Function:** Decreased libido or impotence—rare to infrequent.

Natural Diseases or Disorders That May Be Activated by This Drug

Latent diabetes, latent urinary tract infections.

Possible Effects on Laboratory Tests

Complete blood counts: decreased red cells, hemoglobin, white cells, and platelets.

Blood HDL cholesterol levels: increased.

Blood triglyceride levels: decreased.

Liver function tests: increased liver enzymes (ALT/GPT, AST/GOT, and alkaline phosphatase), increased bilirubin.

CAUTION

1. Gemfibrozil is used only after diet has NOT worked to lower triglyceride levels.
2. If you used the drug clofibrate (Atromid-S) in the past, tell your physician fully about how this worked or affected you.
3. Periodic triglyceride and cholesterol levels are critical.

Precautions for Use

By Infants and Children: Safety and effectiveness for those under 12 years of age are not established.

By Those Over 60 Years of Age: Watch for increased tendency to infection; treat all infections promptly.

▷ **Advisability of Use During Pregnancy**

Pregnancy Category: C. See Pregnancy Risk Categories at the back of this book.

Animal Studies: Produces adverse effects in rabbits and rats.

Human Studies: Adequate studies of pregnant women are not available.

Ask your physician for guidance.

Advisability of Use If Breast-Feeding

Presence of this drug in breast milk: Yes.

Avoid drug or refrain from nursing.

Habit-Forming Potential: None.

Effects of Overdose: Abdominal pain, nausea, vomiting, diarrhea.

Possible Effects of Long-Term Use: Formation of gallstones.

Suggested Periodic Examinations While Taking This Drug (at physician's discretion)

Complete blood cell counts (during the first year of treatment then periodically) and liver function tests.

Measurements of blood levels of total cholesterol, HDL and LDL cholesterol fractions, triglycerides, and sugar.

▷ **While Taking This Drug, Observe the Following**

Foods: Follow the diet prescribed by your physician. Your doctor may also recommend some specific foods such as increased vegetables or functional foods such as Benecol. Three well-designed studies found that both in women and men and before and after a heart attack, people who ate more fish (2–4 servings a week) appeared to avoid heart disease. Additionally, using Omega 3 polyunsaturated fatty acids (PUFA) also appeared to protect against abnormal heart rhythms and sudden death from heart attack.

Herbal Medicines or Minerals: No data exist from well-designed clinical studies about garlic and gemfibrozil combinations and cannot presently be recommended. The FDA allowed one dietary supplement called Cholestin to continue to be sold. This preparation actually contains lovastatin. Since use of an HMG-CoA inhibitor with gemfibrozil may increase risk of rhabdomyolysis or myopathy, the combination is NOT advised. Policosanol has a beneficial effect on cholesterol. Talk to your doctor before combining any herbal products with this medicine.

Beverages: No restrictions. May be taken with milk.

▷ *Alcohol:* No interactions expected.

Tobacco Smoking: No interactions expected. I advise everyone to quit smoking.

▷ *Other Drugs*

Gemfibrozil *taken concurrently* with
- ezetimibe (Zetia) may risk muscle damage or rhabdomyolysis. Combination is not recommended, but if combined, careful monitoring and CK levels are required.
- ritonavir (Norvir) may risk gemfibrozil toxicity.

Gemfibrozil may *increase* the effects of
- glyburide (Micronase) and other oral antidiabetic drugs (see Drug Classes).
- lovastatin and other HMG-CoA-type drugs (see Drug Classes), which may increase muscle damage risk (myopathy) if taken at the same time.
- warfarin (Coumadin) and increase the risk of bleeding; increased frequency of INR (prothrombin time, or protime) measurements and dose changes based on results are critical.

Gemfibrozil may *decrease* the effects of
- chenodiol (Chenix), reducing its benefit in gallstone therapy.
- colestipol (Colestid); separate doses by two hours.

▷ *Driving, Hazardous Activities:* This drug may cause dizziness and blurred vision. Restrict activities as necessary.

Aviation Note: The use of this drug *is usually not a disqualification* for piloting. Consult a designated Aviation Medical Examiner.

Exposure to Sun: No restrictions.

Discontinuation: If triglyceride-lowering does not occur after 3 months, this drug should be stopped.

GLIMEPIRIDE (glim EP er ide)

Introduced: 1996   **Class:**   Antidiabetic, sulfonylureas   **Prescription:**   USA: Yes   **Controlled Drug:**   USA: No   **Available as Generic:** No

Brand Name: Amaryl

BENEFITS versus RISKS

Possible Benefits	*Possible Risks*
TIGHTER CONTROL OF BLOOD SUGAR (added to by appropriate diet and weight control)	Allergic skin reactions
	Possible increased risk of heart (cardiovascular) mortality
DECREASED RISK OF HEART DISEASE, KIDNEY DISEASE, ETC., BY ATTAINING TIGHTER CONTROL OF BLOOD SUGAR	
ONCE-A-DAY DOSING	
DECREASED RISK OF INCREASED INSULIN LEVELS	
DECREASED RISK OF HYPOGLYCEMIA	
MAY BE COMBINED WITH METFORMIN IF BLOOD SUGAR GOALS ARE NOT ACHIEVED WITH SINGLE MEDICINE TREATMENT	
MAY BE USED IN COMBINATION WITH INSULIN (IN SECONDARY FAILURE)	
Inhibits platelet aggregation and probably decreases risk of abnormal clots	

▷ **Principal Uses**

As a Single Drug Product: Uses currently included in FDA-approved labeling: (1) Used in type 2 diabetes (adult, maturity-onset) not requiring insulin, but not adequately controlled by diet alone; (2) approved for combination use with insulin or metformin if diet and exercise and this drug are not adequate and in secondary failures (USED WITH INSULIN).

Other (unlabeled) generally accepted uses: None at present.

How This Drug Works: This drug (1) stimulates insulin secretion from the pancreas; (2) enhances use of insulin by tissues (increased sensitivity); and (3) binds to a receptor on the pancreas (beta cell sulfonylurea-inhibiting K-ATP) and activating the L-type calcium channel. Glimepiride works on platelets to inhibit collagen and ADP-caused aggregation. The effect possibly lowers blood vessel complications such as blood clots. One study showed a beneficial effect on Homocysteine and LP(a), but the cause and effect relationship is uncertain.

▷ **Widely Used Guidelines That Involve This Medicine (representative sample):** Please look at the section at the very beginning of this profile called "Class." Next, turn to Table 22 and you will find guidelines listed by the class involved!

Available Dosage Forms and Strengths

Tablets — 1 mg, 2 mg, 3 mg (Switzerland), 4 mg, 6 mg

▷ **Usual Adult Dosage Ranges:** Started with 1 or 2 mg once daily, with breakfast or the first meal. Once a dose of 2 mg is reached, further dose increases should be made at 1- to 2-week intervals in increments of no more than 2 mg;

the maximum daily dose is 8 mg. Typical ongoing doses have ranged from 1 to 4 mg a day. If target blood sugar goals are not met, combination treatment with metformin (glucophage) used. The minimum effective dose of both medicines should be used. In patients who fail treatment with an oral blood sugar–lowering agent, consideration given to combined glimepiride and insulin therapy. If fasting blood sugar (glucose) is greater than 150 mg/dL and insulin/glimepiride is used, 8 mg is taken with the first main meal. Low-dose insulin is started and adjusted as needed/tolerated weekly based on blood sugar and A1C results.

Note: Actual dose and schedule must be determined for each patient individually.

Conditions Requiring Dosing Adjustments

Liver Function: Starting dose is 1 mg daily in mild liver failure. Further dose changes are based on results of blood sugar testing. No data on use in more severe liver compromise.

Kidney Function: Starting dose is 1 mg daily. Further dose changes are based on results of blood sugar testing.

▷ **Dosing Instructions:** The tablet may be crushed. Follow closely doctor's instructions about dosing and diet. If meals are skipped, hypoglycemia may result. Know the signs and symptoms of hypoglycemia (such as confusion, drowsiness, shakiness, weakness, hunger, blurred vision, headache, and fast heartbeat).

Usual Duration of Use: Use on a regular schedule for 1 to 2 weeks determines effectiveness in controlling diabetes. Failure to respond to maximal doses within 1 month constitutes a primary failure. Insulin or metformin may then be combined with glimepiride to reach blood sugar goals. Blood sugars must be measured, and your doctor will decide if the drug should be continued. If you forget a dose: take it as soon as you remember it, unless it's nearly time for your next dose—if that is the case, skip the missed dose and return to taking the medicine on your usual schedule. DO NOT double doses. Call your doctor if you find yourself missing doses. There are reminder services (beeper-based) that can help.

Typical Treatment Goals and Measurements (Outcomes and Markers)

Blood sugar: The general goal for blood sugar is to return it to the usual "normal" range (generally 80–120 mg/dL), while avoiding risks of excessively low blood sugar. One study (UKPDS) used a fasting plasma sugar (glucose) of less than 108 mg/dL. This medicine generally decreases fasting blood sugar by 60 mg per deciliter.

Fructosamine and glycosylated hemoglobin: Fructosamine levels (a measure of the past 2 to 3 weeks of blood sugar control) should be less than or equal to 310 micromoles per liter. Glycosylated hemoglobin or hemoglobin A1C (a measure of the past 2–3 months of blood sugar control) should be less than or equal to 7.0%. Some clinicians advocate still lower targets. This medicine generally decreases A1C by 1.5% to 2%.

Possible Advantages of This Drug

Effective with once-daily dosing.

May be less likely to cause excessive lowering of the blood sugar (hypoglycemia).

May cause less excessive insulin in the bloodstream (hyperinsulinemia).

May be combined with insulin in secondary failure. Works on platelets to inhibit aggregation, and probably decreases the risk of blood vessel (vascular) complications.

May beneficially change homocysteine and Lp(a) (risk factors for heart disease), but the direct effect of the medicine in the study that found this result is uncertain.

▷ **This Drug Should Not Be Taken If**
- you have had an allergic reaction to it previously.
- you have diabetic ketoacidosis (insulin is the drug of choice).

▷ **Inform Your Physician Before Taking This Drug If**
- you are allergic to other sulfonylurea drugs or to sulfa drugs.
- you have been experiencing prolonged vomiting.
- you are pregnant or are breast-feeding your infant.
- you do not know how to recognize or treat hypoglycemia (see Glossary).
- you will have surgery or have had trauma.
- you have a history of congestive heart failure, peptic ulcer disease, cirrhosis of the liver, kidney disease, or hypothyroidism.
- your blood sugar starts to trend upward (may be a sign of secondary failure).
- you are malnourished or have a high fever, infection, or pituitary or adrenal insufficiency.

Possible Side Effects (natural, expected, and unavoidable drug actions)
Hypoglycemia will occur if drug dose is excessive or if meals are missed or inadequate. The risk of hypoglycemia may be increased if this medicine is combined with insulin.

▷ **Possible Adverse Effects** (unusual, unexpected, and infrequent reactions)
If any of the following develop, consult your physician promptly for guidance.

Mild Adverse Effects
Allergic reactions: skin rash, hives, itching (may subside over time).
Headache, dizziness, or blurred vision—rare.
Nausea—rare.
Increased liver enzymes—infrequent.

Serious Adverse Effects
Allergic reactions: not reported to date.
Lowering of sodium—case reports.
Low blood sugar (hypoglycemia)—possible.

▷ **Possible Effects on Sexual Function:** None reported. Diabetes is a possible cause of impotence.

▷ **Adverse Effects That May Mimic Natural Diseases or Disorders**
Increased liver enzymes may suggest viral hepatitis.

Possible Effects on Laboratory Tests
Hemoglobin A1C (glycosylated hemoglobin): trending toward normal if tight control of blood sugar has been achieved.
Glycated hemoglobin (fructosamine) checks will trend toward normal.
Blood glucose levels: decreased.
Liver function tests: increased liver enzymes (ALT/GPT, AST/GOT, and alkaline phosphatase), increased bilirubin.

CAUTION
1. This drug is only one part of a diabetes program. It is not a substitute for a proper diet and regular exercise.
2. Over time (usually several months) this drug may not work. Periodic follow-up examinations are mandatory.

3. Checking your blood sugar by getting blood from your finger or forearm has become a standard of care. A device called a GlucoWatch is also available. (See Table 18, Patient Power and Home Test Kits.)

4. The American Diabetes Association (ADA) now says that a person is considered diabetic if two fasting blood sugars in a row are more than 125 mg/dL. This more conservative approach reflects current thinking saying that complications start at lower blood sugar levels than previously thought. The concept of pre-diabetes (formerly impaired glucose tolerance) is described in the Glossary. Some British clinicians advocate that statin-type medicines could cut the risk of heart attack and stroke by a third (even in people with "normal" cholesterol)—yet these medicines are underused in diabetics. Talk to your doctor about this.

Precautions for Use

By Infants and Children: Safety and effectiveness in pediatrics have not been established.

By Those Over 60 Years of Age: Use with caution, and start with 1 mg/day. Dose should be increased slowly as needed and tolerated and glucose checked often. Repeated hypoglycemia in the elderly can cause brain damage.

▷ **Advisability of Use During Pregnancy**

Pregnancy Category: C. See Pregnancy Risk Categories at the back of this book.

Human Studies: Adequate studies of pregnant women are not available.

Because uncontrolled blood sugar levels during pregnancy are dangerous for the fetus, many experts recommend insulin instead of an oral agent.

Advisability of Use If Breast-Feeding

Presence of this drug in breast milk: Yes, in animal data; unknown in humans. Avoid drug or refrain from nursing.

Habit-Forming Potential: None.

Effects of Overdose: Symptoms of mild to severe hypoglycemia: headache, light-headedness, faintness, nervousness, confusion, tremor, sweating, heart palpitation, weakness, hunger, nausea, vomiting, stupor progressing to coma.

Possible Effects of Long-Term Use: Reports of increased frequency and severity of heart and blood vessel diseases with long-term use of this class of drugs are highly controversial and inconclusive. A direct cause-and-effect relationship (see Glossary) is tenuous—yet all carry this boxed warning. Ask your doctor for help.

Suggested Periodic Examinations While Taking This Drug (at physician's discretion)

Hemoglobin A1C and/or fructosamine.

Liver function tests.

Evaluation of heart and circulatory system.

Blood sugar levels (via finger sticks and periodic lab checks).

▷ **While Taking This Drug, Observe the Following**

Foods: Follow the diabetic diet and portion control. Rice bran has been checked in a small (57-subject) study of type 1 and type 2 diabetics. The benefit was a 30% lowering of sugar. This might be a complementary care option.

Herbal Medicines or Minerals: Using chromium may change the way your body is able to use sugar. Some health food stores advocate vanadium as mimicking the actions of insulin, but possible toxicity and need for rigorous studies presently preclude recommending it. Caution: St. John's wort may lower blood sugar and also cause photosensitivity, and this drug may also have these effects. Caution is advised in overlapping.

DHEA may change sensitivity to insulin or insulin resistance. Fenugreek, aloe, bitter orange, hawthorn, ginger, garlic, ginseng, glucomannan, guar gum, licorice, nettle, and yohimbe may change blood sugar. Since this may require adjustment of hypoglycemic medicine dosing, talk to your doctor BEFORE combining any herbal medicines with this medicine. Echinacea pupurea (injectable) and blonde psyllium seed or husk should NOT be taken by people living with diabetes. Psyllium increases risk of excessively low blood sugar. Surprisingly, boiled stems of the prickly pear cactus (Optuntia streptacantha) appear to be able to lower blood sugar. Ongoing effects and effects on A1C are not known. Red sage is used for blood sugar effects, but is unproven. Rice bran has been checked in a small study of type 1 and type 2 diabetics. The benefit was a 30% lowering of sugar. This might be a complementary care option.

Beverages: As directed in the diabetic diet. May be taken with milk.

▷ *Alcohol:* Use with extreme caution—alcohol can prolong this drug's hypo-glycemic effect. Other drugs in this class can also cause a disulfiramlike reaction (see Glossary).

Tobacco Smoking: No interactions expected. I advise everyone to quit smoking.

▷ *Other Drugs*

The following drugs may **increase** the effects of glimepiride:
- aspirin and other salicylates.
- chloramphenicol.
- cotrimoxazole (Septra).
- fenfluramine (Pondimin).
- miconazole (Lotrimin).
- monoamine oxidase (MAO) type A inhibitors (see Drug Classes).
- NSAIDs (see Drug Classes).
- probenecid (SK-Probenecid).
- sulfa drugs such as Septra.

The following drugs may **decrease** the effects of glimepiride:
- beta-blocker drugs (see Drug Classes).
- bumetanide (Bumex).
- diazoxide (Proglycem).
- ethacrynic acid (Edecrin).
- furosemide (Lasix).
- phenothiazines (see Drug Classes).
- phenytoin (Dilantin) or fosphenytoin (Cerebyx).
- rifampin (Rifadin, others).
- steroids (betamethasone, prednisone, others).
- thiazide diuretics (see Drug Classes).

Glimepiride **taken concurrently** with
- antacids (magnesium hydroxide–containing) may result in increased risk of excessively lowered blood sugar.
- antifungal agents (such as itraconazole or other azoles) may result in severe lowering of blood sugar.
- calcium channel blockers (see Drug Classes) may cause excessive lowering of blood glucose.
- gatifloxacin (Tequin) or levofloxacin (Levaquin) may result in blood sugar changes. Careful checks of blood sugar and dosing adjustments in response to changes are prudent.

▷ *Driving, Hazardous Activities:* Dosing schedule, eating schedule, and physical activities must be coordinated to prevent hypoglycemia. Know the early symptoms of hypoglycemia so that you can avoid hazardous activities and take corrective measures.

Aviation Note: Diabetes ***is a disqualification*** for piloting. Consult a designated Aviation Medical Examiner.

Exposure to Sun: Some drugs of this class can cause photosensitivity (see Glossary).

Occurrence of Unrelated Illness: Acute infections, vomiting or diarrhea, serious injuries, and surgical procedures can worsen diabetic control and may require insulin. If any of these conditions occur, call your doctor.

Discontinuation: Because of secondary failures, the continued benefit of this drug should be evaluated every 6 months.

GLIPIZIDE (GLIP i zide)

Introduced: 1972 **Class:** Antidiabetic, sulfonylureas **Prescription:** USA: Yes **Controlled Drug:** USA: No **Available as Generic:** Yes

Brand Names: Glucotrol, Glucotrol XL, Metaglip [CD]

BENEFITS versus RISKS

Possible Benefits	*Possible Risks*
TIGHTER CONTROL OF BLOOD SUGAR (adjunctive to appropriate diet and weight control)	HYPOGLYCEMIA, extent varies with patient status
DECREASED RISK OF HEART DISEASE, KIDNEY DISEASE, ETC., BY ATTAINING TIGHTER CONTROL OF BLOOD SUGAR	Allergic skin reactions (some severe)
	Blood cell and bone marrow disorders
ONCE-A-DAY DOSING	Possible increased risk of heart (cardiovascular) mortality (a warning label that all sulfonylureas carry based on a different medicine)
COMBINATION FORM WITH METFORMIN OFFERS TIGHTER SUGAR CONTROL AND LESS RISK OF LOW BLOOD SUGAR	

▷ **Principal Uses**

As a Single Drug Product: Uses currently included in FDA-approved labeling: (1) Type 2 diabetes (adult, maturity-onset) not requiring insulin but not adequately controlled by diet alone; (2) combination form (Metaglip or glipizide/metformin) is used in people who do not meet blood sugar goals using diet and single medicine treatment with metformin or a sulfonylurea.

Other (unlabeled) generally accepted uses: (1) may help reverse abnormal changes in capillaries (very small blood vessels) if given early in diabetes.

As a Combination Drug Product [CD]: When combined with metformin (Metaglip) the pill offers the added benefits/mechanism of action (how it works) of metformin in controlling blood sugar.

How This Drug Works: This drug (1) stimulates the secretion of insulin and (2) enhances the use of insulin by appropriate tissues. The combination form

(Metaglip) also decreases sugar (glucose) production in the liver and increases sensitivity of the body to insulin.

▷ **Widely Used Guidelines That Involve This Medicine (representative sample):** Please look at the section at the very beginning of this profile called "Class." Next, turn to Table 22 and you will find guidelines listed by the class involved!

Available Dosage Forms and Strengths

Tablets, combination (Metaglip) — 2.5 mg glipizide and 250 mg or 500 mg of metformin, 5 mg glipizide and 500 mg metformin

Tablets — 5 mg, 10 mg

Tablets, extended release — 2.5 mg, 5 mg, 10 mg

▷ **Usual Adult Dosage Ranges:** Immediate release form: Starts with 5 mg daily—taken 30 minutes before a meal. At 3- to 7-day intervals, dose may be increased (by 2.5 to 5 mg daily) as needed and tolerated. Daily maximum is 40 mg. If the daily dose is more than 15 mg, it should be divided into two equal doses given twice a day (immediate release form). Extended release form starts at 5 mg, taken with breakfast. Dose increases are made at 7-day intervals. Most patients have a favorable response to 10 mg daily. Maximum daily extended release–form dose is 20 mg. Combination form (Metaglip) is started at 2.5/250 mg once a day with a meal. If the starting blood sugar is 280–320 mg/dL, the starting dose is 2.5/500 mg. The dose is increased as needed and tolerated every 14 days to 10/2000 in equally divided doses with morning and evening meals.

Note: Actual dose and schedule must be determined for each patient individually.

Conditions Requiring Dosing Adjustments

Liver Function: Patients with liver failure should take a starting dose of 2.5 mg and be closely followed. The combination form SHOULD NOT be used in liver compromise (hepatic insufficiency) because of increased risk of lactic acidosis.

Kidney Function: Patients should be monitored closely if the drug is used in mild to moderate renal (kidney) compromise. It is a rare cause of kidney stones. The combination form SHOULD NOT be taken in kidney compromise because the risk of lactic acidosis increases.

▷ **Dosing Instructions:** If the daily maintenance dose is found to be 15 mg or more (immediate release form), the total dose should be divided into two equal doses—the first taken with the morning meal, the second with the evening meal. The immediate release–form tablet may be crushed. If you forget a dose: take it as soon as you remember it, unless it's nearly time for your next dose—if that is the case, skip the missed dose and return to taking the medicine on your usual schedule. DO NOT double doses. Call your doctor if you find yourself missing doses because the best results are achieved by taking exactly the right dose and keeping your blood sugar in "tight" control.

Usual Duration of Use: Use on a regular schedule for 1 to 2 weeks determines effectiveness in controlling diabetes. Failure to respond to maximal doses within 1 month constitutes a primary failure. Up to 10% who respond initially may fail later (secondary failure). Blood sugars must be checked. Better (tight) sugar control is best!

Typical Treatment Goals and Measurements (Outcomes and Markers)

Blood sugar: The general goal for blood sugar is to return it to the usual "normal" range (generally 80–120 mg/dL), while avoiding risks of excessively low blood sugar. One study (UKPDS) used a fasting plasma sugar (glucose) of less than 108 mg/dL.

Fructosamine and glycosylated hemoglobin: Fructosamine levels (a measure of the past 2 to 3 weeks of blood sugar control) should be less than or equal to 310 micromoles per liter. Glycosylated hemoglobin or hemoglobin A1C (a measure of the past 2–3 months of blood sugar control) should be less than or equal to 7.0%. Some clinicians advocate lower.

Possible Advantages of This Drug
Effective with once-daily dosing.

Onset of action within 30 minutes. Near-normal insulin response to eating.

Well tolerated by the elderly diabetic. No substantiated reports of liver toxicity.

Combination form offers fewer pills (better adherence to taking the medicine) and two different mechanisms of action for better blood sugar control.

Advantages of the combination form with metformin may confer:
Overcoming insulin resistance
Avoidance of weight gain

▷ This Drug Should Not Be Taken If
- you have had an allergic reaction to it previously.
- you have diabetic ketoacidosis.

For the Metaglip form:
- you had an allergic reaction to it previously.
- you have impaired kidneys (serum creatinine greater than 1.4 for females or 1.5 for males) as this potentially increases risk of lactic acidosis.
- you have congestive heart failure (CHF) and take medicines to treat it (increases risk of lactic acidosis).
- you have liver disease.
- you are an alcoholic.
- you have a heart or lung insufficiency (increased lactic acidosis risk).
- you are going to have a radiology test that uses iodinated contrast media (ask your doctor).
- you have chronic metabolic acidosis or ketoacidosis.
- you are breast-feeding your infant.

▷ Inform Your Physician Before Taking This Drug If
- you are allergic to other sulfonylurea drugs or to sulfa drugs.
- your diabetes has been unstable or "brittle" in the past.
- you do not know how to recognize or treat hypoglycemia (see Glossary).
- you have severe impairment of liver or kidney function.
- you have an infection or fever or are going to have surgery. Insulin may be required.
- you are pregnant.
- you have a history of congestive heart failure, peptic ulcer disease, cirrhosis of the liver, bone marrow depression, hypothyroidism, or porphyria.

For Metaglip form:
- you are planning to have surgery soon.
- you have a serious infection (increases risk of lactic acidosis).
- you drink excessive amounts of alcohol (talk with your doctor) or are elderly (increases lactic acidosis risk).
- you have a history of megaloblastic anemia.
- you are pregnant (insulin is the drug of choice).
- you have seen another doctor and ketoacidosis was diagnosed.
- you are unsure how much to take or how often to take it.

Possible Side Effects (natural, expected, and unavoidable drug actions)

If drug dose is excessive or if meals are missed or inadequate, abnormally low blood sugar (hypoglycemia) will occur as a drug effect.

▷ **Possible Adverse Effects** (unusual, unexpected, and infrequent reactions)

If any of the following develop, consult your physician promptly for guidance.

Mild Adverse Effects

Allergic reactions: skin rash, hives, itching.

Headache, drowsiness, dizziness, fatigue, sweating—rare to infrequent.

Indigestion, nausea, vomiting, diarrhea—rare to infrequent.

Increased liver enzymes—case reports (questionable causation).

Serious Adverse Effects

Allergic reactions: severe skin reactions—case reports.

Idiosyncratic reaction: hemolytic anemia (see Glossary).

Disulfiramlike reaction (see Glossary) with alcohol use.

Low blood sodium or drug-induced urinary stones—possible.

Bone marrow depression (see Glossary): fatigue, weakness, fever, sore throat, abnormal bleeding or bruising—case reports.

Risk of cardiovascular mortality (based on an old study—UGDP—with a different drug)—possible.

For Metaglip form additional possibilities include:

Lactic acidosis—very rare. (Less than 0.1%, but more likely if used in patients with kidney disease or congestive heart failure that requires medicines, which is why current FDA labeling warns against use in those patients. Lactic acidosis is usually not dramatic in signs or symptoms—breathing difficulty [respiratory distress], low body temp [hypothermia], vague abdominal pain, muscle aches [myalgias], and/or increasing sleepiness.)

Lowered vitamin B12 levels and resultant anemia (megaloblastic)—rare.

Destruction of red blood cells (hemolysis)—case report.

Drug-induced porphyria—case reports.

Liver toxicity—two case reports.

▷ **Possible Effects on Sexual Function:** None reported.

▷ **Adverse Effects That May Mimic Natural Diseases or Disorders**

Liver reaction may suggest viral hepatitis.

Possible Effects on Laboratory Tests

Complete blood counts: decreased red cells, hemoglobin, white cells, and platelets.

Glycated hemoglobin or protein: trending toward normal.

Blood glucose levels: decreased.

Liver function tests: increased liver enzymes (ALT/GPT, AST/GOT, and alkaline phosphatase), increased bilirubin.

CAUTION

1. This drug is only part of a diabetes program, not a substitute for a proper diet and regular exercise.

2. Over time (usually months), this drug may not work. Periodic follow-up examinations are needed.

3. If you develop an infection, insulin may be required to control your blood sugar.

4. The American Diabetic Association (ADA) now says that a person is considered diabetic if 2 fasting blood sugars in a row are more than 125 mg/dL. This more conservative approach reflecting the fact that complications start at lower blood sugar levels than previously thought. The concept of

pre-diabetes (formerly impaired glucose tolerance) is described in the Glossary. Some British clinicians advocate that statin-type medicines could cut the risk of heart attack and stroke by a third (even in people with "normal" cholesterol)—yet comment that these medicines are underused in diabetics. Talk to your doctor about this.

Precautions for Use

By Infants and Children: This drug does not work in type 1 (juvenile, growth-onset) insulin-dependent diabetes.

By Those Over 60 Years of Age: Use with caution, and start with 2.5 mg/day. Dose should be increased slowly and glucose checked often. Repeated hypoglycemia in the elderly can cause brain damage.

▷ **Advisability of Use During Pregnancy**

Pregnancy Category: C. See Pregnancy Risk Categories at the back of this book.

Animal Studies: No birth defects reported in rats and rabbits.

Human Studies: Adequate studies of pregnant women are not available.

Because uncontrolled blood sugar levels during pregnancy are associated with a higher incidence of birth defects, many experts recommend that insulin (instead of an oral agent) be used as necessary to control diabetes during the entire pregnancy.

Advisability of Use If Breast-Feeding

Presence of this drug in breast milk: Unknown.

Avoid drug or refrain from nursing.

Habit-Forming Potential: None.

Effects of Overdose: Symptoms of mild to severe hypoglycemia: headache, light-headedness, faintness, nervousness, confusion, tremor, sweating, heart palpitation, weakness, hunger, nausea, vomiting, stupor progressing to coma.

Possible Effects of Long-Term Use: Reduced thyroid function (hypothyroidism). Reports of increased frequency and severity of heart and blood vessel diseases with long-term use of this class of drugs are highly controversial and inconclusive. A direct cause-and-effect relationship (see Glossary) is tenuous. Ask your doctor for help.

Suggested Periodic Examinations While Taking This Drug (at physician's discretion)

Hemoglobin A1C and/or fructosamine.

Blood sugar checks (via finger stick and periodically in the laboratory).

Complete blood cell counts.

Liver function tests.

Thyroid function tests.

Periodic evaluation of heart and circulatory system (diabetes is a large risk factor for heart and blood vessel disease).

▷ **While Taking This Drug, Observe the Following**

Foods: Follow the diabetic diet prescribed by your physician. Rice bran has been checked in a small (57-subject) study of type 1 and type 2 diabetics. The benefit was a 30% lowering of sugar. This might be a complementary care option.

Herbal Medicines or Minerals: Using chromium may change the way your body is able to use sugar. Some health food stores advocate vanadium as mimicking the actions of insulin, but possible toxicity and need for rigorous studies presently preclude recommending it. Caution: St. John's wort may cause photosensitivity, and this drug may too. DHEA may change sensitivity to insulin or insulin resistance. Fenugreek, hawthorn, bitter melon, bitter orange, ginger, garlic, ginseng, guar gum, licorice, nettle, and yohimbe may change blood sugar. Since this may require adjustment of hypoglycemic medicine dosing, talk to your doctor BEFORE combining any of these herbal medicines with this medicine. Echinacea pupurea (injectable) and blonde psyllium seed or husk should NOT be taken by people living with diabetes. Psyllium increases risk of excessively low blood sugar. Surprisingly, boiled stems of the Optuntia streptacantha form of prickly pear cactus appear to be able to lower blood sugar. Ongoing effects and effects on A1C are not known. Red sage is used for blood sugar effects, but is unproven. Rice bran has been checked in a small (57-subject) study of type 1 and type 2 diabetics. The benefit was a 30% lowering of sugar. This might be a complementary care option.

Beverages: As directed in the diabetic diet. May be taken with milk.

▷ *Alcohol:* Use with extreme caution—alcohol can prolong this drug's hypoglycemic effect. This drug can also cause a disulfiramlike reaction (see Glossary): facial flushing, sweating, palpitation.

Tobacco Smoking: No interactions expected. I advise everyone to quit smoking.

▷ *Other Drugs*

The following drugs may ***increase*** the effects of glipizide:
• acarbose (Precose) may increase risk of excessive lowering of blood sugar.
• aspirin and other salicylates.
• chloramphenicol (Chloromycetin).
• cimetidine (Tagamet).
• clofibrate (Atromid-S).
• cotrimoxazole (Septra).
• fenfluramine (Pondimin).
• itraconazole (Sporanox) and other azole antifungal medicines.
• levothyroxine (and other thyroid products).
• magnesium (increased absorption into the body).
• monoamine oxidase (MAO) type A inhibitors (see Drug Classes).
• NSAIDs (see Drug Classes).
• probenecid (Benemid).
• ranitidine (Zantac).
• sulfa drugs such as trimethoprim/sulfamethoxazole (Septra) or erythromycin/sulfisoxazole (Pediazole).

The following drugs may ***decrease*** the effects of glipizide:
• beta-blocker drugs (see Drug Classes).
• bumetanide (Bumex).
• cholestyramine (Questran).
• diazoxide (Proglycem).
• ethacrynic acid (Edecrin).
• furosemide (Lasix).
• phenothiazines (see Drug Classes).
• phenytoin (Dilantin).
• rifampin (Rifadin, others).
• ritonavir (Norvir).
• steroids (betamethasone, prednisone, others).
• thiazide diuretics (see Drug Classes).

Glipizide ***taken concurrently*** with
• antacids (containing magnesium hydroxide) may result in increased risk of excessively lowered blood sugar.
• antifungal agents (such as itraconazole or other azoles) may result in severe lowering of blood sugar.

- calcium channel blockers (see Drug Classes) may cause excessive lowering of blood glucose.
- cyclosporine (Sandimmune) may result in cyclosporine toxicity.
- gatifloxacin (Tequin) or levofloxacin (Levaquin) may result in blood sugar changes. Careful checks of blood sugar and dosing adjustments in response to changes are prudent.
- sildenafil (Viagra) one case report of an interaction. Talk to your doctor about current data regarding combined use.
- warfarin (Coumadin) can cause an increased hypoglycemic effect.

Metaglip form *taken concurrently* with

- cationic drugs (cotrimoxazole, digoxin [Lanoxin], dofetilide [Tikosyn], procainamide, quinidine, quinine, vancomycin, and others) may increase risk of lactic acidosis.
- contrast media for certain X-ray studies may increase risk of lactic acidosis. Metformin should not be combined with these agents. Some clinicians substitute a different agent to control blood sugar, stop the metformin 48 hours before the X-ray, and then stop the substituted agent and restart metformin once kidney function is tested and found to be normal.
- cotrimoxazole (Bactrim, others) may increase risk of lactic acidosis.
- dofetilide (Tikosyn) may pose a problem because it is a cationic drug and uses the same removal (elimination) pathway that metformin does. This may lead to increased risk of dofetilide toxicity.

▷ *Driving, Hazardous Activities:* Dosing schedule, eating schedule, and physical activities must be coordinated to prevent hypoglycemia. Know the early symptoms of hypoglycemia so that you can avoid hazardous activities and take corrective measures.

Aviation Note: Diabetes *is a disqualification* for piloting. Consult a designated Aviation Medical Examiner.

Exposure to Sun: Some drugs of this class can cause photosensitivity (see Glossary).

Occurrence of Unrelated Illness: Acute infections, vomiting or diarrhea, serious injuries, and surgical procedures can worsen diabetic control and may require insulin. If any of these conditions occur, call your doctor.

Discontinuation: Because of secondary failures, the continued benefit of this drug should be evaluated every 6 months.

GLYBURIDE (GLI byoor ide)

Other Name: Glibenclamide   **Introduced:**   1970   **Class:**   Antidiabetic, sulfonylureas   **Prescription:**   USA: Yes   **Controlled Drug:** USA: No; Canada: No   **Available as Generic:**   Yes

Brand Names: ✤Albert-Glyburide, ✤Apo-Glyburide, Diabeta, ✤Euglucon, ✤Gen-Glybe, Glubate, Glucovance [CD], Glynase Prestab, Micronase, ✤Novo-Glyburide

```
┌─────────────────────────────────────────────────────────────────┐
│                      BENEFITS versus RISKS                        │
│      Possible Benefits              Possible Risks                │
│ HELPS REGULATE BLOOD SUGAR     HYPOGLYCEMIA, SEVERE AND           │
│   IN TYPE 2 DIABETES (NON-       PROLONGED                         │
│   INSULIN DEPENDENT            LACTIC ACIDOSIS (A RARE RISK       │
│   DIABETES) ADJUNCTIVE TO        WITH GLUCOVANCE FORM)            │
│   APPROPRIATE DIET AND         Possible anemia with long-term use │
│   WEIGHT CONTROL                 (added as a rare risk with       │
│ COMBINED WITH METFORMIN IN       Glucovance form)                 │
│   THE GLUCOVANCE FORM TO       Liver damage                       │
│   GIVE ADDED AND TIGHTER       Blood cell and bone marrow disorders│
│   BLOOD SUGAR (GLUCOSE)        Allergic skin reactions (some severe)│
│   CONTROL                      Possible increased risk of heart   │
│                                  (cardiovascular) mortality based on│
│                                  an old study with a different drug│
└─────────────────────────────────────────────────────────────────┘
```

▷ **Principal Uses**

As a Single Drug Product: Uses currently included in FDA-approved labeling: (1) Type 2 diabetes mellitus (adult, maturity-onset) that does not require insulin but can't be adequately controlled by diet alone; (2) combination form (Glucovance or glyburide/metformin) is used in people who do not meet blood sugar goals using diet and single medicine treatment with metformin or a sulfonylurea.

Other (unlabeled) generally accepted uses: None.

How This Drug Works: This drug (1) stimulates the secretion of insulin, (2) decreases glucose production in the liver, and (3) enhances insulin use. The combination form (with metformin): overlaps in some of the way that it works and also increases sensitivity of the body to insulin.

▷ **Widely Used Guidelines That Involve This Medicine (representative sample):** Please look at the section at the very beginning of this profile called "Class." Next, turn to Table 22 and you will find guidelines listed by the class involved!

Available Dosage Forms and Strengths

Tablets — 1.25 mg, 1.5 mg, 2.5 mg, 3 mg, 5 mg, 6 mg

Tablets, combination — 250 mg metformin and 1.25 mg glyburide, 500 mg metformin, and 2.5 or 5.0 mg glyburide (Glucovance form).

▷ **Usual Adult Dosage Ranges:** *Regular-release products:* 2.5 to 5 mg daily with breakfast. At 7-day intervals the dose may be increased by increments of 2.5 mg daily as needed and tolerated. Total daily dose should not exceed 20 mg. Prudent to start sensitive patients on 1.25 mg daily.

Micronized products: 1.5 to 3 mg daily taken with breakfast. (Patients more sensitive to oral agents should be started at 0.75 mg daily.) If the daily dose required is more than 6 mg daily, twice daily dosing may be needed. Maximum dose is 12 mg daily.

Combination form (Glucovance): For people who do not meet blood sugar goals with their existing regimen of exercise and medicine: the beginning dose is 1.25 mg glyburide/250 mg metformin once a day. If patients have fasting plasma blood sugar (glucose) greater than 200 mg/dL or a hemoglobin A1C (glycosylated hemoglobin) more than 9%, the 1.25 mg/250 mg dose can be given with the morning and evening meals. Dosing can be increased as

needed and tolerated until goals of treatment are met up to a maximum of 10 mg glyburide/2000 mg metformin.
Note: Actual dose and schedule must be determined for each patient individually.

Conditions Requiring Dosing Adjustments

Liver Function: Glyburide may cause catastrophic hypoglycemia (low blood sugar) if it is used by patients with liver disease. Very low starting doses should be taken and the patient closely followed. It is also a rare cause of hepatitis and cholestatic jaundice. The Glucovance combination form SHOULD NOT be used in liver compromise (hepatic insufficiency) because of increased risk of lactic acidosis.

Kidney Function: Glyburide should be used with caution in mild renal compromise, with low initial doses and careful patient monitoring. The drug SHOULD NOT be used by patients with moderate kidney failure (creatinine clearances less than 50 mL/min) or in severe kidney failure. The combination form SHOULD NOT be taken in kidney compromise because the risk of lactic acidosis increases.

▷ **Dosing Instructions:** If the daily maintenance dose is 10 mg or more, the total dose should be divided into two equal doses: the first taken with the morning meal, the second with the evening meal. The tablet may be crushed. If you forget a dose: take it as soon as you remember it, unless it's nearly time for your next dose—if that is the case, skip the missed dose and return to taking the medicine on your usual schedule. DO NOT double doses. Call your doctor if you find yourself missing doses—the best results are achieved by taking exactly the right dose and keeping your blood sugar in "tight" control.

Usual Duration of Use: Use on a regular schedule for 1 to 2 weeks determines effectiveness in controlling diabetes. No response to peak doses in 1 month constitutes a primary failure. Up to 10% of those who respond initially may develop secondary failure. The duration of effective use can only be determined by periodic measurement of the blood sugar.

Typical Treatment Goals and Measurements (Outcomes and Markers)

Blood sugar: The general goal for blood sugar is to return it to the usual "normal" range (generally 80–120 mg/dL), while avoiding risks of excessively low blood sugar. One study (UKPDS) used a fasting plasma sugar (glucose) of less than 108 mg/dL.

Fructosamine and glycosylated hemoglobin: Fructosamine levels (a measure of the past 2 to 3 weeks of blood sugar control) should be less than or equal to 310 micromoles per liter. Glycosylated hemoglobin or hemoglobin A1C (a measure of the past 2–3 months of blood sugar control) should be less than or equal to 7.0%. Some clinicians recommend 6.5%.

Possible Advantages of This Drug

Advantages of the combination form with metformin may confer:
Overcoming insulin resistance
Improved glucose control and adherence with a single pill.

▷ **This Drug Should Not Be Taken If**
- you have had an allergic reaction to it previously.
- you have severe impairment of liver and kidney function.
- you have diabetic ketoacidosis.
- you are pregnant.

For the Glucovance form:
- you had an allergic reaction to it previously.

- you have impaired kidneys (serum creatinine greater than 1.4 for females or 1.5 for males) as this potentially increases risk of lactic acidosis.
- you have congestive heart failure (CHF) and take medicines to treat it (increases risk of lactic acidosis).
- you have liver disease.
- you are an alcoholic.
- you have a heart or lung insufficiency (increased lactic acidosis risk).
- you are going to have a radiology test that uses iodinated contrast media (ask your doctor).
- you have chronic metabolic acidosis or ketoacidosis.
- you are breast-feeding your infant.

▷ **Inform Your Physician Before Taking This Drug If**
- you are allergic to other sulfonylurea drugs or to "sulfa" drugs.
- your diabetes has been unstable or "brittle" in the past.
- you do not know how to recognize or treat hypoglycemia (see Glossary).
- you have a history of problems with blood clotting or have a glucose-6-phosphate dehydrogenase (G6PD) deficiency.
- you have a history of congestive heart failure, peptic ulcer disease, cirrhosis of the liver, hypothyroidism, or porphyria.
- you have an infection or a fever.

For the Glucovance form:
- you are planning to have surgery soon.
- you have a serious infection (increases risk of lactic acidosis).
- you drink excessive amounts of alcohol (talk with your doctor) or are elderly (increases lactic acidosis risk).
- you have a history of megaloblastic anemia.
- you are pregnant (insulin is the drug of choice).
- you have seen another doctor and ketoacidosis was diagnosed.
- you are unsure how much to take or how often to take it.

Possible Side Effects (natural, expected, and unavoidable drug actions)

If drug dose is excessive or food intake is delayed or inadequate, abnormally low blood sugar (hypoglycemia) will occur as a predictable drug effect.

▷ **Possible Adverse Effects** (unusual, unexpected, and infrequent reactions)

If any of the following develop, consult your physician promptly for guidance.

Mild Adverse Effects

Allergic reactions: skin rash, hives, itching.

Headache, drowsiness, dizziness, fatigue—possible.

Indigestion, heartburn, nausea—rare.

Bed-wetting at night (nocturnal enuresis), especially in young adults—case reports.

Serious Adverse Effects

Allergic reactions: hepatitis with jaundice (see Glossary), severe skin reactions (exfoliative dermatitis)—case reports.

Idiosyncratic reaction: hemolytic anemia (see Glossary).

Disulfiramlike reaction with concurrent use of alcohol (see Glossary)—possible.

Bone marrow depression (see Glossary): fatigue, fever, sore throat, abnormal bleeding—case reports.

Thrombocytopenic purpura—case report.

Liver toxicity (granulomatous or intrahepatic cholestasis)—case reports.

Blood clotting defects (coagulation)—rare.

Cardiovascular mortality (based on an old study of a different medicine)—increased risk.

For Metaglip form additional possibilities include:

Lactic acidosis—very rare. (Less than 0.1%, but more likely if used in patients with kidney disease or congestive heart failure that requires medicines, which is why current FDA labeling warns against use in those patients. Lactic acidosis is usually not dramatic in signs or symptoms—breathing difficulty [respiratory distress], low body temp [hypothermia], vague abdominal pain, muscle aches [myalgias], and/or increasing sleepiness.)

Lowered vitamin B_{12} levels and resultant anemia (megaloblastic)—rare.

Destruction of red blood cells (hemolysis)—case report.

Drug-induced porphyria—case reports.

Liver toxicity—two case reports (metformin component).

▷ **Possible Effects on Sexual Function:** None reported.

▷ **Adverse Effects That May Mimic Natural Diseases or Disorders**
Liver reactions may suggest viral hepatitis.

Possible Effects on Laboratory Tests
Blood platelet counts: decreased.
Blood cholesterol and triglyceride levels: decreased.
Glycated hemoglobin or protein: trending toward normal.
Blood glucose levels: decreased.
Liver function tests: increased liver enzymes (ALT/GPT, AST/GOT, and alkaline phosphatase).

CAUTION
1. This drug is only part of diabetes management. Much of the damage from diabetes can be delayed or avoided if you keep your blood sugar in the normal range. Ask your doctor about a proper diet and regular exercise.
2. Over time (usually many months), this drug may not work. Periodic follow-up examinations are necessary.
3. The American Diabetic Association (ADA) now says that a person is considered diabetic if 2 fasting blood sugars in a row are more than 125 mg/dL. This more conservative approach reflects information saying that complications start at lower blood sugar levels than previously thought. The concept of pre-diabetes (formerly impaired glucose tolerance) is described in the Glossary. Some British clinicians advocate that statin-type medicines could cut the risk of heart attack and stroke by a third (even in people with "normal" cholesterol)—yet these medicines are underused in diabetics. Talk to your doctor about this.

Precautions for Use
By Infants and Children: This drug does not work in type 1 (juvenile, growth-onset) insulin-dependent diabetes.
By Those Over 60 Years of Age: Use with caution, and start with 1.25 mg/day of the regular form. Dose should be slowly increased and glucose closely followed. Repeated hypoglycemia in the elderly can cause brain damage.

▷ **Advisability of Use During Pregnancy**
Pregnancy Category: C: Glyburide, B: Glyburide/metformin. See Pregnancy Risk Categories at the back of this book.
Animal Studies: No birth defects reported in rats and rabbits.
Human Studies: Adequate studies of pregnant women are not available.
Uncontrolled blood sugar levels during pregnancy are associated with a higher incidence of birth defects, so many experts recommend insulin (instead of an oral agent) to control diabetes during the entire pregnancy.

Advisability of Use If Breast-Feeding

Presence of this drug in breast milk: Unknown.

Avoid drug or refrain from nursing.

Habit-Forming Potential: None.

Effects of Overdose: Symptoms of mild to severe hypoglycemia: headache, light-headedness, faintness, nervousness, confusion, tremor, sweating, heart palpitation, weakness, hunger, nausea, vomiting, stupor progressing to coma.

Possible Effects of Long-Term Use: Reduced thyroid gland function (hypothyroidism). Reports of increased frequency and severity of heart and blood vessel diseases associated with long-term use of this class of drugs are highly controversial and inconclusive. A direct cause-and-effect relationship (see Glossary) is tenuous. Ask your physician for guidance.

Suggested Periodic Examinations While Taking This Drug (at physician's discretion)

Complete blood cell counts.

Liver function tests.

Thyroid function tests.

Periodic evaluation of heart and circulatory system (diabetes is a large risk factor for heart and blood vessel disease).

Self-assessment (finger stick) of blood sugar is prudent as well as periodic glycosylated hemoglobin and/or fructosamine tests.

▷ **While Taking This Drug, Observe the Following**

Foods: Follow the diabetic diet prescribed by your physician.

Herbal Medicines or Minerals: Using chromium may change the way your body is able to use sugar. Some health food stores advocate vanadium as mimicking the actions of insulin, but possible toxicity and need for rigorous studies presently preclude recommending it. Caution: St. John's wort may cause photosensitivity, and this drug may too.

DHEA may change sensitivity to insulin or insulin resistance. Fenugreek, glucomannan, hawthorn, ginger, garlic, ginseng guar gum, licorice, nettle, and yohimbe may change blood sugar. Since this may require adjustment of hypoglycemic medicine dosing, talk to your doctor BEFORE combining any of these herbal medicines with this medicine. Echinacea pupurea (injectable) and blonde psyllium seed or husk should NOT be taken by people living with diabetes. Psyllium increases risk of excessively low blood sugar. Surprisingly, boiled stems of the Optuntia streptacantha, or prickly pear cactus, appear to be able to lower blood sugar. Ongoing effects and effects on A1C are not known. Red sage is used for blood sugar effects, but is unproven. Rice bran has been checked in a small (57-subject) study of type 1 and type 2 diabetics. The benefit was a 30% lowering of sugar. This might be a complementary care option.

Beverages: As directed in the diabetic diet. May be taken with milk.

▷ *Alcohol:* Use with extreme caution—alcohol can exaggerate this drug's hypoglycemic effect. This drug can cause a disulfiramlike reaction (see Glossary): facial flushing, sweating, palpitation.

Tobacco Smoking: No interactions expected. I advise everyone to quit smoking.

▷ *Other Drugs*

The following drugs may ***increase*** the effects of glyburide:

• acarbose (Precose).

• aspirin and other salicylates (aspirin may also block disulfiram effect).

• chloramphenicol (Chloromycetin).

- cimetidine (Tagamet).
- ciprofloxacin (Cipro).
- clofibrate (Atromid-S).
- cotrimoxazole (various).
- fenfluramine (Pondimin).
- gemfibrozil (Lopid).
- monoamine oxidase (MAO) type A inhibitors (see Drug Classes).
- phenylbutazone (Butazolidin).
- ranitidine (Zantac).
- ritonavir (Norvir).
- sulfa drugs such as trimethoprim/sulfamethoxazole (Septra) or erythromycin/sulfisoxazole (Pediazole).

The following drugs may *decrease* the effects of glyburide:
- beta-blocker drugs (see Drug Classes).
- bumetanide (Bumex).
- diazoxide (Proglycem).
- ethacrynic acid (Edecrin).
- furosemide (Lasix).
- phenytoin (Dilantin).
- rifampin (Rifadin, others) and rifabutin (Mycobutin).
- thiazide diuretics (see Drug Classes).
- thyroid hormones (see Drug Classes).

Glyburide *taken concurrently* with
- antacids (containing magnesium hydroxide) or magnesium supplements may result in increased risk of excessively lowered blood sugar.
- antifungal agents (such as itraconazole, voriconazole [Vfend], or other azoles) may result in severe lowering of blood sugar.
- cyclosporine (Sandimmune) may increase cyclosporine levels by up to 57%.
- enalapril (Vasotec) may enhance blood sugar–lowering effect.
- gatifloxacin (Tequin) or levofloxacin (Levaquin) may result in blood sugar changes. Careful checks of blood sugar and dosing adjustments in response to changes are prudent.
- MAO inhibitors (see Drug Classes) may increase risk of hyperglycemia.
- steroids (betamethasone, prednisone, others) blunt glyburide benefits.
- warfarin (Coumadin) may result in bleeding; more frequent INR (prothrombin time) testing is needed.

Glucovance form *taken concurrently* with
- cationic drugs (cotrimoxazole, digoxin [Lanoxin], dofetilide [Tikosyn], procainamide, quinidine, quinine, vancomycin, and others) may increase risk of lactic acidosis.
- contrast media for certain X-ray studies may increase risk of lactic acidosis. Metformin should not be combined with these agents. Some clinicians substitute a different agent to control blood sugar, stop the metformin 48 hours before the X-ray, and then stop the substituted agent and restart metformin once kidney function is tested and found to be normal.
- cotrimoxazole (Bactrim, others) may increase risk of lactic acidosis.
- dofetilide (Tikosyn) may pose a problem because it is a cationic drug and uses the same removal (elimination) pathway that metformin does. This may lead to increased risk of dofetilide toxicity.

▷ *Driving, Hazardous Activities:* Regulate dosing, eating, and physical activities carefully to prevent hypoglycemia. Know the early symptoms of hypoglycemia so that you can avoid hazardous activities and take corrective measures.

Aviation Note: Diabetes *is a disqualification* for piloting. Consult a designated Aviation Medical Examiner.

Exposure to Sun: Use caution until sensitivity has been determined. Some drugs of this class can cause photosensitivity (see Glossary).

Occurrence of Unrelated Illness: Acute infections, vomiting or diarrhea, serious injuries, and surgical procedures can worsen diabetic control and may require insulin. If any of these conditions occur, consult your physician promptly.

Discontinuation: Because of the possibility of secondary failure, it is advisable to evaluate the continued benefit of this drug every 6 months.

GUANFACINE (GWAHN fa seen)

Introduced: 1980   **Class:**   Antihypertensive   **Prescription:**   USA: Yes   **Controlled Drug:**   USA: No   **Available as Generic:**   USA: Yes
Brand Name: Tenex

Author's Note: Information in this profile has been shortened to make room for more widely used medicines.

HALOPERIDOL (hal oh PER i dohl)

Introduced: 1958   **Class:**   Antipsychotic; tranquilizer, strong   **Prescription:**   USA: Yes   **Controlled Drug:**   USA: No; Canada: No   **Available as Generic:**   USA: Yes; Canada: Yes

Brand Names: ✤Alti-Haloperidol, ✤Apo-Haloperidol, Haldol, ✤Haldol LA, Halperon, ✤Novo-Peridol, ✤Peridol, ✤PMS Haloperidol

BENEFITS versus RISKS	
Possible Benefits	*Possible Risks*
EFFECTIVE CONTROL OF PSYCHOSES	FREQUENT PARKINSONLIKE SIDE EFFECTS
BENEFICIAL EFFECTS ON THINKING, MOOD, AND BEHAVIOR	SERIOUS TOXIC EFFECTS ON BRAIN with long-term use
EFFECTIVE CONTROL OF SOME CASES OF TOURETTE'S SYNDROME	Rare blood cell disorders
Beneficial in management of some hyperactive children	Abnormally low white blood cell count
Decanoate form treats schizophrenia for a month with a single injection	

▷ **Principal Uses**

As a Single Drug Product: Uses currently included in FDA-approved labeling: (1) Helps control psychotic thinking and abnormal behavior in acute psychosis of unknown nature, acute schizophrenia, paranoid states, and the manic phase of manic-depressive disorders; (2) helps control outbursts of aggression and agitation; (3) used to treat Tourette's syndrome; (4) approved for use in children 3 years old or older who have unexplained (unprovoked) explosive and combative hyperexcitability.

Other (unlabeled) generally accepted uses: (1) Helps control refractory hiccups; (2) used to lessen delirium in LSD flashbacks and phencyclidine intoxication; (3) used as combination (adjuvant) therapy in chronic pain syndromes; (4) may be helpful in autistic patients; (5) may have a role in refractory vomiting caused by cancer chemotherapy; (6) can ease symptoms in refractory sneezing; (7) may be helpful as adjunctive therapy in stuttering.

How This Drug Works: By interfering with a nerve impulse transmitter (dopamine), this drug reduces anxiety and agitation, improves coherence and thinking, and abolishes delusions and hallucinations.

▷ **Widely Used Guidelines That Involve This Medicine (representative sample):** Please look at the section at the very beginning of this profile called "Class." Next, turn to Table 22 and you will find guidelines listed by the class involved!

Available Dosage Forms and Strengths

Concentrate — 2 mg/mL, 10 mg/mL in some countries

Injection — 5 mg/mL, 50 mg/mL, 100 mg/mL

Tablets — 0.5 mg (Canada), 1 mg, 1.5 mg, 2 mg, 5 mg, 10 mg, 20 mg

▷ **Usual Adult Dosage Ranges:** Initially this medicine can be started at 1 to 6 milligrams a day to help control moderate symptoms and at 6 to 15 mg a day in severe cases. Doses are divided into equal amounts and given 2 to 3 times a day. Dosing is increased as needed and tolerated. Some patients require increases of up to 100 mg a day. Ongoing doses are highly individualized. Decanoate form may relieve schizophrenia for a month with a single injection. The typical change (conversion) to the decanoate form is 10 to 20 times the previous dose (in oral haloperidol equivalents), but not more than a maximum starting decanoate-form dose of 100 mg. If in some cases, the starting conversion dose is greater than 100 mg, the first dose should be 100 mg of decanoate, followed by the rest of the dose in 3 to 7 days.

Note: Actual dose and schedule must be determined for each patient individually.

Conditions Requiring Dosing Adjustments

Liver Function: The dose, dosing interval and titration interval (time to adjust the drug to desired effect) should be adjusted for liver compromise.

Kidney Function: High doses used with caution in kidney compromise.

▷ **Dosing Instructions:** The tablet may be crushed and taken with or following food to reduce stomach irritation. The concentrate may be diluted in 2 ounces of water or fruit juice (do not add it to coffee or tea), and should be measured using a medicine spoon or calibrated dose cup. If you forget a dose: take it as soon as you remember it, unless it's nearly time for your next dose—if that is the case, skip the missed dose and return to taking the medicine on your usual schedule. DO NOT double doses. Call your doctor if you find yourself forgetting doses.

Usual Duration of Use: Use on a regular schedule for several weeks determines this drug's effectiveness in controlling psychotic behavior. If it doesn't provide significant benefit in 6 weeks, it should be stopped. Long-term use requires supervision and periodic physician evaluation.

Typical Treatment Goals and Measurements (Outcomes and Markers)

Psychosis: The general goal: to lessen the degree and severity of abnormal thinking, letting patients return to their daily lives. Specific measures of psychosis may involve testing or inventories and can be valuable in helping check benefits from this medicine.

This Drug Should Not Be Taken If

- you had an allergic reaction to it previously.
- you are experiencing severe mental depression.
- you have any form of Parkinson's disease.
- you have severe active liver disease.
- you are presently experiencing central nervous system (CNS) depression due to alcohol or narcotics.
- you currently have a bone marrow or blood cell disorder.

▷ **Inform Your Physician Before Taking This Drug If**

- you are allergic or abnormally sensitive to phenothiazine drugs.
- you have a history of mental depression.
- you have any type of heart disease.
- you have impaired liver or kidney function.
- you have cancer of the breast.
- you have thyroid disease.
- you are allergic to the dye tartrazine.
- you are pregnant or are planning pregnancy.
- you have a history of neuroleptic malignant syndrome.
- you have low blood pressure, epilepsy, or glaucoma.
- you are taking any drugs with a sedative effect.
- you plan to have surgery and general or spinal anesthesia soon.

Possible Side Effects (natural, expected, and unavoidable drug actions)

Mild drowsiness, low blood pressure, blurred vision, dry mouth, constipation, marked and frequent Parkinson-like reactions (see Glossary).

▷ **Possible Adverse Effects** (unusual, unexpected, and infrequent reactions)

If any of the following develop, consult your physician promptly for guidance.

Mild Adverse Effects

Allergic reactions: skin rash, hives.

Dizziness, weakness, agitation, insomnia—case reports to infrequent.

Loss of appetite, indigestion, nausea, vomiting, diarrhea—case reports.

Decreased white blood cell count—possible.

Serious Adverse Effects

Allergic reactions: rare liver reaction with jaundice, asthma, spasm of vocal cords.

Idiosyncratic reactions: Neuroleptic malignant syndrome (see Glossary).

Nervous system reactions: rigidity of extremities, tremors, seizures, constant movement, facial grimacing, eye-rolling, spasm of neck muscles, tardive dyskinesia (see Glossary)—case reports to infrequent.

Rhabdomyolysis—case report.

Abnormal heartbeat (premature ventricular contractions)—possible with aggressive dosing.

Torsades de Pointes—possible.

Worsening of psychosis—possible.

Low blood sugar or abnormal and frequent urination (SIADH)—case reports.

Liver toxicity—possible.

Bronchospasm or myasthenia gravis—case reports.

▷ **Possible Effects on Sexual Function:** Decreased libido; impotence—infrequent to frequent; painful ejaculation; priapism (see Glossary). Tender and enlarged breast tissue in men (gynecomastia); breast enlargement with milk production in women.

Altered timing and pattern of menstruation—case reports.

▷ **Adverse Effects That May Mimic Natural Diseases or Disorders**

Liver reaction may suggest viral hepatitis. Nervous system reactions may suggest Parkinson's disease or Reye's syndrome.

Natural Diseases or Disorders That May Be Activated by This Drug

Latent epilepsy, glaucoma, diabetes.

Possible Effects on Laboratory Tests

Complete blood counts: decreased red cells, hemoglobin, and white cells; increased eosinophils.

INR (prothrombin time): decreased.

Blood cholesterol level: decreased.

Blood glucose level: increased.

Liver function tests: increased liver enzymes (ALT/GPT, AST/GOT, and alkaline phosphatase), increased bilirubin.

CAUTION

1 The smallest effective dose should be used for long-term therapy.
2. Use with extreme caution in epilepsy; can alter seizure patterns.
3. Those with lupus erythematosus or who are taking prednisone have more nervous system reactions.
4. Levodopa should not be used to treat Parkinson-like reactions; it can cause agitation and worsening of the psychotic disorder.
5. Obtain prompt evaluation of any change or disturbance in vision.

Precautions for Use

By Infants and Children: This drug should not be used in children under 3 years of age or 15 kg in weight. While the dose is not well established in children 3–6 years old, 0.05–0.15 mg per kg of body weight daily for psychotic disorders is the usual range. The total daily dose is separated into 2 or 3 equal oral doses. Avoid this drug in the presence of symptoms suggestive of Reye's syndrome. Side effects are usually similar to the ones seen in adults.

By Those Over 60 Years of Age: Small doses are indicated when therapy is started. This drug can cause significant changes in mood and behavior; watch for confusion, disorientation, agitation, restlessness, aggression, and paranoia. You may be more susceptible to the development of drowsiness, lethargy, orthostatic hypotension (see Glossary), hypothermia (see Glossary), Parkinson-like reactions, and prostatism (see Glossary).

▷ **Advisability of Use During Pregnancy**

Pregnancy Category: C. See Pregnancy Risk Categories at the back of this book.

Animal Studies: Cleft palate reported in mouse studies.

Human Studies: No increase in birth defects reported in 100 exposures. Adequate studies of pregnant women are not available.

Avoid during the first 3 months (trimester). Use only if clearly needed. Ask your physician for guidance.

Advisability of Use If Breast-Feeding

Presence of this drug in breast milk: Yes.

Use is controversial. Monitor nursing infant closely and discontinue drug or nursing if adverse effects develop.

Habit-Forming Potential: Reports of recreational use have been made. If the drug is stopped suddenly, patients may experience a withdrawal syndrome.

Effects of Overdose: Marked drowsiness, weakness, tremor, unsteadiness, agitation, stupor, coma, convulsions.

Possible Effects of Long-Term Use: Eye damage—deposits in cornea, lens, or retina; tardive dyskinesia (see Glossary).

Suggested Periodic Examinations While Taking This Drug (at physician's discretion)
Complete blood counts.
Liver function tests.
Eye examinations.
Electrocardiograms.
The tongue should be watched for fine, involuntary, wavelike movements that could be the beginning of tardive dyskinesia. The Abnormal Involuntary Movement Scale (AIMS) should be checked every 6 months.

▷ **While Taking This Drug, Observe the Following**
Foods: No restrictions.
Herbal Medicines or Minerals: St. John's wort may also lead to increased sensitivity to the sun—DO NOT COMBINE. Evening primrose oil may work to lower the threshold for seizures. Combination with haloperidol may increase seizure risk—DO NOT COMBINE. Since part of the way ginseng works may be as an MAO inhibitor, do not combine. Because chasteberry acts as a dopamine agonist, it may actually work against the action of haloperidol—caution is advised. Betel nut appeared to increase movement problems (extrapyramidal side effects) when it was chewed by patients taking a similar medicine—combination is not advisable.
Beverages: No restrictions. May be taken with milk.
▷ *Alcohol:* Avoid completely. Alcohol can increase the sedative action of haloperidol and accentuate its depressant effects on brain function. Haloperidol can increase the intoxicating effects of alcohol.
Tobacco Smoking: Combination with nicotine actually increased suppression of tics in Tourette's syndrome in one study. I advise everyone to quit smoking.
Marijuana Smoking: Moderate increase in drowsiness; accentuation of orthostatic hypotension; increased risk of precipitating latent psychosis, confusing interpretation of mental status, and drug response.
▷ *Other Drugs*
Haloperidol may *increase* the effects of
• all drugs with sedative actions and cause excessive sedation.
• some antihypertensive drugs and cause excessive lowering of blood pressure; monitor the combined effects carefully.
• fluvoxamine (Luvox) and result in toxicity (altered mental status, GI side effects).
Haloperidol may *decrease* the effects of
• guanethidine (Esimil, Ismelin) and reduce its antihypertensive effect.
Haloperidol *taken concurrently* with
• anticholinergic drugs (see Drug Classes) can cause additive anticholinergic effects (dry mouth, constipation, or sedation).
• beta-blocker drugs may cause excessive lowering of blood pressure.
• bupropion (Zyban, Wellbutrin) can be cautiously combined, but careful patient follow-up and lower haloperidol doses are required.

- buspirone (Buspar) may gradually increase haloperidol levels and lead to toxicity. Careful patient follow-up and adjustment of dose is prudent.
- dextromethorphan (**common cough suppressant in cough medicines**) may lead to dextromethorphan toxicity.
- fluoxetine (Prozac) can result in an increased risk of haloperidol toxicity.
- fluvoxamine (Luvox) can result in an increased risk of haloperidol toxicity.
- lithium (Lithobid, others) may cause toxic effects on the brain and nervous system.
- MAO inhibitors (see Drug Classes) may exaggerate low blood pressure and brain (CNS) effects.
- methyldopa (Aldomet) may cause serious dementia.
- olanzapine (Zyprexa) may lead to Parkinson-like symptoms.
- paroxetine (Paxil) may lead to haloperidol toxicity.
- quinidine (Quinaglute, others) may lead to haloperidol toxicity.
- QT interval–prolonging medicines (see Glossary) such as some fluoro-quinolone antibiotics, quinidine (Quinaglute), Ziprasidone (Geodon), and others (including a number of antiarrhythmic medicines) should NOT be combined.
- ritonavir (Norvir) and perhaps other protease inhibitors (see Drug Classes) may lead to toxicity.
- sertraline (Zoloft) may lead to haloperidol toxicity.
- sparfloxacin (Zagam) may lead to abnormal heartbeats.
- tacrine (Cognex) may lead to Parkinson-like symptoms.
- tramadol (Ultram) may lead to seizures.
- venlafaxine (Effexor) may lead to haloperidol toxicity.
- zotepine (Nipolept) may lead to seizures.

The following drugs may *decrease* the effects of haloperidol:

- antacids containing aluminum and/or magnesium, which may reduce its absorption.
- barbiturates.
- benztropine (Cogentin).
- carbamazepine (Tegretol).
- phenytoin (Dilantin) or fosphenytoin (Cerebyx).
- rifampin (Rifater, others).
- trihexyphenidyl (Artane).

▷ *Driving, Hazardous Activities:* This drug may impair mental alertness, judgment, and physical coordination. Restrict activities as necessary.

Aviation Note: The use of this drug *is a disqualification* for piloting. Consult a designated Aviation Medical Examiner.

Exposure to Sun: Use caution—this drug can cause photosensitivity. See Herbal Medicines note on St. John's wort.

Exposure to Heat: Use caution in hot environments. This drug may impair the regulation of body temperature and increase the risk of heatstroke.

Exposure to Cold: This drug can increase the risk of hypothermia (see Glossary) in the elderly.

Discontinuation: This drug should not be stopped abruptly following long-term use. Gradual withdrawal over a period of 2 to 3 weeks is advised. Ask your doctor for help.

HISTAMINE (H2)-BLOCKING DRUG FAMILY

Cimetidine (si MET i deen)   **Famotidine** (fa MOH te deen)   **Nizatidine** (ni ZA te deen)   **Ranitidine** (ra NI te deen)

Introduced: 1977, 1986, 1988, 1983, respectively **Class:** Histamine (H2)-blocking drugs **Prescription:** USA: Yes **Controlled Drug:** USA: No; Canada: No **Available as Generic:** USA: Yes (prescription forms cimetidine and ranitidine) and Tagamet HB; Canada: Yes

Brand Names: *Cimetidine:* ✤Apo-Cimetidine, ✤Enlon, ✤Novo-Cimetine, ✤Nu-Cimet, ✤Peptol, Tagamet [nonprescription: Tagamet HB 200, Acid Reducer 200, Acid Reducer Cimetidine, Heartburn 200, Heartburn Relief 200]; *Famotidine:* Pepcid [nonprescription: Pepcid AC, Pepcid Complete (CD), ✤Acid Control, Acid Controller], ✤Alti-famotidine; *Nizatidine:* ✤Apo-Nizatidine, Axid, ✤Novo-Nizatidine [nonprescription: Axid AR]; *Ranitidine:* ✤Alti-ranitidine, ✤ Apo-Ranitidine, Novo-Ranidine, Nu-Ranit, Zantac, ✤Zantac-C [nonprescription: Zantac 75, Zantac 75 EFFER-dose, Acid Reducer]

Warning: The brand names Zantac and Xanax are similar and can be mistaken. These are very different drugs, and a mix-up can lead to serious problems. Check the color chart insert of drugs and verify that you are taking the correct drug.

BENEFITS versus RISKS

Possible Benefits

EFFECTIVE TREATMENT OF GERD AND PEPTIC ULCERS IN CHILDREN (FAMOTIDINE ONLY)
EFFECTIVE TREATMENT OF PEPTIC ULCER DISEASE: relief of symptoms, acceleration of healing, prevention of recurrence
CONTROL OF HYPERSECRETORY STOMACH DISORDERS
TREATMENT OF REFLUX ESOPHAGITIS
TREATMENT OF HEARTBURN
PREVENTION OF HEARTBURN (cimetidine, ranitidine, famotidine, and nizatidine)

Possible Risks

Drug-induced hepatitis
Bone marrow depression (lowered white blood cells or hemoglobin)
Confusion (particularly in compromised elderly with some of these drugs)
Low blood platelet counts
(All of the above are case report to rare effects for prescription forms; occasional use of nonprescription forms makes them even less likely)

Author's Note: The nonprescription heartburn-preventing or treating forms of these medicines have, in general, side effects or adverse effects that occur less frequently or not at all when compared to the already well-tolerated prescription forms. Some doctors are using proton pump inhibitors (see Drug Classes) during the day combined with a dose of a histamine H2 blocker at night in order to gain improved acid control.

▷ **Principal Uses**

As a Single Drug Product: Uses currently included in FDA-approved labeling: (1) Treatment and prevention of repeat (recurrence) of peptic ulcer in adults; (2) all are used for both duodenal and gastric ulcers; (3) cimetidine,

ranitidine, and famotidine are used in conditions where extreme production of stomach acid occurs (Zollinger-Ellison syndrome); (4) all four medicines are used to control excess acid moving from the stomach into the
lower throat (gastroesophageal reflux disease—GERD); (5) cimetidine is
approved for use in preventing upper stomach/intestinal bleeding (stress
ulcer prophylaxis); (6) all have been used with antibiotics and bismuth
compounds (Pepto-Bismol and others) in refractory ulcers where *Helicobacter pylori* has been found; (7) cimetidine is approved to prevent ulcers
caused by stress (stress ulcer prophylaxis); (8) all are approved in nonprescription forms for treatment of heartburn—cimetidine (Tagamet HB
200), famotidine (Pepcid AC), and nizatidine (Axid AR) are also approved
for prevention of heartburn; (9) famotidine, ranitidine are approved for
treatment of stomach (peptic) ulcers and GERD in children; (10) cimetidine if approved to treat abnormal growths, which can increase acid
release (multiple endocrine adenomas, systemic mastocytosis).

Other (unlabeled) generally accepted uses: (1) Ranitidine, famotidine, and
nizatidine have been used in the prevention of upper stomach/intestinal
bleeding; (2) cimetidine has been used prior to surgery to prevent aspiration pneumonitis caused by anesthesia, and ranitidine has shown some
benefit here as well; (3) ranitidine and famotidine have been used to help
prevent ulcers that may occur in acutely and seriously ill patients; (4)
cimetidine appears to have a role in helping patients with colorectal cancer and some other cancers live longer, but further research is needed; (5)
famotidine may have a role in treating anaphylactic reactions; (6) cimetidine also may have a role in helping recurrent and resistant warts in some
children; (7) cimetidine intravenously has been helpful in some cases of
severe drug reactions (resistant drug-induced anaphylactic shock); (8)
nizatidine may help by inhibiting weight gain (earlier plateau) in people
taking olanzapine (Zyprexa).

How These Drugs Work: They block the action of histamine and, by doing this,
inhibit the ability of the stomach to make acid. Once acid is decreased, the
body is able to heal itself. Ulcers resistant to healing have now been shown
to have an infectious component (*Helicobacter pylori*), and antibiotics
combined with a histamine (H2)-blocking drug can work.

▷ **Widely Used Guidelines That Involve This Medicine (representative sample):** Please look at the section at the very beginning of this profile called
"Class." Next, turn to Table 22 and you will find guidelines listed by the
class involved!

Available Dosage Forms and Strengths
  Cimetidine:
                    Injection — 300 mg/2 mL, 300 mg/50 mL (single dose in
                          0.9% sodium chloride)
                    Liquid — 300 mg/5 mL (2.8% alcohol)
              Oral solution — 300 mg/5 mL
                    Tablets — 100 mg, 200 mg, 300 mg, 400 mg, 600 mg,
                          800 mg
      Tablets (nonprescription) — 200 mg
  Famotidine:
                    Injection — 10 mg/mL (in 2- and 4-mL vials)
              Oral suspension — 40 mg/5 mL
                    Tablets — 20 mg, 40 mg
      Tablets (nonprescription) — 10 mg

Nizatidine:
     Pulvules (capsules) — 75 mg, 150 mg, 300 mg
  Tablets (nonprescription) — 75 mg
Ranitidine:
          Gelcap — 168 mg, 336 mg (Canada only)
   GELdose capsules — 150 mg, 300 mg
          Injection — 0.5 mg/mL (single dose in 100 mL)
                  25 mg/mL (in 2-, 10-, and 40-mL vials and 2-mL
                  syringes)
  Oral solution (Canada) — 84 mg/5 mL
          Syrup — 15 mg/mL (7.5% alcohol)
          Tablets — 150 mg, 300 mg (effervescent)
                  150 mg
  Tablets (nonprescription) — 5 mg

▷ **Recommended Dosage Ranges** (Actual dose and schedule must be determined
   for each patient individually.)
   Infants and Children:
   Cimetidine: Routine use is not recommended in those less than 16 years old.
     Doses of 20 to 40 mg per kg of body mass per day have been used.
   Famotidine: GERD—1 mg per kg per day separated into two equal daily doses.
     Peptic ulcer—0.5 mg per kg of body mass at bedtime or divided into two
     equal doses up to a total of 40 mg per day (children).
   Nizatidine: No data.
   Ranitidine: GERD: For those 2 to 18 years old—1.25 to 2 mg per kg of body
     mass per dose given every 12 hours, or 37.5 mg per dose.
   16 to 60 Years of Age:
   Peptic ulcer and hypersecretory states:
   Cimetidine: 300 mg by mouth 4 times daily, taken with meals and at bedtime,
     or 800 mg at bedtime. A maintenance dose of 400 mg at bedtime is useful
     for some patients.
   Famotidine: 40 mg by mouth at bedtime for 4 or up to 8 weeks. Maintenance
     doses of 20 mg at bedtime have been used. Up to 640 mg daily for hyper-
     secretory states.
   Nizatidine: 300 mg by mouth at bedtime, or 150 mg twice a day for up to 8
     weeks. A maintenance dose of 150 mg at bedtime is useful for some
     patients. Not used for hypersecretory states.
   Ranitidine: 150 mg by mouth twice daily. Maintenance doses of 150 mg at bed-
     time may be of benefit for some patients. Up to 6 g in hypersecretory states.
   Heartburn (nonprescription forms):
   Cimetidine: 200 mg by mouth 30 minutes or less before eating foods or drink-
     ing liquids that cause you problems. May also be taken once heartburn has
     started.
   Famotidine: 10 mg by mouth before eating foods or drinking liquids that
     cause you problems or once heartburn has started.
   Nizatidine: 75 mg up to twice daily before eating foods or drinking liquids
     that cause you problems, or once heartburn has started.
   Ranitidine: 75 mg by mouth.
   Over 60 Years of Age:
   Cimetidine: Half the usual adult dose to start. Cimetidine may be more likely
     to cause confusion in the elderly than the other medicines in this family.
   Ranitidine, famotidine, and nizatidine: Same dose as 16 to 60 years of age. All
     pose a risk for formation of masses (phytobezoars) of undigested vegetable

fibers. Watch for nervousness, confusion, loss of appetite, stomach fullness, nausea, and vomiting.

Conditions Requiring Dosing Adjustments:
Liver Function: Cimetidine and famotidine are most dependent on the liver for elimination. Dose must be decreased in liver failure.
Kidney Function: All of these H2 blockers are primarily eliminated by the kidneys. Doses must be decreased in moderate kidney failure.

▷ **Dosing Instructions:** Cimetidine and ranitidine should be taken immediately after meals to obtain the longest decrease in stomach acid when treating peptic ulcers. Cimetidine, ranitidine, and famotidine should be taken after meals when used in hypersecretory states. If you forget a dose: take it as soon as you remember it, unless it's nearly time for your next dose—if that is the case, skip the missed dose and return to taking the medicine on your usual schedule. DO NOT double doses. Call your doctor if you find yourself forgetting doses.

Usual Duration of Use: Use on a regular schedule for 4 to 6 weeks usually determines effectiveness in healing active peptic ulcer disease. Long-term use (months to years) for prevention requires periodic individualized consideration by your physician. Continual use for 6 to 12 weeks is needed to heal the esophagus when cimetidine, ranitidine, famotidine, or nizatidine are used in gastroesophageal reflux disease (GERD). Since nonprescription forms are available for heartburn, if heartburn relief has not occurred in 2 hours, call your doctor, as there may be another medical reason for your signs and symptoms.

Typical Treatment Goals and Measurements (Outcomes and Markers)
Ulcers: The role of *Helicobacter pylori* in ulcers is no longer controversial—and omeprazole (a proton pump inhibitor) is widely recognized as the standard for short-term treatment of stomach ulcers. When *H. pylori* is present, single-medicine therapy is not recommended. Additionally, an antibiotic is often used with other agents. The goal is to heal the ulcer area and prevent re-occurrence of the ulceration. Sign and symptom relief as well as endoscopic examination help define success of treatment.
Heartburn: The general goal: to lessen the degree or severity of or to prevent heartburn. Some patients take the nonprescription forms BEFORE they eat foods that historically have given them heartburn. This issue of self-treatment should be discussed with your doctor, and if heartburn continues beyond the time you and your doctor have decided is reasonable, call your doctor.

Possible Advantages of These Drugs: Nonprescription forms offer relief of heartburn discomfort and the opportunity for effective self-care.

These Drugs Should Not Be Taken If
• you had an allergic reaction to the medicine itself or to the ingredients in the pill previously.

▷ **Inform Your Physician Before Taking These Drugs If**
• you have impaired liver or kidney function.
• you have a low sperm count (cimetidine).
• you are taking any anticoagulant drug.
• you do not tolerate or should not take phenylalanine (ranitidine EFFER-dose tablets or granules).
• you have had low white blood cell counts.
• you have a history of acute porphyria (ranitidine).

Possible Side Effects (natural, expected, and unavoidable drug actions)
None reported.

▷ **Possible Adverse Effects** (unusual, unexpected, and infrequent reactions)
If any of the following develop, consult your physician promptly for guidance.

Mild Adverse Effects
Allergic reactions: skin rash, hives.
Headache: ranitidine—rare; cimetidine—rare; famotidine—infrequent; nizatidine—frequent.
Abnormal dreams: nizatidine—rare.
Diarrhea: ranitidine, nizatidine, cimetidine, famotidine—all rare.
Joint pain (arthralgia): cimetidine, ranitidine, famotidine—all rare.
Depression: cimetidine—case reports.
Muscle pain: cimetidine, nizatidine, famotidine—rare.

Serious Adverse Effects
Allergic reactions: cimetidine and ranitidine can be rare causes of pancreatitis and anemia. Cimetidine and nizatidine can cause exfoliative dermatitis. There have been some case reports of serious skin rashes with all of these medicines, including toxic epidermal necrolysis (TEN).
Anaphylactic reactions: cimetidine, nizatidine—rare.
Idiosyncratic reactions: nervousness, confusion, hallucinations.
Worsening of Alzheimer's: cimetidine—case reports.
Liver damage—case reports.
Abnormal heart rhythm changes (slow heartbeat or atrioventricular block)—case reports.
Bone marrow depression: cimetidine, ranitidine, famotidine—rare.
Decreased platelets: cimetidine, ranitidine, nizatidine—rare; famotidine—case reports.
Bronchospasm: cimetidine and ranitidine—rare; famotidine—rare and questionable.

▷ **Possible Effects on Sexual Function:** Impotence: ranitidine, famotidine, cimetidine, nizatidine—case reports.
Decreased libido: cimetidine—rare.
Male breast enlargement (gynecomastia): nizatidine, cimetidine—case reports.

Possible Delayed Adverse Effects: Male breast enlargement (nizatidine and cimetidine).

▷ **Adverse Effects That May Mimic Natural Diseases or Disorders**
Liver changes may mimic viral hepatitis. Mental status changes from cimetidine in older patients may mimic organic causes.

Possible Effects on Laboratory Tests
Blood platelet counts: may be decreased by all histamine (H2) blockers.
Complete blood counts: rare white blood cell (granulocytes) decrease by cimetidine, ranitidine, and famotidine.
Urine protein tests (Multistix): false positive with ranitidine use.
Urine urobilinogen: false positive with nizatidine.
Thyroid hormones: T4, free T4 may be low with ranitidine use.
Liver enzymes (SGPT, OT, etc.): can be increased with liver damage.
Sperm count: decreased with cimetidine.

CAUTION
1. Ulcer rebound/perforation may occur if you stop these drugs abruptly when they are being used to treat ulcers.

2. Once medicines are stopped, call your doctor promptly if symptoms recur.

3. Use of these medicines and symptom relief does not absolutely remove possibility of cancer of the stomach (gastric malignancy).

4. The nonprescription forms of these medicines should NOT be used to treat ulcers.

5. Some of cimetidine is removed by hemodialysis. Additional doses are needed.

6. Cimetidine may worsen thinking ability (mental status) in those older patients with pre-existing mental status problems.

Precautions for Use

By Infants and Children:

Cimetidine: Routine use is not recommended in those less than 16 years old. Doses of 20 to 40 mg per kg of body mass per day have been used.

Famotidine: 0.5 mg per kg of body mass twice a day for 8 weeks in those 6 to 15 years old.

Nizatidine: No data.

Ranitidine: For those 2 to 18 years old—1.25 to 2 mg per kg of body mass per dose given every 12 hours, or 37.5 mg per dose.

By Those Over 60 Years of Age: Increased risk of masses of partially digested vegetable fibers (phytobezoars), especially in people who can't chew well. Watch closely for decreased appetite, stomach fullness, nausea, and vomiting. Watch those in this age range who are taking cimetidine for changes in thinking (mental status changes).

▷ **Advisability of Use During Pregnancy**

Pregnancy Category: B for all. See Pregnancy Risk Categories at the back of this book.

Animal Studies: No birth defects for cimetidine, ranitidine, and famotidine. Rabbit studies of nizatidine showed abortions, while rat studies showed no effects.

Human Studies: Adequate studies of pregnant women are not available. Use only if clearly needed. Ask your doctor for advice.

Advisability of Use If Breast-Feeding

Presence of these drugs in breast milk: Yes.

Avoid drugs or refrain from nursing.

Habit-Forming Potential: None.

Effects of Overdose:

Cimetidine (rarely documented): confusion, tachycardia, sweating, drowsiness, muscle twitching, seizures, respiratory failure, severe CNS symptoms such as coma (after 20–40 g).

Nizatidine (rarely documented): increased tearing of the eyes, salivation, vomiting, and diarrhea.

Ranitidine and famotidine: no documentation of overdose changes. Adverse effects of the usual dose. Symptomatic and supportive care would be indicated (nonprescription forms do not have documentation of overdoses).

Possible Effects of Long-Term Use: Rare liver damage with cimetidine, ranitidine, and nizatidine. Swelling and tenderness of breast tissue with cimetidine, ranitidine, and nizatidine.

Suggested Periodic Examinations While Taking These Drugs (at physician's discretion)

Complete blood counts.

Liver and kidney function tests.

More frequent tests of INR (prothrombin time) if an anticoagulant is also taken.

Sperm counts (cimetidine).

Thinking ability (mental status check).

▷ **While Taking These Drugs, Observe the Following**

Foods: Protein-rich foods increase stomach acid secretion (even milk). Garlic, onions, citrus fruits, and tomatoes may also increase acid secretion. Many people know the kinds of foods that are likely to result in significant heartburn. Ask your doctor or pharmacist for help in timing the dose of a nonprescription agent for heartburn.

Herbal Medicines or Minerals: Kola, cranberry, and ma huang (no longer on the market as a weight loss agent) may increase stomach acid, blunting the benefits of these medicines. Black cohosh root, ginkgo, and squill are contraindicated in gastrointestinal disturbances. Licorice root has a German Commission E monograph indication for gastrointestinal ulcers, but use with H2 blockers has not been studied. Some members of this family have increased sun sensitivity. Caution is advised if St. John's wort is being considered. Talk to your doctor BEFORE adding any herbals to these medicines.

Nutritional Support: Diet as prescribed by your doctor.

Beverages: The caffeine in caffeine-containing beverages such as coffee, tea, and some sodas may stay in the body up to 50% longer than usual with cimetidine (Tagamet) use. Milk may increase acid secretion.

▷ *Alcohol:* Stomach acidity is increased by alcohol—avoid use. Cimetidine may produce a drug interaction with higher-than-expected levels.

Tobacco Smoking: Smoking is a clear risk factor for peptic ulcer disease. I advise everyone to quit smoking.

Marijuana Smoking: Possible additive reduction in sperm counts with cimetidine use.

▷ *Other Drugs*

Cimetidine may *increase* the effects of

- amiodarone (Cordarone).
- amitriptyline (Elavil) and perhaps other tricyclic antidepressants (see Drug Classes). Decreased doses may be needed if the medicines are to be combined.
- amoxapine (Ascendin).
- amprenavir (Agenerase).
- benzodiazepines (Librium, Valium, etc.; see Drug Classes).
- carbamazepine (Tegretol), with increased toxicity risk. Blood level checks are recommended and ongoing carbamazepine doses adjusted to blood levels.
- carvedilol (Coreg) and increased patient monitoring is prudent.
- cyclosporine (Sandimmune, others) may result in increased blood levels and cyclosporine toxicity.
- dofetilide (Tikosyn) may result in increased blood levels and dofetilide toxicity.
- flecainide (Tambocor) and require dosing changes and more frequent blood level checks.
- loratadine (Claritin), by causing a large increase in blood levels. A study did NOT report any adverse effects on the heart from these levels, but since excessive blood levels of any medicine may be more likely to cause undesirable effects, it appears prudent to lower loratadine doses if these medicines are to be combined.

- meperidine (Demerol, others) and result in toxicity with potential respiratory depression, and low blood pressure.
- metformin (Glucophage) (increasing risk of lactic acidosis)—reduced doses are prudent.
- metoprolol (Lopressor, others), and perhaps other beta-blockers (see Drug Classes), and result in very slow heartbeat and excessively low blood pressure.
- morphine (MS Contin, MSIR, others) and result in central nervous system depression and respiratory depression.
- oral anticoagulants, with increased risk of bleeding; increased frequency of INR testing is recommended.
- pentoxifylline (Trental) (excessively low blood pressure, sweating, seizures).
- phenytoin (Dilantin).
- procainamide (Procan, Pronestyl).
- propranolol (Inderal).
- quetiapine (Seroquel).
- quinidine (Quinaglute).
- sertraline (Zoloft).
- sildenafil (Viagra) may increase blood levels of sildenafil by up to 56% (800 mg cimetidine dose). Talk to your doctor about this BEFORE using these medicines together.
- sirolimus (Rapamune) may result in increased blood levels and sirolimus toxicity.
- some statin-type medicines for cholesterol (fluvastatin-Lescol and perhaps others removed from the body in similar fashion) may result in increased blood levels and fluvastatin toxicity. Watch for unexplained muscle ache, weakness, and call your doctor if these occur.
- tacrolimus (Prograf) may result in increased blood levels and tacrolimus toxicity.
- tamsulosin (Flomax) may result in increased blood levels and tamsulosin.
- terbinafine (Lamisil).
- theophylline (Theo-Dur, etc.).
- venlafaxine (Effexor).
- warfarin (Coumadin).
- zaleplon (Sonata) may result in increased blood levels and zaleplon toxicity. A 5 mg dose of zaleplon is prudent in people who require both medicines.
- zolmitriptan (Zomig) may result in increased blood levels and zolmitriptan toxicity.

Ranitidine may *increase* the effects of
- diazepam (Valium).
- fluvastatin (Lescol).
- glipizide (Glucotrol) and perhaps other oral antidiabetic drugs (see Drug Classes).
- metformin (Glucophage).
- midazolam (Versed).
- procainamide (Procan, Pronestyl).
- theophylline (Theo-Dur, etc.).
- warfarin (Coumadin)—rarely; increased INR testing is recommended.

Nizatidine, ranitidine and famotidine (prescription forms) may *increase* the effects of
- amoxicillin.
- high-dose aspirin (may increase level and toxicity risk).

- pentoxifylline (Trental); however, this interaction has only been documented with cimetidine.
- theophylline (Theo-Dur, others); ongoing theophylline dosing should be based on more frequent blood levels if these medicines are to be taken together.

Cimetidine *taken concurrently* with

- most calcium channel blockers (see Drug Classes) may result in increased blood levels of the calcium channel blockers and potential toxicity; decreased calcium channel–blocker doses may be needed. This may also occur with other H2 blockers, and caution is advised.
- carmustine (BiCNU) may cause severe bone marrow depression.
- carvedilol (Coreg) may result in increased blood levels and carvedilol toxicity.
- chloroquine may result in toxicity and may cause cardiac arrest.
- cisapride (Propulsid) may result in increased cisapride levels and a potentially serious increase in heart rate.
- clozapine (Clozaril) may result in increased blood levels and clozapine toxicity.
- digoxin (Lanoxin) may result in changes in digoxin levels.
- oral hypoglycemic agents such as glipizide (Glucotrol), glyburide (DiaBeta, Micronase), and tolbutamide (Tolinase, others) may result in severe low blood sugars and seizures.
- paroxetine (Paxil) and perhaps other SSRI antidepressants (see Drug Classes) may result in increased blood levels of the SSRI and require dosing changes.
- pentoxifylline (Trental) may result in increases in blood levels of pentoxifylline; pentoxifylline dose changes may be needed.
- ritonavir (Norvir), amprenavir (Agenerase), atazanavir (Reyataz), and perhaps other protease inhibitors may result in increased cimetidine levels.
- zalcitabine (Hivid) may result in increased blood levels of zalcitabine and result in toxicity; decreased doses of zalcitabine may be needed.

Cimetidine, ranitidine, famotidine, and nizatidine *taken concurrently* with

- antacids will result in a decreased histamine-blocker level; it may be prudent to separate the dosing of these medicines (prescription forms) by an hour.
- delavirdine (Rescriptor) will result in a decreased amount of delavirdine getting into the body. Ongoing use of this combination of medicines is not advisable.

Cimetidine may *decrease* the effects of

- indomethacin (Indocin) and perhaps other NSAIDs, by decreasing absorption.
- iron salts, by decreasing absorption.
- ketoconazole, itraconazole, and fluconazole—taking cimetidine two hours after these medicines coupled with careful patient follow-up is prudent. The uncomplicated way to address this is to talk to your doctor about taking the antifungal with a cola beverage (low pH).
- tetracyclines, by decreasing absorption.

Ranitidine, nizatidine, and famotidine may *decrease* the effects of

- indomethacin, by decreasing absorption.
- ketoconazole, itraconazole, and fluconazole. The uncomplicated way to address this is to talk to your doctor about taking the antifungal with a cola beverage (low pH).
- sucralfate (Carafate).

▷ *Driving, Hazardous Activities:* Use caution until the degree of confusion, dizziness, or other effect is seen.

Aviation Note: The use of these drugs (prescription forms) *may be a disqualification* for piloting. Consult a designated Aviation Medical Examiner.

Exposure to Sun: Rare and questionable association with some medicines in this family. Use caution with sun exposure when first starting this medicine.

Occurrence of Unrelated Illness: Idiopathic thrombocytopenic purpura (ITP), a rare lowering of blood platelets, is a contraindication for use of any of these medicines. Aplastic anemia, whatever the cause, may be worsened by cimetidine. If symptoms of heartburn get worse, you experience unexplained weight loss and are over 45 years old, talk with your doctor—this may be an indication of stomach cancer.

Discontinuation: **Do not stop these medicines suddenly if they are being taken for peptic ulcer disease.** Ask your doctor for withdrawal instructions. Be alert to the recurrence of ulcers any time after these drugs are stopped. Recurrent or refractory ulcers may also represent an infectious disease caused by *Helicobacter pylori*. If this is the case, combination therapy with an antibiotic may be indicated.

HYDRALAZINE (hi DRAL a zeen)

Introduced: 1950   **Class:** Antihypertensive   **Prescription:** USA: Yes   **Controlled Drug:** USA: No; Canada: No   **Available as Generic:** USA: Yes; Canada: No

Brand Names: Alazine, Alphapress, Apo-Hydralazine, Apresazide [CD], Apresoline, Apresoline-Esidrix [CD], Cam-Ap-Es, Dralserp, Dralzine, H-H-R, Hydroserpine [CD], Hyserp [CD], Lo-Ten, Marpres, Novo-Hylazin, Nu-Hydral, Ser-A-Gen [CD], Ser-Ap-Es [CD], Serpasil-Apresoline [CD], Serprex [CD], Supres [CD], Tri-Hydroserpine, Unipres [CD], Uniserp [CD]

Author's Note: The information in this profile has been shortened to make room for more widely used medicines.

HYDROCHLOROTHIAZIDE (hi droh klor oh THI a zide)

Please see the thiazide diuretics family profile.

HYDROCODONE (hi droh KOH dohn)

Other Name: Dihydrocodeinone   **Introduced:** 1951   **Class:** Analgesic, strong; cough suppressant; opioid   **Prescription:** USA: Yes   **Controlled Drug:** USA: C-III*; Canada: Yes   **Available as Generic:** USA: Yes, hydrocodone/APAP; Canada: No

Brand Names: Allay [CD], Alor 5/500 [CD], Anaplex, Anexsia [CD], Anexsia 7.5 [CD], Anolor DH5, Atuss [CD], Azdone [CD], Ban-Tuss-HC [CD], ✿Biohisdex DHC [CD], ✿Biohisdine DHC [CD], Chemdal-HD [CD], Codone, Detussin [CD], DHC Plus, Dicoril, Dimetane Expectorant-DC [CD], Dolacet [CD], Duocet [CD], Duratuss HD [CD], Endagen HD [CD], Endal-HD, Entuss-D, Histinex-HC [CD], Histussin HC [CD], ✿Hycodan, Hycodan

*See Schedules of Controlled Drugs at the back of this book.

[CD], ✤Hycomine [CD], Hycomine Compound [CD], Hycomine Pediatric Syrup [CD], ✤Hycomine-S [CD], Hycomine Syrup [CD], Hyco-tuss Expectorant [CD], Lorcet-HD [CD], Lorcet Plus [CD], Lortab [CD], Lortab ASA [CD], Medipain 5, Norcet 7 [CD], ✤Novahistex DH [CD], ✤Novahistine DH [CD], Polygesic, Protuss, ✤Robidone, Ru-Tuss [CD], T-Gesic [CD], Triaminic Expectorant DH [CD], ✤Tussaminic Expectorant DH [CD], Tussend [CD], Tussend Expectorant [CD], Tussionex [CD], Tycolet [CD], Vanex [CD], Vicodin [CD], Vicodin ES [CD], Vicoprofen [CD], Zydone [CD]

BENEFITS versus RISKS

Possible Benefits	Possible Risks
EFFECTIVE RELIEF OF MILD TO MODERATE PAIN	Mild allergic reactions—infrequent
	Nausea, constipation
EFFECTIVE CONTROL OF COUGH	Potential for addiction apparently greater than codeine

---

▷ **Principal Uses**

As a Single Drug Product: Uses currently included in FDA-approved labeling: (1) Controls cough; (2) relieves mild to moderate pain.

Other (unlabeled) generally accepted uses: May be a benefit for some patients with chronic obstructive lung disease (COPD).

As a Combination Drug Product [CD]: Often added to cough mixtures containing antihistamines, decongestants, and expectorants to increase effectiveness in reducing cough. Also combined with analgesics, such as acetaminophen and aspirin and other nonsteroidal anti-inflammatory (NSAID) compounds, to enhance pain relief.

Author's Note: Information in this profile has been shortened to make room for more widely used medicines.

HYDROXYCHLOROQUINE (hi drox ee KLOR oh kwin)

Introduced: 1967 **Class:** Antimalarial, immunosuppressant **Prescription:** USA: Yes **Controlled Drug:** USA: No; Canada: No **Available as Generic:** USA: Yes; Canada: No

Brand Names: ✤Dermoplast, Plaquenil

BENEFITS versus RISKS

Possible Benefits	Possible Risks
EFFECTIVE PREVENTION AND TREATMENT OF CERTAIN FORMS OF MALARIA	INFREQUENT DAMAGE OF CORNEAL AND RETINAL EYE TISSUES
Effective in the management of acute and chronic rheumatoid arthritis in adults who have not responded to less toxic medicines	BONE MARROW DEPRESSION
	Heart muscle damage
	Ear damage: hearing loss, ringing in ears
Possibly effective in management of chronic discoid and systemic lupus erythematosus	

▷ **Principal Uses**
   As a Single Drug Product: Uses currently included in FDA-approved labeling:
      (1) Prevention and therapy of acute attacks of certain types of malaria; (2)
      reduces disease activity in rheumatoid arthritis in adults who have not
      responded to less toxic medicines; (3) suppresses disease activity in
      chronic discoid and systemic lupus erythematosus.
   Other (unlabeled) generally accepted uses: (1) Treatment of Sjögren's syn-
      drome; (2) treats refractory Lyme arthritis; (3) therapy of sarcoidosis, poly-
      morphous light eruption, porphyria, solar urticaria, and chronic vasculitis;
      (4) may help decrease steroid requirements in asthma; (5) can help
      decrease insulin needs when an oral hypoglycemic agent is taken with
      insulin; (6) combination therapy of Weber-Christian disease.

How This Drug Works: In malaria, this drug impairs DNA in the organisms. As
   an antiarthritic and antilupus drug, acts as a mild immunosuppressant.
   Accumulates in white blood cells and inhibits many enzymes involved in
   tissue destruction.

▷ **Widely Used Guidelines That Involve This Medicine (representative sample):** Please look at the section at the very beginning of this profile called
   "Class." Next, turn to Table 22 and you will find guidelines listed by the
   class involved!

Available Dosage Forms and Strengths
   Tablets — 200 mg

▷ **Usual Adult Dosage Ranges**
   For malaria suppression: 400 mg once every 7 days. Treatment starts 2 weeks
      before entering an area where malaria is present and continues for
      8 weeks after returning. If treatment is not started before going into an
      area where malaria is likely (endemic), 800 mg should be the initial dose
      (can be given as two 400 mg doses 6 hours apart).
   For malaria treatment: (1) 800 mg as a single dose or (2) initially 800 mg, fol-
      lowed by 400 mg in 6 to 8 hours; then 400 mg once a day on the second
      and third days.
   For pediatric malaria treatment: 10 mg per kg of body mass followed in 6 hours
      by 5 mg per kg of body mass, with 5 mg per kg of body mass given 18 hours
      after the second dose; then 5 mg per kg of body mass taken 24 hours after
      the first dose.
   For lupus erythematosus: 400 mg once or twice daily. This is used for several
      weeks or cautiously until remission. Ongoing dose is 200–400 mg daily.
   For rheumatoid arthritis: Starting dose of 400 to 600 mg and an ongoing dose of
      200–400 mg a day.
   **Note: Actual dose and schedule must be determined for each patient
   individually.**

Conditions Requiring Dosing Adjustments
   Liver Function: Benefit-to-risk decision by patients with liver compromise or
      who take liver-toxic drugs.
   Kidney Function: Use with caution in kidney compromise.

▷ **Dosing Instructions:** Take with food or milk to reduce stomach irritation. The
   tablet may be crushed and mixed with jam, jelly, or gelatin. Take it exactly
   as prescribed.
   **Author's Note: For malaria prevention, begin medication 2 weeks
   before entering malarious area; continue medication while in the
   area and for 8 weeks after leaving the area.**

For treating arthritis and lupus, take medication on a regular schedule daily; continual use for 6 months may be necessary to determine maximal benefit. If you forget a dose: take it as soon as you remember it, unless it's nearly time for your next dose—if that is the case, skip the missed dose and return to taking the medicine on your usual schedule. DO NOT double doses. If you only take one dose a week, call your doctor for instructions.

Usual Duration of Use: Use on a regular schedule for 2 weeks before exposure, during period of exposure and 8 weeks after exposure determines this drug's effectiveness in preventing attacks of malaria. Use on a regular schedule for up to 6 months may be required to evaluate benefits in reducing rheumatoid arthritis and lupus erythematosus. If significant improvement is not achieved in 6 months of treatment in rheumatoid arthritis, this drug should be stopped. Long-term use (months to years) requires periodic physician evaluation.

Possible Advantages of This Drug
Considered to have less potential for retinal toxicity than chloroquine.

Typical Treatment Goals and Measurements (Outcomes and Markers)
Rheumatoid arthritis: Most rheumatologists use sign and symptom control, joint mobility and pain as indicators of success of therapy. For clinicians treating pain, a device called an algometer is used to check your pain. This looks like a small ruler, but lets the clinician better understand your pain. The goals of treatment then relate to where the level of pain started (for example, a rating of 7 on a 0 to 10 scale) and what the cause of the pain was. Pain medicines may also be used together (in combination) in order to get the best result or outcome. If your pain control is not acceptable to YOU (remember, in hospitals and outpatient settings, etc. pain control is a patient right) and if results are not acceptable, be sure to call your doctor as you may need a different medicine or combination.

Currently a Drug of Choice
For the treatment of chronic discoid and systemic lupus erythematosus.

▷ This Drug Should Not Be Taken If
- you had past allergies to chloroquine or hydroxychloroquine.
- you have an active bone marrow or blood cell disorder.
- it was prescribed for long-term treatment in children (should not be used in that way).

▷ Inform Your Physician Before Taking This Drug If
- you are pregnant or planning pregnancy.
- you have had bone marrow depression or a blood cell disorder.
- you have a deficiency of glucose-6-phosphate dehydrogenase (G6PD)—talk with your doctor.
- you have any disorder of the eyes, especially disease of the cornea or retina or visual field changes.
- you have impaired hearing or ringing in the ears.
- you have a seizure disorder of any kind.
- you have a history of peripheral neuritis.
- you have low blood pressure or a heart rhythm disorder.
- you have peptic ulcer disease, Crohn's disease, or ulcerative colitis.
- you have impaired liver or kidney function.
- you have a history of porphyria.
- you have any form of psoriasis.
- you are taking antacids, cimetidine, digoxin, or penicillamine.

Possible Side Effects (natural, expected, and unavoidable drug actions)
> Light-headedness (low blood pressure); blue-black discoloration of skin, fingernails, or mouth lining with long-term use.

▷ **Possible Adverse Effects** (unusual, unexpected, and infrequent reactions)
If any of the following develop, consult your physician promptly for guidance.

Mild Adverse Effects
> Allergic reactions: skin rash, itching (more common in African Americans).
> Loss of hair color, loss of hair.
> Headache, blurring of near vision (reading), ringing in ears—possible to infrequent.
> Loss of appetite, nausea, vomiting, stomach cramps, diarrhea—infrequent.
> Dizziness—case reports.

Serious Adverse Effects
> Allergic reactions: severe skin rash, exfoliative dermatitis.
> Idiosyncratic reactions: hemolytic anemia in those with glucose-6-phosphate dehydrogenase (G6PD) deficiency in red blood cells.
> Emotional or psychotic mental changes; seizures—case reports.
> Loss of hearing, porphyria—case reports.
> Eye tissue damage, specifically cornea and retina, with significant impairment of vision—case reports.
> Aplastic anemia (see Glossary): abnormally low red blood cell counts (fatigue and weakness); abnormally low white blood cell counts (fever, sore throat, infections); abnormally low platelet counts (abnormal bruising or bleeding)—case reports.
> Muscle damage (myopathy)—case report.

▷ **Possible Effects on Sexual Function:** None reported.

Possible Delayed Adverse Effects: Irreversible eye (retinal) damage has developed 7 years after discontinuation of chloroquine, a closely related drug. Retinal damage is more likely to occur following high-dose and/or long-term use.

▷ **Adverse Effects That May Mimic Natural Diseases or Disorders**
> Central nervous system toxicity may suggest unrelated neuropsychiatric disorder. Seizures may suggest the onset of epilepsy.

Natural Diseases or Disorders That May Be Activated by This Drug
> Porphyria, psoriasis.

Possible Effects on Laboratory Tests
> Complete blood cell counts: decreased red cells, hemoglobin, white cells, and platelets.
> Liver function tests: increased liver enzymes (ALT/GPT, AST/GOT, and alkaline phosphatase), increased bilirubin.
> Electrocardiogram: conduction abnormalities, prolonged QRS interval, T-wave changes, and heart block have all been reported for chloroquine, a closely related drug.

CAUTION
1. Does not prevent relapses of certain types of malaria.
2. High-dose and/or long-term use of this drug may cause irreversible retinal damage, significant visual impairment, or hearing loss due to nerve damage. Report promptly any changes in vision or hearing so appropriate evaluation can be made.

3. If toxic signs and symptoms happen, ammonium chloride in a dose of 8 grams a day divided into equal doses may help removal of this drug in adults.

Precautions for Use

By Infants and Children: This age group is very sensitive to the effects of this drug. Doses should be determined and therapy should be monitored by a qualified pediatrician.

By Those Over 60 Years of Age: Tolerance for this drug may be reduced. Watch for behavioral changes, low blood pressure, heart rhythm disturbances, muscle weakness, and changes in vision or hearing.

▷ **Advisability of Use During Pregnancy**

Pregnancy Category: C. See Pregnancy Risk Categories at the back of this book.

Animal Studies: No information available.

Human Studies: Adequate studies of pregnant women are not available. However, closely related drugs of this class are known to cause abnormal retinal pigmentation and hemorrhage and congenital deafness in the fetus.

Avoid use during pregnancy except for the suppression or treatment of malaria. Other use is a benefit-to-risk decision.

Advisability of Use If Breast-Feeding

Presence of this drug in breast milk: Yes.

Avoid drug or refrain from nursing (controversial).

Habit-Forming Potential: None.

Effects of Overdose: Drowsiness, headache, blurred vision, excitability, low blood pressure, seizures, coma.

Possible Effects of Long-Term Use: Irreversible eye damage (cornea and retina), hearing loss, muscle weakness, aplastic anemia.

Suggested Periodic Examinations While Taking This Drug (at physician's discretion)

Complete blood cell counts.

Liver and kidney function tests.

Serial blood pressure readings and electrocardiograms.

Neurological examinations for significant muscle weakness.

Complete eye examinations before starting high-dose and/or long-term treatment and every 3 to 6 months during drug use.

Hearing tests as indicated.

▷ **While Taking This Drug, Observe the Following**

Foods: No restrictions.

Herbal Medicines or Minerals: Caution: St. John's wort may also cause extreme reactions to the sun. Additive photosensitivity may be possible. Hay flower, mistletoe herb, and white mustard seed carry German Commission E monograph indications for arthritis, but have not been studied with this medicine. Talk to your doctor BEFORE combining any herb with hydroxychloroquine.

Beverages: No restrictions. May be taken with milk.

▷ *Alcohol:* Use sparingly to minimize stomach irritation.

Tobacco Smoking: No interactions expected, but I advise everyone to quit smoking.

▷ *Other Drugs*

Hydroxychloroquine may **increase** the effects of
• aurothioglucose (Solganol), which increases risk of blood problems.
• digoxin (Lanoxin) and increase its toxic potential.

- metoprolol (Lopressor). Close follow-up of blood pressure and potential decrease in dose is prudent.
- penicillamine (Cuprimine, Depen) and increase its toxic potential.

The following drug may *increase* the effects of hydroxychloroquine:

- cimetidine (Tagamet).

The following drugs may **decrease** the effects of hydroxychloroquine:

- magnesium salts and antacids.

▷ *Driving, Hazardous Activities:* This drug may cause light-headedness, blurred vision, or impaired hearing. Restrict activities as necessary.

Aviation Note: The use of this drug *may be a disqualification* for piloting. Consult a designated Aviation Medical Examiner.

Exposure to Sun: Use caution until sensitivity has been determined. Closely related drugs of this class may cause photosensitivity (see Glossary and Herbal Medicines note on St. John's wort).

Discontinuation: This drug should be stopped and prompt evaluation should be made if any of the following develop—changes in vision or hearing, seizures, unusual muscle weakness, indications of infection (fever, sore throat, etc.), abnormal bruising or bleeding.

HYDROXYUREA (hi DROX EE yur ia)

Introduced: 1995 (AIDS or sickle cell)   **Class:**   Anti-AIDS, anticancer, anti-sickle-cell anemia   **Prescription:**   USA: Yes   **Controlled Drug:** USA: No; Canada: No   **Available as Generic:**   USA: Yes; Canada: No

Brand Names: Droxia, Hydrea, Mylocel

Warning: This drug is a cytotoxic agent. Appropriate precautions must be taken, as with other chemotherapy.

BENEFITS versus RISKS	
Possible Benefits	*Possible Risks*
COMBINATION TREATMENT OF AIDS	BONE MARROW SUPPRESSION
	Hepatitis
DECREASED SEVERITY AND FREQUENCY OF SICKLE-CELL CRISES	Possible secondary leukemia-causing agent (long-term 7–10 years of therapy)
Treatment of chronic myelocytic leukemia, melanoma, and other cancers	

▷ **Principal Uses**

As a Single Drug Product: Uses currently included in FDA-approved labeling: (1) Blast crisis; (2) chronic myelogenous leukemia; (3) head, neck, and ovarian cancers; (4) chronic leukemias; (5) cancers of certain cell types (squamous cell); (6) decreases frequency and severity of sickle-cell crises; (7) malignant melanoma.

Other (unlabeled) generally accepted uses: (1) Used to treat certain diseases of the red blood cells (polycythemia vera); (2) used in combination with other medicines to treat HIV-positive patients (possible first-line or salvage therapy); (3) brain cancer.

Author's Note: Combination therapy has become a standard of care. NIAID antiretroviral therapy guidelines take into account how easily HIV therapy can fit into a patient's life. The ATIS Guidelines tell us that therapy should be supervised by an expert and cover considerations of when to start therapy in both asymptomatic and established HIV infections. Adherence or taking medicines for HIV exactly on time and in the right amount is ABSOLUTELY critical to getting the best possible results or outcomes. Structured therapy interruptions (STI) or structured interruptions of therapy (SIT) are still controversial.

How This Drug Works: When used in cancer, this medicine is a cell-cycle-specific drug. It works in the S phase of mitosis. When used in HIV-positive patients, the exact mechanism of action is not fully understood. When used in sickle-cell patients, the specific mechanism has not been identified.

▷ **Widely Used Guidelines That Involve This Medicine (representative sample):** Please look at the section at the very beginning of this profile called "Class." Next, turn to Table 22 and you will find guidelines listed by the class involved!

Available Dosage Forms and Strengths
   Capsules (Droxia) — 200 mg, 300 mg, 400 mg
   Capsule (Hydrea) — 500 mg
   Tablet (Mylocel) — 1,000 mg

▷ **Recommended Dosage Ranges** (Actual dose and schedule must be determined for each patient individually.)
   Infants and Children: Safety and effectiveness have not been defined in this age group.
   18 to 60 Years of Age: All doses are decided based on ideal or actual body mass, whichever is less.
   Oral dosing: Usual oral doses range from 20 to 30 mg per kg of body mass per day, which is given as a single daily dose. Some centers give 80 mg per kg of body mass every third day. If a patient is in blast crisis, up to 12 g per day has been given to rapidly decrease white blood cell counts.
   In sickle-cell anemia: Starting dose of 15 mg per kg of body mass. Depending on the blood (hematologic) response, the dose is increased by 5 mg per kg of body mass every 12 weeks (unless toxicity occurs) to the maximum dose of 35 mg per kg of body mass per day or to the maximum dose less than 35 mg per kg that is tolerated.
   In HIV/AIDS: The protocols are still changing.
   Over 60 Years of Age: Same as 18 to 60 years of age.

Conditions Requiring Dosing Adjustments
   Liver Function: No changes in dosing are anticipated.
   Kidney Function: The dose must be decreased for patients with kidney compromise. Decreases of up to 80% are needed in severe compromise.

▷ **Dosing Instructions:** This medicine is best taken on an empty stomach. Do not crush, open, or alter the capsules. Call your doctor if you vomit after taking this medicine. If you forget a dose: take it as soon as you remember it, unless it's nearly time for your next dose—if that is the case, skip the missed dose and return to taking the medicine on your usual schedule. DO NOT double doses. Adherence with this medicine is very important. Follow-up with required laboratory testing is also critical. Call your doctor if you find yourself forgetting doses.

Usual Duration of Use: Continual use on a regular schedule for up to 16 weeks may be needed to treat cancers of the head and neck. Treatment in sickle-cell disease is ongoing, using the lowest effective dose.

Treatment in HIV-positive patients is yet to be defined.

Long-term use (months to years) requires periodic evaluation of response and dose adjustment. Consult your physician on a regular basis.

Typical Treatment Goals and Measurements (Outcomes and Markers)

Sickle-cell anemia: The severity and number of sickle-cell attacks is used as a marker for success when treating sickle-cell anemia. This medicine can also help decrease the number of sudden (acute) visits to the emergency room and subsequent hospitalizations for sickle-cell crisis.

Currently a Drug of Choice

For reducing the frequency and severity of sickle-cell crises in patients with sickle-cell disease.

▷ **This Drug Should Not Be Taken If**
- you had an allergic reaction to it previously.
- you have severely depressed bone marrow. This is seen in very low white blood cell, platelet, or hemoglobin levels (neutrophils less than 2,000, platelets less than 100,000 or severe anemia).

▷ **Inform Your Physician Before Taking This Drug If**
- you have signs or symptoms of cancer.
- you are considering pregnancy (males or females).
- you have had chemotherapy or radiation therapy previously.
- you have compromised kidneys.
- you have herpes zoster (shingles).
- you have recently been exposed to chicken pox.
- you are having unusual bruising or bleeding.
- you are unsure how to dispose of urine or vomit.
- you are unsure how much to take or how often to take it.
- you plan to breast-feed your baby.
- you take prescription or nonprescription medicines not discussed when hydroxyurea was prescribed.

Possible Side Effects (natural, expected, and unavoidable drug actions)

Hair loss, painful mouth sores, sensitivity to the sun, hair loss—rare.

▷ **Possible Adverse Effects** (unusual, unexpected, and infrequent reactions)

If any of the following develop, consult your physician promptly for guidance.

Mild Adverse Effects

Allergic reactions: skin rash and itching or fever.

Dizziness, disorientation, headaches, or fever—rare.

Nausea, vomiting, or diarrhea—frequent (vomiting usually mild).

Difficulty urinating—rare.

Ulceration of the skin—rare.

Serious Adverse Effects

Allergic reactions: skin ulceration—case reports.

Idiosyncratic reactions: not reported.

Bone marrow depression—possible.

Convulsions or hallucinations—rare.

Hepatitis or kidney problems—rare.

Drug-induced lupus erythematosus—case report.

Lung problems (acute interstitial lung disease)—rare.
Squamous cancer (carcinoma) or leukemia—possible increased risk.

▷ **Possible Effects on Sexual Function:** None reported.

Possible Delayed Adverse Effects: Bone marrow suppression, temporary decrease in kidney function.

▷ **Adverse Effects That May Mimic Natural Diseases or Disorders**
Liver toxicity may be similar to acute hepatitis.

Natural Diseases or Disorders That May Be Activated by This Drug
Not defined.

Possible Effects on Laboratory Tests
Liver function tests: increased.
Complete blood counts: decreases in several components.

CAUTION
1. This medicine is toxic to cells. Be certain your doctor has carefully explained how to dispose of urine or vomit.
2. Call your doctor at once if you have a seizure.
3. Both women and men should avoid conception for several months after taking this medicine.
4. Wash your hands after taking this medicine before you touch your eyes or your nose.

Precautions for Use
By Infants and Children: Safety and effectiveness for use by those under 18 years of age have not been established.
By Those Over 60 Years of Age: Lower doses are prudent, as increased sensitivity to any dose may occur. Natural declines in kidney function may require dose decrease.

▷ **Advisability of Use During Pregnancy**
Pregnancy Category: D. See Pregnancy Risk Categories at the back of this book.
Animal Studies: Causes birth defects in animals.
Human Studies: Adequate studies of pregnant women are not available.
Talk with your doctor about this benefit-to-risk decision.

Advisability of Use If Breast-Feeding
Presence of this drug in breast milk: Yes.
Avoid drug or refrain from nursing.

Habit-Forming Potential: None.

Effects of Overdose: Bone marrow depression, increased heart rate, liver cell and testicular damage.

Possible Effects of Long-Term Use: Bone marrow depression.

Suggested Periodic Examinations While Taking This Drug (at physician's discretion)
Complete blood cell counts.
Dental exams.

▷ **While Taking This Drug, Observe the Following**
Foods: No restrictions, but folic acid is recommended with Droxia treatment.
Herbal Medicines or Minerals: Some patients use echinacea to attempt to boost their immune systems. Unfortunately, use of echinacea is not recommended in people with damaged immune systems. This herb may also actually weaken any immune system if it is used too often or for too long a time. **Caution:** St. John's wort may also cause extreme reactions to the sun. Additive photosensitivity may be possible.
Beverages: No restrictions. May be taken with milk.

▷ *Alcohol:* Do not drink alcohol.

Tobacco Smoking: No interactions expected. I advise everyone to quit smoking.

▷ *Other Drugs*

Hydroxyurea *taken concurrently* with

- amphotericin (Abelcet) may increase risk of kidney toxicity and spasm of bronchi.
- didanosine (DDI) may increase risk of lactic acidosis.
- fluorouracil (Efudil) may increase toxicity to nerves.
- other medicines that cause bone marrow depression (see Table 5, Section Six) may lead to additive toxicity to bone marrow.
- stavudine (Zerit) may increase risk of lactic acidosis.
- vaccines (live virus, such as smallpox vaccine) may result in undesirable or life-threatening effects if immune system is depressed.

▷ *Driving, Hazardous Activities:* This drug may cause light-headedness, blurred vision, or impaired hearing. Restrict activities as necessary.

Aviation Note: The use of this drug *may be a disqualification* for piloting. Consult a designated Aviation Medical Examiner.

Exposure to Sun: Use caution until sensitivity has been determined. Closely related drugs of this class may cause photosensitivity (see Glossary). See Herbal Medicines caution on St. John's wort above.

Discontinuation: This drug should be stopped and prompt evaluation should be made if any of the following develop—changes in vision or hearing, seizures, unusual muscle weakness, indications of infection (fever, sore throat, etc.), abnormal bruising or bleeding.

IBANDRONATE (ih BAN droh nate)

Recently approved by the FDA for once-daily treatment of osteoporosis with the original name of Boniva (being changed due to a similarity in name with a different medicine at the time of this writing). Further research is being undertaken by the company to see if giving this medicine less often (such as every 14–21 days) will have beneficial effects. This profile will be broadened in future editions as clinical research warrants.

IBUPROFEN (i byu PROH fen is official pronunciation, EYE byu proh fen is the common one)

Please see the propionic acid (nonsteroidal anti-inflammatory drug) family profile.

IMATINIB (im ah TIN ib)

Introduced: 2001, February 2002 for GIST tumors   **Class:**   Protein-tyrosine kinase inhibitor, signal transduction inhibitor, pharmacogenomic, anticancer   **Prescription:**   USA: Yes   **Controlled Drug:**   USA: No; Canada: No   **Available as Generic:**   No

Brand Name: Gleevec

```
┌─────────────────────────────────────────────────────────────────┐
│                    BENEFITS versus RISKS                          │
│     Possible Benefits              Possible Risks                 │
│ EFFECTIVE TREATMENT OF         HEMATOLOGICAL TOXICITY             │
│   CHRONIC MYELOID LEUKEMIA     EDEMA (MAY BE SEVERE)              │
│   (IN BLAST CRISIS,            Liver toxicity                     │
│   ACCELERATED PHASE OR IN      Opportunistic infections (with long-│
│   CHRONIC PHASE AFTER            term use in animals)            │
│   FAILURE OF INTERFERON-                                          │
│   ALPHA THERAPY)                                                  │
│ APPROVED FOR TREATING KIT                                         │
│   (CD117) POSITIVE                                                │
│   GASTROINTESTINAL STROMAL                                        │
│   TUMORS (GIST) THAT ARE NOT                                      │
│   RESECTABLE OR HAVE SPREAD                                       │
│   (METASTATIC)                                                    │
│ TREATS PEDIATRIC PATIENTS                                         │
│   WITH Ph+ (PHILADELPHIA                                          │
│   POSITIVE) CHRONIC MYELOID                                       │
│   LEUKEMIA IN CHRONIC PHASE                                       │
└─────────────────────────────────────────────────────────────────┘
```

▷ **Principal Uses**

As a Single Drug Product: Uses currently included in FDA-approved labeling: (1) Treats patients with chronic myeloid leukemia (CML) who are in blast crisis, accelerated phase or who are in chronic phase after failure of interferon-alpha therapy; (2) works in gastrointestinal stromal tumors (GIST) that are unresectable or that have spread (metastasized); (3) Treats pediatric patients who are Ph+ (Philadelphia chromosome positive) in chronic phase (for children who have had the disease happen again [recur]) after stem cell transplant or in those children who are resistant to interferon treatment.

Other (unlabeled) generally accepted uses: (1) One small study in people with resistant (refractory) rheumatoid arthritis with further study needed.

In the Pipeline: In leukemia patients treated with imatinib (Gleevec), filgrastim was successfully used to mobilize peripheral blood stem cells (PBSC) in people who achieved complete cytogenetic response (CCR). The yield of CD 34+ cells was improved when imatinib was withheld temporarily (see Hui, C.H. in Sources).

How This Drug Works: By inhibiting protein kinase, this medicine inhibits the Bcr-Abl abnormal kinase required by Philadelphia chromosome–positive chronic myelogenous leukemia cells. This works to stop the abnormal and excessive number of white blood cells seen in that kind of leukemia. In GIST tumors, this signal transduction inhibitor (STI) interferes with a gene named c-kit, which makes cells divide and multiply when the gene is stuck in the "on" position.

▷ **Widely Used Guidelines That Involve This Medicine (representative sample):** Please look at the section at the very beginning of this profile called "Class." Next, turn to Table 22 and you will find guidelines listed by the class involved!

Available Dosage Forms and Strengths

Capsules — 50 mg (Canada), 100 mg, 400 mg

▷ **Usual Adult Dosage Ranges**

Chronic phase chronic myelogenous leukemia (CML): 400 mg is given daily. This dose should be taken at the same time each day with a meal and a large glass of water. In patients who do not get an acceptable initial response (see below) dose increases have been used, with ongoing chronic phase dose of 600 mg once daily.

Blast crisis or accelerated phase CML: 600 mg daily. The dose should be taken at the same time each day with a meal and a large glass of water. If patients fail to get an acceptable response, dose increase to 800 mg (given as 400 mg twice a day) has been used by some clinicians.

Unresectable and/or metastatic, malignant GIST: CD 117–positive patients are given 400 mg to 600 mg a day as a starting dose. Careful dosing adjustment should be made by a qualified specialist (for example, in people also getting medicines that increase the liver enzymes that remove this drug-CYP 450 3A4 inducers).

Note: Actual dose and schedule must be determined for each patient individually.

Conditions Requiring Dosing Adjustments

Liver Function: Not studied in patients with compromised liver function. If liver bilirubin increases by 3 times the upper limit of normal (ULN), or if other liver function tests (liver transaminases) increase by 5 times the ULN, imatinib should be held until bilirubin levels have lowered to 1.5 ULN or transaminase levels to less than 2.5 ULN. Once those conditions are met, therapy can continue at a reduced daily dose.

Kidney Function: Not studied in patients with decreased kidney (renal) function. Clinical trials specifically excluded those with serum creatinine levels more than 2 times the upper limit of normal. Metabolites and imatinib itself are not significantly removed by the kidney.

▷ **Dosing Instructions:** Doses should be taken at the same time each day with a meal and a large glass of water (lessens stomach and intestine-gastrointestinal tract–irritation). If increases in bilirubin or liver enzymes develop, dosing instructions above should be followed. If severe lowering of white blood cells (neutropenia) or severe lowering of platelets happens, specific steps MUST be taken (see Caution). If you forget a dose: take it as soon as you remember it, unless it's nearly time for your next dose—if that is the case, skip the missed dose and return to taking the medicine on your usual schedule. DO NOT double doses. Call your doctor for instructions if you miss more than one dose.

Usual Duration of Use: Duration of use will be decided by your doctor based on response of the condition being treated. For example, in CML, resolution of blast crisis and lowering of abnormally elevated white blood cell counts as well as development of any adverse effects will determine the course of therapy. In GIST, tumor response and adverse effect development will determine therapy steps to be taken. The medicine is generally continued as long as the patient continues to have benefits from it. Long-term safety information of treatment with this medicine is still emerging. Talk to your doctor on a regular basis.

Typical Treatment Goals and Measurements (Outcomes and Markers)

CML: The number and type of white blood cells are used to describe the kind of leukemia. For example, in blast crisis, a certain amount and a certain kind of white blood cell predominates the cells seen in the blood/bone marrow. Resolution of the kind and number of cells toward normal levels indicates response of the condition to the medicine. Usual terms used are: no evidence of leukemia (NEL) or return to chronic phase of CML.

GIST: Shrinkage of the tumor and lack of tumor progression are indicators that the situation is resolving.

Possible Advantages of This Drug

Response of GIST where responses to other chemotherapy were poor. Response of CML where other treatment has failed and blast crisis resulted and return to chronic phase is an excellent result.

Currently a "Drug of Choice"

For use in CML in blast crisis, accelerated phase or chronic phase after interferon-alpha failure. For kit (CD 117)-positive GIST tumors.

▷ **This Drug Should Not Be Taken If**

- you have had an allergic reaction to it previously.
- your absolute neutrophil count and/or platelets have dropped or bilirubin or liver transaminases have increased to unacceptable levels.

▷ **Inform Your Physician Before Taking This Drug If**

- you have an increase in bilirubin or liver transaminases that your doctor is not aware of.
- your white blood cells (neutrophils) have lowered to less than 1.0×10^9 per liter or your platelets have dropped to less than 50×10^9 per liter.
- you are taking medicines that change or are removed by cytochrome P450 3A4 or 2C9.
- you have any type of heart disease, especially congestive heart failure that may be worsened by fluid accumulation.
- you have impaired liver or kidney function.
- you are pregnant or are breast-feeding your infant.
- you develop swelling of the ankles while taking this medicine.
- you have a history of alcoholism.

Possible Side Effects (natural, expected, and unavoidable drug actions)

Weakness and headache—possible (may be more pronounced in women). Weight gain (because of fluid retention). Rapid increases in weight should be promptly evaluated, probably represent fluid increases in the body and are generally treated with water pills (diuretics) and/or decreases in doses. Return of hair color (repigmentation).

▷ **Possible Adverse Effects** (unusual, unexpected, and infrequent reactions)

If any of the following develop, consult your physician promptly for guidance.

Mild Adverse Effects

Allergic reactions—possible.
Nausea, vomiting, diarrhea—possible to infrequent.
Fluid retention/edema—may be frequent.
Blurred vision—infrequent.
Muscle cramps—frequent.
Fever—infrequent.

Serious Adverse Effects

Allergic reactions—possible.
Idiosyncratic reactions—not reported as yet.
Liver or kidney toxicity—infrequent.
Rupture of the spleen (splenic rupture)—case reports.
Carcinogenicity studies not yet performed, but positive genotoxic effects were seen in an in vitro mammalian cell assay (Chinese hamster ovary).
Fluid retention/edema (including rapid weight gain, and/or pulmonary edema, and/or fluid around the eye-periorbital edema—possible (some cases have been life threatening). Periorbital edema may be frequent and require surgery.

Abnormally low white blood cell and platelet counts: fever, sore throat, infections, abnormal bleeding or bruising—possible and dose-related.

▷ **Possible Effects on Sexual Function:** Not reported.

▷ **Adverse Effects That May Mimic Natural Diseases or Disorders**
Liver toxicity may suggest viral hepatitis.

Natural Diseases or Disorders That May Be Activated by This Drug
Not defined.

Possible Effects on Laboratory Tests
Complete blood cell counts: decreased white cells (neutropenia) and platelets (depends on the stage of the disease).
Kidney function tests: increased BUN or creatinine.
Liver function tests: increased liver enzymes (ALT/GPT, AST/GOT, and alkaline phosphatase), increased bilirubin.

CAUTION
1. Look for early signs of liver, kidney, or hematologic toxicity.
2. If a different doctor than the one prescribing imatinib wants to start a new prescription medicine, make certain you tell him or her that you are taking this medicine.
3. Talk to your doctor if you have an unexplained weight gain or swelling of the ankles.
4. Be certain to keep appointments for any follow-up laboratory testing that your doctor orders.
5. Specific interruptions of therapy steps should be taken if platelet counts or the absolute neutrophil count (ANC) are in the range of: white blood cells (neutrophils) have lowered to less than 1.0×10^9 per liter or your platelets have dropped to less than 50×10^9 per liter.

Precautions for Use
By Infants and Children: Indicated for pediatrics in Ph+ (Philadelphia chromosome—positive) patients with chronic myeloid leukemia who have had their disease come back (recur) after stem cell transplant or in those who are resistant to interferon treatment.
By Those Over 60 Years of Age: Results (efficacy) were similar to younger patients. Edema happened more often in older patients than younger ones.

▷ **Advisability of Use During Pregnancy**
Pregnancy Category: D. See Pregnancy Risk Categories at the back of this book.
Human Studies: Information from adequate studies of pregnant women is not available.
Talk to your doctor if you become pregnant while taking this medicine and ask your doctor for guidance about the risk of fetal damage versus the benefits this medicine brings to you.

Advisability of Use If Breast-Feeding
Presence of this drug in breast milk: Yes, estimated at 1.5%.
Breast-feeding is NOT recommended.

Habit-Forming Potential: Not defined, not expected.

Effects of Overdose: Limited experience. An oral dose of 2.5 times the human dose given to rats was not lethal after 14 days. A dose equal to 7.5 times the human dose was lethal to rats after 7–10 days.

Possible Effects of Long-Term Use: Hematologic toxicity—possible; immunosuppression, liver or kidney toxicity.

Suggested Periodic Examinations While Taking This Drug (at physician's dis-
cretion)
Complete blood cell counts.
Liver and kidney function tests.
Weight.
Pedal edema checks.
Check of GIST tumor progression or regression.

▷ **While Taking This Drug, Observe the Following**
Foods: No specific restrictions, and food may help lessen GI irritation.
Herbal Medicines or Minerals: Some people take echinacea or mistletoe to try to
boost their immune systems. Since neither herb was studied with imatinib,
this is NOT recommended. Because St. John's wort acts on the cytochrome
P450 system, DO NOT COMBINE. Talk to your doctor BEFORE combining
any herbal medicine with imatinib.
Beverages: No restrictions. Should be taken with a full glass of water.
▷ *Alcohol:* May increase stomach and intestinal irritation that can be caused by
this drug. Talk to your doctor about this.
Tobacco Smoking: No specific interactions, but I advise everyone to quit.
Marijuana Smoking: Increased chance of opportunistic fungal infections and
possible drug level changes.
▷ *Other Drugs*
Imatinib may *increase* the effects of
• aprepitant (Emend).
• carbamazepine (Tegretol).
• dihydropyridine calcium channel blockers.
• dofetilide (Tikosyn).
• medicines removed by cytochrome P450 2C9.
• triazole benzodiazepines.
• warfarin (Coumadin). Patients who require a blood thinner (anticoagulant) would more prudently be given a low molecular weight heparin (see
Drug Classes).
Imatinib *taken concurrently* with
• all drugs requiring cytochrome P450 3A4 for removal from the body or
inhibiting (such as clarithromycin and voriconazole) or inducing (such as
phenytoin-Dilantin) that enzyme would be expected to increase or
decrease blood levels of imatinib.
• anticonvulsants requires careful monitoring for changes in seizure patterns and need to adjust anticonvulsant dose.
• cyclosporine (Sandimmune) should have more frequent cyclosporine
blood levels and dosing adjusted to blood levels.
• fosphenytoin (Cerebyx) or phenytoin (Dilantin) may excessively lower the
blood level of imatinib.
• medicines with hematologic toxicity may lead to additive toxicity if combined with imatinib.
• ritonavir (Norvir) and perhaps other protease inhibitors (see Drug Classes)
may lead to toxicity.
• "statin"-type medicines (see Drug Classes)—such as simvastatin or
Zocor—may lead to toxicity. Lower doses of all are prudent. Pravastatin
(Pravachol) may be a drug of choice if a statin is needed because it does
not rely on the P450 3A4 system.

The following drugs may *increase* the effects of imatinib:
- azole antifungals (such as fluconazole, itraconazole, and ketoconazole) may lead to higher-than-expected imatinib blood levels and increased risk of adverse effects.
- macrolide antibiotics (Erythromycin [various] or clarithromycin [Biaxin]).

The following drugs may *decrease* the effects of imatinib:
- barbiturates (see Drug Classes).
- carbamazepine (Tegretol).
- dexamethasone (various).
- fosphenytoin (Cerebyx) or phenytoin (Dilantin) may excessively lower the blood level of imatinib.
- rifampin (various).

▷ *Driving, Hazardous Activities:* Fatigue from this medicine or from the underlying condition may make operating hazardous equipment dangerous. Restrict activities as necessary.

Aviation Note: The use of this drug *is probably a disqualification* for piloting. Consult a designated Aviation Medical Examiner.

Exposure to Heat: Use caution. This drug can cause temperature increases.

Discontinuation: Talk to your doctor before stopping this medicine for any reason.

IMIPRAMINE (im IP ra meen)

Introduced: 1955 **Class:** Antidepressant **Prescription:** USA: Yes
Controlled Drug: USA: No; Canada: No **Available as Generic:** USA: Yes; Canada: Yes

Brand Names: Antipress, ✚Apo-Imipramine, ✚Impril, Imprin, Janimine, ✚Novo-Pramine, ✚PMS Imipramine, Presamoine, SK-Pramine, Tipramine, Tofranil, Tofranil-PM, W.D.D.

BENEFITS versus RISKS

Possible Benefits	*Possible Risks*
EFFECTIVE RELIEF OF NEUROSES AND PSYCHOTIC DEPRESSION	ADVERSE BEHAVIORAL EFFECTS
EFFECTIVE TREATMENT FOR CHILDHOOD BED-WETTING (enuresis)	CONVERSION OF DEPRESSION TO MANIA in manic-depressive (bipolar) disorders
Helps manage chronic, severe pain	Aggravation of schizophrenia and paranoia
Aids cocaine withdrawal	Induction of serious heart rhythm abnormalities
Relieves symptoms of attention deficit disorder	Abnormally low white blood cell and platelet counts
Helps prevent panic attacks	
Helps control binge eating and purging in bulimia	

▷ **Principal Uses**

As a Single Drug Product: Uses currently included in FDA-approved labeling: (1) Relieves severe emotional depression and initiates gradual restoration of normal mood; (2) helps prevent childhood bed-wetting in children over 6 years of age; (3) used to treat delusions.

Author's Note: Information in this profile has been shortened to make room for more widely used medicines.

INDAPAMIDE (in DAP a mide)

Introduced: 1974   **Class:** Antihypertensive, diuretic   **Prescription:** USA: Yes   **Controlled Drug:** USA: No; Canada: No   **Available as Generic:** Yes

Brand Names: ♣Apo-Indapamide, ♣Biprel [CD] indapamide and perindopril, Dom-Indapamide, ♣Dom-Indapamide, ♣Gen-Indapamide, ♣Lozide, Lozol, ♣PMS-Indapamide

---

BENEFITS versus RISKS

Possible Benefits	*Possible Risks*
EFFECTIVE ONCE-A-DAY TREATMENT OF MILD TO MODERATE HYPERTENSION	Excessive loss of blood potassium or magnesium
EFFECTIVE, MILD DIURETIC	Increased blood sugar level
COMBINATION USE WITH AN ACE INHIBITOR (PERINDOPRIL OR ACEON) REDUCED RISK OF RECURRENT STROKE BY NEARLY HALF IN ONE STUDY	Increased blood uric acid level

---

▷ **Principal Uses**

As a Single Drug Product: Uses currently included in FDA-approved labeling: (1) Increases urine output (diuresis) to correct fluid retention seen in congestive heart failure (edema); (2) used as starting therapy in high blood pressure (hypertension).

Other (unlabeled) generally accepted uses: (1) Helps ease the excessive elimination of calcium in the urine (hypercalciuria); (2) may help protect the heart after blood-flow problems (preserves ischemic heart from reperfusion injury); (3) combination use with perindopril (Aceon) reduced risk of repeat stroke by nearly 50% in one study.

As a Combination Drug Product [CD]: Available in combination with the ACE inhibitor perindopril in Canada.

How This Drug Works: Increases elimination of salt and water (through increased urine production). Also works directly on the blood vessel walls and relaxes the walls of smaller arteries and decreases pressure reactions (calcium channel action). The combined effects lower blood pressure.

▷ **Widely Used Guidelines That Involve This Medicine (representative sample):** Please look at the section at the very beginning of this profile called "Class." Next, turn to Table 22 and you will find guidelines listed by the class involved!

Available Dosage Forms and Strengths

Tablets — 1.25 mg, 2.5 mg

Tablets, combination — 1.25 mg indapamide, 4 mg perindopril

▷ **Usual Adult Dosage Ranges:** *Hypertension:* 1.25 mg per day, as a single dose in the morning. If needed, the dose may be increased to 2.5 mg/day after 4 weeks, and up to 5 mg if needed and tolerated. Use in treating edema may require a starting dose of 2.5 mg. Maximum total daily dose is 5 mg. (In Canada, the total daily dose limit is given as 2.5 mg.)

Note: Actual dose and dosing schedule must be determined for each individual patient.

Conditions Requiring Dosing Adjustments

Liver Function: Should be used with caution and in decreased doses by patients with liver problems. Blood chemistry (electrolytes) should be closely followed.

Kidney Function: Used with caution and must be stopped if kidney failure progresses after indapamide is started.

▷ **Dosing Instructions:** The immediate release tablet may be crushed and taken with or following food to reduce stomach upset. Sustained release forms should never be crushed. This medicine is best taken in the morning to avoid nighttime urination. If you forget a dose: take it as soon as you remember it, unless it's nearly time for your next dose—if that is the case, skip the missed dose and return to taking the medicine on your usual schedule. DO NOT double doses. Call your doctor for instructions if you miss more than one dose.

Usual Duration of Use: Use on a regular schedule for 2 to 4 weeks determines peak effect in lowering blood pressure. Long-term use (months to years) requires periodic physician evaluation. Make certain you maintain pre-hypertension or hypertension goals!

Typical Treatment Goals and Measurements (Outcomes and Markers)

Blood Pressure: Guidelines (JNC VII) define normal blood pressure (BP) as **less than** 120/80 and **pre-hypertension** as 120/80 to 139/89. This new range is intended to help doctors encourage lifestyle changes (or in the case of people with a risk factor for high blood pressure, start treatment) much earlier—so that damage to blood vessels, heart, kidneys, sexual potency, or eyes might be minimized or avoided altogether. Stage 1 hypertension is 140/90 to 159/99 and stage 2 hypertension equal to or greater than: 160/100 mm Hg. These guidelines also recommend that clinicians work with their patients to agree on the goals and a plan of treatment. The first-ever guidelines for blood pressure (hypertension) in African Americans recommends that MOST black patients be started on TWO antihypertensive medicines with the goal of lowering blood pressure to 130/80 for those with high risk for heart and blood vessel disease or with diabetes. The American Diabetes Association also recommends 130/80 as the target for diabetics and less than 125/75 for those who spill more than one gram of protein into their urine. Most clinicians try to achieve a BP that confers the best balance of lower cardiovascular risk and avoids the problem of too low a blood pressure. Blood pressure duration is generally increased with beneficial restriction of sodium. If goals are not met, it is not unusual to intensify doses or add on medicines.

Possible Advantages of This Drug

Causes no significant increase in blood cholesterol levels. Less likely to cause significant loss of potassium. Increases good cholesterol (HDL). ONCE-DAILY DOSING will encourage people to take this medicine regularly. Works directly on blood vessels while also working as a "water pill," or diuretic. If there are no compelling reasons for other medicines, diuretics are drugs of choice for starting high blood pressure treatment according to JNC VII.

▷ **This Drug Should Not Be Taken If**
- you have had an allergic reaction to it previously or to a sulfonamide-type medicine or chemical.
- your kidneys are not making any urine.

▷ **Inform Your Physician Before Taking This Drug If**
- you are allergic to any form of "sulfa" drug.
- you are pregnant or planning pregnancy.
- you presently have an excessively low blood potassium.
- you have a history of kidney or liver disease.
- you have diabetes, gout, or systemic lupus erythematosus.
- you take any form of cortisone, digoxin, oral antidiabetic drug, or insulin.
- you have had a sympathectomy.
- you plan to have surgery under general anesthesia in the near future.

Possible Side Effects (natural, expected, and unavoidable drug actions)
Light-headedness on rising from sitting or lying position (see orthostatic hypotension in Glossary). Increase in blood sugar level, affecting control of diabetes. Increase in blood uric acid level, affecting control of gout. Decrease in blood potassium level, causing muscle weakness and cramping. Low blood sodium and magnesium.

▷ **Possible Adverse Effects** (unusual, unexpected, and infrequent reactions)
If any of the following develop, consult your physician promptly for guidance.
Mild Adverse Effects
Allergic reactions: skin rashes, hives, itching—infrequent.
Headache, dizziness, drowsiness, weakness, lethargy, visual disturbance—case reports.
Reduced appetite, indigestion, nausea, vomiting, diarrhea—rare.
Paresthesias—rare.
Urination at night—possible, especially with evening dosing.
Serious Adverse Effects
Serious skin rashes (Stevens-Johnson syndrome, toxic epidermal necrolysis)—case reports.
Abnormal heartbeat (premature ventricular contractions)—rare.
Liver or kidney toxicity—rare.
Inhibition of platelet aggregation—possible.

▷ **Possible Effects on Sexual Function:** Decreased libido—infrequent; impotence—rare.

Natural Diseases or Disorders That May Be Activated by This Drug
Diabetes, gout, systemic lupus erythematosus.

Possible Effects on Laboratory Tests
Total cholesterol and LDL cholesterol levels: no effect or slightly decreased.
Blood HDL cholesterol level: increased.
Blood potassium, magnesium, or sodium level: decreased.
Blood uric acid level or blood sugar (glucose): increased.

CAUTION
1. Take exactly as prescribed—excessive doses can cause excessive sodium and potassium loss (decreased appetite, nausea, fatigue, confusion, or tingling extremities).
2. If you take a digitalis preparation (digitoxin, digoxin), ensure intake of high-potassium foods to help avoid digitalis toxicity (see Table 13,

High-Potassium Foods). Magnesium should also be checked and replaced as needed.

Precautions for Use

By Infants and Children: Safety and effectiveness for those under 12 years of age are not established.

By Those Over 60 Years of Age: It is best to start with small doses. You may be more susceptible to impaired thinking, orthostatic hypotension, potassium loss, and blood sugar increase. Overdose or extended use causes excessive loss of body water, thickening (increased viscosity) of blood, and an increased tendency for the blood to clot—predisposing to stroke, heart attack, or thrombophlebitis (vein inflammation with blood clot).

▷ ### Advisability of Use During Pregnancy

Pregnancy Category: B. D by one researcher. See Pregnancy Risk Categories at the back of this book.

Animal Studies: No birth defects reported.

Human Studies: Data from studies of pregnant women are not available.

This drug should not be used during pregnancy unless a very serious complication occurs for which this drug is significantly beneficial. Ask your physician for guidance.

Advisability of Use If Breast-Feeding

Presence of this drug in breast milk: Unknown.

Avoid drug or refrain from nursing.

Habit-Forming Potential: None.

Effects of Overdose: Dry mouth, thirst, lethargy, weakness, muscle cramping, nausea, vomiting, drowsiness progressing to stupor or coma.

Possible Effects of Long-Term Use: Impaired balance of water, salt, and potassium in blood and body tissues. Development of diabetes in predisposed individuals.

Suggested Periodic Examinations While Taking This Drug (at physician's discretion)

Measurements of blood levels of sodium, potassium, chloride, sugar, and uric acid.

▷ ### While Taking This Drug, Observe the Following

Foods: Ask your doctor about a high-potassium diet. If so advised, see Table 13, High-Potassium Foods, in Section Six. Follow your doctor's advice about salt use.

Herbal Medicines or Minerals: Ginseng, bitter orange, country mallow, hawthorn, saw palmetto, ma huang (no longer on the market for weight control), guarana and mate (caffeine), goldenseal, yohimbe, and licorice may also cause increased blood pressure. Calcium and garlic may help lower blood pressure. Ginkgo benefits in helping peripheral artery disease are, as yet, unproven. Indian snakeroot has a German Commission E monograph indication for hypertension—talk to your doctor. Eleuthero root and ephedra (ma huang) should be avoided by people living with hypertension. Magnesium and potassium replacement may be needed.

Beverages: No restrictions. This drug may be taken with milk.

▷ *Alcohol:* Alcohol may exaggerate the blood pressure–lowering effects of this drug and cause orthostatic hypotension.

Tobacco Smoking: No interactions expected. I advise everyone to quit smoking.

▷ *Other Drugs*

Indapamide may ***increase*** the effects of
- ACE inhibitors (see Drug Classes) and cause SEVERE lowering of blood pressure on standing (postural hypotension).
- other antihypertensive drugs; dose adjustments may be necessary to prevent excessive lowering of blood pressure.
- lithium (Lithobid, others) and cause lithium toxicity.

Indapamide may ***decrease*** the effects of
- oral antidiabetic drugs (sulfonylureas); dose adjustments may be needed for proper control of blood sugar.

Indapamide ***taken concurrently*** with
- digitalis preparations (digitoxin, digoxin) must be followed closely and adjustments made to prevent fluctuations of blood potassium levels and serious disturbances of heart rhythm.
- NSAIDs (see Drug Classes) may blunt the therapeutic benefit of indapamide.

The following drugs may ***decrease*** the effects of indapamide:
- cholestyramine (Cuemid, Questran)—may interfere with its absorption.
- colestipol (Colestid)—may interfere with its absorption.

Take cholestyramine and colestipol 1 hour before any oral diuretic.

▷ *Driving, Hazardous Activities:* Use caution until the possible occurrence of orthostatic hypotension, drowsiness, dizziness, or impaired vision has been determined.

Aviation Note: The use of this drug ***may be a disqualification*** for piloting. Consult a designated Aviation Medical Examiner.

Exposure to Sun: No restrictions.

Exposure to Heat: Excessive perspiring could cause additional loss of salt and water.

Heavy Exercise or Exertion: Isometric exercises can raise blood pressure significantly. Ask your physician for help.

Occurrence of Unrelated Illness: Vomiting or diarrhea can produce a serious imbalance of important body chemistry. Consult your physician for guidance.

Discontinuation: It may be advisable to discontinue this drug 5 to 7 days before major surgery. Ask your physician, surgeon and/or anesthesiologist for guidance.

INDOMETHACIN (in doh METH a sin)

Please see the acetic acid (nonsteroidal anti-inflammatory drug) family profile.

INFLIXIMAB (IN FLIX ih mab)

Other Names: Anti-TNF monoclonal antibody, chimeric monoclonal antibody to TNF alpha, cA2

Introduced: 1998 Crohn's, 1999 rheumatoid arthritis combination approval, 2002 improved function in RA   **Class:**   Disease-modifying antirheumatic drug (DMARD), biologic response modifier   **Prescription:**   USA: Yes   **Controlled Drug:**   USA: No; Canada: No   **Available as Generic:**   No   **Brand Name:**   Remicade

BENEFITS versus RISKS

Possible Benefits	*Possible Risks*
GIVEN ORPHAN PRODUCT DESIGNATION FOR USE IN CROHN'S DISEASE	POSSIBLE LOWERED RESISTANCE TO INFECTIONS AND OPPORTUNISTIC INFECTIONS
EASES RHEUMATOID ARTHRITIS (RA) IN COMBINATION WITH METHOTREXATE	Injection site reactions
	Possible development of antibodies
MAY GIVE A RESPONSE IN RA WHERE OTHER AGENTS HAVE FAILED	May have a role in causing lymphoma
COULD HAVE A ROLE IN CONGESTIVE HEART FAILURE AND IN DECREASING RISK OF REPEAT HEART ATTACKS	
FIRST MEDICINE APPROVED TO IMPROVE PHYSICAL FUNCTION IN RA	

▷ **Principal Uses**

As a Single Drug Product: Uses currently included in FDA-approved labeling: (1) Treatment of moderately to severely active Crohn's disease or fistulizing Crohn's disease; (2) Use in combination with methotrexate in rheumatoid arthritis (RA) patients to lower signs and symptoms when patients have not responded to methotrexate alone; (3) improves physical function in RA.

Other (unlabeled) generally accepted uses: (1) May have a role in some kinds of wasting (cachexia) where tumor necrosis factor (TNF) is involved; (2) data from the cholesterol and recurrent events (CARE) trial found that decreasing tumor necrosis factor (TNF) (see How This Drug Works, below) reduces risk of repeat heart attacks; (3) may ease congestive heart failure.

How This Drug Works: Binds with both soluble and transmembrane tumor necrosis factor alpha (TNF alpha) in the body. Inhibits binding of existing TNF alpha to p55 and p75 receptors. Both effects act to stop the biologic actions of TNF alpha. Works to change the body's responses that are caused or regulated by TNF, such as increased levels of matrix metalloproteinase-3, serum levels of cytokines, and release of substances that control white blood cell migration.

Author's Note: The company that makes this product has added a more stringent (black-box) warning about opportunistic infections to the product label. Information in this profile may be broadened in subsequent editions if warranted. Members of an FDA advisory panel found that more data was required for the 3 existing TNF blockers (adalimumab-Humira, etanercept-Enbrel, and infliximab-Remicade) relative to their possible role in causing lymphoma in patients who use them.

INFLUENZA VACCINE (IN flu en za VAX ceen)

Other Name: Flu vaccine

Introduced: Specific formulation for each year. 2003 for FluMist   **Class:** Antiviral **Prescription:**   USA: Yes   **Controlled Drug:**   USA: No; Canada: No   **Available as Generic:**   USA: No; Canada: No

Brand Names: Flu-Immune, FluMist, Fluoge, Flu-Shield, Fluzone

Author's Note: There was significant controversy over coverage of the vaccine in the last flu season. For the 2004–2005 flu season, the shot (vaccine) will have 3 strains: H1N1, A/New Caledonia/20/99; A/Fujian/411/2002, which is an H3N2-like, and finally, a B/Shanghai/361/2002-like. Manufacturers can use the A/Kumamoto/102/2002 (H3N2) or the A/Wyoming/3/2003 (H3N2) for the A/Fujian component. The B/Jilin/20/2003 may be substituted for the B/Shanghai. Between 90 and 100 million doses are anticipated. Like last year, the Advisory Committee suggests that people ages 50–64 get a flu shot. From 20,000 to 40,000 people die from the flu each year. Don't become a statistic. Data from nearly 150,000 patients found that *elderly people who got flu shots benefited from fewer admissions to the hospital for heart disease and stroke* **(see Nichol, K.L. in Sources)! The American Diabetes Association (***www.diabetes.org* **or 1-877-CDC-DIAB for more information) recommends that people living with diabetes get both a flu and pneumococcal shot (vaccine). If you would like a copy of the ACIP recommendations, call 1-888-232-3228. Information on current general shot (vaccine) recommendations can be found at** *www.cdc.gov/nip/recs/child-schedule.htm.* **As in past years, additional concerns about SARS make it especially prudent to get a flu shot to help ease fears that an emerging case of the flu might be SARS. This year, the ACIP recommends: flu shots for: all infants and children aged 6–23 months, all women who will be pregnant for the flu season.**

BENEFITS versus RISKS

Possible Benefits	*Possible Risks*
PREVENTION OF INFLUENZA CAUSED BY THE MOST SERIOUS OR PREVALENT VIRAL STRAINS IDENTIFIED FOR A GIVEN YEAR	GUILLAIN-BARRÉ SYNDROME (questionable causation for previous shot form)
FLUMIST FORM AVOIDS INJECTION AND IS A NASAL SPRAY	Hypersensitivity
Possible cross-protection from other similar virus strains	

▷ **Principal Uses**

As a Single Drug Product: Uses currently included in FDA-approved labeling: Prevention of influenza.

Other (unlabeled) generally accepted uses: (1) Used in patients with compromised immune systems (such as HIV-positive, cancer, and bone marrow transplant patients); (2) can be of use in isolated outbreaks such as in nursing homes or military camps; (3) may decrease the number of middle ear infections in children who attend day-care centers; (4) FluMist form is approved for those 5–49 years old to prevent types A and B influenza.

How This Drug Works: Vaccine made of purified parts of the virus surface, split virus or whole virus, which has been inactivated. When injected, it stimulates the immune system to make antibodies. The antibodies (appearing roughly 2 weeks after vaccination) act to reduce disease severity or decrease probability of infection by the expected flu viruses. The FluMist form is a live-virus vaccine that provokes an immune response using the whole virus. It appears that influenza-specific T cells, mucosal antibodies, and serum antibodies also play a role in conferring immunity to the flu.

▷ **Widely Used Guidelines That Involve This Medicine (representative sample):** Please look at the section at the very beginning of this profile called "Class." Next, turn to Table 22 and you will find guidelines listed by the class involved!

Available Dosage Forms and Strengths
Typical split virus: 15 mcg/0.5 mL of each of the 3 selected strains.
Nasal spray live vaccine form (Flumist): Package of 10 single-use sprayers containing 0.5 mL in each.

▷ **Recommended Dosage Ranges** (Actual dose and schedule must be determined for each patient and each flu season individually.)
Infants and Children: For the shot form: Those 6 to 35 months old should be given 0.25 mL of a split-dose vaccine shot. If this is the first vaccination, two doses should be given 1 month apart. Split dose is suggested for children because it tends to cause fewer undesirable effects. For infants and young children, the vaccine is usually given in the thigh muscle.
Children 3 to 8 years old should be given 0.5 mL of the selected split-virus vaccine shot. Children in this age range who have not been previously vaccinated should be given two vaccinations, 1 month apart.
Children: FluMist: For children 5 to 8 years old: For children not previously vaccinated using FluMist for the first time: Two doses of 0.5 mL each (0.25 mL in each nostril) are needed. The first dose is given (0.25 mL in each nostril as in the dosing instruction section), then a second dose (0.25 mL in each nostril) should be given within 14 days of the first one. For children 9 and older for FluMist: 0.25 mL in each nostril each flu season.
For previously available shots (vaccinations): Those 9 years old or older should be given a single vaccination of 0.5 mL of split-virus vaccine in the deltoid muscle.
9 to 49 Years of Age Using FluMist: Should be given 0.5 mL of FluMist as 0.25 mL in each nostril every flu season.
13 to 60 Years of Age Using Shot Form: Should be given 0.5 mL of whole- or split-virus vaccine in the deltoid muscle.
Over 60 Years of Age: Same as 13 to 60 years of age for the shot form. FluMist form should NOT be used.
Note: Dosing for all appropriate patients is best accomplished in October through November of the flu season for which you are seeking protection. A shot from a prior year will NOT protect you.

Conditions Requiring Dosing Adjustments
Liver Function: Not involved.
Kidney Function: Not involved.

▷ **Dosing Instructions:** Prior vaccination **does not** mean you are immune to the current year's virus strains. People at increased risk for complications from the flu (50 or older, those with asthma or other ongoing chronic lung problems, cardiovascular disease, immunosuppression, women in the 6th to 9th months [second or third trimester] of pregnancy, etc.). Some tenderness at the injection site is possible. Because of SARS, it is particularly prudent to get an influenza vaccine in order to help avoid the stress and confusion that may result. Fever and muscular aches or pains are possible from the injected vaccine and may be pretreated and treated with acetaminophen (Tylenol, others)—you don't have to ache. If you forget to get the shot: timing of vaccination (enough time to let your body build up immunity) before the flu season is important. The FluMist form may range from colorless to pale yellow, and the liquid may by clear to slightly cloudy. Half of the dose of FluMist is given to each nostril while the patient sits upright. The person giving the spray inserts the tip of the sprayer just inside the nose, and pushes the plunger to give the spray. Once the first nostril is sprayed, the dose-dividing clip is removed from the sprayer and the second half of the dose is given into the unsprayed nostril. If you get the flu because you did NOT get vaccinated, a neuramidase inhibitor (see drug profiles) may be an option for you. Talk to your doctor.

Usual Duration of Use: Single vaccination confers relative immunity to the expected viral strains in 2 weeks. This does not confer immunity to all strains of virus capable of causing an influenzalike (flu-like) syndrome. Annual vaccination is strongly suggested.

Typical Treatment Goals and Measurements (Outcomes and Markers)

Influenza: Prevention of a serious viral illness. **In a typical season some 20,000 Americans die from influenza. Years with virulent strains can see 40,000 people lose their lives.** This vaccination can help you avoid illness, hospitalization, and death.

Possible Advantages of This Drug

Allows the prevention of a viral syndrome that can cause loss of several weeks of work in younger, otherwise healthy patients or serious illness in older or compromised patients. Given the SARS problem, a flu shot may help avoid stress and confusion. The FluMist form is a nasal spray and will most probably replace an injection for otherwise healthy people. A large review found that elderly people who get a flu shot avoid a significant number of hospitalizations for stroke and heart disease!

Currently a "Drug of Choice"

For prevention of types A and B influenza due to the viral strains that are of the greatest concern in the current flu season.

▷ **This Drug Should Not Be Taken If**

- you have had an allergic reaction to any dose form of it previously or to any vaccine components.
- you are allergic to eggs (the virus is grown on eggs).
- you have an acute illness and a fever.

FluMist Form:

- you have an asthma or reactive airway disease (safety and efficacy not established)
- you are over 50 (safety and efficacy not established)
- you have an ongoing (chronic) medical condition that predisposes you to severe flu infections (injected form of influenza vaccine is needed).
- you have an immunosuppression (either disease such as AIDS or immune deficiency disease or are taking a medicine that causes immunosuppression). Like other live-virus vaccines, FluMist should not be taken.

▷ **Inform Your Physician Before Taking This Drug If**

- you are HIV positive (shot form).
- you have a history of blood disorders or active nerve problem (neurologic disorder).

- you have had Guillain-Barré syndrome.
- you have a history of seizures or of a latex allergy.
- you have been receiving cancer therapy (chemotherapy).

Possible Side Effects (natural, expected, and unavoidable drug actions)
Pain at the vaccination site. Muscle aches, fever, or bothersome tiredness (malaise). This is **not** the flu. The vaccine contains viral fragments or non-infectious (dead) virus. These symptoms are a reaction to the components of the vaccine.

▷ **Possible Adverse Effects** (unusual, unexpected, and infrequent reactions)
If any of the following develop, consult your physician promptly for guidance.
Mild Adverse Effects
Allergic reactions: swelling and redness—possible.
Muscle aches or fever—infrequent.
Fatigue, nausea, and headache—infrequent.
Vasculitis (joint pain, weakness, fever, and rash)—rare.
Serious Adverse Effects
Allergic reactions: anaphylactic reactions.
Low blood platelets or pericarditis—case reports.
Guillain-Barré syndrome (only reported during the 1976–1977 flu season and of questionable causation).
Kidney toxicity—case report.
Vision changes—case report.

▷ **Possible Effects on Sexual Function:** None reported.

Possible Delayed Adverse Effects: Guillain-Barré syndrome during one flu season.

▷ **Adverse Effects That May Mimic Natural Diseases or Disorders**
Reaction to vaccine contents may mimic the flu.

Natural Diseases or Disorders That May Be Activated by This Drug
None reported.

Possible Effects on Laboratory Tests
Hepatitis B test: false positive.
Hepatitis C test: false positive.
HTLV-1 test: false positive.

CAUTION
1. A vaccine in the previous year **does not** confer immunity to the flu in following years.
2. The flu vaccine confers immunity to viruses predicted to cause influenza in a particular flu season. Vaccine does not confer immunity to all strains of virus capable of causing a flu-like syndrome.
3. If muscle aches or fever occur after vaccination, acetaminophen (Tylenol, others) is recommended. **Do not** take aspirin, and especially do not give aspirin to children. It may be prudent to take acetaminophen BEFORE vaccination to prevent such reactions.
4. Call your doctor immediately if you develop hives, facial swelling, or difficulty breathing after the vaccination.
5. It is ALWAYS better to prevent a disease or condition than to have to treat it. Additionally, **when the type A flu is prevalent, some 20,000 people usually die** from the flu or its complications in that particular flu season. Talk with your doctor or pharmacist. If you do not have a medical reason

for avoiding flu vaccination—get the shot! In many states, your pharmacist can actually give you a flu shot.

Precautions for Use

By Infants and Children: Safety and effectiveness for use by those under 6 months of age have not been established.

By Those Over 60 Years of Age: The vaccine is especially **valuable** in this age group, as the effects of the flu may be devastating.

▷ **Advisability of Use During Pregnancy**

Pregnancy Category: C. See Pregnancy Risk Categories at the back of this book.

Animal Studies: Animal studies have not been conducted.

Human Studies: Information from adequate studies of pregnant women is not available.

Ask your doctor for guidance.

Advisability of Use If Breast-Feeding

Presence of this drug in breast milk: Not defined.

Monitor nursing infant closely and contact your doctor if adverse effects develop. The CDC has not listed breast-feeding as a precaution against receiving this vaccine.

Habit-Forming Potential: None.

Effects of Overdose: No specific cases reported. Treatment would be consistent with any symptoms of the patient.

Possible Effects of Long-Term Use: Not indicated for long-term use.

Suggested Periodic Examinations While Taking This Drug (at physician's discretion)

None indicated.

▷ **While Taking This Drug, Observe the Following**

Foods: No restrictions.

Herbal Medicines or Minerals: Some patients use echinacea to attempt to boost their immune systems. Unfortunately, use of echinacea is not recommended in people with damaged immune systems. This herb may also actually weaken any immune system if it is used too often or for too long a time.

Beverages: No restrictions.

▷   *Alcohol:* No restrictions.

Tobacco Smoking: No interactions expected. I advise everyone to quit smoking.

▷   *Other Drugs*

Influenza vaccine may ***increase*** the effects of

- carbamazepine (Tegretol), by decreasing the elimination of the drug.
- phenobarbital, by increasing the half-life of the drug.
- theophylline (Theo-Dur, others), by increasing the blood level of the drug.
- warfarin (Coumadin) and pose an increased risk of bleeding; more frequent INR (prothrombin time or protime) testing is suggested.

Influenza vaccine ***taken concurrently*** with

- cyclosporine (Sandimmune) can cause blunting of the immune response to the vaccine.
- immunosuppressive agents (chemotherapy, corticosteroids) may impair or blunt immune response to the vaccine.
- medicines for which use of live-virus vaccine is not recommended (talk with your doctor), such as medicines that suppress the immune system. **FluMist form should not be given (is contraindicated).**
- methotrexate (Rheumatrex) can result in blunting of the immune response to the shot.

- neuramidase inhibitors (see Drug Classes) have not been found to cause differences in hemagglutination inhibition antibody levels (titers).
- phenytoin (Dilantin) and fosphenytoin (Cerebyx) have had variable effects on the blood levels of this drug.

▷ *Driving, Hazardous Activities:* This drug may cause excessive tiredness and muscle aches. Restrict activities as necessary.

Aviation Note: The use of this drug **may be a short-term disqualification** for piloting. Consult a designated Aviation Medical Examiner.

Exposure to Sun: No restrictions.

Exposure to Heat: Since this vaccine may cause short-duration fevers, it is wise to avoid hot environments for a day after vaccination.

Heavy Exercise or Exertion: A fever may result, and it is wise to avoid strenuous exercise for a day after vaccination.

Special Storage Instructions: This vaccine is ideally stored in the refrigerator. If this is how storage is accomplished, the outdate specified by the manufacturer is valid. If the vaccine is stored at room temperature, it is stable for up to 7 days.

Observe the Following Expiration Times: If the vaccine is stored at room temperature, it is stable for up to 7 days.

Author's Note: There is a Vaccine Adverse Event Reporting System (VAERS). The toll-free number is 1-800-822-7967.

INSULIN (IN suh lin)

Introduced: 1922; insulin lispro, 1996; insulin glargine, 2000; insulin aspart, 2000, insulin glulisine (Apidra)—investigational 2004   **Class:**   Antidiabetic **Prescription:**   USA: No   **Controlled Drug:**   USA: No; Canada: No **Available as Generic:**   Yes

Brand Names: Apidra (investigational),   Humalog, Humalog Mix 75/25, Humulin BR, Humulin L, Humulin N, Humulin R, Humulin 70/30, Humulin 30/70, Humulin U, Humulin U Ultralente, Iletin I NPH, Iletin II Pork, Iletin U—40, Iletin U—500, ✤Initard, Insulatard NPH, insulin aspart (NovoLog), ✤Insulin Human, ✤Insulin-Toronto, Lantus (insulin glargine), Lente Iletin I, Lente Iletin II Pork, Lente Insulin, Lente Purified Pork, Mixtard, Mixtard Human 70/30, NovoLog, Novolin L, ✤Novolin-Lente, Novolin N, ✤Novolin-NPH, NovolinPen, Novolin R, ✤Novolinset, ✤Novolinset NPH, ✤Novolinset 30/70, ✤Novolinset Toronto, Novolin—70/30, Novolin 70/30, Novolin 70/30 Penfill, Novolin 30/70, ✤Novolin-Toronto, ✤Novolin-Ultralente, NPH Iletin I, NPH Iletin II Pork, NPH Insulin, NPH Purified Pork, Protamine, Zinc & Iletin I, Protamine, Protamine, Zinc & Iletin II Pork, Regular Concentrated Iletin II, Regular Iletin I, Regular Iletin II Pork, Regular Iletin II U—500, Regular Insulin, Regular Purified Pork Insulin, Semilente Iletin I, Semilente Insulin, Semilente Purified Pork, Ultralente Iletin I, Ultralente Insulin, Velosulin, ✤Velosulin Cartridge, Velosulin Human

Author's Note: Not all listed forms may still be available in the United States.

```
┌─────────────────────────────────────────────────────────────────┐
│                     BENEFITS versus RISKS                         │
│      Possible Benefits                    Possible Risks          │
│ EFFECTIVE CONTROL OF TYPE 1      HYPOGLYCEMIA WITH EXCESSIVE       │
│   (INSULIN-DEPENDENT)              DOSE                            │
│   DIABETES MELLITUS              Infrequent allergic reactions    │
│ EFFECTIVE COMBINATION OF         Lipodystrophy                    │
│   TYPE 2 DIABETES THAT DOES                                       │
│   NOT RESPOND (MEET BLOOD                                         │
│   SUGAR GOALS) TO DIET AND                                        │
│   ORAL HYPOGLYCEMIC AGENT                                         │
│   ALONE                                                           │
│ EXTREMELY QUICK ONSET                                             │
│   (ASPART FORM)                                                   │
│ EFFECTIVE CONTROL OF A TYPE                                       │
│   OF BLOOD SUGAR PROBLEM                                          │
│   (GESTATIONAL DIABETES) THAT                                     │
│   HAPPENS IN PREGNANCY                                            │
│ TIGHT CONTROL OF BLOOD                                            │
│   SUGAR MAY AVOID OR DELAY                                        │
│   DEVELOPMENT OF HIGH                                             │
│   BLOOD PRESSURE AND KIDNEY,                                      │
│   HEART, NERVE, EYE, OR OTHER                                     │
│   DAMAGE THAT HAPPENS WHEN                                        │
│   BLOOD SUGAR IS OUT OF                                           │
│   CONTROL                                                         │
│ INTENSIVE INSULIN THERAPY                                         │
│   THAT ACHIEVES NEAR NORMAL                                       │
│   A1C LOWERED MICROVASCULAR                                       │
│   PROBLEMS IN TYPE 1                                              │
│   DAIBETICS                                                       │
│ ONCE-DAILY DOSING (Lantus                                         │
│   form—insulin glargine only)                                     │
│ NOVOLOG FORM APPROVED FOR                                         │
│   USE IN INSULIN PUMPS                                            │
└─────────────────────────────────────────────────────────────────┘
```

▷ **Principal Uses**

As a Single Drug Product: Uses currently included in FDA-approved labeling: (1) Used in diabetes mellitus that is insulin-dependent and by people who have non-insulin-dependent diabetes who are experiencing stress such as illness or who do not meet blood sugar goals; (2) used to control blood sugar in critically ill patients who are being fed by intravenous nutrient mixtures; (3) used to control blood sugar in pregnancy (gestational diabetes as a drug of choice).

Other (unlabeled) generally accepted uses: (1) Insulin in combination with glucagon has been used in alcoholic hepatitis; (2) may have a role in combination therapy with an oral hypoglycemic agent in some diabetics; (3) helps diabetic ketoacidosis; (4) can help diabetic neuropathy and retinopathy; (5) can be of help in critically ill patients with maple syrup urine disease; (6) used in implantable pumps to control blood sugar; (7) intensive therapy (more than 3 injections daily) may decrease risk of small blood vessel disease, retinopathy, and kidney problems (nephropathy); (8) one study used a combination of insulin and sugar (glucose) intravenously after a heart attack and found that death decreased by 30% in the following year.

Author's Note: Controversies in Medicines: Some clinicians are advocating use of insulin in type 2 diabetics. The clear goal is to help keep blood sugar in the normal range and avoid complications of diabetes. Perhaps the first best hope for realistically having patients accept this concept is a "mouth spray insulin" (buccal) that is in clinical trials (see Insulin, Oral in the Leading Edge section).

How This Drug Works: Insulin is a hormone that is made in a body organ called the pancreas. It helps sugar get through the cell wall to the inside of the cell (it actually interacts with an insulin receptor [a glycoprotein complex in the cell membrane]) and then: a) the activated receptor turns on a messenger protein inside the cell, b) the activated messenger bumps into a glucose transporter four (GLUT-4), c) the GLUT-4 vesicle goes (translocates) to the cell surface and actually unfolds into the cell and acts like a taxi to bring sugar into the cell where it is used for energy.

▷ **Widely Used Guidelines That Involve This Medicine (representative sample):** Please look at the section at the very beginning of this profile called "Class." Next, turn to Table 22 and you will find guidelines listed by the class involved!

Available Dosage Forms and Strengths
Buccal (mouth) spray — still investigational
Injections — 40, 100, 500 units per mL
Penfill cartridges — 100 units per mL

▷ **Usual Adult Dosage Ranges:** According to individual requirements for the best regulation of blood sugar on a 24-hour basis. It is not unusual to use a long-acting insulin to provide what is called basal insulin, in addition to a rapidly acting insulin to "cover" and food or sugar that is eaten.

Note: Actual dose and schedule must be determined for each patient individually.

Conditions Requiring Dosing Adjustments
Liver Function: Specific adjustment guidelines are not available.
Kidney Function: Caution should be used by patients with compromised kidneys. Requirements become extremely variable.
Thyrotoxicosis: Glucose utilization is typically increased, and insulin requirements may actually decrease.

▷ **Dosing Instructions:** Inject insulin subcutaneously according to the schedule prescribed by your physician. The timing and frequency of injections will vary with the type of insulin prescribed. The following table of insulin actions (according to type) will help you understand the treatment schedule prescribed for you. If you forget a dose: Please call your doctor. People with type 1 diabetes must also use a long-acting insulin if NovoLog is prescribed. If you are combining a longer-acting insulin with insulin aspart, draw up the insulin aspart into the syringe first. If you are using an insulin pump, make certain you understand how to program it. It is critical that this medicine be taken exactly as prescribed.

Insulin Type	Action Onset	Peak	Duration
Insulin aspart	0.15 hr	0.45–1.5 hrs	3–5 hrs
Insulin (buccal)	hr	hrs	hrs
Insulin glargine	1.0 hr	none	24 hrs
Insulin lispro	0.25 hr	0.5–1.5 hrs	3–4 hrs

Insulin Type	Action Onset	Peak	Duration
Regular	0.5–1 hr	2–4 hrs	5–7 hrs
Isophane (NPH)	3–4 hrs	6–12 hrs	18–28 hrs
Regular 30%/NPH 70%	0.5 hr	4–8 hrs	24 hrs
Semilente	1–3 hrs	2–8 hrs	12–16 hrs
Lente	1–3 hrs	8–12 hrs	18–28 hrs
Ultralente	4–6 hrs	18–24 hrs	36 hrs
Protamine Zinc	4–6 hrs	14–24 hrs	36 hrs

Usual Duration of Use: In type 1 insulin-dependent (juvenile-onset) diabetes mellitus, insulin therapy is usually required for life. Type 2 non-insulin-dependent (maturity-onset) diabetes may be controlled by oral antidiabetic drugs and/or diet, but can require insulin when you have a serious infection, injuries, burns, surgical procedures, and other physical stress. The advent of buccal insulin may find increased use of insulin in type 2 diabetes based on patient acceptance. Type 4, or diabetes in pregnancy (gestational), often finds insulin being stopped as appropriate after the baby is born. See your doctor on a regular basis.

Typical Treatment Goals and Measurements (Outcomes and Markers)

Blood sugar: The general goal for blood sugar is to return it to the usual "normal" range (generally 80–120 mg/dL), while avoiding risks of excessively low blood sugar. One study (UKPDS) used a fasting plasma sugar (glucose) of less than 108 mg/dL.

Fructosamine and glycosylated hemoglobin: Fructosamine levels (a measure of the past 2 to 3 weeks of blood sugar control) should be less than or equal to 310 micromoles per liter. Glycosylated hemoglobin or hemoglobin A1C (a measure of the past 2–3 months of blood sugar control) should be less than or equal to 7.0%. Some clinicians are advocating less than this as the target. Others note an increased risk of hypoglycemia with this very strict target.

Possible Advantages of This Drug: Allows tight control of blood sugar that can help avoid microvascular, visual, kidney, and cardiovascular effects of diabetes. The insulin lispro provides a rapid onset, which may be more forgiving in the sense of timing of the shot itself (goes to work faster) as well as offering a more physiologic response to blood sugar. The insulin aspart (NovoLog) has the quickest onset of all. Insulin glargine actually does NOT have a peak effect. The kinetics of that insulin glargine offer a great advantage in providing a relatively constant (baseline) insulin level. Some prescribers use Lantus as a baseline insulin and Humalog with meals—avoiding use of a pump in some patients. An experimental form of insulin sprayed into the mouth (Oralin) is now poised to enter phase three studies (see Insulin, Oral in the Leading Edge section). The Diabetes Control and Complications Trial (DCCT) showed that intensive insulin treatment that attains a near normal A1C lowers risk of microvascular problems in type 1 diabetics.

▷ **This Drug Should Not Be Taken If**
- the need for insulin and its dose schedule have not been established by a qualified clinician.
- you are hypoglycemic.
- you are using insulin aspart and it is cloudy or thickened.

▷ **Inform Your Physician Before Taking This Drug If**
- you have an insulin allergy.
- you do not know how to recognize and treat abnormally low blood sugar (see hypoglycemia in Glossary).

- you have been newly diagnosed with kidney or liver disease or low thyroid (hypothyroidism).
- you are pregnant.
- you have an illness that is causing diarrhea or vomiting.
- you take aspirin, beta-blockers, fenfluramine (Pondimin), or monoamine oxidase (MAO) type A inhibitors (see Drug Classes).

Possible Side Effects (natural, expected, and unavoidable drug actions)

Hypoglycemia is the most common side effect of insulin treatment. This effect is made more likely when diet, physical activity, and other factors are incorrectly balanced and maintained. In unstable ("brittle") diabetes, unexpected drops in blood sugar levels can occur, resulting in hypoglycemia (see Glossary). Weight gain.

▷ **Possible Adverse Effects** (unusual, unexpected, and infrequent reactions)

If any of the following develop, consult your physician promptly for guidance.

Mild Adverse Effects

Allergic reactions: local redness, swelling, and itching at site of injection or hives—infrequent.

Taste disorders—possible.

Thinning of subcutaneous tissue at sites of injection (lipodystrophy)—infrequent.

Serious Adverse Effects

Allergic reaction: anaphylactic reactions (see Glossary).

Severe, prolonged hypoglycemia—possible to infrequent.

Inflammation of the parotid (parotitis)—case reports.

Hemolytic anemia or porphyria—case reports.

Arrhythmias (such as premature ventricular contractions)—associated with hypoglycemia) or very fast heart rate (with intravenous use)—case reports.

Insulin resistance—possible to rare.

▷ **Possible Effects on Sexual Function:** May resolve sexual problems (dysfunction) in patients who have this prior to starting insulin therapy. May also cause decrease in libido and erectile dysfunction—case reports (may also be a result of nerve/blood vessel damage as part of diabetes progressive effect).

▷ **Adverse Effects That May Mimic Natural Diseases or Disorders**

The early signs of hypoglycemia may be mistaken for alcoholic intoxication.

Possible Effects on Laboratory Tests

Blood cholesterol level: decreased.

Blood glucose level: decreased.

Blood potassium level: decreased.

Glycosylated hemoglobin (hemoglobin A1C) or fructosamine: decreased.

CAUTION

1. Carry a card in your purse or wallet saying that you have diabetes and are taking insulin.
2. Know how to recognize hypoglycemia and how to treat it. Always carry a readily available form of sugar, such as hard candy or sugar cubes. Report any hypoglycemia to your doctor.
3. Your vision may improve during the first few weeks of insulin therapy. Postpone eye exams for eyeglasses for 6 weeks after starting insulin.
4. Insulin is absorbed more quickly or slowly depending on where it is injected. Absorption is 80% greater from the abdominal wall than from

the leg and 30% greater than from the arm. It is advisable to rotate the injection site within the same body region than from one site to another.

5. Insulin glargine is CLEAR, not cloudy. This may be confusing to some patients because in the past, diabetics have been taught that short-acting insulins are clear and long-acting insulins are cloudy. Lantus form should NOT be mixed with other insulins. Insulin aspart is clear and colorless.

6. The American Diabetic Association (ADA) says diabetes is diagnosed when two fasting blood sugars in a row are more than 125 mg/dL. This more conservative approach reflects that complications start at lower blood sugar levels than previously thought. The concept of pre-diabetes (formerly impaired glucose tolerance) is described in the Glossary. Some British clinicians advocates that statin-type medicines could cut the risk of heart attack and stroke by a third (even in people with "normal" cholesterol), yet these medicines are underused in diabetics. Talk to your doctor about this.

7. If metformin is used in combination with insulin (added to existing insulin treatment), the insulin dose is continued at the level used prior to adding metformin. When fasting plasma sugar (glucose) falls below 120 mg/deciliter, the insulin dose should be lowered by 10 to 25%. Ongoing dose adjustments will be determined by goals and blood sugar checks.

8. Newer targets of A1C (glycosylated hemoglobin) of 6.5 are prudent in helping to avoid complications, but also carry the increased risk of excessively low blood sugar (hypoglycemia). Make sure you understand the signs and symptoms of hypoglycemia if more aggressive goals have been chosen.

9. Diabetes IS A RISK FACTOR FOR HEART DISEASE. Talk to your doctor about preventing a first heart attack (primary prevention). There are crucial steps to take involving lifestyle choices, exercise, and proven preventive medicines!

Precautions for Use

By Infants and Children: Insulin doses and schedules are modified according to patient's size. Adhere strictly to the physician's prescribed routine. Some of the insulins, such as insulin aspart (NovoLog), are NOT approved in children.

By Those Over 60 Years of Age: Insulin needs may change with age. Periodic individual evaluation is needed to identify the best dose and schedule. The aging brain adapts well to higher blood sugar levels. Rigid attempts at "tight" sugar control may result in hypoglycemia that shows as confusion and abnormal behavior. Repeated hypoglycemia (especially if severe) may cause brain damage.

▷ Advisability of Use During Pregnancy

Pregnancy Category: B. See Pregnancy Risk Categories at the back of this book.

Animal studies: Inconclusive.

Human studies: Adequate studies of pregnant women are not available. Birth defects occur 2 to 4 times more frequently in infants of diabetic mothers than in infants of mothers who do not have diabetes. The exact causes of this are not known.

Insulin is the drug of choice for managing diabetes during pregnancy. To preserve the health of the mother and fetus, every effort must be made to establish the best dose of insulin necessary for "good control" and to prevent episodes of hypoglycemia.

Advisability of Use If Breast-Feeding
    Presence of this drug in breast milk: No data.
    Insulin treatment of the mother has no adverse effect on the nursing infant. Breast-feeding may decrease insulin requirements; dose adjustment may be necessary.

Habit-Forming Potential: None, but cases of surreptitious insulin injection have been reported.

Effects of Overdose: Hypoglycemia: fatigue, weakness, headache, nervousness, irritability, sweating, tremors, hunger, confusion, delirium, abnormal behavior (resembling alcoholic intoxication), loss of consciousness, seizures.

Possible Effects of Long-Term Use: Thinning of subcutaneous fat tissue at sites of insulin injection. Insulin resistance.

Suggested Periodic Examinations While Taking This Drug (at physician's discretion)
    Routine testing of blood sugar levels at intervals recommended by your physician is prudent. Historically, estimates of blood sugar were obtained by checking urine sugar. This method has been replaced by finger stick testing of blood glucose. Finger stick testing accurately reflects the blood sugar and helps ensure better control (tighter control) of blood glucose. One novel device uses a laser to "stick" the finger (see *www.cellrobotics. com*). The laser is painless and appears to avoid toughening the skin like a lancet. One blood sugar machine can also test glycated protein (fructosamine). If you are ill, increased frequency of finger stick blood glucose testing may be indicated. A handheld machine called A1cNow enables pharmacists and physicians to check hemoglobin A1C in the office or pharmacy in 8 minutes! Additionally, a device called a Glucowatch Biographer uses a pad and a watchlike device to painlessly check blood sugar (see *www.cygnus.com*). Periodic evaluation of heart and circulatory system (diabetes is a large risk factor for heart and blood vessel disease).

▷ **While Taking This Drug, Observe the Following**
    Foods: Follow your diabetic diet conscientiously. Taking a diabetes education course is very smart and can teach you about portion control, what to do on sick days, and other important concepts. Blood sugar control can help avoid or delay diabetes problems! Vitamin C in high dose may worsen blood sugar control. Do not omit snack foods in mid-afternoon or at bedtime if they help prevent hypoglycemia. Rice bran has been checked in a small (57-subject) study of type 1 and type 2 diabetics. The benefit was a 30% lowering of sugar. This might be a complementary care option.
    Herbal Medicines or Minerals: Using chromium may change the way your body is able to use sugar. Some health food stores advocate vanadium as mimicking the actions of insulin, but possible toxicity and need for rigorous studies presently preclude recommending it. DHEA may change sensitivity to insulin or insulin resistance. Aloe, bitter melon, eucalyptus, fenugreek, ginger, garlic, ginseng, glucomannan, guar gum, hawthorn, licorice, nettle, and yohimbe may change blood sugar. Surprisingly, boiled stems of the Optuntia streptacantha prickly pear cactus appear to be able to lower blood sugar. Ongoing effects and effects on A1C are not known. Red sage is used for blood sugar effects, but is unproven. Psyllium increases risk of excessively low blood sugar. Since so many of these products may require adjustment of insulin dosing, talk to your doctor BEFORE combining any

of these herbal medicines with this medicine. Echinacea pupurea (injectable) and blonde psyllium seed or husk should NOT be taken by people living with diabetes.

Beverages: Use according to prescribed diabetic diet.

▷ *Alcohol:* Used excessively, alcohol can cause severe hypoglycemia, resulting in brain damage.

Tobacco Smoking: Regular smoking can decrease insulin absorption and increase insulin requirements by 30%. It is advisable to stop smoking altogether.

Marijuana Smoking: Possible increase in blood sugar levels.

▷ *Other Drugs*

The following drugs may ***increase*** the effects of insulin:

- acarbose (Precose)—by decreasing the amount of sugar that insulin has to work on.
- aspirin and other salicylates.
- some beta-blocker drugs (especially the nonselective ones; see Drug Classes)—may prolong insulin-induced hypoglycemia.
- clofibrate (Atromid-S).
- disopyramide (Norpace).
- fenfluramine (Pondimin).
- fluroquinolone antibiotics (see Drug Classes—such as ciprofloxacin and gatifloxacin). Caution and careful checks of blood sugar are prudent.
- monoamine oxidase (MAO) type A inhibitors (see Drug Classes).
- oral antidiabetic drugs (see Drug Classes)—results in additive hypoglycemia.

The following drugs may ***decrease*** the effects of insulin (by raising blood sugar levels):

- birth control pills (oral contraceptives).
- chlorthalidone (Hygroton).
- cortisonelike (corticosteroid) drugs (see Drug Classes).
- furosemide (Lasix).
- phenytoin (Dilantin, etc.) or fosphenytoin (Cerebyx).
- thiazide diuretics (see Drug Classes).
- thyroid preparations (various).

▷ *Driving, Hazardous Activities:* Be prepared to stop and take corrective action if hypoglycemia develops.

Aviation Note: Diabetes and the use of this drug ***are disqualifications*** for piloting. Consult a designated Aviation Medical Examiner.

Exposure to Sun: No restrictions.

Exposure to Heat: Use caution. Sauna baths can significantly increase the rate of insulin absorption and cause hypoglycemia.

Heavy Exercise or Exertion: Use caution. Periods of unusual or unplanned heavy physical activity will use up sugar more quickly and predispose to hypoglycemia.

Occurrence of Unrelated Illness: Omission of meals as a result of nausea, vomiting, or injury may lead to hypoglycemia. Infections can increase insulin needs. Ask your doctor for help.

Discontinuation: Do not stop this drug without asking your doctor. Omission of insulin may result in life-threatening coma.

Special Storage Instructions: Keep in a cool place, preferably in the refrigerator. Protect from freezing. Protect from strong light and high temperatures when not refrigerated.

Observe the Following Expiration Times: Do not use this drug if it is older than the expiration date on the vial. Always use fresh, "within date" insulin.

IPRATROPIUM (i pra TROH pee um)

Introduced: 1975 **Class:** Bronchodilator **Prescription:** USA: Yes **Controlled Drug:** USA: No; Canada: No **Available as Generic:** USA: No; Canada: No

Brand Names: Atrovent (single ingredient U.S.), Atrovent [CD other countries], ✦Alti-Atrovent, ✦Apo-Atrovent, Atrovent Nasal Spray, Combivent [CD], Dom-Ipratropium, Ipratropium Novaplus, PMS-Ipratropium

---

BENEFITS versus RISKS

Possible Benefits	Possible Risks
EFFECTIVE BRONCHODILATOR FOR TREATMENT OF CHRONIC BRONCHITIS AND EMPHYSEMA EFFECTIVE TREATMENT OF RUNNY NOSE (RHINORRHEA) Effective adjunctive treatment in some bronchial asthma	Mild and infrequent adverse effects (see Possible Adverse Effects)

▷ **Principal Uses**

As a Single Drug Product: Uses currently included in FDA-approved labeling: (1) Helps prevent or relieve episodes of difficult breathing in chronic bronchitis, chronic obstructive pulmonary disease (COPD), and emphysema (should not be used to treat acute attacks of asthma because it takes a while to work); (2) used in nasal spray to relieve symptoms of runny nose (rhinorrhea) from allergic or nonallergic perennial rhinitis (including runny nose from colds) in adults and children over 12 years old.

Other (unlabeled) generally accepted uses: (1) Relief of asthma symptoms; (2) lung symptoms of congestive heart failure.

As a Combination Drug Product [CD]: Available in combination with fenoterol (combivent form in other countries), a beta-adrenergic agonist that works in a different way. Also available with albuterol (combivent form in the United States). These combinations are more effective than either drug used alone. Different ingredients with the same brand name are also a good example of how the same name in different countries can contain different active ingredients. This profile will focus on the single-ingredient forms.

How This Drug Works: Through its atropinelike (anticholinergic) action, it blocks bronchial constriction and opens bronchi. Nasal form keeps acetylcholine from working (antagonizes it) and decreases production and secretion of mucus.

▷ **Widely Used Guidelines That Involve This Medicine (representative sample):** Please look at the section at the very beginning of this profile called "Class." Next, turn to Table 22 and you will find guidelines listed by the class involved!

Available Dosage Forms and Strengths

Inhalation aerosol — 14 g metered dose inhaler; 18 mcg per inhalation

Nasal inhaler — 20 mcg per actuation

Nasal spray — 0.03, 0.06%

Nebulizer — 250 mcg/mL solution

▷ **Usual Adult Dosage Ranges:** *Inhalation form:* Initially two inhalations (36 mcg) 4 times a day, 4 hours apart. If needed, the dose may be increased to 4 inhalations (72 mcg) at one time to get the best (optimal) relief. Maintain 4-hour intervals between doses. Maximum daily dose is 12 inhalations (216 mcg in 24 hours). *Nasal spray:* for use in runny nose (rhinorrhea) seen with the common cold: 0.03%—two sprays (21 mcg each) in each nostril 2 to 3 times a day for up to 4 days; 0.06%—2 sprays (42 mcg each) in each nostril 3 to 4 times a day for up to 4 days.

Note: Actual dose and dosing schedule must be determined for each patient individually.

Conditions Requiring Dosing Adjustments
Liver Function: Specific guidelines not developed.
Kidney Function: Used with caution by patients with bladder neck obstructions.

▷ **Dosing Instructions:** Carefully follow the patient instructions provided with the inhaler because a small amount of medicine reaches the lungs with the best technique. Shake well before using. Many people do NOT take the time to learn the best inhaler technique—take the time to do this. Carefully follow the patient instructions on the nasal form: the pump of the nasal form must be primed before the unit is used. Read the package insert carefully, and ask your pharmacist for help if you don't understand the directions. If you forget a dose: use the inhaler or nasal spray as soon as you remember it, unless it's nearly time for your next dose—then skip the missed dose, space the remaining doses for the day at regularly separated times and continue the next day right on schedule. DO NOT double doses. Call your doctor if you find yourself missing doses or if you do not get the usual benefits from this medicine.

Usual Duration of Use:
Inhalation form: Continual use on a regular schedule for 48 to 72 hours is usually necessary to determine this drug's effectiveness. Long-term use (months to years) requires check of response and dose adjustment. See your doctor.
Nasal spray: The nasal form helps some people feel better right away and may take a week or so for others. The nasal spray may only be used for up to 4 days.

Typical Treatment Goals and Measurements (Outcomes and Markers)
Asthma: Frequency and severity of asthma attacks should ease. Some clinicians also use decreased frequency of rescue inhaler use as a further clinical indicator. Lung function (pulmonary function) tests such as FEV1 are typical for more involved testing. It is critical that this medicine is used regularly to get the best results. If the usual benefit is not realized, call your doctor.
Runny nose (rhinorrhea) from a cold: Decreased need to blow your nose. Resolution of runny nose.

Possible Advantages of This Drug
Inhalation form produces a greater degree of bronchodilation than theophylline in patients with chronic bronchitis and emphysema. Causes minimal adverse effects. Repeated use does not appear to lead to tolerance and loss of effectiveness. Suitable for long-term maintenance therapy.
Nasal spray eases a very annoying symptom (rhinorrhea, or runny nose) seen with common cold.

Currently a "Drug of Choice"
For difficult breathing associated with chronic bronchitis and emphysema. Nasal form makes a common cold more manageable.

▷ **This Drug Should Not Be Taken If**
- you have had an allergic reaction to it previously.
- you are allergic to soybeans or peanuts (inhalation form).
- you are allergic to atropine or to aerosol propellants (fluorocarbons) (inhalation form).
- you are allergic to benzalkonium chloride or edetate disodium (nasal spray).

▷ **Inform Your Physician Before Taking This Drug If**
- you have had an adverse effect from any belladonna-type chemical (derivative) previously.
- you have a history of glaucoma.
- you have any form of urinary retention or prostatism (see Glossary).

Possible Side Effects (natural, expected, and unavoidable drug actions)
Throat dryness, cough, irritation from aerosol—rare.
Blurred vision, dry mouth.
Bad or bitter taste—frequent.

▷ **Possible Adverse Effects** (unusual, unexpected, and infrequent reactions)
If any of the following develop, consult your physician promptly for guidance.
Mild Adverse Effects
Allergic reactions: skin rash, hives—rare.
Headache, dizziness, nervousness—rare.
Palpitations—rare.
Nosebleeds (with nasal spray)—infrequent to frequent.
Serious Adverse Effects
Allergic reactions: rare first-dose angioedema or bronchospasm.
Author's Note: Other than the rare allergic reactions, the nasal spray does not appear to have any serious adverse effects.
Abnormal heartbeat (supraventricular tachycardia)—case report.
Intraocular pressure changes—rare.

▷ **Possible Effects on Sexual Function:** None reported.

Natural Diseases or Disorders That May Be Activated by This Drug
Angle-closure glaucoma, prostatism (see Glossary).

Possible Effects on Laboratory Tests: None reported.

CAUTION
1. This drug won't start to work for 5 to 15 minutes. It should not be used alone to treat acute attacks of asthma needing a fast result.
2. When used as combination therapy with beta-adrenergic antiasthmatic drugs (albuterol, terbutaline, metaproterenol, etc.), the beta-adrenergic aerosol should be used about 5 minutes before using ipratropium to prevent fluorocarbon toxicity.
3. When used as an adjunct to steroid or cromolyn aerosols (beclomethasone, Intal), ipratropium should be used about 5 minutes before using the steroid or cromolyn aerosol to prevent fluorocarbon toxicity.
4. Contact with the eyes can cause temporary blurring of vision.
5. Call your doctor if you are using the nasal spray and your runny nose (rhinorrhea) continues or gets worse and you develop a fever.

Precautions for Use
By Infants and Children: Nasal spray is now approved for use for those 6 to 11 years old. Dosing is the same as for adults for the 0.03% form. Safety and effectiveness for those under 6 are not established.

By Those Over 60 Years of Age: Watch for possible development of prostatism and adjust dose as necessary.

▷ **Advisability of Use During Pregnancy**
Pregnancy Category: B. See Pregnancy Risk Categories at the back of this book.
Animal studies: No drug-induced birth defects in mouse, rat, or rabbit studies.
Human studies: Adequate studies of pregnant women are not available.
Use this drug during pregnancy only if clearly needed.

Advisability of Use If Breast-Feeding
Presence of this drug in breast milk: Possibly yes, but in very small amounts. Watch nursing infant closely and stop drug or nursing if adverse effects start.

Habit-Forming Potential: None.

Effects of Overdose: This drug is not well absorbed into the circulation when it is taken by aerosol inhalation. No systemic effects of overdose are expected.

Possible Effects of Long-Term Use: Drying of the nose with nasal form.

Suggested Periodic Examinations While Taking This Drug (at physician's discretion)
Internal eye pressure measurements if appropriate.

▷ **While Taking This Drug, Observe the Following**
Foods: No restrictions.
Herbal Medicines or Minerals: Fir or pine needle oil should NOT be used by asthmatics. Betel nut may lower the beneficial effects of ipratropium in treating asthma. Ephedra alone does carry a German Commission E monograph indication for asthma treatment. If you are allergic to plants in the Asteraceae family (aster, chrysanthemum, daisy, or ragweed), you may also be allergic to echinacea, chamomile, feverfew, and St. John's wort. Talk to your doctor BEFORE adding any herbals to this medicine.
Beverages: No restrictions.
▷ *Alcohol:* No interactions expected.
Tobacco Smoking: No interactions expected, but smoking should be avoided completely if you have chronic bronchitis or emphysema. I advise everyone to quit smoking.
Marijuana Smoking: Possible excessive increase in heart rate (tachycardia).
▷ *Other Drugs*
Ipratropium may ***increase*** the effects of
• albuterol (Proventil, others).
• other atropinelike drugs (see Drug Classes).
Ipratropium ***taken concurrently*** with
• belladonna (various) may lead to excessive anticholinergic action (fast heart rate, blurred vision, constipation, weakness, etc.).
• cisapride (Propulsid) may lessen benefits of cisapride.
• procainamide (Procan, others) may lead to additive effects on the vagal nerve and heart conduction (atrioventricular).
• tricyclic antidepressants (see Drug Classes) may result in additive anticholinergic effects.
▷ *Driving, Hazardous Activities:* May cause dizziness or blurred vision. Restrict activities as necessary.
Aviation Note: The use of this drug ***may be a disqualification*** for piloting. Consult a designated Aviation Medical Examiner.
Exposure to Sun: No restrictions.
Exposure to Cold: Inhaling cold air may cause bronchospasm and induce asthmatic breathing and cough; dose adjustment of this drug may be necessary.

Heavy Exercise or Exertion: This drug is not considered to be consistently effective in preventing or treating exercise-induced asthma.

Discontinuation: Ask your doctor for help. Substitute medication may be advisable.

IRINOTECAN (ear in oh TEE kan)

Other Name: Camptothecin-11   **Introduced:**   2000   **Class:**   Antineoplastic, chemotherapy, topoisomerase I inhibitor   **Prescription:**   USA: Yes   **Controlled Drug:**   USA: No; Canada: No   **Available as Generic:** USA: No; Canada: No

Brand Name: Camptosar

Warning: You may not expect a non-prescription herbal product to create a problem, but St. John's wort lowered blood levels of irinotecan by 40% in a small study in the Netherlands. Make sure you are getting the most from your chemotherapy and avoid even combination products that have hypericin, hypericum, hypervorin, or similar ingredients. If a generic name of an herbal "shotgun" product sounds similar, talk to your doctor or pharmacist to be sure that an innocent-sounding treatment for depression isn't blocking your "chemo" and letting the cancer continue.

Author's Note: Irinotecan is a first-line treatment for colorectal cancer and is the first such agent to be FDA approved in more than 40 years. It is approved for use in combination with 5-FU/LV to treat colorectal cancer that has spread (metastatic) and for people who have had their cancer recur or progress after being given 5-FU-based treatment. Information in this profile will be broadened in subsequent editions as data warrants.

ISONIAZID (i soh NI a zid)

Other Names: Isonicotinic acid hydrazide, INH

Introduced: 1956   **Class:**   Antituberculosis   **Prescription:** USA: Yes   **Controlled Drug:**   USA: No; Canada: No   **Available as Generic:**   USA: Yes; Canada: Yes

Brand Names: INH, ✤Isotamine, Laniazid, Nydrazid, Pasna Tri-Pack 300 [CD], P-I-N Forte [CD], ✤PMS-Isoniazid, Rifamate [CD], Rifater [CD], Rimactane/INH Dual Pack [CD], Seromycin w/Isoniazid [CD], Teebaconin, Teebaconin and Vitamin B_6 [CD]

BENEFITS versus RISKS	
Possible Benefits	*Possible Risks*
EFFECTIVE PREVENTION AND TREATMENT OF ACTIVE TUBERCULOSIS (TREATS TB IN COMBINATION)	ALLERGIC LIVER REACTION— RARE
	Peripheral neuropathy (see Glossary)
	Bone marrow depression (see Glossary)
	Mental and behavioral disturbances

Principal Uses

As a Single Drug Product: Uses currently included in FDA-approved labeling: (1) Used alone to prevent the development of tuberculous infection (prophylaxis) in people who are at high risk because of exposure to infection or recent conversion of a negative tuberculin skin test to positive; (2) used in combination with other drugs to treat tuberculosis in a variety of body sites.

Other (unlabeled) generally accepted uses: (1) Could have a role in some high-risk patients as part of a methadone maintenance designed to prevent tuberculosis in high-risk patients; (2) may have a role in part of a regimen used to treat local (superficial) bladder cancer (Bacillus Calmette-Guerin—BCG).

As a Combination Drug Product [CD]: Available in combination with rifampin, another antitubercular drug that works in a different way. This combination is more effective than either drug used alone and also encourages patients to take their medicine (adherence). Isoniazid can cause low pyridoxine (vitamin B_6); for this reason, a combination of the two drugs is available in tablet and granule form.

How This Drug Works: By interfering with metabolism or cell walls, this drug kills (bactericidal) or inhibits (bacteriostatic) susceptible tuberculosis organisms.

▷ **Widely Used Guidelines That Involve This Medicine (representative sample):** Please look at the section at the very beginning of this profile called "Class." Next, turn to Table 22 and you will find guidelines listed by the class involved!

Available Dosage Forms and Strengths

Injection — 100 mg/mL

Packet — 100 mg pyridoxine, 10 mg pyridoxine, 4.5 grams aminosalicylate

Syrup — 50 mg/5 mL

Tablets — 50 mg, 100 mg, 300 mg

▷ **Usual Adult Dosage Ranges:** *For prevention:* 300 mg once daily (usually for 6 to 12 months). *For treatment:* 5 mg per kg of body mass daily. The total daily dose should not exceed 300 mg. Some clinicians use 5 mg/kg daily (up to 300 mg) for 2 weeks and then give 15 mg per kg (up to 900 mg) 2 to 3 times weekly. *Latent TB:* 5 mg per kg of body mass once a day (up to 300 mg a day) for 9 months is suggested by the American Thoracic Society to treat latent TB in HIV-negative or HIV-positive patients.

Note: Actual dose and dosing schedule must be determined on an individual basis.

Conditions Requiring Dosing Adjustments

Liver Function: This drug should not be used in sudden (acute) liver disease. It should be discontinued if liver function tests become increased to 3 times the normal value.

Kidney Function: This drug is a rare cause of nephrosis. For severe kidney failure (creatinine clearance less than 10 mL/min), daily dose is lowered by 50%.

▷ **Dosing Instructions:** The tablet may be crushed and taken with food to prevent stomach irritation. Make sure you use a measuring cup or spoon if you are taking the liquid form. If you forget a dose: take the missed dose as soon as you remember it, unless it's nearly time for your next dose, then skip the missed dose and take the next dose right on schedule. DO NOT double doses. Call your doctor if you find yourself missing doses.

Usual Duration of Use: Use on a regular schedule for 1 year or more is often necessary, depending upon the nature of the infection. Shorter courses of intermittent high doses may work, but the medicine must be taken for months. See your doctor regularly.

Typical Treatment Goals and Measurements (Outcomes and Markers)

Infections: The most commonly used measures of serious infections are white blood cell counts and differentials (the kind of blood cells that occur most often in your blood) and temperature or night sweats. Because of the nature of this infection, therapy will be long-term. NEVER stop a medicine for tuberculosis because you start to feel better. The goals and time frame should be discussed with you when the prescription is written.

▷ **This Drug Should Not Be Taken If**
- you have had an allergic reaction (especially a liver reaction) to any dose form of it previously.
- you have active liver disease.

▷ **Inform Your Physician Before Taking This Drug If**
- you have serious impairment of liver or kidney function.
- you drink an alcoholic beverage daily.
- you are an alcoholic.
- you are pregnant or breast-feeding your baby.
- you have a seizure disorder.
- you take other drugs on a long-term basis, especially phenytoin (Dilantin).
- you plan to have surgery under general anesthesia in the near future.

Possible Side Effects (natural, expected, and unavoidable drug actions)
Toxic fever—rare.

▷ **Possible Adverse Effects** (unusual, unexpected, and infrequent reactions)
If any of the following develop, consult your physician promptly for guidance.

Mild Adverse Effects

Allergic reactions: skin rash, fever, swollen glands, painful muscles and joints.

Dizziness, indigestion, nausea, vomiting.

Peripheral neuritis (see Glossary): numbness, tingling, pain, weakness in hands and/or feet—frequent in adults, rare in children (may be prevented with pyridoxine).

Serious Adverse Effects

Allergic reactions: drug-induced hepatitis (see Glossary) (loss of appetite, nausea, fatigue, itching, dark-colored urine, yellowing of eyes and skin)—may be fulminant and fatal, hypersensitivity, meningitis—case reports.

Severe skin reactions (Stevens-Johnson syndrome, pellagra)—case reports.

Acute mental/behavioral disturbances, psychosis, impaired vision, increase in epileptic seizures—rare.

Movement disorders (ataxia)—case reports in patients not receiving supplemental pyridoxine.

High or low blood sugars (hyperglycemia or hypoglycemia)—possible.

Porphyria, pancreatitis, or kidney toxicity—case reports.

Lupus erythematosus–like syndrome or abnormal muscle changes (rhabdomyolysis)—case reports.

Pellagra—rare.

Disseminated intravascular coagulation (DIC)—case report.

Bone marrow depression (see Glossary): fatigue, weakness, fever, sore throat, abnormal bleeding or bruising—case reports.

▷ **Possible Effects on Sexual Function:** Male breast enlargement and tenderness (gynecomastia)—rare.

Possible Delayed Adverse Effects: Increased frequency of liver cirrhosis has been reported.

▷ **Adverse Effects That May Mimic Natural Diseases or Disorders**
Drug-induced hepatitis may suggest viral hepatitis. Collagen vascular changes may mimic rheumatoid arthritis or systemic lupus erythematosus. Pseudolymphoma may occur.

Natural Diseases or Disorders That May Be Activated by This Drug
Latent epilepsy, systemic lupus erythematosus (questionable).

Possible Effects on Laboratory Tests
Complete blood cell counts: decreased red cells, hemoglobin, white cells, and platelets; increased eosinophils (allergic reaction).
Blood amylase level: increased (possible pancreatitis).
Blood antinuclear antibodies (ANA): positive.
Blood lupus erythematosus (LE) cells: positive.
Blood glucose level: increased (with large doses).
Liver function tests: increased liver enzymes (ALT/GPT, AST/GOT, and alkaline phosphatase), increased bilirubin.
Urine sugar tests: increased; false positive results with Benedict's solution and Clinitest.

CAUTION
1. **The FDA requires an updated warning for Laniazid: "A recent report suggests an increased risk of fatal hepatitis associated with isoniazid among women, particularly African American and Hispanic women. The risk may also be increased during the postpartum period."** Increased laboratory testing is also suggested in this case.
2. Ask your doctor about determining if you are a "slow" or "rapid" inactivator (acetylator) of isoniazid. This has a bearing on your predisposition to developing adverse effects.
3. Copper sulfate tests for urine sugar may give a false-positive test result. (Diabetics, please note.)
4. Because multidrug-resistant (MDR) tuberculosis is now more common in many areas, four-drug combination therapy (isoniazid, pyrazinamide, ethambutol, and rifampin) is often used.

Precautions for Use
By Infants and Children: Use with caution in children with seizure disorders. "Slow acetylators" are more prone to adverse drug effects. It is advisable to give supplemental pyridoxine (vitamin B_6).
Prevention: Infants and children are given 10 mg per kg per day up to 300 mg for 6–12 months.
By Those Over 60 Years of Age: There is a greater incidence of liver damage in this age group, and liver status should be closely watched. Watch for any indications of an "acute brain syndrome," which will show up as confusion, delirium, and seizures.

▷ **Advisability of Use During Pregnancy**
Pregnancy Category: C. See Pregnancy Risk Categories at the back of this book.
Animal Studies: No birth defects reported in mice, rats, or rabbits.
Human Studies: Data from adequate studies of pregnant women are not available.
If clearly needed, this drug is now used at any time during pregnancy. Ask your physician for guidance.

Advisability of Use If Breast-Feeding
Presence of this drug in breast milk: Yes.
Talk to your doctor about benefits and risks.

Habit-Forming Potential: None.

Effects of Overdose: Nausea, vomiting, dizziness, blurred vision, hallucinations, slurred speech, stupor, coma, seizures.

Possible Effects of Long-Term Use: Peripheral neuritis due to a deficiency of pyridoxine (vitamin B$_6$).

Suggested Periodic Examinations While Taking This Drug (at physician's discretion)
Complete blood cell counts.
Liver function tests.
Complete eye examinations, repeat sputum cultures. Chest X-rays.

▷ **While Taking This Drug, Observe the Following**
Foods: Eat the following foods cautiously until your tolerance determined: Swiss and Cheshire cheeses, tuna fish, skipjack fish, and Sardinella species. These may interact with the drug to produce skin rash, itching, sweating, chills, headache, light-headedness, or rapid heart rate. Taking this drug with food also acts to decrease absorption and lessen therapeutic benefits. Some red wines and aged cheeses also contain high levels of tyramine and might result in an undesirable increase in blood pressure. Avoid this combination.
Nutritional Support: It is advisable to take a supplement of pyridoxine (vitamin B$_6$) to prevent peripheral neuritis. Ask your physician for help.
Herbal Medicines or Minerals: Echinacea: Some patients use echinacea to attempt to boost their immune systems. Unfortunately, use of echinacea is not recommended in people with damaged immune systems. This herb may also actually weaken any immune system if it is used too often or for too long a time (more than 8 weeks). DO NOT take mistletoe herb, oak bark, F.C. of marshmallow root, and licorice.
Beverages: No restrictions. May be taken with milk.
▷ *Alcohol:* Alcohol may reduce the effectiveness of this drug and increase the risk of liver toxicity, and possibly lead to disulfiram reactions.
Tobacco Smoking: No interactions expected. I advise everyone to quit smoking.
▷ *Other Drugs*
Isoniazid may ***increase*** the effects of
• carbamazepine (Tegretol) and cause toxicity.
• disulfiram (Antabuse) and change behavior.
• phenytoin (Dilantin) or fosphenytoin (Cerebyx) and cause toxicity.
The following drugs may ***decrease*** the effects of isoniazid:
• cortisonelike drugs (see Drug Classes).
Isoniazid ***taken concurrently*** with
• acetaminophen (Tylenol) may increase the risk of liver damage (hepatoxicity).
• antacids may decrease the absorption. Separate antacid dosing by 2 hours from dosing this medicine.
• BCG vaccine will result in decreased vaccine effectiveness.
• cyclosporine (Sandimmune) may blunt cyclosporine benefits.
• diazepam and perhaps other benzodiazepines (see Drug Classes) may result in increased blood levels and toxicity.
• ketoconazole, itraconazole, voriconazole (Vfend), or related compounds may result in decreased therapeutic benefits of the antifungal.

- meperidine (Demerol) may result in excessive lowering of blood pressure.
- niacin (various) may lead to a need for increased niacin.
- oral antidiabetic drugs (see Drug Classes) may result in loss of control of blood glucose.
- propranolol (Inderal, others) may lead to isoniazid toxicity.
- rifampin (Rifadin, others) can result in a serious increased risk of liver toxicity.
- theophylline (Theodur, others) may result in theophylline toxicity.
- valproic acid (Depakene) can result in isoniazid or valproic acid toxicity.
- warfarin (Coumadin) may result in increased bleeding risk; more frequent INR (prothrombin time or protime) testing is needed.

▷ *Driving, Hazardous Activities:* This drug may cause dizziness. Restrict activities as necessary.

Aviation Note: The use of this drug **may be a disqualification** for piloting. Consult a designated Aviation Medical Examiner.

Exposure to Sun: No restrictions.

Discontinuation: Long-term treatment is required. Do not stop this drug without asking your physician.

ISOSORBIDE DINITRATE (i soh SOHR bide di NI trayt)

Other Name: Sorbide nitrate   **Introduced:**   1959   **Class:**   Antianginal, nitrates   **Prescription:**   USA: Yes   **Controlled Drug:**   USA: No; Canada: No   **Available as Generic:**   USA: Yes; Canada: No

Brand Names: Angipec, ✚Apo-ISDN, ✚Cedocard-SR, ✚Coradur, ✚Coronex, Dilatrate-SR, Iso-BID, Isochron, Isonate, Isordil, Isordil Tembids, Isordil Titradose, Isotrate Timecelles, ✚Novo-Sorbide, Sorbitrate, Sorbitrate-SA

Warning: The brand names Isordil and Isuprel sound similar; this can lead to serious errors. Isordil is isosorbide dinitrate, used to treat angina. Isuprel is isoproterenol, used for asthma. Make sure you are taking the correct drug.

BENEFITS versus RISKS	
Possible Benefits	*Possible Risks*
EFFECTIVE RELIEF AND PREVENTION OF ANGINA	Orthostatic hypotension (see Glossary)
EFFECTIVE ADJUNCTIVE TREATMENT IN SOME CASES OF CONGESTIVE HEART FAILURE	Rare skin reactions (severe peeling)

▷ **Principal Uses**

As a Single Drug Product: Uses currently included in FDA-approved labeling: (1) The sublingual (under-the-tongue) tablets and the chewable tablets are used to prevent and relieve acute attacks of anginal pain; (2) the longer-acting tablets and capsules are used to prevent the development of angina, but are not effective in relieving acute episodes of anginal pain (nitroglycerin is the drug of choice in those cases).

Other (unlabeled) generally accepted uses: (1) This drug is also used to improve heart function in selected cases of congestive heart failure; (2) can help ease the pressure in esophageal varices in alcoholics; (3) can help painful leg cramping (intermittent claudication); (4) may be of use topically as an ointment to avoid surgery (sphincterotomy) or to ease symptoms of anal fissures; (5) may help diagnose syndrome X (angina resulting from exercise in people with normal epicardial coronary arteries); (6) used after a heart attack intravenously to help address congestive heart failure; (7) under the tongue (sublingual) dosing may help achalasia.

How This Drug Works: This drug relaxes and dilates arteries and veins. Benefits in treating angina and heart failure are due to dilation of coronary arteries and dilation of systemic veins. Net effects are improved heart blood flow and reduced workload.

▷ **Widely Used Guidelines That Involve This Medicine (representative sample):** Please look at the section at the very beginning of this profile called "Class." Next, turn to Table 22 and you will find guidelines listed by the class involved!

Available Dosage Forms and Strengths

Capsules — 40 mg

Capsules, prolonged action — 40 mg

Tablets — 5 mg, 10 mg, 20 mg, 30 mg, 40 mg

Tablets, chewable — 5 mg, 10 mg

Tablets, prolonged action — 20 mg, 40 mg

Tablets, sublingual — 2.5 mg, 5 mg, 10 mg

▷ **Recommended Dosage Ranges** (Actual dose and schedule must be determined for each patient individually.)

Infants and Children: Dose not established.

12 to 60 Years of Age:

Sublingual tablets: 5 to 10 mg dissolved under tongue every 2 to 3 hours; use for relief of acute attack and for prevention of anticipated attack.

Chewable tablets: initially 5 mg chewed to evaluate tolerance; increase dose to 5 or 10 mg every 2 to 3 hours as needed and tolerated. Use for relief of acute attack and for prevention of anticipated attack.

Tablets: 5 to 20 mg 4 times daily to prevent acute attack, with at least a 12-hour nitrate-free period.

Prolonged-action capsules and tablets: 40 mg to start and then 40–80 mg every 8 to 12 hours as needed to prevent acute attacks.

Author's Note: Dosing for all forms is set up to give a 12-hour nitrate-free period in order to avoid tolerance to the therapeutic benefits of this medicine.

Over 60 Years of Age: Same as 12 to 60 years of age, although excessive lowering of blood pressure on standing (postural hypotension) may be more likely in this population.

Conditions Requiring Dosing Adjustments

Liver Function: Used with caution and in decreased doses by patients with liver compromise, as increased blood levels will occur.

Kidney Function: No specific dosing changes are needed for compromised kidneys. This drug can discolor urine (brown to black).

▷ **Dosing Instructions:** Capsules and tablets to be swallowed are best taken on an empty stomach to achieve maximal blood levels. Regular tablets may be crushed; prolonged-action capsules and tablets should be taken whole, NOT chewed, crushed, or altered. If you forget a dose: take the missed dose as soon as you remember it, unless it's nearly time for your next dose—if this is the case, skip the missed dose, take the next dose right on schedule. DO NOT double doses. Call your doctor if you find yourself missing doses.

Usual Duration of Use: Use on a regular schedule for 3 to 7 days is needed to (1) identify this drug's peak effect in preventing or relieving acute anginal pain and (2) to find the optimal dose schedule. Long-term use (months to years) requires physician supervision. Ask your doctor what he or she wants you to do if the frequency or severity of angina increases or is not relieved by previously effective doses.

Typical Treatment Goals and Measurements (Outcomes and Markers)

Angina: The most commonly used markers are prevention or relief of chest pain (angina). Many cardiologists look for easing of frequency and severity of angina attacks as well as pulmonary capillary wedge pressure as measures of successful therapy. If your chest pain does not go away after using the maximum dose at the recommended time interval, have someone drive you to the hospital or call 911. Ask your doctor on the next office visit if it would make sense for you to chew a regular release full-dose aspirin prior to going to the hospital if that situation occurs.

▷ **This Drug Should Not Be Taken If**
- you had an allergic reaction to any form of it previously.
- you have severe anemia.
- you have increased intraocular pressure.
- you have suffered trauma to the head.
- you have an overactive thyroid gland.
- you have abnormal growth of the heart muscle (hypertrophic cardiomyopathy).
- you have already taken or take sildenafil (Viagra), vardenafil (Levitra), or tadalafil (Cialis).
- you have had a very recent heart attack (myocardial infarction) and have elevated blood pressure or very rapid heart rate (tachycardia).

▷ **Inform Your Physician Before Taking This Drug If**
- you have had an unfavorable response to other nitrate drugs or vasodilators in the past or have an allergy to tartrazine dye (in some forms of this medicine).
- you have a history of low blood pressure.
- you are anemic and are being prescribed the under-the-tongue (sublingual) form.
- you have any form of glaucoma.
- you have had a cerebral hemorrhage recently.
- you are pregnant or are planning pregnancy.
- you are allergic to the dye tartrazine.
- you have a glucose-6-phosphate dehydrogenase (G6PD) deficiency (ask your doctor).
- you have excessive thyroid function (hyperthyroidism), cardiomyopathy, or have suffered head trauma.

Possible Side Effects (natural, expected, and unavoidable drug actions)

Flushing of face, throbbing in head, palpitation, rapid heart rate, orthostatic hypotension (see Glossary).

▷ **Possible Adverse Effects** (unusual, unexpected, and infrequent reactions)

If any of the following develop, consult your physician promptly for guidance.

Mild Adverse Effects

Allergic reaction: skin rash.

Headache (may be severe and persistent)—infrequent to frequent.

Dizziness, fainting—possible.

Nausea, vomiting—possible.

Bad breath (halitosis)—case reports.

Urine discoloration—possible and not clinically significant.

Serious Adverse Effects

Allergic reaction: severe dermatitis with peeling of skin—case reports.

Transient ischemic attacks (TIAs) in presence of impaired circulation within the brain: dizziness, fainting, impaired vision or speech, localized numbness or weakness—possible.

Anemia (in those with G6PD deficiency)—possible.

Abnormal heart rates or conduction—case reports.

Abnormally low blood pressure on standing (postural hypotension)—possible.

Myocardial ischemia (with abrupt withdrawal) or infarction—possible.

Methemoglobinemia—case report.

Tolerance—possible with 24-hour use (daily 12-hour drug-free period is used to prevent this).

▷ **Possible Effects on Sexual Function:** None reported.

▷ **Adverse Effects That May Mimic Natural Diseases or Disorders**

Spells of low blood pressure (due to this drug) may mimic late-onset epilepsy.

Possible Effects on Laboratory Tests

Methemoglobin: increased.

CAUTION

1. Tolerance (see Glossary) to long-acting forms of nitrates may cause sublingual tablets of nitroglycerin to be less effective in relieving acute anginal attacks. Anti-anginal effectiveness is restored after 1 week of abstinence from long-acting nitrates. Daily 12-hour periods without use of the drug are needed.

2. Many over-the-counter (OTC) medicines for allergies, colds, and coughs contain drugs that may counteract the desired drug effects. Ask your physician or pharmacist for help before using such medicines.

Precautions for Use

By Those Over 60 Years of Age: Small starting doses are advisable. You may be more susceptible to the development of low blood pressure and associated "blackout" spells, fainting, and falling. Throbbing headaches and flushing may be more apparent.

▷ **Advisability of Use During Pregnancy**

Pregnancy Category: C. See Pregnancy Risk Categories at the back of this book.

Animal Studies: No information available.

Human Studies: Adequate studies of pregnant women are not available.

Use this drug only if clearly needed.

Advisability of Use If Breast-Feeding

Presence of this drug in breast milk: Unknown.

If this drug is thought to be necessary, monitor the nursing infant for low blood pressure and poor feeding.

Habit-Forming Potential: None.

Effects of Overdose: Headache, dizziness, marked flushing of face and skin, vomiting, weakness, fainting, difficult breathing, coma.

Possible Effects of Long-Term Use: Development of tolerance with temporary loss of effectiveness at recommended doses. Development of abnormal hemoglobin (red blood cell pigment).

Suggested Periodic Examinations While Taking This Drug (at physician's discretion)

Measurement of internal eye pressure.

Red cell counts and hemoglobin and methemoglobin tests.

▷ **While Taking This Drug, Observe the Following**

Foods: Oral doses are best taken on an empty stomach to ensure quick absorption. Vitamin C may help ease nitrate tolerance. More study is needed. Your doctor may also recommend some specific foods such as increased vegetables or functional foods such as Benecol. Three well-designed studies found that both in women and men and before and after a heart attack, people who ate more fish (2–4 servings a week) appeared to avoid heart disease. Additionally, taking supplements containing Omega 3 polyunsaturated fatty acids (PUFA) also appeared to protect against abnormal heart rhythms and sudden death from heart attack. Increasing oat bran in the diet may be of additional help in lowering cholesterol, but might decrease the amount of medicine that gets into your body. Take oat bran 2 hours before or 4 to 6 hours after. Your doctor may also recommend increasing B vitamins. See Tables 19 and 20 about lifestyle changes and risk factors you can fix!

Herbal Medicines or Minerals: Hawthorn and co-enzyme Q10 (co-Q10) can affect the way the heart works. Co-Q10 has a limited number of reports of decreasing INR in people taking warfarin. Soy (milk, tofu, etc.) contains phytoestrogens that have led to an FDA-approved health claim for reducing risk of heart disease (if they have at least 6.25 grams of soy protein per serving). Couch grass or nettle should NOT be taken by patients who have increased fluid (edema) caused by heart weakness. Hawthorn (Crataegus variety) has been used to help heart failure, but should not be combined with heart medicines as combination use has not been studied. BE CERTAIN to tell your doctor that you are taking or are considering taking these herbs if you are taking a nitrate.

Beverages: No restrictions. May be taken with milk.

▷ *Alcohol:* Use extreme caution and avoid alcohol completely in the presence of any side effects or adverse effects of this drug. Alcohol may exaggerate the blood pressure–lowering effect of this drug.

Tobacco Smoking: Nicotine can reduce benefits. Avoid all forms of tobacco.

Marijuana Smoking: Possible reduced effectiveness of this drug; mild to moderate increase in angina; possible changes in electrocardiogram, confusing interpretation.

▷ *Other Drugs*

Isosorbide dinitrate *taken concurrently* with

- antihypertensive drugs may cause excessive lowering of blood pressure; dose adjustments may be necessary.
- hydralazine (Apresoline) may work well to help control angina.
- propranolol (Inderal) can help improve exercise time without angina.
- sildenafil (Viagra), vardenafil (Levitra), or tadalafil (Cialis) may result in LIFE-THREATENING lowering of blood pressure. NEVER COMBINE.

▷ *Driving, Hazardous Activities:* Usually no restrictions. This drug may cause dizziness or spells of low blood pressure. Restrict activities as necessary.

Aviation Note: Coronary artery disease *is a disqualification* for piloting. Consult a designated Aviation Medical Examiner.

Exposure to Sun: No restrictions.

Exposure to Heat: Use caution. Hot environments can cause a significant drop in blood pressure.

Exposure to Cold: Cold environments can increase the need for this drug and limit its benefits.

Heavy Exercise or Exertion: This drug may improve your ability to be more active without anginal pain. Use caution and avoid excessive exertion.

Discontinuation: It is advisable to gradually withdraw this drug after long-term use. DO NOT abruptly withdraw this medicine. Dose and frequency of prolonged-action dose forms should be reduced gradually over a period of 4 to 6 weeks.

ISOSORBIDE MONONITRATE (i soh SOHR bide mon oh NI trayt)

Introduced: 1983 **Class:** Anti-anginal, nitrates **Prescription:** USA: Yes **Controlled Drug:** USA: No **Available as Generic:** USA: Yes

Brand Names: Elan (Italy), Elantan, Imdur, Ismo, Monoket

BENEFITS versus RISKS	
Possible Benefits	*Possible Risks*
EFFECTIVE PREVENTION OF ANGINA	Orthostatic hypotension (see Glossary) Headache

▷ **Principal Uses**

As a Single Drug Product: Uses currently included in FDA-approved labeling: (1) To reduce the frequency and severity of recurrent angina; not effective in acute anginal pain.

Other (unlabeled) generally accepted uses: (1) May have a role in treating congestive heart failure (intravenous); (2) can help in decreasing the number of attacks and time spent in silent myocardial ischemia; (3) may be of help in heart attacks (myocardial infarction); (4) may help stomach bleeding in people with cirrhosis of the liver.

How This Drug Works: Relaxes and dilates arteries and veins. Benefits in angina are due to dilation of coronary arteries and dilation of systemic veins. Net effects are improved blood flow to the heart and reduced workload of the heart.

▷ **Widely Used Guidelines That Involve This Medicine (representative sample):** Please look at the section at the very beginning of this profile called "Class." Next, turn to Table 22 and you will find guidelines listed by the class involved!

Available Dosage Forms and Strengths

Capsules, sustained release — 60 mg

Capsules, sustained release (Italy) — 50 mg

Tablets — 10 mg, 20 mg

Tablets, sustained release — 30 mg, 60 mg, 120 mg

▷ **Recommended Dosage Ranges** (Actual dose and schedule must be determined for each patient individually.)

Infants and Children: Dose not established.

12 to 60 Years of Age:

Regular release: 20 mg (one tablet), taken twice daily. Take the first tablet when you wake up; take the second tablet 7 hours later. Do not take additional doses during the balance of the day. Total daily dose should not exceed 40 mg.

Author's Note: Dosing is set up to give a 12-hour nitrate-free period to avoid tolerance to the therapeutic benefits of this medicine.

Sustained release: 30 mg (one half-tablet) or 60 mg (a whole tablet) once daily, taken in the morning when you get up. The dose can be increased in steps over several days to 120 mg once a day, and then increased farther if needed and tolerated. Total daily dose should not exceed 240 mg.

Over 60 Years of Age: Same as 12 to 60 years of age.

Conditions Requiring Dosing Adjustments

Liver Function: This drug should be used with caution by patients with liver compromise. No specific guidelines for dose reduction are available.

Kidney Function: No dosing changes in kidney compromise. Drug turns urine brown to black in color.

▷ **Dosing Instructions:** The immediate release tablet may be crushed and is preferably taken on an empty stomach to achieve the best blood levels. Sustained release forms should not be chewed or crushed. If you forget a dose: take the missed dose as soon as you remember it, unless it's nearly time for your next dose, then skip the missed dose and take the next dose right on schedule. DO NOT double doses. Call your doctor if you find yourself missing doses.

Usual Duration of Use: Use on a regular schedule for 3 to 7 days is needed to (1) identify this drug's peak effect in preventing or relieving acute anginal pain and (2) to find the optimal dose schedule. Long-term use (months to years) requires physician supervision.

Typical Treatment Goals and Measurements (Outcomes and Markers)

Angina: The most commonly used markers are prevention or relief of chest pain (angina). Many cardiologists look for easing of frequency and severity of angina attacks as well as pulmonary capillary wedge pressure as measures of successful therapy. If your chest pain does not go away after using the maximum dose at the recommended time interval, have someone drive you to the hospital or call 911. Plan for this possibility and ask your doctor on the next office visit if it would make sense for you to chew a regular release full-dose aspirin prior to going to the hospital if you do not get relief from maximum nitrate doses and have to go to the hospital.

Possible Advantages of This Drug

Designed to provide the best possible prevention of acute angina with minimal development of tolerance (loss of effectiveness—see Glossary). The nitrate-free interval during the evening and night prevents the development of tolerance.

▷ **This Drug Should Not Be Taken If**
- you have had an allergic reaction to it previously.
- you currently have congestive heart failure or a severe anemia.
- you have taken or are currently taking sildenafil (Viagra).
- your thyroid is overactive.
- you have a hypertrophic cardiomyopathy.

▷ **Inform Your Physician Before Taking This Drug If**
- you have had an unfavorable response to other nitrate drugs or vasodilators in the past.

- you have a history of low blood pressure or your body is fluid depleted (hypovolemic).
- you have had a very recent heart attack (myocardial infarction) and your heart is beating quickly (tachycardia) or your blood pressure is excessively high.
- you have had a cerebral hemorrhage recently.
- you are pregnant or planning pregnancy or breast-feeding your baby.
- you have any form of glaucoma.
- you have excessive thyroid function (hyperthyroidism) or cardiomyopathy or have suffered head trauma.

Possible Side Effects (natural, expected, and unavoidable drug actions)
Flushing of face, throbbing in head, palpitation, rapid heart rate, orthostatic hypotension (see Glossary).

▷ **Possible Adverse Effects** (unusual, unexpected, and infrequent reactions)
If any of the following develop, consult your physician promptly for guidance.
Mild Adverse Effects
Allergic reactions: skin rash, itching—infrequent.
Headache—frequent, but decreases over time.
Dizziness, fainting, or blurred vision—possible.
Nausea, vomiting, or bad breath (halitosis seen with isosorbide dinitrate)—possible.
Urine discoloration—possible and not clinically significant.
Increased liver enzymes—possible.
Serious Adverse Effects
Transient ischemic attacks (TIAs) in presence of impaired circulation within the brain: dizziness, fainting, impaired vision or speech, localized numbness or weakness—possible.
Bone marrow depression—infrequent and of uncertain relationship.
Anemia (in patients with glucose-6-phosphate dehydrogenase [G6PD] deficiency)—possible.
Abnormally low blood pressure—possible.
Abnormal heartbeat—case reports.
Tolerance—possible with 24-hour use (daily 12-hour drug-free period is used to prevent this).
Worsening of angina or abnormal heartbeats—case reports.

▷ **Possible Effects on Sexual Function:** Decreased libido and impotence—infrequent.

▷ **Adverse Effects That May Mimic Natural Diseases or Disorders**
Spells of low blood pressure with fainting (due to this drug) may be mistaken for late-onset epilepsy.

Possible Effects on Laboratory Tests
Liver function tests: increased.

CAUTION
1. Take this drug exactly as prescribed. If headaches are frequent or troublesome, call your doctor. Aspirin or acetaminophen may be taken to relieve headaches.
2. Many over-the-counter (OTC) medicines for allergies, colds, and coughs contain drugs that may counteract the desired effects of this drug. Ask your doctor or pharmacist for help.

Precautions for Use

By Those Over 60 Years of Age: Small starting doses are advisable. Increased risk of low blood pressure and associated "blackout" spells, fainting, and falling. Throbbing headaches and flushing may be more apparent.

▷ **Advisability of Use During Pregnancy**

Pregnancy Category: Ismo: C. Imdur: B. Monoket: B. See Pregnancy Risk Categories at the back of this book.

Animal Studies: Rat and rabbit studies reveal embryo deaths due to large doses of Ismo. Rat and rabbit studies did not reveal embryo deaths from Imdur.

Human Studies: Adequate studies of pregnant women are not available. Use this drug only if clearly needed. Ask your physician for guidance.

Advisability of Use If Breast-Feeding

Presence of this drug in breast milk: Unknown.

If this drug is thought to be necessary, watch the nursing infant for low blood pressure and poor feeding.

Habit-Forming Potential: None.

Effects of Overdose: Headache, dizziness, marked flushing of face and skin, vomiting, weakness, fainting, difficult breathing, coma.

Possible Effects of Long-Term Use: Development of abnormal hemoglobin (red blood cell pigment).

Suggested Periodic Examinations While Taking This Drug (at physician's discretion)

Measurement of internal eye pressure.

▷ **While Taking This Drug, Observe the Following**

Foods: No restrictions. Vitamin C may help ease nitrate tolerance. More study is needed. Your doctor may also recommend specific foods such as increased vegetables or functional foods such as Benecol. Three well-designed studies found that both in women and men and before and after a heart attack, people who ate more fish (2–4 servings a week) appeared to avoid heart disease. Additionally, supplements containing Omega 3 polyunsaturated fatty acids (PUFA) appeared to protect against abnormal heart rhythms and sudden death from heart attack. Increasing oat bran in the diet may be of additional help in lowering cholesterol, but may decrease the amount of medicine that gets into your body. Take oat bran 2 hours before or 4 to 6 hours after. Your doctor may also recommend increasing B vitamins. See Tables 19 and 20 about lifestyle changes and risk factors you can fix!

Herbal Medicines or Minerals: Hawthorn and co-enzyme Q10 (co-Q10) can affect the way the heart works. Co-Q10 has a limited number of reports of decreasing INR in people taking warfarin. Soy (milk, tofu, etc.) contains phytoestrogens that have led to an FDA-approved health claim for reducing risk of heart disease (if they have at least 6.25 grams of soy protein per serving). Couch grass or nettle should NOT be taken by patients who have increased fluid (edema) caused by heart weakness. Hawthorn (Crataegus variety) has been used to help heart failure, but should not be combined with heart medicines as combination use has not been studied. BE CERTAIN to tell your doctor that you are taking or are considering taking these herbs if you are taking a nitrate.

Beverages: No restrictions. May be taken with milk.

▷ *Alcohol:* Use extreme caution. Avoid alcohol completely in the presence of any side effects or adverse effects of this drug. Alcohol may exaggerate the blood pressure–lowering effect of this drug.

Tobacco Smoking: Nicotine can reduce effectiveness. Avoid all forms of tobacco.

Marijuana Smoking: Possible reduced effectiveness of this drug; mild to moderate increase in angina and possible changes in electrocardiogram confusing interpretation.

▷ *Other Drugs*

Isosorbide mononitrate *taken concurrently* with

- antihypertensive drugs may cause excessive lowering of blood pressure; dose adjustments may be necessary.
- calcium channel–blocking drugs (see Drug Classes) may cause marked orthostatic hypotension (see Glossary).
- hydralazine (Apresoline) may work well to help control angina.
- propranolol (Inderal) can help improve exercise time without angina.
- sildenafil (Viagra), vardenafil (Levitra), or tadalafil (Cialis) may result in LIFE-THREATENING lowering of blood pressure. NEVER COMBINE.

▷ *Driving, Hazardous Activities:* Usually no restrictions. This drug may cause dizziness or spells of low blood pressure. Restrict activities as necessary.

Aviation Note: Coronary artery disease *is a disqualification* for piloting. Consult a designated Aviation Medical Examiner.

Exposure to Sun: No restrictions.

Exposure to Heat: Use caution. Hot environments can cause a significant drop in blood pressure.

Exposure to Cold: Cold environments can increase the need for this drug and limit its effectiveness.

Heavy Exercise or Exertion: This drug may improve your ability to be more active without anginal pain. Use caution and avoid excessive exertion.

Discontinuation: It is best to withdraw this drug gradually (over a period of 2 to 4 weeks) after long-term use.

ISOTRETINOIN (i soh TRET i noy in)

Introduced: 1979 **Class:** Antiacne, vitamin A analog **Prescription:** USA: Yes **Controlled Drug:** USA: No; Canada: No **Available as Generic:** Yes

Brand Names: Accutane, Amnesteem, Claravis

Author's Note: **This medicine has serious benefit-to-risk considerations. Make CERTAIN that you read the specific Medication Guide that is dispensed with the medicine itself. Guidance for this medicine and specific required patient follow-ups have changed over time; but include such serious adverse effects as possible birth defects if this medicine is taken by pregnant women and cases where patients have developed serious depression while taking or shortly after stopping this medicine. See Possible Adverse Effects for more information and check** *www.fda. gov/medwatch/safety/2002/accutaine_deardoc_10-202.htm.*

```
┌─────────────────────────────────────────────────────────────────┐
│                     BENEFITS versus RISKS                         │
│      Possible Benefits              Possible Risks                │
│  EFFECTIVE TREATMENT OF        DEPRESSION                         │
│    SEVERE CYSTIC ACNE          MAJOR BIRTH DEFECTS                │
│  Treatment of other skin       ELEVATED LIPIDS                    │
│    conditions of serious and     (HYPERTRIGLYCERIDEMIA)           │
│    resistant nature            PANCREATITIS                       │
│                                HEARING IMPAIRMENT                 │
│                                Initial worsening of acne (Transient)│
│                                Dry skin, nose, and mouth          │
│                                Musculoskeletal discomfort         │
│                                Corneal opacities                  │
└─────────────────────────────────────────────────────────────────┘
```

▷ **Principal Uses**

As a Single Drug Product: Uses currently included in FDA-approved labeling: (1) Reserved to treat severe, disfiguring nodular, and cystic acne that has failed to respond to all other forms of therapy—*it should not be used to treat mild forms of acne;* (2) it is also used to treat some less common conditions of the skin that are due to disorders of keratin production.

Other (unlabeled) generally accepted uses: (1) May be helpful in refractory hypertrophic lupus erythematosus; (2) can help control resistant oral leukoplakia; (3) used in Apert's syndrome facial treatment; (4) used adjunctively to surgery in some cervical cancers; (5) treats mycosis fungoides; (6) eases symptoms in Darier's disease; (7) may have a role in treating dysplastic nevi; (8) can help treat the abnormal gum growth (gingival hyperplasia) that can occur with phenytoin therapy; (9) treats severe and refractory rosacea; (10) has been combined with interferon alpha treatment in squamous cell skin cancer.

How This Drug Works: Reduces the size of sebaceous glands and inhibits sebum (skin oil) production. This helps to correct acne and complications.

▷ **Widely Used Guidelines That Involve This Medicine (representative sample):** Please look at the section at the very beginning of this profile called "Class." Next, turn to Table 22 and you will find guidelines listed by the class involved!

Available Dosage Forms and Strengths

Capsules—10 mg, 20 mg, 40 mg

▷ **Usual Adult Dosage Ranges:** Starting dose is based on the patient's weight and severity of acne; the usual dose is 0.5 to 2 mg per kg of body mass daily, taken in 2 divided doses for 15 to 20 weeks. After weeks of treatment, the dose should be adjusted according to response of the acne and the development of adverse effects. After 15 to 20 weeks of therapy, if the cyst count has been lowered by more than 70%, the medicine can be stopped (discuss this with your doctor).

Note: Actual dose and schedule must be determined for each patient individually.

Conditions Requiring Dosing Adjustments

Liver Function: The dose should be empirically decreased when isotretinoin is used by patients with compromised livers.

Kidney Function: Isotretinoin should be used with caution in kidney compromise.

Dosing Instructions: Two forms of contraception should be used at the same time for a month before, during therapy and for a month after treatment with this medicine. Begin treatment only on the second or third day of your next normal menstrual period. Serum pregnancy test should be checked BEFORE treatment is started and monthly while taking this medicine. Take this medicine with meals (morning and evening) to achieve optimal blood levels. The capsule should not be opened for administration. If you forget a dose: take the missed dose as soon as you remember it, unless it's nearly time for your next dose, then skip the missed dose and take the next dose right on schedule. DO NOT double doses. Call your doctor if you find yourself missing doses.

Author's Note: A patient consent form must be filled out before starting this medicine. The form will ask you to tell your doctor if you or family members have had symptoms of depression and/or other psychological symptoms. Female patients will also be reminded about pregnancy risks (severe birth defects) possible if they become pregnant while taking this medicine. *Monthly pregnancy tests are required.* **Only 30 days' worth of this medicine will be dispensed at a time. Stronger warnings are now present in labeling about depression and suicide and aggressive behavior in patients taking Accutane.**

Usual Duration of Use: Use on a regular schedule for 15 to 20 weeks best determines effectiveness in clearing or improving severe cystic acne. The drug may be stopped earlier if the total cyst count is reduced by more than 70%. If a repeat course of treatment is necessary, it should not be started for 2 months. Long-term use (months to years) requires physician supervision.

Typical Treatment Goals and Measurements (Outcomes and Markers)

Acne: Many dermatologists look for improvement or decrease in the lesions being treated as the measure of response (see cyst count above). Blood fat (lipid) levels are tested before isotretinoin is given and then are rechecked periodically until reaction to the medicine is seen (often in a month).

▷ **This Drug Should Not Be Taken If**
- you have had an allergic reaction to it previously.
- you are allergic to parabens (preservatives used in this drug product).
- you have mild acne.
- you are not able or willing to follow contraception measures to avoid pregnancy and have not taken 2 forms of contraception for the previous month (unless abstinence is the way pregnancy is chosen to be avoided or if the patient has had a hysterectomy).
- you have not gotten verbal and written warnings about this medicine and fetal damage. You have not read, understood, and signed the consent form required for this medicine.
- you have not had a negative urine or serum pregnancy test (at least 50 mIU/mL sensitivity) when your doctor decided you were eligible for treatment and you did not have a second pregnancy test that was also negative and that was a urine or serum pregnancy test on the second day of the next usual menstrual period (or 11 days after the last time you had unprotected sexual intercourse). You will not be able to comply with monthly pregnancy tests that are required.
- you are pregnant or planning pregnancy.
- you are not starting treatment on the second or third day of a subsequent normal menstrual period.

▷ **Inform Your Physician Before Taking This Drug If**
- you have a history of depression or become depressed while taking this medicine.
- you start to notice a hearing loss or ringing in the ears while you are taking this medicine. If this happens, stop the medicine and call your doctor.
- you had an allergic reaction to vitamin A in the past.
- you routinely take a nonprescription form of vitamin A.
- you have diabetes mellitus.
- you are considering giving blood (you will NOT be eligible for 1 month after the last isotretinoin dose).
- you have a cholesterol or triglyceride disorder, or if signs and symptoms of pancreatitis start while you are taking this medicine.
- you are considering having a child or are breast-feeding your infant.
- you wear contact lenses (your ability to wear these lenses [tolerance] may decrease while you take this medicine).
- you have a change in vision while taking this medicine. The medicine should be stopped and an eye (ophthalmological) exam obtained immediately.
- you have a history of liver or kidney disease.

Possible Side Effects (natural, expected, and unavoidable drug actions)
Frequent dryness of the nose and mouth (often results in nosebleeds or epistaxis), inflammation of the lips (cheilitis), dryness of the skin with itching, peeling of the palms and soles. Decreased night vision, dose-related irritation of the eye (conjunctivitis) may be frequent. Dose-related increase in triglycerides—frequent. Eruptive xanthomas reported.

▷ **Possible Adverse Effects** (unusual, unexpected, and infrequent reactions)
If any of the following develop, consult your physician promptly for guidance.
Mild Adverse Effects
Allergic reaction: skin rash—may resemble pityriasis rosea.
Thinning of hair, conjunctivitis, intolerance of contact lenses, decreased night vision, muscular aches, headache, fatigue, indigestion—infrequent.
Insomnia—infrequent.
Increased blood sugar—infrequent.
Back or joint pain—frequent.
Chest pain (usually reversible if medicine is stopped)—rare.
Serious Adverse Effects
Depression—case reports to infrequent.
Psychosis—case reports.
Suicidal ideation and suicide attempts—rare.
Skin infections, arthritis flare, inflammatory bowel disorders—case reports.
Abnormal acceleration of bone development/growth arrest in children—possible.
Development of opacities in the cornea of the eye/cataracts, retinopathy—possible.
Reduced red blood cell and white blood cell counts; decreased blood platelet count—infrequent, but medicine should be stopped if significant lowering of the white blood cell count happens.
Seizures—case reports.
Aggressive and/or violent behavior—reported.
Hearing loss—reported.
Myopathy—case reports.
Tendonitis (Achilles)—case reports.

Kidney toxicity, liver toxicity, or pancreatitis—rare.

Inflammatory bowel disease (severe diarrhea, abdominal pain, rectal bleeding)—case reports.

Abnormal blood glucose control—infrequent.

Increased pressure within the head (pseudotumor cerebri-headache, visual disturbances, nausea/vomiting)—case reports.

Increased triglycerides—frequent.

Pancreatitis (secondary to increased triglycerides)—case reports.

▷ **Possible Effects on Sexual Function:** Decreased male or female libido—possible.

Ejaculatory failure—case report.

Decreased vaginal secretions—possible.

Altered timing and pattern of menstruation—case reports.

Possible Effects on Laboratory Tests

Complete blood cell counts: infrequently decreased red cells and white cells.

Blood platelets: increased or decreased.

Sedimentation rate (ESR): increased.

Blood total cholesterol, LDL cholesterol, VLDL cholesterol, and triglyceride levels: increased.

Blood HDL cholesterol levels: decreased.

Blood thyroid hormones (T3, T4, and free T4 index): decreased.

Liver function tests: infrequently increased liver enzymes (ALT/GPT, AST/GOT, and alkaline phosphatase), increased bilirubin.

Blood calcium level: increased.

Protein in the urine: positive, though infrequent.

CAUTION

1. This medicine has caused a number of verified cases of depression and aggressive/violent behavior. Your prescriber should ask you about mood changes at each office visit, and you should call if depression or aggressive behavior starts.
2. This drug should not be used to treat mild forms of acne.
3. Worsening of your acne may occur during the first few weeks of treatment; this will subside with continued use of the drug.
4. Do not take any other form of vitamin A while taking this drug. (Check contents of multiple vitamin preparations.)
5. Women who may become pregnant should have a blood pregnancy test 2 weeks before taking this drug, take 2 forms of contraception for the month prior to starting this medicine, have a repeat negative pregnancy test (see timing mentioned earlier), and need 2 effective forms of contraception simultaneously during its use. Contraception should be continued until normal menstruation resumes after stopping this drug.
6. May increase blood levels of cholesterol and triglycerides. Your doctor must get a supply of Accutane Qualification stickers and read the booklet called the SMART (System to Manage Accutane Related Teratogenicity) guide to best practices.
7. If repeated courses of this drug are prescribed, wait a minimum of 2 months between courses before resuming medication.
8. DO NOT give blood for 1 month after this medicine is stopped.
9. This medicine may lead to bone problems (such as osteoporosis). Caution is to be used if people taking this medicine play sports with repeated impacts.
10. DO NOT share this medicine with anyone else.

Precautions for Use

By Infants and Children: Long-term use (6 to 12 months) may cause abnormal acceleration of bone growth and development. Your physician can monitor this possibility by periodic X-ray examination of long bones.

▷ **Advisability of Use During Pregnancy**

Pregnancy Category: X. See Pregnancy Risk Categories at the back of this book.

Animal Studies: Birth defects of skull, brain, and vertebral column found in rats; skeletal birth defects found in rabbits.

Human Studies: Adequate studies of pregnant women are not available. However, many serious birth defects (thought to be due to this drug) have been reported. These include major abnormalities of the head, brain, heart, blood vessels, and hormone-producing glands.

Avoid this drug completely during entire pregnancy.

Advisability of Use If Breast-Feeding

Presence of this drug in breast milk: Unknown.

Avoid drug or refrain from nursing.

Habit-Forming Potential: None.

Effects of Overdose: Increased blood pressure, lethargy, nausea, vomiting, mild gastrointestinal bleeding, elevated blood calcium, hallucinations, and psychosis.

Suggested Periodic Examinations While Taking This Drug (at physician's discretion)

Monthly pregnancy tests are required by the FDA while taking this medicine.

Complete blood cell counts, including platelet counts.

Measurements of blood cholesterol and triglyceride levels.

Complete eye and hearing examinations.

Growth chart checks in children.

May be prudent to get baseline and periodic Bone Mineral Density tests in high-risk patients.

Assessment of mood/depression an behavior change (aggression increase).

Liver and kidney function tests.

▷ **While Taking This Drug, Observe the Following**

Foods: Increases absorption and may be a good mechanism to maintain blood levels.

Herbal Medicines or Minerals: **Caution:** St. John's wort may also cause extreme reactions to the sun. Additive photosensitivity may be possible. Medicinal yeast has a German Commission E monograph indication for acne, but has not been studied with isotretinoin. Talk to your doctor BEFORE combining any herbals with prescription medicines.

Beverages: No restrictions.

▷   *Alcohol:* A disulfiramlike reaction was described in 1 case report. Heavy alcohol intake may increase the risk of osteoporosis and is not advisable while taking this medicine.

Tobacco Smoking: Smoking may increase risk of osteoporosis and is not advisable while taking this medicine. I advise everyone to quit smoking.

▷   *Other Drugs*

Isotretinoin ***taken concurrently*** with

• carbamazepine (Tegretol) may cause subtherapeutic carbamazepine levels.

• medicines known to increase sensitivity to the sun (see Table 2) as these do may additively increase sun sensitivity if taken with isotretinoin.

- medicines known to increase osteoporosis risk (such as corticosteroids [methylprednisolone, prednisone, and others] and phenytoin-Dilantin) may additively increase risk of osteoporosis if combined with isotretinoin.
- micro-dosed Progesterone (Minipills) for birth control may not be effective enough alone in preventing pregnancy while taking this medicine. Two forms of contraception should be taken at the same time while taking this medicine.
- minocycline may increase risk of severe headache, papilledema, and visual changes.
- tetracyclines may cause increased risk of pseudotumor cerebri.

▷ *Driving, Hazardous Activities:* No restrictions.

Exposure to Sun: Caution: This drug can cause photosensitivity (see Glossary). See "Herbal Medicines" caution above.

ISRADIPINE (is RA di peen)

Introduced: 1984   **Class:**   Antihypertensive, calcium channel blocker
Prescription: USA: Yes   **Controlled Drug:**   USA: No   **Available as**
Generic: USA: No

Brand Names: DynaCirc, DynaCirc CR

Controversies in Medicine: **Medicines in this class have had many conflicting reports. The FDA has held hearings on the calcium channel–blocker (CCB) class. Amlodipine got the first FDA approval to treat high blood pressure or angina in people with congestive heart failure. CCBs are currently second-line agents for high blood pressure according to the JNC VII (see Glossary).**

BENEFITS versus RISKS	
Possible Benefits	*Possible Risks*
EFFECTIVE TREATMENT OF MILD TO MODERATE HYPERTENSION	Headache, dizziness, fluid retention, palpitations
May prevent progression of early atherosclerotic damage in blood vessels	
Might slow how quickly new atherosclerotic lesions are developed	

▷ **Principal Uses**

As a Single Drug Product: Uses currently included in FDA-approved labeling: (1) Treats mild to moderate hypertension, alone or in combination.

Other (unlabeled) generally accepted uses: (1) Treatment of chronic, stable angina; (2) may help prevent progression of early lesions and rate of development of new lesions in atherosclerosis.

How This Drug Works: Blocks passage of calcium through cell walls, inhibiting contraction of coronary arteries and peripheral arterioles. As a result:
- promotes dilation of the coronary arteries (anti-anginal effect);
- reduces the degree of contraction of peripheral arterial walls, resulting in lowering of blood pressure. This further reduces heart workload and helps

prevent angina. Isradipine inhibits platelet clumping and thus may have a protective role against heart attack and stroke.

▷ **Widely Used Guidelines That Involve This Medicine (representative sample):** Please look at the section at the very beginning of this profile called "Class." Next, turn to Table 22 and you will find guidelines listed by the class involved!

Available Dosage Forms and Strengths

Capsules — 2.5 mg, 5 mg

Tablets (timed release) — 5 mg and 10 mg

▷ **Usual Adult Dosage Ranges:** *Hypertension:* Initially 2.5 mg twice daily, 12 hours apart, for a trial period of 2 to 4 weeks. If needed, the dose may be increased by 5 mg per day at intervals of 2 to 4 weeks. The usual maintenance dose is 5 to 10 mg daily. The total daily dose should not exceed 20 mg. Timed release form is started at 5 mg once a day and increased slowly (2- to 4-week intervals) if needed.

Note: Actual dose and dosing schedule must be determined for each patient individually.

Conditions Requiring Dosing Adjustments

Liver Function: Empiric decreases in dosing are prudent in liver damage. Careful patient follow-up is needed.

Kidney Function: Use with caution in kidney compromise. Initial dose should be 2.5 mg twice a day or 5 mg once daily (sustained release), with careful patient follow-up.

▷ **Dosing Instructions:** May be taken with or following food to reduce stomach irritation. Swallow the capsule or tablet whole. Even though you take the sustained release tablets correctly, you may see a shell of the tablet, which no longer has any medicine in it, in your stool. If you forget a dose: take the missed dose as soon as you remember it, unless it's nearly time for your next dose—if that is the case, skip the missed dose and take the next dose right on schedule. DO NOT double doses. Call your doctor if you find yourself missing doses as there are pager and timer reminder systems to help get the right dose on time.

Usual Duration of Use: Use on a regular schedule for 2 to 4 weeks determines this drug's effectiveness in controlling hypertension or in reducing the frequency and severity of angina. The smallest effective dose should be used for long-term (months to years) therapy. Periodic physician evaluation is essential to make sure your blood pressure is lowered into the target range and kept there.

Typical Treatment Goals and Measurements (Outcomes and Markers)

Blood Pressure: Guidelines (JNC VII) define normal blood pressure (BP) as **less than** 120/80 and **pre-hypertension** as 120/80 to 139/89. This new range is intended to help doctors encourage lifestyle changes (or in the case of people with a risk factor for high blood pressure, start treatment) much earlier—so that damage to blood vessels, your heart, kidneys, sexual potency, or eyes might be minimized or avoided altogether. Stage 1 hypertension is 140/90 to 159/99 and stage 2 hypertension equal to or greater than: 160/100 mm Hg. These guidelines also recommend that clinicians work with their patients to agree on the goals and a plan of treatment. The first-ever guidelines for blood pressure (hypertension) in African Americans recommends that MOST black patients be started on TWO antihypertensive medicines with the goal of lowering blood pressure to 130/80 for those with high risk for heart and blood vessel disease or with diabetes. The American Diabetes Association also recommends 130/80 as the target for diabetics and less than 125/75 for those who spill more than one gram of protein into their urine. Most clinicians try to achieve a BP that confers the best balance of lower cardiovascular risk and avoids the problem of too low a blood pressure. Blood pressure duration is generally increased with beneficial restriction of sodium. If goals are not met, it is not unusual to intensify doses or add on medicines.

Possible Advantages of This Drug

Does not cause orthostatic hypotension (see Glossary). Inhibits platelet clumping (aggregation) more than nifedipine and therefore may have the most desirable effect of those 2 calcium channel blockers on preventing undesirable blood clots and thus strokes and heart attacks.

▷ **This Drug Should Not Be Taken If**
- you have had an allergic reaction to it previously.
- you have symptomatic low blood pressure (hypotension).
- you have severe problems in the left side of your heart (left ventricular dysfunction).

▷ **Inform Your Physician Before Taking This Drug If**
- you have had an unfavorable response to any calcium channel–blocker drug (see Drug Classes).
- you take any beta-blocker drug (see Drug Classes).
- you are taking any drugs that lower blood pressure.
- you have a history of congestive heart failure, heart attack, or stroke.
- you have narrowing of the aorta.
- you are subject to disturbances of heart rhythm.
- you have muscular dystrophy or myasthenia gravis.
- you develop a skin reaction while taking this drug (call your doctor as this may be an early sign of a significant skin reaction).
- you have impaired liver or kidney function.
- you will have surgery with general anesthesia in the near future.

Possible Side Effects (natural, expected, and unavoidable drug actions)

Flushing, gum overgrowth—infrequent.
Swelling of the feet and ankles, cough, flushing, and sensation of warmth—infrequent.
Small weight loss—possible.

▷ **Possible Adverse Effects** (unusual, unexpected, and infrequent reactions)
If any of the following develop, consult your physician promptly for guidance.
Mild Adverse Effects
Allergic reactions: skin rash—infrequent; hives, itching—rare.
Headache—frequent.
Dizziness, weakness—infrequent.
Nervousness, blurred vision, or eye pain—rare.
Decreased skin sensation—rare.
Palpitation, shortness of breath—infrequent.
Indigestion, nausea, vomiting, constipation—infrequent.
Increased liver enzymes (usually mild and transient)—possible.
Cramps in legs and feet—rare.
Increased urination—rare.
Abnormal growth of the gums (gingival hyperplasia)—frequent with some drugs in the same class.

Serious Adverse Effects

Allergic reactions: erythema multiforme, exfoliative dermatitis—case reports.
Heart rhythm disturbances—infrequent.
Increased frequency or severity of angina (when therapy is started or dose increased)—possible.
Marked drop in blood pressure with fainting—rare.
Low white blood cell counts—rare.

▷ **Possible Effects on Sexual Function:** Decreased libido, impotence (less than 1%).

▷ **Adverse Effects That May Mimic Natural Diseases or Disorders**
Flushing and warmth may resemble menopausal "hot flashes."

Possible Effects on Laboratory Tests
White blood cell counts: decreased (less than 1% of users).
Liver function tests: increased enzyme levels—infrequent.
Electrocardiogram: slight increase in QT interval.

CAUTION

1. If you check your blood pressure, check it just before each dose and 2 to 3 hours after each dose. Even though high blood pressure usually has no symptoms, high blood pressure MUST be treated to avoid serious complications.
2. Tell health care professionals who treat you that you take this drug. List this drug on a card in your purse or wallet.
3. Nitroglycerin and other nitrate drugs may be used as needed to relieve acute episodes of angina pain. However, if your angina attacks are becoming more frequent or intense, notify your physician promptly.

Precautions for Use
By Infants and Children: Safety and effectiveness under 18 years of age not established.
By Those Over 60 Years of Age: Usually well tolerated by this age group. However, watch for weakness, dizziness, fainting, and falling. Take necessary precautions to prevent injury.

▷ **Advisability of Use During Pregnancy**
Pregnancy Category: C. See Pregnancy Risk Categories at the back of this book.
Animal Studies: Embryo and fetal toxicity reported in small animals, but no birth defects due to this drug.
Human Studies: Adequate studies of pregnant women are not available.
Avoid this drug during the first 3 months. Use during the final 6 months only if clearly needed. Ask your physician for guidance.

Advisability of Use If Breast-Feeding
Presence of this drug in breast milk: Unknown.
Avoid drug or refrain from nursing.

Habit-Forming Potential: None. Abrupt withdrawal has led to an increased frequency of angina if this medicine has been used to treat angina.

Effects of Overdose: Weakness, light-headedness, fainting, fast pulse, low blood pressure, shortness of breath, flushed and warm skin, tremors, abnormal heartbeats.

Possible Effects of Long-Term Use: None reported.

Suggested Periodic Examinations While Taking This Drug (at physician's discretion)
Evaluations of heart function, including electrocardiograms.
Measurements of blood pressure in supine, sitting, and standing positions.

▷ **While Taking This Drug, Observe the Following**

Foods: DO NOT take this medicine with grapefruit or grapefruit juice. Avoid excessive salt intake.

Herbal Medicines or Minerals: Ginseng, guarana, bitter orange, country mallow, hawthorn, saw palmetto, ma huang (no longer on the market for weight loss), goldenseal, yohimbe, and licorice may also increase blood pressure. Calcium and garlic may help lower blood pressure. Indian snakeroot has a German Commission E monograph indication for hypertension—talk to your doctor. Eleuthero root and ephedra (ma huang) should be avoided by people living with hypertension. Talk to your doctor before combining any herbal medicine or mineral with isradipine.

Beverages: DO NOT take this medicine with grapefruit or grapefruit juice. May be taken with milk.

▷ *Alcohol:* Use caution. Alcohol may exaggerate the drop in blood pressure in some people.

Tobacco Smoking: Nicotine may reduce the effectiveness of this drug. I advise everyone to quit smoking.

Marijuana Smoking: Possible reduced effectiveness; mild to moderate increase in angina; possible changes in electrocardiogram, confusing interpretation.

▷ *Other Drugs*

Isradipine *taken concurrently* with

- amiodarone (Cordarone) should be avoided in people with certain kinds of heart conduction problems (partial atrioventricular block or "sick sinus" syndrome).
- amprenavir (Agenerase), atazanavir (Reyataz), ritonavir (Norvir), and perhaps other protease inhibitors may increase blood levels of isradipine. Careful patient follow-up and possible decreased doses are prudent.
- antifungals (triazoles) such as fluconazole (Diflucan), itraconazole (Sporanox), ketoconazole (Nizoral), or voriconazole (Vfend) may lead to toxicity.
- beta-blocker drugs or digitalis preparations (see Drug Classes) may affect heart rate and rhythm adversely. Careful monitoring by your physician is needed if these drugs are taken concurrently.
- carbamazepine (Tegretol) has resulted in decreased blood levels of carbamazepine with calcium channel blockers from the same pharmacological family. Caution is advised.
- cimetidine (Tagamet) may lead to isradipine toxicity, careful patient follow-up is advisable.
- class I, IA, and class III antiarrhythmics (see Drug Classes) may prolong the QT interval and lead to dangerous arrhythmias (such as Torsades de Pointes or even cardiac arrest). DO NOT combine.
- cotrimoxazole (various) may lead to additive QT prolongation and arrhythmias. DO NOT combine.
- delavirdine (Rescriptor) may lead to isradipine toxicity.
- digoxin (Lanoxin) may increase blood levels. Laboratory testing of blood levels should be performed more often if these drugs are combined.
- erythromycin (various and combination erythromycin forms) may increase the free (active) form of isradipine, and may prolong the QT interval. DO NOT combine.
- magnesium (various)—especially in doses used in premature labor—can cause very low and abnormal blood pressure.
- nonsteroidal anti-inflammatory drugs (NSAIDs; see Drug Classes) may blunt benefits of isradipine.

- oral anticoagulant medicines (such as Coumadin or warfarin) may lead to increased risk of bleeding from the stomach or intestines.
- phenytoin (Dilantin) may result in loss of isradipine's effectiveness. Caution is advised.
- quinupristin/dalfopristin (Synercid) may increase blood levels of isradipine. Careful patient follow-up and possible decreased doses are prudent.
- rifampin (Rifadin, others) may result in a decreased therapeutic benefit from isradipine.
- trimethoprim (Septra, various) may lead to QT prolongation and arrhythmias. DO NOT combine.
- vasopressin (various) may lead to QT prolongation and arrhythmias. DO NOT combine.
- zolmitriptan (Zomig) and any other QT prolonging medicines (see Glossary) may lead to QT prolongation and arrhythmias. DO NOT combine.

▷ *Driving, Hazardous Activities:* Usually no restrictions. This drug may cause drowsiness or dizziness. Restrict activities as necessary.

Aviation Note: Coronary artery disease and hypertension *are disqualifications* for piloting. Consult a designated Aviation Medical Examiner.

Exposure to Sun: No restrictions.

Exposure to Heat: Caution is advised. Hot environments can exaggerate the blood pressure–lowering effects of this drug. Observe for light-headedness or weakness.

Heavy Exercise or Exertion: This drug may improve your ability to be more active without resulting in angina pain. Use caution and avoid excessive exercise that could impair heart function in the absence of warning pain.

Discontinuation: Do not stop this drug abruptly. Ask your doctor about gradual withdrawal. Watch for the development of rebound angina.

KETOCONAZOLE (kee toh KOHN a zohl)

Introduced: 1981 **Class:** Antifungal **Prescription:** USA: Yes
Controlled Drug: USA: No; Canada: No **Available as Generic:** USA: Yes; Canada: No

Brand Names: ♣Apo-Ketoconazole, Nizoral, Nizoral A-D, ♣Novo-Ketocon, ♣Nu-Ketocon

---

BENEFITS versus RISKS

Possible Benefits	*Possible Risks*
EFFECTIVE TREATMENT OF THE FOLLOWING FUNGUS INFECTIONS: blastomycosis, candidiasis, chromomycosis, coccidioidomycosis, histoplasmosis, paracoccidioidomycosis, tinea (ringworm) Beneficial short-term treatment of advanced prostate cancer Beneficial auxiliary treatment of Cushing's syndrome	SERIOUS DRUG-INDUCED LIVER DAMAGE Allergic reactions Low blood platelets and anemia Some serious drug interactions

▷ **Principal Uses**

As a Single Drug Product: Uses currently included in FDA-approved labeling: Treatment of (1) lung and systemic blastomycosis; (2) *Candida* (yeast) infections of the skin, mouth, throat, and esophagus (may be AIDS-related); (3) systemic *Candida* infections—pneumonia, peritonitis, urinary tract infections (may be AIDS-related); (4) chromomycosis (auxiliary); (5) lung and systemic coccidioidomycosis; (6) lung and systemic histoplasmosis; (7) paracoccidioidomycosis; (8) tinea infections—groin (jock itch) and feet (athlete's foot) using the cream form; (9) tinea versicolor (pityriasis); (10) fungal dandruff (topical).

Other (unlabeled) generally accepted uses: Treatment of (1) *Candida* infections of the vulva and vagina; (2) alternative short-term prostate cancer treatment combined with prednisone; (3) Cushing's syndrome (excessive adrenal hormones); (4) systemic sporotrichosis; (5) fungal toenail infections; (6) visceral leishmaniasis.

How This Drug Works: As an antifungal: By damaging cell walls and impairing critical cell enzymes, this drug inhibits cell growth and reproduction (with low drug levels) and destroys fungal cells (with high drug concentrations).

In treating prostate cancer: Decreases testosterone (male hormone) levels—and prostate cancer needs testosterone to grow.

In treating Cushing's syndrome: This drug suppresses the excessive production of adrenal corticosteroid hormones.

▷ **Widely Used Guidelines That Involve This Medicine (representative sample):** Please look at the section at the very beginning of this profile called "Class." Next, turn to Table 22 and you will find guidelines listed by the class involved!

Available Dosage Forms and Strengths

Cream — 2% (for local application to *Candida* or tinea skin infections)
Oral suspension — 100 mg/5 mL (Canada)
Shampoo — 2%
Tablets — 200 mg (U.S. and Canada)

▷ **Recommended Dosage Ranges** (Actual dose and schedule must be determined for each patient individually.)

Infants and Children: Up to 2 years of age—Dose not established.

Over 2 years of age—3.3 to 6.6 mg per kg of body mass, once daily; the dose depends upon the nature of the infection.

12 to 60 Years of Age: For fungus infections—200 to 400 mg once daily; 800 mg maximum daily dose.

For prostate cancer—400 mg 3 times daily; 1,200 mg maximum daily dose.

For Cushing's syndrome—600 to 1,200 mg once daily; total daily dose should not exceed 1,200 mg.

Topical for dandruff: 2% shampoo is used twice a week for 4 weeks.

Over 60 Years of Age: Same as 12 to 60 years of age.

Conditions Requiring Dosing Adjustments

Liver Function: Dose empirically decreased for patients with liver compromise.

Kidney Function: Decreased doses are not needed in kidney compromise.

Achlorhydria (lack of acid in the stomach): This medicine requires an acid environment in the stomach to be absorbed. Talk with your doctor about making a dilute acid solution or taking a cola drink (acid pH) prior to taking the tablet form.

▷ **Dosing Instructions:** The tablet may be crushed and is best taken with or after food to enhance absorption and reduce stomach irritation. The bottle of suspension form should be shaken well and a measuring cup or measuring spoon used to get the right dose. Do not take with antacids. Take the full course prescribed. If you forget a dose: Take the missed dose as soon as you remember it, unless it's nearly time for your next dose—if that is the case, skip the missed dose and take the next dose right on schedule. Talk with your doctor if you find yourself missing doses.

Usual Duration of Use: Use on a regular schedule for 2 to 4 weeks determines effectiveness in controlling fungal infections. Actual cures (up to 83 days in one patient with mouth yeast infection [oral candidiasis]) or use for long-term suppression often require continual treatment for many months. Periodic physician evaluation of response and dose adjustment are essential. Fungal cultures take a long time to grow and it is not unusual for anti-fungal sensitivity patterns to take a long time to be reported.

Typical Treatment Goals and Measurements (Outcomes and Markers)
Fungal infections: Resolution of signs and symptoms of infection (such as sore throat and white coloration in candidal throat infections), return of white blood cell count and differential to normal (for systemic infections), and failure of the infection to return in prophylactic use. Blood levels can be used to guide dosing in serious infections or in the case of relapses.

▷ **This Drug Should Not Be Taken If**
  • you have had an allergic reaction to it previously.
  • you have active liver disease.
  • you take astemizole, cisapride, or triazolam.

▷ **Inform Your Physician Before Taking This Drug If**
  • you are allergic to related antifungal drugs: clotrimazole, fluconazole, itra-conazole, or miconazole.
  • you have a liver disease or impaired liver function.
  • you take loratadine. Heart problems have not been reported as with other nonsedating antihistamines, but the blood level does increase if the drugs are combined; the dose of loratadine may need to be decreased.
  • you have a history of adrenal gland problems (adrenal insufficiency).
  • you have a history of low blood platelets or anemia.
  • you have a history of alcoholism.
  • you have a deficiency of stomach hydrochloric acid.
  • you are taking any other drugs currently.

Possible Side Effects (natural, expected, and unavoidable drug actions)
  Suppression of testosterone and adrenal corticosteroid hormone production (more pronounced with high drug doses).

▷ **Possible Adverse Effects** (unusual, unexpected, and infrequent reactions)
  If any of the following develop, consult your physician promptly for guidance.
  Mild Adverse Effects
  Allergic reactions: skin rash, hives, itching—rare.
  Headache, dizziness, drowsiness, photophobia—infrequent.
  Nausea (helped by taking with meals) and vomiting, stomach pain, diar-rhea—rare.
  Increased blood pressure—possible.
  Hair loss (alopecia) or ringing in the ears—case reports.
  Muscle and joint aches—infrequent.

Serious Adverse Effects
> Allergic reactions: anaphylactic reaction (see Glossary).
> Severe liver toxicity: loss of appetite, nausea, yellow skin or eyes, dark urine, light-colored stools (see jaundice in Glossary)—rare.
> Suppression of the adrenal gland or low thyroid function—case reports.
> Mental depression—rare.
> Hemolytic anemia or abnormally low platelet counts (abnormal bruising or bleeding)—rare.

▷ **Possible Effects on Sexual Function:** Decreased testosterone blood levels: reduced sperm counts, decreased libido, impotence, male breast enlargement and tenderness (gynecomastia)—case reports.
> Altered menstrual patterns—case reports.

Possible Delayed Adverse Effects: Deficiency of adrenal corticosteroid hormones (cortisone related); this could be serious during stress resulting from illness or injury and require corticosteroids replacement.

▷ **Adverse Effects That May Mimic Natural Diseases or Disorders**
> Drug-induced liver reaction may suggest viral hepatitis.

Possible Effects on Laboratory Tests
> Complete blood cell counts: decreased red cells, white cells and platelets.
> Liver function tests: increased liver enzymes (ALT/GPT, AST/GOT, and alkaline phosphatase), increased bilirubin.
> Thyroid function tests: decreased—rare.
> Adrenal corticosteroid blood levels: decreased.
> Testosterone blood levels: decreased.
> Cholesterol levels: case report of increases.

CAUTION
> 1. This drug inhibits several liver enzymes (CYP3A4, 1A2, 2C9, and 2C19). If you combine medicines with ketoconazole that are removed by these liver enzymes, there may be serious increases in effect or blood levels (toxicity) of those drugs.

Precautions for Use
> *By Infants and Children:* Safety and effectiveness for under 2 years old not established.
> *By Those Over 60 Years of Age:* This drug requires an acid stomach to enter the body. Talk with your doctor if achlorhydria (gastric) has been diagnosed.

▷ **Advisability of Use During Pregnancy**
> *Pregnancy Category:* C. See Pregnancy Risk Categories at the back of this book.
> *Animal Studies:* Rat studies revealed significant embryo toxicity and birth defects due to this drug.
> *Human Studies:* Adequate studies of pregnant women are not available.
> Use this drug only if clearly needed. Ask your physician for guidance.

Advisability of Use If Breast-Feeding
> Presence of this drug in breast milk: Yes.
> Avoid drug or refrain from nursing.

Habit-Forming Potential: None.

Effects of Overdose: Possible nausea, vomiting, diarrhea.

Possible Effects of Long-Term Use: Suppression of adrenal corticosteroid hormone production, requiring replacement therapy during periods of stress.

Suggested Periodic Examinations While Taking This Drug (at physician's discretion)

Liver function tests should be obtained BEFORE long-term therapy is started and checked monthly during treatment.

Adrenal function tests are prudent with long-term therapy.

Sperm counts.

▷ **While Taking This Drug, Observe the Following**

Foods: No restrictions.

Herbal Medicines or Minerals: Some patients use echinacea to attempt to boost their immune systems. Unfortunately, use of echinacea is not recommended in people with damaged immune systems. This herb may also actually weaken any immune system if it is used too often or for too long a time. If you are considering St. John's wort, caution is advised as it can alter the liver enzymes involved in ketoconazole removal and can also cause sun sensitivity. Herbals that can be toxic to the liver such as kava, valerian, and eucalyptus should NOT be combined with ketoconazole.

Beverages: No restrictions. May be taken with milk.

▷ *Alcohol:* Avoid completely. Alcohol can cause a disulfiramlike reaction (see Glossary). In addition, alcohol may cause liver toxicity.

Tobacco Smoking: No interactions expected. I advise everyone to quit smoking.

▷ *Other Drugs*

Ketoconazole may *increase* the effects of

- almotriptan (Axert) by inhibiting liver enzyme (2D6) removal of almotriptan.
- alprazolam (Xanax) and other benzodiazepines (see Drug Classes).
- carbamazepine (Tegretol).
- cortisonelike drugs (budesonide, fluticasone, prednisone, etc.).
- cyclosporine (Sandimmune).
- delavirdine (Rescriptor).
- dihydropyridine calcium channel blockers (nifedipine, nicardipine, amlodipine, isradipine, and felodipine). Caution is advised.
- donepezil (Aricept) and galantamine (Reminyl)—careful patient follow-up is needed.
- ergot derivatives (Cafergot, others)—DO NOT COMBINE.
- fluticasone (Flonase) patients should be carefully watched for adverse effects from increased ketoconazole levels and unexpectedly great suppression of the adrenal (HPA).
- granisetron (Kytril)—careful patient follow-up is needed.
- HMG-CoA reductase inhibitors (atorvastatin, lovastatin, simvastatin, etc.; see Drug Classes), increasing risk of myopathy. Pravastatin (Pravachol) may be the safest medicine in this class to use with ketoconazole.
- imatinib (Gleevec)—careful patient follow-up is needed, perhaps coupled with decreased imatinib doses.
- irinotecan (Camptosar)—careful patient follow-up and decreased doses are needed.
- loratadine (Claritin) and fexofenadine (Allegra), which are minimally sedating antihistamines, but HAVE NOT been associated with heart rhythm problems when combined with ketoconazole. The blood level does appear to increase, and lower doses of both medicines may be prudent if these medicines are to be combined.
- oral antidiabetic drugs (see Drug Classes) and result in very low blood sugars.
- medicines removed by liver cytochrome P450 3A4 because ketoconazole inhibits this medicine-removing enzyme system. Extreme caution is advised.
- nonsedating antihistamines, such as astemizole (Hismanal) and terfenadine (Seldane) (now removed from the U.S. market), and may cause large

increases in blood levels and result in serious heart rhythm problems. DO NOT COMBINE.
- protease inhibitors (see Drug Classes).
- quetiapine (Seroquel).
- quinidine (Quinaglute) and cause toxicity; blood levels are needed.
- sibutramine (Meridia) can lead to sibutramine toxicity. Caution is advised.
- sildenafil (Viagra), vardenafil (Levitra), or tadalafil (Cialis)—talk to your doctor BEFORE using these medicines together.
- sirolimus (Rapamune) or tacrolimus (Prograf) can lead to sirolimus or tacrolimus toxicity. More frequent blood levels and dosing adjustments are prudent.
- sucralfate (Carafate), which may decrease the blood levels of ketoconazole.
- tolterodine (Detrol) can lead to tolterodine toxicity. Caution is advised.
- tretinoin (Vesanoid), which may increase risk of tretinoin toxicity.
- trimexate (Neutrexin).
- warfarin (Coumadin) and cause bleeding; increased testing of INR (prothrombin time or protime) is needed.
- zolpidem (Ambien) can lead to zolpidem toxicity. Caution is advised.

Ketoconazole may *decrease* the effects of
- amphotericin B (Abelcet).
- didanosine (Videx).
- theophyllines (aminophylline, Theo-Dur, etc.).

The following drugs may *decrease* the effects of ketoconazole:
- antacids; if needed, take antacids 2 hours after ketoconazole.
- didanosine (Videx)—take ketoconazole dose first and separate doses by 2 hours.
- histamine (H2)-blocking drugs: cimetidine, famotidine, nizatidine, ranitidine; if needed, take 2 hours after ketoconazole.
- isoniazid (Laniazid, Nydrazid, etc.).
- lansoprazole (Prevacid).
- omeprazole (Prilosec), or other proton pump inhibitors.
- rifampin (Rifadin, Rifater, Rimactane, etc.).

Ketoconazole *taken concurrently* with
- amprenavir (Agenerase) may increase ketoconazole levels and decrease amprenavir slightly.
- cisapride (Propulsid) can lead to serious heart toxicity. DO NOT COMBINE.
- dofetilide (Tikosyn) can lead to serious heart toxicity. DO NOT COMBINE.
- miconazole (Monistat) may increase the blood levels of ketoconazole or miconazole.
- phenytoin (Dilantin) or fosphenytoin (Cerebyx) may change the levels of both drugs.

▷ *Driving, Hazardous Activities:* This drug may cause dizziness or drowsiness. Restrict activities as necessary.

Aviation Note: The use of this drug *may be a disqualification* for piloting. Consult a designated Aviation Medical Examiner.

Exposure to Sun: This drug may cause photophobia; wear sunglasses if appropriate.

Discontinuation: Take the full course prescribed. Continual treatment for several months may be needed. Ask your doctor when the drug should be stopped.

KETOPROFEN (kee toh PROH fen)

Please see the propionic acid (nonsteroidal anti-inflammatory drug) family profile.

LABETALOL (la BET a lohl)

Introduced: 1978 **Class:** Antihypertensive alpha-and-beta-adrenergic blocker **Prescription:** USA: Yes **Controlled Drug:** USA: No; Canada: No **Available as Generic:** Yes

Brand Names: Normodyne, Normozide [CD], Trandate, Trandate HCT [CD]

BENEFITS versus RISKS	
Possible Benefits	*Possible Risks*
EFFECTIVE, WELL-TOLERATED ANTIHYPERTENSIVE in mild to moderate high blood pressure	CONGESTIVE HEART FAILURE in advanced heart disease
PROLONGS LIFE AFTER A HEART ATTACK	Worsening of angina in coronary heart disease (if drug is abruptly withdrawn)
	Masking of low blood sugar (hypoglycemia) in drug-treated diabetes
	Liver toxicity

▷ **Principal Uses**

As a Single Drug Product: Uses currently included in FDA-approved labeling: (1) Treats mild to moderate high blood pressure.

Other (unlabeled) generally accepted uses: (1) Combination therapy of hypertension in heart attacks (acute MI)—beta blockers have also been shown to decrease the risk of repeat heart attacks, limit the size of the original heart attack damage, and help control arrhythmias; (2) treatment of cocaine overdose; (3) therapy of phobic anxiety reactions; (4) treatment of angina; (5) therapy of pheochromocytoma, a tumor that releases compounds that increase blood pressure (controversial); (6) eases blood pressure in severely high blood pressure (hypertensive emergency).

As a Combination Drug Product [CD]: This drug has been combined with hydrochlorothiazide (a thiazide "water pill" or diuretic) to attack high blood pressure in 2 different ways.

How This Drug Works: By blocking part of the sympathetic nervous system, this drug:

- reduces the rate and contraction force of the heart, thus lowering the ejection pressure of blood leaving the heart.
- reduces the degree of contraction of blood vessel walls, resulting in their expansion and lowering of blood pressure.

▷ **Widely Used Guidelines That Involve This Medicine (representative sample):** Please look at the section at the very beginning of this profile called "Class." Next, turn to Table 22 and you will find guidelines listed by the class involved!

Available Dosage Forms and Strengths
Injection — 5 mg/mL
Tablets — 100 mg, 200 mg, 300 mg
Tablets, combination — 100 mg, 200 mg, 300 mg of labetalol with 25 mg
hydrochlorothiazide

▷ **Usual Adult Dosage Ranges:** *High blood pressure*: Initially 100 mg twice daily,
12 hours apart; the dose may be increased by 100 mg twice daily every 2 to
3 days as needed to reduce blood pressure. The usual ongoing dose is 200
to 400 mg twice daily. Maximum daily dose is 3,200 mg in sudden (acute)
and ongoing high blood pressure. For moderate high blood pressure,
400–800 mg is the usual effective dose.

Stable angina: 100 to 400 mg by mouth 2 to 3 times daily. Low doses (100 mg)
are usually used in people who have normal blood pressure to help avoid
excessively low blood pressure on standing up.

**Note: Actual dose and dosing schedule must be determined individu-
ally.**

Conditions Requiring Dosing Adjustments
Liver Function: The dose must be decreased in liver disease. Average dose for
people with long-standing liver disease is 50% of the usual dose. This drug
is a rare cause of liver injury.

Kidney Function: No changes presently needed (only 1% removal of the medicine).

▷ **Dosing Instructions:** Immediate release tablet may be crushed and is best taken
at the same time daily, ideally following morning and evening meals. Do
not stop this drug abruptly. If you forget a dose: take the missed dose as
soon as you remember it, unless it's within 8 hours of the next scheduled
dose—if that is the case, skip the missed dose and take the next dose right
on schedule. Talk with your doctor if you find yourself missing doses.

Usual Duration of Use: Use on a regular schedule for 10 to 14 days determines
peak effectiveness in lowering blood pressure. Long-term use (months to
years) is determined by individual response to this drug and a program
(weight reduction, salt restriction, smoking cessation, etc.).

Typical Treatment Goals and Measurements (Outcomes and Markers)
Blood Pressure: Guidelines (JNC VII) define normal blood pressure (BP) as **less
than** 120/80 and **pre-hypertension** as 120/80 to 139/89. This new range is
intended to help doctors encourage lifestyle changes (or in the case of people with a risk factor for high blood pressure, start treatment) much
earlier—so that damage to blood vessels, your heart, kidneys, sexual
potency, or eyes might be minimized or avoided altogether. Stage 1 hypertension is 140/90 to 159/99 and stage 2 hypertension equal to or greater
than: 160/100 mm Hg. These guidelines also recommend that clinicians
work with their patients to agree on the goals and a plan of treatment. The
first-ever guidelines for blood pressure (hypertension) in African Americans recommends that MOST black patients be started on TWO antihypertensive medicines with the goal of lowering blood pressure to 130/80 for
those with high risk for heart and blood vessel disease or with diabetes.
The American Diabetes Association also recommends 130/80 as the target
for diabetics and less than 125/75 for those who spill more than one gram
of protein into their urine. Most clinicians try to achieve a BP that confers
the best balance of lower cardiovascular risk and avoids the problem of too
low a blood pressure. Blood pressure duration is generally increased with

beneficial restriction of sodium. If goals are not met, it is not unusual to intensify doses or add on medicines.

Possible Advantages of This Drug

Decreases blood pressure more rapidly than other beta-blocker drugs. Can be used to treat hypertensive emergencies.

▷ **This Drug Should Not Be Taken If**

- you have had an allergic reaction to it previously.
- you have active bronchial asthma.
- you have congestive heart failure.
- you are in cardiogenic shock.
- your blood pressure is very low or you have a condition that causes severe lowering of blood pressure for a long time.
- you have an abnormally slow heart rate (bradycardia) or a serious form of heart block (second- or third-degree AV).

▷ **Inform Your Physician Before Taking This Drug If**

- you have had an adverse reaction to any beta-blocker drug (see Drug Classes).
- you have a history of serious heart disease.
- you have a history of hay fever (allergic rhinitis), asthma, chronic bronchitis, or emphysema.
- you have a history of overactive thyroid function (hyperthyroidism) or pheochromocytoma.
- you have a history of low blood sugar (hypoglycemia).
- you have sporadic cramping of the leg muscles (intermittent claudication).
- you have a history of spasms of the bronchi of the lungs.
- you have impaired liver or kidney function.
- you have diabetes or myasthenia gravis.
- you take any form of digitalis, quinidine, or reserpine or any calcium channel–blocker drug (see Drug Classes).
- you will have surgery with general anesthesia.

Possible Side Effects (natural, expected, and unavoidable drug actions)

Lethargy and fatigability—frequent.

Light-headedness in upright position (see orthostatic hypotension in Glossary).

▷ **Possible Adverse Effects** (unusual, unexpected, and infrequent reactions)

If any of the following develop, consult your physician promptly for guidance.

Mild Adverse Effects

Allergic reactions: skin rash, itching.

Headache, drowsiness, dizziness—frequent.

Scalp tingling (during early treatment)—possible.

Vivid dreams, nightmares, depression—infrequent.

Urine retention, difficulty urinating—case reports.

Indigestion, nausea, diarrhea—infrequent.

Joint and muscle discomfort, carpal tunnel syndrome, fluid retention (edema)—rare.

Serious Adverse Effects

Allergic reactions: anaphylaxis—case reports.

Chest pain, shortness of breath, precipitation of congestive heart failure—possible.

Induction of bronchial asthma (in asthmatic individuals)—possible.

Hypertensive crisis in people with pheochromocytoma—case reports.

Lichen planus—case reports.

Muscle toxicity (toxic myopathy, worsening of intermittent claudication)—possible.

Drug-induced systemic lupus erythematosus—rare.

Aggravation of myasthenia gravis—case reports.

Liver damage with jaundice—rare and often reversible (call your doctor immediately if you have dark urine, loss of appetite, unexplained tiredness, or abdominal pain, jaundice, or light-colored stools).

▷ **Possible Effects on Sexual Function:** Impotence, inhibited ejaculation, prolonged erection following orgasm (related to higher doses), Peyronie's disease (see Glossary)—rare to infrequent.

Decreased vaginal secretions (with low doses), inhibited female orgasm (higher doses)—possible.

Possible Effects on Laboratory Tests

Blood potassium or glucose: slight increase.

Liver function tests: rare increases.

CAUTION

1. **_Do not stop this drug suddenly_** without the knowledge and help of your doctor. Carry a note or wear a labetalol drug-identification bracelet.

2. Ask your physician or pharmacist before using nasal decongestants, which are usually present in over-the-counter cold preparations and nose drops. These can cause sudden increases in blood pressure if combined with labetalol.

3. Report the development of any tendency to emotional depression.

4. Sound-alike errors involving Lamictal have been reported. Lamictal is a seizure medicine. Make certain you have the correct medicine.

5. Dosing is usually started at 100 mg twice a day in order to keep blood pressure from becoming too low when you stand up (orthostatic hypotension).

Precautions for Use

By Infants and Children: Safety and effectiveness for those under 12 years of age are not established. If this drug is used, however, watch for low blood sugar (hypoglycemia) during periods of reduced food intake.

By Those Over 60 Years of Age: Proceed **_cautiously_** with all antihypertensive drugs. Therapy should be started with small doses, with frequent checks of blood pressure. Sudden, rapid, or excessive lowering of blood pressure can increase stroke or heart attack risk. Watch for dizziness, unsteadiness, tendency to fall, confusion, hallucinations, depression, or urinary frequency.

▷ **Advisability of Use During Pregnancy**

Pregnancy Category: C. See Pregnancy Risk Categories at the back of this book.

Animal Studies: No significant increase in birth defects found in rats or rabbits; some increase in fetal deaths reported.

Human Studies: Adequate studies of pregnant women are not available.

Use this drug only if clearly needed. Ask your physician for guidance.

Advisability of Use If Breast-Feeding

Presence of this drug in breast milk: Yes, in very small, but variable amounts. Listed as safe in one source. Talk to your doctor.

Habit-Forming Potential: None. Rebound increases in blood pressure have been reported if the medicine is stopped suddenly. This is a physiologic response, not addiction.

Effects of Overdose: Weakness, slow pulse, low blood pressure, fainting, cold and sweaty skin, congestive heart failure, possible coma, and convulsions.

Possible Effects of Long-Term Use: Reduced heart reserve and eventual heart failure in susceptible individuals with advanced heart disease.

Suggested Periodic Examinations While Taking This Drug (at physician's discretion)

Measurements of blood pressure (take advantage of health fairs or your local pharmacy).

Evaluation of heart and liver function.

Antinuclear antibody (ANA) every 3 months.

May be prudent to check for hidden Peripheral Artery Disease (PAD) by checking ankle brachial index (ABI). ABI check (see Glossary) can help find PAD early, and avoid claudication that may result if this medication is taken by someone who has PAD but does not know it.

▷ **While Taking This Drug, Observe the Following**

Foods: May increase the absorption of labetalol and result in a larger-than-expected blood level. Patients taking this medicine should also avoid excessive salt intake.

Herbal Medicines or Minerals: Ginseng, bitter orange, country mallow, hawthorn, saw palmetto, ma huang (no longer on the market), guarana (caffeine), goldenseal, yohimbe, and licorice may also cause increased blood pressure. Dong quai may block the removal of this medicine from the body, leading to toxic effects with "normal" doses. St. John's wort may increase removal of this medicine from the body, leading to loss of benefits despite appropriate doses. Calcium and garlic may help lower blood pressure. Ginkgo benefits in helping peripheral artery disease are, as yet, unproven. Indian snakeroot has a German Commission E monograph indication for hypertension—talk to your doctor. Eleuthero root and ephedra (ma huang) should be avoided by people living with hypertension.

Beverages: No restrictions. May be taken with milk.

▷ *Alcohol:* Use with caution. Alcohol may exaggerate this drug's ability to lower blood pressure and may increase its mild sedative effect.

Tobacco Smoking: Nicotine may reduce this drug's effectiveness. I advise everyone to quit smoking.

▷ *Other Drugs*

Labetalol may ***increase*** the effects of

* oral antidiabetic drugs (see Drug Classes) and prolong recovery from any hypoglycemia (low blood sugar) that may occur.
* other antihypertensive drugs and cause excessive lowering of blood pressure. Dose adjustments may be necessary.

Labetalol ***taken concurrently*** with

* amiodarone (Cordarone) may result in extremely slow heart rates and cardiac arrest.
* cimetidine (Tagamet) can cause elevated labetalol levels and low blood pressure or heart rate.
* clonidine (Catapres) must be closely watched for rebound high blood pressure if clonidine is withdrawn while labetalol is still being taken.
* digoxin's (Lanoxin) atrioventricular node conduction time extension may cause heart block and digoxin toxicity.
* dihydropyridine calcium channel blockers (nifedipine, others) may lead to impaired heart performance or excessively lowered blood pressure.
* epinephrine may result in severe increases in blood pressure.

- fluoxetine (Prozac) may increase labetalol effects.
- fluvoxamine (Luvox) may result in excessive lowering of blood pressure or slowing of the heart.
- imipramine and other tricyclic antidepressants may result in increases in antidepressant blood levels and toxicity.
- insulin must be watched for development of hypoglycemia (see Glossary).
- NSAIDs (see Drug Classes) may result in blunting of the therapeutic effects of labetalol.
- paroxetine (Paxil) may increase labetalol effects.
- phenothiazines (see Drug Classes) may cause additive lowering of the blood pressure.
- ritodrine (Yutopar) may blunt the beneficial effects of ritodrine.
- venlafaxine (Effexor) may increase labetalol effects.
- zileuton (Zyflo) may increase labetalol effects.

▷ *Driving, Hazardous Activities:* Use caution until the full extent of fatigue, dizziness, and blood pressure change has been determined.

Aviation Note: The use of this drug *is a disqualification* for piloting. Consult a designated Aviation Medical Examiner.

Exposure to Sun: No restrictions.

Exposure to Heat: Caution is advised. Hot environments can lower the blood pressure and exaggerate the effects of this drug.

Exposure to Cold: Caution is advised. Cold environments can increase blood flow problems in the extremities that may occur with beta-blocker drugs. The elderly should take precautions to prevent hypothermia (see Glossary).

Heavy Exercise or Exertion: It is prudent to avoid exertion that produces light-headedness, excessive fatigue, or muscle cramping. Use of this drug may intensify hypertensive response to isometric exercise.

Occurrence of Unrelated Illness: Fever can lower blood pressure and require decreased doses. Nausea or vomiting may interrupt scheduled doses. Ask your doctor for help.

Discontinuation: If possible, gradual reduction of dose over a period of 2 to 3 weeks is recommended—otherwise rebound increases in blood pressure may occur. Ask your doctor for help.

LAMIVUDINE (LAM iv u deen)

Introduced: 1995   **Class:**   Antiviral, antiretroviral, reverse transcriptase inhibitor, nucleoside analog   **Prescription:**   USA: Yes   **Controlled Drug:**   USA: No   **Available as Generic:** No

Brand Names: Combivir [CD], Epivir, Epivir HBV, Trizivir [CD]

BENEFITS versus RISKS

Possible Benefits	*Possible Risks*
IMPRESSIVE SUPPRESSION OF VIRAL LOAD WHEN USED IN COMBINATION THERAPY TREATING HIV	DECREASED WHITE BLOOD CELL COUNTS
	Peripheral neuropathy
	Pancreatitis
DOES NOT LEAD TO SUPPRESSION OF THE BONE MARROW	Lactic acidosis
EFFECTIVE TREATMENT OF HEPATITIS B INFECTION	Because of abacavir in the Trizivir form, caution for severe rash and reporting of any rash are required

---

▷ **Principal Uses**

As a Single Drug Product: Uses currently included in FDA-approved labeling: (1) Used to treat HIV infection. Used in combination because of possible resistance; this medicine is now available in combination with 3 drugs used together in one pill—abacavir, lamivudine, and zidovudine (Trizivir); (2) Used with zidovudine (AZT) and other antiretrovirals to reduce the risk of disease progression and death in HIV; (3) FDA-approved (in a lower dose than that used for treating HIV) to treat hepatitis B.

Author's Note: Combination therapy has become a standard of care. NIAID antiretroviral therapy guidelines take into account how easily HIV therapy can fit into a patient's life. The ATIS Guidelines (AIDS Treatment Information Service) tell us that therapy should be supervised by an expert and cover considerations of when to start therapy in both asymptomatic and established HIV infections. Adherence or taking medicines for HIV exactly on time and in the right amount is ABSOLUTELY critical to getting the best possible results or outcomes. Structured therapy interruptions (STI) or structured interruptions of therapy (SIT) are still controversial.

Other (unlabeled) generally accepted uses: Possible combination use in post-exposure prevention (prophylaxis).

As a Combination Drug Product [CD]: Available in combination with zidovudine, a nucleoside analog. Also in a combination of abacavir, lamivudine, and zidovudine (Trizivir) gives benefits of triple combination therapy and a protease inhibitor sparing effect.

How This Drug Works: Potent reverse transcriptase inhibitor—interferes with ability of HIV and the hepatitis B virus to create genetic material.

▷ **Widely Used Guidelines That Involve This Medicine (representative sample):** Please look at the section at the very beginning of this profile called "Class." Next, turn to Table 22 and you will find guidelines listed by the class involved!

Available Dosage Forms and Strengths

Solution (Epivir) — 10 mg/mL

Solution (Epivir HBV) — 5 mg/mL

Tablets (Combivir) — 150 mg lamivudine and 300 mg zidovudine

Tablets (Trizivir) — 150 mg lamivudine, 300 mg zidovudine, and abacavir 300 mg

Tablets (Epivir) — 150 mg

Tablets (Epivir HBV) — 100 mg

▷ **Recommended Dosage Ranges** (Actual dose and schedule must be determined for each patient individually.)

Infants and Children: 3 months to 12 years old: 4 mg per kg of body mass twice daily (300 mg maximum a day).

Combivir (for those over 12 years old): One tablet twice a day.

12 to 65 Years of Age:

HIV: Usual dose is 150 mg twice daily. Two mg per kg of body mass twice daily for adults weighing less than 110 lb, or 50 kg.

Combivir: One tablet twice a day.

Trizivir: One tablet twice a day.

Hepatitis B (Epivir HBV): 100 mg daily.

Over 65 Years of Age: If decision is made to use it in this population, blood levels may be prudent, as up to 70% is removed by the kidneys.

Conditions Requiring Dosing Adjustments

Liver Function: No changes expected.

Kidney Function: Up to 70% of a given dose is removed by the kidneys. Those with creatinine clearances (see Glossary) of 5 to 14 mL/min should take a first dose of 150 mg and then 50 mg once daily. This will limit use of fixed-dose combination forms.

▷ **Dosing Instructions:** Lamivudine tablets and solution can be taken without regard to meals. A solution is available for patients who can't swallow the tablets. Make certain you use a measuring spoon or calibrated dosing cup for the solution. If you forget a dose: take the missed dose as soon as you remember it, unless it's nearly time for your next dose—if that is the case, skip the missed dose and take the next dose right on schedule. Talk with your doctor if you find yourself missing doses.

Author's Note: Adherence to taking medicines for HIV exactly on time and in the right amount is ABSOLUTELY critical to getting the best possible results or outcomes. The current antiretroviral therapy guidelines from NIAID take into account how easily the medicine treating HIV can fit into a patient's life. Structured therapy interruptions (also known as structured interruptions in therapy) are controversial.

Usual Duration of Use: *HIV*: Measurement of viral load (burden) and/or CD4 counts are used to decide the effectiveness of treatment and help in the decision to continue or change medications.

Hepatitis B: Clinical studies saw use of lamivudine for 1 year. The optimal duration of use is yet decided. The question of combination treatment (such as with interferon) of hepatitis B also has yet to be decided.

Typical Treatment Goals and Measurements (Outcomes and Markers)

HIV: Goals for HIV treatment presently are maximum suppression of viral replication, maximum lowering of the amount of virus in your body (viral load or burden), and maximum patient survival. Markers of successful therapy include durable undetectable viral load, increased CD4 cells, absence of indicator or opportunistic infections (OIs), and in the case of the HIV-positive patient, failure of the infection to progress to AIDS.

Hepatitis B: Hepatitis B antigen, hepatitis B antibodies, and liver function tests such as serum alanine aminotransferase (ALT) are used to show that liver damage is resolving and the body is responding to the beneficial effects of the medicine.

Possible Advantages of This Drug

Offers reasonably durable HIV suppression in retroviral naive patients. May work where other combinations have failed (salvage therapy). Trizivir form can reserve protease inhibitor–containing regimens and avoid their metabolic complications.

Possible Side Effects (natural, expected, and unavoidable drug actions)

Paresthesias and/or peripheral neuropathy (12% in a study in children taking lamivudine monotherapy). Trizivir form has the drug abacavir in the pill. Discuss rash issues with your doctor and what to do if a rash or signs and symptoms of allergy happen if you are taking the Trizivir form.

▷ **Possible Adverse Effects** (unusual, unexpected, and infrequent reactions)

If any of the following develop, consult your physician promptly for guidance.

Mild Adverse Effects

Skin rash—infrequent.

Headache—frequent.

Dizziness—infrequent.

Sleep disorders—infrequent to frequent.

Nausea, vomiting, or diarrhea—infrequent to frequent.

Cough—frequent.

Muscle aches—infrequent.

Serious Adverse Effects

Severe and dangerous skin rashes—possible due to the abacavir present in the Trizivir form.

Lowered white blood cell counts—infrequent in adults, frequent in pediatrics.

Lowered red blood cell counts (pure red cell aplasia)—case reports.

Lactic acid buildup (Lactic acidosis)—possible.

Pancreatitis (more common in children receiving lamivudine monotherapy)—rare to infrequent.

Fat redistribution—possible and associated with this and other antiretroviral treatment.

Liver toxicity—infrequent but may be severe (risk factors appear to involve prolonged nucleoside therapy and obesity). The majority of cases have happened in women.

Seizures—case reports.

▷ **Possible Effects on Sexual Function:** None reported.

Possible Delayed Adverse Effects: Anemia or lowering of white blood cell counts. Pancreatitis. Peripheral neuropathy.

▷ **Adverse Effects That May Mimic Natural Diseases or Disorders:** Seizures may suggest the possibility of epilepsy.

Possible Effects on Laboratory Tests

Complete blood cell counts: decreased red cells.

Increased amylase and lipase (if pancreatitis occurs).

Lactic acidosis—possible.

CAUTION

1. This drug is not a cure for HIV or AIDS; nor does it protect completely against other infections or complications. Follow your doctor's instructions. Take exactly as prescribed.
2. HIV can still be spread through sexual contact or blood. Use of an effective condom is mandatory. Don't share needles.

Precautions for Use

By Infants and Children: Patients from 3 months to 12 years old are dosed on a mg-per-kg-of-body-mass basis.

By Those Over 60 Years of Age: Probable age-related decline in kidney function requires blood levels to check need for dose reduction.

▷ **Advisability of Use During Pregnancy**
Pregnancy Category: C. See Pregnancy Risk Categories at the back of this book.
Animal Studies: Rat and rabbit studies reveal no birth defects.
Human Studies: Adequate studies of pregnant women are not available.
   Your physician should call 1-800-258-4263, if the decision is made to use this medicine while you are pregnant.

Advisability of Use If Breast-Feeding
   Presence of this drug in breast milk: Mean concentration varied from less than 5 mcg/mL to 6.06 mcg/mL.
   Refrain from nursing (HIV may be transferred via breast milk).

Habit-Forming Potential: None.

Effects of Overdose: Nausea, vomiting, diarrhea, bone marrow depression.

Possible Effects of Long-Term Use: Anemia and loss of white blood cells.
   Pancreatitis or peripheral neuropathy.

Suggested Periodic Examinations While Taking This Drug (at physician's discretion)
   Complete blood counts.
   Periodic CD4 counts or viral load tests are needed. Increasing viral load or decreasing CD4 are indicators that therapy is failing and you should demand change of antiretroviral therapy.
   Amylase and lipase. Check for peripheral neuropathy.
   Tests for lactic acidosis. Liver function tests.
   Liver biopsy may need to be taken periodically to assess the success of this medicine in treating hepatitis. Slightly more than half of patients responded in clinical trials.

▷ **While Taking This Drug, Observe the Following**
Foods: No restrictions.
Herbal Medicines or Minerals: Milk thistle has some data to support its role as an antioxidant and may help promote liver cell regeneration. Talk to your doctor if lamivudine is being used to treat the infection of hepatitis B and you are considering milk thistle. Echinacea: Some patients use echinacea to attempt to boost their immune systems. Unfortunately, use of echinacea is not recommended in people with damaged immune systems. This herb may also actually weaken any immune system if it is used too often or for too long a time.
Beverages: No restrictions. May be taken with milk.
▷ *Alcohol:* No interactions expected with lamivudine. The abacavir combination form will find abacavir remaining in the system longer than expected. Careful patient follow-up is needed.
Tobacco Smoking: No interactions expected. I advise everyone to quit smoking.
▷ *Other Drugs*
   Lamivudine *taken concurrently* with
   • cotrimoxazole (Septra, Bactrim) may increase lamivudine blood levels.
   • indinavir (Crixivan) and zidovudine (AZT) resulted in undetectable HIV levels in some HIV-positive patients (beneficial effect of combination treatment).
   • nelfinavir (Viracept) may increase lamivudine levels.
   • other medicines capable of causing pancreatitis may result in increased pancreatitis risk.

- other medicines capable of lowering white or red cell counts may cause additive risks.
- ribavirin (Rebetron) may lead to lactic acidosis. A careful and cautious analysis of the benefit-to-risk aspects of this combination should be considered. Careful patient monitoring is prudent if this combination must be used.
- sulfamethoxazole (various) may increase lamivudine levels.
- trimethoprim (various) may increase lamivudine levels.
- trimexate (Mexate) may cause additive blood (hematological) toxicity.

▷ *Driving, Hazardous Activities:* This drug may cause dizziness or fainting. Restrict activities as necessary.

Aviation Note: The use of this drug ***is a disqualification*** for piloting. Consult a designated Aviation Medical Examiner.

Exposure to Sun: No restrictions.

Discontinuation: Do not stop this drug without your physician's knowledge and guidance.

LAMOTRIGINE (la MOH tri jean)

Introduced: 1995 **Class:** Anticonvulsant, phenyltriazine, mood stabilizer **Prescription:** USA: Yes **Controlled Drug:** USA: No; Canada: No **Available as Generic:** USA: No

Brand Names: ✤Alti-Lamotrigine, ✤Apo-Lamotrigine, Lamictal, ✤PMS-Lamotrigine, ✤Ratio-Lamotrigine

---

BENEFITS versus RISKS

Possible Benefits	*Possible Risks*
EFFECTIVE MANAGEMENT OF SEIZURES THAT RESIST THERAPY	RASHES THAT CAN BE LIFE-THREATENING
INCREASE IN SEIZURE-FREE DAYS	Changes in vision
MANAGEMENT OF PARTIAL SEIZURES	Dizziness
MANAGEMENT OF SEIZURES ASSOCIATED WITH LENNOX-GASTAUT SYNDROME	
TREATMENT OF RAPID CYCLING BIPOLAR DISORDER	

▷ **Principal Uses**

As a Single Drug Product: Uses currently included in FDA-approved labeling: (1) Adjunctive combination therapy of partial seizures in adults who have not responded to treatment with other medicines; (2) used to treat Lennox-Gastaut syndrome as add-on therapy; (3) treatment of rapid cycling bipolar disorder.

Other (unlabeled) generally accepted uses: (1) May have a role in treating epilepsy in children who have not responded to more established treatment; (2) could have a role in treating status epilepticus; (3) could have a role in some pain syndromes (trigeminal neuralgia); (4) case reports of resolving of impotence in epileptic men who took this medicine.

How This Drug Works: The exact mechanism of action is not known, but animal models appear to show that this medicine blocks voltage-dependent sodium channels. This causes a decreased amount of glutamate and aspartate transmitters and a decreased likelihood of seizures.

▷ **Widely Used Guidelines That Involve This Medicine (representative sample):** Please look at the section at the very beginning of this profile called "Class." Next, turn to Table 22 and you will find guidelines listed by the class involved!

Available Dosage Forms and Strengths

Chewable tablets — 2 mg, 5 mg, 25 mg

Tablets — 25 mg, 100 mg, 150 mg, 200 mg

▷ **Recommended Dosage Ranges** (Actual dose and schedule must be determined for each patient individually.)

Infants and Children: Safety and efficacy in those under 16 years old have not been established except for Lennox-Gastaut syndrome patients. Dosing is based on weight and whole tablets (chewable) should be used. Dosing should be rounded DOWN to the nearest whole tablet dose. As in adults, dosing is adjusted if medicines known to interact with lamotrigine are also being taken.

16 to 65 Years of Age: Seizures: In patients receiving medicines known to interact (phenytoin, primidone, carbamazepine, or phenobarbital, but not valproic acid), starting dose is 50 mg a day for 2 weeks and then 50 mg twice a day. As needed or tolerated (increases made at 100 mg a day each 7–4 days) finds most patients end up taking 300–500 mg a day in 2 equal doses. Patients only taking valproic acid and/or the above drugs: 25 mg every other day for 2 weeks and then 25 mg once daily for 2 weeks, with increases of 25 to 50 mg per day at 1- to 2-week intervals as needed and tolerated. Usual ongoing dose is 100–400 mg daily. If taking valproic acid alone with this medicine, dose is usually 100–200 mg a day.

Bipolar disorder: Dosing in people not taking valproic acid or an enzyme inducing seizure medicine: For the first two weeks, 25 mg daily is given, then for the third and fourth week, 50 mg is given. After this, week 5 leads to 100 mg a day and week 6 has the dose increased to the 200 mg target dose. More conservative and slower dosing increases are used where valproic acid is being taken.

Over 65 Years of Age: Same dosing as 16 to 65 (single-dose pharmacokinetics were similar to younger adults). Few patients over 65 were included during premarketing studies.

Conditions Requiring Dosing Adjustments

Liver Function: This drug is mostly changed in the liver. In people with moderate liver (hepatic dysfunction) compromise (Child-Pugh Grade B), the starting dose, dose increases, and ongoing doses should be 50% lower than in people with normal liver function. Caution and clinical response as well as drug levels (even though levels are still not well established) should be used to guide the need for any increases. In severe liver compromise (Child-Pugh C), the beginning dose, step increases and ongoing (maintenance) doses should be lowered by 75%.

Kidney Function: Most of this medicine (once changed or glucuronidated) is removed by the kidneys. Used with caution and with more frequent blood levels (in severe kidney failure).

▷ **Dosing Instructions:** Take this medicine exactly as prescribed. Food does not affect how much medicine gets into your body. Swallow the tablet form whole. In pediatrics, dosing is ROUNDED DOWN to the nearest whole chewable tablet. The chewable form can be swallowed whole or can even be dissolved in a teaspoon of water and swallowed after it is given a minute to dissolve. Talk with your doctor IMMEDIATELY if you get a rash, swollen lymph glands, and fever. If you forget a dose: take the missed dose as soon as you remember it, unless it's nearly time for your next dose—if that is the case, skip the missed dose and take the next dose right on schedule. Talk with your doctor if you find yourself missing doses.

Usual Duration of Use: Regular use for 3 months in children with resistant seizures may be needed to see peak benefits. Long-term use (months to years) will be determined by individual response.

Typical Treatment Goals and Measurements (Outcomes and Markers)

Seizures: The general goal for this medicine is effective seizure control. Neurologists tend to define effective results on a case-by-case basis depending on the seizure type and patient factors.

Possible Advantages of This Drug

May work where single medicines have failed.

▷ **This Drug Should Not Be Taken If**
- you have developed a rash with swollen lymph glands while taking this medicine.
- you are allergic to this medicine or ones similar to it.

▷ **Inform Your Physician Before Taking This Drug If**
- you develop a rash. If this happens, stop the medicine and call your doctor immediately as the rash needs to be evaluated and a different seizure medicine needs to be started right away.
- your heart function is compromised.
- you do not understand how much or how often to take it.
- you have liver or kidney damage.

Possible Side Effects (natural, expected, and unavoidable drug actions)

Somnolence.

Weight gain, blurred vision (may be frequent).

▷ **Possible Adverse Effects** (unusual, unexpected, and infrequent reactions)

If any of the following develop, consult your physician promptly for guidance.

Mild Adverse Effects

Allergic reactions: skin rash (should be reported to your doctor), itching—infrequent.

Dizziness and headache—most common adverse effects.

Problems coordinating movements (ataxia)—infrequent.

Muscle tremor, chills, or nerve tingling (peripheral neuropathy)—infrequent.

Nausea and vomiting—dose-related and may be frequent.

Blurred vision—dose-related

Double vision—frequent.

Increased liver enzymes—case reports.

Serious Adverse Effects

Allergic reactions: anaphylaxis, increased liver enzymes—case reports.

Serious rashes (Stevens-Johnson syndrome, toxic epidermal necrolysis)—case reports.

Hostility—rare.

Lowered blood platelets (thrombocytopenia) or increased platelets (thrombocytosis), low white blood cells (leukopenia), or sudden (acute) disseminated intravascular coagulation—case reports.

Anemia (aplastic and hemolytic)—case reports and questioned cause.

Pure red cell aplasia (PRCA)—case report.

Blood in the urine—infrequent.

Movement problems (ataxia)—infrequent.

Myopathy or rhabdomyolysis—case reports.

Tourette's syndrome—case reports and dose-related.

Peripheral neuropathy—rare and of questionable cause.

Sudden unexplained death (SUDEP). The rate of SUDEP was similar to that of another agent also tested and appears to be a population effect—case reports.

▷ **Possible Effects on Sexual Function:** Case reports of lamotrigine controlling seizures and easing impotence in some epileptic men.

Possible Effects on Laboratory Tests: Blood levels of interacting medicines may be changed, sodium may be lowered.

CAUTION
1. **DO NOT** stop this medicine suddenly, as seizures may occur. If it must be stopped because of a rash, your doctor must be called and another medicine started.
2. Sound-alike errors involving labetalol have been reported. Labetalol is a high blood pressure medicine. Make certain you have the correct medicine.
3. Dosing in children is ROUNDED DOWN to the nearest whole chewable tablet.

Precautions for Use
By Infants and Children: This medicine is approved for add-on therapy in children over 16 years of age.
By Those Over 60 Years of Age: No specific changes.

▷ **Advisability of Use During Pregnancy**
Pregnancy Category: C. See Pregnancy Risk Categories at the back of this book.
Animal Studies: No evidence of drug-related changes were found in mice or rabbits that were given up to 1.2 times the human dose.
Human Studies: This medicine has been shown to cause toxicity to the mother and, because of this, toxicity to the fetus. Adequate studies of pregnant women are not available.
Discuss benefits and risks with your doctor.

Advisability of Use If Breast-Feeding
Presence of this drug in breast milk: Yes.
Avoid drug or refrain from nursing.

Habit-Forming Potential: None.

Effects of Overdose: Sleepiness, changes in muscular reflexes, coma. Keep a seizure diary to check for decrease in seizure frequency.

Possible Effects of Long-Term Use: Weight gain.

Suggested Periodic Examinations While Taking This Drug (at physician's discretion)
Examinations for nystagmus, muscular coordination.
Blood counts.
Check for rash.
Sodium.

▷ **While Taking This Drug, Observe the Following**
Foods: No restrictions. Can be taken with or without food.
Herbal Medicines or Minerals: Using St. John's wort, ma huang (no longer on

the market), guarana, mate, bitter orange, country mallow, or kola may result in unacceptable central nervous system stimulation and worsen possible nervousness as a side effect of lamotrigine. Since part of the way that ginseng may work is as an MAO inhibitor, and because some gingko products have been found to be contaminated with 4'-O-methylpyridoxine, which can increase seizures, combination with this medicine is not recommended. Valerian and kava kava (not recommended in Canada) may interact to increase drowsiness. Evening primrose oil may increase seizure risk and is not recommended.

Beverages: No restrictions. May be taken with milk.

▷ *Alcohol:* Avoid alcohol use, unless you discuss this with your doctor.

Tobacco Smoking: No interactions expected. I advise everyone to quit smoking.

▷ *Other Drugs*

Lamotrigine *taken concurrently* with
- long-standing use of acetaminophen (Tylenol, others) may result in decreases in blood levels caused by this medicine and a potential decrease in seizure control. Periodic use should not cause problems.
- birth control pills (combination forms of oral contraceptives—various) may increase the removal of lamotrigine from the body and require dosing changes in lamotrigine.
- carbamazepine (Tegretol) may increase the removal of lamotrigine from the body and require dosing adjustments.
- phenobarbital may result in faster removal of lamotrigine from the body and require dosing changes.
- phenytoin (Dilantin) and fosphenytoin (Cerebyx) may result in faster removal of lamotrigine from the body and require dosing changes.
- primidone (Mysoline) may result in faster removal of lamotrigine from the body and require dosing changes.
- rifampin (Rifater, others) and ritonavir (Norvir) may lead to decreased lamotrigine levels and increased risk of seizure.
- sertraline (Zoloft) may lead to lamotrigine toxicity.
- tramadol (Ultram) may increase seizure risk and is not recommended.
- valproic acid (Depakene) may slow removal of lamotrigine from the body, requiring lamotrigine dose decreases to avoid toxicity.

▷ *Driving, Hazardous Activities:* Use caution until the full extent of fatigue, dizziness, or coordination or vision changes have been determined.

Aviation Note: The use of this drug *is a disqualification* for piloting. Consult a designated Aviation Medical Examiner.

Exposure to Sun: No restrictions.

Exposure to Heat: Use caution. Muscular coordination problems may be worsened by excessive heat.

Discontinuation: DO NOT stop this medicine abruptly without talking with your doctor first. Abrupt discontinuation without first starting another antiseizure medicine may result in seizures. The dose is usually decreased by half (50%) a week over at least 2 weeks. If there are patient safety concerns, clinicians have withdrawn this medicine more rapidly.

LANSOPRAZOLE (lan SO pra sole)

Introduced: 1995 **Class:** Anti-ulcer, proton pump inhibitor **Prescription:** USA: Yes **Controlled Drug:** USA: No; Canada: No **Available as Generic:** USA: No; Canada: No

Brand Names: Prevacid, Prevacid delayed release oral suspension, Prevpac [CD], NapraPAC

BENEFITS versus RISKS

Possible Benefits	*Possible Risks*
VERY EFFECTIVE TREATMENT OF CONDITIONS ASSOCIATED WITH EXCESSIVE PRODUCTION OF STOMACH (GASTRIC) ACID: ZOLLINGER-ELLISON SYNDROME, MASTOCYTOSIS, ENDOCRINE ADENOMA	Liver enzyme increases Protein in the urine
VERY EFFECTIVE TREATMENT OF REFLUX ESOPHAGITIS	
VERY EFFECTIVE TREATMENT OF DUODENAL ULCER	
DELAYED RELEASE SUSPENSION FORM OFFERS EASIER-TO-SWALLOW MEDICINE	
EFFECTIVE MAINTENANCE THERAPY OF HEALED DUODENAL ULCERS	
COMBINATION PRODUCT (PREVPAC) ENCOURAGES ADHERENCE	

▷ **Principal Uses**

As a Single Drug Product: Uses currently included in FDA-approved labeling: (1) Used to treat duodenal and stomach (gastric) ulcers; (2) treats erosive esophagitis; (3) used in syndromes (such as Zollinger-Ellison) where excessive amounts of stomach acid are produced; (4) maintains healed duodenal ulcers; (5) treats heartburn (gastroesophageal reflux disease, or GERD); (6) part of dual (with amoxicillin) or triple (with amoxicillin and clarithromycin) treatment of *Helicobacter pylori*.

Other (unlabeled) generally accepted uses: (1) may increase fat absorption in cystic fibrosis.

As a Combination Drug Product [CD]: This drug is available in combination with two antibiotics—clarithromycin and amoxicillin (Prevpac). Since refractory ulcers are often actually *Helicobacter pylori* infections, the combination works to kill the bacteria and lower acid production. Also available in a combination PAC with naproxen. This combination gives the arthritis fighting power of naproxen with the protection of lansoprazole.

How This Drug Works: Inhibits an enzyme system (H/K adenosine triphosphate) in the stomach (parietal cells) lining and stops production of stomach acid. By doing this, it eliminates the principal cause of ulcers or esophagitis and creates an environment conducive to healing. Taking this medicine 15–30 minutes before the morning meal makes best use of the fact that this will allow the medicine to be at its peak just when the largest number of proton pumps are working. Use of this drug with 1 or 2 antibiotics attacks *Helicobacter pylori* and also decreases acid. The delayed release oral suspension offers a more convenient dosing form and beneficial release characteristics (kinetics).

▷ **Widely Used Guidelines That Involve This Medicine (representative sample):**
Please look at the section at the very beginning of this profile called "Class."
Next, turn to Table 22 and you will find guidelines listed by the class involved!

Available Dosage Forms and Strengths
Capsules — 15 mg, 30 mg
Capsules (Prevpac) — 30 mg lansoprazole, 500 mg amoxicillin
and clarithromycin
Suspension (Prevacid Delayed — 15 or 30 mg packets
Release Oral Suspension)
NapraPAC: 15 mg lansoprazole and either 375 mg or 500 mg of naproxen

▷ **Recommended Dosage Ranges** (Actual dose and schedule must be determined
for each patient individually.)
Infants and Children: Not studied in this age group.
18 to 60 Years of Age: For duodenal ulcer: 15 mg daily, taken before a meal.
Some patients require 30 mg daily. Four weeks of therapy are needed, and
treatment has been used for 8 weeks in some patients.
For ongoing therapy of healed duodenal ulcers: 15 mg daily.
For erosive esophagitis: 30 mg daily, taken before a meal. Up to 8 weeks of
treatment can be given. If healing does not occur, an additional 8 weeks
may be considered.
For excessive acid production syndromes: Dosing is started at 60 mg daily.
The dose is increased as needed and tolerated. Doses up to 90 mg twice
daily have been used. Once the condition is under control, dose is usually
slowly reduced to 30 mg a day.
For *Helicobacter pylori*: Seven-day regimen for duodenal ulcers and *H. pylori*
of lansoprazole 30 mg twice daily, plus amoxicillin 1,000 mg twice daily,
plus clarithromycin 500 mg twice daily. Three-day quadruple treatment:
bismuth subcitrate, 240 mg; clarithromycin, 500 mg; lansoprazole, 30 mg;
and metronidazole, 400 mg twice a day.
Eradication: The above regimen is used for 14 days.
Over 60 Years of Age: Same as 18 to 60 years of age.

Conditions Requiring Dosing Adjustments
Liver Function: The manufacturer strongly suggests a dose of 15 mg daily for
people with significant liver problems.
Kidney Function: No dosing changes are needed.

▷ **Dosing Instructions:** The capsules contain enteric-coated granules that protect
the medicine in the stomach's acid. Take the capsules whole if possible.
Some studies have found that lansoprazole **taken in the morning** works
best in controlling stomach acid. It should be taken 15–30 minutes before
the morning meal so that the peak level of lansoprazole happens just when
the largest number of proton pumps are working. If swallowing is a problem, the capsule may be opened and the intact granules sprinkled into
applesauce, yogurt, strained pears, and even ENSURE pudding. Once
opened, it should be taken right away. The oral suspension form comes as
15 or 30 mg. The contents of the packet should be emptied into a container
holding 2 tablespoons of water, then stirred well and drunk immediately. If
you forget a dose: take the missed dose as soon as you remember it, unless
it's nearly time for your next dose—if that is the case, skip the missed dose
and take the next dose right on schedule. Talk with your doctor if you find
yourself missing doses.

Usual Duration of Use: Use on a regular schedule for 7 days resulted in a 90–94%
decrease in acid release. Patients with stomach (gastric) or duodenal ulcers

had a decrease in symptoms in about 1 week—this DOES NOT mean that the ulcer is gone: Especially with maintenance of healing of duodenal ulcers, therapy may be ongoing. Eradication regimen with 3 drugs (see previous page) took 14 days. People with reflux esophagitis had decreases in heartburn after 7 to 28 days. Some esophagitis patients needed a second 8-week course to bring symptoms under control. Long-term use requires physician follow-up.

Typical Treatment Goals and Measurements (Outcomes and Markers)
Ulcers: The role of *Helicobacter pylori* in ulcers and a proton pump inhibitor is widely recognized as the standard for short-term treatment of stomach ulcers. When *H. pylori* is present, single-medicine therapy is not recommended (an antibiotic is often used with other agents). The goal is to heal the ulcer area and prevent re-occurrence of the ulceration. Sign and symptom relief (stomach pain, etc.) as well as endoscopic examination help define success of treatment.

▷ **This Drug Should Not Be Taken If**
  • you are allergic to the medicine or any of its components.

▷ **Inform Your Physician Before Taking This Drug If**
  • you have a history of liver disease (or kidney compromise if taking the combination product).
  • you smoke and expect to continue smoking (worsens acid secretion).

Possible Side Effects (natural, expected, and unavoidable drug actions)
  Increased serum gastrin levels (clinical significance is unknown). There have been 6 cases of black tongue and mouth inflammation reported in people who took antibiotics and lansoprazole to treat *Helicobacter pylori*.

▷ **Possible Adverse Effects** (unusual, unexpected, and infrequent reactions)
  If any of the following develop, consult your physician promptly for guidance.
  Mild Adverse Effects
  Allergic reaction: skin rash.
  Headache (may be common), dizziness, or tiredness—infrequent.
  Diarrhea or nausea—infrequent.
  Ringing in the ears—rare.
  Serious Adverse Effects
  Allergic reaction: not defined.
  Protein in the urine—rare.
  Liver toxicity or low blood platelets—rare and of questionable cause.

▷ **Possible Effects on Sexual Function:** None reported.

▷ **Adverse Effects That May Mimic Natural Diseases or Disorders**
  Drug-induced liver reaction may suggest viral hepatitis.

Possible Effects on Laboratory Tests
  Liver function tests: increased.

CAUTION
  1. Follow your doctor's advice on how long to take this drug.
  2. This drug effectively treats ulcers but does not preclude the chance of cancer of the stomach.

Precautions for Use
  By Infants and Children: Not indicated in this age group.
  By Those Over 60 Years of Age: This medicine may cause dizziness. Use caution until you've seen the effects it has on you.

▷ **Advisability of Use During Pregnancy**
Pregnancy Category: B. See Pregnancy Risk Categories at the back of this book.

Advisability of Use If Breast-Feeding
Presence of this drug in breast milk: Unknown.
Avoid drug or refrain from nursing.

Habit-Forming Potential: None.

Effects of Overdose: Possible nausea, vomiting, dizziness, lethargy, and abdominal pain.

Possible Effects of Long-Term Use: Serum gastrin levels are increased by this medicine, but the clinical significance is not known. Presently it is indicated for a maximum of two 8-week courses in erosive esophagitis. Maintenance of healed ulcers will further define effects of longer-term treatment.

Suggested Periodic Examinations While Taking This Drug (at physician's discretion)
Complete blood counts.
Liver function tests.

▷ **While Taking This Drug, Observe the Following**
Foods: Lansoprazole is best taken on an empty stomach. Follow your doctor's instructions regarding the types of foods you eat.
Herbal Medicines or Minerals: Kola, guarana, mate, and ma huang (no longer on the market) may increase stomach acid, blunting the benefits of this medicine. Black cohosh root, ginkgo, and squill are contraindicated in gastrointestinal disturbances. Licorice root has a German Commission E monograph indication for gastrointestinal ulcers, but use with proton pump inhibitors has not been studied. Talk to your doctor BEFORE adding any herbals to a proton pump inhibitor.
Beverages: No restrictions.
▷ *Alcohol:* No specific interactions, but alcohol stimulates the secretion of stomach acid and may lessen the therapeutic benefits of this medicine.
Tobacco Smoking: Smoking can stimulate stomach acid and lessen benefits of this drug. I advise everyone to quit smoking.
▷ *Other Drugs*
Lansoprazole *taken concurrently* with
• antacids may blunt how much lansoprazole gets into your body, blunting lansoprazole benefits.
• antazanavir (Reyataz) may blunt how much atazanavir gets into your body. Do NOT combine.
• clarithromycin (Biaxin) may lead to a blackening of the tongue or stomatitis. Lower lansoprazole doses and stopping the clarithromycin may be required.
• corticosteroids may irritate the stomach and blunt the benefits of lansoprazole.
• itraconazole (Sporonox), ketoconazole (Nizoral) absorption, and blood levels may be changed and benefit of antifungal lost. Careful check of treatment progress is needed.
• ritonavir (Norvir) may change lansoprazole blood levels.
• sucralfate (Carafate) may decrease lansoprazole absorption; separate doses by 2 hours.
• theophylline (Theo-Dur, others) may decrease blood theophylline level, requiring dosing adjustments.

▷ *Driving, Hazardous Activities:* Caution—this medicine may cause drowsiness. Limit activities as necessary.

Aviation Note: The use of this drug *may be a disqualification* for piloting. Consult a designated Aviation Medical Examiner.

Exposure to Sun: No restrictions.

Discontinuation: Talk with your doctor before stopping this medicine for any reason. Taking the medicine for a shorter time than needed may result in incomplete ulcer healing and continuation of the original problem.

LATANOPROST (la TAN oh prost)

Introduced: 1996   **Class:**   Prostaglandin F2-alpha analogue, antiglaucoma agent   **Prescription:**   USA: Yes   **Controlled Drug:**   USA: No; Canada: No   **Available as Generic:**   No

Brand Names: ♣Xalacom [CD], Xalatan

BENEFITS versus RISKS

Possible Benefits	*Possible Risks*
EFFECTIVE REDUCTION OF INTERNAL EYE PRESSURE FOR CONTROL OF ACUTE AND CHRONIC GLAUCOMA CONTROL OF OCULAR HYPERTENSION Formation of eyelashes	Mild side effects with systemic absorption Joint or back pain Minor eye discomfort Altered vision Iris pigmentation

---

▷ **Principal Uses**

As a Single Drug Product: Uses currently included in FDA-approved labeling: (1) Used to manage glaucoma; (2) lowers increased pressure in the eye (intraocular pressure).

Other (unlabeled) generally accepted uses: (1) Used to attempt to encourage eyelash formation in patients who previously did not have any.

As a Combination Drug Product [CD]: This drug is available in combination with a beta blocker called timolol. The combination offers 2 different mechanisms of action to help lower pressure (intraocular pressure) in the eye.

How This Drug Works: This medicine lowers pressure in the eye by increasing outflow from the uveoscleral area without changing aqueous flow.

▷ **Widely Used Guidelines That Involve This Medicine (representative sample):** Please look at the section at the very beginning of this profile called "Class." Next, turn to Table 22 and you will find guidelines listed by the class involved!

Available Dosage Forms and Strengths

Combination Eyedrop solutions — 50 mcg per mL of latanoprost and 5 mg/mL of timolol

Eyedrop solutions — 0.005% or 50 mcg per mL

▷ **Usual Adult Dosage Ranges:** For open-angle glaucoma or ocular hypertension: One drop (0.005%) in the eye each evening.

Note: Actual dose and dosing schedule must be determined for each patient individually.

Conditions Requiring Dosing Adjustments

Liver Function: The drug is changed in the liver and removed by the kidneys. Dose changes in liver disease are not defined.

Kidney Function: Changed drug (metabolites) removed by the kidney, but dosing changes in kidney failure are not defined.

▷ **Dosing Instructions:** Remove contact lenses and do not replace them for at least 15 minutes after putting this medicine into your eye. To avoid excessive absorption into the body, press finger against inner corner of the eye (to close off the tear duct) during and for 1 minute after dropping the medicine in. Be careful not to touch the dropper to the eye. If you forget a dose: Take the missed dose as soon as you remember it, unless it's nearly time for your next dose—if that is the case, skip the missed dose and take the next dose right on schedule. DO NOT double doses. Talk with your doctor and pharmacist if you find yourself missing doses—there are many pill boxes, phone services, and even key fobs to help you remember.

Usual Duration of Use: Use on a regular schedule for a day usually sees an effect in lowering the pressure in the eye. A week may be required for the full benefits of the medicine to be realized. Long-term use (months to years) requires physician supervision and may require combination therapy if pressure rises again.

Typical Treatment Goals and Measurements (Outcomes and Markers)

Glaucoma: Ophthalmologists measure intraocular pressure (IOP), and then check IOP-lowering once this medicine is started. The chamber angle can be checked prior to treatment. A 6–8 mm of HG drop in intraocular pressure is common during ongoing use.

▷ **This Drug Should Not Be Taken If**
- you have had an eye infection with herpes simplex (case report authors suggest avoiding latanoprost).
- you have had an allergic reaction to it previously or to the benzalkonium chloride that is in it.

▷ **Inform Your Physician Before Taking This Drug If**
- you wear contact lenses.
- you have had an eye infection in the last 3 months.
- you have some of the risk factors for fluid accumulation in the macula (macular edema). Talk to your doctor about this.
- you have sudden (acute) angle closure of the eye.

Possible Side Effects (natural, expected, and unavoidable drug actions)

Burning of the eyes or irritation—frequent (usually mild).

Pigmentation of the eye (iridial) has been reported.

Growth of eyelashes in patients who previously did not have any has been reported.

▷ **Possible Adverse Effects** (unusual, unexpected, and infrequent reactions)

If any of the following develop, consult your physician promptly for guidance.

Mild Adverse Effects

Allergic reactions: itching of the eyes, eyelid itching and/or swelling, or rash.

Headache—infrequent.

Nausea—case reports.

Muscle or back pain—rare to infrequent.

Serious Adverse Effects

Pigmentation of the iris—infrequent, though may be frequent (up to 16%) with therapy ongoing for more than a year.

Hypertension—2 case reports.
Choroidal detachment of effusion—case reports.
Angina pectorus and/or chest pain—rare.

▷ **Possible Effects on Sexual Function:** None reported.

Natural Diseases or Disorders That May Be Activated by This Drug
Herpes infection in the skin around the eye may be reactivated in patients who have already had this problem.

Possible Effects on Laboratory Tests
None reported.

Precautions for Use
By Those Over 60 Years of Age: No age-specific changes presently needed.

▷ **Advisability of Use During Pregnancy**
Pregnancy Category: C. See Pregnancy Risk Categories at the end of book.
Human Studies: Adequate studies of pregnant women are not available.
Discuss use with your doctor BEFORE using this drug.

Advisability of Use If Breast-Feeding
Presence of this drug in breast milk: Unknown.
Watch infant closely and stop drug or nursing if adverse effects develop.

Habit-Forming Potential: None.

Effects of Overdose: Not defined.

Possible Effects of Long-Term Use: Pigmentation of the iris.

Suggested Periodic Examinations While Taking This Drug (at physician's discretion)
Measurement of internal eye pressure on a regular basis.
Check for early signs of pigmentation.

▷ **While Taking This Drug, Observe the Following**
Foods: No restrictions.
Herbal Medicines or Minerals: Scopolia root has glaucoma as a possible side effect. DO NOT COMBINE. Henbane, ephedra, and belladonna should also be avoided.
Beverages: No restrictions.
▷ *Alcohol:* No restrictions except prudence in alcohol use.
Tobacco Smoking: No interactions expected. I advise everyone to quit smoking.
Marijuana Smoking: Sustained additional decrease in internal eye pressure.
▷ *Other Drugs*
Latanoprost *taken concurrently* with
• pilocarpine (various) may blunt latanoprost benefits. Dose pilocarpine 1 hour after latanoprost.
• thimerosal (various) can cause a precipitation. DO NOT combine eyedrops containing thimerosal with latanoprost. Separate doses by 5 minutes or more.
▷ *Driving, Hazardous Activities:* This drug may cause blurry vision for a time. Restrict activities as necessary.
Aviation Note: The use of this drug *may be a disqualification* for piloting. Consult a designated Aviation Medical Examiner.
Exposure to Sun: This medicine may make your eyes sensitive to the sun. Wear sunglasses. See the table in the back of this book about other medicines that may cause such sensitivity—effects may be additive if these medicines are combined.
Discontinuation: Do not stop regular use of this drug without consulting your physician.

LEFLUNOMIDE (LEH flew no myde)

Introduced: 1998   **Class:** Disease-modifying antirheumatic drug (DMARD), pyrimidine synthesis inhibitor, immunosuppressant (T cell)   **Prescription:** USA: Yes   **Controlled Drug:** USA: No; Canada: No   **Available as Generic:** No

Brand Name: Arava

Author's Note: Considerable controversy has erupted regarding reports of sudden liver problems (acute hepatotoxicity with liver necrosis). Additional considerations of a very long half-life and possible toxicity as well as other considerations mean that until further data are available regarding incidence, testing strategy and other data are available, the information in this profile has been shortened to make room for more widely used medicines.

LEVODOPA (lee voh DOH pa)

Introduced: 1967   **Class:** Anti-Parkinsonism, dopamine pro-drug   **Prescription:** USA: Yes   **Controlled Drug:** USA: No; Canada: No   **Available as Generic:** USA: Yes; Canada: Yes

Brand Names: ✤Apo-Levocarb, Bendopa, Biodopa, Dopar, Larodopa, ✤Prolopa [CD], Sinemet [CD], Sinemet CR [CD]

BENEFITS versus RISKS	
Possible Benefits	*Possible Risks*
EFFECTIVE SYMPTOM RELIEF IN IDIOPATHIC PARKINSON'S DISEASE	Emotional depression, confusion, abnormal thinking and behavior
Helpful in Parkinsonism after encephalitis	Abnormal involuntary movements
Roughly 6-month benefit in Parkinsonism after manganese poisoning	Heart rhythm disturbance
	Urinary bladder retention
	Induction of peptic ulcer
	Blood abnormalities: hemolytic anemia, reduced white blood cell count

▷ **Principal Uses**

   As a Single Drug Product: Uses currently included in FDA-approved labeling: Treats major types of Parkinson's disease: paralysis agitans ("shaking palsy" of unknown cause), the type that follows encephalitis, Parkinsonism that develops with aging (associated with hardening of the brain arteries) and the Parkinsonism that follows poisoning by carbon monoxide or manganese.

   Other (unlabeled) generally accepted uses: (1) May have a limited role in treating catatonic stupor; (2) can improve conscious level in coma caused by liver failure; (3) can help restless leg or periodic limb movements in sleep; (4) could be helpful in treating severe congestive heart failure.

   As a Combination Drug Product [CD]: This drug is available in combination with carbidopa, a chemical that prevents the breakdown of levodopa before it reaches its site of action. The addition of carbidopa reduces levodopa requirements by 75% and also decreases the frequency and severity of adverse effects. Prolopa form has both levodopa and benserazide (12.5 mg) as a decarboxylase inhibitor to help prevent breakdown of levodopa.

How This Drug Works: Levodopa enters the brain tissue and is converted to dopamine. After sufficient dose, this corrects the dopamine deficiency (thought to be the cause of Parkinsonism) and restores a more normal brain chemistry. Carbidopa blocks an enzyme (decarboxylase) that degrades levodopa before it reaches the brain. This allows a lower dose to have a greater benefit. Products containing carbidopa also have fewer adverse effects.

▷ **Widely Used Guidelines That Involve This Medicine (representative sample):** Please look at the section at the very beginning of this profile called "Class." Next, turn to Table 22 and you will find guidelines listed by the class involved!

Available Dosage Forms and Strengths
Capsules — 100 mg, 250 mg, 500 mg
Sinemet CR, sustained release tablets — 25/100 mg, 50/200 mg
Sinemet tablets — 10/100 mg, 25/100 mg, 25/250 mg
Tablets — 100 mg, 250 mg, 500 mg

▷ **Usual Adult Dosage Ranges:** Initially 250 mg 2 to 4 times daily. Dose may be increased by increments of 100 to 750 mg at 3- to 7-day intervals as needed and tolerated. Total dose should not exceed 8,000 mg daily. If the combination drug Sinemet is used, the total levodopa requirement will be considerably less. For someone who has not taken levodopa before (levodopa-naive and using the sustained release form): one 50/200 mg tablet twice daily, no more frequently than every 6 hours while awake. The dose is then increased as needed and tolerated by either daily or every-other-day dosing of one tablet, to a maximum of 8 tablets daily.
Note: Actual dose and schedule must be determined for each patient individually.

Conditions Requiring Dosing Adjustments
Liver Function: Dosing changes are not indicated in liver compromise.
Kidney Function: Possible urine retention requires that patients with urine outflow problems should be closely watched. No dose decreases are needed in kidney failure.
Intestinal Parasites: A report of large increases in doses needed by patients with Strongyloides stercoralis has been filed. Cure of this intestinal parasite allowed the levodopa dose to be decreased by 33%.

▷ **Dosing Instructions:** Immediate release form may be crushed and is best taken with or following carbohydrate foods to reduce stomach upset. When possible, don't take this drug with high-protein foods. Sustained release tablet (Sinemet CR) may be cut in half, but it should not be crushed or chewed. The last daily dose should be taken before 7 P.M. in order to avoid problems with normal sleeping patterns. "Drug holidays" (periods when no medicine is taken) are controversial, and not all patients benefit from this approach to therapy. If you forget a dose: take the missed dose as soon as you remember it, unless it's nearly time for your next dose—if that is the case, skip the missed dose and take the next dose right on schedule. Talk with your doctor if you find yourself missing doses.

Usual Duration of Use: Use on a regular schedule for 2 to 3 weeks determines effectiveness in relieving the major symptoms of Parkinsonism. Peak benefits may require continual use for 6 months. Long-term use (months to years) requires physician supervision.

Typical Treatment Goals and Measurements (Outcomes and Markers)

Parkinson's disease: The general goal is to minimize symptoms (tremor, slug-gish movements, analysis of walking or gait, etc.) to the fullest extent possible. Additionally, many neurologists use Hahn-Yahr scores and the time it takes to maximum amount of finger tapping as indicators of the benefits of this drug.

Possible Advantages of This Drug

The slow-release formulation of Sinemet CR allows a 25% to 50% reduction in dosing frequency.

The wearing-off phenomenon and end-of-dose failure seen with standard Sinemet may be reduced or eliminated.

▷ **This Drug Should Not Be Taken If**
- you are allergic to any of the brands listed.
- you have narrow-angle glaucoma (inadequately controlled).
- you have a history of melanoma or skin lesions that have not been diagnosed.
- you are taking, or have taken within the past 14 days, any monoamine oxi-dase (MAO) type A inhibitor drug (see Drug Classes).

▷ **Inform Your Physician Before Taking This Drug If**
- you have diabetes, epilepsy, heart disease, high blood pressure, or chronic lung disease.
- you have impaired liver or kidney function.
- you have problems making blood (hematopoiesis).
- you have had a heart attack and have some abnormal heart rhythms.
- you have a history of ongoing (chronic) wide-angle glaucoma.
- you have a history of depression or other mental illness.
- you have a history of peptic ulcer disease or malignant melanoma.
- you will have surgery with general anesthesia.

Possible Side Effects (natural, expected, and unavoidable drug actions)

Fatigue, lethargy.

Altered taste, offensive body odor.

Orthostatic hypotension (see Glossary).

Pink- to red-colored urine, which turns black on exposure to air (of no sig-nificance).

Gout.

▷ **Possible Adverse Effects** (unusual, unexpected, and infrequent reactions)

If any of the following develop, consult your physician promptly for guidance.

Mild Adverse Effects

Allergic reactions: skin rash, itching.

Headache, dizziness, numbness, insomnia, nightmares, blurred or double vision—infrequent.

Nausea and vomiting—frequent.

Dry mouth, difficult swallowing, gas, diarrhea, constipation—infrequent.

Decreased taste sensation—possible.

More rapid rate of nail growth—possible.

Loss of hair or changes in hair color—case reports.

Serious Adverse Effects

Idiosyncratic reactions: hemolytic anemia (see Glossary).

Neuroleptic malignant syndrome (see Glossary), high blood pressure—case reports.

Confusion, hallucinations, paranoia, depression—infrequent to frequent.

Psychotic episodes, seizures—rare.

Congestive heart failure—rare.

Mania or seizures—rare.

Abnormal involuntary movements of the head, face, and extremities—frequent.

Disturbances of heart rhythm—infrequent; low blood pressure—rare.

Development of peptic ulcer, gastrointestinal bleeding—case reports.

Urinary bladder retention—case reports.

Low white blood cell count: increased infection risk, sore throat (transient, but may require you to stop this medicine until the condition clears), low blood platelets, or hemolytic anemia—case reports to rare.

Systemic lupus erythematosus—case reports.

▷ **Possible Effects on Sexual Function:** Increased male or female libido—infrequent.

Inhibited ejaculation, priapism (see Glossary), postmenopausal bleeding—all rare.

▷ **Adverse Effects That May Mimic Natural Diseases or Disorders**

Mental reactions may resemble idiopathic psychosis.

Natural Diseases or Disorders That May Be Activated by This Drug

Latent peptic ulcer, gout.

Possible Effects on Laboratory Tests

Complete blood cell counts: occasionally decreased white cells; occasionally increased eosinophils (without symptoms).

Blood thyroxine (T4) level: increased.

Liver function tests: may be increased.

Urine sugar tests: no effect with Tes-Tape; false negative with Clinistix; false positive with Clinitest.

Urine ketone tests: false positive with Ketostix and Phenistix.

Blood uric acid, growth hormone: increased.

Blood potassium or sodium: may be decreased.

CAUTION

1. It is best to start with small doses, increasing gradually until desired response is achieved.
2. As improvement occurs, avoid excessive and hurried activity (often causes falls and injury).

Precautions for Use

By Infants and Children: This drug can cause precocious puberty in prepubertal boys. Watch for hypersexual behavior and premature growth of genital organs.

By Those Over 60 Years of Age: Therapy should start with half the usual adult dose; dose increases should be made in small increments as needed and tolerated. Watch for significant behavioral changes: depression or inappropriate elation, acute confusion, agitation, paranoia, dementia, nightmares, and hallucinations. Abnormal involuntary movements may also occur.

▷ **Advisability of Use During Pregnancy**

Pregnancy Category: C. See Pregnancy Risk Categories at the back of this book.

Animal Studies: Significant birth defects reported in rodent studies.

Human Studies: Adequate studies of pregnant women are not available.

Avoid use of drug during the first 3 months. Use only if clearly needed during the final 6 months.

Advisability of Use If Breast-Feeding

Presence of this drug in breast milk: Yes, at low levels.

Avoid drug or refrain from nursing.

Habit-Forming Potential: None.

Effects of Overdose: Muscle twitching, spastic closure of eyelids, nausea, vomiting, diarrhea, weakness, fainting, confusion, agitation, hallucinations.

Possible Effects of Long-Term Use: Development of abnormal involuntary movements involving the head, face, mouth, and extremities. May be reversible and gradually subside as the drug is withdrawn.

Suggested Periodic Examinations While Taking This Drug (at physician's discretion)

Complete blood cell counts.

Measurements of internal eye pressure.

Blood pressure measurements in lying, sitting, and standing positions.

▷ **While Taking This Drug, Observe the Following**

Foods: Insofar as possible, do not take concurrently with protein foods; proteins compete for absorption.

Herbal Medicines or Minerals: Calabar bean (chop nut, Fabia, ordeal nut, others) is unsafe when taken by mouth (physostigmine is the active ingredient) and should never be taken by people with Parkinson's disease. Octacosanol (a cousin of vitamin E) can worsen movement problems and should also be avoided.

Nutritional Support: If taken alone (without carbidopa), watch for tingling of the extremities (peripheral neuritis). Small (10 mg or less) doses of pyridoxine (vitamin B_6) may help. Larger doses can decrease the effectiveness of levodopa. If taking Sinemet, supplemental pyridoxine is not required. Rare reports of vitamin C (ascorbic acid) decreasing nausea and other side effects have been made.

Beverages: No restrictions. May be taken with milk.

▷ *Alcohol:* No interactions expected.

Tobacco Smoking: No interactions expected. I advise everyone to quit smoking.

Marijuana Smoking: Increased fatigue and lethargy; possible accentuation of orthostatic hypotension (see Glossary).

▷ *Other Drugs*

Levodopa *taken concurrently* with

- benzodiazepines (see Drug Classes) may blunt the therapeutic benefit of levodopa.
- bromocriptine (Parlodel) may result in decreased blood levels of bromocriptine.
- bupropion (Wellbutrin, Zyban) may increase adverse effects.
- cisapride (Propulsid) may increase adverse effects.
- clonidine (Catapres) can result in decreased therapeutic benefit of levodopa; avoid this combination.
- entacapone (Comtan) may enhance therapeutic effects and be used beneficially.
- fentanyl/droperidol (Innovar) can cause muscular rigidity.
- indinavir (Crixivan) may lead to severe movement problems (dyskinesias).
- isoniazid (INH) may cause flushing, worsening of symptoms, or increased blood pressure. DO NOT COMBINE.
- metoclopramide (Reglan) may increase chance of movement problems (extrapyramidal symptoms). Combination is not recommended.
- monoamine oxidase (MAO) type A inhibitor drugs (see Drug Classes) can cause a dangerous rise in blood pressure and body temperature; do not combine these drugs.

- phenothiazines (see Drug Classes) may blunt therapeutic benefits of levo-dopa. DO NOT COMBINE.
- reserpine (Naquival, others) may blunt the therapeutic benefits of levo-dopa; avoid this combination.
- risperidone (Risperdal) can blunt the therapeutic benefits of levodopa; avoid this combination.
- tolcapone (Tasmar) may lead to vitiligo (skin lesions).
- tricyclic antidepressants (see Drug Classes) may decrease the therapeutic effect of levodopa.
- zotepine (Nipolept) may decrease the therapeutic effect of levodopa.

The following drugs may *decrease* the effects of levodopa:

- amoxapine (Asendin).
- chlordiazepoxide (Librium) or other benzodiazepines (see Drug Classes).
- iron salts.
- olanzapine (Zyprexa) may blunt therapeutic benefits of levodopa, but the clinical degree of this is not known.
- papaverine (Cerespan, Pavabid, Vasospan, etc.).
- phenytoin (Dilantin, etc.) or fosphenytoin (Cerebyx).
- pyridoxine (vitamin B_6).
- risperidone (Risperdal).

▷ *Driving, Hazardous Activities:* May cause dizziness, impaired vision, and ortho-static hypotension. Restrict activities as necessary.

Aviation Note: Parkinson's disease *is a disqualification* for piloting. Consult a designated Aviation Medical Examiner.

Exposure to Sun: No restrictions.

Exposure to Heat: Use caution. This drug can cause flushing and excessive sweating and predispose to heat exhaustion.

Occurrence of Unrelated Illness: Dark-colored skin lesions should be evaluated carefully by your doctor, as they may be malignant melanoma. White blood cell counts should be closely followed if you develop an infection.

LEVOTHYROXINE (lee voh thi ROX een)

Other Names: L-thyroxine, thyroxine, T-4

Introduced: 1953   **Class:**   Thyroid hormones   **Prescription:** USA: Yes   **Controlled Drug:**   USA: No; Canada: No   **Available as Generic:**   USA: Yes; Canada: No

Brand Names: Alti-Thyroxine, Armour Thyroid, ✤Eltroxin, Euthroid [CD], Euthyrox, Levo-T, Levotabs, Levothroid, Levoxine, Levoxyl, L-Thyroxine, ✤Proloid, Synthroid, Synthrox, Syroxine, Thyroid USP, Thyrolar [CD], Unithroid, V-Throid

---

BENEFITS versus RISKS

Possible Benefits	*Possible Risks*
EFFECTIVE REPLACEMENT THERAPY IN STATES OF THYROID HORMONE DEFICIENCY (HYPOTHYROIDISM) EFFECTIVE TREATMENT OF SIMPLE GOITER, CHRONIC THYROIDITIS, AND THYROID GLAND CANCER	Intensification of angina in presence of coronary artery disease Drug-induced hyperthyroidism (with excessive dose) Spasm of the coronary vessels

---

▷ **Principal Uses**

As a Single Drug Product: Uses currently included in FDA-approved labeling: (1) Replacement therapy to correct thyroid deficiency (drug-induced, hypothyroidism, cretinism, myxedema); (2) treatment of simple (nonendemic) goiter and benign thyroid nodules; (3) treatment of Hashimoto's thyroiditis; (4) adjunctive prevention and treatment of thyroid cancer; (5) treats Graves' disease.

Other (unlabeled) generally accepted uses: (1) Helps amenorrhea caused by (secondary to) low thyroid function; (2) may help fetal lung tissue mature in premature babies; (3) could help long-standing (chronic) hives (urticaria); (4) some clinicians use levothyroxine in combination with tri-iodothyronine (10–12.5 mcg of triiodothyronine and lowering the levothyroxine dose by 50 mcg); (5) may have a role in easing carpal tunnel syndrome (CTS) in patients who have underactive thyroid glands; (6) some clinicians use this medicine as a way to intensify treatment for certain psychiatric problems (such as depression).

As a Combination Drug Product [CD]: This thyroid hormone is available in combination with the other principal thyroid hormone, liothyronine, in a preparation (generic name: liotrix) that resembles the natural hormone material produced by the thyroid gland.

How This Drug Works: Alters cellular chemistry, making more energy available and increases metabolism of all tissues. Thyroid hormones are essential to normal growth and development, especially the development of infant brain and nervous systems.

▷ **Widely Used Guidelines That Involve This Medicine (representative sample):** Please look at the section at the very beginning of this profile called "Class." Next, turn to Table 22 and you will find guidelines listed by the class involved!

Available Dosage Forms and Strengths

Injections — 100 mcg/mL, 200 mcg/mL, 500 mcg/mL

Tablets — 0.0125 mg, 0.025 mg, 0.037 mg, 0.05 mg, 0.075 mg, 0.088 mg, 0.1 mg, 0.112 mg, 0.125 mg, 0.15 mg, 0.175 mg, 0.2 mg, 0.3 mg

▷ **Recommended Dosage Ranges** (Actual dose and schedule must be determined for each patient individually.)

Infants and Children: Up to 6 months of age—8 to 10 mcg per kg of body mass, in a single daily dose.

6 to 12 months of age—6 to 8 mcg per kg of body mass, in a single daily dose.

1 to 5 years of age—5 to 6 mcg per kg of body mass, in a single daily dose.

6 to 12 years of age—4 to 5 mcg per kg of body mass, in a single daily dose.

Over 12 years of age—2 to 3 mcg per kg of body mass, in a single daily dose, until the usual adult daily dose is reached (150 to 200 mcg).

12 to 60 Years of Age: In younger patients with heart and blood vessel (cardiovascular) disease or in older patients, dosing is started at 12.5 to 50 mcg once a day. Adjustments to this dose are usually made by 12.5 to 25 micrograms every 3 to 6 weeks as needed and tolerated. Clinicians use TSH becoming normal as a marker. One hundred to 200 mcg per day is the usual ongoing dose range from the maker of Levothroid. For many patients, the dose relates to weight as 1.6 micrograms/kilogram per day. Few people require more than 200 mcg per day. If response is not seen at this level, absorption problems or misunderstanding in taking the medicine (adherence) should be evaluated.

Over 60 Years of Age: Initially 12.5 mcg as a single daily dose; increase gradually at intervals of 3 to 4 weeks, as needed and tolerated. The usual maintenance dose is approximately 75 mcg (0.075 mg) daily.

Author's Note: A University of California Medical Center at San Francisco study found the generic to be as effective as the brand name at savings of 50% of the cost of the brand. One key principle is to keep taking the same generic or brand to avoid fluctuations in blood level.

Conditions Requiring Dosing Adjustments

Liver Function: Dosing changes are not needed.

Kidney Function: Dosing changes are not indicated in kidney compromise.

▷ **Dosing Instructions:** The tablets may be crushed and are best taken in the morning on an empty stomach. Take the medicine at the same time every day. If you forget a dose: take the missed dose as soon as you remember it, unless it's nearly time for your next dose—if that is the case, skip the missed dose and take the next dose right on schedule. Talk with your doctor if you find yourself missing doses.

Usual Duration of Use: Use on a regular schedule for 4 to 6 weeks determines effectiveness in correcting the symptoms of thyroid deficiency. Repeat checks of laboratory tests are required. Long-term use (months to years, possibly for life) requires physician supervision.

Typical Treatment Goals and Measurements (Outcomes and Markers)

Hypothyroidism: The goal is to return the thyroid hormone level to normal or euthyroid. Clinicians check easing of low thyroid signs and symptoms (low energy, weight gain, sluggishness, etc.) as well as checking very specific laboratory tests. Tests often used include the thyroid stimulating hormone (TSH) and T3 and T4 as well as the thyrotropin test. Adjunctive tests include total cholesterol.

Currently a "Drug of Choice"

For treatment of hypothyroidism.

▷ **This Drug Should Not Be Taken If**
- you have had an allergic reaction to it previously.
- you are recovering from a heart attack; ask your doctor for help.
- you have an adrenal insufficiency, angina, high blood pressure, or thyrotoxicosis that has not been corrected.
- you are using it to lose weight and your thyroid function is normal (no deficiency).

▷ **Inform Your Physician Before Taking This Drug If**
- you have high blood pressure, any form of heart disease or diabetes.
- you have a history of Addison's disease or adrenal gland deficiency.

- you are taking any antiasthmatic medications.
- you are taking an anticoagulant.

Possible Side Effects (natural, expected, and unavoidable drug actions)
Aggravation of cardiovascular problems.

▷ **Possible Adverse Effects** (unusual, unexpected, and infrequent reactions)
If any of the following develop, consult your physician promptly for guidance.

Mild Adverse Effects
Allergic reactions: skin rash, hives.
Headache in sensitive people, even with proper dose adjustment—may be frequent.

Serious Adverse Effects
Increased frequency or intensity of angina in people with coronary artery disease—possible.
Spasm of the arteries that supply blood to the heart and heart attack—rare.
Seizures, pseudotumor cerebri, drug-induced porphyria, or myasthenia gravis—case reports to rare.
Decrease in IgA immune concentration—rare.
May be a part of the development of osteoporosis. Bone mineral density testing is recommended.
Note: Other adverse effects are manifestations of excessive dose. See Effects of Overdose on next page.

▷ **Possible Effects on Sexual Function:** Altered menstrual pattern during dose adjustments.
Possibly beneficial in treating impaired sexual function that is associated with true hypothyroidism.

Natural Diseases or Disorders That May Be Activated by This Drug
Latent coronary artery insufficiency (angina), diabetes, osteopenia may progress to osteoporosis.

Possible Effects on Laboratory Tests
Prothrombin time: increased (when taken concurrently with warfarin).
Blood total cholesterol, HDL and LDL cholesterol levels: decreased.
Blood triglyceride levels: no effect.
Blood glucose level: increased.
Blood thyroid hormone levels: increased T3, T4 and free T4.
Blood thyroid-stimulating hormone (TSH) level: decreased.

CAUTION
1. Careful supervision of individual response is needed to identify correct dose. Do not change dosing or drug products without asking your physician.
2. This drug should not be used to treat nonspecific fatigue, obesity, infertility, or slow growth. Such use is inappropriate and could be harmful.
3. If combination levothyroxine and triiodothyronine dosing is used, the levothyroxine dose is lowered by 50 mcg.
4. If a combination levothyroxine and triiodothyronine dosing is used, thyroid extract should be avoided, as it has an elevated amount of T3, which can lead to tremors or palpitations.

Precautions for Use
By Infants and Children: Thyroid-deficient children often require higher doses than adults. Transient hair loss may occur during the early months of treatment. Follow the child's response to thyroid therapy by periodic measurements of bone age, growth and mental and physical development.

By Those Over 60 Years of Age: Usually requirements for thyroid hormone replacement are about 25% lower than in younger adults. Watch closely for any indications of toxicity.

▷ **Advisability of Use During Pregnancy**

Pregnancy Category: A. See Pregnancy Risk Categories at the back of this book.

Animal Studies: Cataract formation reported in rat studies. Other defects reported in rabbit and guinea pig studies.

Human Studies: Thyroid hormones do not reach the fetus (cross the placenta) in significant amounts. Clinical experience has shown that appropriate use of thyroid hormones causes no adverse effects on the fetus.

Use this drug only if clearly needed and with carefully adjusted dose.

Advisability of Use If Breast-Feeding

Presence of this drug in breast milk: Yes, in minimal amounts (roughly 10% of the mother's dose).

Talk to your doctor about the advisability of breast-feeding.

Habit-Forming Potential: None. One case report of abuse of this medicine was made in a bulimic patient. Caution and vigilance for abuse in bulimics is warranted.

Effects of Overdose: Headache, sense of increased body heat, nervousness, increased sweating, hand tremors, insomnia, rapid and irregular heart action, diarrhea, muscle cramping, weight loss, heart attack.

Possible Effects of Long-Term Use: Bone loss (osteoporosis) in the lumbar vertebrae (spine). Worsening of abnormal growth of the left side of the heart.

Suggested Periodic Examinations While Taking This Drug (at physician's discretion)

Measurement of thyroid hormone levels in blood.

Bone mineral density testing.

▷ **While Taking This Drug, Observe the Following**

Foods: Enteral formulas for nutrition support that contain soybeans may increase the fecal elimination of thyroxine.

Herbal Medicines or Minerals: Horseradish root might worsen low thyroid (hypothyroidism) or blunt effectiveness of therapy. Calcium doses (if taken) should be separated from levothyroxine doses by 4 hours. Cabbage and iodine may worsen goiters and exacerbate hypothyroidism. Gamma oryzanol (extracted from rice bran oil) can lower thyroid stimulating hormone (TSH) and change test results. Tiratricol is a naturally occurring metabolite of thyroxine and triiodothyronine. In theory, tiratricol may enhance the adverse action and effects of bungleweed, wild thyme and balm leaf. Soy may decrease the absorption of levothyroxine. Kelp products contain iodine and can change thyroid gland function. Talk to your doctor BEFORE adding any herbal medicines to levothyroxine.

Beverages: No restrictions.

▷ *Alcohol:* No interactions expected.

Tobacco Smoking: No interactions expected. I advise everyone to quit smoking.

Levothyroxine may ***increase*** the effects of

- warfarin (Coumadin) and increase the risk of bleeding; decreased anticoagulant dose is usually needed. More frequent INR testing (prothrombin time or protime) is needed.

Levothyroxine may ***decrease*** the effects of

- digoxin (Lanoxin), when correcting hypothyroidism; a larger dose of digoxin may be needed.

Levothyroxine *taken concurrently* with
- antacids may cause decreased levothyroxine absorption and a decreased therapeutic effect.
- all antidiabetic drugs (insulin and oral hypoglycemic agents) may require an increased dose to obtain proper control of blood sugar levels.
- benzodiazepines (Librium and others) can enhance the toxic or therapeutic effects of both drugs.
- calcium carbonate may cause decreased levothyroxine absorption and a decreased therapeutic effect.
- conjugated estrogens (Premarin) may require an increased levothyroxine dose.
- tricyclic antidepressants (see Drug Classes) may cause an increase in activity of both drugs.

The following drugs may *decrease* the effects of levothyroxine:
- cholestyramine (Cuemid, Questran)—may reduce its absorption; intake of the 2 drugs should be separated by 5 hours.
- colestipol (Colestid).
- iron salts—by decreasing absorption.
- lovastatin (Mevacor).
- phenytoin (Dilantin) or fosphenytoin (Cerebyx)—can increase levothyroxine removal (clearance).
- rifampin (Rifater, others).
- ritonavir (Norvir).
- sodium polystyrene sulfonate (Kayexalate).
- sucralfate (Carafate).

▷ *Driving, Hazardous Activities:* No restrictions.

Aviation Note: The use of this drug is *probably not a disqualification* for piloting. Consult a designated Aviation Medical Examiner.

Exposure to Sun: No restrictions.

Exposure to Heat: This drug may decrease individual tolerance to warm environments, increasing discomfort due to heat. Consult your physician if you develop symptoms of overdose during the warm months of the year.

Heavy Exercise or Exertion: Use caution if you have angina (coronary artery disease). This drug may increase the frequency or severity of angina during physical activity.

Discontinuation: Must be taken continually on a regular schedule to correct thyroid deficiency. Never stop it without talking to your doctor.

LIDOCAINE (LYE doh kane)

Other Names: None

Introduced: Patch form 1999   **Class:**   Analgesic, antiarrhythmic
Prescription: USA: Yes   **Controlled Drug:**   USA: No; Canada: No
Available as Generic: USA: No; Canada: No
Brand Names: Lidoderm

BENEFITS versus RISKS

Possible Benefits	*Possible Risks*
EFFECTIVE TREATMENT/ PREVENTION OF THE PAIN WHICH HAPPENS AFTER SHINGLES (POSTHERPETIC NEURALGIA)	Interactions are possible—drug is used with caution in people who are taking other Class I (such as mexiletine or tocainide) antiarrhythmic drugs
WHEN USED AS DIRECTED, ROUGHLY 2% OF THE APPLIED DOSE REACHES THE BODY CIRCULATION	Skin irritation where the patch is applied
	Possible allergic reaction (rare)

▷ **Principal Uses**

As a Single Drug Product: Uses currently included in FDA-approved labeling:
(1) Pain relief for pain associated with postherpetic neuralgia.
Other (unlabeled) generally accepted uses: None at present.

Author's Note: This brief profile focused on the only specifically FDA-approved treatment for pain after shingles (postherpetic neuralgia)—not the antiarrhythmic use. This profile will be broadened in future editions if warranted.

LIOTHYRONINE (li oh THI roh neen)

Other Names: Triiodothyronine, T-3

Introduced: 1956   **Class:**   Thyroid hormone   **Prescription:**
USA: Yes   **Controlled Drug:**   USA: No; Canada: No   **Available as Generic:**   USA: Yes; Canada: No

Brand Names: Cytomel, Euthroid [CD], ✚Proloid, Thyroid USP, ✚Thyrolar [CD], Thyrolar 1/4, 1/2, 1, 2 and 3 [CD], Triostat

---

BENEFITS versus RISKS

Possible Benefits	*Possible Risks*
EFFECTIVE REPLACEMENT THERAPY IN STATES OF THYROID HORMONE DEFICIENCY (HYPOTHYROIDISM)	Intensification of angina in presence of coronary artery disease
	Drug-induced hyperthyroidism (with excessive dosing)
EFFECTIVE TREATMENT OF SIMPLE GOITER, CHRONIC THYROIDITIS, AND THYROIDGLAND CANCER	Rapid heartbeat
	Heart attack

▷ **Principal Uses**

As a Single Drug Product: Uses currently included in FDA-approved labeling:
(1) Replacement therapy to correct thyroid deficiency (hypothyroidism);
(2) treatment of simple (nonendemic) goiter and benign thyroid nodules;
(3) treatment of Hashimoto's thyroiditis; (4) adjunctive prevention and treatment of thyroid cancer; (5) therapy of cretinism; (6) used to help diagnose different kinds of thyroid problems; (7) treats low thyroid that comes from medicines.

Other (unlabeled) generally accepted uses: (1) Can help infertility caused by low thyroid function; (2) thyroid replacement of choice for thyroid cancer; (3) may have a role in some kinds of heart problems (cardiomyopathy); (4) may have a role in some cases of resistant (refractory) depression; (5) could be helpful in supplementing Selective Serotonin Reuptake Inhibitor–treatment of posttraumatic stress disorder (PTSD).

As a Combination Drug Product [CD]: This thyroid hormone is available in combination with the other principal thyroid hormone, levothyroxine, in a preparation (generic name: liotrix) that resembles the natural hormone material produced by the thyroid gland.

How This Drug Works: Alters cellular chemistry, making more energy available. Increases cellular metabolism in all tissues. Thyroid hormones are essential to normal growth and development, especially the development of the infant's brain and nervous system.

▷ **Widely Used Guidelines That Involve This Medicine (representative sample):** Please look at the section at the very beginning of this profile called "Class." Next, turn to Table 22 and you will find guidelines listed by the class involved!

Available Dosage Forms and Strengths
Injection — 10 mcg/mL
Tablets — 5 mcg, 25 mcg, 50 mcg

▷ **Recommended Dosage Ranges** (Actual dose and schedule must be determined for each patient individually.)

Infants and Children: Infants several months old may need 20 mcg a day. When they reach 1 year, 50 mcg a day may be needed. Children over 3 years old may need the full adult dose.

12 to 60 Years of Age: For mild hypothyroidism—initially 25 mcg daily; increase by 12.5 to 25 mcg every 1 to 2 weeks as needed and tolerated. The usual maintenance dose is 25 to 75 mcg daily.

For severe hypothyroidism—initially 2.5 to 5 mcg daily; increase by 5 to 10 mcg at intervals of 1 to 2 weeks. When a dose of 25 mcg is reached, increase by 12.5 to 25 mcg at intervals of 1 to 2 weeks, as needed and tolerated. The usual maintenance dose is 50 to 100 mcg daily.

For simple goiter—initially 5 mcg daily; increase by 5 to 10 mcg at intervals of 1 to 2 weeks. When a dose of 25 mcg is reached, increase by 12.5 to 25 mcg at intervals of 1 week, as needed and tolerated. The usual maintenance dose is 50 to 100 mcg daily.

Over 60 Years of Age: Initially 5 mcg as a single daily dose; increase by 5 mcg at intervals of 1 to 2 weeks, as needed and tolerated. The usual maintenance dose is 12.5 to 37.5 mcg daily.

Conditions Requiring Dosing Adjustments
Liver Function: Dosing changes are not indicated for patients with liver compromise.
Kidney Function: Dosing changes are not indicated in renal compromise. Caution should be used when increasing the dose of this medicine for those with kidney problems.

▷ **Dosing Instructions:** The tablets may be crushed and are preferably taken in the morning on an empty stomach to ensure maximal absorption and uniform results. If you forget a dose: take the missed dose as soon as you remember it, unless it's nearly time for your next dose—if that is the case, skip the missed dose and take the next dose right on schedule. Talk with your doctor if you find yourself missing doses.

Usual Duration of Use: Use on a regular schedule for 2 to 4 days determines effectiveness in correcting the symptoms of thyroid deficiency. Long-term use (months to years, possibly for life) requires physician supervision and checks of thyroid status.

Typical Treatment Goals and Measurements (Outcomes and Markers)
Hypothyroidism: The goal is to return the thyroid hormone level to normal or euthyroid. Clinicians check easing of low thyroid signs and symptoms (low energy, weight gain, sluggishness, etc.) as well as checking very specific laboratory tests. Tests often used include the thyroid stimulating hormone (TSH) and T3 and T4 as well as the thyrotropin test. Adjunctive tests include total cholesterol.

▷ **This Drug Should Not Be Taken If**
- you have had an allergic reaction to it previously.
- you are recovering from a heart attack; ask your doctor for guidance.
- you have an uncorrected adrenal cortical deficiency.
- you are using it to lose weight and your thyroid function is normal.

▷ **Inform Your Physician Before Taking This Drug If**
- you have high blood pressure, any form of heart disease or diabetes.
- you have a history of Addison's disease, adrenal gland deficiency, or thyrotoxicosis.
- you are taking any antiasthmatic medications.
- you take digoxin.
- you are taking an anticoagulant.

Possible Side Effects (natural, expected, and unavoidable drug actions)
Fast heartbeat (tachycardia).

▷ **Possible Adverse Effects** (unusual, unexpected, and infrequent reactions)
If any of the following develop, consult your physician promptly for guidance.
Mild Adverse Effects
Allergic reactions: skin rash, hives.
Headache in sensitive patients, even with proper dose adjustment—may be frequent.
Rapid heart rate (tachycardia)—infrequent.
Hair loss—case reports.
Serious Adverse Effects
Allergic reactions: erythema, bullae, and papules.
Increased frequency or intensity of angina or abnormal heartbeat—possible to infrequent.
Lowering of blood pressure—rare.
Heart attack—rare.
Osteoporosis—possible increased risk (bone mineral density testing is recommended).
Hyperthyroidism—possible with improper dosing.
Drug fever or drug-induced myasthenia gravis—case reports.
Author's Note: Other adverse effects are manifestations of excessive dose. See Effects of Overdose below.

▷ **Possible Effects on Sexual Function:** Altered menstrual pattern during dose adjustments.
Possibly beneficial in treating impaired sexual function that is associated with true hypothyroidism.

Natural Diseases or Disorders That May Be Activated by This Drug
Latent coronary artery insufficiency (angina), diabetes.

Possible Effects on Laboratory Tests
Prothrombin time: increased (when taken concurrently with warfarin).
Blood total cholesterol, HDL and LDL cholesterol levels: decreased.
Blood triglyceride levels: no effect.
Blood glucose level: increased.
Blood thyroid hormone levels: increased T3.
Blood thyroid stimulating hormone (TSH) level: decreased.

CAUTION
1. Careful supervision of individual response is needed to identify correct dose. Do not change dosing schedule without asking your doctor.
2. This drug should not be used to treat nonspecific fatigue, obesity, infertility, or slow growth. Such use is inappropriate and could be harmful.

Precautions for Use
By Infants and Children: Not recommended for treatment of this age group. It must reach the brain and nervous system, and this drug may not do that. Levothyroxine is the drug of choice to treat thyroid deficiency in infants and children.
By Those Over 60 Years of Age: Needs for thyroid hormone are usually about 25% lower than in younger adults. Watch closely for any toxicity.

▷ **Advisability of Use During Pregnancy**
Pregnancy Category: A. See Pregnancy Risk Categories at the back of this book.
Animal Studies: No information available.
Human Studies: Thyroid hormones do not reach the fetus (cross the placenta) in significant amounts. Clinical experience has shown that appropriate use of thyroid hormones causes no adverse effects on the fetus.
Use this drug only if clearly needed and with carefully adjusted dose.

Advisability of Use If Breast-Feeding
Presence of this drug in breast milk: Yes, in minimal amounts.
Talk to your doctor as this decision must be cautiously made (benefit-to-risk).

Habit-Forming Potential: None.

Effects of Overdose: Headache, sense of increased body heat, nervousness, increased sweating, hand tremors, insomnia, rapid and irregular heart action, diarrhea, muscle cramping, weight loss, heart attack.

Possible Effects of Long-Term Use: Bone loss (osteoporosis) in the lumbar vertebrae (spine). Bone mineral density testing is recommended.

Suggested Periodic Examinations While Taking This Drug (at physician's discretion)
Measurement of thyroid hormone levels in blood.
Bone mineral density testing.

▷ **While Taking This Drug, Observe the Following**
Foods: No restrictions.
Herbal Medicines or Minerals: Horseradish root might worsen low thyroid (hypothyroidism) or blunt effectiveness of therapy. Calcium doses (if taken) should be separated from levothyroxine doses by 4 hours. Cabbage and iodine may worsen goiters and exacerbate hypothyroidism. Gamma oryzanol (extracted from rice bran oil) can lower thyroid stimulating hormone (TSH) and change test results. Tiratricol is a naturally occurring metabolite of thyroxine and triiodothyronine. In theory, tiratricol may

enhance the adverse action and effects of bungleweed, wild thyme, and balm leaf. Soy may decrease the absorption of levothyroxine. Kelp products contain iodine and can change thyroid gland function. Talk to your doctor BEFORE adding any herbal medicines to liothyronine.

Beverages: No restrictions.

▷ *Alcohol:* No interactions expected.

Tobacco Smoking: No interactions expected. I advise everyone to quit smoking.

▷ *Other Drugs*

Liothyronine may *increase* the effects of

- warfarin (Coumadin) and increase the risk of bleeding; more frequent INR (prothrombin time or protime) tests are needed (in general, anticoagulant effect is increased in hyperthyroidism and decreased in hypothyroidism).

Liothyronine may *decrease* the effects of

- digoxin (Lanoxin) when correcting hypothyroidism; a larger dose of digoxin may be needed.

Liothyronine *taken concurrently* with

- all antidiabetic drugs (insulin and oral hypoglycemic agents) may require an increased dose to obtain proper control of blood sugar because liothyronine increases insulin.
- estrogens (including birth control pills and Premarin) may require increased doses of liothyronine.
- monoamine oxidase (MAO) inhibitors (see Drug Classes) may increase the therapeutic benefits of the antidepressant.
- tricyclic antidepressants (see Drug Classes) may cause an increase in the activity of both drugs; watch for signs of toxicity.

The following drugs may *decrease* the effects of liothyronine:

- carbamazepine (Tegretol, others) may decrease free serums T4 and T3.
- cholestyramine (Cuemid, Questran), and perhaps other cholesterol-lowering resins, may reduce its absorption; intake of the two drugs should be separated by 5 hours.

▷ *Driving, Hazardous Activities:* No restrictions.

Aviation Note: The use of this drug is *probably not a disqualification* for piloting. Consult a designated Aviation Medical Examiner.

Exposure to Sun: No restrictions.

Exposure to Heat: This drug may decrease individual tolerance to warm environments, increasing discomfort due to heat. Consult your physician if you develop symptoms of overdose during the warm months of the year.

Heavy Exercise or Exertion: Use caution if you have angina (coronary artery disease). This drug may increase the frequency or severity of angina during physical activity.

Discontinuation: This drug must be taken continually on a regular schedule to correct thyroid deficiency. Do not stop it without consulting your physician.

LISINOPRIL (li SIN oh pril)

Introduced: 1988   **Class:**   Antihypertensive, ACE inhibitor
Please see the angiotensin converting enzyme (ACE) inhibitor family profile.

LITHIUM (LITH i um)

Introduced: 1949 **Class:** Antidepressant, mood stabilizer **Prescription:** USA: Yes **Controlled Drug:** USA: No; Canada: No **Available as Generic:** USA: Yes; Canada: No

Brand Names: ❦Carbolith, Cibalith-S, ❦Duralith, Eskalith, Eskalith CR, Liskonium, Lithane, ❦Lithizine, Lithobid, Lithonate, Lithotabs

BENEFITS versus RISKS	
Possible Benefits	*Possible Risks*
RAPID REVERSAL OF ACUTE MANIA	VERY NARROW MARGIN OF TREATMENT
STABILIZATION OF MOOD	POTENTIALLY FATAL TOXICITY WITH INADEQUATE MONITORING
Prevention of recurrent depression in "responders"	Infrequent induction of diabetes mellitus, hypothyroidism
	Diabetes insipidus–like syndrome (excessive dilute urine)

▷ **Principal Uses**

As a Single Drug Product: Uses currently included in FDA-approved labeling: (1) Manages bipolar disorder (promptly corrects acute mania and also reduces frequency and severity of recurrent manic-depressive mood swings); (2) used to treat mania; (3) helps control mania.

Other (unlabeled) generally accepted uses: (1) May be helpful in chronic hair-pulling (trichotillomania); (2) can help prevent cluster headaches; (3) may help control aggressive behavior; (4) can have a role in treating Fanconi's aplastic anemia; (5) may be of use in patients who have mood problems that also affect their sex drive.

In the Pipeline: The Health and Human Services secretary has identified a group of medicines to be tested for use in children. Lithium was on that list of the 12 highest-priority medicines to be studied in children. A finding published in the *Journal of Molecular Psychiatry* reported a flawed gene (GRK3) as being related to development of bipolar disorder. This may serve as a new target for treatment of the *cause* of bipolar disorder.

How This Drug Works: Lithium changes the way nerve signals are transmitted and interpreted, influencing emotional status and behavior.

▷ **Widely Used Guidelines That Involve This Medicine (representative sample):** Please look at the section at the very beginning of this profile called "Class." Next, turn to Table 22 and you will find guidelines listed by the class involved!

Available Dosage Forms and Strengths
Capsules — 150 mg, 300 mg, 600 mg
Syrup — 8 mEq/5 mL
Tablets — 300 mg
Tablets, prolonged action — 300 mg, 450 mg

▷ **Usual Adult Dosage Ranges:** Mania: 1,800 mg per day, divided into 3 equal doses. Dosing is individualized to get the desired clinical response and a general blood level of 1–1.5 mmol/L.

Usual maintenance dose: When manic symptoms ease, the dose is lowered to obtain blood levels of 0.6 to 1.2 millimole per liter. Typical ongoing doses are 900 to 1,200 mg a day. This total daily dose is divided into equal doses that are given (immediate release forms) 3 or 4 times daily, and sustained release forms are given less often—only TWICE daily.

Note: Actual dose and dosing schedule must be determined for each patient individually.

Conditions Requiring Dosing Adjustments

Liver Function: The liver is minimally involved in the elimination of lithium.

Kidney Function: Frequent and careful side effect monitoring, decreased doses, and more frequent blood levels are prudent. In moderate to severe kidney failure (creatinine clearance of 10–50 mL/min), 50–75% of the usual dose is taken. In severe kidney failure, 25–50% of the usual dose is taken.

▷ **Dosing Instructions:** The capsules may be opened, and regular tablets crushed, and taken with or after meals to reduce stomach upset. The prolonged-action tablets *should be swallowed whole and not altered*. Always use a measuring cup or measuring spoon for the liquid form. If you forget a dose: take the missed dose as soon as you remember it, unless it's nearly time for your next dose—if that is the case, skip the missed dose and take the next dose right on schedule. Talk with your doctor if you find yourself missing doses.

Usual Duration of Use: Use on a regular schedule for 1 to 3 weeks determines effectiveness in correcting acute mania; several months of continual treatment may be required to correct swings in mood. Long-term use (months to years) requires physician supervision and periodic evaluation of blood levels.

Typical Treatment Goals and Measurements (Outcomes and Markers)

Bipolar disorder: Helps even out the highs and lows often seen in bipolar problems. The general goal is to create a situation where excessive highs or lows no longer feel "normal" and patients are able to return to their appropriate quality of life. Blood levels are kept in a tight range (0.6 to 1.5 mmol/L). Levels are usually checked every 2 months. Thyroid function tests are checked every 3 to 6 months.

Currently a "Drug of Choice"

For the treatment of acute mania in bipolar manic-depressive disorders.

Author's Note: The American Psychiatric Association updated their 1994 treatment guidelines for bipolar disorder (see *AMJP* in References). Lithium and valproate are recommended first (first line treatment) for most people.

▷ **This Drug Should Not Be Taken If**
- you had an allergic reaction to it previously.
- you have uncontrolled diabetes or uncorrected hypothyroidism.
- you are breast-feeding your infant.
- you will be unable to comply with the need for regular monitoring of lithium blood levels.
- you have severe kidney failure or heart disease.

▷ **Inform Your Physician Before Taking This Drug If**
- you have a history of a schizophreniclike thought disorder.
- you have any type of organic brain disease or a history of grand mal epilepsy.
- you have diabetes, heart disease, hypothyroidism, or impaired kidney function.
- you are on a salt-restricted diet.

- you are pregnant or planning pregnancy.
- you are taking any diuretic drug or a cortisonelike steroid preparation.
- your blood sodium level is low.
- you will have surgery with general anesthesia or electroconvulsive (ECT) therapy.

Possible Side Effects (natural, expected, and unavoidable drug actions)

Increased thirst and urine volume in 60% of initial users and in 20% of long-term users.

Weight gain in first few months of use.

Drowsiness and lethargy in sensitive individuals.

Metallic taste.

Increased white blood cells—not a sign of infection, but an effect of lithium.

Heart block—frequent but does not usually lead to the medicine being stopped.

Tremor (fine)—frequent (may respond to a beta blocker).

▷ **Possible Adverse Effects** (unusual, unexpected, and infrequent reactions)

If any of the following develop, consult your physician promptly for guidance.

Mild Adverse Effects

Allergic reactions: skin rashes, generalized itching.

Skin dryness, loss of hair—case reports.

Headache, joint pain, dizziness, weakness, blurred vision, ringing in ears, unsteadiness—infrequent.

Sleepwalking or restless leg syndrome—case reports.

Nausea, vomiting, diarrhea—frequent.

Metallic taste—possible.

Edema—possible.

Serious Adverse Effects

"Blackout" spells, confusion, stupor, slurred speech, spasmodic movements of extremities, epilepticlike seizures—case reports to rare.

Abnormal fixed eye position (oculogyric crisis)—case reports.

Abnormal changes in heart rate, rhythm, and wave forms—frequent.

Loss of bladder or rectal control—infrequent.

Diabetes insipidus-like syndrome: excessive dilute urine—infrequent to frequent.

Abnormal movements (may be a sign of toxicity)—rare.

Cerebellar atrophy or neuroleptic malignant syndrome—case reports.

Inflammation of the heart muscle (myocarditis)—case reports.

Pseudotumor cerebri, myasthenia gravis, or systemic lupus erythematosus—case reports.

Increased platelet counts—possible.

Low thyroid function or abnormally high thyroid function—possible to case reports.

Elevated blood calcium or blood sugar—rare.

Porphyria or inflammation of the parotid gland—case reports.

Seizures—case reports and certainly with toxicity.

Drug-induced low or high potassium—possible.

▷ **Possible Effects on Sexual Function:**

Decreased libido (blood level of 0.7 to 0.9 mEq/L in one study)—case reports.

Inhibited erection (0.5 to 0.9 mEq/L in one study)—frequent.

Male infertility.

Female breast swelling with milk production—case reports.

▷ **Adverse Effects That May Mimic Natural Diseases or Disorders**
> Painful discoloration and coldness of the hands and feet may resemble Raynaud's phenomenon.

Natural Diseases or Disorders That May Be Activated by This Drug
> Diabetes mellitus may be worsened. Psoriasis may be intensified. Myasthenia gravis may be induced (one case).

Possible Effects on Laboratory Tests
> White blood cell and platelet counts: increased.
> Blood alkaline phosphatase (bone isoenzyme): markedly increased in up to 66% of users.
> Blood cholesterol level: increased.
> Blood parathyroid hormone level: increased.
> Blood thyroid stimulating hormone (TSH) level: increased.
> Blood thyroid hormone (T3 and T4) levels: decreased.
> Blood uric acid level: decreased.
> Blood bromide, calcium or glucose levels: increased.
> Blood potassium level: increased or decreased.

CAUTION
1. The blood level required for this drug to work is close to the level that can cause toxic effects. Periodic blood lithium levels are mandatory. Follow instructions about drug dose and periodic blood tests.
2. Lithium should be stopped at the first signs of toxicity: drowsiness, sluggishness, unsteadiness, tremor, muscle twitching, vomiting, or diarrhea.
3. Some major causes of lithium toxicity are:
   - accidental overdose (may be due to inadequate blood level checks).
   - impaired kidney function.
   - salt restriction.
   - inadequate fluid intake, dehydration.
   - concurrent use of diuretics.
   - intercurrent illness.
   - childbirth (rapid decrease in kidney clearance of lithium).
   - initiation of treatment with a new drug.
   - over-the-counter preparations that contain iodides (some cough products and vitamin-mineral supplements) should be avoided because of the added antithyroid effect when taken with lithium.
   - low blood sodium can lead to toxic lithium effects with a "normal" lithium level.

Precautions for Use
> *By Infants and Children:* Safety and effectiveness for those under 12 years of age are not established. Follow your physician's instructions exactly.
> *By Those Over 60 Years of Age:* Treatment should start with a "test" dose of 75 to 150 mg daily. Observe closely for early indications of toxic effects, especially if on a low-salt diet and using diuretics. Increased risk of Parkinsonian reactions (abnormal gait and movements); coma can develop without warning symptoms.

▷ **Advisability of Use During Pregnancy**
> *Pregnancy Category:* D. See Pregnancy Risk Categories at the back of this book.
> *Animal Studies:* Cleft palate reported in mice; eye, ear, and palate defects reported in rats.
> *Human Studies:* Adequate studies of pregnant women are not available, but cardiovascular defects and goiter in newborn infants (of mothers using lithium) have been reported. If the infant's blood level of lithium

approaches the toxic range before delivery, the newborn may suffer the "floppy infant" syndrome: weakness, lethargy, unresponsiveness, low body temperature, weak cry, and poor feeding ability.

Avoid use of drug during the first 3 months. Use only if clearly necessary during the final 6 months. Monitor mother's blood lithium levels carefully to avoid possible toxicity.

Advisability of Use If Breast-Feeding
Presence of this drug in breast milk: Yes, in significant amounts.
Avoid drug or refrain from nursing.

Habit-Forming Potential: None.

Effects of Overdose: Drowsiness, weakness, lack of coordination, nausea, vomiting, diarrhea, muscle spasms, blurred vision, dizziness, staggering gait, slurred speech, confusion, stupor, coma, cerebellar atrophy, seizures.

Possible Effects of Long-Term Use: Hypothyroidism (5%), goiter, reduced sugar tolerance, diabetes insipidus–like syndrome, serious kidney damage.

Suggested Periodic Examinations While Taking This Drug (at physician's discretion)
Regular determinations of blood lithium levels are absolutely essential. Time to sample blood for lithium level: 12 hours after evening dose or in the morning, just before next dose. Therapeutic range: 0.8 to 1.5 mEq/L (acute) and 0.6 to 1.2 (maintenance). Levels should be checked every 2 months.
Periodic evaluation of thyroid gland size and function.
Complete blood cell counts.
Kidney function tests.

▷ **While Taking This Drug, Observe the Following**
Foods: Maintain a normal diet; do not restrict your use of salt.
Herbal Medicines or Minerals: This drug may cause increased calcium and bromide. Talk to your doctor BEFORE taking any calcium supplements or bromine. Herbs that have a diuretic or potassium-losing effect may lead to lithium toxicity. Many herbal products are actually combination products: read labels carefully to look for guarana and mate as they contain caffeine which may lower lithium levels.
Beverages: Excessive caffeine may lower lithium levels. It is prudent to drink at least 8 to 12 glasses of water or other liquids daily. This drug may be taken with milk.
▷ *Alcohol:* Use with caution. May have an increased intoxicating effect. Avoid alcohol completely if any symptoms of lithium toxicity develop.
Tobacco Smoking: Lithium may increase sensitivity to nicotine. I advise everyone to quit smoking.
Marijuana Smoking: Possible increase in apathy, lethargy, drowsiness, or sluggishness; accentuation of lithium-induced tremor; possible increased risk of precipitating psychotic behavior.
▷ *Other Drugs*
Lithium may *increase* the effects of
• tricyclic antidepressants and selective serotonin reuptake inhibitors (see Drug Classes) and may also increase lithium levels.
Lithium *taken concurrently* with
• ACE inhibitors (see Drug Classes) such as captopril (Capoten) may increase lithium levels by as much as 3 times the level prior to combination therapy.
• calcium channel blockers (see Drug Classes), such as diltiazem, may cause neurotoxicity or mania.

- carbamazepine (Tegretol) may result in neurotoxicity.
- chlorpromazine (Thorazine, etc.) and other phenothiazines (see Drug Classes) may decrease lithium or phenothiazine therapeutic effects.
- cisplatin may cause changes in lithium levels; level checks are prudent.
- citalopram (Celexa) may enhance the effect of citalopram on serotonin.
- clozapine (Clozaril) may result in serious agranulocytosis, delirium, and neuroleptic malignant syndrome; do not combine these medicines.
- diazepam (Valium) may cause hypothermia.
- diuretics (see Diuretic Drug Classes) may lead to lithium toxicity.
- filgrastim (Neupogen) may result in a greater-than-expected increase in white blood cell numbers.
- fludrocortisone (Florinef) may result in loss of the mineralocorticoid benefits of fludrocortisone.
- fluoxetine (Prozac) may result in neurotoxicity.
- fluvoxamine (Luvox) may result in increased lithium levels and toxicity.
- haloperidol (Haldol) or with other neuroleptics may result in decreased beneficial effects from both medicines.
- levofloxacin (Levaquin) may lead to kidney impairment and increased lithium levels and toxicity.
- methyldopa (Aldomet, etc.) is usually well tolerated; however, it may cause a severe neurotoxic reaction in susceptible individuals. These combinations should be used very cautiously.
- metronidazole (Flagyl) may lead to lithium toxicity.
- monoamine oxidase (MAO) inhibitors (see Drug Classes) may result in serotonin syndrome and potential fatality.
- nicotine (various brands) may cause supersensitivity to nicotine.
- sibutramine (Meridia) may cause an increased risk of serotonin syndrome. DO NOT COMBINE.
- valsartan (Diovan) may cause lithium toxicity. Careful follow-up of lithium levels and patient condition are very important.
- verapamil (Calan, Isoptin) may cause unpredictable effects; both lithium toxicity and decreased lithium blood levels have been reported.

The following drugs may *increase* the effects of lithium:
- aspirin (various).
- bumetanide (Bumex).
- celecoxib (Celebrex), rofecoxib (Vioxx) or valdecoxib (Bextra).
- ethacrynic acid (Edecrin).
- fluoxetine (Prozac).
- furosemide (Lasix, etc.).
- ibuprofen (Motrin, others), indomethacin (Indocin) and other nonsteroidal anti-inflammatory drugs (NSAIDs).
- losartan (Cozaar, Hyzaar) and perhaps other angiotensin II inhibitors.
- piroxicam (Feldene) or any nonsteroidal anti-inflammatory drug (NSAID—see Drug Classes).
- thiazide diuretics (see Drug Classes).

The following drugs may *decrease* the effects of lithium:
- acetazolamide (Diamox, etc.).
- calcitonin (various).
- sodium bicarbonate.
- theophylline (Theo-Dur, etc.) and related drugs.

▷ *Driving, Hazardous Activities:* This drug may impair mental alertness, judgment, physical coordination and reaction time. Restrict activities as necessary.

Aviation Note: The use of this drug *is a disqualification* for piloting. Consult a designated Aviation Medical Examiner.

Exposure to Sun: No restrictions.

Exposure to Heat: Excessive sweating can cause significant depletion of salt and water and resultant lithium toxicity. Avoid sauna baths.

Occurrence of Unrelated Illness: Fever, sweating, vomiting or diarrhea can result in significant alterations of blood and tissue lithium concentrations. Close monitoring of your physical condition and blood lithium levels is needed to prevent serious toxicity.

Discontinuation: Sudden discontinuation does not cause withdrawal symptoms. Avoid premature discontinuation; some individuals may require continual treatment for up to a year to achieve maximal response. Discontinuation by "responders" may result in recurrence of either mania or depression. Lithium should be discontinued if symptoms of brain toxicity appear or if an uncorrectable diabetes insipidus–like syndrome develops.

LOMEFLOXACIN (loh me FLOX a sin)

Please see the fluoroquinolone antibiotic family profile.

LOPERAMIDE (loh PER a mide)

Introduced: 1977 **Class:** Antidiarrheal **Prescription:** USA: Yes **Controlled Drug:** USA: No; Canada: No **Available as Generic:** Yes

Brand Names: Anti-Diarrheal, Apo-loperamide, Diarrid, ✢Dom-Loperamide, Imodium, Imodium AD, ✢Imodium Advanced, Kaopectate 1-D, Maalox A/D, Pepto Diarrhea Control

BENEFITS versus RISKS	
Possible Benefits	*Possible Risks*
EFFECTIVE RELIEF OF INTESTINAL CRAMPING AND DIARRHEA	Drowsiness Constipation May cause serious colon problems (toxic megacolon)

▷ **Principal Uses**

As a Single Drug Product: Uses currently included in FDA-approved labeling: (1) Control of cramping and diarrhea associated with acute gastroenteritis and chronic enteritis and colitis and chronic diarrhea; (2) used to reduce the volume of discharge from ileostomies; (3) irritable bowel syndrome that has failed to respond to dietary supplements; (4) traveler's diarrhea.

Other (unlabeled) generally accepted uses: (1) decreases unformed stools in Shigella diarrhea.

As a Combination Drug Product [CD]: Loperamide is available in Canada combined with simethicone. Simethicone works to decrease gas.

How This Drug Works: Acts directly on the nerve supply of the gastrointestinal tract, decreases secretions and relieves cramping and diarrhea. When combined with simethicone, simethicone acts to stop gas.

▷ **Widely Used Guidelines That Involve This Medicine (representative sample):** Please look at the section at the very beginning of this profile called "Class." Next, turn to Table 22 and you will find guidelines listed by the class involved!

Available Dosage Forms and Strengths
Capsules — 2 mg
Liquid (4.07% alcohol) — 0.2 mg/5 mL
Liquid (5.25% alcohol) — 1 mg/5 mL
Tablets, combination — 2 mg simethicone, 125 mg of simethicone
Tablets — 2 mg

▷ **Recommended Dosage Ranges:** *For acute diarrhea:* 4 mg initially (2 capsules) and then 2 mg after each unformed stool until diarrhea is controlled. Stop the medicine and call your doctor if the diarrhea does not decrease in 48 hours (medicine should be stopped if this happens).
For chronic diarrhea: 4 mg immediately, then 2 mg taken after each unformed stool until the diarrhea is successfully controlled. The dosing should then be individualized. Maximum daily dose is 16 mg. If your diarrhea is not controlled after 10 days of the maximum dose of 16 mg, call your doctor.
Pediatric dosing: NOT recommended for children under 2 years old. Two- to 5-year-olds can be given 1 mg 3 times a day on the first day (13–30 kg); 6- to 8-year-olds can have 2 mg twice daily on the first day (20–30 kg); 8- to 12-year-olds can have 2 mg 3 times daily (greater than 30 kg). Follow-up doses on the next day are 1 mg per 10 kg of body mass, up to the maximum daily doses on day 1. If diarrhea persists, call your doctor.
Note: Actual dose and schedule must be determined for each patient individually.

Conditions Requiring Dosing Adjustments
Liver Function: Dosing adjustments for patients with liver compromise are not needed. Half of a given dose is removed unchanged in the feces.
Kidney Function: Changes in dosing are not indicated in kidney compromise.

▷ **Dosing Instructions:** The capsule may be opened and taken on an empty stomach or with food if stomach upset occurs. Liquid form should be taken using a medicine spoon or calibrated medicine dosing cup. If you forget a dose: Take the missed dose as soon as you remember it, unless it's nearly time for your next dose—if that is the case, skip the missed dose and take the next dose right on schedule. Talk with your doctor if you find yourself missing doses.

Usual Duration of Use: Use on a regular schedule for 48 hours determines effectiveness in controlling acute diarrhea; continual use for 10 days may be needed to evaluate its effectiveness in controlling chronic diarrhea. If diarrhea persists, call your doctor.

Typical Treatment Goals and Measurements (Outcomes and Markers)
Diarrhea: The goal is to at least decrease the frequency of stools and ideally to return "normal" bowel patterns and stool consistency. In patients with ostomies, the amount of drainage should decrease.

▷ **This Drug Should Not Be Taken If**
- you have had an allergic reaction to it previously.
- constipation is never acceptable for you.
- it is prescribed for a child under 2 years of age.

▷ **Inform Your Physician Before Taking This Drug If**
- you have a history of liver disease or impaired liver function.
- you have regional enteritis or ulcerative colitis.

- you have swelling of the abdomen, or become constipated.
- you develop swelling (distention) of the abdomen while taking this medicine.
- you have acute dysentery (increased temperature and blood in the stools).

Possible Side Effects (natural, expected, and unavoidable drug actions)
Drowsiness, constipation. Retention of urine.

▷ **Possible Adverse Effects** (unusual, unexpected, and infrequent reactions)
If any of the following develop, consult your physician promptly for guidance.
Mild Adverse Effects
Allergic reaction: skin rash.
Fatigue, dizziness—rare.
Reduced appetite, cramps, dry mouth, nausea, vomiting, stomach pain, bloating—infrequent.
Serious Adverse Effects
"Toxic megacolon" (distended, immobile colon with fluid retention) may develop while treating acute ulcerative colitis—possible.
Hallucinations—case reports.
Movement disorders (akathisia, tardive dyskinesia, acute dystonia)—case reports.
Increased blood sugar—possible.
Necrotizing enterocolitis or paralytic ileus—rare.

▷ **Possible Effects on Sexual Function:** None reported.

Possible Effects on Laboratory Tests: None reported.

CAUTION
1. Do not exceed recommended doses.
2. If treating chronic diarrhea, promptly report development of bloating, abdominal distention, nausea, vomiting, constipation, or abdominal pain.

Precautions for Use
By Infants and Children: Do not use in those under 2 years of age. Follow your physician's instructions exactly regarding dose. Watch for drowsiness, irritability, personality changes, and altered behavior.
By Those Over 60 Years of Age: Small starting doses are needed, as you may be more sensitive to the sedative and constipating effects of this drug.

▷ **Advisability of Use During Pregnancy**
Pregnancy Category: B. See Pregnancy Risk Categories at the back of this book.
Animal Studies: No birth defects found in rat and rabbit studies.
Human Studies: Adequate studies of pregnant women are not available.
Use sparingly and only if clearly needed. Ask your doctor for help.

Advisability of Use If Breast-Feeding
Presence of this drug in breast milk: Small, clinically insignificant amounts.
Talk with your doctor about the BENEFITS versus RISKS of using this medicine and nursing. Described as safe by one source.

Habit-Forming Potential: Physical dependence has occurred in monkeys, but there have been no reports in humans.

Effects of Overdose: Drowsiness, lethargy, depression, dry mouth.

Possible Effects of Long-Term Use: None identified.

Suggested Periodic Examinations While Taking This Drug (at physician's discretion)

Decreased frequency of stools within 48 hours. Check for movement disorders with chronic use.

▷ **While Taking This Drug, Observe the Following**

Foods: No restrictions. Follow prescribed diet.

Herbal Medicines or Minerals: Numerous herbal medicines have German Commission E monograph indications for diarrhea. Examples include: bilberry fruit, oak bark, psyllium seed husk, tormentil root, and uzara root. Use of these herbals with loperamide has not been studied. Electrolyte replacement (sodium, potassium, etc.) can be critical in ongoing diarrhea, especially if you are taking digoxin and other electrolyte-sensitive medicines. St. John's wort led to a case of delirium in one patient. Talk to your doctor BEFORE adding any herbal medicine to loperamide therapy.

Beverages: No restrictions, other than your doctor's recommendations regarding diet.

▷ *Alcohol:* Use with caution. This drug may increase the depressant action of alcohol on the brain.

Tobacco Smoking: No interactions expected. I advise everyone to quit smoking.

▷ *Other Drugs:* No significant drug interactions reported.

▷ *Driving, Hazardous Activities:* This drug may cause drowsiness or dizziness. Restrict activities as necessary.

Aviation Note: The use of this drug *is a disqualification* for piloting. Consult a designated Aviation Medical Examiner.

Exposure to Sun: No restrictions.

LORATADINE (lor AT a deen)

Introduced: 1992   **Class:**   Antihistamines, nonsedating
Please see the minimally sedating antihistamines family profile.

LORAZEPAM (lor A za pam)

Introduced: 1977   **Class:**   Anxiolytic, mild tranquilizer, hypnotic, benzodiazepine   **Prescription:**   USA: Yes   **Controlled Drug:**   USA: C-IV*; Canada: No   **Available as Generic:**   USA: Yes; Canada: Yes

Brand Names: Alzapam, ✤Apo-Lorazepam, Ativan, ✤Dom-Lorazepam, Loraz, Lorazepam Intensol, ✤Novo-Lorazepam, ✤Nu-Loraz, ✤PMS-Loraz

*See Schedules of Controlled Drugs at the back of this book.

BENEFITS versus RISKS

Possible Benefits	*Possible Risks*
RELIEF OF ANXIETY AND NERVOUS TENSION	Habit-forming potential with prolonged use
NOT CHANGED SIGNIFICANTLY INTO ACTIVE DRUG FORMS IN THE LIVER	Minor impairment of mental functions
Wide margin of safety with therapeutic doses	Blood cell, movement or liver disorders
	Dose-related respiratory depression
	Withdrawal symptoms if abruptly stopped

▷ **Principal Uses**

As a Single Drug Product: Uses currently included in FDA-approved labeling: (1) Helps treat anxiety; (2) used in surgical cases to help in delivering effective anesthesia; (3) used intravenously as a sedative.

Other (unlabeled) generally accepted uses: (1) Used to help prevent the severe symptoms of alcohol detoxification (delirium tremens or DTs); (2) used under the tongue to treat serial seizures in children; (3) can be used to promote amnesia in patients who must take chemotherapy and have suffered vomiting; (4) used to relieve insomnia.

In the Pipeline: The Health and Human Services secretary has identified a group of medicines to be tested for use in children. Lorazepam was on that list of the 12 highest-priority medicines to be studied in children.

How This Drug Works: Attaches to a specific site (GABA-A receptor) in the brain and enables gamma-aminobutyric acid to inhibit activity of nervous tissue. Drugs in this class also reduce the time it takes to fall asleep and the number of awakenings during the night.

▷ **Widely Used Guidelines That Involve This Medicine (representative sample):** Please look at the section at the very beginning of this profile called "Class." Next, turn to Table 22 and you will find guidelines listed by the class involved!

Available Dosage Forms and Strengths
Injection — 2 mg/mL, 4 mg/mL
Oral solution — 2 mg/mL
Sublingual tablet — 0.5 mg, 1 mg, 2 mg
Tablet — 0.5 mg, 1 mg, 2 mg

▷ **Recommended Dosage Ranges** (Actual dose and dosing schedule must be determined for each patient individually.)

Infants and Children: Safety and effectiveness in those under 18 years of age are not established for injection. Has been used in 1- to 4-mg doses under the tongue for treatment of serial seizures in children.

18 to 60 Years of Age:

Sedation and anxiety: Therapy is started with 1 to 2 mg per day in 2 to 3 divided doses. Doses may be increased as needed and tolerated to the usual maintenance dose of 2 to 6 mg daily in divided doses. The maximum dose is 10 mg daily in 2 to 3 divided doses.

Insomnia: 2 to 4 mg at bedtime. (transient use only).

Over 60 Years of Age:

Sedation and anxiety: Therapy is started with 0.5 to 1 mg in divided doses. The initial dose should not exceed 2 mg daily.

Insomnia: 0.5 to 1 mg at bedtime.

Conditions Requiring Dosing Adjustments

Liver Function: The dose must be decreased in liver compromise, and the drug should not be used in liver failure. Use of the lowest effective dose is recommended for those with mild to moderate liver failure.

Kidney Function: The drug should not be used in kidney failure. In mild to moderate kidney compromise, the dose must be decreased and the lowest effective dose is recommended.

▷ **Dosing Instructions:** The tablet may be crushed and taken on an empty stomach or with milk or food. Do not stop this drug abruptly if it has been taken for more than 4 weeks. Oral solution should be dosed using a measured dose cup or measuring spoon. If you forget a dose: take the missed dose as soon as you remember it, unless it's nearly time for your next dose—if that is the case, skip the missed dose and take the next dose right on schedule. DO NOT double doses. Talk with your doctor if you find yourself missing doses.

Usual Duration of Use: Use on a regular schedule for 3 to 5 days usually determines effectiveness in relieving moderate anxiety or insomnia. Continual use should be limited to 1 to 3 weeks. Consult your physician on a regular basis.

Author's Note: The National Institute of Mental Health has a good information page on anxiety. It can be found on the World Wide Web (*www.nimh.nih.gov/anxiety*).

Typical Treatment Goals and Measurements (Outcomes and Markers)

Anxiety: Goals for anxiety tend to be more vague and subjective than hypertension or cholesterol. Frequently, the patient (in conjunction with physician assessment) will largely decide if anxiety has been modified to a successful extent. Sleep patterns typically improve with decreased anxiety. The ability of the patient to return to normal activities is a hallmark of successful treatment.

Possible Advantages of This Drug

More direct elimination and lack of active forms may be of benefit in the elderly. Increased lipid solubility is of benefit when the drug is used to treat acute alcohol withdrawal.

▷ **This Drug Should Not Be Taken If**
- you have had an allergic reaction to any dose form or any component of the dose previously.
- you have a primary depression or psychosis.
- you have excessively low blood pressure.
- you have narrow-angle glaucoma.

▷ **Inform Your Physician Before Taking This Drug If**
- you are allergic to any benzodiazepine (see Drug Classes).
- you have a history of alcoholism or drug abuse.
- you are prone to respiratory depression.
- you are pregnant or planning pregnancy.
- you have impaired liver or kidney function.
- you have a history of low white blood cell counts.
- you have asthma, emphysema, epilepsy, or myasthenia gravis.
- you take other prescription or nonprescription medicines that were not discussed with your doctor when lorazepam was prescribed.

Possible Side Effects (natural, expected, and unavoidable drug actions)

Sedation, "hangover" effects on the day following bedtime use.

▷ **Possible Adverse Effects** (unusual, unexpected, and infrequent reactions)
   If any of the following develop, consult your physician promptly for guidance.

   Mild Adverse Effects
   Allergic reactions: rashes, hives—rare.
   Dizziness, amnesia, insomnia (rebound), fainting, confusion, blurred vision, slurred speech, constipation, and sweating—infrequent.
   Ringing in the ears (associated with withdrawal), decreased hearing ability—infrequent.

   Serious Adverse Effects
   Allergic reactions: liver damage with jaundice (see Glossary)—case reports.
   Low white blood cell counts (leukopenia)—rare.
   Paradoxical excitement and rage—case reports.
   Low blood pressure—rare.
   Hallucinations (transient)—rare.
   Porphyria, seizures, or abnormal body movements—case reports.
   Respiratory depression—dose-related.

▷ **Possible Effects on Sexual Function:** Decreased male libido or impotence—case reports.

Possible Effects on Laboratory Tests
   White blood cell counts: decreased.
   Liver function tests: increased SGPT, SGOT, and LDH.

CAUTION
   1. This drug should **not** be stopped abruptly if it has been taken continually for more than 4 weeks.
   2. Over-the-counter medicines with antihistamines can cause excessive sedation if taken with lorazepam.
   3. Lorazepam should **not** be combined with alcohol. This combination will worsen adverse mental and coordination decreases and increase lorazepam levels.

Precautions for Use
   By Infants and Children: Safety and effectiveness for those under 18 years of age are not established. Lorazepam has been used under the tongue in children with serial seizures.
   By Those Over 60 Years of Age: Small doses are indicated. Watch for lethargy, fatigue, weakness, and paradoxical agitation, anger, hostility, and rage.

▷ **Advisability of Use During Pregnancy**
   Pregnancy Category: D. See Pregnancy Risk Categories at the back of this book.
   Animal Studies: Cleft palate has been reported in mice; skeletal defects in rats with similar drugs in this class.
   Human Studies: Adequate studies of pregnant women are not available.
   Frequent use in late pregnancy can result in "floppy infant" syndrome in the newborn: weakness, depressed breathing, and low body temperature. Avoid use during the entire pregnancy.

Advisability of Use If Breast-Feeding
   Presence of this drug in breast milk: Yes.
   Avoid drug or refrain from nursing. Discuss premedication use with your doctor.

Habit-Forming Potential: This drug can cause psychological and/or physical dependence (see Glossary).

Effects of Overdose: Marked drowsiness, weakness, feeling of drunkenness, staggering gait, depression of breathing, stupor progressing to coma.

Possible Effects of Long-Term Use: Psychological or physical dependence, rare liver toxicity.

Suggested Periodic Examinations While Taking This Drug (at physician's discretion)
　　Liver function tests.
　　Complete blood cell counts. Mental status check. Respiratory status check in children.

▷ **While Taking This Drug, Observe the Following**
　　Foods: No restrictions.
　　Herbal Medicines or Minerals: Kava, danshen, skull cap, and valerian may add to central nervous system depression (avoid this combination). Dong Quai may slow removal of lorazepam from the body and increase risk of central nervous system depression. Kola nut, Siberian ginseng, guarana, mate, ephedra, hawthorn, and ma huang may blunt the benefits of this medicine. While St. John's wort is indicated for anxiety, it is also thought to increase (induce) cytochrome P450 enzymes and will tend to blunt lorazepam effectiveness.
　　Beverages: Avoid excessive caffeine-containing beverages: coffee, tea and cola.
▷　*Alcohol:* Avoid this combination. Alcohol increases depression of mental function, further worsens coordination, and causes increased lorazepam levels.
　　Tobacco Smoking: Heavy smoking may reduce the calming action of this drug. I advise everyone to quit smoking.
　　Marijuana Smoking: Additive drowsiness and impaired physical performance.
▷　*Other Drugs*
　　Lorazepam *taken concurrently* with
　　• clozapine (Clozaril) may result in marked sedation and muscular incoordination.
　　• heparin may result in increased effects of lorazepam (increased free fraction).
　　• lithium (Lithobid, others) may result in a lowering of body temperature (hypothermic reaction).
　　• oxycodone (Percocet, others) and other central nervous system depressants may result in additive CNS or respiratory depression.
　　• phenytoin (Dilantin) or fosphenytoin (Cerebyx) may result in altered phenytoin or lorazepam levels.
　　• pyrimethamine (Daraprim) may increase risk of liver problems (toxicity).
　　• quetiapine (Seroquel) may increase lorazepam levels. Watch for increased drowsiness, dizziness, or movement trouble.
　　The following drugs may *increase* the effects of lorazepam:
　　• macrolide antibiotics (see Drug Classes).
　　• probenecid (Benemid)—may result in a 50% increased lorazepam level; decreased lorazepam doses or an increased time between doses are indicated.
　　• valproic acid (Depakene)—decreased doses or an increased time between doses may be needed.
　　The following drugs may *decrease* the effects of lorazepam:
　　• birth control pills (oral contraceptives).
　　• caffeine, amphetamines, or other stimulants.
　　• theophylline (Theo-Dur, others).
▷　*Driving, Hazardous Activities:* This drug can impair alertness and coordination. Restrict activities as necessary.
　　Aviation Note: The use of this drug *is a disqualification* for piloting. Consult a designated Aviation Medical Examiner.

Exposure to Sun: No restrictions.

Discontinuation: Do **not** stop this drug suddenly if it has been taken for over 4 weeks. Consult your doctor about a gradual tapering of dose.

LOSARTAN (loh SAR tan)

Please see the angiotensin II receptor antagonist family profile.

LOVASTATIN (loh vah STA tin)

Author's Note: Because of the release of the ADVOCATE study (see References) and other data, the niacin/lovastatin (Advicor) will supplant lovastatin.

LOW-MOLECULAR-WEIGHT HEPARINS (HEP ar inz)

Introduced: (Europe 1991) 1998, (includes latest PI approval data)   **Class:** Anticoagulant   **Prescription:**   USA: Yes   **Controlled Drug:**   USA: No; Canada: No   **Available as Generic:**   USA: No; Canada: No

Brand Names: Ardeparin: Normiflo; Dalteparin: Fragmin; Enoxaparin: Lovenox; Tinzaparin: Innohep

Author's Note: Because potential outpatient use trends are increasing, information in this profile will be broadened in subsequent editions. Enoxaparin is favored over previously available (unfractionated) heparins in one set of guidelines (NSTEMI).

MACROLIDE ANTIBIOTIC FAMILY (ma KRO lied)

Azithromycin (a zith roh MY sin) **Clarithromycin** (KLAR ith roh my sin) **Erythromycin** (er ith roh MY sin)

Introduced: 1991, 1991, 1952, respectively   **Class:**   Anti-infective, antibiotic, macrolide antibiotic   **Prescription:**   USA: Yes   **Controlled Drug:**   USA: No; Canada: No   **Available as Generic:**   Azithromycin: No; clarithromycin: No; erythromycin: Yes

Brand Names: Azithromycin: ✤Z-Pak, Zithromax, Zithromax TRI-PAK; Clarithromycin: Biaxin, ✤Biaxin BID, Biaxin XL (Biaxin XL Pac), Prevpac [CD]; Erythromycin: AK-Mycin Ophthalmic, Akne-Mycin, ✤Apo-Erythro Base, ✤Apo-Erythro E-C, ✤Apo-Erythro-ES, ✤Apo-Erythro-S, A/T/S, Benzamycin [CD], C-Solve 2, E.E.S., E.E.S. 200, E.E.S. 400, Emgel, E-Mycin, E-Mycin Controlled Release, E-Mycin E, E-Mycin 333, Eramycin, ✤Erybid, ERYC, Erycette, Eryderm, Erygel, Erymax, EryPed, Eryphar, Ery-Tab, Erythrocin, ✤Erythromid, E-Solve 2, Ethril, ETS-2%, Ilosone, Ilotycin, ✤Novo-Rythro, PCE, Pediamycin, ✤Pediazole [CD], ✤PMS-Erythromycin, Robimycin, Sans-Acne, SK-Erythromycin, Staticin, ✤Stievamycin, T-Stat, ✤Wyamycin E, Wyamycin S

BENEFITS versus RISKS

Possible Benefits	*Possible Risks*
EFFECTIVE TREATMENT OF INFECTIONS due to susceptible microorganisms	Allergic reactions, mild and infrequent
ZITHROMAX TRI-PAK TREATS SOME INFECTIONS WITH A THREE DAY SCHEDULE OF PILLS THAT REMAIN IN THE BODY FOR A FULL 10 DAYS	Liver reaction (most common with erythromycin estolate)
	Mild gastrointestinal symptoms
	Drug-induced colitis
	Superinfections

▷ **Principal Uses**

As a Single Drug Product: Uses currently included in FDA-approved labeling: Treatment of (1) skin and skin structure infections (such as acne and *Streptococcus*); (2) upper and lower respiratory tract infections, including "strep" throat, diphtheria, and several types of pneumonia; (3) gonorrhea and syphilis; (4) amebic dysentery (erythromycin); (5) Legionnaire's disease (erythromycin); (6) long-term prevention of recurrences of rheumatic fever (erythromycin)—effective use requires the precise identification of the causative organism and determination of its sensitivity to a macrolide antibiotic; (7) treatment of mycoplasma pneumonia; (8) listeriosis; (9) neonatal conjunctivitis (erythromycin); (10) treatment of ear infections (otitis media) (all); (11) treatment of AIDS-related *Mycobacterium avium-intracellulare* (all); (12) treatment of *Chlamydia trachomatis* urethritis (azithromycin); (13) therapy of *Helicobacter pylori* duodenal ulcers in combination with amoxicillin and omeprazole (clarithromycin); (14) prevention of bacterial endocarditis in people allergic to penicillin; (15) Zithromax TRI-PAK treats acute bacterial exacerbations of COPD (chronic bronchitis) due to susceptible organisms (such as Haemophilus influenzae, Moraxella catarrhalis or Streptococcus pneuoniae).

Author's Note: An Agency for Health Care Policy and Research (AHCPR) study found that most patients who were 60 or younger obtained the same outcomes and significantly reduced costs when erythromycin was used to treat community-acquired pneumonia versus other antibiotics. Biaxin XL is presently only approved for bronchitis, maxillary sinusitis, and community-acquired pneumonia due to susceptible organisms in adults. Please note that resistant *Streptococcus* is a growing threat. In some areas, half of these bacteria are resistant to macrolide antibiotics.

Other (unlabeled) generally accepted uses: (1) Treatment of early Lyme disease (erythromycin; azithromycin is an alternative drug); (2) erythromycin helps sterilize the bowel before surgical procedures; (3) may help threatened preterm labor if the cause is Ureaplasma organisms (erythromycin); (4) helps impetigo (erythromycin); (5) azithromycin or clarithromycin are second choices for Legionnaire's disease; (6) early azithromycin therapy can reduce severity of gum (gingival) hyperplasia caused by cyclosporine; (7) can help some cases of stomach slowness in diabetics (gastroparesis); (8) may treat or prevent some heart attacks where *Chlamydia pneumoniae* is present; (9) erythromycin has shown some efficacy in cholera; (10)) combination treatment results of azithromycin (Zithromax) taken with chloroquine in malaria patients led to a 96% symptom prevention.

As a Combination Drug Product [CD]: Clarithromycin is available in combination with amoxicillin and lansoprazole. Since refractory ulcers are often actually *Helicobacter pylori* infections, the combination works to kill the bacteria and lower acid production. Erythromycin is available in combination with sulfisoxazole (Pediazole). This combination can be useful in patients who are allergic to penicillin.

In the Pipeline: Clarithromycin in combination with 20 mg of rabeprazole (Aciphex) twice daily worked to eradicate *Helicobacter pylori* in 91.4% of patients in one study (see Mario, F. D. in Sources). A larger study (1,200 patients) will be undertaken by Pfizer to assess the effects of combination therapy of malaria using chloroquine and azithromycin (Zithromax).

How These Drugs Work: They prevent growth and multiplication of susceptible organisms by interfering with their formation of essential proteins.

▷ **Widely Used Guidelines That Involve This Medicine (representative sample):** Please look at the section at the very beginning of this profile called "Class." Next, turn to Table 22 and you will find guidelines listed by the class involved!

Available Dosage Forms and Strengths

Azithromycin:

> Oral suspension — 100 mg/5 mL, 200 mg/5 mL
> Tablet — 500 mg (in package of three for a 3-day course of one infection)
> Tablet — 600 mg

Clarithromycin:

> Oral suspension granules — 125 mg/5 mL, 185.5 mg/5mL or 250 mg/5 mL
> Tablets — 250 mg, 500 mg
> Tablets, extended release — 500 mg

Combination form with lansoprazole is addressed in that profile

Erythromycin:

> Capsules — 125 mg, 250 mg
> Capsules, enteric coated — 125 mg, 250 mg
> Drops — 100 mg/mL
> Eye ointment — 5 mg/g
> Gel — 2%
> Oral suspension — 125 mg/5 mL, 250 mg/5 mL
> Skin ointment — 2%
> Tablets — 250 mg, 500 mg
> Tablets, chewable — 125 mg, 200 mg, 250 mg
> Tablets, delayed release — 250 mg, 333 mg
> Tablets, dispersible (Canada) — 500 mg
> Tablets, enteric coated — 250 mg, 333 mg, 500 mg
> Tablets, film coated — 250 mg, 500 mg
> Topical solution — 1.5%, 2%

▷ **Recommended Dosage Ranges** (Actual dose and schedule must be determined for each patient individually.)

Infants and Children:

Azithromycin: For otitis media (6 months and older)—Newer dosing provides for a single dose regimen of 30 mg per kg of the suspension form. For example: a 22-pound child would be dosed based on a 10 kg weight and would be given a 7.5 mL (one-and-a-half teaspoonful) dose of the 200 mg/5 mL suspension (300 mg total dose); or a 3-day regimen of 10 mg per kg of body mass for 3 days. Other options include 10 mg per kg of body mass as a single dose on the first day (up to 500 mg), followed by 5 mg per kg of body mass (up to 250 mg) on days 2–5. For pharyngitis—12 mg per kg of body mass (up to 500 mg) daily for 5 days.

Clarithromycin: When used to treat otitis media (caused by *Haemophilus influenzae, M. catarrhalis* or *Strep. pneumoniae*) in children, the dose is 7.5 mg per kg of body mass twice daily, up to a maximum of 500 mg twice a day for 10 days. For Mycobacterium avium-intracellulare complex infections in HIV-positive children, the dose is 7.5 mg per kg of body mass twice daily, to a maximum of 500 mg twice a day. If this dose is successful, therapy is continued for life. Extended release (XL) form has not yet been evaluated in children.

Erythromycin: In pediatrics, oral erythromycin is usually given at a dose of 30 to 50 mg per kg of body mass per day and is divided into 3 or 4 doses. For some very severe infections, the dose is doubled.

12 to 60 Years of Age:

Azithromycin (16 to 60 years of age): For pharyngitis/tonsillitis, bronchitis, pneumonia and skin infections—500 mg as a single dose on the first day and then 250 mg once daily on days 2–4 for a total dose of 1.5 g. For *Helicobacter pylori*—500 mg daily for 7 days. For nongonococcal urethritis and cervicitis—a single 1 g (1,000 mg) dose. Tri-Pak gives three 500 mg tablets taken over consecutive days for treatment of sudden (acute) bacterial exacerbations of chronic obstructive pulmonary disease (COPD).

Clarithromycin: For pharyngitis/tonsillitis—250 mg every 12 hours for 10 days. For maxillary sinusitis—500 mg every 12 hours for 14 days. For acute bronchitis—250–500 mg every 12 hours for 7 to 14 days. For pneumonia—250–500 mg every 12 hours for 7 to 14 days. For skin infections—250 mg every 12 hours for 7 to 14 days. Biaxin XL treats bronchitis (sudden or acute exacerbation of chronic bronchitis) in adults with two 500 mg tablets (1,000 mg), once a day for 7 days. Sudden or acute maxillary sinusitis is treated using two 500 mg tablets for 14 days.

Erythromycin: 250 mg every 6 hours, or 500 mg every 12 hours according to nature and severity of infection. Total daily dose should not exceed 4 g. For endocarditis prophylaxis (stearate oral form): 1 gram is given 2 hours before procedure and 500 mg 6 hours later.

Over 60 Years of Age:

Azithromycin: Same as 16 to 60 years of age. If liver or kidney function is limited, the dose must be reduced.

Clarithromycin: Same as 12 to 60 years of age. Dose must be reduced in kidney compromise.

Erythromycin: Same as usual adult dosing range. If liver or kidney function is limited, dose must be reduced.

Conditions Requiring Dosing Adjustments

Liver Function: These drugs are metabolized in the liver and will accumulate in patients with liver compromise. Decreased doses may be needed. They should be used with caution by patients with biliary tract disease. Clarithromycin does not need to be adjusted for patients with liver problems if kidney function is normal.

Kidney Function: No dosing changes are needed for azithromycin. The dose of clarithromycin must be decreased or the time between doses (dosing interval) prolonged for patients with compromised kidneys (for example, if the CrCl is less than 30 mL/min, one-half of the usual dose could be used in the usual dosing interval). Patients with severe kidney failure can take 50–75% of the usual erythromycin dose at the usual time. Azithromycin and erythromycin are rare causes of interstitial nephritis (inflammation of a specific part of the kidney).

▷ **Dosing Instructions:** Nonenteric-coated preparations should be taken 1 hour before or 2 hours after eating. Enteric-coated preparations may be taken without regard to food. Azithromycin may be better tolerated if taken with food. The amount that gets into your body increases if the suspension is taken with food, but decreases if the capsules are taken with food. Do not take azithromycin with antacids containing aluminum or magnesium. Regular uncoated capsules may be opened, and tablets may be crushed; coated and prolonged-action preparations should be swallowed whole. Azithromycin suspension should be shaken before giving a dose and should also be dosed using a measuring cup or measuring spoon. Biaxin XL should be taken WITH food to help increase absorption. Ask your pharmacist for help. If you forget a dose: Take the missed dose as soon as you remember it, unless it's nearly time for your next dose—if that is the case, skip the missed dose and take the next dose right on schedule. Talk with your doctor if you find yourself missing doses.

Usual Duration of Use: Use on a regular schedule for the full schedule is necessary to determine this drug's effectiveness in controlling infections and preventing emergence of resistant bacteria. For streptococcal infections, the full course is very important without interruption of any multiple-day course to reduce the possibility of developing rheumatic fever or glomerulonephritis. The duration of use should not exceed the time required to eliminate the infection.

Typical Treatment Goals and Measurements (Outcomes and Markers)
Infections: The most commonly used measures of serious infections are white blood cell counts, differentials (the kind of blood cells that occur most often in your blood) and temperature. Many clinicians look for positive changes in 24–48 hours. NEVER stop an antibiotic because you start to feel better. For many infections, a full 14 days is REQUIRED to kill the bacteria. (TRI-PAK form of azithromycin is an exception to this guideline). The goals and time frame (see benefits above) should be discussed with you when the prescription is written.

Possible Advantages of These Drugs
Azithromycin and clarithromycin: Broader spectrum of infectious microorganism coverage; equivalent to erythromycin, some penicillins, and some cephalosporins. Effective with fewer doses (only 1 dose for azithromycin, 2 for clarithromycin, and once daily for the Biaxin XL form), which may help pill-taking or adherence. Azithromycin and clarithromycin are very well tolerated; infrequent and minor adverse effects.

▷ **These Drugs Should Not Be Taken If**
• you had an allergic reaction to a macrolide previously.
• you have active liver disease (erythromycin estolate form).
• you are pregnant or planning pregnancy (some forms).
• you are allergic to *para*-aminobenzoic-acid-type anesthetics (intramuscular form of erythromycin).

▷ **Inform Your Physician Before Taking These Drugs If**
• you have a history of a previous "reaction" to any macrolide antibiotic.
• you are allergic by nature: hay fever, asthma, hives, eczema.
• you have a blood disorder.
• you have an abnormal heart rhythm.
• you have a history of porphyria.

- you have a history of kidney disorder.
- you have myasthenia gravis.
- you have a hearing disorder.
- you are taking a blood thinner (oral anticoagulant) (clarithromycin).
- you have a history of low blood platelets (some macrolides).
- you have taken the estolate form of erythromycin previously.

Possible Side Effects (natural, expected, and unavoidable drug actions)
Superinfections (see Glossary).

▷ **Possible Adverse Effects** (unusual, unexpected, and infrequent reactions)
If any of the following develop, consult your physician promptly for guidance.

Mild Adverse Effects
Allergic reactions: skin rash, hives, itching—rare.
Nausea, vomiting, diarrhea, abdominal cramping—infrequent.
Headache—rare.
Visual hallucinations—case report for clarithromycin.
Drug-induced increased liver enzymes (see Jaundice in Glossary)—rare.

Serious Adverse Effects
Allergic reaction: anaphylactic reaction (see Glossary)—rare. Stevens-Johnson Syndrome (erythromycin)—case report.
Idiosyncratic reactions: liver reaction—nausea, vomiting, fever, jaundice (usually, but not exclusively, associated with erythromycin estolate).
Prolonging of the QT interval (Torsade de Pointes or ventricular tachycardia)—possible.
Abnormal heart rhythm—rare.
Decreased white blood cells (erythromycin)—rare.
Hemolytic anemia (erythromycin)—case report.
Lowered blood platelets (clarithromycin)—case report.
Worsening of myasthenia gravis—case reports.
Low body temperature (hypothermia)—rare.
Pseudomembranous colitis—rare.
Pancreatitis (erythromycin)—rare.
Kidney problems (interstitial nephritis) (azithromycin, erythromycin)—case reports.
Abnormal urination (SIADH)—case reports for azithromycin.
Hearing loss (ototoxicity)—case reports.

▷ **Possible Effects on Sexual Function:** None reported.

▷ **Adverse Effects That May Mimic Natural Diseases or Disorders**
Liver toxicity may resemble acute gallbladder disease or viral hepatitis.

Possible Effects on Laboratory Tests
Complete blood cell counts: white cells may increase or decrease; eosinophils increased (allergic reaction); platelets decreased.
INR (prothrombin time): increased (drugs taken concurrently with warfarin).
Liver function tests: liver enzymes increased (ALT/GPT, AST/GOT, and alkaline phosphatase), increased bilirubin.

CAUTION
1. Take the **full dose prescribed** to help prevent resistant bacteria.
2. If you have a history of liver disease or impaired liver function, avoid any form of erythromycin estolate.
3. If diarrhea develops and continues for more than 24 hours, consult your physician promptly.

Precautions for Use

By Infants and Children: Watch allergic children closely for indications of developing allergy to this drug. Observe also for evidence of gastrointestinal irritation. Dosing based on body mass is critical.

By Those Over 60 Years of Age: Watch for itching reactions in the genital and anal regions, often due to yeast superinfections. Observe also for evidence of hearing loss. Report such developments promptly. If liver or kidney function is impaired, dose decreases must be considered.

▷ **Advisability of Use During Pregnancy**

Pregnancy Category: C for clarithromycin. B for others. See Pregnancy Risk Categories at the back of this book.

Animal Studies: Studies of rats are inconclusive for erythromycin. Monkey, rabbit, and rat studies have shown problems in pregnancy outcomes and fetal development.

Human Studies: Information from adequate studies of pregnant women is not available.

Generally thought to be safe during entire pregnancy, except for erythromycin estolate; this form of erythromycin can cause toxic liver reactions during pregnancy and should be avoided. Clarithromycin should be avoided unless no other antibiotic option is available.

Advisability of Use If Breast-Feeding

Presence of this drug in breast milk: Yes for others; clarithromycin unknown. Watch nursing infant closely and discontinue drug or nursing if adverse effects develop.

Habit-Forming Potential: None.

Effects of Overdose: Possible nausea, vomiting, hallucinations (clarithromycin), diarrhea, and abdominal discomfort.

Possible Effects of Long-Term Use: Superinfections (see Glossary).

Suggested Periodic Examinations While Taking These Drugs (at physician's discretion)

Liver function tests if the erythromycin estolate form is used.
Complete blood counts to measure response of infection.

▷ **While Taking These Drugs, Observe the Following**

Foods: Newer formulation absorption is decreased by more than 70% (especially with high-fat meals) and effectiveness may be seriously compromised for erythromycin. Azithromycin suspension is increased, while capsules are decreased. Clarithromycin immediate release is not affected. Biaxin XL form is best taken with food.

Herbal Medicines or Minerals: Echinacea: Some patients use echinacea to attempt to boost their immune systems. Unfortunately, use of echinacea is not recommended in people with damaged immune systems. This herb may also actually weaken any immune system if it is used too often or for too long a time. DO NOT take mistletoe herb, oak bark or F.C. of marshmallow root, and licorice. **Caution:** St. John's wort may also cause extreme reactions to the sun. Additive photosensitivity may be possible.

Beverages: Avoid fruit juices and carbonated beverages for 1 hour after taking any nonenteric-coated preparation of erythromycin. May be taken with milk.

▷ *Alcohol:* Avoid if you have impaired liver function or are taking the estolate form of erythromycin.

Tobacco Smoking: No interactions expected. I advise everyone to quit smoking.

▷ *Other Drugs*

Clarithromycin and erythromycin may ***increase*** the effects of

- amprenavir (Agenerase) or atazanavir (Reyataz. This competition for removal from the body may also lead to increased clarithromycin concentrations. Dose decrease by 50% should be considered if the combination is required in order to avoid possible QTC prolongation.
- benzodiazepines (see Drug Classes).
- buspirone (Buspar) (erythromycin only).
- carbamazepine (Tegretol) and cause toxicity.
- cilostazol (Pletal). Patients should be watched for increased heart rate, blood pressure, and complete blood counts taken in order to check for possible toxicity if these medicines must be combined.
- cisapride (Propulsid).
- clozapine (Clozaril).
- digoxin (Lanoxin) and cause toxicity.
- entacapone (Comtan) leading to increased entacapone adverse effects (movement problems, diarrhea).
- ergotamine (Cafergot, Ergostat, etc.) and cause impaired circulation to extremities/ergotism. DO NOT combine.
- imatinib (Gleevec) and cause excess imatinib effects or toxicity.
- medicines that have an effect on the QTc interval of the heart (see glossary) such as class I, IA or class III antiarrhythmic drugs such as flecainide (Tambocor) and medicines such as ziprasidone (Zyprexa) may lead to serious toxicity such as Torsades de Pointes. DO NOT COMBINE these medicines.
- methylprednisolone (Medrol) and prednisone and cause excess steroid effects.
- phenytoin (Dilantin or fosphenytoin [Cerebyx]).
- quetiapine (Seroquel).
- quinidine (Quinaglute, others).
- sibutramine (Meridia) [erythromycin and clarithromycin].
- sildenafil (Viagra)—reported up to 182% increased blood level (clarithromycin and erythromycin only).
- tacrolimus (Prograf) or sirolimus (Rapamune).
- theophylline (aminophylline, Theo-Dur, etc.) and cause toxicity.
- tretinoin (Vesanoid).
- valproic acid (Depakote).
- vinblastine (Velban) erythromycin and clarithromycin.
- warfarin (Coumadin) and increase the risk of bleeding (azithromycin also).

These medicines may ***decrease*** the effects of

- clindamycin.
- lincomycin.
- penicillins.

These medicines ***taken concurrently*** with

- atorvastatin (Lipitor), pravastatin (Pravachol), simvastatin (Zocor), and other HMG-CoA reductase inhibitors INCREASE RISK OF MYOPATHY (serious muscle damage) if used with erythromycin or clarithromycin. Combination is NOT recommended.
- birth control pills (oral contraceptives) can cause loss of effectiveness and result in pregnancy (erythromycin).
- cyclosporine (Sandimmune) may result in cyclosporine toxicity if taken with erythromycin.

- disopyramide may cause heart (cardiac) arrhythmias.
- dofetilide (Tikosyn) may lead to dofetilide toxicity.
- fluoxetine (Prozac) may lead to fluoxetine toxicity.
- grepafloxacin (Raxar) and perhaps gatifloxacin (Tequin) may lead to heart-beat changes (prolonged QTc interval) if combined with erythromycin.
- lansoprazole (Prevacid) may lead to black tongue if combined with clarithromycin.
- loratadine (Claritin) may result in increased loratadine levels (also with fexofenadine [Allegra]), but it does not appear to cause the serious arrhythmia of some of the other nonsedating antihistamines. Since loratadine or fexofenadine levels may be increased, it may be prudent to decrease doses while taking erythromycin.
- midazolam (and probably other benzodiazepines) (see Drug Classes) may lead to excessive central nervous system depression.
- nevirapine (Viramune), delavirdine (Rescriptor) or efavirenz (Sustiva) may lead to nevirapine, efavirenz or delavirdine toxicity.
- omeprazole, esomepraxole and perhaps other proton pump inhibitors may increase levels of both erythromycin and clarithromycin.
- prednisone and other corticosteroids may lead to corticosteroid toxicity if combined with clarithromycin or erythromycin.
- rifabutin (Mycobutin) increases risk of low white blood cells (neutropenia) if combined with azithromycin or clarithromycin; clarithromycin also increases risk of rifabutin rash.
- ritonavir (Norvir) and perhaps other protease inhibitors (see Drug Classes) may lead to toxicity.
- sparfloxacin (Zagam) may lead to heartbeat changes (prolonged QTc interval) if combined with erythromycin.
- triazolam may cause toxicity.
- trimexate (Mexate) can decrease trimexate metabolism and can lead to toxicity.
- valproic acid (Depakene, Depakote) can lead to toxic blood levels.
- zafirlukast (Accolate) and blunt zafirlukast benefits.
- zidovudine (AZT) may lead to decreased levels and lack of zidovudine effectiveness (clarithromycin and erythromycin).

▷ *Driving, Hazardous Activities:* This drug may cause nausea and/or diarrhea. Restrict activities as necessary.

Aviation Note: The use of these drugs **may be a disqualification** for piloting. Consult a designated Aviation Medical Examiner.

Exposure to Sun: Use caution; some medicines in this class have caused increased sensitivity to the sun (photosensitivity).

Special Storage Instructions: Keep liquid forms refrigerated.

Observe the Following Expiration Times: Freshly mixed oral suspension—14 days for clarithromycin (DO NOT refrigerate). Freshly mixed oral suspensions of erythromycin should be refrigerated to preserve taste. These go bad (outdate) in 14 days. Single-dose azithromycin suspension should be mixed with water and taken right away. Ask your pharmacist for help.

MAPROTILINE (ma PROH ti leen)

Introduced: 1974   **Class:** Antidepressant   **Prescription:** USA: Yes   **Controlled Drug:** USA: No; Canada: No   **Available as Generic:** Yes

Brand Name: Ludiomil

Author's Note: Because use of this medicine has declined in favor of newer medicines, the information in this profile has been abbreviated.

MECLOFENAMATE (me kloh fen AM ayt)

Please see the fenamate (nonsteroidal anti-inflammatory drug) family profile.

MEDROXYPROGESTERONE (me DROX e proh jess te rohn)

Introduced: 1959   **Class:**   Female sex hormones, progestins   **Prescription:**   USA: Yes   **Controlled Drug:**   USA: No; Canada: No   **Available as Generic:**   Yes

Brand Names: ✤Alti-MPA, Amen, Curretab, Cycrin, Depo-Provera, Premphase, Prempro, ✤PMS-Medroxyprogesterone, ✤Premelle, ✤Proclim, Provera, ✤Riva-Medrone

Author's Note: This profile will focus on the single medicine medroxyprogesterone forms.

BENEFITS versus RISKS

Possible Benefits	*Possible Risks*
EFFECTIVE TREATMENT OF ABSENT OR ABNORMAL MENSTRUATION due to hormone imbalance	Thrombophlebitis
	Pulmonary embolism
	Liver reaction with jaundice
EFFECTIVE CONTRACEPTION when given by injection	Drug-induced birth defects
USED IN ADJUNCTIVE AND PALLIATIVE TREATMENT OF INOPERABLE, RECURRING, AND METASTATIC ENDOMETRIAL AND KIDNEY CANCER	

▷ **Principal Uses**

As a Single Drug Product: Uses currently included in FDA-approved labeling: (1) Used to initiate and regulate menstruation and correct abnormal patterns of menstrual bleeding caused by hormonal imbalance (and not by organic disease); (2) used in combination to treat metastatic, inoperable or recurrent endometrial carcinoma; (3) treatment of renal cell carcinoma; (4) used as a contraceptive injected into the muscle, once every 3 months; (5) helps dysfunctional uterine bleeding; (6) used to help infants with alveolar hypoventilation syndrome.

Other (unlabeled) generally accepted uses: (1) Used as a part of combination therapy in breast, refractory prostate, lung and ovarian cancers; (2) therapy of endometriosis; (3) helps abnormal hair growth in women (hirsutism); (4) can help breast pain (mastodynia); (5) used in combination with estrogen to help symptoms of menopause; (6) can be of use in pelvic congestion and pickwickian syndrome; (7) may help severe PMS; (8) can be of use in male hypersexuality.

How This Drug Works: By inducing and maintaining a lining in the uterus that resembles pregnancy, this drug can prevent uterine bleeding until it is withdrawn. By suppressing the release of the pituitary gland hormone that induces ovulation and by stimulating the secretion of mucus by the uterine cervix (to resist the passage of sperm), this drug can prevent pregnancy.

▷ **Widely Used Guidelines That Involve This Medicine (representative sample):** Please look at the section at the very beginning of this profile called "Class." Next, turn to Table 22 and you will find guidelines listed by the class involved!

Available Dosage Forms and Strengths

Injection — 100, 150 and 400 mg/mL
Injection (single-dose vials) — 150 mg
Tablets — 2.5 mg, 5 mg, 10 mg

▷ **Usual Adult Dosage Ranges:** *To initiate menstruation*: 5 to 10 mg daily for 5 to 10 days, started at any time.

To correct abnormal bleeding: 5 to 10 mg daily for 5 to 10 days, started on the 16th day of the menstrual cycle. Withdrawal bleeding usually begins within 3 to 7 days after stopping the drug.

As a contraceptive: Intramuscular injections of 150 mg every 3 months are needed.

Author's Note: Controversy about estrogen therapy (ERT) and use of combination hormone replacement therapy (HRT) is fully outlined in the estrogen profile presented earlier in this book. The Women's Health Initiative raised important questions regarding use of the combined form of estrogen and progestin (Premphase and Prempro forms are listed for completeness).

Conditions Requiring Dosing Adjustments

Liver Function: This drug should be used with caution and the dose empirically decreased, by patients with liver compromise.

Kidney Function: No dosing changes thought to be needed.

▷ **Dosing Instructions:** The tablet may be crushed and taken on an empty stomach or with food to prevent nausea. If you forget a dose: take the missed dose as soon as you remember it, unless it's nearly time for your next dose—if that is the case, skip the missed dose and take the next dose right on schedule. If you miss a contraceptive injection, call your doctor about alternative forms of birth control. Talk with your doctor if you find yourself missing doses.

Usual Duration of Use: Use on a regular schedule for 2 or 3 menstrual cycles determines effectiveness in correcting abnormal patterns of menstrual bleeding. See your doctor on a regular basis.

Typical Treatment Goals and Measurements (Outcomes and Markers)

Contraception: Used to prevent conception with an injection once every 13 weeks. Ongoing use is required to avoid becoming pregnant.

Possible Advantages of This Drug

Effective contraception with a shot once every 13 weeks.

▷ **This Drug Should Not Be Taken If**
• you have had an allergic reaction to it previously.
• you are pregnant.
• you have experienced a missed abortion.
• you have impaired liver function/liver disease.
• you have a history of cancer of the breast or reproductive organs.

- you have a history of thrombophlebitis, embolism or stroke.
- you have abnormal and unexplained vaginal bleeding.

▷ **Inform Your Physician Before Taking This Drug If**
  - you have impaired kidney function.
  - you have any of the following disorders: asthma, diabetes, emotional depression, epilepsy, heart disease, migraine headaches.

Possible Side Effects (natural, expected, and unavoidable drug actions)
  Fluid retention, weight gain (when injected as a contraceptive by increasing deposition of fat), changes in menstrual timing and flow, spotting between periods.

▷ **Possible Adverse Effects** (unusual, unexpected, and infrequent reactions)
  If any of the following develop, consult your physician promptly for guidance.

Mild Adverse Effects
  Allergic reactions: skin rash, hives, itching.
  Fatigue, weakness, nausea—infrequent.
  Conflicting reports on blood lipids.
  Acne, excessive hair growth, hair loss—case reports.

Serious Adverse Effects
  Allergic reaction: anaphylactic reaction (see Glossary)—rare. Stevens-Johnson Syndrome.
  Liver toxicity with jaundice (see Glossary): yellow eyes/skin, dark-colored urine, light-colored stools—possible.
  Thrombophlebitis (inflammation of a vein with blood clot formation): pain or tenderness in thigh or leg, with or without swelling of the foot, ankle, or leg—case reports. Stop medicine immediately and call your doctor.
  Pulmonary embolism (movement of blood clot to lung): sudden shortness of breath, chest pain, cough, bloody sputum—case reports. The medicine should be stopped immediately if this happens.
  Stroke (blood clot in the brain): sudden headache, weakness or paralysis of any part of the body—possible.
  Cushing's Syndrome—case reports.
  Retinal thrombosis (blood clot in the eye): sudden impairment or loss of vision—case reports.
  Drug-induced pseudotumor cerebri—possible.
  Arachnoiditis (with intrathecal injection)—case reports.
  Pneumonitis, especially in patients who have received radiation therapy—case reports.
  Medroxyprogesterone was NOT found to increase risk of breast cancer in a World Health Organization study of 12,759 women. It was also found NOT to increase risk of ovarian or uterine cancer in a study of 5,000 African American women who received it as a contraceptive for 10 years. (Estrogen/progestin combinations did increase breast cancer risk more than the estrogen alone product).
  A study in mice found that when progesterone was used in large doses for prolonged periods, it acted as a co-carcinogen.
  Cervical cancer—weak or no association in case-control studies.

▷ **Possible Effects on Sexual Function:** Altered timing and pattern of menstruation. Female breast tenderness and secretion (galactorrhea). Decreased vaginal secretions. Infertility—case reports.

▷ **Adverse Effects That May Mimic Natural Diseases or Disorders**
  Liver toxicity may suggest viral hepatitis.

Possible Effects on Laboratory Tests

Blood total cholesterol, HDL cholesterol, LDL cholesterol, and triglyceride levels: variable results.

Glucose tolerance test (GTT): decreased.

CAUTION

1. There is an increased risk of birth defects in children whose mothers take this drug during the first 4 months of pregnancy.
2. Inform your physician promptly if you think you may be pregnant.
3. This drug should not be used as a test for pregnancy.

Precautions for Use

By Infants and Children: Not used in this age group.

By Those Over 60 Years of Age: Used as adjunctive therapy in cancer of the breast, uterus, prostate, and kidney. Watch for excessive fluid retention.

▷ **Advisability of Use During Pregnancy**

Pregnancy Category: X. See Pregnancy Risk Categories at the back of this book.

Animal Studies: Genital defects reported in rat and rabbit studies; masculinization of the female rodent fetus; various defects in chick embryos and rabbits.

Human Studies: In a study of 1,016 pregnancies, oral doses of 80–120 mg daily used from the 5th to 7th week of pregnancy up to the 18th week were not associated with teratogenic effects. Other data show masculinization of the female genitals: enlargement of the clitoris, fusion of the labia. Increased risk of heart, nervous system, and limb defects when used in the second and third trimesters of pregnancy.

The drug is used as a benefit-to-risk decision in the first 3 months of pregnancy. Avoid this drug completely during the final 6 months of pregnancy.

Advisability of Use If Breast-Feeding

Presence of this drug in breast milk: Yes.

Avoid drug or refrain from nursing.

Habit-Forming Potential: None.

Effects of Overdose: Nausea, vomiting, fluid retention, breast enlargement and discomfort, abnormal vaginal bleeding.

Possible Effects of Long-Term Use: There has been considerable controversy regarding use of this drug and cancer. The most recent large patient studies do not show an increased relative risk that is statistically significant.

Suggested Periodic Examinations While Taking This Drug (at physician's discretion)

Regular examinations (every 6 to 12 months) of the breasts and reproductive organs (pelvic examination of the uterus and ovaries, including Pap smear).

▷ **While Taking This Drug, Observe the Following**

Foods: No restrictions.

Herbal Medicines or Minerals: Black cohosh appears to work by (1) suppressing luteinizing hormone; (2) binding to estrogen receptors in the pituitary and inhibiting luteinizing hormone release and (3) binding to estrogen receptors in the pituitary. The net effect is that this herb eases symptoms of menopause, but little is known about long-term use or heart and bone protective effects. Talk to your doctor before starting black cohosh if you are currently taking medroxyprogesterone—particularly if you take it for PMS. Calcium may help ease some PMS symptoms.

Beverages: Do not take this medicine with grapefruit juice. Grapefruit juice inhibits CYP3A4, which helps remove this drug from the body.

▷ *Alcohol:* No interactions expected.

Tobacco Smoking: No direct drug interactions expected. I advise everyone to quit smoking.

▷ *Other Drugs*

The following drugs may *decrease* the effects of medroxyprogesterone:
- nevirapine (Viramune).
- rifampin (Rifadin, Rimactane, etc.) may hasten its elimination.

Medroxyprogesterone *taken concurrently* with
- CYP3A4 inhibitors (such as erythromycin, fluoxetine, fluvoxamine, itraconazole, ketoconazole, virconazole, ritonavir, and others) may lead to increased medroxyprogesterone levels.
- digitoxin may result in slightly higher-than-expected digoxin levels.
- estrogens (Premphase, Prempro) have a very different benefit-to-risk profile (see earlier estrogens profile in this book).
- nevirapine (Viramune) may lower medroxyprogesterone levels and blunt contraceptive or other benefits.
- ritonavir (Norvir) and perhaps other protease inhibitors (see Drug Classes) may lead to toxicity.
- tamoxifen (Nolvadex) may result in blunting of the therapeutic benefits of tamoxifen.
- warfarin (Coumadin) may increase warfarin effects; increased lab INR (prothrombin time or protime) testing is needed.

▷ *Driving, Hazardous Activities:* Usually no restrictions. Ask your doctor about your individual risk and for guidance regarding specific restrictions.

Aviation Note: The use of this drug *may be a disqualification* for piloting. Consult a designated Aviation Medical Examiner.

Exposure to Sun: No restrictions.

MEFENAMIC ACID (me FEN am ik A sid)

Please see the fenamate (nonsteroidal anti-inflammatory drug) family profile.

MEMANTINE (MEH maan teen)

Introduced: 2003   **Class:**   Low-affinity N-Methyl-D-aspartate (NMDA) receptor agonist, anti-Alzheimer's drug   **Prescription:**   USA: Yes   **Controlled Drug:**   USA: No; Canada: No   **Available as Generic:**   USA: No, Canada: No

Brand Names: Namenda

```
┌─────────────────────────────────────────────────────────────────────┐
│                      BENEFITS versus RISKS                            │
│      Possible Benefits                      Possible Risks            │
│ IMPROVEMENT OF MEMORY IN        Inner restlessness                    │
│   MODERATE to SEVERE            Nausea                                │
│   ALZHEIMER'S DISEASE           Dizziness                             │
│ IMPROVEMENT OF SYMPTOMS IN      Over excitation                       │
│   MODERATE to SEVERE                                                  │
│   ALZHEIMER'S DISEASE                                                 │
│ MODERATE to SEVERE                                                    │
│   ALZHEIMER'S PATIENTS                                                │
│   BENEFIT FROM ADD ON                                                 │
│   TREATMENT WITH DONEPEZIL                                            │
│   (one study)                                                         │
│ ONCE-DAILY DOSING MAKES IT                                           │
│   EASIER FOR CAREGIVERS AND                                           │
│   PATIENTS TO KEEP TAKING THE                                         │
│   MEDICINE                                                            │
└─────────────────────────────────────────────────────────────────────┘
```

▷ **Principal Uses**

  As a Single Drug Product: Uses currently included in FDA-approved labeling: Treats moderate to severe Alzheimer's disease symptoms.

  Other (unlabeled) generally accepted uses: (1) May have a role in combination treatment with donepezil in patients already being treated with donepezil (see Tariot in Sources).

How This Drug Works: Alzheimer's disease is thought to be contributed to by ongoing (persistent) activation of the central nervous system (NMDA receptors) by a chemical called glutamate. Memantine works by blocking the place (receptor) where the chemical glutamate has its undesirable action.

▷ **Widely Used Guidelines That Involve This Medicine (representative sample):** Please look at the section at the very beginning of this profile called "Class." Next, turn to Table 22 and you will find guidelines listed by the class involved!

Available Dosage Forms and Strengths
            Tablets — 5 mg, 10 mg

▷ **Recommended Dosage Ranges** (Actual dosage and schedule must be determined for each patient individually.)

  Infants and Children: No data are available on use of these drugs in infants and children.

  Adults:

  Dosing is started with 5 mg once daily. After seven days, the dose is increased to 5 mg twice a day. After another seven days, the dose is increased to 10 mg in the morning and 5 mg in the evening. After another seven days, dosing is increased to the target dose of 10 mg twice daily.

  Over 60 Years of Age: Same as adult dosing.

Conditions Requiring Dosing Adjustments

  Liver Function:

  Dose decreases not thought to be needed.

  Kidney Function: Dose decreases in kidney compromise are prudent as most of this medicine is removed by the kidneys.

▷ **Dosing Instructions:** The tablet may be crushed and is not affected by food. If you forget a dose: take it right away unless it's nearly time for your next regular dose. If it IS nearly time, just take the scheduled dose. DO NOT double doses.

Usual Duration of Use: Regular use for 2-3 weeks may be needed to see improvement from this medicine. Dose increases are made at 7-day intervals. Long-term use (months to years) requires periodic evaluation of response and dose. There is no evidence to tell us that this drug stops or slows nerve degeneration in Alzheimer's.

Typical Treatment Goals and Measurements (Outcomes and Markers)
Thinking and cognition: Improvement in the Mini-Mental State Examination (sMMSE), Alzheimer's Disease Assessment Scale (ADAS-cog) and/or global function using the Clinician Interview-Based Assessment of Change Plus Caregiver Input (CIBIC-Plus). Cooperative Studies Activities of Daily Living Inventory modified for severe dementia (ADCS-ADLsev) was used in one add-on study. Assessments should be made periodically as benefits from this medicine will decay over time.

Possible Advantage of This Drug
Improvement of memory and other symptoms of moderate to severe Alzheimer's with a novel mechanism of action. Can be used as add-on therapy in patients already taking donepezil.

▷ **This Drug Should Not Be Taken If**
- you have had an allergic reaction to it previously.

▷ **Inform Your Physician Before Taking These Drugs If**
- you have a history of seizure disorder.
- you have compromised kidney function (remember the age-related decline in kidney function).

Possible Side Effects (natural, expected, and unavoidable drug actions)
Drowsiness.

▷ **Possible Adverse Effects** (unusual, unexpected, and infrequent reactions)
If any of the following develop, consult your physician promptly for guidance.
Mild Adverse Effects
Allergic reactions: skin rash, itching.
Muscle aches—infrequent.
Insomnia—frequent.
Agitation—may be frequent.
Increased blood pressure—infrequent.
Sweating—infrequent.
Blurred vision—infrequent.
Weight gain or loss—infrequent.
Nausea/vomiting, diarrhea, decreased appetite—infrequent.
Dizziness, confusion—infrequent.
Serious Adverse Effects
Allergic reactions: not reported.
Hallucinations—reported in clinical trials.
Feeling of inner motion or need to move (akathisia)—infrequent.

▷ **Possible Effects on Sexual Function:** Not defined as yet.

Possible Delayed Adverse Effects: Not yet defined.

Adverse Effects That May Mimic Natural Diseases or Disorders
Not defined.

Natural Diseases or Disorders That May Be Activated by These Drugs
Not defined.

Possible Effects on Laboratory Tests
Not defined.

CAUTION
1. This drug does **NOT** alter the course of Alzheimer's disease. Over time, benefits may be lost.

Precautions for Use
By Infants and Children: Safety and effectiveness for those under 18 years of age not established.
By Those Over 60 Years of Age: No specific changes are presently indicated.

▷ **Advisability of Use During Pregnancy**
Pregnancy Category: B. See Pregnancy Risk Categories at the back of this book.
Animal Studies: Data not available.
Human Studies: Adequate studies of pregnant women are not available. Consult your doctor.

Advisability of Use If Breast-Feeding
Presence of these drugs in breast milk: Unknown.
Monitor nursing infant closely, and discontinue drug or nursing if adverse effects develop.

Habit-Forming Potential: None.

Effects of Overdose: One case report of 400 mg lead to psychosis, restlessness, stupor and visual hallucinations.

Suggested Periodic Examinations While Taking These Drugs (at physician's discretion)
Assessment of mental status: periodically—check benefits or loss of benefits as Alzheimer's progresses.

▷ **While Taking This Drug, Observe the Following**
Foods: Can be taken without regard to food.
Herbal Medicines or Minerals: Data from appropriate scientific studies about combination of this medicine with ginkgo biloba is not available and cannot be recommended. A well-designed study of ginkgo biloba DID show it to be effective in mild to moderate Alzheimer's.
Beverages: No restrictions.
▷ *Alcohol:* Occasional small amounts of alcohol are okay. Frequent use may worsen memory problems and affect the liver.
Tobacco Smoking: Nicotine uses the same removal system as Memantine. Altered levels of either drug may happen. I advise everyone to quit smoking.
Marijuana Smoking: Additive dizziness may occur.
▷ *Other Drugs*
This medicine may *increase* the effects of
• medicines removed by the kidney using tubular secretion (talk to your doctor and pharmacist).
This medicine may *decrease* the effects of
• hydrochlorothiazide (see Drug Classes).
This medicine *taken concurrently* with
• cimetidine (Tagamet) or ranitidine (Zantac) may change blood levels of either drug.
• dextromethorphan (the DM in many cough and some sinus medicines) has not been evaluated and caution is advised.

- quinidine (various) may change blood levels of either drug.
- urine alkalinizers (sodium bicarbonate, others) will lead to higher than expected blood levels and possible toxicity. Lower memantine doses may be prudent.

▷ *Driving, Hazardous Activities:* This drug may cause sleepiness, confusion or dizziness. Restrict activities as necessary.

Aviation Note: This drug **may be a disqualification** for piloting. See a designated Aviation Medical Examiner.

Exposure to Sun: No restrictions.

Exposure to Heat: Increased sweating may occur. The combination of increased sweating and hot environments may lead to more rapid dehydration.

Discontinuation: No specific recommendations at present.

MEPERIDINE (me PER i deen)

Other Name: Pethidine **Introduced:** 1939 **Class:** Strong analgesic, opioids **Prescription:** USA: Yes **Controlled Drug:** USA: C-II*; Canada: Yes **Available as Generic:** Yes

Brand Names: Demerol, Demerol APAP [CD], Mepergan, Pethadol, ❧Pethidine

---

BENEFITS versus RISKS

Possible Benefits	*Possible Risks*
EFFECTIVE RELIEF OF MODERATE TO SEVERE PAIN NORMEPERIDINE METABOLITE	POTENTIAL FOR HABIT FORMATION (DEPENDENCE) ADVERSE REACTIONS: Weakness, fainting, disorientation, hallucinations, interference with urination, constipation

---

Author's Note: This profile has been shortened to make room for more effective medicines.

MERCAPTOPURINE (mer kap toh PYUR een)

Other Names: 6-mercaptopurine, 6-MP

Introduced: 1960 **Class:** Anticancer (antineoplastic), immunosuppressant **Prescription:** USA: Yes **Controlled Drug:** USA: No; Canada: No **Available as Generic:** USA: No; Canada: No

Brand Names: ❧Alti-Mercaptopurine, Purinethol

*See Schedules of Controlled Drugs at the back of this book.

BENEFITS versus RISKS

Possible Benefits	*Possible Risks*
EFFECTIVE TREATMENT OF CERTAIN ACUTE AND CHRONIC LEUKEMIAS AND LYMPHOMAS	BONE MARROW DEPRESSION (see Glossary)
Effective treatment of polycythemia vera	DRUG-INDUCED LIVER DAMAGE
Possibly effective treatment of Crohn's disease and ulcerative colitis	Rare gastrointestinal ulceration

---

▷ **Principal Uses**

As a Single Drug Product: Uses currently included in FDA-approved labeling: Combination treatment of acute lymphocytic leukemia.

Other (unlabeled) generally accepted uses: Treatment of (1) inflammatory bowel diseases (Crohn's disease and ulcerative colitis).

How This Drug Works: This drug interferes with specific stages of cell reproduction (tissue growth) by inhibiting the formation of DNA and RNA.

▷ **Widely Used Guidelines That Involve This Medicine (representative sample):** Please look at the section at the very beginning of this profile called "Class." Next, turn to Table 22 and you will find guidelines listed by the class involved!

Available Dosage Forms and Strengths

Tablets — 50 mg

▷ **Recommended Dosage Ranges** (Actual dose and schedule must be determined for each patient individually.)

Infants and Children: For acute lymphoblastic leukemia (induction dose)—2.5 mg per kg of body mass (to the nearest 25 mg) daily (roughly 50 mg for the average 5-year-old), in single or divided doses. If the platelets and white blood cell counts do not fall and clinical improvement is not acceptable after 4 weeks of the induction dosing, the dose may be increased to 5 mg per kg of body mass per day. If there is still no response, some centers give mercaptopurine as 75 mg per square meter on days 29–42. This is combined with vincristine, prednisone, and methotrexate. Maintenance therapy then occurs as in adult dosing.

12 to 60 Years of Age: For leukemia (induction)—initially 2.5 mg per kg of body mass (to the nearest 25 mg, usually 100–200 mg) daily, in single or divided doses, for 4 weeks. If the white blood cell or platelet counts do not fall and there is no clinical improvement, the dose may be increased as needed and tolerated to 5 mg per kg of body mass daily. For ongoing dose (maintenance): 1.5 to 2.5 mg per kg of body mass daily.

For inflammatory bowel disease (Crohn's)—1.5 mg per kg of body mass daily. The dose is subsequently adjusted to keep the platelet count above 100,000 and the white blood cell count above 4,500.

Over 60 Years of Age: Same as 12 to 60 years of age.

Author's Note: If mercaptopurine is given with allopurinol, the mercaptopurine dose should be lowered to a fourth or a third of the usual dose.

Conditions Requiring Dosing Adjustments

Liver Function: Used with caution and in decreased doses by patients with liver compromise. It is also a rare cause of liver toxicity.

Kidney Function: Dose should be decreased in kidney (renal) compromise. It is a rare cause of drug crystals in urine.

TPMT Negatives: Some patients do not have an enzyme called thiopurine methyltransferase (TPMT). The mercaptopurine dose is decreased by 10% for these patients.

▷ **Dosing Instructions:** The tablet may be crushed and taken with or following food to reduce stomach upset. Increasing the amount of water that you drink while taking this medicine can help avoid kidney problems. Talk to your doctor about the amount he or she would like you to drink. This medicine can lead to serious harm of a fetus. Talk to your doctor about appropriate contraception if you are a female of child-bearing age. If you forget a dose: take the missed dose as soon as you remember it, unless it's nearly time for your next dose—if that is the case, skip the missed dose and take the next dose right on schedule. DO NOT double doses. Talk with your doctor and pharmacist if you find yourself missing doses.

Usual Duration of Use: Use on a regular schedule for 4 to 6 weeks determines effectiveness in inducing remission in leukemia; continual use for 2 to 3 months determines benefit in treating inflammatory bowel disease. Long-term use requires periodic physician evaluation.

Typical Treatment Goals and Measurements (Outcomes and Markers)
Leukemia: The goal is to improve clinical signs and symptoms, and control leukemia while avoiding myelosuppression and liver toxicity. Checks of blood platelets, hematocrits, and white blood cell counts are required. Periodic checks of liver function tests help detect liver problems early. Bone marrow tests help define changes in peripheral blood.

▷ **This Drug Should Not Be Taken If**
- you have had an allergic reaction to it previously.
- you have a solid tumor or lymphoma (this drug is not indicated).
- you have prior resistance to the drug.
- you are pregnant. (Ask your physician for guidance.)

▷ **Inform Your Physician Before Taking This Drug If**
- you have a history of drug-induced bone marrow depression.
- you have impaired liver or kidney function.
- you are not using any contraception.
- you have gout.
- you are taking allopurinol (the mercaptopurine dose must be reduced).
- you have inflammatory bowel disease.
- you do not understand the steps needed to dispose of any vomit or urine.
- you have been exposed recently to chicken pox or herpes zoster (shingles).
- you are taking any of the following drugs: allopurinol, probenecid, sulfinpyrazone, anticoagulants, immunosuppressants.

Possible Side Effects (natural, expected, and unavoidable drug actions)
Bone marrow depression (see Glossary). Abnormally increased blood uric acid levels; possible urate kidney stones, hyperpigmentation of the skin. Possible drug fever. Serum sickness.

▷ **Possible Adverse Effects** (unusual, unexpected, and infrequent reactions)
If any of the following develop, consult your physician promptly for guidance.
Mild Adverse Effects
Allergic reactions: skin rash, itching, joint pain—case reports.
Headache, weakness—infrequent.

Loss of appetite, mouth and lip sores, nausea, vomiting, diarrhea—infrequent.

Serious Adverse Effects

Liver damage with jaundice (see Glossary)—infrequent.

Kidney damage: fever, cloudy or bloody urine—rare.

Pancreatitis (especially in patients taking this medicine for inflammatory bowel disease)—infrequent.

Gastrointestinal ulceration: stomach pain, bloody or black stools.

Increased cancer risk (carcinogen): one case report of cancer in a patient with bowel disease—possible.

▷ **Possible Effects on Sexual Function:** Suppression of sperm production. Cessation of menstruation—case reports.

Possible Delayed Adverse Effects: Bone marrow depression may not be apparent during early treatment.

▷ **Adverse Effects That May Mimic Natural Diseases or Disorders**

Drug-induced liver damage may suggest viral hepatitis.

Natural Diseases or Disorders That May Be Activated by This Drug

Latent gout, peptic ulcer disease, inflammatory bowel disease.

Possible Effects on Laboratory Tests

Complete blood cell counts: decreased red cells, hemoglobin, white cells, and platelets.

Blood glucose levels: falsely increased with SMA testing.

Blood uric acid levels: increased.

Liver function tests: increased enzymes (ALT/GPT, AST/GOT, and alkaline phosphatase) or bilirubin.

Kidney function tests: increased blood urea nitrogen (BUN) and creatinine.

Sperm counts: decreased.

CAUTION

1. Make sure you get all laboratory tests ordered.
2. Call your doctor at the first sign of infection or abnormal bleeding or bruising.
3. Inform your physician promptly if you become pregnant.
4. It is best to avoid immunizations while taking this drug and to avoid contact with people who have recently taken oral poliovirus vaccine. If possible, the vaccinations can be given BEFORE therapy is started.
5. Call your doctor if you see a different doctor who finds a significant fall in your blood tests (this medicine must usually then be stopped if the test was accurate).

Precautions for Use

By Infants and Children: No specific problems anticipated.

By Those Over 60 Years of Age: Increased risk of bone marrow depression. Periodic blood counts are mandatory.

▷ **Advisability of Use During Pregnancy**

Pregnancy Category: D. See Pregnancy Risk Categories at the back of this book.

Animal Studies: Rat studies reveal toxic effects on the embryo.

Human Studies: Adequate studies of pregnant women are not available. Known to cause abortions and premature births.

Avoid drug during entire pregnancy if possible. Use a nonhormonal method of contraception.

Advisability of Use If Breast-Feeding

Presence of this drug in breast milk: Unknown.

Avoid drug or refrain from nursing.

Habit-Forming Potential: None.

Effects of Overdose: Headache, dizziness, abdominal pain, nausea.

Possible Effects of Long-Term Use: Development of new malignant diseases.

Suggested Periodic Examinations While Taking This Drug (at physician's discretion)
> Complete blood cell counts.
> Blood uric acid levels.
> Amylase and lipase.
> Liver and kidney function tests.

▷ **While Taking This Drug, Observe the Following**
> *Foods:* No restrictions.
> *Herbal Medicines or Minerals:* Echinacea: Some patients use echinacea to attempt to boost their immune systems. Unfortunately, use of echinacea is not recommended in people with damaged immune systems. This herb may also actually weaken any immune system if it is used too often or for too long a time. Herbals that have known toxic effects on the liver (such as kava, eucalyptus, and valerian) should be avoided as they could lead to additive toxicity.
> *Beverages:* No restrictions. Drink liquids liberally, up to 2 quarts daily. Ask your doctor about the specific amount he or she wants you to drink.
> ▷ *Alcohol:* Avoid completely.
> *Tobacco Smoking:* No interactions expected. I advise everyone to quit smoking.
> ▷ *Other Drugs*
> Mercaptopurine may *decrease* the effects of
> • warfarin (Coumadin); the INR (prothrombin time or protime) should be checked more frequently.
> The following drug may *increase* the effects of mercaptopurine:
> • allopurinol (Zyloprim). Doses must be reduced to 33% or even as low as 25% of the usual dose if these two medicines are to be combined.
> Mercaptopurine *taken concurrently* with
> • amphotericin B (Abelcet) may increase risk of kidney toxicity or spasm of the bronchi.
> • live-virus vaccines (such as smallpox) may lead to life-threatening infections.
> • methotrexate (Rheumatrex, Mexate) can result in mercaptopurine toxicity.
> • olsalazine (Dipentum) may increase risk of bone marrow depression.
> ▷ *Driving, Hazardous Activities:* No restrictions.
> *Aviation Note:* The use of this drug *may be a disqualification* for piloting. Consult a designated Aviation Medical Examiner.
> *Exposure to Sun:* No restrictions.
> *Discontinuation:* To be determined by your physician.

MESALAMINE (me SAL a meen)

Other Names: Mesalazine, 5-aminosalicylic acid, 5-ASA

Introduced: 1982 **Class:** Bowel anti-inflammatory **Prescription:** USA: Yes **Controlled Drug:** USA: No; Canada: No **Available as Generic:** USA: No; Canada: No

Brand Names: Asacol, ✤Mesasal, Pentasa, ✤Quintasa, Rowasa, ✤Salofalk

---

BENEFITS versus RISKS

Possible Benefits	*Possible Risks*
EFFECTIVE SUPPRESSION OF INFLAMMATORY BOWEL DISEASE	Allergic reactions: acute intolerance syndrome, drug-induced kidney damage

---

▷ **Principal Uses**

As a Single Drug Product: Uses currently included in FDA-approved labeling: Treatment of active mild to moderate ulcerative colitis, proctosigmoiditis, and proctitis.

Other (unlabeled) generally accepted uses: (1) May help improve semen quality that had been damaged by prior sulfasalazine treatment; (2) can ease canker sores (aphthous ulcers); (3) has a steroid-sparing effect in Crohn's disease; (4) used to maintain remission in ulcerative colitis.

How This Drug Works: Suppresses prostaglandin (and related compounds) formation, chemicals causing inflammation, tissue destruction, and diarrhea— the main problems in ulcerative colitis and proctitis.

▷ **Widely Used Guidelines That Involve This Medicine (representative sample):**
Please look at the section at the very beginning of this profile called "Class." Next, turn to Table 22 and you will find guidelines listed by the class involved!

Available Dosage Forms and Strengths
Capsules, timed release — 400 mg
Rectal suspension — 4 g per 60-mL unit, 1 gram, 2 and 4 gram per 100-mil (Canada)
Suppositories (Canada) — 250 mg
Suppositories — 500 mg (US and Canada)
Tablets, enteric coated — 250 mg, 500 mg
Tablets, sustained release — 250 mg, 500 mg

▷ **Recommended Dosage Ranges** (Actual dose and schedule must be determined for each patient individually.)
Infants and Children: Dose not established.
12 to 60 Years of Age: Active ulcerative colitis: Immediate release (Asacol)—800 mg 3 times a day for 6 weeks. Controlled release (Pentasa)—1,000 mg 4 times a day for up to 8 weeks.
Maintenance of ulcerative colitis remission: Immediate release (Asacol)—1,600 mg divided into equal doses.
Crohn's disease (Pentasa): 1,000 mg taken 3 times a day.
Over 60 Years of Age: Same as 12 to 60 years of age.

Conditions Requiring Dosing Adjustments
Liver Function: Guidelines for dose adjustment not available. Drug changed by the liver and colon wall to Ac-5-ASA.
Kidney Function: This drug should be used with caution in kidney compromise.

▷ **Dosing Instructions**
Rectal suspension: Use as a retention enema at bedtime. If possible, empty the rectum before inserting suspension; try to retain the suspension all night.
Tablets: Best taken with 8 ounces of water on an empty stomach, 1 hour before or 2 hours after eating. Also can be taken with or following food to reduce stomach upset. Sustained release tablet should be swallowed whole without

alteration. If you forget a dose: take the missed dose as soon as you remember it, unless it's nearly time for your next dose—if that is the case, skip the missed dose and take the next dose right on schedule. Talk with your doctor if you find yourself missing doses.

Usual Duration of Use: Regular use for 1 to 3 weeks determines benefits controlling ulcerative colitis. Long-term use (months to years) requires periodic physician evaluation.

Typical Treatment Goals and Measurements (Outcomes and Markers)

Inflammatory bowel disease: The goal is to cause (induce) a remission and maintain it. Symptoms that will resolve include rectal bleeding and diarrhea. More involved exams will reveal an absence of bowel ulceration and easing of friability or granularity of the bowel itself.

Possible Advantages of This Drug

Does not cause bone marrow or blood cell disorders. Does not inhibit sperm production or function. Better side effect profile than sulfasalazine. May actually (5-ASA form) help prevent risk of colorectal cancer.

▷ **This Drug Should Not Be Taken If**
- you have had an allergic reaction to it previously.
- you have severely impaired kidney function.
- you have a known sulfite allergy. (Rectal suspension should NOT be used.)
- you have active ulcer disease.

▷ **Inform Your Physician Before Taking This Drug If**
- you are allergic to aspirin (or other salicylates), olsalazine, or sulfasalazine.
- you are allergic by nature: history of hay fever, asthma, hives, eczema.
- you have impaired liver or kidney function.
- you have a history of a blood-clotting (coagulation) disorder.
- you develop chest pain or trouble while taking this medicine (pericarditis happens rarely).
- you have a history of low white blood cell counts.
- you are taking other medicines that affect the bone marrow. Discuss this with your doctor.
- you are currently taking sulfasalazine (Azulfidine).

Possible Side Effects (natural, expected, and unavoidable drug actions)

Anal irritation (with use of rectal suspension or suppositories). Flu-like syndrome with oral mesalamine use.

▷ **Possible Adverse Effects** (unusual, unexpected, and infrequent reactions)

If any of the following develop, consult your physician promptly for guidance.

Mild Adverse Effects

Allergic reaction: skin rash.

Headache (may be dose related), hair loss—rare.

Blurred vision, ringing in the ears—possible.

Paresthesias, neck and joint pain, dizziness, cough—infrequent.

Nausea, stomach pain, excessive gas—infrequent.

Serious Adverse Effects

Allergic reactions: acute intolerance syndrome (fever, skin rash, severe headache, severe stomach pain, bloody diarrhea).

Depression or confusion—reported.

Kidney damage (nephrosis, interstitial nephritis)—rare.

Peripheral neuropathy—rare.

Pancreatitis, peptic ulcers or hepatitis—rare.

Low white blood cell or platelet counts (thrombocytopenia) or anemia—rare.

Heart toxicity (myocarditis, pericarditis, pericardial effusions)—case reports.

Lung toxicity (interstitial infiltrates)—case report.

▷ **Possible Effects on Sexual Function:** Oligospermia and infertility have been reported with sulfasalazine, but NOT with mesalamine.

Possible Effects on Laboratory Tests

Increased liver function tests.

CAUTION

1. Report promptly any signs of acute intolerance syndrome. Stop taking drug.
2. Shake the rectal suspension thoroughly before administering.
3. This medicine is a salicylate and as such is a cousin of aspirin. Avoid taking this medicine in combination with other medicines or during other conditions in which aspirin is contraindicated. Salicylate toxicity is possible.
4. Mesalamine and other medicines that belong to the sulfasalazine family have been implicated as possible causes of heart toxicity in case reports. Call your doctor if you are taking mesalamine or a medicine related to sulfasalazine and start to have difficulty breathing and/or pain in the chest.

Precautions for Use

By Infants and Children: Safety and effectiveness by those under 12 years of age are not established.

By Those Over 60 Years of Age: None.

▷ **Advisability of Use During Pregnancy**

Pregnancy Category: B. See Pregnancy Risk Categories at the back of this book.

Animal Studies: No drug-induced birth defects found in rat or rabbit studies.

Human Studies: Adequate studies of pregnant women are not available.

Use this drug only if clearly needed. Ask your physician for guidance.

Advisability of Use If Breast-Feeding

Presence of this drug in breast milk: Yes.

Avoid drug or refrain from nursing.

Habit-Forming Potential: None.

Effects of Overdose: Headache, dizziness, nausea, vomiting, abdominal cramping.

Possible Effects of Long-Term Use: None reported.

Suggested Periodic Examinations While Taking This Drug (at physician's discretion)

Kidney function tests.

Urinalysis.

▷ **While Taking This Drug, Observe the Following**

Foods: Decreases 5-ASA levels. Follow prescribed diet.

Herbal Medicines or Minerals: Flaxseed, peppermint oil, and psyllium husk have Commission E monograph indications for irritable bowel syndrome. This is NOT the same as ulcerative colitis, and those products have not been studied in ulcerative colitis. Aloe, buckhorn berry or bark, cascara sagrada bark, rhubarb root, and senna should not be taken by people living with ulcerative colitis.

Beverages: No restrictions. May be taken with milk.

▷ *Alcohol:* No interactions expected.
Tobacco Smoking: No interactions expected. I advise everyone to quit smoking.
▷ *Other Drugs*
Mesalamine *taken concurrently* with
- alendronate (Fosamax) may increase stomach or intestinal upset risks (because of salicylate) and would decrease the alendronate absorbed.
- ardeparin (Normiflo), dalteparin (Fragmin), enoxaparin (Lovenox), or other low molecular weight heparins may increase risk of bleeding (hemorrhage).
- aspirin or other salicylates may increase risk of salicylate toxicity.
- varicella vaccine (Varivax) may result in Reye's syndrome; avoid taking this medicine for 6 weeks following varicella vaccine.
- warfarin (Coumadin) may blunt warfarin effectiveness. More frequent INRs are prudent.
▷ *Driving, Hazardous Activities:* No restrictions.
Aviation Note: The use of this drug is *probably not a disqualification* for piloting. Consult a designated Aviation Medical Examiner.
Exposure to Sun: No restrictions.

METAPROTERENOL (met a proh TER e nohl)

Other Name: Orciprenaline

Introduced: 1964 **Class:** Antiasthmatic, bronchodilator **Prescription:** USA: Yes **Controlled Drug:** USA: No; Canada: No **Available as Generic:** Yes

Brand Names: ✤Alti-Orciprenaline, Alupent, Arm-a-Med, Dey-Dose, Dey-Lute, Metaprel, Metaprel Nasal Inhaler, Prometa

BENEFITS versus RISKS	
Possible Benefits	*Possible Risks*
VERY EFFECTIVE RELIEF OF BRONCHOSPASM	Increased blood pressure Fine hand tremor Fast heart rate Irregular heart rhythm (with excessive use)

▷ **Principal Uses**
As a Single Drug Product: Uses currently included in FDA-approved labeling: (1) Relieves acute bronchial asthma and reduces the frequency and severity of chronic, recurrent asthmatic attacks; (2) used to relieve reversible bronchospasm associated with chronic bronchitis and emphysema; (3) eases symptoms in obstructive bronchial disease.
Other (unlabeled) generally accepted uses: Some use in stopping premature labor (threatened abortion).

How This Drug Works: Dilates those bronchial tubes that are in sustained constriction, increasing the size of airways and improving breathing.

▷ **Widely Used Guidelines That Involve This Medicine (representative sample):** Please look at the section at the very beginning of this profile called "Class." Next, turn to Table 22 and you will find guidelines listed by the class involved!

Available Dosage Forms and Strengths
Nasal inhaler — 0.65 mg per metered dose
Oral suspension — 10 mg/5 mL
Powder for inhalation — 0.65 mg per inhalation
Solution for nebulizer — 0.4%, 0.6%, 5%
Syrup — 10 mg/5 mL
Tablets — 10 mg, 20 mg

▷ **Usual Adult Dosage Ranges:** *Inhaler*: 2 or 3 inhalations as often as every 3 to 4 hours; do not exceed 12 inhalations daily.

Hand nebulizer: 5 to 15 inhalations every 4 hours; do not exceed 40 inhalations daily.

Syrup and tablets: 20 mg up to every 6 to 8 hours.

Note: Actual dose and schedule must be determined for each patient individually.

Conditions Requiring Dosing Adjustments
Liver Function: Specific guidelines for dosing adjustment for patients with liver compromise are not usually indicated.

Kidney Function: Dosing changes are not indicated in kidney compromise.

▷ **Dosing Instructions:** May be taken on empty stomach or with food or milk. Tablets should not be crushed. For aerosol and nebulizer, follow the written instructions carefully in order to get the needed dose. Do not overuse. If symptoms are not controlled with most-frequent dosing, call your doctor. If you forget a dose: take the missed dose as soon as you remember it, then take the remaining daily doses at evenly spaced intervals. If it's nearly time for your next dose, skip the missed dose and take the next dose right on schedule. Talk with your doctor and pharmacist if you find yourself missing doses.

Usual Duration of Use: According to individual requirements. Do not use beyond the time necessary to stop episodes of asthma.

Typical Treatment Goals and Measurements (Outcomes and Markers)
Asthma: Beta-adrenergic medicines like this one are used to prevent or treat reversible spasms of the bronchial tubes. The peak effect happens 2 to 4 hours after dosing. Inhaled use often gives improvement in FEV-1 in 5 to 30 minutes. Patient signs such as wheeze and symptoms (rales and rhonchi) should ease. If the usual benefit is not realized, call your doctor.

▷ **This Drug Should Not Be Taken If**
- you had an allergic reaction to it previously.
- you currently have an irregular heart rhythm.
- you are taking, or have taken within the past 2 weeks, any monoamine oxidase (MAO) type A inhibitor drug (see Drug Classes).

▷ **Inform Your Physician Before Taking This Drug If**
- you are overly sensitive to other sympathetic stimulant drugs.
- you currently use epinephrine (Adrenalin, Primatene Mist, etc.) to relieve asthmatic breathing.
- you have any type of heart or circulatory disorder, especially high blood pressure or coronary heart disease.
- you have diabetes or an overactive thyroid gland (hyperthyroidism).
- you are taking any form of digitalis or any stimulant drug.

Possible Side Effects (natural, expected, and unavoidable drug actions)
Aerosol—dryness or irritation of mouth or throat, altered taste, nervousness. Tablet—nervousness, palpitation.

▷ **Possible Adverse Effects** (unusual, unexpected, and infrequent reactions)

If any of the following develop, consult your physician promptly for guidance.

Mild Adverse Effects
Headache, dizziness, restlessness, insomnia, fine tremor of hands—possible to infrequent.

Increased sweating; muscle cramps in arms and legs—case reports.

Nausea, heartburn, vomiting—possible.

Serious Adverse Effects
Rapid or irregular heart rhythm, intensification of angina, increased blood pressure—possible.

Hallucinations and psychosis—rare.

Paradoxical spasm of the bronchi (bronchospasm)—rare.

▷ **Possible Effects on Sexual Function:** None reported.

Natural Diseases or Disorders That May Be Activated by This Drug
Latent coronary artery disease, diabetes or high blood pressure.

Possible Effects on Laboratory Tests
Urine sugar tests: positive (unreliable results with Benedict's solution).

CAUTION
1. Combined use of this drug by aerosol inhalation with beclomethasone aerosol (Beclovent, Vanceril) may increase the risk of toxicity due to fluorocarbon propellants (these propellants are being phased out). Use this aerosol 20 to 30 minutes before beclomethasone aerosol, as this will reduce the risk of toxicity and enhance the penetration of beclomethasone.
2. *Avoid excessive use of aerosol inhalation.* Excessive or prolonged use of this drug by inhalation can reduce its effectiveness and cause serious heart rhythm disturbances, including cardiac arrest.
3. Do not combine this drug with epinephrine. These 2 drugs may be used alternately if an interval of 4 hours is allowed between doses.
4. If you do not respond to your usually effective dose, ask your doctor for help. Do not increase the size or frequency of the dose without your physician's approval.

Precautions for Use
By Infants and Children: Safety and effectiveness of the aerosol and nebulized solution are not established for children under 12 years of age.

By mouth (oral) dosing in children 2–6 years old—1.3 to 2.6 mg per kg of body mass per day, divided into equal doses and given 3 to 4 times a day. In children 6 to 9 years old or less than 60 pounds—10 mg per dose 3 to 4 times a day. Children over 9 years old or over 60 pounds—20 mg 3 or 4 times a day.

Safety and effectiveness of the syrup and tablet are not established for children under 6 years of age.

By Those Over 60 Years of Age: Avoid excessive and continual use. If acute asthma is not relieved promptly, other drugs will have to be tried. Watch for nervousness, palpitations, irregular heart rhythm, and muscle tremors. Use with extreme caution if you have hardening of the arteries, heart disease, or high blood pressure.

▷ **Advisability of Use During Pregnancy**
Pregnancy Category: C. See Pregnancy Risk Categories at the back of this book.
Animal Studies: Significant birth defects reported in rabbit studies.
Human Studies: Adequate studies of pregnant women are not available.
Avoid during first 3 months. Use in final 6 months only if clearly needed.

Advisability of Use If Breast-Feeding
Presence of this drug in breast milk: Unknown.
Avoid drug or refrain from nursing.

Habit-Forming Potential: None.

Effects of Overdose: Nervousness, palpitation, rapid heart rate, sweating, headache, tremor, vomiting, chest pain.

Possible Effects of Long-Term Use: Loss of effectiveness (see Caution above).

Suggested Periodic Examinations While Taking This Drug (at physician's discretion)
Blood pressure measurements.
Evaluation of heart status.

▷ **While Taking This Drug, Observe the Following**
Foods: No restrictions.
Herbal Medicines or Minerals: Using St. John's wort, guarana, ma huang (no longer on the market), bitter orange, country mallow, ephedrine-like compounds, mate or kola while taking this medicine may result in unacceptable central nervous system stimulation. Fir or pine needle oil should NOT be used by asthmatics. Ephedra alone does carry a German Commission E monograph indication for asthma treatment. If you are allergic to plants in the Asteraceae family (aster, chrysanthemum, daisy, or ragweed), you may also be allergic to echinacea, chamomile, feverfew, and St. John's wort.
Beverages: Avoid excessive use of caffeine-containing beverages: coffee, tea, cola, chocolate.
▷ *Alcohol:* No interactions expected.
Tobacco Smoking: No interactions expected. I advise everyone to quit smoking.
▷ *Other Drugs*
Metaproterenol *taken concurrently* with
• albuterol (Proventil, others) may result in increased heart (cardiovascular) side effects.
• monoamine oxidase (MAO) type A inhibitors (see Drug Classes) may cause excessive increase in blood pressure and undesirable heart stimulation.
• phenothiazines (see Drug Classes) may blunt some effects of this drug.
▷ *Driving, Hazardous Activities:* Usually no restrictions. Use caution if excessive nervousness or dizziness occurs.
Aviation Note: The use of this drug *is a disqualification* for piloting. Consult a designated Aviation Medical Examiner.
Exposure to Sun: No restrictions.
Heavy Exercise or Exertion: Use caution. Excessive exercise can induce asthma in sensitive individuals.

METFORMIN (met FOR min)

Introduced: 1995   **Class:**   Antidiabetes drug, oral; biguanide   **Prescription:**   USA: Yes   **Controlled Drug:**   USA: No; Canada: No   **Available as Generic:**   USA: Yes (Geneva extended release generic); Canada: Yes

Brand Names: ♣Apo-Metformin, Avandamet [CD], ♣Dom-Metformin, Glucophage, Glucophage XR, Glucovance [CD], ♣Glycon, Metaglip [CD], ♣Novo-Metformin, PMS-Metformin, Riomet, Riva-Metformin

Warning: Avoid excessive alcohol. Alcohol can cause lactic acidosis, a condition that metformin can also rarely cause. (See note in Conditions Requiring Dosage Adjustments below.)

BENEFITS versus RISKS

Possible Benefits	*Possible Risks*
USE IN HIGH-RISK PATIENTS MAY ACTUALLY PREVENT DIABETES (31% IN A LARGE STUDY)	LACTIC ACIDOSIS (see Caution below)
COMBINATION USE WITH ROSIGLITAZONE (AVANDIA) MAY SLOW THE PROGRESSION OF DIABETES	Possible anemia with long-term use (most likely due to decreased B_{12})
COMBINATION USE WITH ROSIGLITAZONE MAY PREVENT LONG-TERM COMPLICATIONS OF DIABETES	
EFFECTIVE GLUCOSE CONTROL WITHOUT INSULIN INJECTION	
A PRESENTATION AT AN AMERICAN DIABETES CONFERENCE FOUND EXCELLENT RESULTS WHEN METFORMIN WAS COMBINED WITH AN INSULIN SPRAYED INTO THE MOUTH (ORALIN)	
MAY BE USED CONCURRENTLY WITH A SULFONYLUREA	
DOES NOT LEAD TO WEIGHT GAIN	
TAKEN BY MOUTH, VERSUS INJECTION OF INSULIN	
COMBINATION WITH GLIPIZIDE OFFERS IMPROVED BLOOD SUGAR CONTROL	
Usually avoids excessive lowering of blood sugar	
Favorable effects on lipids	

▷ **Principal Uses**

As a Single Drug Product: Uses currently included in FDA-approved labeling: (1) Used in combination with diet restrictions to treat non-insulin-dependent diabetes (type 2); (2) can be combined with a sulfonylurea (see Drug Classes) for patients who do not have an adequate response to diet restrictions. May also be combined with insulin.

Other (unlabeled) generally accepted uses: (1) May be used as single-agent therapy to overcome insulin resistance; (2) could help nondiabetic, obese women with high blood pressure in helping improve blood pressure and lipid profile; (3) may help insulin-dependent (type 1) diabetics decrease insulin requirements; (4) may have a role in treating polycystic ovary syndrome (PCOS); (5) combination use with rosiglitazone may slow the progression of diabetes; (6) use in patients at risk for diabetes may PREVENT diabetes from happening (31% decrease in a large study—see Knowler, W.C. in Sources).

As a Combination Drug Product [CD]: Metformin is available combined with glyburide (Glucovance) as initial treatment of type 2 diabetes or when blood sugar (glucose) control goals are not met by either medicine alone. Also available combined with glipizide (Metaglip) and rosiglitazone (Avandamet).

How This Drug Works: Decreases sugar (glucose) production in the liver. It also increases sensitivity of the body to insulin.

▷ **Widely Used Guidelines That Involve This Medicine (representative sample):** Please look at the section at the very beginning of this profile called "Class." Next, turn to Table 22 and you will find guidelines listed by the class involved!

Available Dosage Forms and Strengths

Tablets — 500 mg, 850 mg, 1,000 mg

Tablets, combination (Glucovance) — 250 mg metformin and 1.25 mg glyburide, 500 mg metformin and 2.5 or 5.0 mg glyburide

Tablets, combination (Metaglip) — 250 mg metformin and 2.5 mg glipizide, 500 mg metformin and 5.0 mg glipizide

Tablets, combination (Avandamet) — 500 mg metformin and 2 mg rosiglitazone

Tablets, extended release — 500 mg

▷ **Recommended Dosage Ranges** (Actual dose and schedule must be determined for each patient individually.)

Infants and Children: Immediate release metformin is NOT recommended for children under 10 years old. For ages 10 to 16 years, the starting dose is 500 mg twice daily with meals. Dosing can be increased as needed and tolerated by 500 mg every 7 days to a maximum of 2,000 mg a day. Doses of this size are separated into equal doses and given 2 or 3 times a day based on results and patient tolerance. The safety and effectiveness for the XR form have not been established in that population.

16 to 60 Years of Age: Dosing is started at 500 mg twice daily. It is best to take this medicine with the morning and evening meals. Doses can be increased as needed and tolerated by 500 mg increments every 7 days. Some clinicians use 850 mg once daily. If the 850 mg dose is used, dosing is increased as needed and tolerated at 14-day intervals. Maximum dose is 2,500 mg if the 500 mg tablets are used, and 2,550 mg if the 850 mg tablets are used. Doses up to 2,000 mg are separated into 2 doses, but doses higher than this are best divided into 3 daily doses.

Extended Release Form: Dosing is started with 500 mg once daily with the evening meal. With this form, doses can be increased as needed and tolerated by 500 mg a day every 7 days up to a maximum of 2,000 mg a day. If the 2,000 mg daily dose does not achieve goals (see below), some patients benefit from 1,000 mg twice daily. If after 28 days of regular medicine use (good adherence), goals are still not met, a sulfonylurea (see Drug Classes) may be added. Each medicine dose should be carefully changed to obtain the best control of blood sugar. Once again, good control is critical. If 1 to 3 months of maximum metformin and sulfonylurea doses does not meet goals, the next step is to start insulin treatment, with or without metformin.

Combination form: (Avandamet): Fasting plasma sugar (glucose) is checked. For patients not well controlled on metformin alone: Dosing is started with a total daily dose of 4 mg of rosiglitazone plus the previous daily dose of metformin. For example, for people previously getting 1,000 mg of metformin a day, dosing is started with 1 of the 2 mg rosiglitazone/500 mg metformin tablets twice a day.

Combination form: (Glucovance): Dosing is started with the 1.25 glyburide and 250 mg metformin once a day with meals in people who have a fasting blood sugar more than 200 mg/dL or a glycosylated hemoglobin (hemoglobin A1C) more than 9%.

Combination form: (Metaglip): Dosing is started with the 1.25 glyburide and 250 mg metformin once a day with breakfast. The dose is increased as needed and tolerated every 14 days to 10/2000 in equally divided doses with morning and evening meals.

Over 60 Years of Age: Some patients may have acceptable blood sugar control with as little as 500 mg daily. If this dose is used, take it with the morning meal. Dose may be slowly increased if needed.

Conditions Requiring Dosing Adjustments

Liver Function: This drug should not be used by patients with liver compromise. This is a risk factor for lactic acidosis.

Kidney Function: NOT to be used in kidney disease (renal dysfunction) defined as females with steady-state creatinine levels greater than 1.4 or males with levels greater than 1.5.

▷ **Dosing Instructions:** This drug should be taken with the morning and evening meals if it has been prescribed on a twice-daily basis. One study found that use of metformin with insulin at bedtime not only lowered risk of excessively low blood sugar (hypoglycemia), but also prevented weight gain. If you forget a dose: take the missed dose as soon as you remember it, unless it's nearly time for your next dose—if that is the case, skip the missed dose and take the next dose right on schedule. Talk with your doctor if you find yourself missing doses. Follow-up of benefits of this medicine involve finger stick blood sugar testing. Talk to your doctor about how often to check your blood sugar and what to check it with. (See Table 18, Patient Power and Home Test Kits).

Usual Duration of Use: Continual use on a regular schedule for a week is usually necessary to determine this drug's effectiveness in establishing tight glucose control. A month or more of continuous use will be needed before an effect on glycosylated hemoglobin (a measure of past success of glucose control) is seen. Long-term use (months to years) requires periodic evaluation of response and dose adjustment. See your doctor on a regular basis.

Typical Treatment Goals and Measurements (Outcomes and Markers)

Blood sugar: The general goal for blood sugar is to return it to the usual "normal" range (generally 80–120 mg/dL), while avoiding risks of excessively low blood sugar. One study (UKPDS) used a fasting plasma sugar (glucose) of less than 108 mg/dL. DCCT found that tight control of blood sugar helped avoid long-term diabetic complications (see Sources). For Prediabetes (see below): one goal of the use of this medicine may actually be to PREVENT development of diabetes.

Fructosamine and glycosylated hemoglobin: Fructosamine levels (a measure of the past 2 to 3 weeks of blood sugar control) should be less than or equal to 310 micromoles per liter. Glycosylated hemoglobin or hemoglobin A1C (a measure of the past 2–3 months of blood sugar control) should be less than or equal to 7.0%. Some clinicians recommend 6.5% with the caveat that you must be more aware of the signs and symptoms of low blood sugar and know what to do if this happens.

Possible Advantages of This Drug
Does not lead to weight gain.

Can be used (because of its mechanism of action) in combination with a sulfonylurea.

Can be used to overcome insulin resistance.

Can be used in combination with rosiglitazone to slow diabetes progression and help avoid long-term diabetes complications.

Does not cause excessive lowering of blood sugar (hypoglycemia) when used as monotherapy.

Combined with glipizide (Metaglip) to offer better (tighter) blood sugar control while being less likely to lead to prolonged low blood sugar like some other possible combinations.

Data from the Diabetes Prevention Program (DPP) showed that use of metformin in high-risk patients PREVENTED diabetes in 31% of those studied.

Currently a "Drug of Choice"
For helping to PREVENT development of diabetes. Also a "drug of choice" for treatment of hyperglycemia in the elderly.

▷ This Drug Should Not Be Taken If
- you had an allergic reaction to it previously.
- you have impaired kidneys (serum creatinine greater than 1.4 for females or 1.5 for males) as this potentially increases the risk of lactic acidosis).
- you have congestive heart failure (CHF) and take medicines to treat it (increases risk of lactic acidosis).
- you have liver disease.
- you are an alcoholic.
- you have a heart or lung insufficiency (increased lactic acidosis risk).
- you are going to have a radiology test that uses iodinated contrast media (ask your doctor because this medicine should be stopped before or at the time of the test, then kidney function checked and found to be in the normal range; then metformin can be started 48 hours after).
- you have chronic metabolic acidosis or ketoacidosis.
- you are breast-feeding your infant.

▷ Inform Your Physician Before Taking This Drug If
- you are planning to have surgery soon.
- you have a serious infection (increases risk of lactic acidosis).
- you drink excessive amounts of alcohol (talk with your doctor) or are elderly (increases lactic acidosis risk).
- you have a history of megaloblastic anemia.
- you are pregnant (insulin is the drug of choice).
- you have seen another doctor and ketoacidosis was diagnosed.
- you are unsure how much to take or how often to take it.

Possible Side Effects (natural, expected, and unavoidable drug actions)
Low blood sugar (hypoglycemia) if meals are skipped or if you exercise strenuously without eating. Blocking of absorption of vitamin B_{12} and development of anemia (some 7% have lowered B_{12} with no anemia).

▷ Possible Adverse Effects (unusual, unexpected, and infrequent reactions)
If any of the following develop, consult your physician promptly for guidance.

Mild Adverse Effects
Allergic reaction: rare rash.

Metallic taste—infrequent and usually resolves.

Anorexia, nausea, vomiting, or diarrhea—up to 30% when started and then they often subside.

Headache, nervousness, dizziness, or tiredness—infrequent.

Serious Adverse Effects

Allergic reactions: not reported.

Idiosyncratic reactions: liver toxicity—rare.

Lactic acidosis—very rare (Less than 0.1%, but more likely if used in patients with kidney disease or congestive heart failure that requires medicines—which is why current FDA labeling warns against use in those patients. Lactic acidosis is usually not dramatic in signs or symptoms—breathing difficulty [respiratory distress], low body temp [hypothermia], vague abdominal pain, muscle aches [myalgias], and/or increasing sleepiness).

Lowered vitamin B_{12} levels and resultant anemia (megaloblastic)—rare.

Destruction of red blood cells (hemolysis)—case report.

Drug-induced porphyria—case reports.

All oral hypoglycemic agents carry a label indicating that they may increase risk of cardiovascular death (based on a 1975 study of tolbutamide and phenformin)—possible.

Liver toxicity—2 case reports.

▷ **Possible Effects on Sexual Function:** None reported.

Possible Delayed Adverse Effects: Low vitamin B_{12} levels and anemia (megaloblastic).

▷ **Adverse Effects That May Mimic Natural Diseases or Disorders**

Acidosis may mimic ketoacidosis, which is seen in diabetics.

Natural Diseases or Disorders That May Be Activated by This Drug

None reported.

Possible Effects on Laboratory Tests

Blood glucose: decreased.

A1C: trending toward 7 or 6.5 %—a beneficial effect.

Vitamin B_{12}: lowered.

Liver function tests: possibly increased.

CAUTION

1. This drug may cause lactic acidosis. Ask your doctor for signs or symptoms that may occur.
2. Drugs in this class (phenformin or tolbutamide) were reported to increase risk of cardiovascular death based on an old study. Although there is no data to support that effect for this medicine, patients should be closely followed.
3. The risk of lactic acidosis is increased if this medicine is used in patients with kidney disease or heart failure that requires medicine. The current drug label says that metformin should not be used in those patients (black box warning).
4. You should know the signs and symptoms of lactic acidosis (breathing difficulty [respiratory distress], low body temp [hypothermia], vague abdominal pain, muscle aches [myalgias], and/or increasing sleepiness) and should stop the medicine and immediately call your doctor if any develop while taking this medicine.
5. The American Diabetic Association (ADA) now says that diabetes is diagnosed when two fasting blood sugars in a row are more than 125 mg/dL. This more conservative approach reflects current information saying that complications start at lower blood sugar levels than previously thought.

The concept of pre-diabetes (formerly impaired glucose tolerance) is described in the Glossary. Some British clinicians advocate that statin-type medicines could cut the risk of heart attack and stroke by a third (even in people with "normal" cholesterol), yet comment that these medicines are underused in diabetics. Talk to your doctor about this.

Precautions for Use

By Infants and Children: Safety and effectiveness for use by those under 10 years of age have not been established. See dosing information above for those 10 or older for the regular form. Safety and effectiveness for the Metformin XR form in the pediatric population have not been established.

By Those Over 60 Years of Age: Smaller starting doses (500 mg daily) are indicated. People in this age group tend to have an age-related decline in kidney function as well as a more compromised ability to tolerate lower blood sugar levels. Some patients have had great blood sugar control with 500 mg a day, but doses up to 3,000 mg have been used. Patients who are over 80 should have a laboratory test called a MEASURED CREATININE clearance to check how well their kidneys work before this medicine is used. If the test result is within the normal limits, this medicine can be given with the same lower dose caveat described above.

▷ ## Advisability of Use During Pregnancy

Pregnancy Category: B (metformin and glyburide/metformin. See Pregnancy Risk Categories at the back of this book. C for glipizide metformin and rosiglitazone/metformin.

Animal Studies: No birth defects in rats at 2 times the typical human dose.

Human Studies: Information from adequate studies of pregnant women is not available. The manufacturer does not recommend the use of this drug in pregnancy.

Insulin is still considered the "drug of choice" to control blood sugar in pregnancy.

Advisability of Use If Breast-Feeding

Presence of this drug in breast milk: Unknown.

Avoid drug or refrain from nursing.

Habit-Forming Potential: None.

Effects of Overdose:
Nausea and vomiting, pulmonary edema, hemorrhage from the stomach, lactic acidosis, seizures, intractable lowering of blood pressure, coma.

Possible Effects of Long-Term Use:
Lowering of vitamin B_{12} and resultant anemia (megaloblastic). Possible malabsorption of folic acid and amino acids.

Suggested Periodic Examinations While Taking This Drug (at physician's discretion)

Vitamin B_{12} levels (particularly in those likely to have low B_{12}), but at least every 2 to 3 years. Annual complete blood count (CBC).

Tests of kidney and liver function before treatment is started and yearly at least. Hemoglobin A1C.

▷ ## While Taking This Drug, Observe the Following

Foods: Follow the ADA diet your doctor recommends. Taking a well-formulated multivitamin that contains B_{12} is prudent. Rice bran has been checked in a small (57-subject) study of type 1 and type 2 diabetics. The benefit was a 30% lowering of sugar. This might be a complementary care option.

Herbal Medicines or Minerals: Using chromium may change the way your body is able to use sugar. Some health food stores advocate vanadium as mimicking the actions of insulin, but possible toxicity and need for rigorous studies presently preclude recommending it. DHEA may change sensitivity to insulin or insulin resistance. Aloe, bitter melon, eucalyptus, fenugreek, ginger, garlic, ginseng, glucomannan, guar gum, hawthorn, licorice, nettle, and yohimbe may change blood sugar. Surprisingly, boiled stems of the Optuntia streptacantha prickly pear cactus appear to be able to lower blood sugar. Ongoing effects and effects on A1C are not known. Red sage is used for blood sugar effects, but is unproven. Psyllium increases risk of excessively low blood sugar. Since so many of these products may require adjustment of insulin dosing, talk to your doctor BEFORE combining any of these herbal medicines with this medicine. Echinacea pupurea (injectable) and blonde psyllium seed or husk should NOT be taken by people living with diabetes.

Nutritional Support: Diet as prescribed by your doctor. Check of vitamin B_{12} levels determines need for support. A multivitamin that has B_{12} in it may be prudent.

Beverages: No restrictions.

▷ *Alcohol:* Use with extreme caution. Alcohol worsens the effect of metformin on lactate. Avoid alcohol in excessive amounts.

Tobacco Smoking: No interactions expected, but I advise everyone to quit smoking.

Marijuana Smoking: May worsen dizziness.

▷ *Other Drugs*

Metformin may ***increase*** the effects of
- insulin, in the sense that the lowering of blood sugar will be increased; this may be used to therapeutic advantage in some insulin-dependent diabetics.

Metformin ***taken concurrently*** with
- ACE inhibitors (see Drug Classes) may increase lowering of blood sugar to an undesirable extent.
- azole antifungals (see Drug Classes) may increase lowering of blood sugar to an undesirable extent.
- beta blockers (see Drug Classes) may slow recovery from any hypoglycemia that occurs and can also block symptoms of low blood sugar.
- cationic drugs (cotrimoxazole, procainamide, quinidine, quinine, vancomycin, and others) may increase risk of lactic acidosis.
- contrast media for certain X-ray studies may increase risk of lactic acidosis. Metformin should not be combined with these agents. Some clinicians substitute a different agent to control blood sugar, stop the metformin 48 hours before the X-ray and then stop the substituted agent and restart metformin once kidney function is tested and found to be normal.
- cotrimoxazole (Bactrim, others) may increase risk of lactic acidosis.
- digoxin (Lanoxin, others) may pose a problem because it is a cationic drug and may lead to excess metformin levels.
- dofetilide (Tikosyn) may pose a problem because it is a cationic drug and uses the same removal (elimination) pathway that metformin does. This may lead to increased risk of dofetilide toxicity.
- gatifloxacin (Tequin), levofloxacin (Levaquin), perhaps other fluoroquinolone antibiotics can have variable effects on blood sugar. Close patient follow-up and blood sugar checks are prudent if these medicines must be combined.
- itraconazole (Sporanox), voriconazole (Vfend), or other azole antifungal agents can result in severe lowering of the blood sugar.
- procainamide (Pronestyl) may lead to toxicity.
- quinidine (Quinaglute) may lead to toxicity.

- thyroid hormones (see Drug Classes) can result in blunting of metformin's therapeutic effect.

The following drugs may *increase* the effects of metformin:

- cimetidine (Tagamet)—may result in toxicity.
- monoamine oxidase inhibitors (see Drug Classes) can result in severe lowering of the blood sugar.
- morphine (various)—may lead to toxicity.
- nifedipine (Adalat)—may lead to toxicity.
- oral antidiabetic drugs (see Drug Classes)—this effect may be used to therapeutic advantage.
- ranitidine (Zantac)—may lead to toxicity.
- trimethoprim (Septra)—may lead to toxicity.

▷ *Driving, Hazardous Activities:* This drug may cause drowsiness or dizziness. Restrict activities as necessary.

Aviation Note: Diabetes *is a disqualification for piloting.* Consult a designated Aviation Medical Examiner.

Exposure to Sun: Use caution. Some medicines that are similar in chemical structure can cause increased sensitivity to the sun.

Heavy Exercise or Exertion: Heavy exercise will tend to use up sugar faster than usual. This drug will have an effect on lowering the blood sugar. Be alert to the symptoms of low blood sugar.

Occurrence of Unrelated Illness: Infections or other illness may still require use of insulin to achieve acceptable blood sugar control.

Discontinuation: Periodic physician evaluations of the continued benefit of this medicine are needed in order to get the best results. It is not unusual to change doses or to combine this medicine with other medicines. Do not stop this medicine without talking to your doctor.

METHOTREXATE (meth oh TREX ayt)

Other Names: Amethopterin, MTX

Introduced: 1948   **Class:**   Chemotherapy, Anticancer drugs, antipsoriasis   **Prescription:**   USA: Yes   **Controlled Drug:**   USA: No; Canada: No   **Available as Generic:**   Yes

Brand Names: Abitrexate, Folex, Folex PFS, Mexate, Mexate AQ, Rheumatrex Dose Pack, Trexall

---

BENEFITS versus RISKS	
Possible Benefits	*Possible Risks*
EFFECTIVE TREATMENT OF SOME CASES OF SEVERE DISABLING PSORIASIS	GASTROINTESTINAL ULCERATION AND BLEEDING MOUTH AND THROAT ULCERATION
EFFECTIVE TREATMENT OF CERTAIN ADULT AND CHILDHOOD CANCERS	SEVERE BONE MARROW DEPRESSION
PREVENTION OF REJECTION OF BONE MARROW TRANSPLANTS	DAMAGE TO LUNGS, LIVER OR KIDNEYS
USEFUL IN RHEUMATOID ARTHRITIS AND RELATED DISORDERS	Loss of hair

▷ **Principal Uses**

As a Single Drug Product: Uses currently included in FDA-approved labeling: (1) Combination therapy of acute lymphocytic leukemia; (2) combination therapy of various types of adult and childhood cancer; (3) severe and widespread forms of disabling psoriasis that have failed to respond to all standard treatment procedures; (4) various types of both adult and childhood cancer; (5) used to prevent rejection of transplanted bone marrow; (6) used in the treatment of connective tissue disorders such as rheumatoid arthritis and related conditions (its use in rheumatoid arthritis is restricted to the treatment of selected adults and children with severe active disease [particular] that has failed to respond to conventional therapy); (7) used in COMBINATION with sulfasalazine or hydroxychloroquin in some cases of refractory rheumatoid arthritis. Also used in combination with infliximab and some of the other DMARDs in rheumatoid arthritis patients who do not have successful response to methotrexate alone.

Other (unlabeled) generally accepted uses: (1) Used in a variety of neoplastic syndromes in combination therapy; (2) may have a role in helping decrease steroid use in steroid-dependent asthma; (3) helps lessen neutropenia in Felty's syndrome; (4) used in combination with misoprostol to cause abortion; (5) can be of help in chronic granulomatous hepatitis of unknown cause (idiopathic); (6) used in some cases of systemic lupus erythematosus.

How This Drug Works: Blocks normal use of folic acid in cell reproduction and slows abnormally rapid tissue growth (as in psoriasis and cancer). How this works in rheumatoid arthritis is not presently known, but probably works by fighting inflammation and by slowing down the immune system (immunosuppression).

▷ **Widely Used Guidelines That Involve This Medicine (representative sample):** Please look at the section at the very beginning of this profile called "Class." Next, turn to Table 22 and you will find guidelines listed by the class involved!

Available Dosage Forms and Strengths

Injections — 2.5 mg/mL, 10 mg/mL, 25 mg/mL

Injections, preservative free — 25 mg/mL, 50 mg/mL, 100 mg/mL, 250 mg/mL

Powder, intrathecal cryodessicated — 20 mg, 50 mg, 100 mg

Tablets — 2.5 mg, 10 mg (Canada)

▷ **Usual Adult Dosage Ranges:** For psoriasis (alternate schedules): (1) 10 to 25 mg once a week taken by mouth (orally); (2) a test dose of 5 to 10 mg is given, then if the laboratory test results are normal, 7 days later, 2.5 to 5 mg every 12 hours for 3 doses per week can be given. Doses can be increased as needed and tolerated by 2.5 to 5 mg every 7 days. The maximum dose is 20 mg per week on this divided schedule.

For rheumatoid arthritis (alternate schedules): (1) single oral dose of 7.5 mg once weekly; (2) divided doses of 2.5 mg every 12 hours given 3 times (doses) a week. Dose may be increased gradually as needed and tolerated. Do not exceed a weekly dose of 20 mg. Intramuscular injections of 7.5 to 15 mg per week have been used. Once people respond to the medicine, the dose should be gradually lowered to the lowest dose that still works. The length of treatment will be determined by your doctor.

For acute lymphocytic leukemia (ALL): Induction—3.3 mg per square meter in combination with corticosteroid treatment is usually taken daily for 4 to 6 weeks. Maintenance—a total weekly dose of 30 mg per square meter is given as 2 divided oral or intramuscular injections. Some centers also use 2.5 mg per kg of body mass intravenously every 14 days. The tablets can be substituted for the solution. Injections beneath the skin (subcutaneous) can be substituted for injection into the muscle (intramuscular).

Note: Actual dose and schedule must be determined for each patient individually.

Conditions Requiring Dosing Adjustments

Liver Function: Used with caution and in decreased dose in liver disease. Some clinicians use laboratory tests as a guide—for example, when dose is due, if bilirubin is less than 3 mg % and AST (SGOT) is less than 180 IU, 100% of the scheduled dose can be given. If bilirubin is greater than 5.0 mg %, dose SHOULD NOT be given.

Kidney Function: Methotrexate is a benefit-to-risk decision. Increased adverse effects are possible with damaged kidneys. Do not take with severe kidney failure (creatinine clearance less than 10 mL/min). For moderate failure, 50% of the usual dose should be taken in the usual dosing interval.

▷ **Dosing Instructions:** The tablet may be crushed and taken with food to reduce stomach irritation. Drink at least 2 to 3 quarts of liquids daily. Many clinicians using methotrexate in rheumatoid arthritis also give folic acid in order to minimize methotrexate toxicity. If you forget a dose: take the missed dose as soon as you remember it, unless it's nearly time for your next dose—if that is the case, skip the missed dose and take the next dose right on schedule. Two forms of birth control should be used by women who can have children while they are taking this medicine and for 3 months after treatment ends. Talk with your doctor if you find yourself missing doses of methotrexate. Ask your doctor BEFORE getting any vaccinations. Some shots can be given before treatment is started, others should be avoided.

Usual Duration of Use: Use on a regular schedule for several weeks determines benefit in reducing the severity and extent of psoriasis. Response in rheumatoid arthritis usually begins after 3 to 6 weeks of treatment. Dose should be reduced to smallest amount that will maintain acceptable improvement. Long-term use (months to years) requires physician supervision. The ideal length of treatment is not presently known for rheumatoid arthritis.

Typical Treatment Goals and Measurements (Outcomes and Markers)

Rheumatoid arthritis: Control of arthritis symptoms (severity of pain, number of swollen joints, loss of mobility, decreased ability to accomplish activities of daily living, range of motion, early morning stiffness [EMS], etc.) is paramount in returning patient quality of life and to checking the results (beneficial outcomes) from this medicine. A scale called the ACR response is widely used (see Glossary). Many arthritis management or pain centers use interdisciplinary teams (physicians from several specialties, nurses, physician's assistants, physical and occupational therapists, pharmacotherapists, psychotherapists, social workers, and others) to get the best results. Blood levels of methotrexate are used to help avoid toxicity. In rheumatoid arthritis, C-reactive protein, or sedimentation rate also measures results.

▷ **This Drug Should Not Be Taken If**
- you have had an allergic reaction to it previously.
- you currently have, or have had a recent exposure to, either chicken pox or shingles (herpes zoster).

- you are pregnant or planning pregnancy in the near future and you are taking this drug to treat psoriasis or rheumatoid arthritis.
- you are breast-feeding your infant.
- you have alcoholic liver disease.
- you have an immune deficiency.
- you have fluid in the pleura of the lung (pleural effusions).
- you have active liver disease, peptic ulcer, regional enteritis, or ulcerative colitis.
- you are making very small amounts of urine or your creatinine clearance (see Glossary) is less than 40 mL/min.
- you currently have a blood cell or bone marrow disorder.

▷ **Inform Your Physician Before Taking This Drug If**
- you have a chronic infection of any kind.
- you do not understand how to handle vomit or urine while taking chemotherapy.
- you have impaired liver or kidney function.
- you have a history of bone marrow impairment of any kind, especially drug-induced bone marrow depression.
- your white blood cell count is less than 1,500 or your platelet count is less than 75,000.
- you start to have a skin reaction while taking this drug.
- you are dehydrated.
- you have a history of gout, peptic ulcer disease, regional enteritis, or ulcerative colitis.

Possible Side Effects (natural, expected, and unavoidable drug actions)
> The following are due to the pharmacological actions of this drug. **Report such developments to your physician promptly.**
> Sores on the lips, in the mouth or throat.
> Vomiting.
> Severe reactions (photoxicity) with sun exposure.
> Intestinal cramping.
> Diarrhea (may be bloody).
> Painful urination.
> Eye irritation (conjunctivitis).
> Bloody urine.
> Superinfections (may be lung/respiratory: pneumocystis pneumonia, or PCP. Case reports of histoplasmosis).
> Reduced resistance to infection, fatigue, weakness, fever, abnormal bleeding or bruising (bone marrow depression).

▷ **Possible Adverse Effects** (unusual, unexpected, and infrequent reactions)
> **If any of the following develop, consult your physician promptly for guidance.**

Mild Adverse Effects
> Allergic reactions: skin rash, hives, itching.
> Headache, drowsiness, blurred vision, conjunctivitis—infrequent.
> Loss of appetite, nausea, vomiting—infrequent to frequent.
> Muscle pain—rare.
> Loss of hair, loss of skin pigmentation, acne—infrequent.
> Impaired sense of smell or taste—possible.

Serious Adverse Effects
> Allergic reactions: drug-induced pneumonia (cough, chest pain, shortness of breath).

Anaphylaxis.

Asthma-like reaction—possible (may require dosing interval extensions).

Nervous system toxicity: speech disturbances, paralysis, seizures—infrequent.

Liver toxicity with jaundice (see Glossary)—case reports.

Kidney toxicity: reduced urine volume, kidney failure—more likely with higher doses.

Accumulation of fluid around the heart (pericardial effusion and pericarditis)—possible and some may require leucovorin rescue.

Clogging of the arteries (atherosclerotic vascular disease)—possibly increased.

Colitis or toxic megacolon—case report.

Tumor lysis syndrome: uric acid nephropathy; very low potassium, magnesium, and calcium—possible.

Fluid buildup in the lung pleura (pleural effusion)—possible.

Immune suppression and subsequent infection with Pneumocystis carinii pneumonia—possible.

Bone toxicity (osteopathy)—case reports (6 month- to 8.5-year onset with usual or even low-dose treatment).

Severe skin reactions (toxic epidermal necrolysis)—case reports.

Chromosomal damage (from occupational exposure)—possible.

▷ **Possible Effects on Sexual Function:** Altered timing and pattern of menstruation. Swelling and tenderness of the male breast tissue (gynecomastia)—case reports. Impotence—case reports.

Possible Delayed Adverse Effects: Some reports suggest that methotrexate therapy may contribute to the later development of secondary cancers. Other studies have not confirmed this.

Possible Effects on Laboratory Tests

Complete blood cell counts: decreased red cells, hemoglobin, white cells, and platelets.

Blood uric acid level: increased.

Liver function tests: increased liver enzymes (ALT/GPT, AST/GOT, and alkaline phosphatase) or bilirubin.

Kidney function tests: increased blood urea nitrogen (BUN) level; increased urine creatinine.

Fecal occult blood test: positive.

Sperm count: decreased.

CAUTION

1. This drug must be monitored carefully by a qualified physician. Request the Patient Package Insert (Rheumatrex Dose Pack) and read it thoroughly.
2. When methotrexate is used to treat rheumatoid arthritis, folic acid can minimize toxicity.
3. Appropriate laboratory examinations, performed before and during the use of this drug, are mandatory.
4. Women with potential for pregnancy should have a pregnancy test before taking this drug and should use 2 forms of birth control while taking this medicine and for 3 months after stopping it.
5. Live-virus vaccines should be avoided during use of this drug. Live-virus vaccines could actually produce infection rather than stimulate an immune response.
6. Try to avoid people with obvious infections like the flu or colds because this medicine lowers the strength of your immune system and you will be more likely to catch them.

Precautions for Use
By Those Over 60 Years of Age: Careful evaluation of kidney function should be made before starting treatment and during the entire course of therapy.

▷ **Advisability of Use During Pregnancy**
Pregnancy Category: X. See Pregnancy Risk Categories at the back of this book.
Animal Studies: Skull and facial defects reported in mice.
Human Studies: This drug is known to cause fetal deaths and birth defects. Its use during pregnancy to treat psoriasis or rheumatoid arthritis cannot be justified.

Advisability of Use If Breast-Feeding
Presence of this drug in breast milk: Yes.
Avoid drug or refrain from nursing.

Habit-Forming Potential: None.

Effects of Overdose: The side effects and adverse effects listed on the previous page develop earlier and with greater severity.

Possible Effects of Long-Term Use: Liver compromise (fibrosis and cirrhosis) occurs in 3–5% of long-term users (35 to 49 months).

Suggested Periodic Examinations While Taking This Drug (at physician's discretion)
Complete blood cell counts (CBCs). When methotrexate is used in rheumatoid arthritis, complete blood counts are checked after the first, second and fourth weeks of use. If the CBC is acceptable, after 2 weeks, the dose can be increased to 7.5 mg a week. Usually the CBC is checked each month after this. ACR response should be checked as there are more medicines available for rheumatoid arthritis now (RA).
Liver and kidney function tests.
Blood uric acid levels.
Blood methotrexate levels in high-risk patients (some examples include those with dehydration, compromised kidneys, pleural effusion, prior treatment with cysplatin and acites).
Chest X-ray examinations.

▷ **While Taking This Drug, Observe the Following**
Foods: Avoid highly seasoned foods that could be irritating. Between courses of treatment, eat liberally of the following foods: beef, chicken, lamb, and pork liver, asparagus, navy beans, kale, and spinach. Any food will reduce the peak methotrexate level obtained. Folic acid supplementation is suggested for people who will take this medicine on an ongoing basis.
Herbal Medicines or Minerals: Some patients use echinacea to attempt to boost their immune systems. Unfortunately, use of echinacea is not recommended in people with damaged immune systems (even if a medicine caused the damage). This herb may also actually weaken any immune system if it is used too often or for too long a time. Like methotrexate, St. John's wort may cause sensitivity to the sun. Avoid this combination. There are no data regarding combined use of hay flower, mistletoe herb, or white mustard seed with methotrexate in rheumatoid arthritis. Herbals such as kava, valerian, and eucalyptus may have additive effects on liver toxicity and should be avoided.
Beverages: No restrictions. This drug may be taken with milk.
Alcohol: Markedly lower how much you drink or avoid completely (increases risk of liver damage).

Tobacco Smoking: No interactions expected. I advise everyone to quit smoking.
Marijuana Smoking: May cause additional impairment of immunity.
▷   *Other Drugs*
Methotrexate may ***decrease*** the effects of
- digoxin (Lanoxin).
- folate (various) by blocking the change (conversion) of folate to folic acid.
- phenytoin (Dilantin) or fosphenytoin (Cerebyx).

The following drugs may ***increase*** the effects of methotrexate and enhance its toxicity:
- aspirin and other salicylates.
- diuretics (see Drug Classes) may result in methotrexate-enhanced lowering of granulocyte-type white blood cells (myelosuppression).
- NSAIDs (see Drug Classes) (especially with higher NSAID doses).
- omeprazole (Prilosec).
- probenecid (Benemid).
- rofecoxib (Vioxx).

Methotrexate ***taken concurrently*** with
- amiodarone (Cordarone) may result in methotrexate toxicity.
- asparaginase (Elspar, others) may result in blunted methotrexate activity.
- bismuth subsalicylate (Pepto-Bismol, others) may result in methotrexate toxicity.
- carbenicillin (Geocillin, others) and other penicillins (see Drug Classes) may lead to methotrexate toxicity.
- cholestyramine (Questran, others) and other cholesterol-lowering resins may result in decreased methotrexate effectiveness.
- cotrimoxazole (Bactrim) may result in lowering of all blood cells (pancytopenia).
- cyclosporine (Sandimmune) can result in increased toxicity from both drugs. This combination should be avoided.
- doxycycline (various) may result in methotrexate toxicity.
- etretinate (Tegison) results in increased liver toxicity.
- influenzae (flu) vaccine may blunt benefits of the vaccine.
- leflunomide (Arava) may result in liver toxicity.
- live-virus vaccines (such as MMWR) may lead to severe infections.
- mercaptopurine (Purinethol) may lead to mercaptopurine toxicity.
- neomycin (various) may result in decreased methotrexate benefits.
- penicillins (see Drug Classes) may result in serious methotrexate toxicity. If these medicines must be combined, lower methotrexate doses, blood levels of methotrexate and extremely careful patient follow-up are required.
- pneumococcal or smallpox vaccine may result in decreased immune response to the vaccine.
- sulfa drugs, such as sulfamethoxazole, can result in increased hematological toxicity.
- tamoxifen (Nolvadex) may increase risk of blood clots (thromboembolism)—part of a combination regimen that leads to this.
- thiazide diuretics (see Drug Classes) may increase risk of myelosuppression.
- theophylline (Theo-Dur, others) may result in theophylline toxicity; decreased theophylline doses may be needed.
- triamterene (Dyazide, others) may increase risk of bone marrow problems (myelosuppression).
- trimethoprim (Septra, others) may increase risk of toxicity.
- yellow fever vaccine can result in blunted response and benefit from the vaccine.

▷ *Driving, Hazardous Activities:* This drug may cause drowsiness, dizziness, or blurred vision. Restrict activities as necessary.

Aviation Note: The use of this drug **is a disqualification** for piloting. Consult a designated Aviation Medical Examiner.

Exposure to Sun: Use caution—this drug can cause photosensitivity. Avoid ultraviolet lamps.

METHYCLOTHIAZIDE (METH i kloh thi a zide)

Please see the thiazide diuretics family profile.

METHYLPHENIDATE (meth il FEN i dayt)

Introduced: 1956 **Class:** Amphetaminelike drug, anti–attention deficit disorder drug **Prescription:** USA: Yes **Controlled Drug:** USA: C-II*; Canada: Yes **Available as Generic:** USA: Yes; Canada: Yes

Brand Names: Concerta, Metadate CD and ER, Methylin ER, ✤PMS-Methylphenidate, Ritalin, Ritalin-LA and SR

Author's Note: Focalin is a relatively new treatment for ADHD. This medicine is NOT the same as methylphenidate. This drug is DEX-methylphenidate. The usual dose is only half of the methylphenidate dose. Information on Focalin will be included in a broader dexmethylphenidate profile if ongoing studies and results warrant this.

BENEFITS versus RISKS	
Possible Benefits	*Possible Risks*
EFFECTIVE CONTROL OF NARCOLEPSY	POTENTIAL FOR SERIOUS PSYCHOLOGICAL DEPENDENCE (oral dosing reaches brain levels slowly and appears to avoid this effect)
USEFUL AS ADJUNCTIVE TREATMENT IN ATTENTION DEFICIT DISORDERS	
CONCERTA FORM OFFERS ONCE-DAILY DOSING	SUPPRESSION OF GROWTH IN CHILDHOOD (recovers when medicine is stopped)
Adjunctive treatment in ADHD	Abnormal behavior
Useful in treatment of mild to moderate depression	Rare blood cell disorders
Useful in some cases of emotional withdrawal in the elderly	
May have a role in some chronic pain cases	

*See Schedules of Controlled Drugs at the back of this book.

▷ **Principal Uses**

As a Single Drug Product: Uses currently included in FDA-approved labeling: Treats (1) narcolepsy—recurrent spells of uncontrollable drowsiness and sleep; (2) attention deficit disorders of childhood, formerly known as the hyperactive child syndrome, with minimal brain damage and minimal brain dysfunction.

Other (unlabeled) generally accepted uses: (1) Treats mild to moderate depression; (2) manages apathetic and withdrawal states in the elderly; (3) combination therapy of chronic pain, particularly cancer pain; (4) could have a role in autism; (5) may help passing out (recurrent neurocardiogenic syncope).

How This Drug Works: Activates the brain stem, improves alertness and concentration, increases learning ability and attention span. A study in *Science* found that levels of the nerve transmitter serotonin are increased by this medicine, restoring a proper balance between serotonin and other brain chemicals.

▷ **Widely Used Guidelines That Involve This Medicine (representative sample):** Please look at the section at the very beginning of this profile called "Class." Next, turn to Table 22 and you will find guidelines listed by the class involved!

Available Dosage Forms and Strengths

Capsule, extended release (Metadate CD) — 20 mg

Tablets — 5 mg, 10 mg, 20 mg

Tablets, prolonged action — 20 mg, 30 mg and 40 mg

Tablet, extended osmotic release (Concerta) — 18 mg, 27 mg, 36 mg, 54 mg

Tablet, extended release (Metadate ER) — 10 mg, 20 mg

▷ **Recommended Dosage Ranges:** *Narcolepsy*: 10 to 60 mg daily, divided into equal doses, given 2 to 3 times daily. Ideally, given 30 to 45 minutes before meals.

Attention deficit disorder: Pediatric dosing: Children over 6 years old (regular release form)—5 mg before breakfast and lunch (twice daily). Some clinicians use 0.25 mg per kg per day divided into 2 doses as a starting dose. Dose is increased as needed and tolerated (weekly intervals) to daily maximum of dose of 60 mg. Sustained release form lasts 8 hours. The Metadate CD form is started at 20 mg once a day before breakfast. Osmotic release form (Concerta) is given once daily in the morning. A specific conversion table is used when people are changed from the immediate release forms to the Concerta form. For example: If 5 mg of immediate release (IR) was being taken 2 or 3 times daily or if 20 mg of the SR form was being taken daily, 18 mg of the Concerta form is taken in the morning.

Pain management: Some clinicians use methylphenidate added onto opioid pain relievers (analgesics) using 10 mg in the morning and 5 mg at lunch.

Note: Actual dose and schedule must be determined for each patient individually.

Conditions Requiring Dosing Adjustments

Liver Function: Used with caution and prudent to decrease dose in liver disease.

Kidney Function: No changes currently thought to be needed.

▷ **Dosing Instructions:** The regular tablet may be crushed and taken 30 to 45 minutes before meals. The prolonged-action tablet, the osmotic controlled release form (Concerta) and any other extended release forms should be taken whole, not crushed. Best to take this medicine with a full glass of water, juice, or milk. The Ritalin LA capsules can be opened and the contents sprinkled over a spoonful of room temperature or cold (not warm) applesauce. Once so prepared, ALL of the applesauce/ritalin mixture should be taken right away. If you forget a dose: take the missed dose as soon as you remember it, unless it's nearly time for your next dose—if that is the case, skip the missed dose and take the next dose right on schedule. Talk with your doctor if you find yourself missing doses.

Usual Duration of Use: Regular use for 3 to 4 weeks determines benefits in easing the symptoms of narcolepsy or improving behavior of attention deficit children. If there is no improvement after this time, the drug should be stopped. Long-term use (months to years) requires supervision by your doctor.

Typical Treatment Goals and Measurements (Outcomes and Markers)
Attention Deficit: The general goal is to achieve the ability to "stay on task." This medicine can also help decrease impulsiveness and increase socially appropriate behavior. Specific measures of cognitive function, motor performance, and educational tasking may help assess response. Treatment guidelines from AHCPR and DSM-IV criteria from the American Psychiatric Association are widely used. The American Academy of Pediatricians has an important set of guidelines. Please remember that these are guidelines and therapy must still be individualized. The guidelines can be found at *www.pediatrics.org* (see also Sources and American Academy of Pediatrics).

▷ **This Drug Should Not Be Taken If**
- you have had an allergic reaction to it previously.
- you have glaucoma.
- you have taken a monoamine oxidase inhibitor (MAOI—see Drug Classes) in the last 14 days.
- you have Tourette's syndrome or experience tics while using this medicine.
- you are experiencing a period of severe anxiety, nervous tension, or emotional depression.

▷ **Inform Your Physician Before Taking This Drug If**
- you have a history of mental illness.
- you have a seizure disorder.
- you have a history of abnormal heartbeats.
- you have high blood pressure, angina, or epilepsy.
- you are under 6 years old (usually avoided).

Possible Side Effects (natural, expected, and unavoidable drug actions)
Nervousness, excitement, insomnia. Reduced appetite. Growth suppression (stopping the medicine in the summer is used to allow a growth spurt). Slight increase in heart rate.

▷ **Possible Adverse Effects** (unusual, unexpected, and infrequent reactions)
If any of the following develop, consult your physician promptly for guidance.
Mild Adverse Effects
Allergic reactions: skin rash, hives, drug fever, joint pains—possible.
Headache, dizziness, rapid and forceful heart palpitation—infrequent.
Nausea, abdominal discomfort—infrequent.
Stuttering and hallucinations—case reports.
Serious Adverse Effects
Allergic reactions: severe skin reactions, extensive bruising (allergic destruction of platelets)—case reports.
Idiosyncratic reactions: abnormal patterns of behavior.

Cerebral vasculitis (tingling and numbness followed by movement disorders)—case report.

Porphyria or muscle damage (rhabdomyolysis)—rare.

Liver toxicity—case reports.

Precipitation of Tourette's syndrome—case reports.

▷ **Possible Effects on Sexual Function:** None reported.

Natural Diseases or Disorders That May Be Activated by This Drug

Latent epilepsy. Increased eye pressure unmasking glaucoma.

Possible Effects on Laboratory Tests

Eosinophils: Increased (IV abuse).

CAUTION

1. This drug should be used ONLY AFTER a careful assessment by a qualified specialist is made. True attention deficit disorder requires careful assessment to differentiate it from behavior problems arising from family tensions or other conditions that do not require methylphenidate therapy.

2. A February 2000 study of 200,000 children coordinated by the University of Maryland found a large increase in Ritalin, Prozac, and clonidine prescriptions in patients under 4 years old. This retrospective review of Medicaid and HMO records may represent better ability to diagnose, but may also reflect excessive use. The American Academy of Pediatricians has an important set of guidelines. Please remember that these are guidelines and therapy must still be individualized. The guidelines can be found at *www.pediatrics.org* (see also Sources and American Academy of Pediatrics).

3. Careful dose adjustments on an individual basis are mandatory.

4. Paradoxical reactions (see Glossary) can occur, causing aggravation of initial symptoms for which this drug was prescribed.

Precautions for Use

By Infants and Children: Safety and effectiveness for those under 6 years of age are not established. If this drug is not beneficial in managing attention deficit disorder after a trial of 1 month, it should be stopped. During long-term use, monitor the child for normal growth and development.

By Those Over 60 Years of Age: Start with small doses. Those in this group may be at increased risk for nervousness, agitation, insomnia, high blood pressure, angina, or disturbance of heart rhythm.

▷ **Advisability of Use During Pregnancy**

Pregnancy Category: C. See Pregnancy Risk Categories at the back of this book.

Animal Studies: No birth defects found in mouse studies.

Human Studies: Adequate studies of pregnant women are not available.

Ask your physician for guidance.

Advisability of Use If Breast-Feeding

Presence of this drug in breast milk: Unknown.

Avoid drug or refrain from nursing.

Habit-Forming Potential: This drug can produce tolerance and cause serious psychological dependence (see Glossary), a potentially dangerous characteristic of amphetaminelike drugs (see Drug Classes). The street name for this medicine is R-ball or Vitamin-R. It is one of the top prescription drugs stolen in the United States for recreational use. Caution is needed. If you start to feel like the medicine is not working, call your doctor. One study of abuse of methylphenidate on a college campus described this as a potentially serious public health issue (see Teter, C.J. in Sources).

Effects of Overdose: Headache, vomiting, agitation, tremors, dry mouth, sweating, fever, confusion, hallucinations, seizures, coma.

Possible Effects of Long-Term Use: Suppression of growth (in weight and/or height) occurs. Many patients are taken off the drug during summer vacations.

Suggested Periodic Examinations While Taking This Drug (at physician's discretion)

Complete blood cell counts.

Blood pressure measurements.

Height and weight.

Follow-up evaluation for beneficial effects of treatment.

▷ **While Taking This Drug, Observe the Following**

Herbal Medicines or Minerals: Using St. John's wort, guarana, mate, ma huang (no longer on the market for weight loss), bitter orange, country mallow or kola while taking this medicine may result in unacceptable central nervous system stimulation. Tyrosine may increase risk of adverse effects.

Beverages: Avoid beverages prepared from meat or meat extracts. This drug may be taken with milk.

▷ *Alcohol:* Avoid beer, Chianti wines and vermouth (may have high tyramine contents).

Tobacco Smoking: No interactions expected. I advise everyone to quit smoking.

▷ *Other Drugs*

Methylphenidate may ***increase*** the effects of

• tricyclic antidepressants (see Drug Classes) and enhance their toxic effects.

Methylphenidate may ***decrease*** the effects of

• guanethidine (Ismelin) and impair its ability to lower blood pressure.

Methylphenidate ***taken concurrently*** with

• anticonvulsants (such as carbamazepine or fosphenytoin or phenytoin) may cause a significant change in the pattern of epileptic seizures; dose adjustments may be necessary for proper control.

• monoamine oxidase (MAO) type A inhibitors (see Drug Classes) may cause a significant rise in blood pressure; avoid the concurrent use of these drugs.

• morphine may be used to great therapeutic benefit to increase alertness, especially if high doses of morphine must be used.

• tricyclic antidepressants (see Drug Classes) may result in undesirable increases in blood pressure.

▷ *Driving, Hazardous Activities:* This drug may cause dizziness or drowsiness. Restrict activities as necessary.

Aviation Note: The use of this drug ***is a disqualification*** for piloting. Consult a designated Aviation Medical Examiner.

Exposure to Sun: No restrictions.

Discontinuation: If the drug has been taken for a long time, do not stop it abruptly. Talk to your doctor about how to slowly decrease doses.

METHYLPREDNISOLONE (meth il pred NIS oh lohn)

Introduced: 1957 **Class:** Cortisonelike drugs **Prescription:** USA: Yes **Controlled Drug:** USA: No; Canada: No **Available as Generic:** USA: Yes; Canada: Yes

Brand Names: A-Methapred, Depmedalone-40, Depmedalone-80, Depo-Medrol, Enpak Refill, Mar-Pred 40, Medrol, ✤Medrol Acne Lotion, Medrol Enpak, ✤Medrol Veriderm Cream, Meprolone, ✤Neo-Medrol Acne Lotion, ✤Neo-Medrol Veriderm, Pre-Dep 40, 80, Rep-Pred 80, Solu-Medrol

---

BENEFITS versus RISKS

Possible Benefits	*Possible Risks*
EFFECTIVE RELIEF OF SYMPTOMS IN A WIDE VARIETY OF INFLAMMATORY AND ALLERGIC DISORDERS	Ongoing systemic use or exposure (variable onset) can be associated with increased possible emergence of effects such as:
EFFECTIVE IMMUNO-SUPPRESSION IN SELECTED BENIGN AND MALIGNANT DISORDERS	ALTERED MOOD AND PERSONALITY
	CATARACTS, GLAUCOMA
	HYPERTENSION
	OSTEOPOROSIS
	INCREASED SUSCEPTIBILITY TO INFECTIONS, AND OTHERS
	ASCEPTIC BONE NECROSIS (OSTEONECROSIS) IS AN AREA OF CONTROVERSY, UNCLEAR ONSET. PATIENT RISK FACTORS AND CORRELATION VERSUS CAUSATION (SEE "CONTROVERSIES IN MEDICINE" ON PAGE 716)

▷ **Principal Uses**

As a Single Drug Product: Uses currently included in FDA-approved labeling: (1) Treats a wide variety of allergic and inflammatory conditions (used most commonly in the management of serious skin disorders, asthma, regional enteritis, multiple sclerosis, lupus erythematosus, ulcerative colitis, and all types of major rheumatic disorders including bursitis, tendonitis, and most forms of arthritis); (2) helps treat low platelet counts of unknown cause (idiopathic thrombocytopenic purpura); (3) treats shock due to adrenal gland insufficiency—Addisonian shock; (4) plays an adjunctive role in anaphylactic shock; (5) used in acute lymphocytic leukemia as part of chemotherapy treatment.

Other (unlabeled) generally accepted uses: (1) Treats refractory anemia; (2) used in therapy of chronic obstructive pulmonary disease; (3) used in combination therapy of severe vomiting caused by chemotherapy; (4) helps prevent rejection of transplanted organs; (5) combination therapy of *Pneumocystis carinii* pneumonia in AIDS patients; (6) helps treat bone cysts in children; (7) has a role in treating croup; (8) can help symptoms in Still's disease; (9) used by intramuscular injection to treat polymyalgia rheumatica and some carpal tunnel cases; (10) used to help control cancer pain, especially where inflammation is involved.

How This Drug Works: Anti-inflammatory effect is due to its ability to block normal defensive functions of certain white blood cells. Immunosuppressant effect comes from reduced production of lymphocytes (a kind of white blood cell) and antibodies.

▷ **Widely Used Guidelines That Involve This Medicine (representative sample):** Please look at the section at the very beginning of this profile called "Class." Next, turn to Table 22 and you will find guidelines listed by the class involved!

Available Dosage Forms and Strengths

Injection, solution (per vial) — 40 mg, 125 mg, 500 mg, 1 g

Injection, suspension — 40 mg/mL, 80 mg/mL

Ointment — 0.25%, 1%

Retention enema (per bottle) — 40 mg

Tablets — 2 mg, 4 mg, 8 mg, 16 mg, 24 mg, 32 mg

▷ **Usual Adult Dosage Ranges:** 4 to 48 mg daily as a single (oral) dose or in divided doses. Medrol dosepaks are a card with 4 mg tablets of methylprednisolone in them. On the first day, 2 tablets are taken before breakfast, 1 tablet after the noon and evening meals and then 2 tablets are taken at bedtime. Patients should then follow the ongoing instructions on the card for the remaining days (6 days total).

Note: Actual dose and schedule must be determined for each patient individually.

Conditions Requiring Dosing Adjustments

Liver Function: Specific dose adjustments in liver compromise are not defined. This drug is a rare cause of liver changes (hepatomegaly).

Kidney Function: This drug can worsen existing kidney compromise. A benefit-to-risk decision must be made regarding the use of methylprednisolone by these patients.

Obesity: The amount of time this medicine stays in the body is extended in obese patients. Dosing should be calculated based on ideal body weight.

▷ **Dosing Instructions:** The tablet may be crushed and taken with or following food to prevent stomach irritation, preferably in the morning. If you forget a dose: Call your doctor for instructions. Follow the specific instructions from your doctor and as outlined on the Medrol Dose Pak if that form is used.

Usual Duration of Use: For sudden (acute) disorders, 4 to 10 days. Need for tapering, patient reaction, possible disease flare are all factors to be considered. Medrol Dose Paks are a pre-planned 6-day course. For long-standing (chronic) disorders, this medicine is used according to individual and condition requirements. Duration of use should not exceed the time necessary to obtain adequate symptomatic relief in acute self-limiting conditions, then permit appropriate withdrawal or the time required to stabilize a chronic condition and permit appropriate withdrawal. Because of its intermediate duration of action, this drug may be appropriate for alternate-day use in some cases. See your doctor on a regular basis.

Typical Treatment Goals and Measurements (Outcomes and Markers)

Inflammation: The general goal is to decrease inflammation. Physical signs and symptoms such as hives (urticaria), rash, difficulty breathing, and swelling should ease. Representative tests may include sedimentation rate, cortisol, peak expiratory flow rate, FEV1 for respiratory conditions.

Asthma: Frequency and severity of asthma attacks should ease. Some clinicians also use decreased frequency of rescue inhaler use as a further clinical indicator. It is critical that this medicine is used regularly to get the best results. An additional goal of therapy is to use the lowest effective dose. Some people keep their improvements when doses are lowered, while others relapse. Specific testing goals include improvement in PEFR, FEV1, and other lung (pulmonary) function tests. Wheezing and difficulty breathing (dyspnea) should ease as well as asthma caused (induced) by exercise. If the usual benefit is not realized, call your doctor.

▷ **This Drug Should Not Be Taken If**
- you had an allergic reaction to it previously.
- you have active peptic ulcer disease.
- you have had recent bowel surgery where an anastomosis was performed (ask your doctor).
- you have a premature infant and the injection form is ordered (contains benzyl alcohol).
- you have an active eye infection from herpes simplex virus.
- you have active tuberculosis or a full-body (systemic) fungus infection.

▷ **Inform Your Physician Before Taking This Drug If**
- you have had a reaction to any cortisonelike drug.
- you have a history of peptic ulcer disease, colitis, thrombophlebitis, or tuberculosis.
- you have diabetes, glaucoma, high blood pressure, deficient thyroid function, or myasthenia gravis.
- you have been exposed to measles or chicken pox or other viral illness.
- you have osteoporosis, kidney disease, or have a history of threadworm (Strongyloides) infection.
- you start to have restricted motion, increased and/or unexplained pain (such as in the knees, hips, or shoulders), fever, or swelling of joints while taking or after taking this medicine—these may be early signs of aseptic necrosis (osteonecrosis). Call your doctor right away.
- you plan to have surgery of any kind in the near future.
- you have liver compromise.

Possible Side Effects (natural, expected, and unavoidable drug actions)

Increased appetite, weight gain, retention of salt and water, excretion of potassium, increased susceptibility to infection. Decreased wound healing. Adrenal gland suppression. Growth retardation with chronic use in children. Increased eye pressure (intraocular). Easy bruising (ecchymosis). Increased white blood cell count (not a sign of infection, but an effect of the medicine). Suppression of the immune system leading to possible opportunistic infections or increased chance of infections in general.

▷ **Possible Adverse Effects** (unusual, unexpected, and infrequent reactions)
If any of the following develop, consult your physician promptly for guidance.

Mild Adverse Effects
Allergic reaction: skin rash.
Headache, dizziness, insomnia—infrequent.
Acid indigestion, abdominal distention—infrequent.
Muscle cramping, weakness, and joint pain—possible.
Acne, excessive growth of facial hair—case reports.

Serious Adverse Effects
Allergic reactions: anaphylaxis.
Mental and emotional disturbances—infrequent.
Reactivation of latent tuberculosis, *Pneumocystis carinii* pneumonia—possible, case reports.
Development of peptic ulcer—case reports.
Seizures—possible.
Toxic megacolon—case reports.
Liver or kidney compromise—rare.

Blindness, opportunistic infections of the eye, cataracts—case reports.

Changes in white blood cell counts—possible.

Cushing's syndrome with chronic use (central obesity, "buffalo hump," and moon-shaped face)—possible.

Osteoporosis—possible with long-term use.

Bone death (aseptic necrosis, osteonecrosis, or avascular necrosis)—questions remain as to correlation versus causation, but may be more likely with high initial doses, long-term treatment, and cumulative doses of 4.32 grams. May also happen after short-term modest use. Individual patient risk factors appear to be important. See Controversies in Medicine below. Call your doctor if unexplained joint pain happens.

Increased blood sugar (hyperglycemia)—possible and dose-related.

Muscle changes (myopathy) or pancreatitis—case reports.

Increased blood pressure—case reports.

Abnormal heartbeat (arrhythmias)—case reports.

Development of inflammation of the pancreas—case reports.

Thrombophlebitis (inflammation of a vein with the formation of blood clot): pain or tenderness in thigh or leg, with or without swelling of the foot, ankle, or leg—case reports.

Pulmonary embolism (movement of a blood clot to the lung): sudden shortness of breath, pain in the chest, coughing, bloody sputum—case reports.

▷ **Possible Effects on Sexual Function:** Altered timing and pattern of menstruation—infrequent.

▷ **Adverse Effects That May Mimic Natural Diseases or Disorders**

Pattern of symptoms and signs resembling Cushing's syndrome.

Natural Diseases or Disorders That May Be Activated by This Drug

Latent diabetes, glaucoma, peptic ulcer disease, tuberculosis.

Possible Effects on Laboratory Tests

Blood amylase and lipase levels: increased (possible pancreatitis).

Glucose tolerance test (GTT): decreased.

Blood potassium or testosterone level: decreased.

Cholesterol and LDL: increased.

HDL: decreased.

CAUTION

1. If your treatment will exceed 1 week, carry a card in your purse or wallet that says you take this drug. Suppression of the adrenal gland may continue for months even after this medicine is stopped (adrenocortical insufficiency), and replacement therapy (with quick-acting steroids) can be needed during stress (such as serious illness or surgery).

2. You have an increased risk of severe infection from viral illnesses, such as measles or chicken pox. Try to avoid being exposed, and call your doctor if exposure occurs.

3. Growth and development of children receiving chronic steroids should be carefully followed.

4. Do not stop this drug abruptly after long-term treatment (the medicine should be slowly tapered).

5. If vaccination against measles, rabies, smallpox, or yellow fever is required, stop drug 72 hours before vaccination and do not resume it for at least 14 days.

6. Dermatitis around the mouth may occur. Talk with your doctor if this happens.

7. A variety of patient risk factors appear to be important in possible development of osteonecrosis. Talk to your doctor about the current list.

**Controversies in Medicine: Medicines in this class have had conflicting re-
ports regarding correlation with or causation of aseptic bone necrosis
(osteonecrosis, or ON). There appear to be patient risk factors, possible
delayed onset with occurrence even after the medicine is stopped, and
some diseases or conditions where corticosteroids are often used and
ON is more frequent than the general population. It is unclear if this is
because of the disease or condition or the use of corticosteroids. Previous data regarding cumulative dosing (4.32 grams) appears controversial, with more recent case reports of 6 days of treatment with some
doses being associated with ON. Some existing and emerging patient
risk factors include alcohol use versus abuse, initial high doses, HIV-
positive patients who weight trained, Systemic Lupus Erythematosus,
some clotting disorders, and high homocysteine levels amongst others
appear to increase risk. Early research regarding use of alendronate
(Fosamax) to treat ON appears to show that it is important for patients
to quickly return to their doctors if unexplained joint pain (such as in
the hip or knee) happens. Some centers note that ON has been poorly
studied, and while the weight of data is growing, it is yet too early to
say more than that ON is correlated with corticosteroid use.**

Precautions for Use
By Infants and Children: Avoid prolonged use if possible. Watch for growth suppression. Long-term use also increases risk of adrenal gland deficiency
during stress (up to 18 months after drug is stopped). Pressure in the brain
may increase.

By Those Over 60 Years of Age: Cortisonelike drugs should be used very sparingly after 60 and only when the disorder under treatment is unresponsive
to adequate trials of unrelated drugs. Avoid prolonged use of this drug
where possible. Continual use (even in small doses) can increase the severity of diabetes, enhance fluid retention, raise blood pressure, weaken resistance to infection, induce stomach ulcer, and accelerate the development
of cataract and osteoporosis or other bone problems.

▷ ### Advisability of Use During Pregnancy
Pregnancy Category: C. See Pregnancy Risk Categories at the back of this book.
Animal Studies: Birth defects reported in mice, rats, and rabbits.
Human Studies: Adequate studies of pregnant women are not available. Avoid
completely during the first 3 months. Limit use during the final 6 months
as much as possible. If used, the infant should be examined for possible
deficiency of adrenal gland function.

Advisability of Use If Breast-Feeding
Presence of this drug in breast milk: Yes.
The amount that the infant is exposed to can be decreased by avoiding
breast-feeding for 3 to 4 hours after methylprednisolone is given. Talk to
your doctor about this benefit-to-risk decision.

Habit-Forming Potential: Use of this drug over an extended period of time may
produce a state of functional dependence (see Glossary). Treating asthma
and rheumatoid arthritis, the dose should be kept as small as possible, and
withdrawal should be attempted after periods of reasonable improvement.
Such procedures may reduce "steroid rebound"—return of symptoms as
the drug is withdrawn.

Effects of Overdose: Fatigue, muscle weakness, stomach irritation, acid indigestion, excessive sweating, facial flushing, fluid retention, swelling of extremities, increased blood pressure.

Possible Effects of Long-Term Use: Increased blood sugar (possible diabetes), increased fat deposits on the trunk of the body ("buffalo hump"), rounding of the face ("moon face"), thinning and fragility of skin, loss of texture and strength of bones (osteoporosis, aseptic necrosis—questionable causation versus correlation), cataracts, glaucoma, retarded growth and development in children.

Suggested Periodic Examinations While Taking This Drug (at physician's discretion)

Measurements of blood pressure.

Blood sugar and potassium levels.

Complete eye examinations at regular intervals.

Chest X-ray if history of tuberculosis.

Determination of the rate of development of the growing child to detect retardation of normal growth.

Bone mineral density testing to assess osteoporosis and fracture risk. Any unexplained joint pain (such as knee, hip, or shoulder) should be evaluated (possible ON and need for MRI).

Homocysteine levels are prudent (appear to be a risk factor for osteonecrosis).

▷ **While Taking This Drug, Observe the Following**

Foods: See grapefruit note under "Beverages." Ask your physician regarding need to restrict salt intake or to eat potassium-rich foods. During long-term use, higher protein diet may be prudent.

Herbal Medicines or Minerals: Hawthorn, ginger, garlic, ma huang (no longer on the market for weight loss), ginseng, guar gum, fenugreek, and nettle may change blood sugar. Since methylprednisolone may also change blood sugar control, caution is advised. Fir or pine needle oil should NOT be used by asthmatics. Ephedra alone does carry a German Commission E monograph indication for asthma treatment, and may blunt benefits of this drug. If you are allergic to plants in the Asteraceae family (aster, chrysanthemum, daisy, or ragweed), you may also be allergic to echinacea, chamomile, feverfew, and St. John's wort. Licorice may increase methylprednisolone blood levels and lead to excessive effects. Added calcium and vitamin D while taking this medicine is prudent. Combination use of glucosamine has not been studied, but the combined use in cases of post-traumatic osteoarthritis may be beneficial. During wound repair, zinc supplementation may be prudent. Using echinacea or ginseng may boost the immune system and blunt the benefits of methylprednisolone. Talk to your doctor BEFORE adding any herbals to this medicine.

Beverages: Grapefruit juice will increase the plasma levels of methylprednisolone—water is a better liquid to take this medicine with. Drink all forms of milk liberally (as a calcium and vitamin D source).

▷ *Alcohol:* Alcohol use is a risk factor seen in osteonecrosis cases. Talk to your doctor about how he or she would like you to approach any alcohol use. Caution needed as well if you are prone to peptic ulcer disease.

Tobacco Smoking: Nicotine increases the blood levels of naturally produced cortisone and related hormones. I advise everyone to quit smoking.

Marijuana Smoking: May cause additional impairment of immunity.

▷ *Other Drugs*

Methylprednisolone may *decrease* the effects of
- insulin and require higher doses.
- isoniazid (INH, Niconyl, etc.).
- salicylates (aspirin, sodium salicylate, etc.).
- vaccines by blunting immune response to them.

Methylprednisolone *taken concurrently* with
- amphotericin B (Fungizone) may increase risk of potassium loss.
- aprepitant (Emend) may increase risk of methylprednisolone toxicity. Doses should be decreased by 50% (pill form) and 25% if intravenous.
- carbamazepine (Tegretol) may blunt methylprednisolone benefits.
- cholestyramine (Questran) may decrease the amount of medicine that is absorbed into your body.
- clarithromycin (Biaxin) can result in increased methylprednisolone levels and toxicity.
- cyclosporine (Sandimmune) can result in increased steroid levels and cyclosporine toxicity.
- ketoconazole (Nizoral) (and other azole antifungals) may increase blood levels of methylprednisolone and result in toxicity (abnormal heartbeats or psychiatric reactions).
- loop diuretics, such as furosemide (Lasix) or bumetanide (Bumex), may result in increased risk of potassium loss.
- neuromuscular blocking agents (such as pancuronium [Pavulon], vecuronium [Norcuron], others) can result in increased risk and/or severity of muscle problems (myopathy and flaccid paralysis) and can also antagonize blockade from these medicines. Caution and unparalyzed periods are prudent.
- NSAIDs (such as aspirin, ibuprofen or others—see Drug Classes) may cause increased risk of ulceration of the stomach or intestine.
- oral anticoagulants (warfarin [Coumadin]) may either increase or decrease their effectiveness; consult your physician regarding the need for prothrombin time testing and dose adjustment.
- oral antidiabetic drugs (see Drug Classes) or insulin may result in loss of control of blood sugar and require higher doses or more frequent dosing of oral hypoglycemics or insulin in order to control blood sugar.
- primidone (Mysoline) may lead to increased metabolism of methylprednisolone and decreased therapeutic benefits of methylprednisolone.
- quinupristin/dalfopristin (Synercid) can result in increased steroid levels and toxicity.
- rifampin (Rifadin, others) may lead to increased metabolism of methylprednisolone and decreased therapeutic benefits of methylprednisolone.
- ritonavir (Norvir) and perhaps other protease inhibitors (see Drug Classes) may change therapeutic benefits of methylprednisolone.
- tacrolimus (Prograf) can result in increased tacrolimus levels and tacrolimus toxicity.
- theophylline (Theo-Dur) results in variable changes in blood levels; more frequent theophylline blood levels are indicated.
- thiazide diuretics (see Drug Classes) can result in additive potassium loss.
- vaccines (such as flu or pneumococcal) may result in a blunting of the immune response to the vaccine.

The following drugs may *decrease* the effects of methylprednisolone:
- antacids—may reduce its absorption.
- barbiturates (Amytal, Butisol, phenobarbital, etc.).

- phenytoin (Dilantin, etc.) or fosphenytoin (Cerebyx).
- rifampin (Rifadin, Rimactane, etc.).

▷ *Driving, Hazardous Activities:* Usually no restrictions. Be alert to the rare occurrence of dizziness.

Aviation Note: The use of this drug **may be a disqualification** for piloting. Consult a designated Aviation Medical Examiner.

Exposure to Sun: No restrictions.

Occurrence of Unrelated Illness: Decreases resistance to infection. Tell your doctor if you get an infection of any kind. May also reduce ability to respond to stress of acute illness, injury or surgery. Tell your doctor about any significant changes in your state of health.

Discontinuation: Do not stop this drug abruptly after chronic use. Ask your doctor for help with gradual, individualized withdrawal. Some clinicians change from daily to every-other-day therapy for 4 weeks BEFORE starting to lower the dose in a stepwise fashion. Many patients tolerate dose reductions of 2.5 mg of prednisone (other steroids are calculated on the basis of prednisone equivalents) with those decreases made every 3–7 days. If a disease flare occurs (worsening of symptoms), the dose should be increased to the last dose before the disease flare and should be tapered more slowly down to 5–10 mg or lower. Some clinicians use 8 A.M. predose plasma cortisol to guide tapering. If this lab test is less than 10 mcg/deciliter, tapering is continued until the daily prednisone equivalent is 2–5 mg. In general, if long-term treatment or high doses were used, prednisone equivalents should be tapered over 9–12 months. For up to 2 years after stopping this drug, you may require it again if you have an injury, surgery or an illness.

METHYSERGIDE (meth i SER jide)

Introduced: 1961   **Class:**   Antimigraine drug, ergot derivative   **Prescription:**   USA: Yes   **Controlled Drug:**   USA: No; Canada: No
Available as Generic: USA: No; Canada: No
Brand Name: Sansert

BENEFITS versus RISKS

Possible Benefits	*Possible Risks*
EFFECTIVE PREVENTION OF MIGRAINE AND CLUSTER HEADACHES	FIBROSIS (SCARRING) INSIDE CHEST AND ABDOMINAL CAVITIES, OF HEART AND LUNG TISSUES, ADJACENT TO MAJOR BLOOD VESSELS AND INTERNAL ORGANS (see "Possible Effects of Long-Term Use" below)
	Aggravation of hypertension, coronary artery disease and peripheral vascular disease

---

▷ **Principal Uses**

As a Single Drug Product: Uses currently included in FDA-approved labeling: Prevention of frequent and/or disabling vascular headaches (migraine and cluster neuralgia) that have not responded to other conventional treatment.

Other (unlabeled) generally accepted uses: None at present.

How This Drug Works: Blocks serotonin inflammatory and vasoconstrictor effects, easing blood vessel constriction that causes vascular headaches. (Competitive 5-HT blocker and also stabilizes platelet release of 5-HT.)

▷ **Widely Used Guidelines That Involve This Medicine (representative sample):** Please look at the section at the very beginning of this profile called "Class." Next, turn to Table 22 and you will find guidelines listed by the class involved!

Available Dosage Forms and Strengths

Tablets — 2 mg

▷ **Recommended Dosage Ranges** (Actual dose and schedule must be determined for each patient individually.)

Infants and Children: Safety and efficacy are not established — use of this drug is not recommended.

18 to 60 Years of Age: 4 to 8 mg daily, in divided doses with meals. A medication-free period of 3 to 4 weeks is *REQUIRED* after every 6-month course.

Over 60 Years of Age: 2 to 4 mg daily, in divided doses. Use very cautiously, with frequent monitoring for adverse effects.

Conditions Requiring Dosing Adjustments

Liver Function: This drug should not be used by patients with liver compromise.

Kidney Function: This drug should not be used by patients with renal compromise.

▷ **Dosing Instructions:** The tablet may be crushed and taken with food or milk to reduce stomach irritation. Uninterrupted use is limited to 6 months; avoid drug completely for 3 to 4 weeks between courses. If you forget a dose: Call your doctor. **It is extremely important that you take this medicine exactly as directed.**

▷ **Usual Duration of Use:** Use on a regular schedule for 3 weeks usually determines effectiveness in preventing recurrence of vascular headache. If significant benefit does not occur during this trial, this drug should be stopped. None of this medicine can be given for 3 to 4 weeks after every 6-month course of treatment. Periodic long-term use (months to years) requires periodic physician evaluation.

Typical Treatment Goals and Measurements (Outcomes and Markers)

Pain: Most clinicians treating pain use a device called an algometer to check your pain. This looks like a small ruler, but lets the clinician better understand your pain. The goals of treatment then relate to where the level of pain started (for example, a rating of 7 on a 0 to 10 scale) and what the cause of the pain was. Specific results in migraine therapy and this medicine relate to decreasing the frequency and/or severity of headaches or avoiding them altogether.

▷ **This Drug Should Not Be Taken If**

- you have had an allergic reaction to it previously.
- you are pregnant.
- you currently have a severe infection.
- you have any of the following conditions:
  - angina pectoris
  - Buerger's disease

- cellulitis of the lower legs
- chronic lung disease
- connective tissue (collagen) disease
- coronary artery disease
- hardening of the arteries (arteriosclerosis)
- heart valve disease
- high blood pressure (significant hypertension)
- kidney disease or significantly impaired kidney function
- liver disease or significantly impaired liver function
- active peptic ulcer disease
- peripheral vascular disease
- phlebitis of any kind
- Raynaud's disease or phenomenon

▷ **Inform Your Physician Before Taking This Drug If**
- you had an adverse reaction to any ergot.
- you have a history of peptic ulcer disease or heart disease.

Possible Side Effects (natural, expected, and unavoidable drug actions)
Fluid retention, weight gain. Impaired circulation to the extremities (peripheral ischemia).

▷ **Possible Adverse Effects** (unusual, unexpected, and infrequent reactions)
If any of the following develop, consult your physician promptly for guidance.

Mild Adverse Effects
Allergic reactions: skin rashes, flushing of the face, transient loss of scalp hair.
Dizziness, drowsiness, agitation, unsteadiness, altered vision—infrequent to frequent.
Heartburn, nausea, vomiting, diarrhea—infrequent.
Transient muscle and joint pains—infrequent.

Serious Adverse Effects
Idiosyncratic reactions: nightmares, hallucinations, acute mental disturbances.
Fibrosis (scar tissue formation) involving the chest and/or abdominal cavities, heart, heart valves, lungs, kidneys, major blood vessels—case reports.
Spasm and narrowing of coronary and peripheral arteries: anginal chest pain, cold and painful extremities, leg cramps on walking—case reports.
Hemolytic anemia (see Glossary) or abnormally low platelet or white blood cell counts—case reports.
Heart attack (myocardial infarction)—case reports.

▷ **Possible Effects on Sexual Function:** Fibrosis of penile tissues—case reports.

▷ **Adverse Effects That May Mimic Natural Diseases or Disorders**
Swelling of the hands, lower legs, feet, and ankles (peripheral edema) may suggest heart or kidney dysfunction.

Natural Diseases or Disorders That May Be Activated by This Drug
Latent coronary artery insufficiency (angina), Buerger's disease, Raynaud's disease, peptic ulcer disease.

Possible Effects on Laboratory Tests
Complete blood cell counts: decreased white cells (lymphocytes).
Stomach hydrochloric acid: increased.
Kidney function tests: increased blood urea nitrogen (BUN).

CAUTION

1. Continual use limited to 6 months. Gradual dose reduction is prudent during last 2 to 3 weeks of each course to prevent headache rebound. Omit drug for a period of 3 to 4 weeks before resuming. Mandatory "drug-free" period reduces fibrosis risk.
2. Promptly report fatigue, fever, chest pain, difficult breathing, stomach/flank pain, or urinary changes.
3. Useful only for prevention of recurring vascular headaches. NOT recommended for sudden (acute) headaches. Not effective for tension headaches.

Precautions for Use

By Infants and Children: Use of this drug is not recommended.

By Those Over 60 Years of Age: The age-related changes in blood vessels, circulatory functions and kidney function can make you more susceptible to the serious adverse effects of this drug. See the list of diseases and disorders on the previous page that are contraindications to the use of this drug. Ask your doctor for help.

▷ Advisability of Use During Pregnancy

Pregnancy Category: X. See Pregnancy Risk Categories at the back of this book.

Animal Studies: No information is available.

Human Studies: Adequate studies of pregnant women are not available.

The manufacturer states that this drug is contraindicated during entire pregnancy.

Advisability of Use If Breast-Feeding

Presence of this drug in breast milk: Yes.

Avoid drug or refrain from nursing.

Habit-Forming Potential: None.

Effects of Overdose: Nausea, vomiting, stomach pain, diarrhea, dizziness, excitement, cold hands and feet.

Possible Effects of Long-Term Use: Formation of scar tissue (fibrosis) inside chest cavity and/or abdominal cavity, on heart valves, in lung tissues and surrounding major blood vessels and internal organs. Requires close and continual medical supervision.

Suggested Periodic Examinations While Taking This Drug (at physician's discretion)

Careful examination at regular intervals (6 to 12 months) for scar tissue formation or circulatory complications.

Complete blood cell counts.

Kidney function tests.

▷ While Taking This Drug, Observe the Following

Foods: No restrictions except foods you are allergic to. Some vascular headaches are due to food allergy, or have specific food triggers. A headache diary can help you identify triggers and then avoid them.

Herbal Medicines or Minerals: Since methysergide and St. John's wort may act on serotonin, the combination is not advised. Using ma huang or ephedrine-like (bitter orange or country mallow) compounds (ephedra- no longer on the market for weight loss) may result in additive and undesirable vasoconstriction. If you are allergic to plants in the *Asteraceae* family (aster, chrysanthemum, daisy, or ragweed), you may also be allergic to echinacea, chamomile, feverfew, and St. John's wort. St. John's wort can cause changes in the liver enzymes that help remove this medicine—talk to your doctor before combining any herbal medicine or mineral with methysergide.

Beverages: No restrictions.

▷ *Alcohol:* No interactions expected. Observe closely to determine if alcoholic beverages can initiate a migrainelike headache.

Tobacco Smoking: Avoid completely.

▷ *Other Drugs*

Methysergide **taken concurrently** with

- beta-blocker drugs (see Drug Classes) may cause hazardous constriction of peripheral arteries; watch combined effects on circulation in the extremities. Careful patient monitoring and a selective beta blocker (such as atenolol) are prudent.
- clarithromycin, erythromcin (macrolide antibiotics) may lead to egotism. DO NOT combine.
- efavirenz (Sustiva) increases risk of methysergide toxicity.
- medicines removed by the cytochrome P450 3A4 enzymes (atazanavir (Reyataz), others as well as those that inhibit CYP 3A4 may lead to methysergide toxicity. Medicines that increase CYP3A4 will blunt methysergide benefits.
- sibutramine (Meridia) increases serotonin syndrome risk.
- sildenafil (Viagra) may increase risk of methysergide toxicity.
- sumatriptan (Imitrex) and other triptans, such as naratriptan, zolmitriptan, almotriptan, or rizatriptan, may cause prolonged spasm of blood vessels—DO NOT COMBINE or use within 24 hours of a "triptan" dose.

▷ *Driving, Hazardous Activities:* This drug may cause dizziness, drowsiness, or impaired vision. Restrict activities as necessary.

Aviation Note: The use of this drug **is a disqualification** for piloting. Consult a designated Aviation Medical Examiner.

Exposure to Sun: No restrictions.

Exposure to Cold: Use caution. Cold environments may increase the occurrence of reduced circulation (blood flow) to the extremities.

Discontinuation: Do not stop it abruptly if drug has been taken for a long time. Slowly lowering (tapering) the dose over 2 to 3 weeks can prevent rebound vascular headaches.

METOCLOPRAMIDE (met oh KLOH pra mide)

Introduced: 1973   **Class:** Gastrointestinal drug, antinausea (antiemetic)
Prescription: USA: Yes   **Controlled Drug:** USA: No; Canada: No
Available as Generic: Yes

Brand Names: ♣Apo-Metoclop, ♣Clopra, ♣Emex, ♣Gastrobid, ♣Maxeran, Maxolon, Octamide, Reclomide, Reglan

---

BENEFITS versus RISKS

Possible Benefits	*Possible Risks*
EFFECTIVE STOMACH STIMULANT FOR CORRECTING DELAYED EMPTYING	Sedation and fatigue
	Parkinson-like reactions
	Tardive dyskinesia
Symptomatic relief in reflux esophagitis	
Relief of nausea and vomiting associated with migraine headache	

▷ **Principal Uses**

As a Single Drug Product: Uses currently included in FDA-approved labeling: Helps (1) stomach retention (gastroparesis) associated with diabetes; (2) acid reflux from the stomach into the esophagus (esophagitis); (3) nausea and vomiting associated with migraine headaches; (4) nausea and vomiting induced by anticancer drugs (chemotherapy); (5) decrease the time needed to place a tube in the intestine; (6) used prior to cesarean section to decrease postdelivery or postsurgical nausea or vomiting; (7) used in some X-ray (radiologic) tests or tube placements (intubations).

Other (unlabeled) generally accepted uses: (1) Used as a preparatory drug in stomach hemorrhage; (2) may help gastrointestinal symptoms in anorexia nervosa; (3) eases drug-induced slowed functioning of the intestine (adynamic ileus); (4) decreases the frequency of accumulations of food in the stomach (bezoars); (5) can be of benefit in migraine attacks; (6) can help tongue protrusion in resistant tardive dyskinesia cases.

How This Drug Works: Inhibits relaxation of stomach muscles and enhances parasympathetic nervous system (responsible for stomach muscle contractions) stimulation, which accelerates emptying of stomach contents into the intestine.

▷ **Widely Used Guidelines That Involve This Medicine (representative sample):** Please look at the section at the very beginning of this profile called "Class." Next, turn to Table 22 and you will find guidelines listed by the class involved!

Available Dosage Forms and Strengths

Injection — 5 mg/mL, 10 mg/mL
Intranasal — available in Italy as Pramdin (investigational in the U.S.)
Solution — 10 mg/mL
    Syrup — 5 mg/5 mL
Tablets — 5 mg, 10 mg

▷ **Usual Adult Dosage Ranges:** *Diabetic gastroparesis:* 10 mg, taken 30 minutes before breakfast, lunch, and dinner and at bedtime (4 times a day) for 2 to 8 weeks. Daily maximum is 0.5 mg per kg of body mass.

Note: Actual dose and schedule must be determined for each patient individually.

Conditions Requiring Dosing Adjustments

Liver Function: No changes appear to be needed.

Kidney Function: For patients with moderate kidney failure, 75% of the usual dose can be taken at the usual dosing interval. In severe kidney failure, 50% of the usual dose can be taken at the usual dosing interval. A benefit-to-risk decision must be made.

▷ **Dosing Instructions:** Take tablet or syrup 30 minutes before each meal and at bedtime. The tablet may be crushed. Use a calibrated medication spoon or dosing cup for the liquid form. If you forget a dose: take the missed dose as soon as you remember it, unless it's nearly time for your next dose—if that is the case, skip the missed dose and take the next dose right on schedule. Talk with your doctor if you find yourself missing doses.

Usual Duration of Use: Use on a regular schedule for 5 to 7 days determines benefit in accelerating stomach emptying and relieving symptoms of heartburn, fullness and belching. Long-term use (2 to 8 weeks) requires physician supervision. Repeat cycles of the medicine are possible.

Typical Treatment Goals and Measurements (Outcomes and Markers)
Gastroparesis: The general goal is to decrease feeling of stomach fullness by increasing stomach (gastric) emptying. For other uses, nausea and vomiting are decreased.

▷ **This Drug Should Not Be Taken If**
• you have had an allergic reaction to it previously.
• you have a seizure disorder of any kind.
• you have active gastrointestinal bleeding.
• you are taking, or have taken within the last 14 days, an MAO inhibitor (see Drug Classes).
• you are taking tricyclic antidepressants.
• you have a pheochromocytoma (adrenaline-producing tumor).

▷ **Inform Your Physician Before Taking This Drug If**
• you are allergic or overly sensitive to procaine or procainamide.
• you have impaired liver or kidney function.
• you have Parkinson's disease.
• you have epilepsy.
• you have high blood pressure.
• you have a history of depression.
• you are taking atropinelike drugs, antipsychotics, or opioid analgesics (see Drug Classes).

Possible Side Effects (natural, expected, and unavoidable drug actions)
Drowsiness and lethargy, breast tenderness and swelling, milk production.

▷ **Possible Adverse Effects** (unusual, unexpected, and infrequent reactions)
If any of the following develop, consult your physician promptly for guidance.
Mild Adverse Effects
Allergic reaction: skin rash. Mild decreases in blood pressure.
Headache, dizziness, restlessness, depression, insomnia—infrequent.
Dry mouth, nausea, diarrhea, constipation—infrequent to frequent.
Urinary retention or incontinence—possible.
Serious Adverse Effects
Idiosyncratic reactions: neuroleptic malignant syndrome (see Glossary), bronchospastic reactions in asthmatics.
Parkinson-like reactions (see Glossary) or tardive dyskinesia (see Glossary—may be more likely in females and with longer treatment)—case reports.
Abnormal fixed positioning of the eyes (oculogyric crisis)—case reports.
Movement disorders (extrapyramidal symptoms)—rare.
Depression—case reports.
Severe decrease in white blood cells (agranulocytosis)—case report.

Abnormal heartbeat—possible, case reports with intravenous use.
Severe increases in blood pressure (hypertensive crisis)—case reports.
Drug-induced porphyria—case reports.
Methemoglobinemia—case report in an overdose case.

▷ **Possible Effects on Sexual Function:** Decreased libido, impaired erection, decreased sperm count, sustained painful erection (priapism). Sudden milk production by a non-pregnant woman (galactorrhea)—case reports. Altered timing and pattern of menstruation—case reports to infrequent.

Possible Effects on Laboratory Tests
Blood lithium level: increased.
Blood thyroid stimulating hormone (TSH) level: increased.

Precautions for Use
By Infants and Children: Watch for development of Parkinson-like reactions soon after starting therapy. Use of the smallest effective dose can minimize such reactions. For diabetic gastroparesis, 0.5 mg per kg of body mass per day, divided into 3 equal doses given every 8 hours has been used. Children under 6 years old should NOT receive single doses more than 0.1 mg per kg of body mass.
By Those Over 60 Years of Age: Parkinson-like reactions and tardive dyskinesias are more likely to occur with the use of high doses over an extended period of time. The smallest effective dose should be identified and used only when clearly needed.

▷ **Advisability of Use During Pregnancy**
Pregnancy Category: B. See Pregnancy Risk Categories at the back of this book.
Animal Studies: No birth defects found due to this drug.
Human Studies: Adequate studies of pregnant women are not available.
Use this drug only if clearly needed.

Advisability of Use If Breast-Feeding
Presence of this drug in breast milk: Yes.
But blood levels appear to avoid therapeutic 500 mcg/kg/day in children. Talk to your doctor about BENEFITS versus RISKS and watch your infant closely.

Habit-Forming Potential: None.

Effects of Overdose: Marked drowsiness, confusion, muscle spasms, jerking movements of head and face, tremors, shuffling gait. Methemoglobinemia.

Possible Effects of Long-Term Use: Parkinson-like reactions may appear within several months of use. Tardive dyskinesias usually occur after a year of continual use; they may persist after this drug is discontinued.

Suggested Periodic Examinations While Taking This Drug (at physician's discretion)
During long-term use, observe for the development of fine, wormlike movements on the surface of the tongue; these may be the first indications of an emerging tardive dyskinesia.

▷ **While Taking This Drug, Observe the Following**
Foods: No restrictions.
Herbal Medicines or Minerals: Valerian and kava kava may intensify drowsi-

ness (no longer recommended because of liver toxicity questions. Aloe, cascara, and senna may increase possibility of diarrhea. Using chromium may change the way your body is able to use sugar. Some health food stores advocate vanadium as mimicking the actions of insulin, but possible toxicity and need for rigorous studies presently preclude recommending it. DHEA may change sensitivity to insulin or insulin resistance. Hawthorn, ginger, garlic, ginseng and licorice, nettle, and yohimbe may change blood sugar. Since this may require adjustment of hypoglycemic medicine dosing, talk to your doctor BEFORE combining any of these herbal medicines with metoclopramide. Echinacea pupurea (injectable) and blonde psyllium seed or husk should NOT be taken by people living with diabetes.

Beverages: No restrictions. May be taken with milk.

▷ *Alcohol:* Combined effects can result in excessive sedation and marked intoxication because of increased alcohol absorption. Alcohol is best avoided.

Tobacco Smoking: No interactions expected. I advise everyone to quit smoking.

▷ *Other Drugs*

Metoclopramide may ***decrease*** the effects of
- cimetidine (Tagamet).
- digoxin (slow-dissolving dose forms) and reduce their effectiveness.

Metoclopramide ***taken concurrently*** with
- acetaminophen may increase the absorption of this drug; decreased doses are prudent if chronic acetaminophen use will continue with metoclopramide therapy.
- major antipsychotic drugs (phenothiazines, thiothixenes, haloperidol, etc.) may increase the risk of developing Parkinson-like reactions.
- cyclosporine (Sandimmune) may result in increased cyclosporine levels and toxicity.
- morphine (slow release) may result in faster onset and increased sedation.
- neuromuscular blocking agents (such as pancuronium-Pavulon, vecuronium-Norcuron, others) can result in extended recovery times from blockade. Caution is prudent.
- penicillin may result in decreased therapeutic benefits of the antibiotic; increased doses may be needed.
- quinidine (Quinaglute, others) may result in decreased therapeutic benefits from quinidine; increased blood level testing and adjustment of dosing to levels is indicated.
- sirolimus (Rapamune) or tacrolimus (Prograf) may result in toxicity. Checks of sirolimus or tacrolimus levels are prudent.
- sertraline (Zoloft) may increase risk of movement disorders.
- zalcitabine (Hivid) may blunt zalcitabine levels and benefits.

The following drugs may ***decrease*** the effects of metoclopramide:
- atropinelike drugs.
- opioid analgesics (see Drug Classes).
- ritonavir (Norvir).

▷ *Driving, Hazardous Activities:* This drug may cause drowsiness and dizziness. Restrict activities as necessary.

Aviation Note: The use of this drug ***may be a disqualification*** for piloting. Consult a designated Aviation Medical Examiner.

Exposure to Sun: No restrictions.

METOLAZONE (me TOHL a zohn)

Please see the thiazide diuretics family profile.

METOPROLOL (me TOH proh lohl)

Introduced: 1974   **Class:** Antihypertensive, beta-adrenergic blocker
Prescription: USA: Yes   **Controlled Drug:** USA: No; Canada: No
Available as Generic: Yes

Brand Names: ♣Apo-Metoprolol, ♣Betaloc, ♣Co-Betaloc [CD], ♣Logimax [CD], Lopressor, Lopressor Delayed-Release, Lopressor HCT [CD], Lopressor OROS, ♣Novo-Metoprol, ♣Nu-Metop, Toprol, Toprol XL

BENEFITS versus RISKS

Possible Benefits	*Possible Risks*
EFFECTIVE, WELL-TOLERATED ANTIHYPERTENSIVE in mild to moderate high blood pressure	Worsening of angina in coronary heart disease (abrupt withdrawal)
MAY HELP REDUCE DEATH FROM HEART ATTACKS	Masking of low blood sugar (hypoglycemia) in drug-treated diabetes
APPROVED (Toprol XL form) TO TREAT CONGESTIVE HEART FAILURE	Provocation of asthma (with high doses in asthmatics)
REDUCES DEATH AND DISABILITY AFTER A HEART ATTACK	
EFFECTIVE TREATMENT OF ANGINA	

▷ **Principal Uses**

As a Single Drug Product: Uses currently included in FDA-approved labeling: (1) Treats mild to moderate high blood pressure, alone or with other drugs; (2) helps reduce the frequency and severity of angina; (3) used to reduce the risk of a second heart attack; (4) approved (Toprol XL form) to treat congestive heart failure (carvedilol, or Coreg, is the only other beta blocker approved for this use).

Other (unlabeled) generally accepted uses: (1) Reduces symptoms of heart muscle damage (dilated cardiomyopathy); (2) second-line drug in panic attacks; (3) used to decrease pressure in the eye (intraocular pressure) in open-angle glaucoma; (4) helps prevent migraine headaches; (5) a May 2002 study from Duke (see Ferguson, et al. in Sources) found that people who get beta blockers before heart bypass surgery (CABG) have better results than those who do not take those medicines.

As a Combination Drug Product [CD]: Metoprolol is available combined with hydrochlorothiazide (Lopressor HCT) which gives the benefits of both a beta blocker and a thiazide diuretic. Also available as Logimax in Canada which offers the benefits of metoprolol and a calcium channel blocker called felodipine.

In the Pipeline: The COMET (Carvedilol or Metoprolol European Trial) was the first study to make a head to head (drug to drug) comparison of two beta blockers in people with ongoing (chronic) heart failure (CHF) and looked at the effect of the two medicines on survival. CARVEDILOL showed a significant preferential lowering of death from heart and blood vessel disease (cardiovascular mortality) as well as all-cause mortality versus metoprolol.

How This Drug Works: Blocks some actions of the sympathetic nervous system:
- reducing rate, contraction force and ejection pressure of the heart.
- reducing contraction of blood vessels, resulting in lowering of blood pressure.
- prolonging conduction time of nerve impulses through the heart, managing certain heart rhythm disorders.

In heart failure, lowered remodeling of the left side of the heart (left ventricular remodeling) as well as lowered heart rate and action of the renin-angiotensin system may all work to help.

▷ **Widely Used Guidelines That Involve This Medicine (representative sample):** Please look at the section at the very beginning of this profile called "Class." Next, turn to Table 22 and you will find guidelines listed by the class involved!

Available Dosage Forms and Strengths

Injection — 1 mg/mL

Tablets — 50 mg, 100 mg

Tablets, prolonged action — 25 mg, 50 mg, 100 mg, 200 mg

▷ **Usual Adult Dosage Ranges:** *Hypertension:* Starts with 50 mg once or twice daily (12 hours apart). Dose may be increased gradually at intervals of 7 to 10 days as needed and tolerated, up to 300 mg/day. For ongoing use (maintenance), 100 mg twice a day. The total daily dose should not exceed 450 mg. The sustained release form is given once daily.

Angina: Dosing is started at 50 mg twice a day taken with meals or right after eating. The XL form is a sustained release dosage and can be taken as 100 mg once a day. Doses can be carefully increased as needed and tolerated to 400 mg a day. The selectiveness of this medicine for the heart goes away as the dose increases.

Migraine prevention: 50 to 200 mg a day.

Heart failure (NYHA Class II or III—once symptoms are stable for 2–4 weeks): Clinicians may start patients with the Toprol XL form (plus other evidence-based medicines such as ACE inhibitors, water pills—diuretics and digoxin) on a low dose such as 25 mg once a day for 14 days in class II patients. For more severe heart failure, 12.5 mg once a day. The dose then can be doubled every 2 weeks as needed and tolerated up to 200 mg a day. Other medicines used in combination should be adjusted as needed and tolerated.

After an Unstable Angina or one kind of heart attack (UA/NSTEMI): Intravenous (IV) dosing is started with 5 mg every 1-2 minutes with careful checks of heart rate, blood pressure and ECG. People who are able to handle (tolerate) the full 15 mg intravenous dosing are started on the by mouth (oral) form. 25-50 mg is then given fifteen minutes after the last intravenous dose. This dosing is continued every 6 hours for 48 hours. Ongoing doses are 100 mg twice a day.

Note: Actual dose and schedule must be determined for each patient individually.

Conditions Requiring Dosing Adjustments

Liver Function: Used with caution by patients with liver compromise.

Kidney Function: No changes thought to be needed.

▷ **Dosing Instructions:** The regular tablet may be crushed and taken without regard to eating. In general, prolonged-action forms should be swallowed whole (not altered). Toprol XL comes in a 25 mg form that is scored so that heart failure patients can take a 12.5 mg dose (talk to your doctor about this). While it is OK to split the scored XL tablet, do not crush the half-tablet to take it as it will change how quickly the medicine is released into your body. Do not stop this drug abruptly. If you forget a dose: take the missed dose as soon as you remember it, unless it's within 4 hours (regular release) or 8 hours (extended release form) of your next dose—if that is the case, skip the missed dose and take the next dose right on schedule. Talk with your doctor and pharmacist if you find yourself missing doses.

Usual Duration of Use: Regular use for 10 to 14 days determines benefits in lowering blood pressure. Long-term use in controlling blood pressure will be determined by your response to a treatment and risk factor control program (weight reduction, restricted salt, smoking cessation, etc.). Secondary cardiovascular disease prevention use (after a heart attack) and use in heart failure will be ongoing. See your doctor regularly.

Typical Treatment Goals and Measurements (Outcomes and Markers)

Blood Pressure: Guidelines (JNC VII) define normal blood pressure (BP) as **less than** 120/80 and **pre-hypertension** as 120/80 to 139/89. This new range is intended to help doctors encourage lifestyle changes (or in the case of people with a risk factor for high blood pressure, start treatment) much earlier—so that damage to blood vessels, heart, kidneys, sexual potency, or eyes might be minimized or avoided altogether. Stage 1 hypertension is 140/90 to 159/99 and stage 2 hypertension equal to or greater than 160/100 mm Hg. These guidelines also recommend that clinicians work with their patients to agree on the goals and a plan of treatment. The first-ever guidelines for blood pressure (hypertension) in African Americans recommends that MOST black patients be started on TWO antihypertensive medicines with the goal of lowering blood pressure to 130/80 for those with high risk for heart and blood vessel disease or with diabetes. The American Diabetes Association also recommends 130/80 as the target for diabetics and less than 125/75 for those who spill more than one gram of protein into their urine. Most clinicians try to achieve a BP that confers the best balance of lower cardiovascular risk and avoids the problem of too low a blood pressure. Blood pressure duration is generally increased with beneficial restriction of sodium. If goals are not met, it is not unusual to intensify doses or add on medicines.

Migraine prevention: Specific results in migraine therapy and this medicine relate to decreasing the frequency and/or severity of headaches or avoiding them altogether.

Possible Advantages of This Drug: Generic form offers beta-blocker advantages at a lower cost than some other medicines in the same class. A small study in the journal *Circulation* found no difference between the generic version of metoprolol and the more expensive carvedilol. The Oros brand of metoprolol works to reduce exercise-induced angina and daily lowering of heart blood flow (ischemia). The Toprol XL form is FDA-approved for use in heart failure.

Currently a "Drug of Choice"

For starting hypertension therapy with one drug, especially for those with bronchial asthma or diabetes and to lower cardiovascular morbidity and mortality.

▷ **This Drug Should Not Be Taken If**
  - you have had an allergic reaction to it previously.
  - you have had a heart attack and your heart rate is less than 45 beats/min.
  - you have an abnormally slow heart rate or a serious form of heart block (second or third degree).
  - you are in cardiogenic shock.
  - you took any monoamine oxidase (MAO) type A drug (see Drug Classes) in the last 14 days.

▷ **Inform Your Physician Before Taking This Drug If**
  - you had an adverse reaction to any beta blocker (see Drug Classes).
  - you have a history of serious heart disease.
  - you have a history of hay fever (allergic rhinitis), asthma, chronic bronchitis or emphysema. (People with bronchial asthma should generally not take beta blockers. This drug is somewhat heart selective and may be used with caution by asthmatics.)
  - you have a history of overactive thyroid function (hyperthyroidism).
  - you have a history of low blood sugar (hypoglycemia).
  - you have impaired liver or kidney function.
  - you have diabetes or myasthenia gravis.
  - you currently take digitalis, quinidine or reserpine or any calcium channel–blocker drug (see Drug Classes).
  - you have a history of poor circulation to the extremities (peripheral vascular disease).
  - you have a history of periodic cramps of your legs (intermittent claudication).
  - you will have surgery with general anesthesia.

Possible Side Effects (natural, expected, and unavoidable drug actions)
  Lethargy and fatigability, cold extremities, slow heart rate, light-headedness in upright position (see orthostatic hypotension in Glossary). Abnormally slow heartbeat (bradycardia). Mild increase in potassium.

▷ **Possible Adverse Effects** (unusual, unexpected, and infrequent reactions)
  If any of the following develop, consult your physician promptly for guidance.
  Mild Adverse Effects
  Allergic reactions: skin rash, itching.
  Worsening of psoriasis—case reports.
  Headache, fatigue, dizziness, insomnia, abnormal dreams—infrequent.
  Indigestion, nausea, vomiting, constipation, diarrhea—infrequent.
  Eye and joint pain—case reports.
  Joint and muscle discomfort, fluid retention (edema)—possible.
  Serious Adverse Effects
  Mental depression, hallucinations, anxiety—infrequent.
  Chest pain, shortness of breath, precipitation of congestive heart failure—case reports.
  Intermittent claudication—possible. May be prudent to check for hidden peripheral artery disease (PAD) by checking ankle brachial index (ABI). ABI check (see Glossary) can help find PAD early, and avoid claudication that may result if this medication is taken by someone who has PAD but does not know it.
  Induction of bronchial asthma (in asthmatic patients)—possible.
  Rebound hypertension—if the drug is abruptly stopped.
  Precipitation of myasthenia gravis—case reports.

Carpal tunnel syndrome—case reports.

Low or high blood sugar (hypoglycemia or hyperglycemia)—possible and more likely in type 1 diabetics.

Liver compromise (hepatitis)—case report.

▷ **Possible Effects on Sexual Function:** Decreased libido (4 times more common in men); impaired erection (less common with this drug than with most other beta blockers); Peyronie's disease (see Glossary)—case reports.

Possible Effects on Laboratory Tests

Blood HDL cholesterol level: decreased.

Blood LDL and VLDL cholesterol level: decreased.

Blood glucose level: increased.

Blood triglyceride levels: increased.

CAUTION

1. *Do not stop this drug suddenly* without the knowledge and help of your physician. Carry a note with you that says you take this drug.
2. Ask your doctor or pharmacist before using any nasal decongestants. These are often found in nonprescription cold medicines and nose drops. They may increase blood pressure.
3. Report development of emotional depression.
4. When patients are changed from an immediate release to a sustained release form, the same total dose is used and is then increased as needed and tolerated.
5. As the dose of this medicine is increased, the heart (beta one) selectivity is lost.

Precautions for Use

By Infants and Children: Safety and effectiveness for use by those under 12 years of age have not been established, but if this drug is used, observe for the development of low blood sugar (hypoglycemia) during periods of reduced food intake.

By Those Over 60 Years of Age: Proceed cautiously with all antihypertensive drugs. Unacceptably high blood pressure should be reduced slowly, to avoid the risks associated with excessively low blood pressure. Therapy should be started with small doses and the blood pressure checked often. Sudden, rapid, and excessive reduction of blood pressure can predispose to stroke or heart attack. Watch for dizziness, unsteadiness, tendency to fall, confusion, hallucinations, depression, or urinary frequency.

▷ **Advisability of Use During Pregnancy**

Pregnancy Category: C. C/D from one researcher. See Pregnancy Risk Categories at the back of this book.

Animal Studies: No significant increase in birth defects due to this drug.

Human Studies: Adequate studies of pregnant women are not available.

Use this drug only if clearly needed. Ask your physician for guidance.

Advisability of Use If Breast-Feeding

Presence of this drug in breast milk: Yes.

Discuss BENEFITS versus RISKS with your doctor.

Habit-Forming Potential: None.

Effects of Overdose: Weakness, slow pulse, low blood pressure, cold and sweaty skin, congestive heart failure, possible coma, and convulsions.

Possible Effects of Long-Term Use: Reduced heart reserve and eventual heart failure in susceptible individuals with advanced heart disease.

Suggested Periodic Examinations While Taking This Drug (at physician's discretion)
Measurements of blood pressure.
Evaluation of heart function, check of frequency of angina. When used after a heart attack, the function of the left side of the heart, size of the damaged area (infarct size), and heart rate should be checked.

▷ **While Taking This Drug, Observe the Following**
Foods: Peak drug concentration and peak effect will increase if taken with food. Avoid excessive salt intake. Migraines often have specific food triggers. Keep a headache diary, and then avoid the triggering foods.
Herbal Medicines or Minerals: Valerian and kava kava (no longer recommended in Canada) may intensify drowsiness. Ginseng, guarana, bitter orange, country mallow, mate, hawthorn, saw palmetto, ma huang (do not take if hypertensive), goldenseal, yohimbe, and licorice may also increase blood pressure. Calcium and garlic may help lower blood pressure and could be part of complementary care. Use of calcium to excess (7.5 to 10 grams) with combination thiazide diuretics can lead to excessive calcium levels. Talk to your doctor about how much calcium to take. Indian snakeroot has a German Commission E monograph indication for hypertension—talk to your doctor. Eleuthero root and ephedra should be avoided by people living with hypertension. St. John's wort may blunt benefits of this medicine.
Beverages: No restrictions. May be taken with milk.
▷ *Alcohol:* Use with caution. Alcohol may exaggerate this drug's ability to lower the blood pressure and may increase its mild sedative effect.
Tobacco Smoking: Nicotine may reduce this drug's benefit in treating high blood pressure. I advise everyone to quit smoking.
▷ *Other Drugs*
Metoprolol may ***increase*** the effects of
• other antihypertensive drugs, causing excessive lowering of blood pressure; dose adjustments may be necessary.
• reserpine (Ser-Ap-Es, etc.) and cause sedation, depression, slowing of the heart rate, and lowering of the blood pressure.
• verapamil (Calan, Isoptin) and cause excessive depression of heart function; monitor this combination closely.
Metoprolol ***taken concurrently*** with
• amiodarone (Cordarone) may result in extremely slow heartbeat and cardiac arrest—NOT ADVISED.
• clonidine (Catapres) requires close monitoring for rebound high blood pressure if clonidine is withdrawn while metoprolol is still being taken.
• digoxin (Lanoxin, others) may increase heart slowing.
• fluoxetine (Prozac) may cause metoprolol toxicity.
• fluvoxamine (Luvox) may lead to metoprolol toxicity.
• insulin requires close monitoring to avoid undetected hypoglycemia (see Glossary).
• lidocaine can lead to lidocaine toxicity (cardiac arrest).
• methyldopa (Aldomet, others) can have a rare paradoxical hypertensive response—caution is advised.
• nifedipine (Adalat, Procardia, others) may result in heart failure.
• oral antidiabetic drugs (see Drug Classes) can result in prolonged hypoglycemia if it occurs.
• phenothiazines (see Drug Classes) can result in low blood pressure or toxicity due to the phenothiazine.

- quinidine (Quinaglute, others) can lead to abnormally slow heartbeat and shortness of breath.
- ritonavir (Norvir) and perhaps other protease inhibitors (see Drug Classes) may cause toxicity.
- tocainide (Tonocard) may lead to depressed contraction ability of the heart (myocardial contractility).
- venlafaxine (Effexor) may lead to metabolic changes and toxic blood levels of both medicines.

The following drugs may *increase* the effects of metoprolol:
- alpha one adrenergic blockers, such as prazosin (Minipres).
- bupropion (Zyban). Metoprolol doses at the lower end of the dosing range are prudent if these drugs must be used together.
- cimetidine (Tagamet).
- ciprofloxacin (Cipro).
- diltiazem (Cardizem) and other dihydroperidine calcium blockers—especially in people with decreased function of the left ventricle.
- MAO inhibitors (see Drug Classes).
- methimazole (Tapazole).
- oral contraceptives (birth control pills); a different (non–first pass) beta blocker is advisable.
- propafenone (Rythmol).
- propoxyphene (Darvocet, others).
- propylthiouracil (Propacil).
- zafirlukast (Accolate) or zileuton (Zyflo): dose decreases of metoprolol may be needed.

The following drugs may *decrease* the effects of metoprolol:
- barbiturates (phenobarbital, etc.).
- indomethacin (Indocin) and possibly other aspirin substitutes or NSAIDs—may impair metoprolol's antihypertensive effect.
- rifampin (Rifadin, Rimactane).

▷ *Driving, Hazardous Activities:* Use caution until the full extent of drowsiness, lethargy and blood pressure change has been determined.

Aviation Note: The use of this drug *is a disqualification* for piloting. Consult a designated Aviation Medical Examiner.

Exposure to Sun: No restrictions.

Exposure to Heat: Caution is advised. Hot environments can lower the blood pressure and exaggerate the effects of this drug.

Exposure to Cold: Caution: Cold environments can increase circulatory deficiency in extremities. The elderly should take care to prevent hypothermia (see Glossary).

Heavy Exercise or Exertion: Best to avoid exertion that produces light-headedness, excessive fatigue or muscle cramping. This drug may intensify the blood pressure response to isometric exercise.

Occurrence of Unrelated Illness: Fever can lower the blood pressure and require adjustment of dose. Nausea or vomiting may interrupt the regular dose schedule. Ask your doctor for help.

Discontinuation: **Do not stop this drug suddenly.** Gradual dose lowering over 1 to 2 weeks is recommended. Ask your doctor for help.

METRONIDAZOLE (me troh NI da zohl)

Introduced: 1960   **Class:** Anti-infective   **Prescription:** USA: Yes
Controlled Drug: USA: No; Canada: No   **Available as Generic:** Yes
Brand Names: ♣Apo-Metronidazole, Femazole, Flagyl, Flagyl ER (extended release form), Flagystatin [CD], Helidac [CD], Lagyl, Losec Helicopak [CD], Metizol, MetroGel, MetroLotion, Metro IV, Metryl, ♣Neo-Tric, ♣Noritate cream, ♣Novo-Nidazole, ♣PMS-Metronidazole, Protostat, ♣Rho-Metrostatin, SK-Metronidazole, ♣Trikacide

---

BENEFITS versus RISKS

Possible Benefits	*Possible Risks*
EFFECTIVE TREATMENT FOR *TRICHOMONAS* INFECTIONS, AMEBIC DYSENTERY AND GIARDIASIS AND SOME ANAEROBIC BACTERIAL INFECTIONS	Superinfection with yeast organisms
	Peripheral neuropathy
	Abnormally low white blood cell count (transient)
	Colitis
	Aggravation of epilepsy
TREATMENT OF BACTERIAL VAGINOSIS (ER FORM)	
EFFECTIVE LOCAL TREATMENT (TOPICAL) FOR ROSACEA	

▷ **Principal Uses**

As a Single Drug Product: Uses currently included in FDA-approved labeling: (1) Treats *Trichomonas* infections of the vaginal canal and cervix and of the male urethra; (2) also used to treat amebic dysentery and liver abscess, *Giardia* infections of the intestine, and serious infections caused by certain strains of anaerobic bacteria; (3) treats *Gardnerella* infections of the vagina; (4) treatment of acne rosacea with local application of a gel dose form; (5) used in therapy of pseudomembranous colitis in adults; (6) has a role in treating bed sores (decubitus ulcers); (7) can help prevent infection (prophylaxis) in gynecological, appendectomy or colorectal surgery; (8) ER form used in bacterial vaginosis.

Other (unlabeled) generally accepted uses: (1) Combination therapy with gentamicin in treating intra-abdominal infections; (2) combination antibiotic treatment of duodenal ulcers caused by *Helicobacter pylori;* (3) can help treat infections caused by *Giardia lamblia;* (4) used to help heal the lesions in Crohn's disease; (5) may help abnormal gum growth (gingival hyperplasia) caused by cyclosporine; (6) often used to treat pseudomembranous colitis.

As a Combination Drug Product [CD]: Metronidazole is available combined with 20 mg of omeprazole, 500 mg of amoxicillin and 400 mg of metronidazole for combination treatment of *Helicobacter pylori.* Also available in Canada combined with nystatin for yeast infections as a vaginal insert.

How This Drug Works: Interacts with DNA, destroying essential component (nucleus) that is needed for life and growth of infecting organisms.

▷ **Widely Used Guidelines That Involve This Medicine (representative sample):** Please look at the section at the very beginning of this profile called "Class." Next, turn to Table 22 and you will find guidelines listed by the class involved!

Available Dosage Forms and Strengths

Capsules — 375 mg

Gel — 0.75%

Injection — 500 mg/100 mL

Tablets — 250 mg, 500 mg

Tablets, extended release — 750 mg

Vaginal cream — 10%

Vaginal insert — 500 mg/100,000 U (Canada)

▷ **Usual Adult Dosage Ranges:** *For bacterial vaginosis* (ER form): 750 mg once a day for 7 days in a row.

For trichomoniasis: 1-day course — 2 g as a single dose or 1 g for 2 doses 12 hours apart. 7-day course — 250 mg 3 times a day for 7 consecutive days. (The 7-day course is preferred.)

For amebiasis: 500 to 750 mg 3 times a day for 5 to 10 consecutive days.

For giardiasis: 2 g once daily for 3 days, or 250 to 500 mg 3 times a day for 5 to 7 days.

For Helicobacter pylori: The Helidac kit has 14 blister cards. One metronidazole and tetracycline tablet are taken once a day and 2 bismuth subsalicylate tablets are taken 4 times daily for a total regimen of 14 consecutive days. An H2 antagonist is also added to this combination. The total daily dose should not exceed 4 g (4,000 mg).

Note: Actual dose and schedule must be determined for each patient individually.

Conditions Requiring Dosing Adjustments

Liver Function: Dose is decreased by one-third in mild to moderate liver disease. Should not be used in severe liver compromise.

Kidney Function: In severe kidney failure, 50% of the normal dose can be taken at the usual dosing interval. A benefit-to-risk decision must be made for these patients, as there is a risk of systemic lupus erythematosus (SLE) from the metabolites of this drug.

▷ **Dosing Instructions:** The tablet may be crushed and taken with or following food to reduce stomach irritation. If you forget a dose: take the missed dose as soon as you remember it, unless it's nearly time for your next dose—if that is the case, skip the missed dose and take the next dose right on schedule. Talk with your doctor if you find yourself missing doses. Continue to take the full course of this medicine as prescribed even if you start to feel better.

Usual Duration of Use: Use on a regular schedule as outlined is needed to ensure effectiveness. Do not repeat the course of treatment without your physician's approval.

Typical Treatment Goals and Measurements (Outcomes and Markers)

Infections: The most commonly used measures of serious infections are white blood cell counts and differentials (the kind of blood cells that occur most often in your blood), and temperature. Many clinicians look for positive changes in 24–48 hours. NEVER stop an antibiotic because you start to feel better. For many infections, a full 14 days is REQUIRED to kill the bacteria. The goals and time frame should be discussed with you when the prescription is written.

▷ **This Drug Should Not Be Taken If**

- you have had an allergic reaction to it or any of the parabens contained in the gel form.
- you are pregnant (first 3 months).

- you currently have a bone marrow or blood cell disorder.
- you have any type of central nervous system disorder, including epilepsy.

▷ **Inform Your Physician Before Taking This Drug If**
- you have a history of any type of blood cell disorder, especially one caused by drugs.
- you have a history of seizures or peripheral neuropathy.
- you have impaired liver or kidney function.
- you are taking a form applied on the skin (topical) and develop a rash after applying it.
- you have a history of alcoholism.
- you are pregnant or breast-feeding.

Possible Side Effects (natural, expected, and unavoidable drug actions)
> A sharp, metallic, unpleasant taste. Dark discoloration of the urine (of no clinical significance). Superinfection (see Glossary) by yeast organisms in the mouth or vagina. Pseudomembranous colitis.

▷ **Possible Adverse Effects** (unusual, unexpected, and infrequent reactions)
> **If any of the following develop, consult your physician promptly for guidance.**
>
> *Mild Adverse Effects*
> Allergic reactions: skin rash, hives, flushing, itching.
> Headache, dizziness, incoordination, unsteadiness, incontinence—infrequent.
> Loss of appetite, nausea, vomiting, abdominal cramps, diarrhea—infrequent.
> Irritation of mouth and tongue, possibly due to yeast infection—possible.
>
> *Serious Adverse Effects*
> Idiosyncratic reactions: abnormal behavior; confusion; depression; Jarisch-Herxheimer's reaction (sweating, diarrhea, vomiting, scalding urination, joint pain, and itching)—case reports.
> Peripheral neuropathy (see Glossary)—case reports.
> Abnormally low white blood cell count (transient): fever, sore throat, infections—case reports.
> Disulfiram-type reaction (nausea, vomiting) if alcoholic beverages are consumed—possible.
> Seizures—case reports.
> Drug-induced pneumonitis, porphyria or pancreatitis—case reports.
> Hemolytic-uremic syndrome—case reports.

▷ **Possible Effects on Sexual Function:** Decreased libido; decreased vaginal secretions (difficult or painful intercourse)—case reports. Abnormal swelling of male breast tissue (gynecomastia)—case report.

Possible Delayed Adverse Effects: Studies have shown that this drug can cause cancer in mice and possibly in rats. Two researchers concluded that the carcinogenic risk is low in doses used to treat episodic vaginitis. High-dose, long-term use may carry increased cancer risk. Follow your doctor's instructions exactly. Avoid unnecessary or prolonged use.

▷ **Adverse Effects That May Mimic Natural Diseases or Disorders**
> Behavioral changes may suggest spontaneous psychosis.

Natural Diseases or Disorders That May Be Activated by This Drug
> Latent yeast infections.

Possible Effects on Laboratory Tests
> White blood cell counts: decreased.
> INR (prothrombin time): increased.
> Blood theophylline levels: falsely increased by some methods.

CAUTION
1. Troublesome and persistent diarrhea can develop. If diarrhea persists for more than 24 hours, stop this drug and call your physician.
2. Stop this drug immediately if you develop any signs of toxic effects on the brain or nervous system: confusion, irritability, dizziness, incoordination, unsteady stance or gait, muscle jerking or twitching, numbness or weakness in the extremities.
3. Don't get the topical cream form in your eyes.
4. If this medicine is being taken for an infection of the genitals, it is important to make certain that your partner(s) also get treated.
5. Do not drink alcoholic beverages while taking this medicine. The combination of alcohol and this medicine leads to flushing, vomiting, and other signs and symptoms (disulfiram reaction).

Precautions for Use
By Infants and Children: Avoid use in those with a history of bone marrow or blood cell disorders.

By Those Over 60 Years of Age: Natural changes in the skin may predispose to yeast infections in the genital and anal regions. Report the development of rashes and itching promptly.

▷ **Advisability of Use During Pregnancy**
Pregnancy Category: B. See Pregnancy Risk Categories at the back of this book.

Animal Studies: No birth defects reported in rat studies, but this drug is known to cause cancer in mice and possibly in rats.

Human Studies: No increase in birth defects reported in 206 exposures to this drug during the first 3 months. However, information from adequate studies of pregnant women is not available.

The manufacturer advises against the use of this drug during the first 3 months. Use during the final 6 months is not advised unless it is absolutely essential to the mother's health.

Advisability of Use If Breast-Feeding
Presence of this drug in breast milk: Yes.
Avoid drug or refrain from nursing.

Habit-Forming Potential: None.

Effects of Overdose: Weakness, stomach irritation, nausea, vomiting, confusion, disorientation.

Possible Effects of Long-Term Use: None reported. Avoid long-term use.

Suggested Periodic Examinations While Taking This Drug (at physician's discretion)
Complete blood cell counts.

▷ **While Taking This Drug, Observe the Following**
Foods: No restrictions.

Herbal Medicines or Minerals: Some patients use echinacea to attempt to boost their immune systems. Unfortunately, use of echinacea is not recommended in people with damaged immune systems (even if a medicine caused the damage). This herb may also actually weaken any immune system if it is used too often or for too long a time. DO NOT take mistletoe herb, oak bark or F.C. of marshmallow root, and licorice.

Beverages: No restrictions. May be taken with milk.

▷ *Alcohol:* A disulfiramlike reaction has been reported (see Glossary). It is NOT advisable to drink alcohol while taking metronidazole.

Tobacco Smoking: No interactions expected. I advise everyone to quit smoking.

▷   *Other Drugs*
Metronidazole may *increase* the effects of
  • amprenavir (Agenerase) oral solution (contains a lot of propylene glycol). Pill form does not have this.
  • carbamazepine (Tegretol) and lead to toxicity.
  • warfarin (Coumadin, etc.) and cause abnormal bleeding; the INR (prothrombin time or protime) should be monitored closely, especially during the first 10 days of concurrent use.
Metronidazole *taken concurrently* with
  • antacids may decrease absorption of metronidazole.
  • birth control pills (oral contraceptives) may block the effectiveness of contraception and result in pregnancy.
  • cholestyramine (Questran) or other cholesterol-lowering resins may decrease metronidazole absorption and lower its therapeutic effect.
  • cotrimoxazole or other sulfa drugs may result in a disulfiramlike effect.
  • cyclosporine (Sandimmune) can lead to cyclosporine toxicity.
  • disulfiram (Antabuse) may cause severe emotional and behavioral disturbances.
  • lithium (Lithobid, others) can cause lithium toxicity.
  • phenytoin (Dilantin) or fosphenytoin (Cerebyx) may result in increased blood levels of phenytoin; more frequent blood level testing is needed, and the phenytoin dose should be adjusted to blood levels.
  • ritonavir (Norvir) may increase blood levels of metronidazole.
  • sirolimus (Rapamune) or tacrolimus (Prograf) may increase risk of sirolimus toxicity.
  • sulfamethoxazole (Septra, others) and perhaps other sulfa drugs may lead to a disulfiramlike reaction.
  • trimethoprim (Septra, others) and perhaps other sulfa drugs may lead to a disulfiramlike reaction.
▷   *Driving, Hazardous Activities:* This drug may cause dizziness or incoordination. Restrict activities as necessary.
Aviation Note: The use of this drug *may be a disqualification* for piloting. Consult a designated Aviation Medical Examiner.
Exposure to Sun: No restrictions.

MEXILETINE (mex IL e teen)

Introduced: 1973 **Class:** Antiarrhythmic (Class or Group One)
Prescription: USA: Yes **Controlled Drug:** USA: No; Canada: No
Available as **Generic:** Yes
Brand Name: Mexitil

BENEFITS versus RISKS	
Possible Benefits	*Possible Risks*
EFFECTIVE TREATMENT IN SELECTED HEART RHYTHM DISORDERS	NARROW TREATMENT RANGE FREQUENT ADVERSE EFFECTS WORSENING OF SOME ARRHYTHMIAS (class one antiarrhythmics have increased risk of death when used in non–life threatening arrhythmias) Rare seizures, liver injury, and reduced white blood cell count

▷ **Principal Uses**

As a Single Drug Product: Uses currently included in FDA-approved labeling: Helps correct premature beats that arise in the ventricles (lower heart chambers).

Other (unlabeled) generally accepted uses: (1) Used before breast cancer surgery in one small study before surgery (preemptive analgesia) and was found to decrease pain medicine requirements (analgesic) after surgery; (2) useful in some patients for diabetic nerve damage pain (diabetic neuropathy).

How This Drug Works: Slows transmission of electrical impulses in the heart, restoring normal heart rate and rhythm in selected types of arrhythmia.

▷ **Widely Used Guidelines That Involve This Medicine (representative sample):** Please look at the section at the very beginning of this profile called "Class." Next, turn to Table 22 and you will find guidelines listed by the class involved!

Available Dosage Forms and Strengths

Capsules — 150 mg, 200 mg, 250 mg

Gelcap — 100 mg

Gelcap (Canada) — 200 mg

Tablet — 250 mg

▷ **Usual Adult Dosage Ranges:** When rapid control of life-threatening ventricular arrhythmias is required, the manufacturer suggests a loading dose of 400 mg, then 200 mg every 8 hours. Dose can be increased (every 2 to 3 days), as needed and tolerated in 50- or 100-mg steps. Daily maximum is 1,200 mg (doses greater than this can have undesirable central nervous system side effects). If rapid control of abnormal heartbeats is not required, starting doses of 200 mg given every eight hours can be used. Some clinicians try to improve how well patients take this medicine by using an every-12-hours dosing strategy. The strategy is to arrive at an every-8-hours approach (for example, 300 mg every 8 hours). If that dose (or less) works to control abnormal heartbeats, the same dose is given every 12 hours with careful follow-up for rhythm control. Dosing can then be adjusted as needed and tolerated based on individual patient response as far as 450 mg every 12 hours. Testing blood levels is advised to guide dosing.

Note: Actual dose and schedule must be determined for each patient individually.

Conditions Requiring Dosing Adjustments

Liver Function: Dose should be decreased by one-fourth to one-third in liver disease.

Kidney Function: Dose is decreased and blood levels obtained more often.

▷ **Dosing Instructions:** The capsule may be opened and taken with food or antacid to reduce stomach irritation. DO NOT change extended release forms (Britain). Take at same times each day to obtain uniform results (even blood levels). If you forget a dose: and you take this medicine twice a day, take the missed dose as soon as you remember it, unless you are more than 6 hours late—if that is the case, skip the missed dose and take the next dose right on schedule. If you take the mexiletine three times a day, take the missed dose once you remember it, unless you are more than 4 hours late—if that is the case, skip the missed dose and return to your usual schedule. Talk with your doctor if you find yourself missing doses.

Usual Duration of Use: Effect of the loading dose strategy is usually seen in 30 to 120 minutes. Use on a regular schedule for 1 to 2 weeks determines effectiveness in correcting or preventing responsive rhythm disorders—particularly if a loading dose approach is used. Long-term use requires physician supervision.

Typical Treatment Goals and Measurements (Outcomes and Markers)

Abnormal Heartbeats: The general goal is to return the heart to a normal rhythm or at least to markedly reduce the occurrence of abnormal heartbeats. For example, when a loading dose is used to help control ventricular arrhythmias, the effect is usually seen in 30 to 150 minutes. In life-threatening arrhythmias, the goal is to abort the abnormal beats and return the heart rhythm pattern to normal. 24-hour heart monitors such as Holter monitors are often used to check success over a full day in controlling abnormal heartbeats. An early study found that sudden and short-term benefits of this medicine in controlling rapid heartbeat rate (ventricular tachycardia), was predictive of long-term results of this medicine.

▷ **This Drug Should Not Be Taken If**
- you have had an allergic reaction to it previously.
- you have shock resulting from the heart (cardiogenic shock).
- you have second- or third-degree heart block (determined by electrocardiogram), uncorrected by a pacemaker.

▷ **Inform Your Physician Before Taking This Drug If**
- you had adverse reactions to other antiarrhythmic drugs.
- you have a history of heart disease of any kind, especially "heart block" or heart failure AND YOU DO NOT HAVE A PACEMAKER.
- you have a blood disorder that lowers white blood cells (agranulocytosis or leukopenia) or platelets (thrombocytopenia).
- you have impaired liver function.
- you have Parkinson's disease.
- another doctor has prescribed a medicine to make your urine basic (alkalinization) as this can keep mexiletine in your body longer.
- you are prone to low blood pressure or have a seizure disorder of any kind.
- you take digitalis, a potassium supplement or any diuretic drug that can cause potassium loss (ask your doctor).

Possible Side Effects (natural, expected, and unavoidable drug actions)
Nervousness, light-headedness. Unpleasant taste.

▷ **Possible Adverse Effects** (unusual, unexpected, and infrequent reactions)
If any of the following develop, consult your physician promptly for guidance.
Mild Adverse Effects
Allergic reaction: skin rash.

Headache, dizziness, visual disturbance, fatigue, weakness, tremor—infrequent.

Loss of appetite, indigestion, nausea, vomiting, constipation, diarrhea, joint or abdominal pain—rare.

Hesitation of urine stream (urinary hesitancy)—case reports.

Serious Adverse Effects

Idiosyncratic reactions: depression, confusion, amnesia, hallucinations, seizures—all rare.

Drug-induced heart rhythm disorders: shortness of breath, palpitations, chest pain, swelling—rare.

Myelofibrosis—case reports.

Systemic lupus erythematosus (SLE)—(increased ANA rarely [two in 10,000 patients] and SLE in roughly 4 of 10,000 patients—rare.

Seizures—case reports.

Psychological changes (depression, hallucinations, or psychosis)—reported.

Ataxia and confusion—reported.

Congestive heart failure and sinus arrest—rare.

Urinary retention—possible.

Bleeding in the stomach or intestines (gastrointestinal tract)—rare.

Liver damage with jaundice (see Glossary)—case reports.

Low white blood cell or platelet counts: fever, sore throat, abnormal bleeding/bruising—case reports.

▷ **Possible Effects on Sexual Function:** Decreased libido, impotence—rare.

▷ **Adverse Effects That May Mimic Natural Diseases or Disorders**

Liver toxicity may suggest viral hepatitis.

Natural Diseases or Disorders That May Be Activated by This Drug

Latent epilepsy.

Possible Effects on Laboratory Tests

Blood white cell and platelet counts: decreased.

Liver function tests: increased liver enzymes (ALT/GPT, AST/GOT)—increased in less than 1% of users.

CAUTION

1. Thorough evaluation of your heart function (including electrocardiograms) is necessary prior to using this drug.
2. Periodic evaluation of your heart function is needed to determine your response to this drug. Some individuals may experience worsening of their heart rhythm disorder and/or deterioration of heart function. Close monitoring of heart rate, rhythm, and overall performance is essential.
3. Dose must be adjusted carefully for each person. Do not change your dose without talking to your doctor.
4. Do not take any other antiarrhythmic drug while taking this drug unless you are directed to do so by your physician.
5. Carry a card in your purse or wallet saying that you take this drug. Tell health care providers that you take it.

Precautions for Use

By Infants and Children: Safety and effectiveness for those under 12 years of age are not established. Initial use of this drug requires hospitalization and supervision by a qualified cardiologist.

By Those Over 60 Years of Age: Reduced liver function may require reduction in dose. Watch carefully for light-headedness, dizziness, unsteadiness, and tendency to fall.

▷ **Advisability of Use During Pregnancy**
Pregnancy Category: C. See Pregnancy Risk Categories at the back of this book.
Animal Studies: No birth defects reported in mice, rats, or rabbits, but an increased rate of fetal resorption was found.
Human Studies: Adequate studies of pregnant women are not available. Avoid during first 3 months. Use this drug only if clearly needed. Ask your physician for guidance.

Advisability of Use If Breast-Feeding
Presence of this drug in breast milk: Yes.
Avoid drug or refrain from nursing.

Habit-Forming Potential: None.

Effects of Overdose: Impaired urination, constipation, marked drop in blood pressure, abnormal heart rhythms, congestive heart failure, dizziness, incoordination, seizures.

Possible Effects of Long-Term Use: None reported.

Suggested Periodic Examinations While Taking This Drug (at physician's discretion)
Electrocardiograms.
Complete blood cell counts.
Liver function tests.
Mexiletine blood levels. Check of beneficial outcomes on the heart with 24-hour monitoring (such as Holter monitors).

▷ **While Taking This Drug, Observe the Following**
Foods: No restrictions. Ask your physician regarding need for salt restriction.
Herbal Medicines or Minerals: Using St. John's wort, bitter orange, country mallow, ma huang, ephedra (no longer on the market as a weight loss medicine), guarana, mate, or kola while taking this medicine may result in unacceptable heart stimulation. Belladonna, henbane, scopolia, pheasant's eye extract or lily-of-the-valley, or squill powdered extracts should NOT be taken if you have abnormal heart rhythms.
Beverages: Caffeine may have an effect on heart rate and may not be desirable. Talk to your doctor about caffeine. Can be taken with milk.
▷ *Alcohol:* Use caution. Alcohol can increase the blood pressure–lowering effects of this drug.
Tobacco Smoking: Nicotine irritates the heart, reducing drug effectiveness. I advise everyone to quit smoking.
▷ *Other Drugs*
Mexiletine may ***increase*** the effects of
- antihypertensive drugs and cause excessive lowering of blood pressure.
- beta-blocker drugs (see Drug Classes).
- disopyramide (Norpace).
- lidocaine (various).
- quinidine (Quinaglute, various).
- theophylline (Theo-Dur, others), leading to theophylline toxicity and seizures.

Mexiletine ***taken concurrently*** with
- amiodarone (Cordarone) may lead to abnormal heartbeat or rhythm (QT changes and torsades de pointes).
- dofetilide (Tikosyn) and other medicines such as class I, IA or III antiarrhythmics, clarithromycin, cotrimoxazole, ondansetron, ziprazidone, and others may lead to prolongation of the QTc interval and undesirable effects. Combination is not recommended.

- drugs that inhibit or are removed by CYP 2D6 (talk to your doctor) may increase mexiletine effects.
- ritonavir (Norvir) and perhaps other protease inhibitors (see Drug Classes) may lead to toxicity.

The following drugs may *decrease* the effects of mexiletine:

- phenytoin (Dilantin, etc.) or fosphenytoin (Cerebyx).
- rifampin (Rifadin, Rimactane).

▷ *Driving, Hazardous Activities:* This drug may cause weakness, dizziness, or blurred vision. Restrict activities as necessary.

Aviation Note: The use of this drug *may be a disqualification* for piloting. Consult a designated Aviation Medical Examiner.

Exposure to Sun: No restrictions.

Occurrence of Unrelated Illness: Vomiting, diarrhea, or dehydration can affect this drug's action adversely. Report such developments promptly.

Discontinuation: Should not be stopped abruptly after long-term use. Ask your doctor about slowly reducing the dose.

MIGLITOL (MIG lit all)

Introduced: 1999   **Class:** Antidiabetic, Second generation alpha-glucosidase inhibitor   **Prescription:** USA: Yes   **Controlled Drug:** USA: No; Canada: No   **Available as Generic:** No

Brand Name: Glyset

BENEFITS versus RISKS

Possible Benefits	*Possible Risks*
EFFECTIVE LOWERING OF BLOOD SUGAR	Gas and abdominal pain (often decreases over time)
USE IN TYPE 1 OR TYPE 2 DIABETICS	
DECREASED RISK OF HIGH BLOOD PRESSURE, HEART DISEASE, OR OTHER LONG-TERM DAMAGE OF HIGH BLOOD SUGAR (WITH BETTER GLUCOSE CONTROL)	
COMBINED TREATMENT WITH SULFONYLUREA IF NEEDED	

▷ **Principal Uses**

As a Single Drug Product: Uses currently included in FDA-approved labeling: (1) Used with diet in diabetics who don't require insulin, yet don't have good blood sugar control with diet alone; (2) can be combined with a sulfonylurea (see Drug Classes) if diet plus miglitol or diet and sulfonylurea do not control blood sugar as well as needed.

Other (unlabeled) generally accepted uses: None at present.

How This Drug Works: By blocking intestinal alpha glucosidase and pancreatic alpha amylase (two enzymes), this medicine impairs sugar digestion and actually keeps sugar low after meals.

▷ **Widely Used Guidelines That Involve This Medicine (representative sample):**
Please look at the section at the very beginning of this profile called "Class." Next, turn to Table 22 and you will find guidelines listed by the class involved!

Available Dosage Forms and Strengths
Tablets — 25 mg, 50 mg, 100 mg (Canada)
Tablets, coated — 25 mg, 50 mg, 100 mg

▷ **Recommended Dosage Ranges** (Actual dose and schedule must be determined individually for each patient.)

Infants and Children: Safety and effectiveness not established in those less than 18 years old.

18 to 65 Years of Age: The most conservative starting dose is 25 mg once a day with the first bite of the first meal of the day. Subsequently, as needed and tolerated, the dose can be increased to 25 mg three times daily, taken at the start of each meal (after first bite). Dose increases are made at 4- to 8-week intervals to achieve blood sugar control while minimizing intestinal side effects (using 50 mg three times daily at the start of each meal). If response is not acceptable, dose may be increased to 50 mg three times daily. After three months of therapy, an A1C (glycosylated hemoglobin) should be checked. If this is still abnormal, dose may be increased to 100 mg three times daily. If a dose increase doesn't give better sugar control, dose decreases are usually considered because side effects tend to increase with increasing doses. 50-100 mg three times daily is often successful when this medicine is used by itself (monotherapy).

Over 65 Years of Age: No specific recommendations unless kidney function is very limited. Smaller doses are prudent.

Conditions Requiring Dosing Adjustments
Liver Function: Specific dosing changes do not appear to be needed.
Kidney Function: Use NOT recommended in kidney disease.

▷ **Dosing Instructions:** Take this pill after starting breakfast, lunch, and dinner—after the first bite of a meal has been eaten. Gas (flatulence) and diarrhea are common side effects but often decrease over time. Limiting the sugar sucrose can also help. If dose changes are made at 4- to 8-week intervals, the best sugar response and the least potential gas (flatulence) or diarrhea are realized. Often blood sugar is checked one hour after a meal (1 hr postprandial) and the dose adjusted to get the best balance of blood sugar and side effects. If you forget a dose: Take the missed dose as soon as you remember it, if you are still eating your meal. If you've finished eating, the most conservative course is to check your blood sugar and ask the doctor what to do. DO NOT double doses. Return to the next dose right on schedule. Talk with your doctor if you find yourself missing doses.

Usual Duration of Use: Dosing must be individualized. Peak drug response happens in about an hour. Dosing changes are made at 4- to 8-week intervals if needed. Regular use required to give better blood glucose control. Since non-insulin–dependent diabetes is a chronic condition, use of miglitol will be ongoing. Periodic hemoglobin A1C (glycosylated hemoglobin) tests and physician follow-up are needed. Keeping the sugar close to normal can minimize diabetic problems.

Typical Treatment Goals and Measurements (Outcomes and Markers)
Blood Sugar: The general goal for blood sugar is to return it to the usual "normal" range (generally 80–120 mg/dL), while avoiding risks of excessively low blood sugar. One study (UKPDS) used a fasting plasma sugar (glucose)

of less than 108 mg/dL. Fasting plasma sugar (glucose) is generally decreased by 20–30 mg/dL.

Fructosamine and Glycosylated Hemoglobin: Fructosamine levels (a measure of the past 2–3 WEEKS of blood sugar control) should be less than or equal to 310 micromoles per liter. Glycosylated hemoglobin or hemoglobin A1C (a measure of the past 2–3 months of blood sugar control) should be less than or equal to 7.0%. Some clinicians are advocating much lower targets, but others note an increased risk of hypoglycemia. A1C is often lowered by 0.7 to 1% by miglitol.

Possible Advantages of This Drug

May be used in combination with sulfonylurea oral hypoglycemics (see Drug Classes) to get the best control of blood sugar. This second generation alpha-glucosidase inhibitor has a chemical structure similar to sugar (glucose) and is well absorbed by the body—generally upsetting the stomach and intestines to a lesser degree. May also be more potent than acarbose (Precose) on a mg-to-mg basis.

▷ **This Drug Should Not Be Taken If**
- you have had an allergic reaction to it previously.
- you are in diabetic ketoacidosis.
- your history includes intestinal obstruction or you have a partial obstruction of the intestine.
- you have inflammatory bowel disease or colon ulceration.
- you have an intestinal condition that may worsen (such as a megacolon or bowel obstruction) if increased gas (flatus) forms.
- you have a long-standing (chronic) intestinal disease altering digestion or your ability to absorb materials from the intestine.

▷ **Inform Your Physician Before Taking This Drug If**
- you do not know what the symptoms of hypoglycemia are.
- you have an infection (insulin may be required).
- you are pregnant or are breast-feeding your infant (no data exists on use in pregnancy or breast-feeding).
- you have a history of kidney or liver disease.
- you will have surgery with general anesthesia or have a serious infection (insulin may be required).
- you forgot to tell your doctor about all the drugs you take.
- you are unsure of how much to take or how often to take it.

Possible Side Effects (natural, expected, and unavoidable drug actions)

Gas (flatulence) or diarrhea results from bacterial action on sugars and tends to decrease over time.

▷ **Possible Adverse Effects** (unusual, unexpected, and infrequent reactions)
If any of the following develop, consult your physician promptly for guidance.

Mild Adverse Effects
Allergic reactions: skin rash, itching.
Sleepiness, headache, dizziness—of questionable causation.
Pain or swelling of the belly (abdomen)—frequent.
Gas (flatulence) or diarrhea—frequent (often eases).
Low serum iron—infrequent.

Serious Adverse Effects
Low blood sugar if combined with sulfonylureas—possible.
Anemia—possible.
Ileus—case reports and in those with prior bowel blockage history.

▷ **Possible Effects on Sexual Function:** None reported.

Possible Effects on Laboratory Tests

Hemoglobin A1C: trending more toward normal (good effect).

Blood sugar one hour after eating (postprandial): decreased.

Liver enzymes: no change in one short-term study.

CAUTION

1. This medicine itself does not cause hypoglycemia. Low sugar may result if combined with insulin or sulfonylureas.
2. Infections may cause loss of sugar control and require temporary insulin use.
3. This medicine is part of the total management of diabetes. A properly prescribed diet and regular exercise are still required for best control of blood sugar.
4. If your kidneys fail or worsen, tell your doctor. This drug is generally not used if serum creatinine is greater than 2 mg/dL.

Precautions for Use

By Infants and Children: Safety and effectiveness for those under 18 not established.

By Those Over 60 Years of Age: Specific recommendations are not made at this time.

▷ **Advisability of Use During Pregnancy**

Pregnancy Category: B. See Pregnancy Risk Categories at the back of this book.

Human Studies: Adequate studies of pregnant women are not available.

Insulin is often the drug of first choice for blood sugar control in pregnancy. Ask your doctor for help.

Advisability of Use If Breast-Feeding

Presence of this drug in breast milk: Yes, in very small amounts.

Avoid drug or refrain from nursing.

Habit-Forming Potential: None.

Effects of Overdose: Temporary gas (flatus), abdominal discomfort, and diarrhea.

Possible Effects of Long-Term Use: Beneficial effects on blood sugar and A1C.

Suggested Periodic Examinations While Taking This Drug (at physician's discretion)

Routine testing of blood sugar levels at intervals recommended by your physician is prudent. Historically, estimates of blood sugar were obtained by checking urine sugar. This method has been replaced by finger stick testing of blood glucose. Finger stick testing accurately reflects the blood sugar and helps ensure better control (tighter control) of blood glucose. One blood sugar machine can also test glycated protein (fructosamine). If you are ill, increased frequency of finger stick blood glucose testing may be indicated. Periodic checks of blood sugar one hour after eating are prudent. A device called a Glucowatch Biographer uses a pad and a watch-like device to painlessly check blood sugar (see *www. cygnus.com*).

Because diabetes is a clear risk factor for heart and blood vessel disease, periodic checks are prudent (also Peripheral Artery Disease check). With this medicine a periodic complete blood count is prudent—with serum iron or iron-binding capacity if anemia develops. Liver function tests (transaminases) do not appear to be required based on one study.

▷ **While Taking This Drug, Observe the Following**

Foods: Follow your diabetic diet conscientiously. Taking a diabetes education course is very smart and can teach you about portion control, what to do on sick days and other important concepts. Blood sugar control can help avoid or delay diabetes problems. Vitamin C in high dose may worsen blood sugar control. Do not omit snack foods in mid-afternoon or at bedtime if they help prevent hypoglycemia. Rice bran has been checked in a small (57 subject) study of type 1 and type 2 diabetics. The benefit was a 30% lowering of sugar. This might be a new complementary care option.

Herbal Medicines or Minerals: Using chromium may change the way your body is able to use sugar. Some health food stores advocate vanadium as mimicking the actions of insulin, but possible toxicity and need for rigorous studies presently preclude recommending it. DHEA may change sensitivity to insulin or insulin resistance. Aloe, eucalyptus, fenugreek, ginger, garlic, ginseng, glucomannan, guar gum, hawthorn, licorice, nettle, and yohimbe may change blood sugar. Surprisingly, boiled stems of the Optuntia streptacantha prickly pear cactus appears to be able to lower blood sugar. Ongoing effects and effects on A1C are not known. Red sage is used for blood sugar effects, but is unproven. Psyllium increases risk of excessively low blood sugar. Since so many of these products may require adjustment of insulin dosing, talk to your doctor BEFORE combining any of these herbal medicines with this medicine. Echinacea pupurea (injectable) and blonde psyllium seed or husk should NOT be taken by people living with diabetes.

Beverages: No restrictions. May be taken with milk.

▷ *Alcohol:* No interaction with miglitol. If you also take a sulfonylurea (see Drug Classes), alcohol can exaggerate lowering of blood sugar or cause a disulfiramlike (see Glossary) reaction.

Tobacco Smoking: No interactions expected. I advise everyone to stop smoking.

▷ *Other Drugs*

Miglitol may *increase* the effects of
- sulfonylureas (see Drug Classes), causing a lower blood sugar (not a miglitol effect); this may be used for therapeutic benefit.

Miglitol *taken concurrently* with
- clofibrate (Atromid-S) may result in hypoglycemia.
- digestive enzyme products that contain amylase or lipase may result in loss of blood sugar control.
- digoxin (Lanoxin) may lead to low digoxin levels and benefits.
- disopyramide (Norpace) may result in hypoglycemia.
- gatifloxacin (Tequin) or levofloxacin (Levaquin) may increase or decrease blood sugar. Caution and close follow-up on blood sugar are required.
- high-dose aspirin or other salicylates and some NSAIDs (see Drug Classes) may result in hypoglycemia.
- insulin (see profile) increases risk of low blood sugar.
- ranitidine (Zantac) may blunt the benefits of ranitidine.
- sulfonamide antibiotics (see Drug Classes) may pose an increased risk for low blood sugar (hypoglycemia).

The following drugs may *decrease* the effects of miglitol:
- adrenocorticosteroids (see Drug Classes).
- beta blockers (see Drug Classes).
- calcium channel blockers (see Drug Classes).
- furosemide (Lasix) and bumetanide (Bumex).
- isoniazid (INH).

- monoamine oxidase (MAO) inhibitors (see Drug Classes).
- nicotinic acid.
- pancreatin (various).
- phenytoin (Dilantin).
- rifampin (Rifadin, others).
- theophylline (Theo-Dur, others).
- thiazide diuretics (see Drug Classes).
- thyroid hormones (see Drug Classes).

▷ *Driving, Hazardous Activities:* Use caution until degree of drowsiness you may experience is known.

Aviation Note: Diabetes *is a disqualification* for piloting. Consult a designated Aviation Medical Examiner.

Exposure to Sun: No restrictions.

Heavy Exercise or Exertion: Caution advised because this drug lowers peak in blood sugar after meals. Talk over dosing changes with your doctor.

Occurrence of Unrelated Illness: Illness can change blood sugar control. Temporary use of insulin may be required.

Discontinuation: Never stop miglitol before calling your doctor.

MINIMALLY SEDATING ANTIHISTAMINES

Cetirizine   (sa TEER a zeen)   **Desloratadine**   (DEZ lor AT a deen)
Fexofenadine   (fex oh FEN a deen)   **Loratadine**   (lor AT a deen)

Introduced: 1996, 2002, 1996, 1992, respectively   **Class:**   Antihistamines, minimally sedating   **Prescription:**   USA: Yes   **Controlled Drug:** USA: No; Canada: No   **Available as Generic:**   U.S.: cetirizine: No; desloratidine: No; fexofenadine: No; loratadine: Yes; Canada: Same as USA.

Brand Names: *Cetirizine:* ✤Apo-Cetirizine, ✤Reactine Zyrtec, Zyrtec D [CD], *Desloratadine:* Clarinex, *Fexofenadine:* Allegra, Allegra-D [CD], *Loratadine:* Alavert (nonprescription), ✤Allertin, ✤Chlor-Tripolon ND [CD], ✤Claritin Extra, Claritin Reditabs [CD], ✤Novo-Loratadine.

Author's Note: Loratadine is now available as Alavert in a nonprescription 10 mg orally disintegrating tablet form (can be taken with or without water). Fexofenadine (Allegra) still requires a prescription at the time of this writing. Information on desloratadine (Clarinex) is included in this edition.

BENEFITS versus RISKS

Possible Benefits	*Possible Risks*
EFFECTIVE AND LONG-LASTING RELIEF OF ALLERGIC RHINITIS	Change in heart wave (QTc increased) fexofenadine has one case report
EFFECTIVE RELIEF OF SOME ALLERGIC SKIN DISORDERS	Low white blood cell count (leukopenia) (1.8% of fexofenadine patients)
MINIMAL DROWSINESS	
MINOR TO NO ANTICHOLINERGIC SIDE EFFECTS	Slight atropinelike effects (some medicines in this class)
	Aggressive reactions and possible seizures (cetirizine)
	Mild sedation or fatigue

▷ **Principal Uses**

As a Single Drug Product: Uses currently included in FDA-approved labeling: (1) Used to treat non-nasal and nasal symptoms of seasonal allergic rhinitis (hay fever); (2) helps ease symptoms of rhinitis; (3) used to treat swellings of unknown origin (idiopathic urticaria) (cetirizine, loratadine); (4) helps ease symptoms of pollen-induced asthma (cetirizine, loratadine). Other (unlabeled) generally accepted uses: (1) chronic idiopathic urticaria (loratadine); (4) food allergies (cetirizine).

As a Combination Drug Product [CD]: Allegra-D, Claritin-D and Zyrtec-D contain the original minimally sedating antihistamine and add the benefits of pseudoephedrine. Caution should be used when taking the "D" forms if you are also taking a medicine that interacts with pseudoephedrine.

How These Drugs Work: These medicines block histamine, stopping symptoms (caused by histamine), such as swelling and itching of the eyes.

▷ **Widely Used Guidelines That Involve This Medicine (representative sample):** Please look at the section at the very beginning of this profile called "Class." Next, turn to Table 22 and you will find guidelines listed by the class involved!

Available Dosage Forms and Strengths

Cetirizine:

Solution — 5 mg/mL
Tablets — 5 mg, 10 mg
Tablets (Canada only) — 20 mg

Desloratadine:

Tablets — 5 mg

Fexofenadine:

Capsules — 60 mg
Tablet — 30 mg, 60 mg, 180 mg
Tablets, extended-release — 60 mg fexofenadine, 120 mg pseudoephedrine

Loratadine:

Syrup — 1 mg/mL
Tablets — 10 mg
Tablets, extended-release (Claritin-D 24-Hour) — 10 mg loratadine, 240 mg pseudoephedrine
Tablets, rapidly disintegrating (micronized — 10 mg loratadine)
Tablets, repeat-action (Claritin-D [CD]) — 5 mg loratadine, 120 mg pseudoephedrine

▷ **Recommended Dosage Ranges** (Actual dose and schedule must be determined for each patient individually.)

Infants and Children: **Safety and efficacy in children younger than 12 years old have been established only for fexofenadine and cetirizine, not for the rest of the medicines in this family.**

Cetirizine (Zyrtec) is approved for children 2 to 5 years old who have seasonal or perennial allergic rhinitis or hives (idiopathic urticaria) of unknown cause.

Fexofenadine (Allegra) is approved for children 6 to 11 years old who have seasonal or perennial allergic rhinitis or hives (idiopathic urticaria) of unknown cause using 30 mg twice daily.

12 to 60 Years of Age:

Cetirizine: The starting dose is 5 mg (depending on severity, may be 10 mg) and is increased as needed and tolerated to a maximum of 20 mg daily.

Desloratadine: A single 5-mg tablet once a day. (5 mg every other day if liver or kidneys are impaired).

Fexofenadine:

  Seasonal allergic rhinitis: 60 mg twice daily or 180 mg once daily.

  Chronic idiopathic urticaria: 60 mg twice daily.

Loratadine: A single 10-mg tablet (of the nonrepeat action, noncombination product) is taken once daily.

Loratadine/pseudoephedrine (5 mg/120 mg nonrepeat action): One tablet twice daily.

Loratadine/pseudoephedrine (10 mg/240 mg repeat action): One tablet daily.

Over 60 Years of Age:

  Dosing changes for fexofenadine and loratadine (Claritin-D and Claritin-D 24-hour forms) do not appear to be needed. Prudent to decrease cetirizine doses, as it is slowly removed from the body at this age.

Conditions Requiring Dosing Adjustments

Liver Function: Cetirizine: A 5-mg dose is recommended.

  Fexofenadine: Dosing changes do not appear to be needed.

  Desloratadine: 5 mg every other day.

  Loratadine: Patients with liver compromise take a dose of 10 mg (of the non-repeat action, noncombination product) every other day.

Kidney Function: Cetirizine: Patients with moderate kidney decline (creatinine clearance 11–31 mL/min) may take 5 mg daily.

  Desloratadine: 5 mg every other day.

  Fexofenadine: A daily dose of 60 mg once daily is recommended.

  Loratadine: Patients with moderate kidney failure (creatinine clearance less than 30 mL/min) get a starting dose of 10 mg (of nonrepeat action, non-combination product) every other day.

▷ **Dosing Instructions:** Loratadine is best taken on an empty stomach. Once the rapidly disintegrating (Reditab) form has dissolved, water may be used to help patients swallow the contents of the pill. The other medicines in this class may be taken with food. Extended-release forms of these medicines should never be crushed. If you forget a dose: Take the missed dose as soon as you remember it, unless it's nearly time for your next dose—if that is the case, skip the missed dose and take the next dose right on schedule. DO NOT double doses. Talk with your doctor if you find yourself missing doses.

Usual Duration of Use: Although all of these medicines may go to work immediately, regular use for up to 1 day (fexofenadine), up to 2 days (astemizole or cetirizine) or up to 3 days (loratadine) may be needed to see substantial symptom improvement. Long-term use requires evaluation of response by your doctor.

Typical Treatment Goals and Measurements (Outcomes and Markers):

Seasonal Allergic Rhinitis: The general goal is to decrease or eliminate hay fever symptoms such as watery eyes, sneezing, and itchy feelings in the throat or eyes, and runny nose.

Possible Advantages of These Drugs: Less sedating than previously available antihistamines. Once-daily dosing for some agents in this class. Some medicines in this class do not interact with certain antifungals and macrolide antibiotics (see Drug Classes) or do interact but do not appear to cause side effects on the heart or change the safety profile. Cetirizine has NOT had ANY case reports of QTc prolongation. Tachyphylaxis or tolerance may be less likely to occur to these medicines than with earlier agents. Reditabs do not require water to take them. Fexofenadine did NOT exhibit any driving performance decrease in one small study of 24 healthy men. Once a day dosing is a distinct advantage.

Currently "Drugs of Choice"

For patients who must take antihistamine-type medicines and require the best possible balance of symptom relief and minimal sedation.

▷ **These Drugs Should Not Be Taken If**
- you have had an allergic reaction to any dose form of these medicines or any of the ingredients in them previously.
- you are presently being tested (using skin tests) for allergies.
- you are taking medicines that prolong the QT interval, such as quinidine, pentamidine, disopyramide, or others (for fexofenadine).
- you have urinary retention, liver disease, severe disease of the arteries of the heart (coronary artery disease), or narrow-angle glaucoma (loratadine combination products that contain pseudoephedrine).

▷ **Inform Your Physician Before Taking These Drugs If**
- you have asthma.
- you are at risk for drowsiness or fainting (syncope).
- you have a history of a heart rhythm disorder.
- your electrolytes are not in balance.
- you are taking other medicines metabolized by or that change CYP 3A4 levels (ask your doctor) and one of these medicines is removed by that enzyme.
- you are taking other medicines (especially antifungal or macrolide antibiotics). Blood levels of loratadine or fexofenadine may be increased. Decreases in loratadine and fexofenadine doses may be prudent.
- you have a history of liver or kidney compromise.
- you are pregnant.
- your work REQUIRES mental alertness.

Possible Side Effects (natural, expected, and unavoidable drug actions)

Dry nose, mouth, or throat, somnolence (drowsiness): cetirizine—frequent, fexofenadine—rare, loratadine—infrequent.

▷ **Possible Adverse Effects** (unusual, unexpected, and infrequent reactions)
If any of the following develop, consult your physician promptly for guidance.

Mild Adverse Effects

Allergic reactions: skin rash, itching.

Headache, fatigue or dizziness—infrequent to frequent, depending on the agent.

Dry mouth—possible to infrequent.

Leg cramps, muscle aches (loratadine)—rare.

Weight gain (cetirizine)—uncommon.

Fast heart rate (tachycardia) (loratadine)—rare.

Prolonged QTc interval (fexofenadine)—possible if used in people with existing heart disease, case report(s).

Lowering of the blood pressure (loratadine)—rare.

Vision changes (loratadine)—rare.

Serious Adverse Effects

Allergic reactions: anaphylaxis (loratadine)—rare.

Idiosyncratic reactions: not reported.

Aggressive reactions (cetirizine)—possible.

Seizure (cetirizine)—possible.

Serious heart rhythm disorders: fexofenadine—case report.

Tachycardia—rare.

Lowering of the white blood cell count (fexofenadine)—rare.
Abnormal liver function (loratadine)—case reports.
Depression, confusion, paresthesias—rare.
Passing out (syncope)—rare.

▷ **Possible Effects on Sexual Function:** Vaginitis, painful menses (dysmenorrhea), breast enlargement or breast pain (loratadine)—case reports.
Menstrual disorders (loratadine, fexofenadine)—case reports to rare.
Galactorrhea (loratadine)—case reports.
Impotence (loratadine)—case reports.

Possible Delayed Adverse Effects: None reported.

▷ **Adverse Effects That May Mimic Natural Diseases or Disorders**
Increased liver enzymes may mimic hepatitis of infectious origin.

Natural Diseases or Disorders That May Be Activated by These Drugs
None reported.

Possible Effects on Laboratory Tests
Skin tests for allergies will be blunted and less diagnostic.
Liver function tests: may be increased (loratadine, fexofenadine [mildly]).
White blood cell counts: decreased (leukopenia)—rare in clinical trials (fexofenadine).

CAUTION
1. Loratadine does interact with some antifungals and some macrolide antibiotics—but appears to be free of the heart (cardiac) effects, even though blood levels of loratadine may increase if it is taken with these interacting medicines. Talk to your doctor or pharmacist before taking any medicines that were not discussed when loratadine was prescribed.
2. Some of these medicines HAVE LIFE-THREATENING DRUG INTERACTIONS. Talk to your doctor or pharmacist BEFORE combining any prescription, nonprescription or herbal remedies with medicines in this class.
3. Report dizziness, heart palpitation, or chest pain promptly when using any of these medicines.
4. Fexofenadine (Allegra) levels may be decreased by roughly 70% if it is taken with orange, apple, or grapefruit juice. Current thinking holds that this is due to fruit juice inhibiting a drug "taxi" (transporter) called OATP.

Precautions for Use
By Infants and Children: Safety and effectiveness for use by those under 12 years of age have not been established.
By Those Over 60 Years of Age: Smaller starting and maintenance doses are needed. Longer dosing intervals may be needed as well.

▷ **Advisability of Use During Pregnancy**
Pregnancy Category: B (cetirizine, loratadine); C (fexofenadine). See Pregnancy Risk Categories at the back of this book.
Animal Studies: No birth defects reported.
Human Studies: Information from adequate studies of pregnant women is not available. **These medicines should be used during pregnancy only if clearly needed. Discuss the BENEFITS versus RISKS with your doctor.**

Advisability of Use If Breast-Feeding
Presence of this drug in breast milk: No data (cetirizine, fexofenadine); yes (loratadine).
Ask your doctor for guidance regarding stopping the drug or stopping nursing (cetirizine, fexofenadine, or loratadine).

Habit-Forming Potential: None.

Effects of Overdose: With overdoses greater than 10 mg (40–80 mg): tachycardia, somnolence, and headache (loratadine). Usual antihistamine protocols (cetirizine or fexofenadine).

Possible Effects of Long-Term Use: None defined.

Suggested Periodic Examinations While Taking These Drugs (at physician's discretion)

Examination for relief of the condition(s) being treated.

If palpitations, unexplained dizziness, or chest pain or discomfort happens, an electrocardiogram (ECG) and heart pattern (QT interval, etc.) should be checked.

▷ **While Taking These Drugs, Observe the Following**

Foods: Loratadine is best taken on an empty stomach. DO NOT combine with grapefruit.

Herbal Medicines or Minerals: Valerian and kava kava may intensify drowsiness. St. John's wort may lead to photosensitivity. Combination with medicines in this class that also cause photosensitivity is NOT advised. If you are allergic to plants in the *Asteraceae* family (aster, chrysanthemum, daisy, or ragweed), you may also be allergic to echinacea, chamomile, feverfew, and St. John's wort. A well-designed study of 125 patients (see Schapowal in Sources) found that an herb called butterbur was comparable to cetirizine in seasonal allergic rhinitis. Talk to your doctor to see if this makes sense for you.

Beverages: Grapefruit juice may lead to increased blood levels of loratadine, leading to toxicity. Fexofenadine (Allegra) levels may be decreased by roughly 70% if it is taken with orange, apple, or grapefruit juice. Current thinking holds that this is due to fruit juice inhibiting a drug "taxi" (transporter) called OATP. Water is the best liquid to use to take the medicines in this family.

▷ *Alcohol:* May cause excessive drowsiness (central nervous system depression).

Tobacco Smoking: No interactions expected. I advise everyone to quit smoking.

Marijuana Smoking: May cause additive drowsiness or lethargy.

▷ *Other Drugs*

These medicines *taken concurrently* with

- cimetidine (Tagamet) may produce a significant increase in loratadine blood levels. No serious drug effects have been reported, but since in general the frequency of adverse effects increases with increasing blood levels, it appears prudent to decrease the dose of loratadine if these medicines are to be taken at the same time because of possible loratadine toxicity. The loratadine dose should certainly be decreased if increased frequency of adverse effects occurs if these medicines are combined in usual doses. Cetirizine is mostly removed by the kidneys.
- fluvoxamine (Luvox) may result in increased blood levels of cetirizine or loratadine. Caution is advised.
- indinavir (Crixivan) and perhaps ritonavir, saquinavir or nelfinavir may decrease metabolism of astemizole and should NEVER BE COMBINED. Loratadine levels may be increased, and doses may need to be lowered. Other drugs in this family may also be affected.
- itraconazole (and perhaps other similarly structured antifungals, such as ketoconazole) should NEVER BE COMBINED with astemizole. These drugs may cause increased blood levels of loratadine or fexofenadine.

Although no serious heart rhythm toxicity has been reported to date with this medicine, caution is advised, and it appears prudent to lower the dose of loratadine or fexofenadine.

- macrolide antibiotics such as clarithromycin or erythromycin—while no serious heart rhythm toxicity has been reported to date with loratadine or fexofenadine, caution is advised, as excessive blood levels of any medicine may increase risk of adverse effects; it may be prudent to lower the dose of loratadine.
- medicines that prolong the QT interval possibly should be avoided with fexofenadine. Examples of QT changing medicines are: disopyramide, ibutilide, quinolones (grepafloxacin, sparfloxacin), sotalol (Betapace, others); cetirizine and loratadine and desloratadine are the drugs in this chemical family without any reports of QTc interval changes.
- nefazodone (Serzone) may lead to life-threatening heart problems if combined with astemizole.
- paroxetine (Paxil) may inhibit the enzymes needed to remove cetirizine or loratadine. Caution is advised.
- quinidine (Quinaglute, others) may result in a change in the effect of quinidine and result in undesirable effects on the heart. Caution is advised.
- ritonavir (Norvir) and perhaps other protease inhibitors (see Drug Classes) may increase blood levels and toxicity.
- sertraline (Zoloft) may lead to life-threatening heart problems if combined with astemizole. DO NOT COMBINE.
- theophylline (Theo-Dur, others) may decrease cetirizine clearance. Patients should be closely followed for signs of excessive cetirizine levels.
- zafirlukast (Accolate), and perhaps zileuton (Zyflo) if combined with astemizole, may decrease zafirlukast levels and blunt the therapeutic benefits of zafirlukast.

▷ *Driving, Hazardous Activities:* Although these medicines are much less likely than earlier antihistamines to cause drowsiness, caution should be used until your individual reaction to these medicines is determined. Restrict activities as necessary.

Aviation Note: The use of these drugs **is probably not a disqualification** for piloting. Consult a designated Aviation Medical Examiner.

Exposure to Sun: Rare cases of photosensitivity have been reported with some medicines (astemizole, loratadine) in this class. Use caution.

MINOXIDIL (min OX i dil)

Introduced: 1972   **Class:** Antihypertensive, hair growth stimulant
Prescription: USA: Yes   **Controlled Drug:** USA: No; Canada: No
Available as Generic: Yes

Brand Names: Alostil, ✤Apo-Gain, ✤Hairgro, Kresse, Loniten, ✤Med-Minoxidil, Minocalve 5, Minodyl, Minoximen, Rogaine, Rogaine Extra Strength, Rogaine 5

Author's Note: Rogaine treatment for baldness is available without a prescription.

BENEFITS versus RISKS

Possible Benefits	*Possible Risks*
POTENT, LONG-ACTING ANTIHYPERTENSIVE	EXCESSIVE BODY HAIR GROWTH
EFFECTIVE IN CASES OF SEVERE HYPERTENSION, ACCELERATED AND MALIGNANT HYPERTENSION	SALT AND WATER RETENTION
	Excessively rapid heart rate
	Aggravation of angina
Moderately effective in treating male pattern baldness and female baldness (alopecia androgenica)	Local scalp irritation (topical use)

▷ **Principal Uses**

As a Single Drug Product: Uses currently included in FDA-approved labeling: (1) Treats severe high blood pressure not controlled by conventional therapy; (2) treats female androgenic baldness or male pattern baldness; (3) effective in patients with high blood pressure and kidney failure.

Other (unlabeled) generally accepted uses: (1) Supportive therapy in hair transplants.

How This Drug Works: (1) Relaxes constricted muscles in walls of small arteries and permits expansion of the arteries and lower blood pressure. (2) May act directly on the hair follicle, may increase size of previously closed small scalp blood vessels, restoring blood flow and returning small hair follicles to normal size and activity.

▷ **Widely Used Guidelines That Involve This Medicine (representative sample):**

Please look at the section at the very beginning of this profile called "Class." Next, turn to Table 22 and you will find guidelines listed by the class involved!

Available Dosage Forms and Strengths

Tablets — 2.5 mg, 10 mg

Topical solution — 2%

— 5% (Extra-Strength)

▷ **Usual Adult Dosage Ranges:** *For hypertension:* In severe cases, initially 5 mg once a day. The dose is then gradually increased as needed and tolerated to 10 mg, 20 mg and then 40 mg every 24 hours, taken in one or two divided doses daily. The usual ongoing dose is 10 to 40 mg daily.

For Male Pattern Baldness: Apply thinly 1 mL of topical solution to the balding area of the scalp twice a day (for example in the morning and at bedtime). The total daily dose should not exceed 2 mL.

Note: Actual dose and schedule must be determined for each patient individually.

Conditions Requiring Dosing Adjustments

Liver Function: This drug is metabolized (90%) in the liver. It should be used with caution by patients with liver compromise.

Kidney Function: In moderate kidney failure, the dose should be decreased empirically.

▷ **Dosing Instructions:** For hypertension: Tablets may be crushed and taken with or following food to prevent nausea. Take at the same time each day. If you forget a dose: Take or apply the missed dose as soon as you remember it, unless it's nearly time for your next dose—if that is the case, skip the missed dose and take or apply the next dose right on schedule. Talk with your doctor and pharmacist if you find yourself missing doses.

For baldness: The topical solution is for external, local use only; it is not to be swallowed. Begin application at the center of the bald area; apply thinly to cover the entire area. The scalp and hair must be dry at the time of application. Follow instructions carefully.

Usual Duration of Use: Use on a regular schedule for 3 to 7 days usually determines effectiveness in controlling severe hypertension. Continual use of the topical solution for at least 4 months is needed to determine its ability to promote hair growth. Growth usually continues for up to a year of treatment. Long-term use (months to years) of both dose forms requires physician supervision.

Typical Treatment Goals and Measurements (Outcomes and Markers)

Baldness: The goal is to regain hair and maintain existing hair. Some dermatologists use hair counts to assess progress and peak benefits. Initial regrowth may be uncolored and soft in texture. Continued use of topical form finds development of hair of the same texture and color as the original hair.

Blood Pressure: Guidelines (JNC VII) define normal blood pressure (BP) as **less than** 120/80 and **pre-hypertension** as 120/80 to 139/89. This new range is intended to help doctors encourage lifestyle changes (or in the case of people with a risk factor for high blood pressure, start treatment) much earlier—so that damage to blood vessels, your heart, kidneys, sexual potency, or eyes might be minimized or avoided altogether. Stage 1 hypertension is 140/90 to 159/99 and stage 2 hypertension equal to or greater than: 160/100 mm Hg. These guidelines also recommend that clinicians work with their patients to agree on the goals and a plan of treatment. The first-ever guidelines for blood pressure (hypertension) in African Americans recommends that MOST black patients be started on TWO antihypertensive medicines with the goal of lowering blood pressure to 130/80 for those with high risk for heart and blood vessel disease or with diabetes. The American Diabetes Association also recommends 130/80 as the target for diabetics and less than 125/75 for those who spill more than one gram of protein into their urine. Most clinicians try to achieve a BP that confers the best balance of lower cardiovascular risk and avoids the problem of too low a blood pressure. Blood pressure duration is generally increased with beneficial restriction of sodium. If goals are not met, it is not unusual to intensify doses or add on medicines.

▷ **This Drug Should Not Be Taken If**
- you have had an allergic reaction to it previously.
- you are known to have a pheochromocytoma (an adrenaline-producing tumor).
- you have pulmonary hypertension due to mitral valve stenosis.
- the topical dosing form should not be used with products that can increase absorption in the skin. Combined use of Vasoline (petrolatum), retinoids, and topical corticosteroids should be avoided.

▷ **Inform Your Physician Before Taking This Drug If**
- you are pregnant or planning pregnancy.
- you are breast-feeding your infant.
- you have had a heart attack in the last month or have swelling around the heart (pericarditis).
- you have angina attacks.

- you have existing blood vessel disease in your head (cerebrovascular disease).
- you have a history of coronary artery disease (and are not taking a water pill–diuretic) or impaired heart function.
- you have a history of stroke or impaired brain circulation.
- you have impaired liver or kidney function.

Possible Side Effects (natural, expected, and unavoidable drug actions)

Increased heart rate, fluid retention with weight gain, excessive hair growth on face, arms, legs, and back (frequent).

▷ **Possible Adverse Effects** (unusual, unexpected, and infrequent reactions)

If any of the following develop, consult your physician promptly for guidance.

Mild Adverse Effects

Allergic reaction: skin rash.

Localized dermatitis at site of application of topical solution—rare.

Headache, dizziness, fainting—rare.

Nausea, increased thirst—infrequent.

Hair growth and changes in hair color—case reports.

Weight gain—possible (may be due to fluid if this drug is used without a water pill (diuretic).

Mild increase in liver enzymes—infrequent.

Serious Adverse Effects

Allergic reactions: serious skin rash (Stevens-Johnson syndrome).

Idiosyncratic reaction: fluid formation around the heart (pericardial effusion).

Development of angina pectoris; high blood pressure in the lungs (pulmonary hypertension)—case reports.

Systemic lupus erythematosus—case reports.

Low white blood cells or platelets—rare and transient.

Author's Note: Topical use of this medicine for hair growth avoids most of these adverse effects.

▷ **Possible Effects on Sexual Function:** Male breast tenderness (gynecomastia)—case reports. Some data to support that this drug balances the male ability to ejaculate and have a healthy sex drive that may have been blunted by other drugs that treat high blood pressure.

Natural Diseases or Disorders That May Be Activated by This Drug

Latent coronary artery disease with symptomatic angina (systemic form).

Possible Effects on Laboratory Tests

Blood HDL cholesterol level: increased.

Blood LDL cholesterol level: decreased.

CAUTION

1. Long-term use for hypertension usually requires use of a diuretic to counteract salt and water retention.
2. The long-term use of this drug for hypertension may require concurrent use of a beta-blocker drug to control excessive acceleration of the heart.
3. It is best to avoid combining this drug and guanethidine; the combination can cause severe orthostatic hypotension (see Glossary).
4. Consult your physician regarding the advisability of using a "no-salt-added" diet.
5. Little of this drug is absorbed into the general circulation when the topical solution is applied to the scalp. However, some systemic effects have been reported. Inform your physician promptly if you experience any unusual symptoms while using the topical solution.

6. The topical form contains alcohol. Avoid getting this baldness medicine into your eyes.

Precautions for Use

By Infants and Children: Dose schedules should be determined by a qualified pediatrician. In children under 12 years old, starting dose is 0.2 mg per kg of body mass in a single dose. Dose is then increased as needed and tolerated by 0.1 to 0.2 mg per kg per day at 3-day intervals. Children over 12 are given the adult dose. Monitor closely for salt and water retention.

By Those Over 60 Years of Age: Treatment with small doses and a limit of total daily dose to 75 mg is indicated. Headache, palpitation, and rapid heart rate due to this drug are more common in this age group and can mimic acute anxiety states. Observe for dizziness, unsteadiness, fainting, and falling.

▷ **Advisability of Use During Pregnancy**

Pregnancy Category: C. See Pregnancy Risk Categories at the back of this book.

Animal Studies: No birth defects reported in rats or rabbits, but studies did reveal decreased fertility and increased fetal deaths.

Human Studies: Adequate studies of pregnant women are not available.

Avoid during the first 3 months. Use only if clearly needed during the final 6 months.

Advisability of Use If Breast-Feeding

Presence of this drug in breast milk: Yes.

Avoid drug or refrain from nursing.

Habit-Forming Potential: None.

Effects of Overdose: Headache, dizziness, weakness, nausea, marked low blood pressure, weak and rapid pulse, loss of consciousness.

Possible Effects of Long-Term Use: Excessive growth of body hair occurs in 80% of users after 1 to 2 months of continual treatment for hypertension. Close to 100% of users will experience this effect after 1 year of continual treatment. This may be accompanied by darkening of the skin and coarsening of facial features.

Suggested Periodic Examinations While Taking This Drug (at physician's discretion)

Body weight measurement for insidious gain due to water retention.

Electrocardiographic and echocardiographic heart examinations.

▷ **While Taking This Drug, Observe the Following**

Foods: Avoid excessive salt and heavily salted foods.

Herbal Medicines or Minerals: Hawthorn, bitter orange, country mallow, ginseng, saw palmetto, ma huang (no longer available for weight loss), guarana, mate, goldenseal, yohimbe, and licorice may cause increased blood pressure, blunting the benefits of this medicine. St. John's wort can change liver removal of medicines. Careful patient follow-up for decreased benefit from minoxidil is prudent. Calcium and garlic may help lower blood pressure, and the dose has to be individualized with a standardized extract. Dong quai can change the removal of medicines by the liver—caution is advised for excessive lowering of blood pressure. Indian snakeroot has a German Commission E monograph indication for hypertension—talk to your doctor. Eleuthero root and ephedra should be avoided by people living with hypertension. Talk to your doctor BEFORE adding any herbals. Autumn crocus should be avoided in alopecia.

Beverages: No restrictions. May be taken with milk.

▷ *Alcohol:* Use with extreme caution. Alcohol can exaggerate the blood pressure–lowering effects of this drug when it is taken orally.

Tobacco Smoking: Best avoided. Nicotine can contribute significantly to angina. I advise everyone to quit smoking.

▷ *Other Drugs*

Minoxidil may *increase* the effects of
• all other antihypertensive drugs; careful dose adjustments are mandatory.

Minoxidil *taken concurrently* with
• clonidine (Catapres TTS, others) may help ease fast heart rate and increased sympathetic nervous system activity caused by minoxidil.
• guanethidine (Ismelin, Esimil) may cause severe orthostatic hypotension; avoid this combination.
• NSAIDs may blunt the therapeutic benefit of minoxidil.
• vitamin E (one report of high-dose use) reversing hair growth.

▷ *Driving, Hazardous Activities:* This drug may cause dizziness and fatigue. Restrict activities as necessary.

Aviation Note: The use of this drug *is a disqualification* for piloting. Consult a designated Aviation Medical Examiner.

Exposure to Sun: No restrictions.

Discontinuation: This drug should not be stopped abruptly. If it is to be discontinued, consult your physician regarding gradual reduction in dose and appropriate replacement with other drugs for the management of hypertension. Following discontinuation of the topical solution, the pretreatment pattern of baldness may return within 3 to 4 months.

MIRTAZAPINE (mur TAZ a peen)

Introduced: 1996 **Class:** Antidepressant, piperazinoazepine, norepinephrine, serotonin reuptake inhibitor **Prescription:** USA: Yes **Controlled Drug:** USA: No; Canada: No **Available as Generic:** USA: Yes; Canada: Yes

Brand Names: Remeron, Remeron Sol Tab

BENEFITS versus RISKS	
Possible Benefits	*Possible Risks*
EFFECTIVE TREATMENT OF DEPRESSION	Sleepiness
BENEFICIAL ACTION ON SLEEP	Weight gain
HELPS PATIENTS WITH DEPRESSION WHO ALSO HAVE PROBLEMS SLEEPING AND ARE ANXIOUS	Lowering of white blood cells
AVAILABLE IN A TABLET THAT MELTS ON THE TONGUE AND CAN BE TAKEN EASILY	

▷ **Principal Uses**

As a Single Drug Product: Uses currently included in FDA-approved labeling: Treatment of depression.

Other (unlabeled) generally accepted uses: (1) Eases presurgical insomnia; (2) may help antidepressant (SSRI–see Drug Classes)-induced sexual problems (dysfunction); (3) could be useful in tremor or pain syndromes; (4) helpful in a small study of post–traumatic stress disorder (PTSD); (5) has antianxiety effects which need to be further studied.

How This Drug Works: Works on antihistaminic (H1) and subtypes of the serotonin receptor (5-HT2 and 5-HT-3). Works to decrease the time it takes to fall asleep (sleep latency), but the mechanism isn't clear at present.

▷ **Widely Used Guidelines That Involve This Medicine (representative sample):** Please look at the section at the very beginning of this profile called "Class." Next, turn to Table 22 and you will find guidelines listed by the class involved!

Available Dosage Forms and Strengths
Tablets — 15 mg, 30 mg, 45 mg
Tablets (orally disintegrating) — 15 mg, 30 mg

▷ **Recommended Dosage Ranges** (Actual dose and schedule must be determined for each patient individually.)
Infants and Children: Dose not established.
Adults to Age 60: For treatment of adult depression, 15 to 45 mg at bedtime. Dosing is started at 15 mg. Increases in dose (as needed and tolerated) are made at seven- to fourteen-day intervals.
Over 60 Years of Age: Removed more slowly from the body, and slower still by males versus females. Lower doses are prudent.

Conditions Requiring Dosing Adjustments
Liver Function: Lower doses and slow dose increases are needed. Doses may need to be decreased by half of the usual dose in severe liver compromise.
Kidney Function: Lower doses and slow dose increases are needed. Patients should be closely followed.

▷ **Dosing Instructions:** The original tablet form may be crushed and can be taken with or without food. Take it at the same time daily. The Soltab is made to fall apart in your mouth and should NOT be crushed or chewed. This dosage form does not need to be taken with water. Make certain to take it once you remove it from the compartment (blister pack). Because any form of this medicine can cause drowsiness, it is usually taken at bedtime. If you forget a dose: Take the missed dose as soon as you remember it, unless it's morning when you remember it—if that is the case, skip the missed dose and take the next dose right on schedule. Talk with your doctor if you find yourself missing doses. Continue to take this medicine after you start to feel better.

Usual Duration of Use: Use on a regular schedule for 1 week will usually start to show benefits in relieving depression. Peak effect may take several weeks to be seen. Long-term use (months to years) requires follow-up by your doctor. Controversy exists as to the length of time to take an antidepressant once problems resolve, but many clinicians advocate 4–9 months and individualized treatment.

Typical Treatment Goals and Measurements (Outcomes and Markers)
Depression: The general goal: to lessen the degree and severity of depression, letting patients return to their daily lives. Specific measures of depression (Hamilton Depression or Ham-D) involve testing or inventories and can be valuable in helping check benefits from this medicine.
Pain Syndromes: The general goal: to decrease pain to a manageable level. Pain should be appropriately checked, and progress defined based on lowering of overall pain level.

Possible Advantages of This Drug

Less likely to cause dry mouth, constipation, urinary retention, orthostatic hypotension (see Glossary), and heart rhythm disturbances than tricyclic antidepressants. Does not cause Parkinson-like reactions. Has been successfully used in people who were depressed, had sexual problems from medicines in the selective serotonin reuptake inhibitor (SSRI) family. The Soltab form can be taken without water. May go to work faster than other medicines for depression.

▷ This Drug Should Not Be Taken If

- you have had an allergic reaction to it previously.
- you are currently taking, or have taken within the past 14 days, any monoamine oxidase (MAO) type A inhibitor drug (see Drug Classes).

▷ Inform Your Physician Before Taking This Drug If

- you have experienced any adverse effects from antidepressant drugs.
- you have impaired liver or kidney function.
- you have Parkinson's disease.
- you have had a recent heart attack or have heart disease.
- you have a seizure disorder.
- you have phenylketonuria (PKU) as the Soltab has 2.6 mg of phenylalanine in each 15 mg tablet.
- you are pregnant or plan pregnancy while taking this drug.

Possible Side Effects (natural, expected, and unavoidable drug actions)

Increased appetite, weight gain. Lower blood pressure on standing (see postural hypotension in Glossary).

▷ Possible Adverse Effects (unusual, unexpected, and infrequent reactions)

If any of the following develop, consult your physician promptly for guidance.

Mild Adverse Effects

Allergic reactions: skin rash, itching—rare.

Headache, nervousness, insomnia—rare to infrequent.

Somnolence—frequent (may be up to 54%—this is why the medicine is taken at night).

Ringing in the ears, excessive noise sensitivity, and decreased hearing ability—reported.

Fatigue and dry mouth or constipation—frequent.

Tremor, dizziness, abnormal dreams—rare.

Muscle or joint pain—rare.

Abnormal vision, numbness and tingling—rare.

Confusion—rare.

Fluid accumulation (edema)—rare.

Chest pain and increased blood pressure—rare.

Increased heart rate—infrequent.

Altered taste, nausea, vomiting, diarrhea—rare to infrequent.

Serious Adverse Effects

Allergic reactions: dermatitis (various forms)—rare.

Drug—induced seizures—case reports.

Hallucinations, paranoid reactions—rare.

Movement problems (akathisia [feeling that you have to keep moving], dysarthrias)—infrequent.

Diabetes or thyroid problems—rare.

Increased blood cholesterol (hypercholesterolemia)—infrequent.

Liver cirrhosis or pancreatitis—rare in controlled studies.
Agranulocytosis—case reports.

▷ **Possible Effects on Sexual Function:** Male sexual dysfunction: delayed ejaculation—infrequent. Has been successfully used in people who could not tolerate SSRIs due to sexual dysfunction caused by the drug itself.
Female sexual dysfunction: inhibited orgasm—rare.
Swelling and tenderness of male and female breast tissue—case reports.
Dysmenorrhea—rare.

Natural Diseases or Disorders That May Be Activated by This Drug
Latent epilepsy.

Possible Effects on Laboratory Tests
Blood total cholesterol and triglyceride levels: increased—infrequent.
Liver function tests: increased liver enzymes (ALT/GPT, AST/GOT, and alkaline phosphatase).
Blood cell counts: decreased (aplastic anemia)—case reports.
Blood sodium: decreased (with rare SIADH).

CAUTION
1. If any type of skin reaction develops (rash, hives, etc.), discontinue this drug and inform your physician promptly.
2. Ask your dentist for help if dryness of the mouth starts and persists for more than 2 weeks.
3. Ask your doctor or pharmacist before taking any other prescription or over-the-counter drug while taking mirtazapine.
4. If you are advised to take any monoamine oxidase (MAO) type A inhibitor (see Drug Classes), allow an interval of 5 weeks after discontinuing this drug before starting the MAO inhibitor.
5. It is advisable to withhold this drug if electroconvulsive therapy (ECT, or "shock" treatment) is to be used to treat your depression.

Precautions for Use
By Infants and Children: Safety and effectiveness for those under 12 years of age are not established.
By Those Over 60 Years of Age: The lowest effective dose should be used for maintenance treatment and adjusted as needed for reduced kidney function.

▷ **Advisability of Use During Pregnancy**
Pregnancy Category: C. See Pregnancy Risk Categories at the back of this book.
Animal Studies: Delayed bone development due to this drug found in rat and rabbit studies.
Human Studies: Adequate studies of pregnant women are not available.
Use this drug only if clearly needed. Ask your physician for guidance.

Advisability of Use If Breast-Feeding
Presence of this drug in breast milk: Unknown.
Avoid drug or refrain from nursing.

Habit-Forming Potential: None, however, a withdrawal syndrome (nausea, anxiety, paresthesia, and panic attack) has been reported after abrupt discontinuation.

Effects of Overdose: Agitation, restlessness, excitement, nausea, vomiting, seizures.

Possible Effects of Long-Term Use: None reported.

Suggested Periodic Examinations While Taking This Drug (at physician's discretion)

Periodic complete blood counts and liver function tests. Because of lipid effects, a baseline lipid panel and periodic checks appear prudent.

▷ **While Taking This Drug, Observe the Following**

Foods: No restrictions.

Herbal Medicines or Minerals: Since part of the way ginseng works may be as a MAO inhibitor, do not combine ginseng with mirtazapine. Valerian and kava kava may interact additively (drowsiness). Avoid these combinations. St. John's wort may lead to dangerously increased serotonin activity as well as additive sensitivity to the sun. Indian snakeroot, ma huang, and yohimbe are also best avoided while taking this medicine.

Beverages: No restrictions. May be taken with milk.

▷ *Alcohol:* Avoid completely.

Tobacco Smoking: No interactions expected. I advise everyone to quit smoking.

▷ *Other Drugs*

Mirtazapine *taken concurrently* with

- diazepam (Valium) and perhaps other benzodiazepines (see Drug Classes) may impair movement ability.
- inhibitors of cytochrome CYP 2D6, such as amiodarone, fluoxetine, and zileuton, may lead to excessive blood levels and mirtazapine toxicity.
- monoamine oxidase (MAO) type A inhibitor drugs may cause confusion, agitation, high fever, seizures, and dangerous elevations of blood pressure; avoid the concurrent use of these drugs.
- ritonavir (Norvir) and perhaps other protease inhibitors (see Drug Classes) may lead to toxicity.

▷ *Driving, Hazardous Activities:* This drug may cause drowsiness, dizziness, impaired judgment and altered vision. Restrict activities as necessary.

Aviation Note: The use of this drug *is a disqualification* for piloting. Consult a designated Aviation Medical Examiner.

Exposure to Sun: Use caution—this drug may (rarely) cause photosensitivity (see Glossary).

Discontinuation: The slow elimination of this drug from the body makes it unlikely that any withdrawal effects will result from abrupt discontinuation. However, case reports of a withdrawal syndrome have been made. It appears prudent to slowly decrease (taper) the dose if you and your doctor have decided to stop this medicine. Call your doctor if you plan to stop this drug for any reason.

MISOPROSTOL (mi soh PROH stohl)

Introduced: 1987   **Class:** Gastrointestinal drug (ulcer preventive), prostaglandin analog   **Prescription:** USA: Yes   **Controlled Drug:** USA: No; Canada: No   **Available as Generic:** USA: No; Canada: No

Brand Names: ♣Apo-Misoprostol, Arthrotec [CD], Cytotec, ♣Novo-Misoprostol, ♣PMS-Misoprostol

---

BENEFITS versus RISKS

Possible Benefits	*Possible Risks*
EFFECTIVE PREVENTION OF STOMACH ULCERATION WHILE TAKING ANTI-INFLAMMATORY DRUGS	INCREASED RISK OF ABORTION (IF USED DURING PREGNANCY) Diarrhea (transient) Neuropathy
GEL FORM IS USED TO "RIPEN" THE CERVIX DURING LABOR	
Effective treatment of duodenal ulcer	

▷ **Principal Uses**

As a Single Drug Product: Uses currently included in FDA-approved labeling: (1) Prevents development of stomach ulcers during long-term use of anti-inflammatory drugs as therapy for arthritis and related conditions; (2) treatment of duodenal ulcers.

Other (unlabeled) generally accepted uses: (1) Used (in Canada and other countries) for treatment of active duodenal ulcer unrelated to use of anti-inflammatory drugs; (2) has some use in inducing abortions; (3) used in combination with cyclosporine or prednisone to decrease transplanted organ rejection; (4) widely used to help "ripen" or prime the cervix in preparation for a vaginal delivery.

As a Combination Drug Product [CD]: Available in combination with diclofenac, a NSAID (see Drug Classes). The misoprostol is used to prevent stomach (gastric) irritation or ulceration from the NSAID.

How This Drug Works: Protects lining of the stomach and duodenum by (1) replacing tissue prostaglandins depleted by anti-inflammatory drugs; (2) inhibiting secretion of stomach acid; (3) increasing local production of bicarbonate (to neutralize acids) and mucus (to protect stomach and duodenal tissues). Combined effects prevent new ulcers and promote healing of existing ulcer(s).

Arthrotec form: This combination uses the above mechanism of misoprostol to protect from possible ulcers caused by the NSAID diclofenac.

▷ **Widely Used Guidelines That Involve This Medicine (representative sample):** Please look at the section at the very beginning of this profile called "Class." Next, turn to Table 22 and you will find guidelines listed by the class involved!

Available Dosage Forms and Strengths

Tablets — 100 mcg, 200 mcg

Tablets (Arthrotec) — misoprostol 0.2 mg (200 mcg) and diclofenac 50 mg

Conditions Requiring Dosing Adjustments

Liver Function: Specific dose adjustments in liver compromise are not defined.

Kidney Function: The dose of misoprostol should be decreased in kidney disease. (See the diclofenac profile for information on diclofenac.)

▷ **Usual Adult Dosage Ranges:** *Prevention of stomach ulcer:* 200 mcg four times daily with food, taken concurrently during the use of any anti-inflammatory drug (see Antiarthritic or NSAIDs Drug Classes).

Treatment of Duodenal Ulcer: 200 mcg four times daily for 4 to 8 weeks.

Combination Abortions: RU-496 600 mg taken once, followed by 400–600 mcg of misoprostol in one dose or two equal doses.

Rheumatoid Arthritis (Arthrotec Form): one tablet 2 to 4 times daily.

Cervical Ripening: 100 mcg of extemporaneous gel vaginally with repeat doses of 100 mcg by mouth every two hours until they have 3 contractions in ten minutes.

Note: Actual dose and schedule must be determined for each patient individually.

▷ **Dosing Instructions:** The regular, noncombination tablet may be crushed and taken with each of three daily meals; take the last (fourth) dose of the day with food at bedtime. Arthrotec form should be taken right after a meal or with food or milk. DO NOT crush or alter. If you forget a dose: Take the missed dose as soon as you remember it, unless it's nearly time for your next dose—if that is the case, skip the missed dose and take the next dose right on schedule. DO NOT double doses. Talk with your doctor and pharmacist if you find yourself missing doses. The intravaginal gel is made in the hospital.

Usual Duration of Use: For prevention of stomach ulcer, use is recommended for the entire period of anti-inflammatory drug use. For treatment of duodenal ulcer, continual use on a regular schedule for 4 weeks is recommended; if ulcer healing is not complete, a second course of 4 weeks is advised. Long-term use (months to years) requires periodic physician evaluation of response and dose adjustment.

Typical Treatment Goals and Measurements (Outcomes and Markers)

Prevention of ulcers: The goal is to prevent ulceration from anti-inflammatory drug use, or to heal the ulcer area and prevent re-occurrence of the ulceration. Sign and symptom prevention or relief as well as endoscopic examination help define success of ulcer treatment or prevention.

Induction of labor: In an early comparative study of causing (inducing) labor, 100 mcg of misoprostol versus intravenous oxytocin (one miliunit per minute) were compared in 126 pregnant women. Misoprostol shortened the time until labor more effectively than oxytocin.

Possible Advantages of This Drug: Significantly more effective than histamine (H2) blocking drugs (cimetidine, famotidine, nizatidine, ranitidine) or sucralfate in preventing the development of stomach ulcers. Arthrotec form may increase adherence (having people take it as directed). Use to help ripen the cervix shortens the time until labor better than a previously used medicine called oxytocin.

▷ **This Drug Should Not Be Taken If**
• you have had an allergic reaction to it previously.
• you are allergic to any type of prostaglandin.
• you are pregnant (unless this medicine is being used in the hospital to help "ripen" the cervix).
• you are breast-feeding your infant.
• you are not able or willing to use effective contraception (oral contraceptives or intrauterine device) while taking this drug.

▷ **Inform Your Physician Before Taking This Drug If**
• you have a history of peptic ulcer disease or Crohn's disease.
• you have inflammatory bowel disease.
• you have impaired kidney function.
• you have a seizure disorder.

Possible Side Effects (natural, expected, and unavoidable drug actions)

Diarrhea (14–40% of users), usually beginning after 13 days of use and subsiding spontaneously after 8 days.

Abortion (miscarriage) of pregnancy (11% of users); this is often incomplete and accompanied by serious uterine bleeding that may require hospitalization and urgent treatment.

▷ **Possible Adverse Effects** (unusual, unexpected, and infrequent reactions)
   If any of the following develop, consult your physician promptly for guidance.
   Mild Adverse Effects
   Allergic reaction: skin rash.
   Headache, dizziness—infrequent.
   Anxiety, depression—rare.
   Hair loss with long-term use—case reports.
   Ringing in the ears (tinnitus)—case reports.
   Joint pain and muscle aches—rare.
   Passing out (syncope)—rare.
   Abdominal pain, indigestion, nausea, vomiting, flatulence, constipation—rare to infrequent.
   Serious Adverse Effects
   Allergic reactions: anaphylaxis—rare.
   Anemia and low blood platelets—rare.
   Blood in the urine—rare.
   Uterine complications (excessive action of the uterus or tachysystole)—frequent.
   Bronchospasm—rare.
   Neuropathy—rare.
   Autonomic dysreflexia (Arthotec form)—case reports.
   Abortion (if taken while pregnant—NOT for cervical ripening).

▷ **Possible Effects on Sexual Function:** Menstrual irregularity, menstrual cramps, heavy menstrual flow, spotting between periods—all rare.
   Postmenopausal vaginal bleeding; this may require further evaluation.
   Reduced libido and impotence—rare and causal relationship not established.

▷ **Natural Diseases or Disorders That May Be Activated by This Drug**
   Latent epilepsy.

Possible Effects on Laboratory Tests
   Mild increase in liver function enzymes.

CAUTION
   1. Do not take this drug if you are pregnant. It can cause abortion (see cervical ripening note).
   2. Do not make this drug available to others who may be pregnant or who may become pregnant.
   3. If this drug is prescribed, it is advisable that you have a negative serum pregnancy test within 2 weeks before starting treatment.
   4. Start taking this drug only on the second or third day of your next normal menstrual period.
   5. Initiate effective contraceptive measures when you begin to take this drug. Discuss the use of oral contraceptives or intrauterine devices with your physician.
   6. Should you become pregnant, stop the drug immediately and call your doctor.

Precautions for Use
   By Infants and Children: Safety and effectiveness for those less than 18 years of age not established.

By Those Over 60 Years of Age: This drug is usually well tolerated by this age group, but some forms of prostaglandins can cause drops in blood pressure; watch for light-headedness or faintness that may indicate low blood pressure. Report any such development to your physician.

▷ **Advisability of Use During Pregnancy**
Pregnancy Category: X. See Pregnancy Risk Categories at the back of this book.
Animal Studies: No birth defects due to this drug found in rat or rabbit studies.
Human Studies: Information from studies of pregnant women confirms that this drug can cause abortion, sometimes incomplete; unpassed products of conception can cause life-threatening complications.
Avoid this drug completely.
Author's Note: Because of widespread use of a specific dosage (intra-vaginal gel) form of this medicine to ripen the cervix, labeling regarding use in pregnancy was modified by the FDA.

Advisability of Use If Breast-Feeding
Presence of this drug in breast milk: Unknown.
Avoid drug or refrain from nursing.

Habit-Forming Potential: None.

Effects of Overdose: Abdominal pain, diarrhea, fever, drowsiness, weakness, tremor, convulsions, difficult breathing.

Possible Effects of Long-Term Use: Unknown at this time.

Suggested Periodic Examinations While Taking This Drug (at physician's discretion)
Monitoring for accidental pregnancy.

▷ **While Taking This Drug, Observe the Following**
Foods: High-fat meals may reduce peak blood concentration.
Herbal Medicines or Minerals: Kola, guarana, mate and ma huang may increase stomach acid, blunting the benefits of the combination use in Arthrotec form. Black cohosh root, ginkgo, and squill are contraindicated in gastrointestinal disturbances. Licorice root has a Commission E monograph indication for gastrointestinal ulcers, but use with misoprostol has not been studied. Talk to your doctor BEFORE adding any herbals to this medicine.
Beverages: No restrictions. May be taken with milk.
▷ *Alcohol:* No interactions expected, but alcohol can promote the development of stomach ulcer and reduce the effectiveness of this drug.
Tobacco Smoking: No interactions expected. Nicotine is conducive to stomach ulcers. I advise everyone to quit smoking.
▷ *Other Drugs*
Misoprostol *taken concurrently* with
  • antacids that contain magnesium may increase the risk of diarrhea; avoid this combination. Antacids in general may decrease misoprostol absorption and lessen its therapeutic benefits.
  • phenylbutazone may result in neurosensory problems (movement problems, tingling, etc.).
▷ *Driving, Hazardous Activities:* This drug may cause dizziness, light-headedness, stomach pain, or diarrhea. Restrict activities as necessary.
Aviation Note: The use of this drug *may be a disqualification* for piloting. Consult a designated Aviation Medical Examiner.
Exposure to Sun: No restrictions.
Discontinuation: This drug should be taken as combination therapy while you are taking antiarthritic/anti-inflammatory drugs that can cause stomach ulceration. Call your doctor if you have reason to stop it prematurely.

MODAFINIL (moh DAF in ihl)

Introduced: 1998 **Class:** Central nervous system stimulant **Prescription:** USA: Yes **Controlled Drug:** USA: Yes C-IV*; Canada: Yes **Available as Generic:** No

Brand Name: Provigil

Author's Note: Information in this profile will be broadened in subsequent editions if warranted.

MOLINDONE (moh LIN dohn)

Introduced: 1971 **Class:** Antipsychotic **Prescription:** USA: Yes **Controlled Drug:** USA: No; Canada: No **Available as Generic:** No

Brand Name: Moban

Author's Note: Information in this profile has been truncated to make room for more widely used medicines.

MORPHINE (MOR feen)

Other Name: MS (morphine sulfate)

Introduced: 1806, Avinza form 2002 **Class:** Strong analgesic, opioids **Prescription:** USA: Yes **Controlled Drug:** USA: C-II*; Canada: Yes **Available as Generic:** Yes

Brand Names: ✦Alti-Morphine, Astramorph, Astramorph PF, Avinza, Duramorph, ✦Epimorph, Infumorph, Kadian, ✦M-Eslon, ✦Morphine H.P., ✦Morphitec, ✦M.O.S., ✦M.O.S.-S.R., MS Contin, MS-IR, OMS Concentrate, Opium Tincture, Oramorph SR, Paregoric, RMS Uniserts, Roxanol, Roxanol 100, Roxanol SR, ✦Statex

---

BENEFITS versus RISKS

Possible Benefits	*Possible Risks*
EFFECTIVE RELIEF OF MODERATE TO SEVERE PAIN WHEN IT IS DOSED CORRECTLY	POTENTIAL FOR HABIT FORMATION (DEPENDENCE)
EXTENDED-RELEASE FORMS OFFER TWICE OR ONCE DAILY DOSES AND INCREASED ADHERENCE	Respiratory depression (dose and patient dependent)
	Disorientation, hallucinations
	Constipation
	Problems urinating

▷ **Principal Uses**

As a Single Drug Product: Uses currently included in FDA-approved labeling: (1) Given by mouth, suppository or injection to relieve moderate to severe pain of heart attack, cancer, surgical procedures/operations, fluid on the lungs, and other causes; (2) used as an adjunct to anesthesia; (3) used in treatment-resistant (intractable) cough.

*See Schedules of Controlled Drugs at the back of this book.

Other (unlabeled) generally accepted uses: (1) Therapy of pain in sickle cell crisis; (2) used in patient-controlled analgesia pumps to fight pain.

Author's Note: The FDA and Purdue Pharmaceuticals have worked together to strengthen warnings for a related strong opioid called OxyContin because of continuing reports of abuse and diversion of this medicine. An important factor that MUST be considered when OxyContin is prescribed is the severity of the pain that is being treated, not simply the disease that is the root cause of the painful symptoms. Because ALL opioids (like morphine) are subject to abuse, the FDA is also encouraging all makers of opioids sold in the US to voluntarily review and revise product labeling to help ensure adequate warnings and precautions regarding risks of abuse, misuse, and diversion are presented and that responsible prescribing practices are promoted.

How This Drug Works: Acting primarily as a depressant of certain brain functions, this drug suppresses the perception of pain and calms the emotional response to pain. There are a variety of brain places (receptors) where morphine works to have both beneficial and undesirable effects. Widely quoted is the mu receptor where much like endorphins, morphine acts to block pain. Avinza form actually has two components. One part goes to work right away (immediate release), and the second part is an extended-release form (Spheroidal Oral Drug Absorption System or SODAS).

▷ **Widely Used Guidelines That Involve This Medicine (representative sample):** Please look at the section at the very beginning of this profile called "Class." Next, turn to Table 22 and you will find guidelines listed by the class involved!

Available Dosage Forms and Strengths

Capsules, extended-release (Avinza) — 30 mg, 60 mg, 90 mg and 120 mg

Capsules, sustained-release (Kadian) — 20 mg, 30 mg, 50 mg, 60 mg, 100 mg

Injection — 0.5 mg/mL, 1 mg/mL, 2 mg/mL, 4 mg/mL, 5 mg/mL, 8 mg/mL, 10 mg/mL, 15 mg/mL, 25 mg/mL, 50 mg/mL

Oral solution — 20 mg/mL; 10 mg/5 mL, 20 mg/5 mL, 100 mg/5 mL

Suppositories — 5 mg, 10 mg, 20 mg, 30 mg

Syrup — 1 mg/mL, 5 mg/mL, 10 mg/mL, 20 mg/mL

Syrup (Canada only) — 50 mg/mL

Tablets — 5 mg, 10 mg, 15 mg, 25 mg, 30 mg, 50 mg

Tablets, soluble — 10 mg, 15 mg, 30 mg

Tablets, sustained-release — 15 mg, 30 mg, 60 mg, 100 mg, 200 mg

Tablets, timed-release — 15 mg, 30 mg, 60 mg, 100 mg, 200 mg

▷ **Recommended Dosage Ranges** (Actual dose and schedule must be determined for each patient individually.)

Infants and Children: 0.05 to 0.1 mg per kg of body mass have been used every 4 hours for the immediate-release form. Single dose should not exceed 15 mg, and dosing is adjusted (titrated to pain control goals). Infants and small children should be approached cautiously as they are generally more sensitive to narcotic (opioid) medicines dosed on a body weight basis.

17 to 60 Years of Age: By injection (IV form is used where naloxone [Narcan] and assisted breathing are available): Requirements for analgesia vary with the patient and with the painful condition being treated. For example: After a heart attack (Acute Myocardial Infarction or MI). When patient symptoms are not helped by 3 appropriately spaced nitroglycerin tablets taken under the tongue or in patients who have symptoms come back (recur) after such treatment: IV morphine 1–5 mg is given every 5 to 30 minutes until the pain is controlled. Limiting factors include patient intolerance or excessive lowering of blood pressure. For general intravenous pain relief (analgesia): 2–10 mg given over 4–5 minutes. Repeat dosing is guided by pain control goals and patient effects. In sickle cell crisis some clinicians have used Patient-Controlled Analgesia (PCA) with or without a constant IV infusion. Constant infusions of 10 to 75 mg per hour were detailed in one case study where the patient had not responded to IV injections. PCA dosing usually combines a loading dose (determined by patient weight, pain being treated and other individual factors) and subsequent patient-administered doses (usually a lesser amount than the loading dose with a lock out interval [such as fifteen minutes] to allow for the peak effect of the prior dose to be reached before another dose is given).

By mouth (regular solution, syrup and tablets)—5 to 30 mg every 4 hours.

By mouth (sustained-release forms)—30 mg every 12 hours.

By mouth (Kadian brand sustained-release form and the Avinza extended-released form)—once daily. Dosing here is usually made after pain relief requirements are defined by an immediate-release form of morphine. An immediate-release form should still be made available in order to ease pain (rescue dose) which is used to check daily requirements for medicine (and is added back into the daily dose if such rescue dose use continues).

By suppository—10 to 30 mg every 4 hours.

Over 60 Years of Age: Same as 12 to 60 years of age, using smaller doses to start. Dose is slowly increased if needed. Many clinicians treat constipation in this age group once the morphine is started.

Author's Note: Current pain treatment theory calls for timed or scheduled dosing. This tends to prevent pain, rather than allowing pain and then treating it. Some clinicians will use timed dosing immediately after surgery and then change to regular pain assessment with Patient-Controlled Analgesia (PCA), then to regular pain assessment with oral dosing once the most severe period of pain has passed. Pain is the fifth vital sign and should be checked regularly.

Conditions Requiring Dosing Adjustments

Liver Function: The dose and frequency **must** be adjusted (decreased) with liver compromise. This medicine is removed (metabolized) by the liver to morphine-6-glucuronide.

Kidney Function: Dose and frequency are prudently reduced in kidney compromise.

▷ **Dosing Instructions:** The regular tablet may be crushed and taken with or following food to reduce stomach irritation or nausea. Extended-release (such as Kadian or Avinza) or sustained-release forms should be swallowed whole; do not break, crush, or chew them. Oral liquid form may be mixed with fruit juice to improve taste. If you forget a dose: Take the missed dose as soon as you remember it, unless it's nearly time for your next dose—if that is the case, skip the missed dose and take the next dose right on schedule. DO NOT double dose. Talk with your doctor if you find yourself missing doses. If you are uncertain about any dose, call your doctor.

Usual Duration of Use: Used to control pain, hence the duration will be determined by the source of the pain. For short-term, self-limiting conditions, continual use should not exceed 5 to 7 days without reassessment of need. For the long-term management of severe chronic pain, it is advisable to determine a fixed dose schedule with rescue dose contingency schedule. It is not unusual for additional (adjuvant) medicines such as those usually used for seizures or for depression to be combined with morphine in chronic pain situations.

Typical Treatment Goals and Measurements (Outcomes and Markers)

Pain: Most clinicians treating pain use a device called an algometer to check your pain. This looks like a small ruler, but lets the clinician better understand your pain. The goals of treatment then relate to where the level of pain started (for example, a rating of 7 on a 0–10 scale) and what the cause of the pain was. I use the PQRSTBG (see Glossary) system. Pain medicines may also be used together (in combination) in order to get the best result or outcome. If your pain control is not acceptable to YOU (remember, in hospitals and outpatient settings, etc. pain control is a patient right and the fifth vital sign), call your doctor. It is not unusual to have an immediate-release rescue dose available and then some percentage of previous-day use added back to an extended-release form. Pain can be dynamic and adjustments are often required.

▷ **This Drug Should Not Be Taken If**
- you had an allergic reaction to it previously.
- you are having an acute attack of asthma or your upper airway is blocked (obstructed).
- you have a specific bowel problem (paralytic ileus).
- you have acute respiratory depression.

▷ **Inform Your Physician Before Taking This Drug If**
- you took a monoamine oxidase (MAO) type A inhibitor drug (see Drug Classes) in the last 14 days.
- you are taking atropinelike drugs, antihypertensives, metoclopramide (Reglan), or zidovudine (AZT).
- you are taking any other drugs that have a sedative effect.
- you have a history of drug abuse or alcoholism.
- you have impaired liver, bile tract, or kidney function.
- you have prostate gland enlargement (see prostatism in Glossary).
- you have a history of asthma, emphysema, epilepsy, gallbladder disease, or inflammatory bowel disease.
- you are dehydrated.
- you have a tendency toward constipation.
- you have a history of head injury or a seizure disorder.
- you have a history of sickle cell anemia.
- you have a history of low blood pressure.
- you plan to have surgery under general anesthesia in the near future.

Possible Side Effects (natural, expected, and unavoidable drug actions)

Drowsiness, light-headedness, weakness, euphoria, dry mouth, urinary retention, dose-related constipation. Temperature changes. Miosis or pinpoint pupils. Histamine release if morphine is injected too quickly.

▷ **Possible Adverse Effects** (unusual, unexpected, and infrequent reactions)
  If any of the following develop, consult your physician promptly for guidance.
  Mild Adverse Effects
  Allergic reactions: skin rash, hives, itching (especially if the intravenous form is injected too quickly).
  Headache, dizziness, impaired concentration, sensation of drunkenness, confusion, depression, blurred or double vision—infrequent to frequent and may be dose-related.
  Facial flushing, sweating, heart palpitation—possible.
  Nausea, vomiting—possible and may be dose-related.
  Spasm of the biliary tract—possible.
  Urine retention—possible.
  Serious Adverse Effects
  Allergic reactions: swelling of throat or vocal cords, spasm of larynx or bronchial tubes—rare.
  Hallucinations, psychosis—case reports.
  Drop in blood pressure, causing severe weakness and fainting—possible.
  Disorientation, hallucinations, unstable gait, tremor, muscle twitching—possible.
  Drug-induced myasthenia gravis—case reports.
  Respiratory depression—dose-related.
  Seizures—possible.

▷ **Possible Effects on Sexual Function:** Reduced libido and/or potency.
  Amenorrhea and disruption of ovulation—case reports.

▷ **Adverse Effects That May Mimic Natural Diseases or Disorders**
  Paradoxical behavioral disturbances may suggest psychotic disorder.

Possible Effects on Laboratory Tests
  Blood amylase and lipase levels: increased (natural side effects).
  Liver function tests: increased liver enzymes (ALT/GPT, AST/GOT, and alkaline phosphatase), increased bilirubin.
  Urine screening tests for drug abuse: may be positive. (Test results depend upon amount of drug taken and testing method used.)

CAUTION
  1. If you have asthma, chronic bronchitis, or emphysema, excessive use of this drug may cause significant respiratory difficulty, thickening of bronchial secretions, and suppression of coughing.
  2. Taking this drug with atropinelike drugs can increase the risk of urinary retention and reduced intestinal function.
  3. Constipation can be a serious problem, particularly in older patients (as bowel function tends to slow down). Many clinicians prescribe a medicine (such as Senokot-S) to promote bowel movements at the same time that morphine is prescribed.
  4. Do not take this drug following acute head injury.

Precautions for Use
  By Infants and Children: Use very cautiously in infants under 2 years of age because of their vulnerability to life-threatening respiratory depression. Watch for paradoxical excitement in this age group.
  By Those Over 60 Years of Age: Small doses and short-term use are indicated. There may be increased risk of drowsiness, dizziness, unsteadiness, falling, urinary retention, and constipation (often leading to fecal impaction).

▷ **Advisability of Use During Pregnancy**

Pregnancy Category: C. D if used long-term or in high doses at term. See Pregnancy Risk Categories at the back of this book.

Animal Studies: Significant skeletal birth defects reported in mouse and hamster studies.

Human Studies: Adequate studies of pregnant women are not available, but no significant increase in birth defects was found in one report of 448 exposures to this drug.

Avoid during the first 3 months. Use sparingly and in small doses during the final 6 months only if clearly needed.

Advisability of Use If Breast-Feeding

Presence of this drug in breast milk: Yes.

Avoid drug or refrain from nursing.

Habit-Forming Potential: This drug can cause psychological and physical dependence (see Glossary).

Effects of Overdose: Marked drowsiness, dizziness, confusion, restlessness, depressed breathing, tremors, convulsions, stupor progressing to coma.

Possible Effects of Long-Term Use: Psychological and physical dependence, chronic constipation.

Suggested Periodic Examinations While Taking This Drug (at physician's discretion)

Ask the patient about his or her bowel habits.

▷ **While Taking This Drug, Observe the Following**

Foods: No restrictions.

Herbal Medicines or Minerals: Valerian and kava kava (no longer recommended in Canada) may interact additively (drowsiness). Avoid these combinations. St. John's wort can change (inducing or increasing) P450 3A4 enzymes, blunting the effects of morphine. Yohimbe may increase adverse effects as well as increase the pain-relieving effects of morphine. Talk to your doctor BEFORE you combine any herbal medicines with morphine.

Beverages: No restrictions. May be taken with milk.

▷ *Alcohol:* Alcohol is best avoided. Opioid analgesics can intensify the intoxicating effects of alcohol and alcohol can intensify the depressant effects of opioids on brain function, breathing and circulation.

Tobacco Smoking: No interactions expected. I advise everyone to quit smoking.

Marijuana Smoking: Increase in drowsiness and pain relief; impairment of mental and physical performance.

▷ *Other Drugs*

Morphine may ***increase*** the effects of
- antihypertensives and cause excessive lowering of blood pressure.
- atropinelike drugs and increase the risk of constipation and urinary retention.
- metformin (Glucophage).
- other drugs with sedative effects.

Morphine may ***decrease*** the effects of
- metoclopramide (Reglan).

Morphine ***taken concurrently*** with
- benzodiazepines (see Drug Classes) may result in increased risk of respiratory depression.
- cimetidine (Tagamet) may result in morphine toxicity.

- fluoxetine (Prozac) may antagonize morphine's pain-relieving effect.
- gabapentin (Neurontin) can increase gabapentin levels (watch for arm cogging and increased sleepiness.
- hydroxyzine (Vistaril) can increase pain relief but carries the risk of increased respiratory depression.
- medicines that increase CYP 3A4 will blunt morphine benefits and those that inhibit or use 3A4 for removal from the body may increase morphine blood levels. Caution and dosing adjustments are prudent.
- metoclopramide (Reglan) may lead to increased morphine effects.
- monoamine oxidase (MAO) type A inhibitors (see Drug Classes) may cause the equivalent of an acute narcotic overdose: unconsciousness and severe depression of breathing, heart rate and circulation. A variation can be excitability, convulsions, high fever and rapid heart action.
- naltrexone (ReVia or Narcan) may lead to sudden withdrawal symptoms.
- phenothiazines (see Drug Classes) may cause excessive and prolonged depression of brain functions, breathing and circulation.
- rifampin (Rifater, others) may lower morphine benefits.
- ritonavir (Norvir) may lead to lower morphine benefits.
- tramadol (Ultram) may increase CNS side effects.
- trovafloxacin (Trovan) may blunt trovafloxacin benefits.
- zidovudine (AZT) may increase the toxicity of both drugs; avoid concurrent use.

▷ *Driving, Hazardous Activities:* This drug can impair mental alertness, judgment, reaction time and physical coordination. Avoid hazardous activities.

Aviation Note: The use of this drug **is a disqualification** for piloting. Consult a designated Aviation Medical Examiner.

Exposure to Sun: No restrictions.

Discontinuation: Where possible, it is advisable to limit this drug to short-term use. Longer-term use requires gradual tapering (decreasing) of doses to minimize possible effects of withdrawal: body aches, fever, sweating, nervousness, trembling, weakness, runny nose, sneezing, rapid heart rate, nausea, vomiting, stomach cramps, diarrhea.

MUPIROCIN (myu PEER oh sin)

Introduced: 1987   **Class:** Antibiotic, topical   **Prescription:** USA: Yes   **Controlled Drug:** USA: No; Canada: No   **Available as Generic:** USA: No; Canada: No

Brand Names: Bactroban, Bactroban Nasal

BENEFITS versus RISKS	
Possible Benefits	*Possible Risks*
EFFECTIVE TOPICAL TREATMENT OF *STAPHYLOCOCCUS* AND *STREPTOCOCCUS* SKIN INFECTIONS	Skin irritation
EFFECTIVE ERADICATION OF *STAPHYLOCOCCUS AUREUS* FROM THE NOSE	

▷ **Principal Uses**

As a Single Drug Product: Uses currently included in FDA-approved labeling: (1) Used to treat skin infections caused by staphylococcal and streptococcal infections such as ecthyma or impetigo; (2) the intranasal form is specifically formulated to kill *Staphylococcus aureus* bacteria that are living (have colonized) in the nasal passages; (3) treats secondary skin infections caused by strep or staph; (4) treats skin lesions that are traumatic.

Other (unlabeled) generally accepted uses: (1) Used in burns where resistant *Staphylococcus aureus* is causing infection; (2) helps prevent opportunistic infections of venous access devices, such as intravascular cannulas; (3) treats cellulitis caused by Gram-positive organisms; (4) has been used in some specific situations in skin surgery to prevent infections; (5) used to eradicate vaginal *Staphylococcus* infections.

How This Drug Works: Binds to an enzyme (isoleucyl transfer-RNA synthetase) and stops susceptible bacteria from being able to make critical proteins and kills them.

▷ **Widely Used Guidelines That Involve This Medicine (representative sample):** Please look at the section at the very beginning of this profile called "Class." Next, turn to Table 22 and you will find guidelines listed by the class involved!

Available Dosage Forms and Strengths

Intranasal form (Bactroban Nasal) — 2%

Topical cream — 2.15%

Topical ointment (Bactroban) — 2%

Topical ointment (Bactroban, Canada) — 20 mg/g

▷ **Recommended Dosage Ranges** (Actual dose and schedule must be determined for each patient individually.)

Infants and Children: Cream (3 months to 16 years)—follow your pediatrician's recommendations.

Nasal (children 12 or over)—one-half of the ointment from the single-use tube of mupirocin is applied into one nostril and the other half is applied to the second nostril, twice daily, in the morning and evening, for 5 consecutive days. One study found that application of this medicine to both nostrils (nares) three times daily for up to 21 days removed resistant staph (methicillin-resistant *Staphylococcus aureus* [MRSA]) in 62.5% of infants in a small study.

16 to 60 Years of Age: 2% ointment—apply three times daily for 5 to 14 days. Some more involved or extensive infections have been treated for longer periods. If the infection in question has not resolved after the initial course of the ointment, the site should be evaluated by a physician and full body (systemic) antibiotics or other treatment considered.

2% topical cream—for traumatic skin infections caused by *Strep pyogenes* or *Staph aureus*, apply (small amount) three times daily for 10 days (and the infection is rechecked).

Intranasal—one-half of the ointment from the single-use tube of mupirocin is applied into one nostril and the other half is applied into the second nostril, twice daily in the morning and evening for 5 consecutive days.

Over 60 Years of Age: Same as 16 to 60 years of age.

Conditions Requiring Dosing Adjustments

Liver Function: Little of this ointment is usually absorbed into the body. No guidelines exist for liver disease adjustments.

Kidney Function: A substance in this formulation (polyethylene glycol) may be toxic to the kidneys if the ointment is applied over an extensive burn or wound area.

▷ **Dosing Instructions:** This medicine should be applied as a thin film or as described by your doctor. Call your doctor if the condition has not improved or worsens during the course of treatment. Do not combine this medicine with other ointments or treatments unless your doctor has prescribed this approach. Please remember that if you are going to use this medicine in the nose, you should have Bactroban Nasal. Using the Bactroban ointment in the nose (polyethylene glycol base) is more likely to cause irritation. As with other medicines, applying this medicine right on time is critical. If you forget a dose: Apply the missed dose as soon as you remember it, unless it's nearly time for your next dose—if that is the case, skip the missed dose and apply the next dose right on schedule. Talk with your doctor and pharmacist if you find yourself missing doses.

Usual Duration of Use: Continual use on a regular schedule for several days is usually necessary to determine this drug's effectiveness in treating skin infections. Wounds not responding in 3 to 5 days must be evaluated by your doctor. Longer-term use requires physician evaluation.

Typical Treatment Goals and Measurements (Outcomes and Markers)
Staph Colonization or Other Infection: The goal is to kill the colonizing or infecting organism. Markers for improvement include improvement in signs and symptoms of the infection or in the case of colonization—negative rechecks (repeat cultures).

Possible Advantages of This Drug
Effective topical treatment of skin infections. Intranasal form can help people who have been colonized by infectious bacteria stop spreading it to other people.

▷ **This Drug Should Not Be Taken If**
• you had an allergic reaction to any form of it previously.
• you have extensive burns or open wounds.

▷ **Inform Your Physician Before Taking This Drug If**
• several days have passed after starting this medicine and there has been no change or the wound has worsened.
• pain at the site of the infection or severe irritation occurs.
• you are unsure how much to apply or how often to apply mupirocin.

Possible Side Effects (natural, expected, and unavoidable drug actions)
Irritation at the site of infection caused by the polyethylene glycol component.

▷ **Possible Adverse Effects** (unusual, unexpected, and infrequent reactions)
If any of the following develop, consult your physician promptly for guidance.
Mild Adverse Effects
Allergic reactions: skin rash and irritation at the infection site.
Soreness, stinging or pain at the infection site—possible.
Headache or taste changes—infrequent (intranasal is higher than cream).
Serious Adverse Effects
Allergic reactions: contact dermatitis—rare.
If this medicine is applied to an extensive skin area, polyethylene glycol may be absorbed and cause kidney toxicity—possible.

▷ **Possible Effects on Sexual Function:** Not reported.

Possible Delayed Adverse Effects: This medicine is indicated for short-term use.

▷ **Adverse Effects That May Mimic Natural Diseases or Disorders**
   None reported.

Natural Diseases or Disorders That May Be Activated by This Drug
   None reported.

Possible Effects on Laboratory Tests
   None reported.

CAUTION
   1. Do not apply this medicine to an area of skin larger than what your doctor prescribed.
   2. Because the Bactroban ointment uses a polyethylene glycol base and may cause irritation, the calcium mupirocin (Bactroban Nasal) is recommended for intranasal use.

Precautions for Use
   By Infants and Children: Safety and effectiveness for use by some age groups varies with the product.
   By Those Over 60 Years of Age: No special changes are needed.

▷ **Advisability of Use During Pregnancy**
   Pregnancy Category: B. See Pregnancy Risk Categories at the back of this book.
   Animal Studies: No fetal problems defined.
   Human Studies: Information from adequate studies of pregnant women is not available.

Advisability of Use If Breast-Feeding
   Presence of this drug in breast milk: Unknown.
   Avoid drug or refrain from nursing.

Habit-Forming Potential: None.

Effects of Overdose: If this medicine is applied to an extensive area of skin, excessive amounts of polyethylene glycol may be absorbed and cause kidney toxicity.

Possible Effects of Long-Term Use: None defined.

Suggested Periodic Examinations While Taking This Drug (at physician's discretion)
   Follow-up bacterial cultures of the nose with intranasal form.

▷ **While Taking This Drug, Observe the Following**
   Foods: No restrictions.
   Herbal Medicines or Minerals: Echinacea: Some patients use echinacea to attempt to boost their immune systems. Unfortunately, use of echinacea is not recommended in people with damaged immune systems. This herb may also actually weaken any immune system if it is used too often or for too long a time. DO NOT take mistletoe herb, oak bark or F.C. of marshmallow root, and licorice.
   Beverages: No restrictions.
▷ *Alcohol:* No restrictions.
   Tobacco Smoking: No interactions expected. I advise everyone to quit smoking.
▷ *Other Drugs*
   Mupirocin *taken concurrently* with
   • other medications that are toxic to the kidneys may result in additive kidney toxicity if mupirocin is applied to a large area of skin.
   Aviation Note: The use of this drug *does not appear to be a restriction* for piloting. Consult a designated Aviation Medical Examiner.

Exposure to Sun: Increased sensitivity (photosensitivity) has NOT been reported with topical application. No restrictions.

NABUMETONE (na BYU me tohn)

Please see the acetic acid (nonsteroidal anti-inflammatory drug) family profile.

NADOLOL (NAY doh lohl)

Introduced: 1976   **Class:**   Antianginal, antihypertensive, beta blocker
Prescription: USA: Yes   **Controlled Drug:**   USA: No; Canada: No
Available as Generic: Yes
Brand Names: ✤Alti-Nadol, ✤Apo-Nadol, Corgard, Corzide [CD], ✤Novo-Nadolol, ✤Ratio-Nadol, Syn-Nadol

BENEFITS versus RISKS	
Possible Benefits	*Possible Risks*
EFFECTIVE, WELL-TOLERATED ANTIHYPERTENSIVE for mild to moderate high blood pressure	CONGESTIVE HEART FAILURE in advanced heart disease
EFFECTIVE ANTIANGINAL DRUG IN CLASSIC CORONARY ARTERY DISEASE with moderate to severe angina	Provocation of asthma (in predisposed patients)
	Masking of hypoglycemia in drug-dependent diabetes
	Worsening of angina following abrupt withdrawal

▷ **Principal Uses**

As a Single Drug Product: Uses currently included in FDA-approved labeling: (1) Treats high blood pressure; (2) helps prevent attacks of effort-induced angina (should not be used in Prinzmetal's vasospastic angina).

Other (unlabeled) generally accepted uses: (1) Helps prevent hemorrhage from bulging veins (esophageal varices) in cirrhosis; (2) may have an adjunctive role in helping prevent and reduce migraine severity; (3) may have a role in helping prevent death after a heart attack (myocardial infarction) similar to other beta blockers; (4) may help ease tremor in patients taking lithium; (5) helps decrease risk of ruptured blood vessels in the esophagus (esophageal varices) in patients with cirrhosis; (6) can ease aggressive behavior for some patients (BPRS scores improve).

As a Combination Drug Product [CD]: Available in combination with bendroflumethiazide, a diuretic antihypertensive drug. This combination product works better and is more convenient for long-term use.

How This Drug Works: By blocking certain actions of the sympathetic nervous system, this drug:

- reduces the rate and contraction force of the heart, lowering oxygen needs of heart muscle and reducing ejection pressure of blood leaving the heart. This reduces frequency of angina and lowers blood pressure.
- reduces contraction of blood vessel walls, lowering blood pressure.
- prolongs conduction time of nerve impulses through the heart, which is of benefit in the management of certain heart rhythm disorders.

May use a vasodilating effect (possible involving dopamine) to preserve kidney blood flow and glomerular filtration.

▷ **Widely Used Guidelines That Involve This Medicine (representative sample):** Please look at the section at the very beginning of this profile called "Class." Next, turn to Table 22 and you will find guidelines listed by the class involved!

Available Dosage Forms and Strengths
Tablets — 20 mg, 40 mg, 80 mg, 100 mg, 120 mg, 160 mg
Tablets, combination — 40 mg or 80 mg of nadolol with 5 mg
bendroflumethiazide

▷ **Usual Adult Dosage Ranges:** For hypertension: Start with 40 mg daily; this may be increased gradually (in steps of 40–80 mg at 14-day intervals) as needed and tolerated, up to 320 mg daily. Many people meet blood pressure goals with 40 to 80 mg a day—but some require up to 320 mg daily. Daily maximum is 320 mg.
For Angina: Initially 40 mg daily; increased gradually at intervals of 3 to 7 days as needed and tolerated until the best control is achieved or there is unacceptable slowing of the heart (to 240 mg daily). Usual ongoing dose is 80 to 240 mg every 24 hours. Daily maximum is 240 mg of nadolol when treating angina.

Note: Actual dose and schedule must be determined for each patient individually.

Conditions Requiring Dosing Adjustments
Liver Function: No dosing changes needed.
Kidney Function: For patients with moderate kidney failure, the usual dose should be taken every 24 to 36 hours. For patients with severe kidney failure, the dose can be taken every 40 to 60 hours.

▷ **Dosing Instructions:** Immediate-release tablet may be crushed and taken without regard to eating. Do not stop this drug abruptly. If you forget a dose: Take the missed dose as soon as you remember it, unless it's 8 hours or less until your next scheduled dose—if that is the case, skip the missed dose and take the next dose right on schedule. Talk with your doctor if you find yourself missing doses.

Usual Duration of Use: Use on a regular schedule for up to 14 days determines this drug's effectiveness in lowering blood pressure and preventing angina. The long-term use of this drug (months to years) will be determined by your response to an overall treatment program (weight reduction, salt restriction, smoking cessation, etc.). Keep follow-up appointments with your doctor.

Typical Treatment Goals and Measurements (Outcomes and Markers)
Blood Pressure: Guidelines (JNC VII) define normal blood pressure (BP) as **less than** 120/80 and **pre-hypertension** as 120/80 to 139/89. This new range is intended to help doctors encourage lifestyle changes (or in the case of people with a risk factor for high blood pressure, start treatment) much earlier—so that damage to blood vessels, heart, kidneys, sexual potency, or eyes might be minimized or avoided altogether. Stage 1 hypertension is 140/90 to 159/99 and stage 2 hypertension equal to or greater than: 160/100 mm Hg. These guidelines also recommend that clinicians work with their patients to agree on the goals and a plan of treatment. The first-ever guidelines for blood pressure (hypertension) in African Americans recommends that MOST black patients be started on TWO antihypertensive medicines with the goal of lowering blood pressure to 130/80 for those with high risk for heart and blood vessel disease or with diabetes. The American Diabetes Association also recommends 130/80 as the target for diabetics and less than 125/75 for those

who spill more than one gram of protein into their urine. Most clinicians try to achieve a BP that confers the best balance of lower cardiovascular risk and avoids the problem of too low a blood pressure. Blood pressure duration is generally increased with beneficial restriction of sodium. If goals are not met, it is not unusual to intensify doses or add on medicines.

Possible Advantages of This Drug
Does not reduce blood flow to the kidney. Can be used with other drugs that may reduce blood flow to the kidney (such as most anti-inflammatory aspirin substitutes). May be taken without regard to meals. Once-daily dosing encourages patients to take their medicine (adherence). May have positive effects on lipid peroxidation which then could block processes leading to atherosclerosis.

▷ **This Drug Should Not Be Taken If**
- you have had an allergic reaction to it previously.
- you have heart shock (cardiogenic).
- you have an abnormally slow heart rate or a serious form of heart block (2nd or 3rd degree AV).
- you have ongoing obstructive lung disease (COPD) or bronchial asthma.

▷ **Inform Your Physician Before Taking This Drug If**
- you have had an adverse reaction to any beta blocker (see Drug Classes).
- you have a history of serious heart disease/heart failure.
- you have a history of hay fever (allergic rhinitis), asthma, chronic bronchitis, or emphysema.
- you have a history of overactive thyroid function (hyperthyroidism).
- you have a history of low blood sugar (hypoglycemia).
- you have impaired liver or kidney function.
- you have diabetes or myasthenia gravis.
- you are pregnant or breast-feeding your infant.
- you have difficulty with blood circulation to the periphery (peripheral vascular disease).
- you are currently taking any form of digitalis, quinidine, or reserpine, or any calcium-channel-blocker drug (see Drug Classes).
- you will have surgery with general anesthesia.

Possible Side Effects (natural, expected, and unavoidable drug actions)
Lethargy and fatigability, cold extremities, slow heart rate, light-headedness in upright position (see orthostatic hypotension in Glossary).

▷ **Possible Adverse Effects** (unusual, unexpected, and infrequent reactions)
If any of the following develop, consult your physician promptly for guidance.

Mild Adverse Effects
Allergic reactions: skin rash, itching, drug fever.
Headache, dizziness, vivid dreaming, visual disturbances, ringing in ears, slurred speech, paresthesia—case reports to infrequent.
Hair loss and sweating—case reports to infrequent.
Bleeding gums (gingival bleeding)—case report.
Cough, indigestion, nausea, vomiting, diarrhea, abdominal pain—infrequent.
Increased blood potassium—possible.
Numbness and tingling of extremities—case reports.

Serious Adverse Effects
Allergic reactions: facial swelling, anaphylaxis.
Chest pain, shortness of breath, precipitation of congestive heart failure—possible.

Intensification of heart block or severe slowing of the heart—case reports and may be dose-related.

Bronchospasm—rare.

Carpal tunnel syndrome or pancreatitis—case reports.

Precipitation of bronchial asthma (in people already living with asthma)—possible and dose-related.

Masking of warning indications of acute hypoglycemia in drug-treated diabetes—possible.

May precipitate cramping when walking (intermittent claudication)—possible. May be prudent to check for hidden Peripheral Artery Disease (PAD) by checking ankle brachial index (ABI). ABI check (see Glossary) can help find PAD early, and avoid claudication that may result if this medication is taken by someone who has PAD but does not know it.

Excessively low blood pressure—possible.

▷ **Possible Effects on Sexual Function:** Decreased libido, impotence, impaired erection—case reports to frequent.

▷ **Adverse Effects That May Mimic Natural Diseases or Disorders**

Impaired circulation to the extremities may resemble Raynaud's phenomenon.

Natural Diseases or Disorders That May Be Activated by This Drug

Bronchial asthma, Prinzmetal's variant (vasospastic) angina, latent Raynaud's disease, myasthenia gravis (questionable).

Possible Effects on Laboratory Tests

Blood HDL cholesterol level: decreased.

Blood VLDL cholesterol level: increased.

Blood triglyceride levels: increased.

CAUTION

1. ***Do not stop this drug suddenly*** without the knowledge and help of your doctor. Carry a note saying you are taking this drug.
2. Ask your physician or pharmacist before using nasal decongestants, which are usually present in over-the-counter cold preparations and nose drops. These can cause rapid blood pressure increases when combined with beta-blocker drugs.
3. Report the development of any tendency to emotional depression.

Precautions for Use

By Infants and Children: Safety and effectiveness for those under 12 years of age are not established. However, if this drug is used, observe for the development of low blood sugar (hypoglycemia) during periods of reduced food intake.

By Those Over 60 Years of Age: Unacceptably high blood pressure should be reduced without creating the risks associated with excessively low blood pressure. Small doses and frequent blood pressure checks are needed. Sudden, rapid, and excessive reduction of blood pressure can predispose to stroke or heart attack. Watch for dizziness, unsteadiness, tendency to fall, confusion, hallucinations, depression, or urinary frequency.

▷ **Advisability of Use During Pregnancy**

Pregnancy Category: C. See Pregnancy Risk Categories at the back of this book.

Animal Studies: No significant increase in birth defects due to this drug, but embryotoxicity reported in rabbits.

Human Studies: Adequate studies of pregnant women are not available. Avoid use during the first 3 months if possible. Use this drug only if clearly needed. Ask your physician for guidance.

Advisability of Use If Breast-Feeding
Presence of this drug in breast milk: Yes.
Avoid drug or refrain from nursing.

Habit-Forming Potential: None.

Effects of Overdose: Weakness, slow pulse, low blood pressure, fainting, cold and sweaty skin, congestive heart failure, possible coma, and convulsions.

Possible Effects of Long-Term Use: Reduced heart reserve and possible heart failure in susceptible individuals with advanced heart disease.

Suggested Periodic Examinations While Taking This Drug (at physician's discretion)
Measurements of blood pressure.
Evaluation of heart function, check of lipid panel.

▷ **While Taking This Drug, Observe the Following**
Foods: Follow the diet your doctor prescribes. Avoid excessive salt intake.
Herbal Medicines or Minerals: Valerian and kava kava (no longer recommended in Canada) may intensify drowsiness. Dong quai may make this medicine stay in the body longer than expected, while St. John's wort may increase removal of this medicine from the body, blunting the benefit. Ginseng, guarana, bitter orange, country mallow, hawthorn, saw palmetto, ma huang (do not take if hypertensive), goldenseal, yohimbe, and licorice may also increase blood pressure. Calcium and garlic may help lower blood pressure and could be part of complementary care. Use of calcium to excess (7.5 to 10 grams) with combination thiazide diuretics can lead to excessive calcium levels. Talk to your doctor about how much calcium to take. Indian snakeroot has a German Commission E monograph indication for hypertension—talk to your doctor. Eleuthero root and ephedra should be avoided by people living with hypertension.
Beverages: No restrictions. May be taken with milk.
▷ *Alcohol:* Use with caution. Alcohol may exaggerate this drug's ability to lower blood pressure and may increase its mild sedative effect.
Tobacco Smoking: Nicotine may reduce this drug's effectiveness. I advise everyone to quit smoking.
▷ *Other Drugs*
Nadolol may ***increase*** the effects of
• other antihypertensive drugs and cause excessive lowering of blood pressure; dose adjustments may be necessary.
• reserpine (Ser-Ap-Es, etc.) and cause sedation, depression, slowing of the heart rate, and lowering of blood pressure.
• verapamil (Calan, Isoptin) or other calcium channel blockers (see Drug Classes) and cause excessive depression of heart function; monitor this combination closely.
Nadolol may ***decrease*** the effects of
• ritodrine (Yutopar), and may result in undesirable heart effects.
• theophyllines (Aminophyllin, Theo-Dur, etc.) and reduce their effectiveness in treating asthma.
Nadolol ***taken concurrently*** with
• amiodarone (Cordarone) can cause severe slowing of the heart and potentially stop the heart (cardiac arrest).
• antacids containing aluminum can block absorption of this medicine and lessen therapeutic nadolol effects.
• clonidine (Catapres) requires close monitoring for rebound high blood pressure if clonidine is withdrawn while nadolol is still being taken.

- digoxin (Lanoxin) may result in undesirable heart effects.
- dihydropyridine calcium channel blockers may result in undesirable heart effects (bradycardia) or excessively low blood pressure.
- epinephrine can cause serious hypertension and slowing of the heart and, should anaphylaxis occur, epinephrine resistance.
- ergot derivatives (see Drug Classes) can cause decreased blood flow to the extremities (peripheral ischemia).
- insulin requires close monitoring to avoid undetected hypoglycemia (see Glossary).
- lidocaine can lead to lidocaine toxicity (depressed heart function, cardiac arrest).
- oral antidiabetic drugs (see Drug Classes) can cause slowed recovery from any hypoglycemia that may occur.

The following drug may *decrease* the effects of nadolol:
- indomethacin (Indocin), and possibly other "aspirin substitutes," or NSAIDs, and may impair nadolol's antihypertensive effect.

▷ *Driving, Hazardous Activities:* Use caution until the full extent of drowsiness, lethargy, and blood pressure change has been determined.

Aviation Note: The use of this drug *is a disqualification* for piloting. Consult a designated Aviation Medical Examiner.

Exposure to Sun: No restrictions.

Exposure to Heat: Caution is advised. Hot environments can lower blood pressure and exaggerate the effects of this drug.

Exposure to Cold: Caution is advised. Cold environments can enhance the circulatory deficiency in the extremities that may occur with this drug. The elderly should take precautions to prevent hypothermia (see Glossary).

Heavy Exercise or Exertion: Prudent to avoid exertion that produces light-headedness, excessive fatigue, or muscle cramping.

Occurrence of Unrelated Illness: Fever can lower blood pressure, requiring dose decreases. Nausea or vomiting may interrupt dosing. Ask your doctor for help.

Discontinuation: Best not to stop this drug suddenly. Gradual lowering of doses (tapering) over 2 to 3 weeks is recommended.

NAFARELIN (NAF a re lin)

Introduced: 1984 **Class:** Hormones, miscellaneous **Prescription:** USA: Yes **Controlled Drug:** USA: No; Canada: No **Available as Generic:** USA: No

Brand Name: Synarel

BENEFITS versus RISKS	
Possible Benefits	*Possible Risks*
VERY EFFECTIVE TREATMENT OF ENDOMETRIOSIS (alternative to oophorectomy)	Symptoms of estrogen deficiency (during treatment)
	Masculinizing effects (during treatment)
	Loss of bone density
	White blood cell count lowering

▷ **Principal Uses**

As a Single Drug Product: Uses currently included in FDA-approved labeling: (1) Treats endometriosis: reduction in the size and activity of endometrial implants within the pelvis; relief of pelvic pain associated with menstruation; (2) also used to treat precocious puberty due to excessive production of gonadotropic hormones.

Other (unlabeled) generally accepted uses: (1) Intranasal dosing helps control abnormal hair growth in women; (2) can be injected below the skin (subcutaneously) to help benign prostatic hyperplasia; (3) may be used before surgery to help decrease size of some tumors (myomas); (4) low-dose use for in vitro fertilization.

How This Drug Works: Stimulates the pituitary gland to release two additional hormones that regulate production of estrogen by the ovaries. With continued use, estrogen levels suppress (by a feedback mechanism) ovary-stimulating hormones—thereby lowering estrogen levels. The implants of endometrium (from the lining of the uterus) that are attached to the pelvic wall are stimulated by the rise and fall of estrogen in menstruation. When this drug suppresses estrogen production, the displaced endometrial tissue (endometriosis) becomes dormant and the premenstrual and menstrual pain no longer happens.

▷ **Widely Used Guidelines That Involve This Medicine (representative sample):** Please look at the section at the very beginning of this profile called "Class." Next, turn to Table 22 and you will find guidelines listed by the class involved!

Available Dosage Forms and Strengths

Nasal solution (10-mL bottle) — 2 mg/mL

▷ **Usual Adult Dosage Ranges:** Endometriosis: Pregnancy MUST be excluded prior to starting therapy. Dosing starts with 400 mcg daily. Spray one dose of 200 mcg into one nostril in the morning and one dose of 200 mcg into the other nostril in the evening, 12 hours apart. Start taking this medicine between days 2 and 4 of the menstrual cycle. If menstruation persists after 2 months of treatment, the dose may be increased to 800 mcg daily: one spray into each nostril (a total of two sprays, 400 mcg) in the morning and again in the evening.

Note: Actual dose and schedule must be determined for each patient individually.

Conditions Requiring Dosing Adjustments

Liver Function: No dosing changes needed.

Kidney Function: Specific guidelines are not available for dosing. Decreases may be needed in kidney compromise.

▷ **Dosing Instructions:** Carefully read and follow the patient instructions provided with this drug. The solution is to be sprayed directly into the nostrils; it is not to be swallowed. Time the start of therapy and daily dosing exactly as directed. A nasal decongestant (spray or drops) should not be used for at least 30 minutes after dosing with the nafarelin spray; earlier use could impair absorption of nafarelin. If you forget a dose: Take the missed dose as soon as you remember it, unless it's nearly time for your next dose—if that is the case, skip the missed dose and take the next dose right on schedule. DO NOT double doses. Talk with your doctor and pharmacist if you find yourself missing doses.

Usual Duration of Use: Regular use for 2 to 3 months usually determines benefits in easing endometriosis symptoms. The standard course of treatment is limited to 6 months. Safety data does not exist for re-treatment and is not advised by the maker.

Typical Treatment Goals and Measurements (Outcomes and Markers)

Endometriosis: The goal most gynecologists use is the resolution of active endometriosis lesions as well as patient relief from pelvic pain, difficulty having intercourse, and painful menstruation (dysmenorrhea). A laboratory test (estradiol levels) can be used (when they go below 30 pg/mL) as a guide to expecting patient response.

Possible Advantages of This Drug

Causes fewer masculinizing effects than danazol. Less tendency than danazol to increase blood cholesterol levels. Unlike danazol, this drug does not cause abnormally low HDL cholesterol levels or abnormally high LDL cholesterol levels. Superb alternative to oophorectomy.

Currently a Drug of Choice

For management of symptoms associated with endometriosis.

▷ This Drug Should Not Be Taken If

- you have had an allergic reaction to it previously.
- you are pregnant or breast-feeding.
- you have abnormal vaginal bleeding of unknown cause.

▷ Inform Your Physician Before Taking This Drug If

- you have used this drug, danazol, or similar drugs previously.
- you are taking any type of estrogen, progesterone, or oral contraceptive.
- you are planning pregnancy in the near future.
- you have a family history of osteoporosis or have low bone mass (osteopenia).
- you use alcohol or tobacco regularly.
- you have a history of low white blood cells.
- you are using anticonvulsants or cortisonelike drugs.
- you are subject to allergic or infectious rhinitis and use nasal decongestants frequently.

Possible Side Effects (natural, expected, and unavoidable drug actions)

Effects due to reduced estrogen production: hot flashes (90%), headaches, emotional lability, insomnia. Masculinizing effects: acne, muscle aches, fluid retention, increased skin oil, weight gain, excessive hair growth—rare.

▷ Possible Adverse Effects (unusual, unexpected, and infrequent reactions)

If any of the following develop, consult your physician promptly for guidance.

Mild Adverse Effects

Allergic reactions: skin rash, hives—rare.
Nasal irritation—frequent.
Vaginal dryness—infrequent to frequent.
Depression—rare.
Hot flashes—when used in men with prostate problems (BPH).

Serious Adverse Effects

Loss of vertebral bone density: at completion of 6 months of treatment, bone density decreases an average of 8.7% and bone mass decreases an average of 4.3%; partial recovery during the post treatment period restores bone density loss to 4.9% and bone mass loss to 3.3% (prudent to talk to your doctor about preventing this).
Lowering of the white blood cell count (leukopenia)—case reports.
Transient prostate enlargement—possible.
Uterine bleeding—case report.

▷ **Possible Effects on Sexual Function:** Decreased libido, vaginal dryness, reduced breast size—infrequent to frequent. Milk production in women who are not pregnant (galactorrhea)—case reports. Uterine bleeding—case reports. Impotence occurred in all men in one study using this drug for prostate problems; hot flashes also occurred in all of them.

Natural Diseases or Disorders That May Be Activated by This Drug
Worsening or increased progression of osteoporosis.

Possible Effects on Laboratory Tests
Blood testosterone level: decreased in men with benign enlargement of prostate gland.
Blood estradiol: decreased.
Blood progesterone: decreased to less than 4 mg/mL.
Alkaline phosphatase: increased.
Serum estrone: decreased.

CAUTION
1. With continual use of this drug, menstruation will stop. If regular menstruation persists, call your doctor. Dose changes may be needed.
2. Use this drug consistently on a regular basis. Missed doses can result in breakthrough bleeding and ovulation.
3. It is advisable to avoid pregnancy during the course of treatment. Use a nonhormonal method of birth control; do not use oral contraceptives. Inform your physician promptly if you think you may be pregnant.
4. If you need to use nasal decongestant sprays or drops, delay their use for at least 30 minutes after the intranasal spray of nafarelin.

Precautions for Use
By Infants and Children: Safety and effectiveness for those less than 18 years of age are not established.
By Those Over 60 Years of Age: If used for prostatism, impotence is a common side effect. Depression and hot flashes were also often reported.

▷ **Advisability of Use During Pregnancy**
Pregnancy Category: X. See Pregnancy Risk Categories at the back of this book.
Animal Studies: Major fetal abnormalities and increased fetal deaths due to this drug have been demonstrated in rat studies.
Human Studies: Adequate studies of pregnant women are not available.
Avoid this drug during entire pregnancy.

Advisability of Use If Breast-Feeding
Presence of this drug in breast milk: Unknown.
Avoid drug or refrain from nursing.

Habit-Forming Potential: None.

Effects of Overdose: No significant effects expected.

Possible Effects of Long-Term Use: Continual use should be limited to 6 months.

Suggested Periodic Examinations While Taking This Drug (at physician's discretion)
Blood cholesterol and triglyceride profiles.
Bone mineral density measurements.

▷ **While Taking This Drug, Observe the Following**
Foods: No restrictions.
Herbal Medicines or Minerals: Black cohosh appears to work by: (1) suppressing luteinizing hormone; (2) binding to estrogen receptors in the pituitary and inhibiting luteinizing hormone release; and (3) binding to estrogen

receptors in the pituitary. Talk to your doctor before starting black cohosh or any other herbal products if you are currently taking nafarelin.

Beverages: No restrictions.

▷ *Alcohol:* No interactions expected.

Tobacco Smoking: No interactions expected. I advise everyone to quit smoking.

▷ *Other Drugs*

The following drugs will ***decrease*** the effects of nafarelin:
- birth control pills (oral contraceptives).
- estrogens.

▷ *Driving, Hazardous Activities:* No restrictions.

Aviation Note: The use of this drug ***is not a disqualification*** for piloting. Consult a designated Aviation Medical Examiner for confirmation.

Exposure to Sun: No restrictions.

Special Storage Instructions: Store in an upright position at room temperature. Protect from light.

Discontinuation: Normal ovarian function (ovulation, menstruation, etc.) is usually restored within 4 to 8 weeks after discontinuation of this drug.

NALTREXONE (nahl TREX ohn)

Introduced: 1995   **Class:** Antialcoholism, opioid antagonist   **Prescription:** USA: Yes   **Controlled Drug:** USA: No; Canada: No   **Available as Generic:** USA: Yes; Canada: Yes

Brand Names: Depade, Trexan, ReVia

Warning: This medication can cause liver damage if taken in excessive doses. If abdominal pain, white stools, or yellowing of the eyes or skin occurs, call your doctor immediately.

BENEFITS versus RISKS

Possible Benefits	*Possible Risks*
CONTROL OF CRAVING FOR ALCOHOL	LIVER DAMAGE IF EXCESSIVE DOSES TAKEN
PART OF AN EFFECTIVE COMBINATION APPROACH TO ALCOHOLISM	
ONCE-DAILY DOSING	

▷ **Principal Uses**

As a Single Drug Product: Uses currently included in FDA-approved labeling: (1) Used as part of a comprehensive program to help alcohol dependence; (2) used to treat narcotic addiction.

Other (unlabeled) generally accepted uses: (1) May help women with a specific type of cessation of menstruation (hypothalamic amenorrhea); (2) helps itching in hemodialysis patients; (3) incidental reports from a detoxification program may yield a use for this drug in smoking cessation.

How This Drug Works: In narcotic addiction, this medicine antagonizes the effects of opioid medicines and blocks the perceived benefit of the drug to the addicted patient. In alcohol addiction, it may interfere with the body's own opioids that are released in response to drinking alcoholic beverages.

If the effect of the body's own opioids (endogenous) is blocked, the craving for alcohol is then reduced.

▷ **Widely Used Guidelines That Involve This Medicine (representative sample):** Please look at the section at the very beginning of this profile called "Class." Next, turn to Table 22 and you will find guidelines listed by the class involved!

Available Dosage Forms and Strengths
Tablets — 50 mg

▷ **Recommended Dosage Ranges** (Actual dose and schedule must be determined for each patient individually.)
Infants and Children: Not indicated.
18 to 60 Years of Age: 50 mg daily. The best results are gained when this medicine is used as part of a comprehensive approach to curbing alcohol use.
Over 60 Years of Age: Same as 18 to 60 years of age.

Conditions Requiring Dosing Adjustments
Liver Function: This drug is extensively metabolized in the liver and is contraindicated in acute hepatitis or liver failure.
Kidney Function: Metabolites of this drug are removed by the kidneys, but specific guidelines for dosing changes are not available.

▷ **Dosing Instructions:** If there is any question of opioid dependence, a Narcan challenge test must be performed. Naltrexone is almost completely absorbed after oral dosing. This medicine may be taken with or without food. If you forget a dose: Take the missed dose as soon as you remember it, unless it's nearly time for your next dose—if that is the case, skip the missed dose and take the next dose right on schedule. Talk with your doctor and pharmacist if you find yourself missing doses.

Usual Duration of Use: Continual use on a regular schedule for 12 weeks is usually necessary to determine this drug's effectiveness in treating alcoholism. This drug should be a part of a comprehensive alcohol treatment program. Long-term use (months to years) requires periodic evaluation of response and dose adjustment. Consult your physician on a regular basis.

Typical Treatment Goals and Measurements (Outcomes and Markers)
Alcohol or Narcotic Abuse: The general goal is to gain a patient defined (subjective) decrease in desire for alcohol or narcotics (opioids). Specific markers may include an alcohol abstinence diary or specific urine or blood tests for narcotics.

Possible Advantages of This Drug
Actually decreases the craving for alcohol versus aversive therapy with antabuse (leads to vomiting).

▷ **This Drug Should Not Be Taken If**
• you had an allergic reaction to any form of it previously.
• you have liver failure or acute hepatitis.
• you are in opioid withdrawal.
• you are physically dependent on narcotics.

▷ **Inform Your Physician Before Taking This Drug If**
• you have a history of viral hepatitis.
• you are planning surgery or a diagnostic procedure requiring anesthesia.
• you are unsure how much to take or how often to take it.
• you take prescription or nonprescription medicines not discussed with your doctor when naltrexone was prescribed.

Possible Side Effects (natural, expected, and unavoidable drug actions)
None.

▷ **Possible Adverse Effects** (unusual, unexpected, and infrequent reactions)
If any of the following develop, consult your physician promptly for guidance.

Mild Adverse Effects
Allergic reaction: rash.
Oily skin, itching, hair loss—case reports.
Nosebleeds—possible.
Joint and muscle pain—infrequent to frequent.
Anorexia, weight loss, fatigue, anxiety, nervousness—case reports to frequent.
Sleep disturbances—infrequent.
Depression—case reports.

Serious Adverse Effects
Allergic reactions: none reported.
Idiosyncratic reactions: none reported.
Liver toxicity (hepatocellular injury)—case reports and reported with large doses.
Muscle damage (rhabdomyolysis)—case report.
Precipitation of acute withdrawal syndrome in patients dependent on narcotics.
Suicidal ideation—case reports.
Abnormal platelet function (idiopathic thrombocytopenic purpura)—case reports.

▷ **Possible Effects on Sexual Function:** Delayed ejaculation—infrequent.

Possible Delayed Adverse Effects: None reported.

▷ **Adverse Effects That May Mimic Natural Diseases or Disorders**
Liver problems may mimic acute hepatitis.

Natural Diseases or Disorders That May Be Activated by This Drug
None.

Possible Effects on Laboratory Tests
Liver function tests: increased.
Gonadotropins (LH, FSH, ACTH, catecholamines, and cortisol): increased.

CAUTION
1. The therapeutic dose and doses that can cause liver damage may be fairly close in some patients. Make certain that you understand how much to take and how often to take it.
2. Self-administration of any narcotic drug may be fatal.
3. If you are taking ongoing narcotic or opioid treatment for pain, this drug could precipitate an acute withdrawal syndrome.

Precautions for Use
By Infants and Children: Safety and effectiveness for use by those under 18 years of age have not been established.
By Those Over 60 Years of Age: None.

▷ **Advisability of Use During Pregnancy**
Pregnancy Category: C. See Pregnancy Risk Categories at the back of this book.
Animal Studies: This drug has been shown to be embryocidal in rats and rabbits at roughly 140 times the typical human dose.
Human Studies: Information from adequate studies of pregnant women is not available.
Ask your doctor for help with this benefit-to-risk decision.

Advisability of Use If Breast-Feeding
    Presence of this drug in breast milk: Unknown.
    Avoid drug or refrain from nursing.

Habit-Forming Potential: None.

Effects of Overdose: Human subjects who received over 800 mg daily for a week showed no adverse effects.

Possible Effects of Long-Term Use: None defined.

Suggested Periodic Examinations While Taking This Drug (at physician's discretion)
    Liver function tests.

▷ **While Taking This Drug, Observe the Following**
    Foods: No restrictions.
    Herbal Medicines or Minerals: Ephedra (no longer on the market for weight loss), guarana, mate, kola, or yohimbe may worsen anxiety associated with abstaining from alcohol. Valerian or kava kava (no longer recommended in Canada because of possible toxic liver effects) may ease anxiety or difficulty falling asleep, but has not been studied with naltrexone. Given the possible effects on the liver of those herbs and naltrexone, this combination is not recommended. Talk to your doctor BEFORE you add any herbal medicine.
    Beverages: No restrictions.
▷   *Alcohol:* Obviously not recommended, as this medication is part of a combination approach to help problem drinkers.
    Tobacco Smoking: No interactions expected. I advise everyone to quit smoking.
    Marijuana Smoking: Should not be attempted.
▷   *Other Drugs*
        Naltrexone *taken concurrently* with
        • narcotic medicines (opioids) may result in a severe reaction.
        • other drugs that are toxic to the liver may result in increased risk of liver toxicity.
        • thioridazine (Mellaril) may result in somnolence and lethargy.
▷   *Driving, Hazardous Activities:* This drug may cause fatigue. Restrict activities as necessary.
    Aviation Note: Alcoholism *is a disqualification* for piloting. Consult a designated Aviation Medical Examiner.
    Exposure to Sun: No restrictions.
    Discontinuation: Do not stop this medicine without the knowledge of your doctor.

NAPROXEN (na PROX en)

Please see the propionic acid (nonsteroidal anti-inflammatory drug) family profile.

NATEGLINIDE (na TAG lyn ide)

Introduced: 2000 **Class:** Antidiabetic, D-phenylalanine derivative
Prescription: USA: Yes **Controlled Drug:** USA: No; Canada: No
Available as Generic: No
Brand Name: Starlix

```
┌─────────────────────────────────────────────────────────────────────┐
│                      BENEFITS versus RISKS                            │
│      Possible Benefits                     Possible Risks             │
│  HELPS REGULATE BLOOD SUGAR      Hypoglycemia (less common than       │
│    in TYPE 2 DIABETES (adjunctive    repaglinide or sulfonylureas)    │
│    to appropriate diet and weight  Possible increased risk of heart   │
│    control)                          (cardiovascular) problems (based │
│  MAY BE COMBINED WITH                on a 1970 UGDP study)            │
│    METFORMIN IF BLOOD SUGAR                                           │
│    CONTROL IS NOT ACCEPTABLE                                          │
│  Absorbed well and cleared quickly                                    │
│    from the blood                                                     │
│  More selective for beta cells in the                                 │
│    pancreas than nateglinide                                          │
└─────────────────────────────────────────────────────────────────────┘
```

▷ **Principal Uses**

 As a Single Drug Product: Uses currently included in FDA-approved labeling: (1) Type 2 diabetes mellitus (adult, maturity-onset) that does not require insulin but can't be adequately controlled by diet alone; (2) combination treatment with metformin in people who do not have an adequate blood sugar response from nateglinide alone.

 Other (unlabeled) generally accepted uses: (1) One small study of combined use with rosiglitazone found very favorable results in controlling blood sugar and A1C.

How This Drug Works: Stimulates secretion of insulin by the pancreas (closes ATP-sensitive potassium channels in beta cells leading to an influx of calcium and increased release of insulin). This mechanism is like the sulfonylureas, but nateglinide works faster.

▷ **Widely Used Guidelines That Involve This Medicine (representative sample):** Please look at the section at the very beginning of this profile called "Class." Next, turn to Table 22 and you will find guidelines listed by the class involved!

Available Dosage Forms and Strengths

 Tablets — 60 mg, 120 mg, 180 mg

▷ **Usual Adult Dosage Ranges:** Dosing is started at 120 mg given three times a day between one and 30 minutes before meals (ten minutes before works well). *People with a hemoglobin A1C (HGB A1C or glycosylated hemoglobin) who are near the treatment goal can be started on 60 mg taken before meals as above.* If goals are not met with the 60 mg dose, it can be increased to 120 mg as above. If goals are still not met, this medicine can be combined with metformin.

 Note: Actual dose and schedule must be determined for each patient individually.

Conditions Requiring Dosing Adjustments

 Liver Function: Current thinking is that dosing changes are not needed in mild liver compromise. Studies are limited in more severe compromise (moderate to severe), but generally, dosing changes are not thought to be needed for mild to moderate liver compromised people. More frequent blood sugar checks are prudent in this patient population until the full effects are individually known.

 Kidney Function: Dosing changes are not required in mild to severe kidney compromise.

▷ **Dosing Instructions:** It is important to take this medicine before meals. You can take it up to 30 minutes before a meal, but ten appears to be best. If you skip a meal, then skip the dose of nateglinide. This medicine rarely causes low blood sugar (hypoglycemia), and you should talk to your doctor about what he wants you to do if symptoms (unexplained weakness, tiredness, nervousness, sweating, trouble concentrating, and headache) occur. At present there is no sustained-release form, so the immediate-release tablet may be crushed. If you forget a dose: Skip the missed dose and take the next dose right on schedule. DO NOT double doses. Talk with your doctor if you find yourself missing doses. Staying on schedule helps keep tight blood sugar control and can help you avoid diabetic complications.

Usual Duration of Use: This medicine goes to work quickly (about 15 minutes). Use on a regular schedule for 1 to 2 weeks determines effectiveness in controlling diabetes. Checking blood sugar by finger stick is the best way to make sure you are getting the best results from this medicine. Some patients will have control of their blood sugar for a while and then the medicine will not continue to work and will need to be changed. Diabetes is now recognized as a risk factor for cardiovascular disease. Take control of your blood sugar and help your heart.

Typical Treatment Goals and Measurements (Outcomes and Markers)
Blood Sugar: The general goal for blood sugar is to return it to the usual "normal" range (generally 80–120 mg/dL), while avoiding risks of excessively low blood sugar. One study (UKPDS) used a fasting plasma sugar (glucose) of less than 108 mg/dL. Tight control helps avoid diabetic complications.
Fructosamine and glycosylated hemoglobin: Fructosamine levels (a measure of the past two to three weeks of blood sugar control) should be less than or equal to 310 micromoles per liter. Glycosylated hemoglobin or hemoglobin A1C (a measure of the past 2–3 months of blood sugar control) should be less than or equal to 7.0%. Some clinicians advocate less than or equal to 6.5% as a target. This approach carries an increased risk of too low a blood sugar, but may give other benefits.

Possible Advantages of This Drug
The risk of excessively low blood sugar (hypoglycemia) is expected to be less than with other agents. Goes to work more quickly than repaglinide. Safety and results (efficacy) in patients more than 65 years old is the same as in younger patients. A study of combined use with rosiglitasone found improvement in insulin release and lower increases in sugar after meals (postprandial).

▷ **This Drug Should Not Be Taken If**
- you have had an allergic reaction to it previously.
- you have diabetic ketoacidosis.
- you are pregnant.
- you have the kind of diabetes that requires insulin.

▷ **Inform Your Physician Before Taking This Drug If**
- your blood sugar begins to drift up. This may be a sign of failure and require a change in medicine.
- you do not know how to recognize or treat hypoglycemia (see Glossary).
- you have a history of congestive heart failure, cirrhosis of the liver, or hypothyroidism.
- you have an infection or a fever—insulin may be required.

Possible Side Effects (natural, expected, and unavoidable drug actions)

If drug dose is excessive or food intake is delayed or inadequate, abnormally low blood sugar (hypoglycemia) will occur. Mild hypoglycemia happened in 2–3% of people using this medicine in reported studies.

▷ **Possible Adverse Effects** (unusual, unexpected, and infrequent reactions)

If any of the following develop, consult your physician promptly for guidance.

Mild Adverse Effects

Allergic reactions: skin rash, hives, itching.

Headache, drowsiness, dizziness, fatigue—possible.

Nausea, vomiting, diarrhea, heartburn—infrequent.

Serious Adverse Effects

Allergic reactions: not defined.

Idiosyncratic reactions: not reported.

Hypoglycemia—possible but less than sulfonylureas such as glyburide.

Cardiovascular mortality (based on an old study of a different medicine)—possible increased risk.

▷ **Possible Effects on Sexual Function:** None reported.

▷ **Adverse Effects That May Mimic Natural Diseases or Disorders**

Not defined.

Possible Effects on Laboratory Tests

Blood glucose levels: decreased.

Glycosylated hemoglobin (A1C) or protein: trending toward normal.

CAUTION

1. This drug is only part of diabetes management. Much of the damage from diabetes can be delayed or avoided if you keep your blood sugar in the normal range. Ask your doctor about a proper diet and regular exercise.
2. Over time, this drug, like other oral medicines for type 2 diabetes may not work. Periodic follow-up examinations are necessary.
3. If you develop an infection, insulin may be required to control your blood sugar.

Precautions for Use

By Infants and Children: Safety and efficacy not defined.

By Those Over 65 Years of Age: No differences in pharmacokinetics in this age group in clinical trials. People in this population may be more sensitive to this medicine, and careful patient follow-up and more frequent blood sugar checks are prudent when nateglinide is started.

▷ **Advisability of Use During Pregnancy**

Pregnancy Category: C. See Pregnancy Risk Categories at the back of this book.

Animal Studies: No birth defects reported in rats and rabbits.

Human Studies: Adequate studies of pregnant women are not available.

Uncontrolled blood sugar levels during pregnancy are associated with a higher incidence of birth defects, so many experts recommend insulin (instead of an oral agent) to control diabetes during the entire pregnancy.

Advisability of Use If Breast-Feeding

Presence of this drug in breast milk: Unknown.

Avoid drug or refrain from nursing.

Habit-Forming Potential: None.

Effects of Overdose: Symptoms of mild to severe hypoglycemia: headache, light-headedness, faintness, nervousness, confusion, tremor, sweating, heart palpitation, weakness, hunger, nausea, vomiting, stupor progressing to coma.

Possible Effects of Long-Term Use: More normal hemoglobin A1C.

Suggested Periodic Examinations While Taking This Drug (at physician's discretion)

Periodic evaluation of heart and circulatory system. Check of lipid panel (because diabetes is a significant risk factor for heart disease).

Self-assessment of blood sugar is prudent as well as periodic glycosylated hemoglobin tests and/or fructosamine tests.

▷ **While Taking This Drug, Observe the Following**

Foods: Follow your diabetic diet conscientiously. Taking a diabetes education course is very smart and can teach you about portion control, what to do on sick days and other important concepts. Blood sugar control can help avoid or delay diabetes problems. Vitamin C in high dose may worsen blood sugar control. Do not omit snack foods in mid-afternoon or at bedtime if they help prevent hypoglycemia. Rice bran has been checked in a small (57 subject) study of type 1 and type 2 diabetics. The benefit was a 30% lowering of sugar. This might be a new complementary care option.

Herbal Medicines or Minerals: Using chromium may change the way your body is able to use sugar. Some health food stores advocate vanadium as mimicking the actions of insulin, but possible toxicity and need for rigorous studies presently preclude recommending it. DHEA may change sensitivity to insulin or insulin resistance. Aloe, bitter melon, eucalyptus, fenugreek, ginger, garlic, ginseng, glucomannan, guar gum, hawthorn, licorice, nettle, and yohimbe may change blood sugar. Surprisingly, boiled stems of the Optuntia streptacantha prickly pear cactus appears to be able to lower blood sugar. Ongoing effects and effects on A1C are not known. Red sage is used for blood sugar effects, but is unproven. Psyllium increases risk of excessively low blood sugar. Since so many of these products may require adjustment of insulin dosing, talk to your doctor BEFORE combining any of these herbal medicines with this medicine. Echinacea purpura (injectable) and blonde psyllium seed or husk should NOT be taken by people living with diabetes.

Beverages: As directed in the diabetic diet. May be taken with milk.

▷ *Alcohol:* Use with extreme caution—alcohol can exaggerate this drug's hypoglycemic effect.

Tobacco Smoking: No interactions expected. I advise everyone to quit smoking.

▷ *Other Drugs*

The following drugs may ***increase*** the effects of nateglinide:

- cimetidine (Tagamet).
- erythromycins (see Drug Classes).
- itraconazole (Sporanox).
- ketoconazole (Nizoral).
- medicines that inhibit or compete for CYP3A4 or 2C9 (liver enzymes) may increase nateglinide because it is removed by that enzyme.
- nelfinavir (Viracept) and perhaps other protease inhibitors (see Drug Classes)—may increase blood levels.
- sildenafil (Viagra), since both drugs are removed by CYP3A4.
- Any medicine that interferes with cytochrome CYP3A4 or 2C9—will potentially increase nateglinide blood levels; in some cases, I expect that nateglinide dosing will need to be adjusted.

The following drugs may ***decrease*** the effects of nateglinide:

- carbamazepine (Tegretol), since it induces CYP3A4, which removes nateglinide from the body.
- corticosteroids (see Drug Classes).

- rifabutin (Mycobutin).
- rifampin (Rifadin, Rimactane).

▷ *Driving, Hazardous Activities:* This drug may cause dizziness, drowsiness, impaired vision, and impaired hearing. Restrict activities as necessary.

Aviation Note: Diabetes *is a disqualification* for piloting. Consult a designated Aviation Medical Examiner.

Exposure to Sun: No restrictions.

Discontinuation: It is advisable not to interrupt or stop this drug without consulting your physician.

NEDOCROMIL (na DOK ra mil)

Introduced: 1992   **Class:** Antiasthmatic, preventive   **Prescription:**
USA: Yes   **Controlled Drug:** USA: No; Canada: No   **Available as**
Generic: USA: No; Canada: No

Brand Names: Alocril, Tilade, Tilade Nebulizer Solution

BENEFITS versus RISKS	
Possible Benefits	*Possible Risks*
EFFECTIVE PREVENTION OF RECURRENT ASTHMA	Acute bronchospasm—rare
Prevention of exercise-induced asthma	Taste disorder

▷ **Principal Uses**

As a Single Drug Product: Uses currently included in FDA-approved labeling: (1) Ongoing therapy of mild to moderate asthma; (2) steroid-sparing effect that may allow reduction or elimination of oral steroids; (3) helps manage asthmatic bronchitis; (4) eases allergic conjunctivitis.

Other (unlabeled) generally accepted uses: (1) May have a role in helping ease allergic rhinitis.

How This Drug Works: Inhibits release of inflammatory chemical mediators such as histamine, prostaglandins and leukotrienes that constrict the bronchi and cause inflammation seen in acute asthma.

Author's Note: Information in this profile has been shortened to make room for more widely used medicines.

NEFAZODONE (na FAZ oh dohn)

Introduced: 1994   **Class:** Antidepressant   **Prescription:** USA:
Yes   **Controlled Drug:** USA: No; Canada: No   **Available as Generic:**
USA: No; Canada: No

Brand Names: ✤Lin-Nefazodone, Serzone, ✤Serzone 5HT2

Author's Note: Revisions have been made to the label for this medicine noting a thorough benefit-to-risk analysis when deciding between this medicine and other antidepressants.

NEOSTIGMINE (nee oh STIG meen)

Introduced: 1931   **Class:** Antimyasthenic   **Prescription:** USA:
Yes   **Controlled Drug:**   USA: No; Canada: No   **Available as Generic:**
USA: Yes; Canada: Yes

Brand Names: ✚PMS-Neostigmine, Prostigmin

BENEFITS versus RISKS

Possible Benefits	*Possible Risks*
MODERATELY EFFECTIVE TREATMENT OF OCULAR AND MILD FORMS OF MYASTHENIA GRAVIS (symptomatic relief of muscle weakness) Eases postoperative bowel slowing or block (paralytic ileus)	Cholinergic crisis (overdose): excessive salivation, nausea, vomiting, stomach cramps, diarrhea, shortness of breath (asthmalike wheezing), weakness.

**Author's Note: Information in this profile has been shortened to make
room for more widely used medicines.**

NESIRITIDE (Neh SEAR ih tyde)

Introduced: 2001   **Class:** Cardiac hormone   **Prescription:** USA:
Yes   **Controlled Drug:**   USA: No; Canada: No   **Available as Generic:**
No

Brand Name: Natrecor (NAH trah core)

BENEFITS versus RISKS

Possible Benefits	*Possible Risks*
EFFECTIVE TREATMENT IN CONGESTIVE HEART FAILURE EFFECTIVE PREVENTION AND TREATMENT OF CERTAIN HEART RHYTHM DISORDERS	Lowering of blood pressure (hypotension) Mild increase in heart rate

---

▷ **Principal Uses**

As a Single Drug Product: Uses in current FDA-approved labeling: (1) Treats
congestive heart failure.

Other (unlabeled) generally accepted uses: (1) None at present.

How This Drug Works: Binds to specific receptors (guanylate cyclase linked
natriuretic peptide A/B) which works to increase specific beneficial chemicals such as guanosine 3, 5-cyclic monophosphate (cGMP). The overall
effect is to cause both coronary conductance and resistance vessels to
dilate. This leads to an increase in blood flow and uptake of oxygen in the
heart.

▷ **Widely Used Guidelines That Involve This Medicine (representative sample):** Please look at the section at the very beginning of this profile called
"Class." Next, turn to Table 22 and you will find guidelines listed by the
class involved!

Available Dosage Forms and Strengths
Injection — 1.5 mg/vial
Author's Note: Information in this profile will be broadened as more
information and clinical studies become available. A study of this
medicine called FUSION (Management of Patients with CHF After
Hospitalization with Follow Up Serial Infusions Of Natrecor should
provide an excellent opportunity to further define the use of this
medicine.

NEURAMIDASE INHIBITOR FAMILY (Nur AM ih dayce)

Oseltamivir   (Oss uhl TAM ih veer)   **Zanamivir**   (Zah NAM ih veer)
Introduced: 1999   **Class:**   Antiviral, anti-influenza   **Prescription:**
USA: Yes   **Controlled Drug:**   USA: No; Canada: No   **Available as**
Generic: USA: No; Canada: No
Brand Names: Oseltamivir: Tamiflu, Zanamivir: Relenza

BENEFITS versus RISKS	
Possible Benefits	*Possible Risks*
DECREASED COMPLICATIONS FROM TYPE A OR B FLU (INFLUENZA) DECREASED FLU SEVERITY	Triggering of bronchospasm by zanamivir (may be more likely in those with underlying airway diseases)

▷ **Principal Uses**
As a Single Drug Product: Uses currently included in FDA-approved labeling:
(1) Treatment or prevention of type A or B influenza in people 13 or older
(for oseltamivir) or people 7 or older (for zanamivir).
Other (unlabeled) generally accepted uses: (1) oseltamivir reduced complications (secondary) from the flu in one study.

How These Drugs Work: These medicines preferentially inhibit a critical chemical called neuramidase in type A or B flu (influenza) viruses. When neuramidase is blocked, newly formed virus is not released from infected cells
(because sialic acid cleavage is inhibited from cell surface glycoconju-
gates) and the flu virus is kept from spreading across the respiratory tract
(mucous lining). Oseltamivir is the ester prodrug of GS 4071.

▷ **Widely Used Guidelines That Involve This Medicine (representative sample):** Please look at the section at the very beginning of this profile called
"Class." Next, turn to Table 22 and you will find guidelines listed by the
class involved!

Available Dosage Forms and Strengths
Oseltamivir
Capsule — 75 mg
Solution — see dosing in mg per mL to get the total dose needed
Suspension — see dosing in mg per mL to get the total dose needed (Canada)
Zanamivir
Dry powder inhaler — 5 mg per inhalation

▷ **Usual Adult Dosage Ranges:**
Oseltamivir: Treatment: Adults: 75 mg is taken twice a day (BID) for 5 days.
Best if started within 24 hours of flu symptoms (up to 48 hours still

helps/confers benefits). For the solution or suspension form: children as young as one year old based on weight.

Prevention *(Prophylaxis):* FDA-approved for patients 13 or older (following close contact with an infected person) is 75 mg once daily for at least seven days. During a community outbreak, 75 mg once a day for up to six weeks has been used.

Zanamivir: Treatment of adults or children more than 7 years old: Two doses are used on the first day that this medicine is started. Take the first dose once you get the medicine, then wait at least two hours and inhale the second dose. After this, take two inhalations (5 mg each, total 10 mg) twice a day (12 hours apart) for a total of 5 days. Better started within 30 hours after symptoms start and in patients who have a fever (are febrile).

Note: Actual dose and schedule must be determined for each patient individually.

Conditions Requiring Dosing Adjustments

Liver Function: No dosing changes currently thought to be needed.

Kidney Function: Oseltamivir: Must be carefully adjusted in people with kidney problems. Those with creatinine clearances of less than 30 mL/min should receive 75 mg daily for five days. Those with clearances less than 10 mL/min have not been studied and can not be recommended.

Zanamivir: This medicine is absorbed into the body (systemically) to a limited extent—therefore even though it is primarily removed by the kidneys, dosing changes probably are not needed.

▷ **Dosing Instructions:** May be taken with or following meals. Can open the oseltamivir capsule to take it. The oseltamivir suspension should be shaken well before dosing. Both suspension and solution should be given using the dosing syringe to measure the correct dose. Zanamivir is used with a device called a Diskhaler. Make sure you understand how to use this product in order to get the medicine into your lungs. If your symptoms worsen or do not improve, call your doctor. If you forget a dose: Take or use the missed dose as soon as you remember it, unless it's nearly time for your next dose—if that is the case, skip the missed dose and take the next dose right on schedule. DO NOT double doses. Talk with your doctor and pharmacist if you find yourself missing doses.

Usual Duration of Use: Best results come from starting oseltamivir or zanamivir within a day of flu symptoms, but benefits are gained if started within 48 hours. Use as prescribed for five days is REQUIRED to get results. During influenza epidemics (for example, if flu vaccine is NOT available), oseltamivir was given for 6 weeks in one study.

Typical Treatment Goals and Measurements (Outcomes and Markers)

Influenza: The general goal is to ease the severity of the flu (lessening of muscle aches, headache, vomiting, sore throat, fever, and others). Prophylactic use of oseltamivir or zanamivir (investigational) seeks to avoid or prevent a "full blown" case of the flu if possible. **If you would like a copy of the ACIP (flu shot and other) recommendations, call 1-888-232-3228.**

▷ **These Drugs Should Not Be Taken If**
  • you have had an allergic reaction to them previously.

▷ **Inform Your Physician Before Taking This Drug If**
  • you have a history of kidney impairment (oseltamivir).
  • you have high-risk medical conditions (zanamivir).

- you have a compromised immune system.
- you have severe or decompensated ongoing and obstructive lung disease (COPD) or asthma (zanamivir).
- you are pregnant (oseltamivir and zanamivir).

Possible Side Effects (natural, expected, and unavoidable drug actions)
Not defined.

▷ **Possible Adverse Effects** (unusual, unexpected, and infrequent reactions)
If any of the following develop, consult your physician promptly for guidance.

Mild Adverse Effects
Allergic reaction: Not defined.
Headache, nervousness, irritability, inability to concentrate, insomnia—rare to infrequent (oseltamivir).
Unsteadiness, dizziness—infrequent (oseltamivir).
Loss of appetite, nausea, vomiting—infrequent to frequent (oseltamivir).

Serious Adverse Effects
Allergic reaction—toxic epidermal necrolysis (questionable causality—oseltamivir).
Arrhythmia—causality not defined (oseltamivir).
Aggravation of existing diabetes—case reports—causality not defined (oseltamivir).
Bronchospasm/respiratory distress—reported for zanamivir and in people with underlying COPD or asthma.

▷ **Possible Effects on Sexual Function:** None reported.

Adverse Effects That May Mimic Natural Diseases or Disorders
Not defined.

Natural Diseases or Disorders That May Be Activated by These Drugs
Possible aggravation of diabetes and change in heart rhythm for oseltamivir, but of questionable causation. Underlying respiratory disease such as COPD or asthma may be associated with an increased risk of bronchospasm or decline in lung function (zanamivir).

Possible Effects on Laboratory Tests
Not defined.

CAUTION
1. These medicines may be very helpful for high-risk patients who are unable to prevent the flu with a shot and need to decrease the amount of time that they have the flu and also to decrease adverse outcomes from the flu.
2. Zanamivir may not work in Chronic Obstructive Pulmonary Disease (COPD) and can pose a safety risk in asthmatics.

Precautions for Use
By Infants and Children: Safety and effectiveness for those under 13 (oseltamivir) for prophylaxis have not been established. Prophylactic dosing: for those 13 or older is 75 mg daily for 7 days. Flu treatment using oseltamivir for children one year and older (must be started within 48 hours): based on body weight. For example—Less than 15 kg: 30 mg, twice daily for seven days. For influenza treatment using zanamavir: Dosing for those under 7 (zanamivir) not established. For those 7 or over, see adult dosing above. For prevention (prophylaxis): zanamavir is not FDA-approved.
By Those Over 60 Years of Age: Special considerations not defined at present.

▷ **Advisability of Use During Pregnancy**

Pregnancy Category: C for both medicines. See Pregnancy Risk Categories at the back of this book.

Human Studies: Adequate studies of pregnant women (both drugs) are not available. Ask your doctor for help.

Advisability of Use If Breast-Feeding

Presence of this drug in breast milk: Yes in animals for oseltamivir; unknown for zanamivir.

Talk to your doctor about this benefit-to-risk decision.

Habit-Forming Potential: None.

Effects of Overdose: Single doses of roughly 1,000 mg of oseltamivir have resulted in vomiting. No data for zanamivir. Supportive care and contact of a poison control center are indicated for both medicines.

Possible Effects of Long-Term Use: Not defined.

Suggested Periodic Examinations While Taking This Drug (at physician's discretion)

Rapid influenza test.

▷ **While Taking This Drug, Observe the Following**

Foods: No restrictions.

Herbal Medicines or Minerals: Echinacea: Some patients use echinacea to attempt to boost their immune systems. Unfortunately, use of echinacea is not recommended in people with damaged immune systems. This herb may also actually weaken any immune system if it is used too often or for too long a time.

Beverages: No restrictions. May be taken with milk.

▷ *Alcohol:* No interactions expected.

Tobacco Smoking: No interactions expected, but smoking may further irritate airways. I advise everyone to quit smoking.

Marijuana Smoking: Added dizziness (oseltamivir).

▷ *Other Drugs*

Oseltamivir *taken concurrently* with

• Probenecid (various) may increase blood levels of oseltamivir, but adverse effects are not defined.

Zanamivir *taken concurrently* with

• other inhaled medicines has NOT been studied.

▷ *Driving, Hazardous Activities:* Oseltamivir may cause dizziness. Avoid hazardous activities until the extent of this effect is known.

Aviation Note: The use of this drug *may be a disqualification* for piloting. Consult a designated Aviation Medical Examiner.

Exposure to Sun: No restrictions.

NIACIN (NI a sin)

Other Names: Nicotinic acid, vitamin B3

Introduced: 1937   **Class:**   Anticholesterol, vasodilator   **Prescription:** USA: tablets and liquid: No; capsules: Yes   **Controlled Drug:**   USA: No; Canada: No   **Available as Generic:**   USA: Yes; Canada: Yes

Brand Names: ✤Antivert [CD], Endur-Acin, Niac, Niacels, Niacin SR, Niacin TR, Niacor, Niacor-B, Nia-Bid, Niaplus, Niaspan, Nicobid, Nico-400, Nicolar,

Nicotinex, ✤Novoniacin, SK-Niacin, Slo-Niacin, Span-Niacin-150, Tega-Span, Tri-B3

Author's Note: Because of the ADVOCATE study and other data, the combination product Advicor (extended-release niacin/lovastatin has replaced the niacin profile.

NICARDIPINE (ni KAR de peen)

Introduced: 1984   Class: Antianginal, antihypertensive, calcium channel blocker   Prescription: USA: Yes   Controlled Drug: USA: No; Canada: No   Available as Generic: USA: Yes

Brand Names: Cardene, Cardene SR

Controversies in Medicine: Medicines in this class have had many conflicting reports. The FDA has held hearings on the calcium channel blocker (CCB) class. Research at New York University found that nifedipine (a member of the same class) is a cause of reversible male infertility. CCBs are currently second-line agents for high blood pressure according to the JNC VII (see Glossary).

Author's Note: Information in this profile has been truncated in order to make room for more widely used medicines.

NICOTINE (NIK oh teen)

Introduced: 1992, 1996, 1997   Class: Smoking cessation adjunct, nicotine replacement therapy   Prescription: USA: Both Nicorettes (2 mg and 4 mg) are now available without a prescription for those over 18 years old. Nicotine patches are FDA-approved for nonprescription use. The nicotine inhaler and nasal spray are only available with a prescription.   Controlled Drug: USA: No; Canada: No   Available as Generic: USA: Yes; Canada: Yes

Brand Names: Habitrol, Clear Nicoderm CQ, ✤Nicoderm, Nicorette, Nicorette DS, Nicotine Transdermal System, Nicotrol, Nicotrol Inhaler, Nicotrol NS, Prostep, Prostep Transdermal System

Author's Note: A medicine in clinical trials called rimonabant (see the Leading Edge section of this book) works in different ways to help smokers quit smoking.

BENEFITS versus RISKS	
Possible Benefits	*Possible Risks*
EFFECTIVE REDUCTION OF NICOTINE CRAVING AND WITHDRAWAL EFFECTS WHEN USED ADJUNCTIVELY IN SMOKING-CESSATION TREATMENT PROGRAMS	Aggravation of existing angina, heart rhythm disorders, hypertension, insulin-dependent diabetes, peptic ulcer, and vascular diseases Increased risk of abortion (if used during pregnancy)

▷ Principal Uses
    As a Single Drug Product: Uses currently included in FDA-approved labeling: Nicotine chewing gum, nicotine transdermal systems, inhaler, and nasal spray are used adjunctively in behavior modification programs to help cigarette smokers who wish to stop smoking.

Author's Note: The American Lung Association has an excellent resource called the "Quit Smoking Action Plan." If you are planning to stop smoking (and I hope that you are), call them at 1-800-LUNG-USA (1-800-586-4872) or find them at the Web site listed in Table 17 at the back of this book. The American Heart Association guidelines for primary and secondary prevention of cardiovascular disease once again tell people that smoking is a risk factor for heart attacks and that you should immediately STOP. Visit *www.americanheart.org* for more information.

Other (unlabeled) generally accepted uses: (1) Gum and nasal spray have been used to increase nicotine levels in the blood and help ease sudden cravings; (2) a study using nicotine patches along with haloperidol (see drug profile) lead to better overall results in children with Tourette's syndrome compared to haloperidol alone (Yale Global Tic Severity Scale-YGTSS).

How This Drug Works: By providing an alternate source of nicotine (for nicotine-dependent smokers), the appropriate use of these drug products can reduce nicotine craving and lessen smoking withdrawal effects, such as irritability, nervousness, headache, fatigue, sleep disturbances, and drowsiness.

▷ **Widely Used Guidelines That Involve This Medicine (representative sample):** Please look at the section at the very beginning of this profile called "Class." Next, turn to Table 22 and you will find guidelines listed by the class involved!

Available Dosage Forms and Strengths
Inhaler (per cartridge) — 10 mg
Nasal spray (10-mL bottle) — 10 mg/mL
Nicotine chewing gum tablets — 2 mg (nonprescription)
Nicorette (U.S., Canada) — 2 mg
Nicorette (Canada) — 4 mg
Nicorette DS (U.S., Canada) — 4 mg
Transdermal systems:
16-hour systems, U.S. only — 5 mg, 10 mg, 15 mg
24-hour systems — 7 mg (U.S., Canada), 11 mg (U.S.), 14 mg (U.S., Canada), 21 mg (U.S., Canada), 22 mg (U.S.)

How to Store
Store nicotine gum at room temperature and protect from light. Store nicotine patches at room temperature and be especially careful to avoid exposing the patches to temperatures greater than 86 degrees F. (30 degrees C.). Do not store unpouched. Once opened, patches should be used promptly because they may lose their strength.

▷ **Recommended Dosage Ranges** (Actual dose and schedule must be determined for each patient individually.)
Infants and Children: Avoid use completely in children. Avoid accidental exposure to patches.
18 to 60 Years of Age: For chewing gum tablets: Initially one piece every hour while awake (10 to 12 pieces daily); supplement with one additional piece if and when needed to control urge to smoke. Total daily dose should not exceed 30 pieces (60 mg).
For inhaler form: Dosing is divided into two parts (phases). At first (weeks one to 12), 6–16 cartridges a day. Dosing is individualized to control smoking

urges, excess nicotine, or withdrawal. During the second phase (weeks 13–24), a quit date is set, patients are told to use the inhaler less often, and the dose is gradually decreased. Maximum daily dose is 16 cartridges. If a particular patient is not able to quit smoking after 4 weeks, treatment should be stopped, and a "break" (therapeutic holiday) given before another attempt to stop smoking is made.

For nasal spray: Two sprays, one in each nostril. Starting dose is usually two to four sprays each hour. Dosing follows a 14-week pattern: In the weeks one to eight, one or two doses are used per hour and at least 8 doses daily. When weeks 9–14 are reached: dosing is gradually reduced (as in second phase of the inhaler form protocol). Maximum is 5 doses per hour (5 mg) and 40 doses per day (40 mg or 80 sprays).

For transdermal systems: Dose depends upon patient characteristics and product used:

For those weighing 100 lb. or more, smoking 10 or more cigarettes daily, and without cardiovascular disease: The 16-hour system (Nicotrol) is started with one 15-mg patch applied for 16 hours daily for 6 weeks. The patch is taken off at bedtime. The 24-hour system (Nicoderm CQ) is started with one 21-mg patch applied daily for weeks one to 6. For those who have abstained from smoking, reduce dose to one 14-mg patch daily for the next 2 weeks and then to one 7-mg patch daily for weeks 9–10.

For those weighing less than 100 lb. smoking less than 10 cigarettes daily, or with cardiovascular disease: The 24-hour system (Habitrol) is started with one 14-mg patch applied daily for 1 to 6 weeks. For those who have abstained from smoking, reduce dose to one 7-mg patch daily for the next 2 weeks.

Over 60 Years of Age: Same as 12 to 60 years of age in those without diseases that pose as risk factors (such as cardiovascular problems—see cautions).

Conditions Requiring Dosing Adjustments

Liver Function: Lower starting doses are prudent in liver disease.

Kidney Function: Doses are decreased in severe kidney compromise.

Cardiovascular Disease: See above.

▷ **Dosing Instructions:** Carefully follow the manufacturer's directions provided with each product.

For Chewing Gum: Limit use to one piece of gum at a time. While it is called gum, it is much harder than typical chewing gum to chew. Be careful of any dental work that you should not put much pressure on. Chew each piece slowly and intermittently for 30 minutes. A tingling of your gum tissue or peppery taste means the nicotine is being released. Try to gradually reduce the number of pieces chewed each day by using it only when there is an urge to smoke. When trying to quit smoking, always have the gum available.

For Transdermal Systems: Apply a new patch at the same time each day. Do not alter the patch in any way. Apply the patch to the upper arm or body where the skin is clean, dry, and free of hair, oil, scars, and irritation of any kind; alternate sites of application. Press the patch firmly in place for 10 seconds; ensure good contact throughout. Wash your hands when you have finished applying the patch. Replace patches that are dislodged by showering, bathing, or swimming.

For Spray: DO NOT swallow, inhale, or sniff when spraying the spray. The nasal route may best mimic the effect of using a cigarette to deliver nicotine.

For the Inhaler: Follow the patient package insert exactly. Make sure you understand how to use this product.

For All: If you can't quit by the fourth week, treatment should be stopped. It's best to have a therapeutic holiday before trying to quit again.

If you Forget a Dose: Take the missed dose as soon as you remember it, unless it's nearly time for your next dose—if that is the case, skip the missed dose and take the next dose right on schedule. DO NOT double doses. Talk with your doctor if you find yourself missing doses.

Usual Duration of Use: Use on a regular schedule as described above determines effectiveness in achieving lasting cessation of smoking. Nicotine chewing gum should not be used for more than 6 months; transdermal systems, nasal spray, and inhaler form are used according to the guidelines (protocols). It's smart to involve your family and friends to help in this difficult process. Use of the prescription forms requires periodic physician evaluation of response and dose adjustment. It's smart to involve your doctor in the use and selection for the nonprescription forms as well.

Typical Treatment Goals and Measurements (Outcomes and Markers)

Smoking Cessation: The goal is to ease or eliminate signs or symptoms of tobacco withdrawal, encouraging patients to stop smoking. Replacing the nicotine that smokers previously received from tobacco products avoids the life-threatening by-products of tobacco smoke while replacing the chemical that a smoker has become addicted to. Once the replacement has occurred, the patch, nasal inhalation, or inhaled nicotine dose can be gradually decreased, and then replacement stopped altogether.

Author's Note: There are NO DATA to show that smoking is good for you. Please make every effort to stop. I firmly believe that my father would be alive today if he had been able to stop smoking. A study in Iceland (Iceland has an abundance of genetic and family data) found that combining two methods of nicotine replacement (such as a patch and the spray) worked better than using a single method. The American Lung Association has a Quit Smoking Action Plan that can be very helpful. Find them on the web at *www.lungusa.org.* **Once again—- please involve your friends, family, pharmacist, and doctor in this critical effort to quit. Be persistent—you can do it!**

Possible Advantages of These Drugs

Provides control and flexibility of gradual nicotine withdrawal for use in supervised smoking-cessation programs. Avoids the cancer-causing components, "excipients," of cigarette smoke.

Currently a "Drug of Choice"

For people who are motivated to stop smoking. Since many forms are now available without a prescription, be sure to talk with your doctor or pharmacist about how to best use these medicines. Many pharmacists also offer programs to help you quit.

▷ **This Drug Should Not Be Taken If**

- you had an allergic reaction to any form of it previously or to any of the ingredients in the dosage form (read the label carefully).
- you have severe or uncontrolled or a pattern of worsening angina (physician's discretion)
- you keep smoking or using other tobacco products (yes, chewing tobacco or tobacco pouches count—in general if it is a product that has nicotine— it should be stopped).
- you have uncontrolled, life-threatening heart rhythm disorders.
- you have had a recent heart attack.

▷ **Inform Your Physician Before Taking This Drug If**
- you have any form of angina (coronary heart disease).
- you have had a heart attack at any time.
- you are subject to heart rhythm disorders.
- you have insulin-dependent diabetes.
- you have hypertension (high blood pressure).
- you have hyperthyroidism (overactive thyroid function).
- you have a pheochromocytoma (adrenaline-producing tumor).
- you have a history of esophagitis or peptic ulcer disease.
- you have a history of Buerger's disease or Raynaud's phenomenon.
- you currently have any dental problems or skin disorders.
- you have a history of kidney or liver disease.
- you have an increase in cardiovascular effects while you are taking this medicine.
- you have already taken a 3-month course of the patch.
- you use birth control pills (oral contraceptives).
- you think you are pregnant or plan to become pregnant.
- you are unsure how much to take or how often to take this medicine.

Possible Side Effects (natural, expected, and unavoidable drug actions)
Increased blood pressure.
For chewing gum: mouth or throat irritation; injury to teeth or dental repairs.
For transdermal systems: redness, itching, or burning at site of application (mild and transient).
For nasal spray: runny nose, nasal irritation.
For inhaler: coughing and nose irritation—frequent.

▷ **Possible Adverse Effects** (unusual, unexpected, and infrequent reactions)
If any of the following develop, consult your physician promptly for guidance.
Mild Adverse Effects
Allergic reactions: skin rash, hives, itching, local or generalized swellings.
Headache, light-headedness, dizziness, drowsiness, irritability, nervousness, insomnia, joint pain, muscle aches, abnormal dreams—possible to infrequent and some may be dose-related.
Rapid heartbeat, palpitation, increased sweating—infrequent to frequent, dose-related.
Increased or decreased appetite, nausea, dry mouth, indigestion, constipation, or diarrhea—infrequent.
Serious Adverse Effects
Irregular heart rhythms, chest pain (angina), edema—infrequent.
Stroke—case report.
Depression—case report.
Worsening of myasthenia gravis—case report.
Heart attack—related in time, but of inconclusive cause.
See Effects of Overdose below.

▷ **Possible Effects on Sexual Function:** There are some data questioning an effect on sperm (diminished penetration), but a distinct demonstration of an effect is lacking.

Natural Diseases or Disorders That May Be Activated by This Drug
Latent angina, atrial fibrillation, hypertension, peptic ulcer disease, temporomandibular joint (TMJ) disorder (by chewing gum).

Possible Effects on Laboratory Tests
Free fatty acids (FFA blood level): increased.

Blood glucose: increased.

Prothrombin time (INR): decreased.

Urine screening test for drug abuse: no effect.

CAUTION

1. For these drug products to be safe and effective, it is mandatory that all smoking be stopped immediately at the beginning of drug treatment.

2. Extended use of chewing gum may cause damage to mouth tissues and teeth, loosen fillings, stick to dentures, and initiate or aggravate TMJ dysfunction.

3. Smoking cessation and the use of these drug products can result in increased blood levels of insulin (in insulin-dependent diabetics); dose reduction of insulin may be necessary to prevent hypoglycemic reactions.

4. If you are taking any of the following drugs, consult your physician regarding the need to reduce their dose while participating in a smoking-cessation program: aminophylline, beta-blocker drugs, imipramine, oxazepam, oxtriphylline, pentazocine, prazosin, propoxyphene, theophylline.

5. If you are taking any of the following drugs, consult your physician regarding the need to increase their dose while participating in a smoking-cessation program: isoproterenol, phenylephrine.

6. Used patches should be folded in half with the adhesive sides sealed together; place them in the original pouch or aluminum foil and dispose of them promptly; keep out of reach of animals and children.

7. Use of antacids, such as Tums, prior to chewing nicotine gum can increase the amount of nicotine absorbed from the gum.

8. Patches have improved benefits when they are part of a complete smoking-cessation program that includes counseling.

9. The Centers for Disease Control (CDC) has many excellent publications available to give you more information on stopping smoking. Call 1-800-232-1311 for more information.

10. The possibility of becoming dependent on these replacement products also exists. The chance of this happening may be greater for the nasal spray than for the transdermal or "gum" products.

Precautions for Use

By Infants and Children: Safety and effectiveness for those less than 12 years of age are not established for the gum, and for those under 18 are not established for other forms.

By Those Over 60 Years of Age: Because of the increased possibility of cardiovascular disorders in this age group, treatment should be cautiously started. Watch closely for adverse effects.

▷ **Advisability of Use During Pregnancy**

Pregnancy Category: For nicotine chewing gum: C. For nicotine transdermal systems, nasal spray, and inhaler: D. See Pregnancy Risk Categories at the back of this book.

Animal Studies: Impaired fertility found in mouse, rat, and rabbit studies. Birth defects found in high-dose studies of mice.

Human Studies: Adequate studies of pregnant women are not available, but it is known that cigarette smoking during pregnancy may cause low birth weight, increased risk of abortion, and increased risk of newborn death.

The use of these drug products is not recommended during pregnancy.

Advisability of Use If Breast-Feeding

Presence of this drug in breast milk: Yes.

Avoid drug or refrain from nursing.

Habit-Forming Potential: The prolonged use of these drug products may perpetuate the physical dependence of nicotine-dependent smokers. Patches should have the lowest potential for dependence. Potential exists for abuse of nonprescription forms of this medicine.

Effects of Overdose: Nausea, vomiting, increased salivation, stomach cramps, diarrhea, headache, dizziness, impaired vision and hearing, weakness, confusion, fainting, difficult breathing, seizures.

Possible Effects of Long-Term Use: If not slowly lowered in dose, perpetuation of nicotine dependence.

Suggested Periodic Examinations While Taking This Drug (at physician's discretion)
Evaluation of patient's ability to abstain from smoking.
Evaluation of patient's blood pressure and heart function.

▷ **While Taking This Drug, Observe the Following**
Foods: Avoid any food with nicotine content.
Herbal Medicines or Minerals: Using ephedra, ma huang, guarana, kola, or similar products may accentuate nervousness and anxiety people have when trying to quit smoking. Talk to your doctor BEFORE combining any herbal medicine with nicotine.
Beverages: No restrictions.
▷ *Alcohol:* May cause an increase in heart and blood vessel (cardiovascular) effects.
Tobacco Smoking: Avoid all forms of tobacco completely.
Marijuana Smoking: Avoid completely.
▷ *Other Drugs*
Nicotine may ***increase*** the effects of
• adenosine.
The following drugs may **increase** the effects of nicotine:
• antacids such as Tums used prior to chewing nicotine-containing gum—may increase the absorption of nicotine from the gum.
• cimetidine (Tagamet).
• lithium (Lithobid).
• ranitidine (Zantac).
Nicotine ***taken concurrently*** with
• memantine (Namenda) can cause changes in blood levels of either drug.
• niacin (Nicobid, others) can cause severe facial flushing.
▷ *Driving, Hazardous Activities:* This drug may cause dizziness or drowsiness. Restrict activities as necessary.
Aviation Note: The use of this drug ***may be a disqualification*** for piloting. Consult a designated Aviation Medical Examiner.
Exposure to Sun: No restrictions.
Exposure to Cold: Use caution until tolerance is determined. Cold environments may enhance the vasospastic action of nicotine.
Heavy Exercise or Exertion: Patients with angina, coronary artery disease, or hypertension should use this drug with caution.
Special Storage Instructions: Store nicotine gum at room temperature and protect from light. Store nicotine patches at room temperature, and be especially careful to avoid exposing the patches to temperatures greater than 86 degrees F. (30 degrees C.). Do not store unpouched. Once opened, patches should be used promptly because they may lose their strength.
Discontinuation: As soon as a lasting cessation of smoking has been achieved, these drugs should be gradually reduced in dose and then discontinued.

Continual use of the chewing gum or inhaler should not exceed 6 months, the nasal spray form no longer than 3 months, and the transdermal system no more than 20 weeks.

NIFEDIPINE (ni FED i peen)

Introduced: 1972   **Class:**   Antianginal, antihypertensive, calcium channel blocker   **Prescription:**   USA: Yes   **Controlled Drug:**   USA: No; Canada: No   **Available as Generic:**   Yes

Brand Names: Adalat, Adalat CC, ✤Adalat FT, XL, ✤Adalat P.A., ✤Apo-Nifed, ✤Gen-Nifedipine, ✤Novo-Nifedin, ✤Nu-Nifed, Procardia, Procardia XL, ✤Scheinpharm Nifedipine XL

Controversies in Medicine: Medicines in this class have had many conflicting reports. The FDA has held hearings on the calcium channel blocker (CCB) class. Research at New York University found that nifedipine is a cause of reversible male infertility. CCBs are currently second-line agents for high blood pressure according to the JNC VII (see Glossary).

BENEFITS versus RISKS

Possible Benefits	*Possible Risks*
EFFECTIVE PREVENTION OF CLASSICAL ANGINA OF EFFORT AND OTHER ANGINA TYPES	Rare increase in angina upon starting treatment
SECOND-LINE TREATMENT OF HYPERTENSION (sustained-release form)	Rare precipitation of congestive heart failure
NIFEDIPINE CR FORM MAY HELP AVOID A MORNING SURGE IN BLOOD PRESSURE IF IT IS TAKEN RIGHT AFTER YOU WAKE UP	Rare anemia and low white blood cell counts
	Very rare drug-induced hepatitis
	Fainting

▷ **Principal Uses**

As a Single Drug Product: Uses currently included in FDA-approved labeling: Treats (1) angina pectoris due to coronary artery spasm (Prinzmetal's variant angina) that occurs spontaneously and is not associated with exertion; (2) classical angina of effort (due to atherosclerotic disease of the coronary arteries) in people who have not responded to or cannot tolerate the nitrates and beta-blocker drugs customarily used to treat this disorder (sustained-release form); (3) mild to moderate hypertension (extended-release forms).

Author's Note: A chart review found the immediate-release form of this medicine IS NOT recommended for use in treating hypertension, heart attack, hypertensive crisis, and Acute Coronary Syndrome (ACS). This lead to FDA label changes (see below).

Other (unlabeled) generally accepted uses: (1) Treats symptoms of Raynaud's phenomenon; (2) may stop some early atherosclerosis; (3) can have a role in treating pulmonary hypertension; (4) helps decrease risk of heart attack after coronary artery bypass grafting; (5) could have a role in some neurologically based pain disorders; (6) can help itching (urticaria) of unknown cause; (7) therapy of achalasia or esophageal spasm; (8) helps intractable hiccups; (9) helps amaurosis fugax; (10) helps abnormal reactions to cold (chilblains).

How This Drug Works: Blocks passage of calcium through certain cell walls (needed for nerve and muscle tissue function), slowing electrical activity through the heart (post excitation phase) and inhibits contraction of coronary arteries and peripheral arterioles. As a result:

- prevents spontaneous spasm of coronary arteries (Prinzmetal's angina).
- reduces heart rate and force during exertion, decreasing oxygen needs of heart muscle and reducing occurrence of effort-induced angina (classical angina pectoris).
- reduces the degree of contraction of peripheral arterial walls, lowering blood pressure. This further reduces the work of the heart during exertion and helps prevent angina.

Some data has shown that this medicine helps red blood cells bend (RBC deformability) by decreasing the amount of calcium in the red cells.

Author's Note: One study found that nifedipine restored the function of the lining of blood vessels (endothelium).

▷ **Widely Used Guidelines That Involve This Medicine (representative sample):** Please look at the section at the very beginning of this profile called "Class." Next, turn to Table 22 and you will find guidelines listed by the class involved!

Available Dosage Forms and Strengths

Capsules — 5 mg (Canada), 10 mg (U.S. and Canada), 20 mg (U.S.)

Tablets — 10 mg, 20 mg (Canada)

Tablets, extended-release — 10 mg, 20 mg (Canada), 30 mg, 60 mg, 90 mg (U.S.)

Tablets, sustained-release — 30 mg, 60 mg, 90 mg

▷ **Recommended Dosage Ranges** (Actual dose and schedule must be determined for each patient individually.)

Infants and Children: Dose not established.

Adults up to 60 Years of Age: Chronic stable angina or vasospastic (Prinzmetal's) angina: Immediate-release form: Dosing is started with 10 mg three times a day. Most people respond to 10–20 mg three times a day. Change to extended-release forms can be accomplished on a same dose to same dose (mg to mg) basis. *Extended-release form for high blood pressure:* Initially 30 mg once daily. Dose may be increased gradually at 7- to 14-day intervals (as needed and tolerated) up to 60 mg. Maximum total daily dose should not exceed 90 mg.

Sublingual for hypertensive crisis: **FDA labeling for the immediate-release form of this medicine says that it is NOT recommended for use in treating acute hypertensive crisis, ongoing (chronic) hypertension, acute myocardial infarction (heart attack), and acute coronary syndrome.**

Over 60 Years of Age: **Nifedipine immediate-release capsules have revised FDA labeling recommendations against use in people with acute coronary syndrome, heart attack (acute myocardial infarction), hypertensive crisis and ongoing (chronic) hypertension. Use of the immediate-release form by those over 71 has been associated with almost a fourfold increase in risk for all-cause death when compared to ACE inhibitors, beta blockers, or other calcium channel blockers. Extended-release tablets adjusted between 10–20 mg twice daily gave significant response rate in that group.**

Conditions Requiring Dosing Adjustments

Liver Function: Lower doses are prudent in liver disease. This drug is also a rare cause of liver toxicity (allergic hepatitis) and should be used with caution. Also a potential cause of portal hypertension and should NOT be used by patients with portal hypertension.

Kidney Function: For patients with compromised kidneys, nifedipine is a benefit-to-risk decision, as it can lead to kidney toxicity.

▷ **Dosing Instructions:** May be taken with or following food to reduce stomach irritation. Take this medicine with water. DO NOT take this medicine with grapefruit juice or eat grapefruit while you are taking this medicine. The capsule and the sustained-release tablet should be swallowed whole (not altered). DO NOT be frightened if you see part of the tablet in your stools—while it looks like something wrong happened, the form that you see is simply what remains after your body has taken out all the medicine. As with other medicines, it is critical to take the right dose, right on time. One study found that the nifedipine CR form helped prevent a surge in blood pressure if it was taken right after the patients woke up. Talk to your doctor about this. If you forget a dose: Take the missed dose as soon as you remember it, unless it's nearly time for your next dose—if that is the case, skip the missed dose and take the next dose right on schedule. DON'T take two doses at the same time. Talk with your doctor if you find yourself missing doses.

Usual Duration of Use: Use on a regular schedule for 2 to 4 weeks determines effectiveness in reducing the frequency and severity of angina and in controlling hypertension. For long-term use (months to years), the smallest effective dose should be used. Supervision and periodic physician evaluation are essential.

Typical Treatment Goals and Measurements (Outcomes and Markers)

Blood Pressure Guidelines (JNC VII) define normal blood pressure (BP) as **less than** 120/80 and **pre-hypertension** as 120/80 to 139/89. This new range is intended to help doctors encourage lifestyle changes (or in the case of people with a risk factor for high blood pressure, start treatment) much earlier—so that damage to blood vessels, your heart, kidneys, sexual potency, or eyes might be minimized or avoided altogether. Stage 1 hypertension is 140/90 to 159/99 and stage 2 hypertension equal to or greater than: 160/100 mm Hg. These guidelines also recommend that clinicians work with their patients to agree on the goals and a plan of treatment. The first-ever guidelines for blood pressure (hypertension) in African Americans recommends that MOST black patients be started on TWO antihypertensive medicines with the goal of lowering blood pressure to 130/80 for those with high risk for heart and blood vessel disease or with diabetes. The American Diabetes Association also recommends 130/80 as the target for diabetics and less than 125/75 for those who spill more than one gram of protein into their urine. Most clinicians try to achieve a BP that confers the best balance of lower cardiovascular risk and avoids the problem of too low a blood pressure. Blood pressure duration is generally increased with beneficial restriction of sodium. If goals are not met, it is not unusual to intensify doses or add on medicines.

Possible Advantages of This Drug

The sustained-release form offers effective once-a-day treatment for both angina and hypertension. Little or no effect on depressing the SA or AV node of the heart. Greater effect as a peripheral vasodilator than other medicines in the same family.

▷ **This Drug Should Not Be Taken If**
- you have had an allergic reaction to it previously.
- you have active liver disease or had a heart attack in the last month.
- you are over 71 and have been prescribed the immediate-release form of nifedipine.
- you have low blood pressure—systolic pressure below 90—or you have had a heart attack in the last 4 weeks.
- you have significant narrowing of your aorta (aortic stenosis). Ask your doctor.
- you have been prescribed nifedipine immediate-release capsules and have acute coronary syndrome, heart attack (acute myocardial infarction), hypertensive crisis, and ongoing hypertension. Ask your doctor.

▷ **Inform Your Physician Before Taking This Drug If**
- you had an adverse response to any calcium channel blocker.
- you take any form of digitalis or a beta blocker (see Drug Classes).
- you are taking any drugs that lower blood pressure.
- you have a history of congestive heart failure, heart attack, or stroke.
- you are subject to disturbances of heart rhythm.
- you have cardiomyopathy (nonobstructive) or aortic stenosis.
- you have impaired liver or kidney function.
- you have abnormal circulation to your fingers.
- you have atrial fibrillation.
- you develop a skin condition while taking this medicine.
- you have diabetes or Duchenne muscular dystrophy.
- you have a history of drug-induced liver damage.

Possible Side Effects (natural, expected, and unavoidable drug actions)
Low blood pressure, rapid heart rate, swelling of the feet and ankles, flushing and sensation of warmth, sweating.

▷ **Possible Adverse Effects:** (unusual, unexpected, and infrequent reactions)
If any of the following develop, consult your physician promptly for guidance.
Mild Adverse Effects
Allergic reactions: skin rash, hives, itching, fever.
Headache, dizziness, weakness, nervousness, blurred vision, eye pain, or swelling around eyes—infrequent.
Pedal edema—frequent.
Depression—rare.
Abnormal growth of the gums (gingival hyperplasia)—rare.
Taste disturbances—possible.
Ringing in the ears (tinnitus)—case reports.
Sleep disturbances or bedwetting—case reports.
Increased or decreased blood potassium—possible.
Palpitation, shortness of breath, wheezing, cough—infrequent.
Impaired sense of smell—possible.
Heartburn, nausea, taste disturbances, cramps, diarrhea—rare.
Tremors, muscle cramps—possible.
Serious Adverse Effects
Allergic reaction: drug-induced hepatitis—very rare; drug eruptions and erysipelaslike reactions and exfoliative dermatitis or erythema multiforme.
Idiosyncratic reactions: joint stiffness and inflammation.
Increased frequency or severity of angina on initiation of treatment following an increase in dose.
Abnormal muscle movements (myoclonus)—case reports.

Kidney toxicity or pulmonary edema—case reports.

Bezoars—rare (seen with sustained-release forms).

Acute psychosis—case report.

Worsening of circulation to the fingers—possible.

Marked drop in blood pressure with fainting—possible.

Low white blood cells, platelets, and hemoglobin—case reports.

▷ **Possible Effects on Sexual Function:** Altered timing and pattern of menstruation; excessive menstrual bleeding. Tenderness and swelling of male breast tissue (gynecomastia)—case reports.

▷ **Adverse Effects That May Mimic Natural Diseases or Disorders**

Allergic rash and swelling of the legs may resemble erysipelas. Drug-induced hepatitis may suggest viral hepatitis. Transient increases in liver function tests may suggest infectious hepatitis.

Possible Effects on Laboratory Tests

Bleeding time: increased.

Liver function tests: transient increases.

Blood total cholesterol level: no effect in those less than 60 years old; decreased in those over 60 years old.

Blood HDL cholesterol level: no effect or lowered slightly.

Blood LDL and VLDL cholesterol levels: no effect.

Blood triglyceride levels: no effect or decreased.

CAUTION

1. Tell health care providers that you take this drug. Note nifedipine use on a card in your purse or wallet.
2. You may use nitroglycerin and other nitrate drugs as needed to relieve acute angina pain. If angina attacks become more frequent or intense, call your doctor.
3. Nifedipine immediate-release capsules have revised FDA labeling recommendations against use in people with acute coronary syndrome, heart attack (acute myocardial infarction), hypertensive crisis, and ongoing hypertension. Use of the immediate-release form by those over 71 has been associated with almost a fourfold increase in risk for all-cause death when compared to ACE inhibitors, beta blockers, or other calcium channel blockers.

Precautions for Use

By Infants and Children: Safety and effectiveness for those less than 12 years of age are not established.

By Those Over 60 Years of Age: You may be more susceptible to the development of weakness, dizziness, fainting, and falling. Take necessary precautions to prevent injury. Report promptly any changes in your pattern of thirst and urination.

▷ **Advisability of Use During Pregnancy**

Pregnancy Category: C. See Pregnancy Risk Categories at the back of this book.

Animal Studies: Embryo and fetal deaths reported in mice, rats, and rabbits; birth defects reported in rats.

Human Studies: Adequate studies of pregnant women are not available. Avoid this drug during the first 3 months. Use during the final 6 months only if clearly needed. Ask your physician for guidance.

Advisability of Use If Breast-Feeding

Presence of this drug in breast milk: Yes.

Avoid drug or refrain from nursing.

Habit-Forming Potential: None.

Effects of Overdose: Weakness, light-headedness, fainting, fast pulse, low blood pressure, shortness of breath, flushed and warm skin, tremors.

Possible Effects of Long-Term Use: None reported.

Suggested Periodic Examinations While Taking This Drug (at physician's discretion)

Evaluations of heart function, including electrocardiograms.

Measurements of blood pressure in supine, sitting, and standing positions.

▷ **While Taking This Drug, Observe the Following**

Foods: Do not eat grapefruit while you are taking this medicine. It is also prudent to avoid excessive salt intake.

Herbal Medicines or Minerals: Valerian and kava kava (no longer recommended in Canada) may intensify drowsiness. Dong quai may make nifedipine stay in the body longer than expected while St. John's wort may increase removal of this medicine from the body, blunting the benefit of this medicine (also increases sun sensitivity). Ginseng, guarana, mate, bitter orange, country mallow, hawthorn, saw palmetto, ma huang (do not take if hypertensive), goldenseal, yohimbe, and licorice may also increase blood pressure. Calcium and garlic may help lower blood pressure and could be part of complementary care. Use of calcium to excess (7.5 to 10 grams) with combination thiazide diuretics can lead to excessive calcium levels. Talk to your doctor about how much calcium to take. Indian snakeroot has a German Commission E monograph indication for hypertension—talk to your doctor. Eleuthero root and ephedra should be avoided by people living with hypertension.

Beverages: Grapefruit juice may greatly increase the absorption (bioavailability) of nifedipine and result in an exaggerated therapeutic effect. Water is the best liquid to take this medicine with. May be taken with milk.

▷ *Alcohol:* Use with caution. Alcohol may exaggerate the drop in blood pressure experienced by some people.

Tobacco Smoking: Nicotine may reduce the effectiveness of this drug. I advise everyone to quit smoking.

Marijuana Smoking: Possible reduced effectiveness of this drug; mild to moderate increase in angina; possible changes in electrocardiogram, confusing interpretation.

▷ *Other Drugs*

Nifedipine *taken* **concurrently** with

- amiodarone (Cordarone) may cause the heart to stop.
- beta-blocker drugs or digitalis preparations (see Drug Classes) may affect heart rate and rhythm adversely; careful monitoring by your physician is necessary if these drugs are taken concurrently.
- cyclosporine (Sandimmune) can lead to nifedipine toxicity.
- digoxin (Lanoxin) may lead to digoxin toxicity.
- diltiazem (Cardizem) may lead to nifedipine toxicity.
- magnesium can cause additive lowering of the blood pressure.
- oral blood thinners (anticoagulant drugs–see Drug Classes) may increase risk of bleeding.
- oral antidiabetic drugs (see Drug Classes) or insulin may result in loss of glucose control.
- phenytoin (Dilantin) or fosphenytoin (Cerebyx) can cause phenytoin or fosphenytoin toxicity.
- quinupristin/dalfopristin (Synercid) can cause nifedipine toxicity.

- rifampin (Rifadin) can decrease nifedipine's effectiveness.
- tacrolimus (Prograf) may lead to tacrolimus toxicity.
- theophylline can reduce the therapeutic benefits of nifedipine and may lead to theophylline toxicity as well.
- vincristine (Oncovin) can cause vincristine toxicity.

The following drugs may *increase* the effects of nifedipine:

- some antifungals (fluconazole, itraconazole, ketoconazole, and voriconazole)—may increase nifedipine blood levels and lead to toxicity.
- cimetidine (Tagamet).
- quinidine (Quinaglute, others)—can lead to nifedipine toxicity as well as decreased quinidine effectiveness.
- ranitidine (Zantac).
- ritonavir (Norvir) and other protease inhibitors (such as amprenavir [Agenerase] or atazanavir [Reyataz] which are removed by the same liver enzyme).

▷ *Driving, Hazardous Activities:* Usually no restrictions. This drug may cause drowsiness or dizziness. Restrict activities as necessary.

Aviation Note: Coronary artery disease *is a disqualification* for piloting. Consult a designated Aviation Medical Examiner.

Exposure to Sun: Caution—rare cases of phototoxicity have been reported.

Exposure to Heat: Caution is advised. Hot environments can exaggerate the blood pressure–lowering effects of this drug. Observe for light-headedness or weakness.

Heavy Exercise or Exertion: This drug may improve your ability to be more active without resulting angina pain. Use caution and avoid excessive exercise that could impair heart function in the absence of warning pain.

Discontinuation: Do not stop this drug abruptly. Consult your physician regarding gradual withdrawal. Observe for the possible development of rebound angina.

NISOLDIPINE (ni SOLD i peen)

Introduced: 1996 **Class:** Antianginal, antihypertensive, calcium channel blocker **Prescription:** USA: Yes **Controlled Drug:** USA: No; Canada: No **Available as Generic:** No

Brand Name: Sular

Author's Note: Information in this profile will be broadened in subsequent editions if data warrant.

NITROGLYCERIN (ni troh GLIS er in)

Introduced: 1847 **Class:** Antianginal, nitrates **Prescription:** USA: Yes **Controlled Drug:** USA: No; Canada: No **Available as Generic:** Yes

Brand Names: Corobid, Deponit, Minitran Transdermal Delivery System, Nitrek, Nitro-Bid, Nitrocap TD, Nitrocine Timecaps, Nitrocine Transdermal, Nitrodisc, Nitro-Dur, Nitro-Dur II, Nitrogard, ✤Nitrogard-SR, Nitroglyn, Nitrol, Nitrolin, Nitrolingual Spray, ✤Nitrol TSAR Kit, Nitrong, ✤Nitrong SR, Nitroquick, Nitrospan, ✤Nitrostabilin, Nitrostat, Nitro Transdermal System, NTS Transdermal Patch, Transderm-Nitro, ✤Trates S.R., Tridil

---

BENEFITS versus RISKS

Possible Benefits	*Possible Risks*
EFFECTIVE RELIEF AND PREVENTION OF ANGINA	Orthostatic hypotension with and without fainting
EFFECTIVE ADJUNCTIVE TREATMENT IN SELECTED CASES OF CONGESTIVE HEART FAILURE	Skin rash—rare
	Altered hemoglobin with large doses—very rare
SPRAY FORM OFFERS NEWER EASE OF DOSING	Low blood platelets—rare

---

▷ **Principal Uses**

As a Single Drug Product: Uses currently included in FDA-approved labeling: (1) Treats symptomatic coronary artery disease (rapid-action forms are used to relieve acute attacks of anginal pain; sustained-action forms prevent development of angina, translingual spray is used in acute treatment and acute prevention); (2) helps improve breathing difficulty caused by heart failure (left ventricle); (3) intravenous form used in surgery to control blood pressure; (4) relieves congestive heart failure after heart attacks. Other (unlabeled) generally accepted uses: (1) May help ease spasms of the Oddi's sphincter; (2) topical use may help in impotence; (3) can help reduce the extent of heart damage if given following a heart attack (myocardial infarction); (4) helps relax cocaine-constricted heart arteries; (5) eases the pain of peripheral neuropathy; (6) may be of help in easing esophageal problems (achalasia); (7) when the anal sphincter does not work correctly, this drug can help reduce the muscle pressure and ease constipation; (8) nitroglycerin in combination with vasopressin may be of use in stopping bleeding esophageal varices; (9) can help loss of vision that has been caused by a clot in the retinal artery; (10) if ergot medications (see Drug Classes) have shut down circulation to the extremities, nitroglycerin can open up the circulation; (11) used to delay contractions in order to rotate an abnormally positioned fetus; (12) may help diabetics with nerve damage (diabetic neuropathy); (13) helps relax the uterus when the placenta has been retained; (14) relaxes the uterus in cases where a fetus's head is trapped or there is a second fetus.

How This Drug Works: Relaxes and dilates both arteries and veins. Beneficial effects in angina are due to (1) dilation of narrowed coronary arteries and (2) dilation of veins in the general circulation, with reduced volume and pressure of blood entering the heart. Net effects are improved blood supply to the heart and reduced work for the heart. Both actions reduce the frequency and severity of angina.

▷ **Widely Used Guidelines That Involve This Medicine (representative sample):** Please look at the section at the very beginning of this profile called "Class." Next, turn to Table 22 and you will find guidelines listed by the class involved!

Available Dosage Forms and Strengths

Canisters, translingual spray — 13.8 g (200 doses), 0.4 mg per metered dose

Capsules, prolonged-action — 2.5 mg, 2.6 mg, 6.5 mg, 9 mg

Ointment — 2%

Tablets, buccal — 1 mg, 2 mg, 3 mg

Tablets, prolonged-action — 2.6 mg, 6.5 mg, 9 mg
Tablets, sublingual — 0.15 mg, 0.3 mg, 0.4 mg, 0.6 mg
Transdermal systems (all per 24 hours) — 2.5 mg, 5 mg, 7.5 mg, 10 mg, 15 mg

▷ **Usual Adult Dosage Ranges:** Translingual spray—one or two metered sprays (0.4 mg) under the tongue every 3 to 5 minutes, up to three doses within 15 minutes, to relieve acute angina. To prevent angina, one spray taken 5 to 10 minutes before exertion.

Sublingual tablets—0.15 to 0.6 mg (150 to 600 mcg) dissolved under tongue at 5-minute intervals to relieve acute angina. Up to three doses can be taken. One tablet can be taken 5–10 minutes BEFORE you participate in an activity that may cause angina in order to try to prevent an attack (prophylactic use).

Prolonged-action tablets—2.5 mg at 6- to 8-hour intervals to prevent angina. Many clinicians give a 6- to 12-hour nitrate-free interval when using this dosage form.

Ointment—0.5 inch or 7.5 mg applied in a thin, even layer of uniform size to hairless skin at 3- to 4-hour intervals to prevent angina. A 10- to 12-hour ointment-free interval is recommended by some clinicians to avoid tolerance.

Buccal tablets—1 to 2 mg every 4 to 5 hours, placed between cheek and gum.

Transdermal patches—5-square-cm to 30-square-cm patch applied to hairless skin once every 24 hours (with a 10- to 12-hour nitrate-free interval to avoid tolerance) when used to prevent angina.

Translingual spray: Once an angina attack starts, one to two metered doses are sprayed under or onto the tongue. Like other immediate-onset forms, repeat doses can be given. Repeat doses can be given every 3-5 minutes for Nitrolingual. No more than three doses should be used in a 15-minute period. Prevention (prophylaxis): The spray is used 5-10 minutes prior to a patient activity which might lead to an attack of angina.

Note: Actual dose and schedule must be determined for each patient individually.

Author's Note: In order to avoid tolerance to the therapeutic effects of this medicine, a nitrate-free interval of 10–12 hours daily is recommended: 24-hour patches are removed after having been applied for 12 hours; dosing of ointment is interrupted for 12 hours a day; oral sustained-release formulations are dosed to give a 6- to 12-hour nitrate-free interval.

Conditions Requiring Dosing Adjustments
Liver Function: Specific dose adjustments in liver compromise are not defined.
Kidney Function: Specific guidelines for dosing changes are not available. This drug can discolor urine.

▷ **Dosing Instructions:** Dosage forms to be swallowed are best taken when stomach is empty (1 hour before or 2 hours after eating) to obtain maximal blood levels. Tablets should not be crushed. Under the tongue tablets (sublingual): Please sit down before you take this medicine, then place the tablet in your mouth and wet it with saliva. After this, move the tablet under your tongue or in your cheek and let it dissolve there. Avoid chewing or swallowing the tablet whole. It's not unusual to feel a tingle or even a burning sensation in your mouth when this medicine dissolves. Capsules may be opened, but contents should not be crushed or chewed before swallowing. Don't inhale if you are using the under- or on-the-tongue (lingual) spray. This form can be used 5-10 minutes before you undertake an activity that usually leads to angina. If you forget a dose: Call your doctor about what to do. Once you have a prescription for an immediate-onset form of this medicine, ask your doctor what he or she wants you to do if the usual dose (such as 3 sublingual tablets or 3 translingual sprays in 15 minutes) does not relieve your chest pain. The usual course is to have someone take you to the hospital immediately for further evaluation.

Usual Duration of Use: Use on a regular schedule for 3 to 5 days is often needed to determine effectiveness in preventing and relieving acute anginal attacks. Individual dose adjustments will be necessary for optimal results. Long-term use (months to years) requires physician supervision.

Typical Treatment Goals and Measurements (Outcomes and Markers)
Angina: The goal is to relieve chest pain with under the tongue (sublingual) forms or spray. If pain is NOT relieved, have someone take you to the hospital and call your doctor. For patch or prolonged action tablets, the frequency and severity of anginal attacks should decrease. Call your doctor if you gain a lowered severity and frequency of angina, and then start to lose that benefit.

▷ **This Drug Should Not Be Taken If**
- you have had an allergic reaction to it or to other components (such as the adhesive in the patch forms) of this medicine.
- you are severely anemic (sublingual form).
- you have had recent head trauma.
- you have had a heart attack and have an increased heart rate or increased blood pressure.
- you are taking sildenafil (Viagra) and this medicine has been newly prescribed.
- you take this medicine and sildenafil (Viagra) has been newly prescribed.
- you have pericarditis (intravenous form).
- you have hyperthyroidism.
- you have increased intraocular pressure.
- you have closed-angle glaucoma (inadequately treated).

▷ **Inform Your Physician Before Taking This Drug If**
- you had an unfavorable response to other nitrates.
- you have low blood pressure.
- you have abnormal growth of the heart muscle in response to vascular disease (hypertrophic cardiomyopathy).
- you have problems absorbing medicines (malabsorption syndromes) or excessive action of your stomach (gastric hypermotility).
- you have any form of glaucoma.
- you have an overactive thyroid or are pregnant.
- you have had recent bleeding or trauma to your head.

Possible Side Effects (natural, expected, and unavoidable drug actions)
Flushing of face, headaches (50%), orthostatic hypotension (see Glossary), rapid heart rate, palpitation.

▷ **Possible Adverse Effects** (unusual, unexpected, and infrequent reactions)
If any of the following develop, consult your physician promptly for guidance.
Mild Adverse Effects
Allergic reaction: skin rash.
Throbbing headaches (may be severe and persistent), dizziness, fainting—possible.
Nausea, vomiting, taste disorders—infrequent.

Serious Adverse Effects

Allergic reactions: severe skin reactions with peeling.

Idiosyncratic reaction: methemoglobinemia—case reports.

Abnormally slow heartbeat (bradycardia)—rare.

Low blood supply to the head (transient ischemic attacks)—case reports.

Increased intracranial pressure—rare.

Low blood platelets or prolonged bleeding time—reported.

▷ **Possible Effects on Sexual Function:** Correction of impotence (one report following sublingual use). Preventive use of nitroglycerin prior to sexual activity has been recommended to eliminate or reduce the risk of angina. Consult your physician for guidance.

▷ **Adverse Effects That May Mimic Natural Diseases or Disorders**

Hypotensive spells (sudden drops in blood pressure) due to this drug may be mistaken for late-onset epilepsy.

Possible Effects on Laboratory Tests

Blood platelet count: decreased—very rare.

Bleeding time: prolonged.

CAUTION

1. This drug can provoke migraine headaches in susceptible individuals.
2. Patients with impaired brain circulation (cerebral arteriosclerosis) have increased risk of transient ischemic attacks—periods of temporary speech impairment, paralysis, numbness, etc.
3. Tolerance to long-acting forms of nitrates will happen in most patients after 24 hours of continuous use. A nitrate-free interval of 10 hours usually restores effectiveness.
4. Many over-the-counter (OTC) nonprescription drug products for allergies, colds, and coughs contain drugs that counteract the benefits of this drug. Ask your doctor or pharmacist for help before using any such medications.

Precautions for Use

By Infants and Children: Limited usefulness and experience in this age group. Dose schedules are not established.

By Those Over 60 Years of Age: Begin treatment with small doses and increase dose cautiously as needed and tolerated. You may be more susceptible to the development of flushing, throbbing headache, dizziness, "blackout" spells, fainting, and falling.

▷ **Advisability of Use During Pregnancy**

Pregnancy Category: C. See Pregnancy Risk Categories at the back of this book.

Animal Studies: No information available.

Human Studies: Adequate studies of pregnant women are not available.

Use this drug only if clearly needed. Ask your physician for guidance.

Advisability of Use If Breast-Feeding

Presence of this drug in breast milk: Unknown.

Watch nursing infant closely, and discontinue drug or nursing if adverse effects develop.

Habit-Forming Potential: None.

Effects of Overdose: Throbbing headache, dizziness, marked flushing, nausea, vomiting, abdominal cramps, confusion, delirium, paralysis, seizures, circulatory collapse.

Possible Effects of Long-Term Use: The development of tolerance (see Glossary) and the temporary loss of effectiveness.

Suggested Periodic Examinations While Taking This Drug (at physician's discretion)

Measurements of blood pressure and internal eye pressures.

Evaluation of hemoglobin.

▷ **While Taking This Drug, Observe the Following**

Foods: No restrictions.

Herbal Medicines or Minerals: Hawthorn and co-enzyme Q10 (co-Q10) can affect the way the heart works. Co-Q10 has a limited number of reports of decreasing INR in people taking warfarin. BE CERTAIN to tell your doctor that you are taking or are considering taking these herbs if you are taking a nitrate.

Beverages: No restrictions. May be taken with milk.

▷ *Alcohol:* Avoid alcohol completely. This combination may result in severe lowering of blood pressure. There is a potential for collapse of the circulation and pumping effectiveness of the heart.

Tobacco Smoking: Nicotine can reduce the effectiveness of this drug. I advise everyone to quit smoking.

Marijuana Smoking: Possible reduced effectiveness of this drug; mild to moderate increase in angina; possible changes in the electrocardiogram, confusing interpretation.

▷ *Other Drugs*

Nitroglycerin *taken concurrently* with

- acetylcysteine (NAC) may reverse tolerance to the intravenous form of this medicine.
- alteplase (Activase) lessens the benefits of alteplase; nitroglycerin and alteplase combination should be avoided if possible.
- antihypertensive drugs may cause excessive lowering of blood pressure; careful dose adjustments may be necessary.
- dihydroergotamine or similar ergot medicines (see Drug Classes) may result in ergotamine toxicity. DO NOT combine.
- diltiazem (Cardizem) can result in abnormally low blood pressure when used with the sustained-release form of nitroglycerin.
- heparin can result in decreased therapeutic benefit of heparin.
- indomethacin (Indocin) can blunt the benefits of nitroglycerin.
- isosorbide dinitrate (Isordil) or mononitrate (Ismo) may result in decreased nitroglycerin therapeutic benefits.
- neuromuscular blocking agents (such as pancuronium-Pavulon, vecuronium-Norcuron, others) can result in increased severity of muscle blockade. Use of lower neuromuscular blocker doses is prudent.
- sildenafil (Viagra), tadalafil (Cialis), vardenafil (Levitra) may cause very low blood pressure—DO NOT combine.

The following drugs may *increase* the effects of nitroglycerin:

- aspirin and perhaps other NSAIDs. May actually be of treatment benefit in patients who have had a heart attack (NSTEMI or STEMI). Talk to your doctor about this benefit-to-risk decision.

▷ *Driving, Hazardous Activities:* Usually no restrictions. This drug may cause dizziness or faintness. Restrict activities as necessary.

Aviation Note: Coronary artery disease *is a disqualification* for piloting. Consult a designated Aviation Medical Examiner.

Exposure to Sun: No restrictions.

Exposure to Heat: Hot environments can cause significant lowering of blood pressure.

Exposure to Cold: Cold environments can increase the need for this drug and limit its effectiveness.

Heavy Exercise or Exertion: This drug can increase your tolerance for exercise. Ask your doctor how much exercise is okay for you.

Special Storage Instructions: For sublingual tablets, to prevent loss of strength:
- keep tablets in the original glass container.
- do not transfer tablets to a plastic or metallic container (such as a pillbox).
- do not place absorbent cotton, paper (such as the prescription label), or other material inside the container.
- do not store other drugs in the same container.
- immediately close the container tightly after each use.
- store at room temperature.

Discontinuation: Do not stop this drug abruptly after long-term use. Best to lower the dose (of prolonged-action forms) slowly over 4 to 6 weeks. Watch for rebound angina.

NIZATIDINE (ni ZA te deen)

Please see the histamine (H2) blocking drug family profile.

NORFLOXACIN (nor FLOX a sin)

Please see the fluoroquinolone antibiotic family profile.

NORTRIPTYLINE (nor TRIP ti leen)

Introduced: 1963 **Class:** Antidepressant **Prescription:** USA: Yes **Controlled Drug:** USA: No; Canada: No **Available as Generic:** USA: Yes; Canada: No
Brand Names: Aventyl, Pamelor

BENEFITS versus RISKS	
Possible Benefits	*Possible Risks*
EFFECTIVE RELIEF OF ENDOGENOUS DEPRESSION	ADVERSE BEHAVIORAL EFFECTS: confusion, disorientation, hallucinations, delusions
Possibly beneficial in other depressive disorders	CONVERSION OF DEPRESSION TO MANIA in manic-depressive (bipolar) disorders
Possibly beneficial in the management of some types of chronic, severe pain	Aggravation of schizophrenia Irregular heart rhythms Rare blood cell abnormalities

Author's Note: The information in this profile has been shortened to make room for more widely used medicines.

OFLOXACIN (oh FLOX a sin)

Please see the fluoroquinolone antibiotic family profile.

OLANZAPINE (oh LAN za peen)

Introduced: 2004, (combination Symbyax form), 1996 **Class:** Antipsychotic; tranquilizer, major; thienobenzodiazepines; atypical antipsychotics **Prescription:** USA: Yes **Controlled Drug:** USA: No; Canada: No **Available as Generic:** USA: No; Canada: No
Brand Names: Symbyax (olanzapine, fluoxetine), Zyprexa, Zyprexa Zydis

---

BENEFITS versus RISKS

Possible Benefits	*Possible Risks*
EFFECTIVE SHORT-TERM CONTROL OF ACUTE MENTAL DISORDERS: beneficial effects on thinking, mood, and behavior	POSSIBLE TARDIVE DYSKINESIA (SERIOUS TOXIC BRAIN EFFECT WITH LONG-TERM USE)
DELIVERS BENEFITS IN EASING MANIA (IN BIPOLAR DISORDER) AS SOON AS IN THE FIRST WEEK OF TREATMENT	Orthostatic hypotension (see Glossary)
COMBINATION FORM TREATS DEPRESSION ASSOCIATED WITH BIPOLAR DISORDER WITH A SINGLE PILL	Increased liver enzymes Weight gain Blood sugar changes (glucose dysregulation)
Zyprexa Zydis form falls apart in the mouth, making it easier to take and preventing resistant patients from "cheeking" the medicine	
Relief of anxiety, agitation, and tension	
Medicines in this class are probably "drugs of choice" in older adults.	

▷ **Principal Uses**

As a Single Drug Product: Uses currently included in FDA-approved labeling: (1) Helps manage thinking problems and other difficulties seen in psychosis (schizophrenia and shizophreniform); (2) treats mania in bipolar disorder (often easing mania symptoms after only one week of treatment); (3) combination form (Symbyax) treats depression associated with bipolar disorder.

Other (unlabeled) generally accepted uses: (1) Works in anorexia; (2) eases anxiety in nursing home patients (Neuropsychiatric Inventory/Nursing Home Instrument or NPI/NH); (3) some data for helping patients with bipolar or mixed presentation who are resistant (refractory) to lithium or valproic acid; (4) eases marijuana (cannabis)-induced psychotic disorder.

How This Drug Works: This drug works as an antipsychotic by inhibiting the action of two primary nerve transmitters (dopamine and serotonin) in certain brain centers and acts to correct an imbalance of nerve impulse transmissions thought to be responsible for certain mental disorders. It also works at histamine, muscarinic, GABA, BZD, and adrenergic sites. The mechanism of action in bipolar disorder is not fully known at present.

▷ **Widely Used Guidelines That Involve This Medicine (representative sample):** Please look at the section at the very beginning of this profile called "Class." Next, turn to Table 22 and you will find guidelines listed by the class involved!

Available Dosage Forms and Strengths

Capsules (combination olanz/fluox) — 6 mg/25 mg, 12 mg/25 mg, 6 mg/50 mg, 12 mg/50 mg

Tablets — 2.5 mg, 5 mg, 7.5 mg,10 mg

Tablets, orally-disintegrating (Zyprexa Zydis) — 5 mg, 10 mg, 15 mg, 20 mg

▷ **Recommended Dosage Ranges** (Actual dose and schedule must be determined for each patient individually.)

Infants and Children: Dose not established, but use is increasing (see Bloch, Y in Sources).

18 to 60 Years of Age: Psychosis: Dosing is started with 5 to 10 mg daily. If the 5-mg dose is used, the dose may be increased to a maximum of 10 mg as needed and tolerated. Dose changes should only be made after seven days at a new dose. Changes in dose are usually done in 5-mg steps.

Sudden (acute) mania: Starting doses of 10 to 15 mg once daily, increased as needed and tolerated in steps of 5 mg daily have been used. Treatment in mania has been up to 4 weeks.

Author's Note: Gender data are now FDA-required for new approvals—it must be noted that the drug is removed (cleared) 30% slower in women than in men. Therefore effects (both desirable and undesirable) caused by the medicine may last longer in women (dose to dose) than in men.

Over 60 Years of Age: 5 mg of olanzapine is taken.

Conditions Requiring Dosing Adjustments

Liver Function: The drug is highly metabolized in the liver. The manufacturer says that even in patients with significantly impaired liver function (Childs Pugh A or B), only a lower (5 mg) initial starting dose should be given. It appears prudent to make any dose increases more slowly and closely follow the patient as well.

Kidney Function: Dosing changes are not thought to be needed.

Seizure Disorders: Seizures happened in 0.9% of patients during clinical trials of olanzapine. Olanzapine should be used with caution by seizure patients. Dose decreases are not defined at present.

▷ **Dosing Instructions:** The tablet may be crushed and taken with food. It is best to take this medicine at the same time every day. The (Zydis) form is an orally disintegrating tablet and does not require water to take it. Make sure your hands are dry, peel back the foil on the blister pack (avoid pushing the tablet through the foil), and put the tablet into your mouth. This form easily falls apart in saliva and water is not needed. If you forget a dose: Take the missed dose as soon as you remember it, unless it's nearly time for your next dose—if that is the case, skip the missed dose and take the next dose right on schedule. DO NOT double doses. Talk with your doctor if you find yourself missing doses.

Usual Duration of Use: Use on a regular schedule for at least 1 week is required to reach steady-state levels and hence determines effectiveness. Clinical benefits in mania of bipolar disorder may be seen in the first week of therapy. Clinical trials that led to FDA approval were conducted for 6 weeks, and the medicine is also approved for long-term use. Ongoing use requires physician supervision and checks of ongoing results.

Typical Treatment Goals and Measurements (Outcomes and Markers)

Schizophrenia: The general goal: to ease the severity of symptoms in order to let the patient resume his or her usual activities. There should be lessened intrusion of abnormal thinking into more normal life. As in depression, scales such as the Brief Psychiatric Rating Scale (BPRS) and the Scale for Assessment of Negative Symptoms (SANS) can help assess the benefits of this medicine. *Mania:* Young Mania Rating Scale (YMRS) is often used to check results in bipolar manic patients.

Possible Advantages of This Drug

Effective reversal of symptoms of psychosis while acting at different sites than previously available agents. Rapid onset in bipolar disorder. Medicines in this class are probably drugs of choice in older adults. Zyprexa Zydis form falls apart in the mouth making it easier to take and prevents noncompliant patients from "cheeking" this medicine. Low probability of movement disorders (extrapyramidal). New Symbyax form treats depression in bipolar disorder.

▷ **This Drug Should Not Be Taken If**
- you have had an allergic reaction to it previously.

▷ **Inform Your Physician Before Taking This Drug If**
- you have a seizure disorder.
- you have had neuroleptic malignant syndrome.
- you are at risk for suicide.
- your liver is compromised.
- you have constitutionally low blood pressure, take medicine to treat high blood pressure, or have cardiovascular or cerebrovascular disease.
- you have had narrow angle glaucoma.
- you are pregnant.
- you have prediabetes or diabetes.
- you have a history of breast cancer.
- you are taking any drug with sedative effects.
- you tend to be constipated.
- you plan to have surgery under general or spinal anesthesia in the near future.
- you have problems swallowing.

Possible Side Effects (natural, expected, and unavoidable drug actions)
Orthostatic hypotension (see Glossary), drowsiness.

▷ **Possible Adverse Effects** (unusual, unexpected, and infrequent reactions)
If any of the following develop, consult your physician promptly for guidance.

Mild Adverse Effects
Allergic reactions: skin rash, itching—rare.
Drowsiness, agitation and insomnia—frequent.
Headache, drowsiness—rare.
Vision changes (such as "lazy eye" or conjunctivitis)—infrequent.
Weight gain—may be frequent (29% in short-term studies had increase of 7% or more). Nizatidine may help (unlabeled use) by inhibiting weight gain (earlier plateau) in people taking olanzapine.

Depression—rare.

Dizziness—rare to infrequent.

Sugar changes (increased-hyperglycemia/diabetes)-possible with all atypical antipsychotics (risk not available).

Somnolence—frequent.

Prolonged QT interval—possible.

Edema—infrequent.

Constipation—infrequent.

Serious Adverse Effects

Allergic reactions: hair loss—rare. Pustular skin eruptions—case report. Hypersensitivity syndrome with fever, toxic hepatitis, and esosinophilia—case report.

Drug-induced increased liver enzymes—rare.

Pancreatitis—case report.

Increased triglycerides—(more likely with those who also gain weight).

Low white blood cell count (neutropenia)—case reports.

Difficulty swallowing (dysphagia)—case reports.

Tardive dyskinesia or other movement disorders—possible (less than other medicines).

Neuroleptic malignant syndrome—case reports.

Seizure—case report.

New-onset diabetes mellitus and/or blood sugar problems (increased sugar or hyperglycemia, glucose dysregulation)—possible with all antipsychotics and possible ketoacidosis—frequency not available.

▷ **Possible Effects on Sexual Function:** Case reports of extended and painful erections (priapism), amenorrhea, and vaginitis.

▷ **Adverse Effects That May Mimic Natural Diseases or Disorders**

Nervous system reactions may suggest true Parkinson's disease. Liver reactions may suggest viral hepatitis. Blood sugar changes resemble diabetes.

Possible Effects on Laboratory Tests

Prolactin levels: increased.

Liver function tests: increased liver enzymes (ALT/GPT, AST/GOT, and alkaline phosphatase).

Triglycerides—increased.

Blood sugar (glucose)—increased.

CAUTION

1. Other medicines (nonprescription or prescription) that can cause drowsiness or central nervous system effects may react unfavorably with this medicine. Talk with your doctor or pharmacist before combining any medicines.

2. Since this medicine can cause orthostatic hypotension, some high blood pressure (antihypertensive) medicines may have a greater than expected effect if taken with olanzapine.

3. Given reports of glucose changes, caution should be used with people already having a problem regulating blood sugar and more careful monitoring undertaken.

4. Pediatric and adult patients treated with this medicine should be closely watched for worsening depression or suicidal thinking. The FDA has required makers of antidepressants such as this one to alert healthcare professionals to the fact that children and adults with major depression may develop worsening depression or suicidal thoughts and behavior whether they take medicine for depression or do not take it. Patients

should be carefully followed for such clinical worsening (particularly when treatment is started or doses are increased or decreased—Symbyax).

Precautions for Use

By Infants and Children: Safety and effectiveness for those under 18 years of age are not established.

By Those Over 60 Years of Age: Lower starting doses should be taken; caution is advised regarding drowsiness, dizziness, and orthostatic hypotension, since olanzapine can cause changes in the ability of the body to regulate changes in temperature and this regulation may be less intact in older patients to begin with. You may also be more susceptible to Parkinson-like reactions and/or tardive dyskinesia (see Glossary). Discuss early indications of these reactions with your doctor, as progression of these reactions may lead to symptoms that are not reversible.

▷ Advisability of Use During Pregnancy

Pregnancy Category: C. See Pregnancy Risk Categories at the back of this book.

Animal Studies: Rat and mouse studies reveal increased mammary gland adenomas (when the animals were given 0.5 and 2 times the mg-per-square-meter human dose) respectively. Increased numbers of nonviable fetuses were seen in one rat study using nine times the maximum human dose.

Human Studies: Adequate studies of pregnant women are not available.

Use of this drug is a benefit-to-risk decision. Ask your doctor for guidance.

Advisability of Use If Breast-Feeding

Presence of this drug in breast milk: Yes—up to 2.5 % of the maternal dose. Avoid drug or refrain from nursing.

Habit-Forming Potential: None. A withdrawal syndrome was reported in one patient. The authors concluded it was a serotonergic rebound.

Effects of Overdose: Reports of 67 overdoses were made during clinical trials. The patient who took the largest dose had drowsiness and slurred speech.

Possible Effects of Long-Term Use: Possible changes in blood sugar regulation.

Suggested Periodic Examinations While Taking This Drug (at physician's discretion)

Liver function tests.

Careful inspection of the tongue for early evidence of fine, involuntary, wave-like movements that could be the beginning of tardive dyskinesia.

Sitting and standing blood pressure checks may be advisable when therapy is started, to assess orthostatic hypotension.

Blood sugar and A1C (glycosylated hemoglobin)—particularly when starting treatment, then periodically.

▷ While Taking This Drug, Observe the Following

Foods: Avoid eating grapefruit while taking this medicine. Follow prescribed diet. See grapefruit warning below.

Herbal Medicines or Minerals: Data from a small study of forty patients (See Emsley, R. in Sources) found that add-on therapy with one of the components of fish oil (eicosapenteanoic acid or EPA) helped schizophrenic patients (Positive and Negative Syndrome Scale scores) and was well-tolerated. Additional research is needed.

Using kola, guarana, mate, bitter orange, country mallow or ma huang may result in unacceptable central nervous system stimulation. Evening primrose oil may increase risk of seizure, adding to the risk that this medicine already has. St. John's wort may impact one of the liver enzymes that helps remove this medicine, leading to reduced benefits. Do not combine. Since part of the way ginkgo and ginseng work may be as a MAO inhibitor, do not combine them with olanzapine. Belladonna may lead to excessive anticholinergic actions. Betel nut may make movement disorders more likely. DHEA use may blunt medicine benefits. Given more recent concerns regarding blood sugar and this medicine: Using chromium may change the way your body is able to use sugar. Some health food stores advocate vanadium as mimicking the actions of insulin, but possible toxicity and need for rigorous studies presently preclude recommending it. DHEA may change sensitivity to insulin or insulin resistance. Aloe, bitter melon, eucalyptus, fenugreek, ginger, garlic, ginseng, glucomannan, guar gum, hawthorn, licorice, nettle, and yohimbe may change blood sugar. Surprisingly, boiled stems of the Optuntia streptacantha prickly pear cactus appears to be able to lower blood sugar. Ongoing effects and effects on A1C are not known. Red sage is used for blood sugar effects, but is unproven. Psyllium increases risk of excessively low blood sugar. Since so many of these products may require adjustment of insulin dosing, talk to your doctor BEFORE combining any of these herbal medicines with this medicine. Echinacea purpurea (injectable) and blonde psyllium seed or husk should NOT be taken by people living with diabetes.

Talk to your doctor before adding ANY herbals.

Beverages: Grapefruit juice may decrease metabolism of olanzapine and lead to toxicity. May be taken with milk or water.

▷ *Alcohol:* Avoid completely.

Tobacco Smoking: Olanzapine is removed from the body up to 40% faster in people who smoke compared to those who do not. Recommendations for dosing changes are not available. I advise everyone to quit smoking.

Marijuana Smoking: Expected to cause an increase in drowsiness; accentuation of orthostatic hypotension; increased risk of precipitating latent psychoses, confusing the interpretation of mental status and drug responses.

▷ *Other Drugs*

Olanzapine **taken concurrently** with

- activated charcoal will decrease absorption of olanzapine. (May be of use in overdoses.)
- any medicine that has central nervous system activity may result in additive effects.
- any medicine that can cause liver damage may result in additive liver problems.
- any sedative drugs (prescription and nonprescription) can cause excessive sedation.
- benzodiazepines (see Drug Classes) may magnify the orthostatic hypotension problem caused by olanzapine.
- carbamazepine (Tegretol) causes up to a 50% increase in removal of olanzapine from the body; dosing increases in olanzapine appear prudent.
- fluoroquinolone antibiotics, such as ciprofloxacin (Cipro) or norfloxacin (Noroxin), may lead to olanzapine toxicity.
- fluvoxamine (Luvox) may lead to olanzapine toxicity.
- lithium (Lithobid, others) may increase risk of serious nerve effects—extreme care should be taken and patients closely monitored for signs of toxicity and movement problems—especially if high doses of antipsychotic drugs and lithium are used. Call your doctor immediately if these signs or symptoms begin.
- medicines that **decrease** or inhibit cytochrome P450 1A2 or glucuronyl transferase enzymes may lead to olanzapine toxicity.

- medicines that *change* or modify blood sugar may lead to additive problems with possible olanzapine changes in blood sugar.
- medicines that *change* or modify the QT interval such as: dofetilide (Tikosyn) and other medicines such as class I, IA, or III antiarrhythmics, clarithromycin, cotrimoxazole, ondansetron, ziprazidone, and others may lead to prolongation of the QTc interval and undesirable effects. Combination is not recommended.

The following drugs may *decrease* the effects of olanzapine:

- medicines that increase (induce) cytochrome P450 1A2 or glucuronyl transferase enzymes may blunt olanzapine benefits.
- omeprazole (Prilosec).
- rifampin (Rifater, others).
- ritonavir (Norvir).

▷ *Driving, Hazardous Activities:* This drug may cause drowsiness or dizziness. Restrict activities as necessary.

Aviation Note: The use of this drug *may be a disqualification* for piloting. Consult a designated Aviation Medical Examiner.

Exposure to Sun: No problems reported.

Exposure to Heat: This medicine can cause problems in regulating body temperature (core temperature homeostasis). If you work or are frequently in a hot environment, be careful to replace enough fluids to avoid dehydration.

Heavy Exercise or Exertion: Since this medicine may cause problems in temperature regulation, caution is advised.

Discontinuation: Do not stop this medicine without first talking to your doctor. May be prudent to slowly decrease the dose (taper) it to help avoid any withdrawal syndrome.

OLSALAZINE (ohl SAL a zeen)

Introduced: 1987   **Class:**   Bowel anti-inflammatory   **Prescription:**
USA: Yes   **Controlled Drug:**   USA: No; Canada: No   **Available as**
Generic: USA: No; Canada: No
Brand Name: Dipentum

BENEFITS versus RISKS	
Possible Benefits	*Possible Risks*
EFFECTIVE SUPPRESSION OF INFLAMMATORY BOWEL DISEASE	RARE BONE MARROW DEPRESSION (see Glossary) Drug-induced hepatitis Occasional aggravation of ulcerative colitis

▷ **Principal Uses**

As a Single Drug Product: Uses currently included in FDA-approved labeling: Used to keep up remission (maintenance) of chronic ulcerative colitis and proctitis in people who do not tolerate sulfasalazine.

Other (unlabeled) generally accepted uses: (1) Has a role in treatment of active ulcerative colitis; (2) works in collagenous colitis in adults.

How This Drug Works: This drug is actually two molecules of 5-aminosalicylic acid (ASA) joined together. In the body, it is converted to the active ASA and then suppresses the formation of prostaglandins (and related compounds), tissue substances that induce inflammation, tissue destruction, and diarrhea—the main features of ulcerative colitis and proctitis.

▷ **Widely Used Guidelines That Involve This Medicine (representative sample):** Please look at the section at the very beginning of this profile called "Class." Next, turn to Table 22 and you will find guidelines listed by the class involved!

Available Dosage Forms and Strengths
Capsules — 250 mg
Tablets (Canada only) — 500 mg

▷ **Recommended Dosage Ranges: Actual dose and schedule must be determined for each patient individually.**
Infants and Children: Dose not established.
12 to 60 Years of Age: 500 mg twice daily, morning and evening.
Over 60 Years of Age: Same as 12 to 60 years of age.

Conditions Requiring Dosing Adjustments
Liver Function: No changes needed in liver disease, but since this drug can be toxic to the liver (granulomatous hepatitis), it should be used with caution by patients with liver problems.
Kidney Function: Some of the metabolites of olsalazine are eliminated by the kidneys. There is potential for kidney damage by one of these compounds, and the drug should be a benefit-to-risk decision by patients with compromised kidneys.

▷ **Dosing Instructions:** The capsule may be opened and taken with food, preferably with breakfast and dinner. If you forget a dose: Take the missed dose as soon as you remember it, unless it's nearly time for your next dose—if that is the case, skip the missed dose and take the next dose right on schedule. DON'T double doses. Talk with your doctor if you find yourself missing doses.

Usual Duration of Use: Use on a regular schedule for 1 to 3 weeks determines effectiveness in controlling the symptoms of ulcerative colitis. Ongoing treatment of up to two years has been successful in preventing relapse of ulcerative colitis. Long-term use (months to years) requires physician supervision.

Typical Treatment Goals and Measurements (Outcomes and Markers)
Ulcerative Colitis: The general goal is to lower the frequency of stools, ease cramping, reduce amount of blood in the stools, and stop fever. More involved exams will reveal an absence of bowel ulceration and easing of friability or granularity of the bowel itself. Use after sudden (acute) cases have resolved seeks to prevent relapse of ulcerative colitis.

▷ **This Drug Should Not Be Taken If**
• you have had an allergic reaction to it previously.
• you have severely impaired kidney function.
• you are allergic to aspirin or aspirinlike compounds (salicylates).

▷ **Inform Your Physician Before Taking This Drug If**
• you are allergic to aspirin (or other salicylates), mesalamine, or sulfasalazine.
• you are allergic by nature: history of hay fever, asthma, hives, eczema.
• you have impaired kidney function.
• you have severe liver disease.
• you are currently taking sulfasalazine (Azulfidine).

Possible Side Effects (natural, expected, and unavoidable drug actions)
None.

▷ **Possible Adverse Effects** (unusual, unexpected, and infrequent reactions)
  If any of the following develop, consult your physician promptly for guidance.
  Mild Adverse Effects
  Allergic reactions: skin rash, itching—rare.
  Headache, drowsiness, depression, dizziness—rare.
  Fever and chills—rare.
  Loss of appetite, indigestion, nausea, vomiting, stomach pain, diarrhea—rare to infrequent.
  Paresthesias or blurred vision—rare.
  Joint aches and pains—infrequent.
  Serious Adverse Effects
  Allergic reactions: dermatitis, hair loss—rare.
  Bone marrow depression (see Glossary): fatigue, fever, sore throat, abnormal bleeding/bruising—case reports.
  Drug-induced hepatitis (see Glossary), pericarditis, pancreatitis, or kidney damage—rare.
  Spasm of the bronchi of the lung—rare.

▷ **Possible Effects on Sexual Function:** Impotence, excessive menstrual flow—case reports.

Possible Effects on Laboratory Tests
  Complete blood cell counts: decreased red cells, hemoglobin, white cells, and platelets; increased eosinophils.
  Liver function tests: increased liver enzymes (ALT/GPT, AST/GOT, and alkaline phosphatase), increased bilirubin.
  Urinalysis: red blood cells and protein present.

CAUTION
  1. Report promptly any signs of infection or unusual bleeding or bruising.
  2. Report promptly any indications of active or intensified ulcerative colitis: abdominal cramping, bloody diarrhea, fever.
  3. Promptly call your doctor if you develop a skin rash, unexplained tiredness, sore throat or unexplained fever.

Precautions for Use
  By Infants and Children: Safety and effectiveness for those less than 12 years of age are not established.
  By Those Over 60 Years of Age: None.

▷ **Advisability of Use During Pregnancy**
  Pregnancy Category: C. See Pregnancy Risk Categories at the back of this book.
  Animal Studies: Rat studies reveal toxic effects on the fetus, retarded bone development, and impaired development of internal organs.
  Human Studies: Adequate studies of pregnant women are not available.
  Use this drug only if clearly needed. Ask your physician for guidance.

Advisability of Use If Breast-Feeding
  Presence of this drug in breast milk: Controversial, has caused diarrhea in some infants.
  Avoid drug or refrain from nursing. Talk to your doctor about a benefit-to-risk decision.

Habit-Forming Potential: None.

Effects of Overdose: Headache, dizziness, nausea, vomiting, abdominal cramping.

Possible Effects of Long-Term Use: Bone marrow depression (impaired production of blood cells).

Suggested Periodic Examinations While Taking This Drug (at physician's discretion)

Complete blood cell counts.
Liver function tests.
Kidney function tests.
Urinalysis.
Number and frequency of stools.

▷ **While Taking This Drug, Observe the Following**

Foods: No restrictions. Follow prescribed diet.

Herbal Medicines or Minerals: Flaxseed, peppermint oil, and psyllium husk have commission E monograph indications for irritable bowel syndrome. This is NOT the same as ulcerative colitis, and those products have not been studied in ulcerative colitis. Aloe, buckhorn berry or bark, cascara sagrada bark, rhubarb root, and senna should not be taken by people living with ulcerative colitis.

Beverages: No restrictions. May be taken with milk.

▷ *Alcohol:* No interactions expected.

Tobacco Smoking: No interactions expected. I advise everyone to quit smoking.

▷ *Other Drugs*

Olsalazine **taken concurrently** with

- alendronate (Fosamax) may increase risk of GI upset.
- low molecular weight heparins enoxaparin (Lovenox), Normiflo, or Fragmin (see Drug Classes) may increase bleeding risk.
- mercaptopurine (Purinethol) may lead to bone marrow depression.
- varicella vaccine (Varivax) may result in an increased risk of Reye's syndrome; this drug should be avoided for 6 weeks after the vaccine is given.
- warfarin (Coumadin) may increase INR; more frequent tests are warranted if these medicines are combined.

▷ *Driving, Hazardous Activities:* This drug may cause drowsiness or dizziness. Restrict activities as necessary.

Aviation Note: The use of this drug **may be a disqualification** for piloting. Consult a designated Aviation Medical Examiner.

Exposure to Sun: Use caution—this drug can cause photosensitization (see Glossary).

OMALIZUMAB (oh MAH liz you mab)

Introduced: 2003 **Class:** Antiasthmatic drug, IgG1kapa monoclonal antibody, IgE blocker **Prescription:** USA: Yes **Controlled Drug:** USA: No; Canada: No **Available as Generic:** USA: Yes; Canada: No

Brand Name: Xolair

Author's Note: This medicine is the first medicine that actually attaches (binds) to an immunoglobulin (IgE) on the surface of cells (mast cells and basophils) involved in releasing chemicals that lead to asthma signs and symptoms. Once omalizumab attaches to these receptors, IgE, a culprit in causing those cells to release chemicals that lead to an asthmatic attack, is not able to attach to those cells to tell them to release the compounds that cause asthma. The medicine is given as a shot under the skin (subcutaneous injection) for people 12 years old or older with moderate to severe persistent asthma. The benefit is that the shot is only given once every 2–4 weeks. The FDA approved the medicine for people who do not

get relief from typical medications, but has asked the manufacturer to continue to study cancer (malignant neoplasm) risk. In clinical trials which lasted less than a year, 0.5% of people getting omalizumab versus 0.2% of people getting a dummy shot (placebo), developed malignant neoplasms.

BENEFITS versus RISKS

Possible Benefits	*Possible Risks*
REDUCTION IN ASTHMA ATTACKS IN MODERATE TO SEVERE PERSISTENT ASTHMA	Allergic reaction
	Unknown relationship to cancer (see author's note above)
Steroid SPARING EFFECT (BENEFIT WITH LOWER DOSES)	Headache
DECREASED HOSPITALIZATIONS FOR SUDDEN ASTHMA ATTACKS	
PREVENTION OF NIGHTTIME (NOCTURNAL) ASTHMA SYMPTOMS	
2–4 WEEK DOSING SCHEDULE	
Improved quality of life	

▷ **Principal Uses**

As a Single Drug Product: Uses currently included in FDA-approved labeling: (1) Reduction of exacerbations of and symptoms of moderate to severe persistent asthma in adults and children over 12 years old who have a positive skin test or outside the body (in vitro) reaction to a perennial allergen and who do not get enough control of asthma symptoms from inhaled corticosteroids. Other (unlabeled) generally accepted uses: (1) None at present.

How This Drug Works: Prevents a substance called IgE from attaching (binding) to specific parts (high-affinity Fc epsilon RI receptor) in cells of the body (mast cells and basophils) that are actually the ones that release many of the chemicals that cause an asthma attack (release mediators of the allergic response). It also decreases the number of receptors in basophils in some patients.

▷ **Widely Used Guidelines That Involve This Medicine (representative sample):** Please look at the section at the very beginning of this profile called "Class." Next, turn to Table 22 and you will find guidelines listed by the class involved!

Available Dosage Forms and Strengths

Single use vial — 150 mg in 5 mL (once reconstituted).

▷ **Recommended Dose Ranges** (Actual dose and schedule must be determined for each patient individually.)

Infants and Children: Safety and efficacy in those less than 12 years of age not established.

12 to 60 Years of Age: Asthma:

Dosing is somewhat complicated in that it is decided by both the weight of the patient and the level of an inflammatory substance called IgE for initial dosing. For example: for a patient with a pretreatment IgE of 30–100 IU/mL who weighs 71–90 kg, 150 mg can be given every 4 weeks. For a patient with a pre-treatment IgE of 201–300 who weighs 71–90 kg, 225 mg is given every 2 weeks.

Over 60 Years of Age: Same as 12 to 60 years of age.

Conditions Requiring Dosing Adjustments
  Liver Function: Not studied in this population.
  Kidney Function: No adjustment defined.

▷ **Dosing Instructions:** Follow written instructions closely. This medicine needs to be prepared according to instructions and injected UNDER THE SKIN (subcutaneously). With the correct technique (aseptic), 1.4 mL of sterile water for injection (SWFI) is injected into a vial that contains the lyophilized medicine. The vial should be swirled (NOT SHAKEN) for about a minute. Once this initial mixing is done, the vial should be swirled for 5–10 seconds every 5 minutes. The medicine usually takes about 20 minutes to dissolve—but some vials may take longer. Talk with your doctor and pharmacist if you find yourself missing doses. Like other medicines, benefits come from using the medicine correctly. Put the next injection date on your calendar.

Usual Duration of Use: May take two to four weeks to lower IgE levels. Use on an ongoing basis requires periodic physician evaluation of response and dose adjustment.

Typical Treatment Goals and Measurements (Outcomes and Markers)
  Asthma: Signs and symptoms of asthma such as difficulty breathing (dyspnea), cough, light-headedness, and wheezing should lessen. Forced expiratory volume at one second (FEV1) and/or peak expiratory flow rate (PEF) are checked by most pulmonologists as indicators of successful treatment. If the usual benefit is not realized, call your doctor.

Possible Advantages of This Drug
  Works in a different way (novel mechanism of action) than previously available medicines. Effect may last 2–4 weeks.

▷ **This Drug Should Not Be Taken If**
  • you had an allergic reaction to it previously.

▷ **Inform Your Physician Before Taking This Drug If**
  • your breathing does not improve after taking this drug.
  • you have a history of compromised liver function (data not available).
  • you are unsure how much to take or how often to take it.

Possible Side Effects (natural, expected, and unavoidable drug actions)
  Irritation at the injection site.

▷ **Possible Adverse Effects** (unusual, unexpected, and infrequent reactions)
  If any of the following develop, consult your physician promptly for guidance.
  Mild Adverse Effects
  Allergic reactions: skin rash—infrequent.
  Headache—frequent.
  Tiredness or dizziness—infrequent.
  Serious Adverse Effects
  Allergic reactions: anaphylactic reactions—possible.
  Paradoxical worsening of asthma –one case report but questionable causation.

▷ **Possible Effects on Sexual Function:** Not defined.

Possible Delayed Adverse Effects: None defined at present.

▷ **Adverse Effects That May Mimic Natural Diseases or Disorders**
  Not defined.

Natural Diseases or Disorders That May Be Activated by This Drug
  See asthma case report above.

Possible Effects on Laboratory Tests
IgE: decreased (beneficial effect).

CAUTION
1. Dosing is adjusted to IgE only for starting dosing.
2. Serious allergic reaction (anaphylaxis) usually happens within 2 hours after a dose.
3. Call your doctor if asthma symptoms appear more often than usual, or if you begin to increase use of your rescue (immediate) bronchodilator.
5. Omalizumab should NOT be used for acute symptoms or asthma exacerbations.

Precautions for Use
By Infants and Children: Safety and effectiveness for those under 12 not established.

By Those Over 60 Years of Age: No specific instructions at present.

▷ ## Advisability of Use During Pregnancy
Pregnancy Category: B. See Pregnancy Risk Categories at the back of this book.
Human Studies: Adequate studies of pregnant women are not available.
Ask your doctor for guidance.

Advisability of Use If Breast-Feeding
Presence of this drug in breast milk: not defined in humans.
Equaled 1.5 percent of the mothers' blood levels in one kind of monkey. Avoid drug or refrain from nursing.

Habit-Forming Potential: None.

Effects of Overdose: Not defined.

Suggested Periodic Examinations While Taking This Drug (at physician's discretion)
Lung function tests such as: FEV-1 and PEFR.
Decrease in asthma attack frequency and decreased severity of symptoms.

▷ ## While Taking This Drug, Observe the Following
Foods: No restrictions.

Herbal Medicines or Minerals: Fir or pine needle oil should NOT be used by asthmatics. Ephedra alone does carry a German Commission E monograph indication for asthma treatment. If you are allergic to plants in the Asteraceae family (aster, chrysanthemum, daisy, or ragweed), you may also be allergic to echinacea, chamomile, feverfew, and St. John's wort.

Beverages: Not defined.

▷ *Alcohol:* No interactions expected.

Tobacco Smoking: Asthma may be worsened by irritation from smoking. I advise everyone to quit smoking.

▷ *Other Drugs*
Omalizumab *taken concurrently* with
• Other medicines has not been defined in the sense of drug interactions at present.

▷ *Driving, Hazardous Activities:* This drug may cause dizziness and fatigue. Restrict activities until the full extent of this effect is understood and then ask your doctor for guidance.

Aviation Note: The use of this drug *may be a disqualification* for piloting. Consult a designated Aviation Medical Examiner.

Exposure to Sun: No restrictions.

Heavy Exercise or Exertion: Use caution—this may stress the protective effects of this drug.

OMEPRAZOLE (oh MEH pra zohl)

Introduced: 1986   **Class:** Proton pump inhibitor   **Prescription:**
USA: Yes   **Controlled Drug:**   USA: No; Canada: No   **Available as**
Generic: USA: Yes; Canada: No
Brand Names: ✣Losec, Prilosec, Risek

**Author's Note: The FDA approved this medicine for nonprescription use in
2003 (see** *www.fda.gov/bbs/topics/news/2003/NEW00916.html*).

BENEFITS versus RISKS

Possible Benefits	*Possible Risks*
VERY EFFECTIVE TREATMENT OF CONDITIONS ASSOCIATED WITH EXCESSIVE PRODUCTION OF GASTRIC ACID: Zollinger-Ellison syndrome, mastocytosis, endocrine adenoma	Rare aplastic anemia Rare liver failure
VERY EFFECTIVE TREATMENT OF REFLUX ESOPHAGITIS, GASTRIC AND DUODENAL ULCERS	
EFFECTIVE IN COMBINATION WITH CLARITHROMYCIN AND AMOXICILLIN in treatment of *Helicobacter pylori* infections	
ONCE DAILY DOSING ENHANCES COMPLIANCE	
EFFECTIVE HEARTBURN TREATMENT (GERD)	
Prevention of NSAID-induced ulcers	

▷ **Principal Uses**

As a Single Drug Product: Uses currently included in FDA-approved labeling: (1) Inhibits stomach acid formation in acute and chronic gastritis, reflux esophagitis, gastroesophageal reflux disease, Zollinger-Ellison syndrome, mastocytosis, endocrine adenomas, and active duodenal ulcer; (2) approved for long-term use in erosive esophagitis; (3) approved for combination treatment (with clarithromycin [Biaxin]) in patients with positive *Helicobacter pylori* cultures (removes the bacteria in up to 92% of patients); (4) helps in the short-term treatment of active and benign stomach (gastric) ulcers; (5) part of a three-drug, 10-day regimen (omeprazole, amoxicillin, and clarithromycin) to treat duodenal ulcers.

Other (unlabeled) generally accepted uses: (1) May have a role in treating severe stomach bleeding (hemorrhagic gastritis); (2) possible use in ulcerative colitis; (3) prevention of ulcers caused by NSAIDs; (4) could be of help in asthma; (5) could help hiccups resistant to other therapy (intractable).

How This Drug Works: Inhibits a specific enzyme system (proton pump H/K ATPase) in the stomach lining, stopping production of stomach acid and thereby (1) eliminates a principal cause of the condition under treatment and (2) creates an environment conducive to healing. Taking this medicine 15–30 minutes before the morning meal makes best use of the fact that this will allow the medicine to be at its peak just when the largest number of proton pumps are working.

▷ **Widely Used Guidelines That Involve This Medicine (representative sample):** Please look at the section at the very beginning of this profile called "Class." Next, turn to Table 22 and you will find guidelines listed by the class involved!

Available Dosage Forms and Strengths
  Capsules, immediate-release — 10 mg, 20 mg, 40 mg (Canada)
    Capsules, delayed-release — 10 mg, 20mg
  Capsules, sustained-release — 10 mg, 20 mg
    Capsules, timed-release — 20 mg

▷ **Usual Adult Dosage Ranges:** *Reflux esophagitis:* 20 mg once daily 15–30 minutes before the morning meal for a duration of 4 to 8 weeks. Excessive stomach acid conditions: 60 mg once daily for as long as necessary. In extreme cases, doses of 120 mg three times a day have been used.
  Gastric and Duodenal Ulcer: 20–30 mg once daily for 4 to 8 weeks.
  Duodenal Ulcer Combination Therapy (28-day regimen): Omeprazole 40 mg daily with clarithromycin 500 mg 3 times a day for days 1–14 and then omeprazole 20 mg daily for days 15–28.
  Helicobacter Pylori: Dual drug approach: 40 mg of omeprazole once a day combined with 500 mg of clarithromycin three times a day. Treatment is continued for two weeks. Triple drug approach: Omeprazole 20 mg twice a day or 40 mg once a day with clarithromycin 500 mg and amoxicillin 1,000 mg, all given twice a day for 10 days. Patients who have (present with) an ulcer when treatment is started also get omeprazole alone at 20 mg a day for another 18 days.
  Note: Actual dose and schedule must be determined for each patient individually.

Conditions Requiring Dosing Adjustments
  Liver Function: Patients should be monitored closely.
  Kidney Function: Dose adjustments do not appear to be needed.

▷ **Dosing Instructions:** Take immediately before eating, preferably 15–30 minutes before the morning meal. The capsule should be swallowed whole without opening; the contents should not be crushed or chewed. This drug may be taken with antacids if they are needed to relieve stomach pain. If swallowing is a problem, the capsules CAN be opened and the intact granules mixed in a fruit juice (such as apple, cranberry, orange, or grape—acidic fruit juices) or a small amount of applesauce just before you take it. Don't mix with milk. If you forget a dose: Take the missed dose as soon as you remember it, unless it's nearly time for your next dose—if that is the case, skip the missed dose and take the next dose right on schedule. DO NOT double doses. Talk with your doctor and pharmacist if you find yourself missing doses.

Usual Duration of Use: Use on a regular schedule for 2 to 3 weeks determines benefit in suppressing stomach acid production. Long-term use (months to years) requires periodic physician evaluation of response, particularly where *Helicobacter pylori* is involved.

Typical Treatment Goals and Measurements (Outcomes and Markers)
  Ulcers: A proton pump inhibitor is widely recognized as the standard for short-term treatment of stomach ulcers. When *H. pylori* is present, single medicine therapy is not recommended and an antibiotic is often used with other agents. The goal is to heal the ulcer area and prevent reoccurrence

of the ulceration. Sign and symptom relief as well as endoscopic examination help define success of treatment. Negative results for *Helicobacter pylori* cultures (eradication) is the goal when that agent is present.

Possible Advantages of This Drug

Effectively inhibits acid secretion at all times: basal conditions (stomach empty and at rest) and following food, alcohol, smoking, or other stimulants. More effective than histamine (H2) receptor blocking drugs in treating severe reflux esophagitis and refractory duodenal ulcer.

Currently a Drug of Choice

For the short-term treatment of severe reflux esophagitis and the long-term treatment of Zollinger-Ellison syndrome and erosive esophagitis. Part of a one-week regimen of choice (comparing outcomes) with clarithromycin and metronidazole for treating *H. pylori*.

▷ **This Drug Should Not Be Taken If**
- you have had an allergic reaction to it previously.
- you have a currently active bone marrow or blood cell disorder.

▷ **Inform Your Physician Before Taking This Drug If**
- you have a history of liver disease or impaired liver function.
- your history includes any bone marrow or blood cell disorder, especially a drug-induced one.
- you take any anticoagulant medication or diazepam (Valium) or phenytoin (Dilantin, etc.).

Possible Side Effects (natural, expected, and unavoidable drug actions)

Acid in the stomach actually works to protect it from some bacterial infections. Since omeprazole is so effective in decreasing acid, it may increase the likelihood of infection by *Campylobacter*. This organism causes gastroenteritis. Symptoms may include mucus, loose stools, and fever. Talk with your doctor if you start to develop these symptoms while taking omeprazole.

▷ **Possible Adverse Effects** (unusual, unexpected, and infrequent reactions)

If any of the following develop, consult your physician promptly for guidance.

Mild Adverse Effects

Allergic reactions: skin rash—rare; itching.

Headache, dizziness, muscle pain or ringing in ears; drowsiness, paresthesias, weakness—rare to infrequent.

Indigestion, nausea, vomiting, diarrhea, constipation—rare to infrequent.

Serious Adverse Effects

Allergic reactions: rare allergic kidney damage (interstitial nephritis), rare anaphylactic reaction. Erythema multiforme—case report.

Bone marrow depression: fatigue, fever, sore throat, infections, abnormal bleeding/bruising—case reports.

Hemolytic anemia—case report.

Liver damage with jaundice (see Glossary)—case reports.

Low blood sugar—case report.

Chest pain or angina—case reports.

Half-facial pain—case reports.

Yeast infection (Candida) of the esophagus—possible.

Kidney inflammation (interstitial nephritis)—case reports.

Possible Effects on Sexual Function: Drug-induced male breast enlargement and tenderness (gynecomastia)—case reports.

Nocturnal erections—case report.

▷ **Adverse Effects That May Mimic Natural Diseases or Disorders**

Persistent infection or bruising may be bone marrow depression; blood counts are advisable.

Liver reactions may suggest viral hepatitis.

Possible Effects on Laboratory Tests

Complete blood cell counts: decreased red cells, hemoglobin, white cells, and platelets.

Blood glucose level: decreased.

Liver function tests: increased liver enzymes (ALT/GPT, AST/GOT, and alkaline phosphatase), increased bilirubin.

CAUTION

1. Take this drug for exactly as long as your doctor prescribed. Do not extend its use without your physician's guidance.
2. Report promptly any indications of infection.
3. Tell your doctor if you plan to take any other medications (prescription or over-the-counter) while taking omeprazole.
4. Acid in the stomach actually works to protect it from some bacterial infections. Since omeprazole is so effective in decreasing acid, it may increase the likelihood of infection by Campylobacter. This organism causes gastroenteritis. Symptoms may include mucus, loose stools, and fever. Call your doctor if this happens to you.
5. Although this drug effectively treats ulcers, it does not preclude the possibility of cancer of the stomach.

Precautions for Use

By Infants and Children: Safety and effectiveness for those less than 12 years of age are not established.

By Those Over 60 Years of Age: Slower elimination of this drug makes it possible to achieve satisfactory response with smaller doses; this reduces the risk of adverse effects. Limit the daily dose to 20 mg if possible.

▷ **Advisability of Use During Pregnancy**

Pregnancy Category: C. See Pregnancy Risk Categories at the back of this book.

Animal Studies: No drug-induced birth defects found in rats; drug-induced embryo and fetal toxicity were demonstrated in rats and rabbits.

Human Studies: Adequate studies of pregnant women are not available.

Avoid use if possible. Use only if clearly necessary and for the shortest possible time.

Advisability of Use If Breast-Feeding

Presence of this drug in breast milk: Yes.

Avoid drug or refrain from nursing.

Habit-Forming Potential: None.

Effects of Overdose: Possible drowsiness, dizziness, lethargy, abdominal pain, nausea.

Possible Effects of Long-Term Use: Some long-term (2-year) studies in rats revealed the development of drug-induced carcinoid tumors in the stomach. To date, long-term use of this drug (more than 5 years) in humans has not revealed any drug-induced tumor potential. Pending more studies of long-term human use, it is advisable to limit the use of this drug to the shortest duration possible.

Suggested Periodic Examinations While Taking This Drug (at physician's discretion)

Complete blood cell counts.

▷ **While Taking This Drug, Observe the Following**

Foods: Follow your doctor's advice.

Herbal Medicines or Minerals: Kola, guarana, mate, and ma huang may increase stomach acid, blunting the benefits of this medicine. Black cohosh root, ginkgo, and squill are contraindicated in gastrointestinal disturbances. Licorice root has a German Commission E monograph indication for gastrointestinal ulcers, but use with proton pump inhibitors has not been studied. St. John's wort has been found to increase sensitivity to the sun like this medicine. The combination is not recommended. Talk to your doctor BEFORE taking any herbals with this medicine.

Beverages: No restrictions. May be taken with milk.

▷ *Alcohol:* No interactions expected, but alcohol is best avoided; it stimulates the secretion of stomach acid.

Tobacco Smoking: Smoking may stimulate the secretion of stomach acid. I advise everyone to quit smoking.

▷ *Other Drugs*

Omeprazole may ***increase*** the effects of
- anticoagulants (warfarin, etc.) and increase the risk of bleeding.
- benzodiazepines [some such as diazepam] (see Drug Classes).
- carbamazepine (Tegretol).
- cilostazol (Pletal) by increasing an active metabolite called 3,4-dehydro cilostazol because of its action in inhibiting cytochrome P450 2C19. A lower dose of cilostazol and careful patient follow-up are prudent if these medicines must be combined.
- clonazepam (Klonopin) and some other benzodiazepines (see Drug Classes) and lead to benzodiazepine toxicity.
- cyclosporine (Sandimmune), by increasing its level (decreased levels also reported).
- diazepam (Valium) and cause excessive sedation.
- digoxin (Lanoxin) and lead to toxicity.
- disulfiram (Antabuse).
- fluvastatin (Lescol).
- methotrexate (Rheumatrex).
- phenytoin (Dilantin, etc.) or fosphenytoin (Cerebyx) and cause phenytoin or fosphenytoin toxicity.
- tacrolimus (Prograf) may increase tacrolimus levels—blood levels and adjustment of tacrolimus dosing is prudent.
- warfarin (Coumadin) and lead to bleeding; more frequent INR (prothrombin time or protime) testing is needed. Warfarin doses should be adjusted according to laboratory results.

Omeprazole ***taken concurrently*** with
- voriconazole (Vfend) or medicines that inhibit a liver enzyme involved in removing this medicine (P450-2C19) will increase the blood levels of omeprazole and make adverse effects from omeprazole more likely.

Omeprazole may ***decrease*** the effects of
- ampicillin (various).
- atazanavir (Reyataz), indinavir (Agenerase) and ritonavir (Norvir).
- clozapine (Clozaril). More frequent checks of clozapine blood levels and adjustment of dosing is prudent.
- iron preparations.
- itraconazole (Sporanox) or ketoconazole (Nizoral) may easily be addressed by taking the antifungals with a low pH cola (talk to your doctor about this).

- olanzapine (Zyprexa).
- trovafloxacin (Trovan).

▷ *Driving, Hazardous Activities:* This drug may cause drowsiness and dizziness. Limit activities as necessary.

Aviation Note: The use of this drug ***may be a disqualification*** for piloting. Consult a designated Aviation Medical Examiner.

Exposure to Sun: Photosensitivity has been reported.

Discontinuation: The duration of use will vary according to the condition under treatment and individual patient response. Premature discontinuation could result in incomplete healing or prompt recurrence of symptoms.

ONDANSETRON (on DAN sa tron)

Introduced: 1993   **Class:** Antiemetic, 5-HT3 antagonist   **Prescription:** USA: Yes   **Controlled Drug:** USA: No; Canada: No   **Available as Generic:** USA: No; Canada: No

Brand Names: Zofran, Zofran ODT, Zofran Oral Solution

BENEFITS versus RISKS	
Possible Benefits	*Possible Risks*
EFFECTIVE ORAL TREATMENT AND RELIEF OR PREVENTION OF SEVERE VOMITING	Bronchospasm
	Grand mal seizures
	Liver toxicity
EFFECTIVE PREVENTION OF VOMITING AFTER CHEMOTHERAPY	Heart rate and rhythm changes
	Low potassium
	(All rare)
EFFECTIVE PREVENTION OF VOMITING AFTER SURGERY	
EFFECTIVE PREVENTION OF VOMITING AFTER RADIATION TREATMENT	
ODT FORM ALLOWS THIS DRUG TO BE CONVENIENTLY TAKEN WITHOUT WATER	

▷ **Principal Uses**

As a Single Drug Product: Uses currently included in FDA-approved labeling: (1) Prevention of nausea and vomiting associated with initial and repeat courses of chemotherapy; (2) treatment or prevention of postoperative nausea and vomiting; (3) prevention or treatment of emesis (vomiting) caused by radiation therapy.

Other (unlabeled) generally accepted uses: (1) Helps patients keep from vomiting up medicines used to treat drug overdoses; (2) may have a role in treating schizophrenia and a movement problem (tardive dyskinesia or TD) seen with some medicines used to treat TD; (3) some data reducing the number of panic attacks; (4) eases some tremor cases.

How This Drug Works: Ondansetron antagonizes 5-HT3 receptors. It appears to block vomiting by blocking serotonin (a chemical causing a signal to the brain via vagal neurons) at 5-HT3 receptors keeping a message to vomit from getting to the brain.

▷ **Widely Used Guidelines That Involve This Medicine (representative sample):** Please look at the section at the very beginning of this profile called "Class." Next, turn to Table 22 and you will find guidelines listed by the class involved!

Available Dosage Forms and Strengths
  Intravenous — 2 mg/mL
  Oral solution — 4 mg/5 mL
      Tablets — 4 mg, 8 mg, 24 mg
  Tablets, ODT — 4 mg, 8 mg

▷ **Recommended Dosage Ranges** (Actual dose and schedule must be determined for each patient individually.)
  Infants and Children: Little information is available regarding use in those less than 3 years old.
  4 to 11 Years of Age: Vomiting from chemotherapy—one 4-mg tablet or 5 mL of the oral solution is given three times by mouth daily. The method and frequency are then the same as for adults.
  12 to 60 Years of Age: One 24-mg tablet for medicines such as cisplatin which is highly likely to lead to vomiting. For *chemotherapy* that poses a moderate risk of vomiting (moderately emetogenic chemo), 8 mg is given twice a day. The first dose should be taken 30 minutes before the start of the chemotherapy. Subsequent doses should be taken 8 hours after the first dose. Further doses of 8 mg every 12 hours are taken for 1–2 days after chemotherapy is finished.
  Vomiting from Radiation Therapy—8 mg three times a day. Doses are started 1–2 hours BEFORE radiation treatment. Doses after radiation are given every 8 hours for 1–2 days.
  Postoperative Nausea and Vomiting—one 16-mg dose one hour before anesthesia is given.
  Panic Attacks: one to two mg twice a day have worked in some cases (more effective than a sugar pill or placebo).
  Over 60 Years of Age: Same as 12 to 60 years of age.

Conditions Requiring Dosing Adjustments
  Liver Function: Maximum dose for people with severe liver failure is 8 mg per day.
  Kidney Function: Studies have not been conducted on patients with impaired kidneys. The decision to use ondansetron must be made by your physician. Only 5 to 10% of the drug is removed unchanged by the kidneys. Based on this small involvement of the kidneys, no changes are expected to be needed with short-term use.

▷ **Dosing Instructions:** May be taken on an empty stomach. DO NOT push the ODT form through the blister pack—simply peel back the foil before you take it. If you forget a dose: Take the missed dose as soon as you remember it, unless it's nearly time for your next dose—if that is the case, skip the missed dose and take the next dose right on schedule. DO NOT double doses. Talk with your doctor if you find yourself missing doses.

Usual Duration of Use: Since chemotherapy can cause vomiting long after it has been given, continual use on a regular schedule for 3 days is usually necessary.

Typical Treatment Goals and Measurements (Outcomes and Markers)
  Vomiting: The goal is to prevent or at least to decrease vomiting (emesis) frequency, amount or severity.

Possible Advantages of This Drug

Effective oral prevention of severe vomiting caused by some kinds of chemotherapy that have been poorly controlled by earlier agents. Orally disintegrating tablets (ODT) form dissolves in a few seconds on the tongue WITHOUT water. If panic attack data stands up to further testing, this medicine will offer a more desirable mental status side effect profile than other medicines for use in children.

Currently a "Drug of Choice"

For control of vomiting secondary to emetogenic (likely to cause vomiting) cancer chemotherapy.

▷ **This Drug Should Not Be Taken If**
- you had an allergic reaction to it or to a different 5HT antagonist (cross sensitivity possible).

▷ **Inform Your Physician Before Taking This Drug If**
- you have a history of liver disease.
- you have a history of kidney disease.
- you have a history of alcoholism.
- you have a history of PKU (ODT form has phenylalanine).
- you are unsure how much to take or how often to take it.

Possible Side Effects (natural, expected, and unavoidable drug actions)
Constipation, sedation.

▷ **Possible Adverse Effects** (unusual, unexpected, and infrequent reactions)
If any of the following develop, consult your physician promptly for guidance.

Mild Adverse Effects
Allergic reactions: skin rash—rare.
Headache—frequent.
Dizziness and light-headedness, constipation, diarrhea, dry mouth—infrequent.

Serious Adverse Effects
Allergic reactions: anaphylaxis—rare.
Extrapyramidal reactions (abnormal body movements) or seizures (intravenous form)—case reports.
Bronchospasm—rare.
Liver failure—one case report in a patient with hepatitis B.
Angina, tachycardia, arrhythmias—all rare.
Hypokalemia (low potassium)—rare (intravenous form).

▷ **Possible Effects on Sexual Function:** None reported.

Possible Delayed Adverse Effects: None reported.

▷ **Adverse Effects That May Mimic Natural Diseases or Disorders**
Changes in liver enzymes may mimic hepatitis, but specific antibodies will not be present. Bronchospasm may mimic asthma.

Natural Diseases or Disorders That May Be Activated by This Drug
Epilepsy, asthma.

Possible Effects on Laboratory Tests
Liver function tests: Transient increases in SGPT, SGOT, and bilirubin.

CAUTION
1. Even though you do not feel an urge to vomit, continue ondansetron for the prescribed length of therapy. The vomit-causing effect of cancer

chemotherapy or radiation therapy continues **after** the medicine or radiation has been given.
2. The ODT form contains phenylalanine.
3. Use after abdominal surgery may hide (mask) swelling of the stomach (gastric distension) and possible progressive intestinal block (ileus).

Precautions for Use

By Infants and Children: Safety and effectiveness for those under 3 years of age are not established.

By Those Over 60 Years of Age: Same as for general adult population.

▷ **Advisability of Use During Pregnancy**

Pregnancy Category: B. See Pregnancy Risk Categories at the back of this book.

Animal Studies: Drug and its metabolites pass into the milk. No adverse effects on gestation, postnatal development, or reproductive performance have been observed in rats.

Human Studies: Adequate studies of pregnant women are not available. Ask your physician for guidance.

Advisability of Use If Breast-Feeding

Presence of this drug in breast milk: This medicine is excreted in the milk of rats; human data is not available.

Caution should be used if this medicine is to be used by nursing mothers.

Habit-Forming Potential: None.

Effects of Overdose: Doses 10 times greater than recommended have not resulted in illness.

Possible Effects of Long-Term Use: Not indicated for long-term use.

Suggested Periodic Examinations While Taking This Drug (at physician's discretion)

Observe for vomiting occurrence and frequency.

▷ **While Taking This Drug, Observe the Following**

Foods: No restrictions.

Herbal Medicines or Minerals: Since St. John's wort may act to increase serotonin, the combination is not advised. Since part of the way ginkgo and ginseng work may be as a MAO inhibitor, do not combine them with ondansetron.

Beverages: No restrictions.

▷ *Alcohol:* Additive sedation and potential additive urge to vomit if alcohol is taken in large doses. Alcohol abuse that has led to liver problems may limit the total dose that can be taken.

Tobacco Smoking: No direct clinical interactions; I advise everyone to quit smoking.

Marijuana Smoking: May induce additive sedation and provide additive antiemetic effects.

▷ *Other Drugs*

The following drugs may ***increase*** the effects of ondansetron:
- allopurinol (Zyloprim).
- cimetidine (Tagamet).
- disulfiram (Antabuse).
- fluconazole (Diflucan).
- isoniazid (Nydrazid).
- macrolide antibiotics (erythromycin, azithromycin, clarithromycin, dirithromycin).

- metronidazole (Flagyl).
- monoamine oxidase (MAO) inhibitor antidepressants (Nardil).
- ritonavir (Norvir) and perhaps other protease inhibitors (see Drug Classes).

Ondansetron *taken concurrently* with:

- amiodarone (Cordarone) may lead to abnormal heartbeat or rhythm (QT changes and torsades de pointes).
- dofetilide (Tikosyn) and other medicines such as class I, IA, or III antiarrhythmics, clarithromycin, cotrimoxazole, ondansetron, ziprazidone, and others may lead to prolongation of the QTc interval and undesirable effects. Combination is not recommended.

The following drugs may *decrease* the effects of ondansetron:

- barbiturates.
- carbamazepine (Tegretol).
- phenylbutazone (Butazolidin, Azolid).
- phenytoin (Dilantin).
- rifabutin (Mycobutin).
- rifampin (Rifadin).
- tolbutamide (Orinase).

▷ *Driving, Hazardous Activities:* This drug may cause drowsiness and dizziness. Restrict activities as necessary.

Aviation Note: The use of this drug *may be a disqualification* for piloting. Consult a designated Aviation Medical Examiner.

Exposure to Sun: No restrictions.

Special Storage Instructions: Keep at room temperature. Avoid exposing this medicine to extreme humidity.

Discontinuation: Ondansetron may be stopped after you've completed the prescribed course (usually 3 days) of therapy.

ORAL CONTRACEPTIVES (or al kon tra SEP tivs)

Other Names: Estrogens/progestins, OCs, birth control pills

Introduced: 1956   **Class:**   Female sex hormones   **Prescription:** USA: Yes   **Controlled Drug:**   USA: No; Canada: No   **Available as Generic:**   USA: Yes, in some forms; Canada: No

Brand Names: Alesse, Brevicon, Cyclessa, Demulen, Desogen, Enovid, Estrostep FE, Genora, Gestodene, Jenest 28, Levlen, Levlite, Levora, Loestrin, Low-Ogestrel, Lo/Ovral, Micronor, ✽Minestrin 1/20, Min-Ovral, Mircette, Modicon, Necon, NEE, Nelova, Nelova 1/50 M, Nelova 10/11, Norcept-E 1/35, Nordette, Norethin 1/35E, Norethin 1/50M, Norinyl, Norlestrin, Nor-Q.D., Ortho-Cept 21, Ortho-Evra (patch form), Ortho Cyclen, Ortho-Novum 777, Ortho Tri-Cyclen, Ovcon, Ovral, Ovrette, Preven, Seasonale, ✽Synphasic, Tri-Levlen, Tri-Norinyl, Triphasil, Triquilar, Trivora, Yasmin, Zovia

---

BENEFITS versus RISKS

Possible Benefits	*Possible Risks*
HIGHLY EFFECTIVE FOR CONTRACEPTIVE PROTECTION	SERIOUS, LIFE-THREATENING THROMBOEMBOLIC DISORDERS in susceptible individuals
SEASONALE FORM PREVENTS CONTRACEPTION AND REDUCES THE NUMBER OF MENSTRUAL PERIODS TO FOUR A YEAR	Hypertension
	Fluid retention
OVCON 25 HAS AN APPROVED CHEWABLE FORM	Intensification of migrainelike headaches and fibrocystic breast changes
Moderately effective as adjunctive treatment in management of excessive menses and endometriosis	Accelerated growth of uterine fibroid tumors
	Drug-induced hepatitis with jaundice
Helps decrease the risk of ovarian cancer while the pill is being taken	Benign liver tumors—rare
Some forms decrease acne (especially Estrostep, Ortho Tri-Cyclen, and Alesse)	

▷ **Principal Uses**

As a Single Drug Product: Uses currently included in FDA-approved labeling: (1) Prevention of conception—the "Mini-Pill" contains only one component, a progestin; this has been shown to be slightly less effective than the combination of estrogen and progestin in preventing pregnancy; (2) used in cases where women do not make enough hormones (female hypogonadism); (3) helps decrease excessive blood flow at menstruation (hypermenorrhea); (4) of use in endometriosis as the combination mestranol and norethynodrel; (5) Estrostep and Ortho Tri-Cyclen are approved to prevent acne.

As a Combination Drug Product [CD]: Uses currently included in FDA-approved labeling: (1) Most oral contraceptives consist of a combination of an estrogen and a progestin; these products are the most effective form of medicinal contraception available; (2) they are sometimes used to treat menstrual irregularity, excessively heavy menstrual flow, and endometriosis; (3) norgestimate and ethinyl estradiol combination product (Ortho Tri-Cyclen) is used to treat acne in females over 15.

Other (unlabeled) generally accepted uses: (1) Gestodene has been reported to inhibit certain breast cancer cell lines (clinical studies are needed); (2) may have a protective effect against osteoporosis; (3) triphasic oral contraceptives can help in the prevention or treatment of menopause symptoms; (4) may have a role in rheumatoid arthritis, but the data are conflicting; (5) sometimes used around the time of menopause (perimenopausally) to provide regularity of menstruation; (6) used to reduce LH surges in order to improve results from in vitro fertilization or embryo transfer; (7) used as emergency contraception or a morning-after pill (MAP) or EC—while Preven is the only dedicated product for this use, Alesse, Ovral, Ovrette, Nordette, Levlen, Levlite, Levora, Lo/Ovral, Trivora, and Tri-Levlen have FDA safe and effective ratings as emergency contraceptives; (8) some forms may benefit osteoporosis; (9) Alesse form has an application pending for use in acne.

Author's Note: Research linked the number of times a woman ovulates to increased risk of ovarian cancer. This finding was associated with

a P-53 gene, which may account for as much as 50% of ovarian cancer. Since birth control pills decrease the number of times that women ovulate, they may have a role in helping prevent cancer in women found to carry the P-53 gene. Further research is required. While the patch form is not technically a "pill," it is a contraceptive. Information has been included in this profile. Ortho Evra offers a novel benefit in ease of taking the product (adherence). Emergency contraception (the morning after pills or EC) have become an area of controversy with some groups advocating that these forms be provided without a prescription. One study in London found pharmacists as a unique and valuable resource for supplying and counseling on those progestogen only emergency contraceptives.

How These Drugs Work: When estrogen and progestin are taken in sufficient doses and on a regular basis, the blood and tissue levels of these hormones increase to resemble those that occur during pregnancy. This results in suppression of the two pituitary gland hormones that normally cause ovulation (the formation and release of an egg by the ovary). In addition, these drugs may (1) alter the cervical mucus so that it resists the passage of sperm and (2) alter the lining of the uterus so that it resists implantation of the egg (if ovulation occurs).

▷ **Widely Used Guidelines That Involve This Medicine (representative sample):** Please look at the section at the very beginning of this profile called "Class." Next, turn to Table 22 and you will find guidelines listed by the class involved!

Available Dosage Forms and Strengths

Tablets: Several combinations of synthetic estrogens and progestins in varying strengths; see the package label of the brand prescribed. Seasonale form is a 91-day dosing approach.

Patch: Ortho-Evra form is a combination of estrogen (ethinyl estradiol) and progestin (norelgestromin).

▷ **Usual Adult Dosage Ranges:** For contraception: Start with the first tablet on the fifth day after the onset of menstruation. Follow with one tablet daily (taken at the same time each day) for 21 consecutive days. Resume treatment on the eighth day following the last tablet taken during the preceding cycle. The schedule is to take the drug daily for 3 weeks and to omit it for 1 week. For the Mini-Pill (progestin only), initiate treatment on the first day of menstruation and take one tablet daily, every day, throughout the year (no interruption). The Mircette brand uses 20 mcg of ethinyl estradiol and 150 mcg of dogesterel for 21 days. Two days of dummy (placebo) tablets are then taken and then five days of 10 mcg ethinyl estradiol. Seasonale form is an extended cycle form (84 active and 7 inactive pills). For the patch form, the system uses a 28-day cycle. Patches are worn for three weeks out of the 28-day cycle followed by a seven day patch-free period (see Dosing Instructions).

Emergency contraception (MAP): This is a critical situation. Talk to your doctor to be certain that you understand the possible side effects (nausea, etc.) and other issues and medical follow-up required for this procedure.

Author's Note: Seasonale form is a combination of ethinyl estradiol and levonorgestrel. Thus the first 91-day dosing (84 active pills and 7 dummy or placebo pills). This reduces the number of menstrual periods to four a year.

Note: Actual dose and schedule must be determined for each patient individually.

Conditions Requiring Dosing Adjustments

Liver Function: Should NOT be taken if you have liver disease.

Kidney Function: Oral contraceptives are not significantly eliminated by the kidneys.

▷ **Dosing Instructions:** Combination products versus biphasic or triphasic forms are started in ways specific to the product. Make certain that you understand this. The tablets may be crushed and taken with or after food to reduce stomach upset. To ensure regular (every day) use and uniform blood levels, it is best to take the tablet at the same time daily. See specific instructions for the Seasonale form. For the patch form, it is best to apply the patch at the same time and on the same day of the week. If you forget a dose (varies with the birth control form): For triphasic forms (Tri-Leven, Tri-Norinyl or Triphasil): Take the missed dose as soon as you remember. If you only remember on the next day, take two pills for the next two days, then return to your regular schedule, but USE ANOTHER TYPE OF BIRTH CONTROL UNTIL YOUR PERIOD BEGINS. Call your doctor for help. If you miss three pills in a row, stop the remaining pills for the month, USE A DIFFERENT KIND OF BIRTH CONTROL UNTIL YOUR PERIOD STARTS, and call your doctor. Your doctor will advise you as to when to re-start (usually just the same as when you first started the pills) with a new dose pack. For other birth control pill forms, if you forget a dose, call your doctor for detailed instructions.

When the patch is first used, a woman should wait until the day that her period (menstruation) starts. Two options are then available: a first day start or a Sunday start. For the first day start, the patch is applied during the first 24 hours of the menstrual period. The day that the patch is applied is day one. If the patch is applied after day one of the menstrual cycle, a backup (nonhormonal) form of contraception should be used at the same time as the patch for the first seven consecutive days that the patch is worn during the first treatment. The "patch change day" will be on the same day every week. Every new patch is applied on the same day and best applied at the same time of day. For example, if the patch is applied on a Tuesday, seven days later, the old patch will be removed and the next patch will be applied—keeping the same Tuesday schedule. Only one patch should be worn at a time. Patches are applied for three weeks in a row, followed by a seven-day patch-free interval. The process then repeats. Patches should be applied to healthy and intact skin which is clean and dry. It can be placed on the abdomen, buttocks, upper arm (outer portion), or upper torso. Never place the patch on the breasts.

Author's Note: One popular women's magazine advocated placing birth control pills in the vagina. This was presented as an option, but unless directed by your doctor, can lead to subtherapeutic benefits (and possible pregnancy) with most pills currently on the market. Talk to your doctor.

Possible Advantages of These Drugs

Effective control of conception. Mircette form may benefit women who have migraines the second week they are "off the pill." A study of 46,000 British women released in early 1999 showed that women who took the pill did not show any increased risk of cancer. These data are important because of the large number of women and also because they were studied for 25 years. A Swedish study showed that oral contraceptives may increase bone density in women who take the pill between the ages of 30 and 40. Patch form

(Ortho Evra) offers great benefits in ease of use (once weekly application for 3 weeks with one week off). Seasonale form reduces the number of periods (menstruation) to four per year.

Usual Duration of Use: According to individual needs and circumstances. Long-term use (months to years) requires physician supervision and evaluation every 6 months.

Typical Treatment Goals and Measurements (Outcomes and Markers)
Contraceptive: The goal is to avoid pregnancy. Serum pregnancy tests (you have to have blood drawn for this) are presently the most sensitive tests to rule out pregnancy.

▷ **These Drugs Should Not Be Taken If**
- you have had an allergic reaction to any dose form of it.
- you have a history of thrombophlebitis, embolism, heart attack, or stroke.
- you have breast cancer.
- you have a weakness of the adrenal gland or impaired kidney function (Yasmin brand).
- you have active liver disease, seriously impaired liver function or a history of liver tumor.
- you have diabetes and have developed circulatory disease.
- you have high blood pressure.
- you have not had any periods (amenorrhea).
- you have abnormal and unexplained vaginal bleeding.
- you have sickle cell disease.
- you are pregnant.

▷ **Inform Your Physician Before Taking These Drugs If**
- you have had an adverse reaction to any oral contraceptive.
- you have a history of cancer of the breast or reproductive organs.
- you have fibrocystic breast changes, uterine fibroid tumors, endometriosis, migrainelike headaches, epilepsy, asthma, elevated lipids, prolapse of the mitral valve of the heart, heart disease, high blood pressure, gallbladder disease, diabetes, or porphyria.
- you are over 40. This was an age-related limit previously, but current thinking says that use of these medicines may be a benefit-to-risk decision.
- you have been prescribed an antibiotic (some antibiotics may blunt the benefits of oral contraceptives and REQUIRE use of an alternative birth control method).
- you are using St. John's wort for depression.
- you have a history of or have kidney (renal disease or dysfunction) and are to take the Yasmin form.
- you smoke tobacco on a regular basis.
- you plan to have surgery in the near future.

Possible Side Effects (natural, expected, and unavoidable drug actions)
Fluid retention, weight gain, "breakthrough" bleeding (spotting in middle of menstrual cycle), altered menstrual pattern, lack of menstruation (during and following cessation of drug), increased susceptibility to yeast infection of the genital tissues. Tannish pigmentation of the face. Modest increases in blood pressure.

▷ **Possible Adverse Effects** (unusual, unexpected, and infrequent reactions)
If any of the following develop, consult your physician promptly for guidance.

Mild Adverse Effects
Allergic reactions: skin rash, hives, itching.
Headache, nervous tension, irritability, accentuation of migraine headaches—infrequent to frequent.
Rise in blood pressure (in some people)—possible.
Nausea, perhaps with vomiting—frequent (related to estrogen) and may ease if taken with evening meals.
Reduced tolerance to contact lenses or impaired color vision: blue tinge to objects, blue halo around lights—possible.

Serious Adverse Effects
Allergic reactions: anaphylaxis, erythema multiforme, and nodosum (skin reactions), loss of scalp hair.
Idiosyncratic reactions: joint and muscle pains.
Emotional depression—frequent.
Eye changes: optic neuritis, retinal thrombosis, altered curvature of the cornea, cataracts—possible.
Gallbladder disease, benign liver tumors, jaundice—case reports.
Ischemic colitis—case report.
Enlargement of uterine fibroid tumors—possible.
Abnormal glucose tolerance (hyperglycemia)—frequent in people with pregnancy (gestational) diabetes.
Thrombophlebitis (inflammation of a vein with formation of blood clot): pain or tenderness in thigh or leg, with or without swelling of foot or leg—increased risk, especially with high estrogen doses.
Drug-induced porphyria or worsening of systemic lupus erythematosus (SLE)—case reports.
Esophageal ulcers (especially if the medicine is taken lying down with no water)—case reports.
Stroke (blood clot in brain): headaches, blackout, sudden weakness or paralysis of any part of the body, severe dizziness, altered vision, slurred speech, inability to speak—possible increased risk (more probable in one study with high-dose estrogen formulations).
Heart attack (blood clot in coronary artery): sudden pain in chest, neck, jaw or arm; weakness; sweating; nausea—increased risk (not seen with low-dose estrogen products)—possible increased risk with use in women having cardiovascular risk factors, taking pills with more than 50 mcg of estrogen and in those who smoke.
Increased potassium—possible (Yasmin form).
Liver cancer—possible increased risk with long-term use.

▷ **Possible Effects on Sexual Function:** Altered character of menstruation; mid-cycle spotting—may be frequent.
Increased or decreased libido—possible.
Breast enlargement and tenderness with milk production—possible.
Absent menstruation and infertility (temporary) after discontinuation of drug.

Possible Delayed Adverse Effects: Estrogens taken during pregnancy can predispose the female child to the later development of cancer of the vagina or cervix following puberty. Nonpregnant use does not increase breast cancer.

▷ **Adverse Effects That May Mimic Natural Diseases or Disorders**
Liver reactions may suggest viral hepatitis. Increased blood pressure may mimic increased blood pressure from other causes.

Natural Diseases or Disorders That May Be Activated by These Drugs

Latent hypertension, diabetes mellitus, clotting factor disorders that favor blood clots, acute intermittent porphyria, lupus erythematosus-like syndrome.

Possible Effects on Laboratory Tests

Blood lupus erythematosus (LE) cells: positive.

Blood-clotting time or INR: decreased.

Blood amylase and lipase levels: increased (very rare pancreatitis).

Blood total cholesterol, HDL, LDL and VLDL cholesterol levels: usually no effects; some variability, depending upon estrogen and progestin content of preparation used.

Blood triglyceride levels: no effect to increased, depending upon estrogen and progestin content of preparation used.

Blood glucose level: increased.

Blood potassium: increased (Yasmin form).

Blood thyroid-stimulating hormone (TSH) level: no effect.

Blood thyroid hormone levels: T3 and T4 increased; free T4 either no effect or decreased.

Liver function tests: increased liver enzymes (ALT/GPT, AST/GOT, alkaline phosphatase) and bilirubin.

CAUTION

1. Serious adverse effects due to these drugs are a very low risk. However, any unusual development should be reported and evaluated promptly by your doctor.

2. Studies indicate that women over 30 years of age who smoke and use oral contraceptives are at significantly greater risk of having a serious cardiovascular event than are nonusers.

3. The risk of thromboembolism increases with the amount of estrogen in the product and the age of the user. Low-estrogen combinations are advised. One larger United Kingdom study failed to find a difference in risk of unknown cause venous thromboembolism when combination oral contraceptives containing less than 50 micrograms of ethinyl estradiol were used. Other data says that combining smoking, asthma history, history of blood clots, increased body mass index with high estrogen combining pills increases risks of thromboembolism.

4. It is advisable to stop these drugs 1 month prior to elective surgery to reduce the risk of postsurgical thromboembolism. If they can't be stopped, preventive use of anticoagulants may be prudent.

5. Investigate promptly any alteration or disturbance of vision that occurs during the use of these drugs.

6. Investigate promptly the nature of recurrent, persistent, or severe headaches that develop while taking these drugs.

7. Observe for significant change of mood. Call your doctor if depression develops.

8. Certain commonly used drugs may reduce the effectiveness of oral contraceptives. Some of these are listed in the category of Other Drugs below.

9. Diarrhea lasting more than a few hours (and occurring during the days the drug is taken) can prevent adequate absorption of these drugs and impair their effectiveness as contraceptives.

10. If two consecutive menstrual periods are missed, ask your doctor if you should get a pregnancy test. Do not continue to use these drugs until you know whether you are pregnant.

11. **Many antibiotics may lower or stop the effectiveness of birth control pills** (oral contraceptives). If your doctor prescribes an antibiotic, ask whether a different method of birth control is needed.
12. One researcher uses the acronym ACHES (A=abdominal pain, C=chest pain, H=headaches, E=eye problems and S=severe leg pain) to list signs of adverse effects that require a patient taking these medicines to call her doctor immediately.
13. One 8-year study found that women who used oral contraceptives IN THE PAST do not have an increased risk of cardiovascular disease.

▷ **Advisability of Use During Pregnancy**
Pregnancy Category: X. See Pregnancy Risk Categories at the back of this book.
Animal Studies: Genital defects reported in mice and guinea pigs; cleft palate reported in rodents.
Human Studies: Information from studies of pregnant women indicates that estrogens can masculinize the female fetus. In addition, limb defects and heart malformations have been reported. It is now known that estrogens taken during pregnancy can predispose the female child to the development of cancer of the vagina or cervix following puberty.
Avoid these drugs completely during entire pregnancy.

Advisability of Use If Breast-Feeding
Presence of these drugs in breast milk: Yes, in minute amounts (ethinyl estradiol or norethindrone). These drugs may suppress milk formation if started early after delivery.
Breast-feeding is considered to be safe during the use of oral contraceptives.

Habit-Forming Potential: None.

Effects of Overdose: Headache, drowsiness, nausea, vomiting, fluid retention, abnormal vaginal bleeding, breast enlargement and discomfort.

Possible Effects of Long-Term Use: High blood pressure, gallbladder disease with stones, accelerated growth of uterine fibroid tumors, absent menstruation, and impaired fertility after discontinuation of drug.

Suggested Periodic Examinations While Taking These Drugs (at physician's discretion)
Regular (every 6 months) evaluation of the breasts and pelvic organs, including Pap smears.
Liver function tests as indicated.

▷ **While Taking These Drugs, Observe the Following**
Foods: Avoid excessive use of salt if fluid retention occurs. Excessive vitamin C may increase risk of contraceptive failure.
Herbal Medicines or Minerals: Black cohosh appears to work by (1) suppressing luteinizing hormone; (2) binding to estrogen receptors in the pituitary and inhibiting luteinizing hormone release and (3) binding to estrogen receptors in the pituitary. The net effect is that this herb eases symptoms of menopause, but little is known about long-term use or heart and bone protective effects. This herb may lower the effectiveness of birth control pills. Talk to your doctor before starting black cohosh if you are currently taking estrogen or an estrogen-containing product. DHEA (dehydroepiandrosterone) may lead to signs and symptoms of too much estrogen. Androstenedione (Triple Stack, Andro-Surge, others) with ongoing use actually increases estrogen levels and should not be combined. Since St. John's wort and this drug may cause increased sun sensitivity, caution is advised. St. John's wort may blunt contraceptive effects and result in unwanted

pregnancy. Ginseng does have actions similar to estrogen. Combined use should be avoided until more data are available.

Beverages: No specific restrictions, but caffeine will stay in the body (increased half-life) longer and caffeine consumption should decrease while patients are on the pill. May be taken with milk.

▷   *Alcohol:* No interactions expected.

Tobacco Smoking: Studies indicate that smoking—especially heavy smoking (15 or more cigarettes daily) while taking oral contraceptives significantly increases the risk of heart attack (coronary thrombosis). Heavy smoking should be considered a contraindication to the use of oral contraceptives. DO NOT SMOKE while taking these medicines. I advise everyone to quit smoking.

▷   *Other Drugs*

Oral contraceptives may ***increase*** the effects of
- alprazolam (Xanax) and other benzodiazepines (see Drug Classes).
- some benzodiazepines (see Drug Classes) and cause excessive sedation.
- cyclosporine (Sandimmune) and cause toxicity.
- metoprolol (Lopressor) and cause excessive beta-blocker effects.
- prednisolone and prednisone and other corticosteroids such as dexamethasone may lead to excessive cortisonelike effects.
- ropinirole (Requip).
- selegiline (Eldepryl, others), leading to increased selegiline adverse effects risk.
- tacrine (Cognex).
- tacrolimus (Prograf). Blood levels and tacrolimus dosing changes may be needed.
- theophyllines (Theo-Dur, others) and increase the risk of toxic effects.

Oral contraceptives ***taken concurrently*** with
- antibiotics (such as amoxicillin or ampicillin) can seriously impair effectiveness and allow pregnancy to occur.
- antidiabetic drugs (oral hypoglycemic agents) may cause unpredictable fluctuations of blood sugar.
- arginine (R-Gene intravenous) may result in falsely increased growth hormone levels during pituitary function testing. Results of the arginine test should be interpreted with caution.
- ascorbic acid (vitamin C) may result in increased levels of ethinyl estradiol and breakthrough bleeding if the vitamin C is stopped.
- atorvastatin (Lipitor) leading to increased ethinyl estradiol and norethindrone levels.
- efavirenz (Sustiva), leading to increased ethinyl estradiol levels.
- liothyronine (Thyrostat) may lower benefits from thyroid supplementation in people with a functional thyroid gland. Liothyronine dosing may need to be adjusted.
- tricyclic antidepressants (Elavil, Sinequan, others) may enhance their adverse effects and reduce their antidepressant effectiveness.
- troleandomycin (TAO) may increase occurrence of liver toxicity and jaundice.
- warfarin (Coumadin) may cause unpredictable alterations of prothrombin activity; more frequent INR (prothrombin time or protime) testing is needed, and warfarin dosing should be adjusted to laboratory test results.
- zolmitriptan (Zomig) or naratriptan (Amerge) may lead to "triptan" toxicity.
- The following drugs may ***decrease*** the effects of oral contraceptives (and impair their effectiveness):

- barbiturates (phenobarbital, etc.; see Drug Classes).
- carbamazepine (Tegretol).
- fluconazole (Diflucan).
- griseofulvin (Fulvicin, etc.).
- nelfinavir (Viracept).
- nevirapine (Viramune).
- penicillins (ampicillin, penicillin V).
- phenytoin (Dilantin) or fosphenytoin (Cerebyx).
- pioglitazone (Actos) may possibly interact.
- primidone (Mysoline).
- rifampin (Rifadin, Rimactane).
- ritonavir (Norvir), amprenavir (Agenerase), atazanavir (Reyataz) and perhaps other protease inhibitors (see Drug Classes).
- tetracyclines (see Drug Classes).
- topiramate (Topamax).

▷ *Driving, Hazardous Activities:* Usually no restrictions. Consult your physician for assessment of individual risk and for guidance regarding specific restrictions.

Aviation Note: Usually no restrictions, but watch for the rare occurrence of disturbed vision and restrict activities accordingly. Consult a designated Aviation Medical Examiner.

Exposure to Sun: Use caution—these drugs can cause photosensitivity (see Glossary).

Discontinuation: Do not stop these drugs if "breakthrough" bleeding occurs. If spotting or bleeding continues, call your doctor. A higher-estrogen pill may be required. Remember: Omitting this drug for only 1 day may allow pregnancy to occur. It is best to avoid pregnancy for 3 to 6 months after stopping these drugs; aborted fetuses from women who became pregnant within 6 months after discontinuation reveal significantly increased chromosome abnormalities.

ORLISTAT (OAR li stat)

Introduced: 1999   **Class:**   Weight loss agent, lipase inhibitor   **Prescription:**   USA: Yes   **Controlled Drug:**   USA: No; Canada: No
Available as Generic: USA: No; Canada: No
Brand Name: Xenical

BENEFITS versus RISKS

Possible Benefits	*Possible Risks*
EFFECTIVE REDUCTION IN WEIGHT WHEN USED IN CONJUNCTION WITH A REDUCED-CALORIE DIET	Reduced absorption of fat-soluble vitamins (A, D, E, K) and beta carotene
HELPS REDUCE RISK FOR WEIGHT GAIN AFTER PREVIOUS WEIGHT LOSS	Fecal incontinence and flatulence
WEIGHT LOSS HELPS DECREASE RISK OF DIABETES AND CORONARY HEART DISEASE	
LOWERED TOTAL CHOLESTEROL	
DECREASED LOW DENSITY LIPOPROTEINS	
INCREASED HIGH DENSITY LIPOPROTEINS	
USED FOR UP TO FOUR YEARS WITH BENEFICIAL EFFECTS	
Possible beneficial decreases in blood pressure	

▷ **Principal Uses**

As a Single Drug Product: Uses currently included in FDA-approved labeling: (1) Reduces weight in patients with a body mass index (BMI) of 30 kg/square meter or greater or in those with a BMI of 27 kg/square meter with other risk factors (such as diabetes, high blood pressure, or high blood lipids); (2) helps maintain weight loss in patients who have already lost weight.

Other (unlabeled) generally accepted uses: (1) May have a role in type 2 diabetes because weight loss was associated with better blood sugar control; (2) could have a role in some cases of elevated lipids (hyperlipidemia); (3) weight loss helps decrease risk of diabetes and coronary heart disease.

How This Drug Works: Inhibits the action of an enzyme called lipase (both in the stomach and pancreas), thereby inhibiting the absorption of fats. Since fats can account for a significant number of daily calories and orlistat blocks roughly 30% of fat absorption, use of orlistat over time leads to weight loss.

▷ **Widely Used Guidelines That Involve This Medicine (representative sample):** Please look at the section at the very beginning of this profile called "Class." Next, turn to Table 22 and you will find guidelines listed by the class involved!

Available Dosage Forms and Strengths

Capsules — 120 mg

▷ **Usual Adult Dosage Ranges:** *Weight Loss:* One capsule three times a day with (or up to an hour after) each main meal that contains fat. If a meal is eaten that has no fat, the capsule should not be taken until the next meal that has fat in it.

Note: Actual dose and schedule must be determined for each patient individually.

Conditions Requiring Dosing Adjustments

Liver Function: This medicine is poorly absorbed, and liver function is not expected to be a factor (removed in the stool). Since the liver IS involved in making clotting factors, possible decreased vitamin K absorption from orlistat may be an issue in patients with liver disease.

Kidney Function: **Minimally** absorbed into the body, and kidney function is not expected to be a factor.

▷ **Dosing Instructions:** This medicine may be taken up to an hour after a meal that contains fat. If you skip a meal or eat a meal without any fat in it, it is okay to skip that dose of orlistat. You should be eating a well-balanced, reduced-carbohydrate diet that has roughly 30% of its calories as fat. This medicine can lower the amount of fat-soluble vitamins (A, D, E, K) and beta carotene that can get into your body from your diet. Over time, this may lead to a deficiency. A multivitamin containing those nutrients is important and should be taken two hours before or after your dose of orlistat. If you forget a dose, but eat a fat-free meal—simply skip the dose you forgot. If you forget a dose and have taken a fatty meal, take the missed dose if it is within an hour of the time the dose should have been taken. If you remember the missed dose more than an hour after the meal, skip the missed dose and wait until your next meal to take this medicine. DO NOT double doses. Talk with your doctor if you find yourself missing doses.

Usual Duration of Use: Regular use is required to get the best results from this medicine. Results (as measured by stool fat) can be seen in as little as 24–48 hours. Measurable weight loss will be determined by the amount of exercise, metabolic rate, adherence to diet, and other factors. Long-term use (months to years) requires ongoing follow-up by your doctor.

Typical Treatment Goals and Measurements (Outcomes and Markers)

Weight Loss: The goal is to lower body weight or maintain weight loss by preventing absorption of fat. Body weight, percent body fat and laboratory tests such as triglycerides, VLDL, LDL, and HDL can be checked to assess successful combination treatment. In some initial clinical data, people who took this medicine for two years lost an average of 4.5% of their starting body weight or about 4 kilograms. Be sure to talk to your doctor about the benefits of losing some weight and keeping it off versus crash or fad diets and weight yo-yoing.

Possible Advantages of This Drug

Works in a novel way compared to previously available medicines for weight loss. Does not have an effect on heart valves. Increases good cholesterol (HDL) and decreases LDL and total cholesterol. Used for up to four years with good results.

▷ **This Drug Should Not Be Taken If**
- you have had an allergic reaction to it previously.
- you have ongoing (chronic) malabsorption.
- you have a cause for obesity (such as hypothyroidism that should be treated) which would then obviate the need for orlistat, and an evaluation of this or other metabolic causes haven't been checked.
- you have stagnation of bile in the small bile ducts in the liver (cholestasis).

▷ **Inform Your Physician Before Taking This Drug If**
- you have significant disease in your stomach or intestine (gastrointestinal or GI tract), especially diseases that make you prone to diarrhea.

- you do not understand that increasing fat in your diet may also increase GI adverse effects from this medicine.
- you have a history of kidney stones (calcium oxalate).
- you have a history of low thyroid function (hypothyroidism).
- you have a known deficiency of vitamin A, D, E, or K or a poor diet that would lead you to tend toward deficiency of those vitamins or of beta carotene.

Possible Side Effects (natural, expected, and unavoidable drug actions)

Interference with normal fat digestion and absorption; reduced absorption of vitamins A, D, E, and K as well as beta carotene.

▷ **Possible Adverse Effects** (unusual, unexpected, and infrequent reactions)

If any of the following develop, consult your physician promptly for guidance.

Mild Adverse Effects

Allergic reaction: skin rash—possible.

Excessive gas (flatus) with or without fecal discharge—possible to frequent and can increase with higher amounts of fat in the diet.

Oily spotting of stool—may be frequent.

Nausea and soft or liquid stools—frequent.

(All of the above effects may decrease over time.)

Headache or dizziness—infrequent to frequent.

Increased blood pressure, edema—infrequent.

Serious Adverse Effects

Allergic reaction: not reported.

Lowering of vitamins A, D, E, and K. Vitamin K lowering may lead to an increased bleeding tendency if not supplemented—possible.

In clinical trials, nine cases of breast neoplasm were reported in patients taking 120 mg three times daily and one case was reported in the placebo group. Causation by orlistat is questionable, as the cases were seen within 6 months of the start of the clinical trials and the drug is minimally absorbed.

Depression—case reports.

Diabetic ketoacidosis—case report (in a diabetic woman taking this drug for weight loss).

Liver toxicity—case report.

▷ **Possible Effects on Sexual Function:** Menstrual irregularity—infrequent.

Natural Diseases or Disorders That May Be Activated by This Drug

Problems with patients who have cholestasis are possible.

Possible Effects on Laboratory Tests

INR (prothrombin time): possibly increased (impaired vitamin K absorption).

LDL and total cholesterol: decreased.

CAUTION

1. Since this medicine may interfere with absorption of fat-soluble vitamins and beta carotene, these compounds should be supplemented while you are taking orlistat and the vitamin dosing separated from orlistat doses by two hours.

2. Causes of obesity that are organic (such as low thyroid function or hypothyroidism) should be evaluated BEFORE orlistat is prescribed.

3. If you have a history of kidney stones made of calcium oxalate (nephrolithiasis), this medicine may worsen this problem.

4. Weight loss may improve how well blood sugar is controlled in people with diabetes—a beneficial effect. Oral hypoglycemic medicines (see Drug Classes) may have to be used in lower doses.

5. No data are available on the combination of orlistat with other weight loss agents, such as sibutramine (Meridia).

Precautions for Use

By Infants and Children: Safety and effectiveness for those less than 16 years of age not established.

By Those Over 60 Years of Age: Studies in special populations were not conducted.

▷ **Advisability of Use During Pregnancy**

Pregnancy Category: B. See Pregnancy Risk Categories at the back of this book.

Animal Studies: No embryotoxicity or teratogenicity in mice or rabbits.

Human Studies: Adequate studies of pregnant women are not available. NOT recommended for use during pregnancy.

Advisability of Use If Breast-Feeding

Presence of this drug in breast milk: Unknown.

Stop nursing or don't take the medicine if breast-feeding is to be undertaken.

Habit-Forming Potential: None, but misuse of the medicine is possible (as in anorexia).

Effects of Overdose: Reports of single 800-mg doses have been studied in people of normal weight without any adverse effects. If a significant overdose of orlistat happens, the patient should be medically observed for at least 24 hours. It is expected that any systemic effects would be rapidly reversible.

Possible Effects of Long-Term Use: Deficiencies of vitamins A, D, E, and K and beta carotene. Calcium deficiency, osteoporosis. Acidosis (excessive retention of chloride).

Suggested Periodic Examinations While Taking This Drug (at physician's discretion)

Measurements of blood levels of total cholesterol, low-density (LDL) cholesterol, and high-density (HDL) cholesterol. Possible bone mineral density tests if vitamin D is not supplemented. Blood levels of vitamins may be prudent to guide supplementation or need for supplementation.

▷ **While Taking This Drug, Observe the Following**

Foods: Follow your doctor's recommended diet and portion control. Avoid foods that have tended to cause gas (flatus) formation previously.

Herbal Medicines or Minerals: A variety of products that promise weight loss has been or is available. Some of these products have contained ma huang or other potentially dangerous ingredients. DO NOT combine any herbal weight loss product with orlistat. No data for use with bitter orange or country mallow. Talk to your doctor if you are considering any herbal weight loss product BEFORE you take it.

Nutritional Support: Ask your doctor about the need for supplements of vitamins A, D, E, and K as well as beta carotene.

Beverages: No restrictions.

▷ *Alcohol:* No interactions expected, but remember, many alcoholic beverages deliver a lot of calories.

Tobacco Smoking: No interactions expected. I advise everyone to quit smoking.

▷ *Other Drugs*

Orlistat may *decrease* the effects of

• beta carotene; take 2 hours before or after orlistat.

• fat-soluble vitamins, such as vitamin A, D, E, or K.

Orlistat *taken concurrently* with

• cyclosporine (Sandimmune, others) may (because of possible variation in

cyclosporine levels with changes in diet) lead to changes in cyclosporine levels. Caution is advised, and study is needed.
- pravastatin (Pravachol) or other HMG-CoA reductase inhibitors work well in further lowering cholesterol. Pravastatin levels may be increased by roughly 30%. Patients taking this combination should be followed more closely for possible adverse effects.
- warfarin (Coumadin, others) may (because of possible decreases in vitamin K over time) lead to increased warfarin effects; more frequent INR testing is prudent.

▷ *Driving, Hazardous Activities:* No restrictions.

Aviation Note: The use of this drug is usually not a disqualification for piloting. Consult a designated Aviation Medical Examiner.

Exposure to Sun: No reports of problems at present.

Discontinuation: The dose of any potentially toxic or narrow therapeutic-window drug (such as warfarin) taken concurrently must be changed appropriately if orlistat is stopped.

OXAPROZIN (OX a proh zin)

Please see the propionic acids (nonsteroidal anti-inflammatory drug) family profile.

OXICAMS (Nonsteroidal Anti-Inflammatory Drug Family)

Piroxicam   (peer OX i kam)

Introduced: 1978   **Class:**   Mild analgesic, anti-inflammatory   **Prescription:**   USA: Yes   **Controlled Drug:**   USA: No; Canada: No   **Available as Generic:**   Yes

Brand Names: ✚Alti-Piroxicam, ✚Apo-Piroxicam, ✚Brexidol, ✚Dom-Piroxicam, Feldene, ✚Fexicam, ✚Med-Pirocam, ✚Novo-Pirocam, ✚Nu-Pirox

BENEFITS versus RISKS	
Possible Benefits	*Possible Risks*
EFFECTIVE RELIEF OF MILD-TO-MODERATE PAIN AND INFLAMMATION	Gastrointestinal pain, ulceration and bleeding
ONCE-A-DAY DOSING HELPS PEOPLE TAKE IT	Drug-induced hepatitis—rare
	Rare kidney damage
	Mild fluid retention
	Reduced white blood cell and platelet counts

▷ **Principal Uses**

As a Single Drug Product: Uses currently included in FDA-approved labeling: Relieves mild to moderately severe pain and inflammation associated with (1) rheumatoid arthritis and (2) osteoarthritis.

Other (unlabeled) generally accepted uses: (1) Treats the morning and evening pain associated with ankylosing spondylitis; (2) helps relieve the pain and inflammation of acute gout; (3) used to treat terminal cancer pain in combination with doxepin; (4) may have a role in easing temporal arteritis;

(5) effective in painful menstruation (primary dysmenorrhea); (6) second-line therapy in acute gout (7) may help in preventing colon cancer and possibly Alzheimer's, but further research is needed.

How This Drug Works: This drug suppresses the formation of prostaglandins (and related compounds), chemicals involved in the production of inflammation and pain. Inhibits platelets from making prostaglandins (PGE1 and 2, etc.). By lowering the number of white blood cells in joints (synovial fluid) and decreasing the chemicals they can use to cause damage, this medicine works to limit joint damage and inflammation.

▷ **Widely Used Guidelines That Involve This Medicine (representative sample):** Please look at the section at the very beginning of this profile called "Class." Next, turn to Table 22 and you will find guidelines listed by the class involved!

Available Dosage Forms and Strengths
Capsules — 10 mg, 20 mg
Rectal suppository — 10 mg, 20 mg

▷ **Usual Adult Dosage Ranges:** *As antiarthritic:* 20 mg once daily. Higher doses may not confer added benefits. This dose may be separated into two equal doses.
Dysmenorrhea: 40 mg (two tablets) in the morning for two days, then 20 mg a day until symptoms ease or menstruation ends.
Note: Actual dose and schedule must be determined for each patient individually.

Conditions Requiring Dosing Adjustments
Liver Function: This drug should be used with caution and in decreased dose by patients with liver compromise.
Kidney Function: Piroxicam should be used with caution in renal compromise and kidney function followed closely.

▷ **Dosing Instructions:** Take with or following food (may also take with an antacid) to prevent stomach irritation. Take with a full glass of water and remain upright (do not lie down) for 30 minutes. The capsule may be opened. If you forget a dose: Take the missed dose as soon as you remember it, unless it's nearly time for your next dose—if that is the case, skip the missed dose and take the next dose right on schedule. DO NOT double doses. Talk with your doctor if you find yourself missing doses.

Usual Duration of Use: Use on a regular schedule for a few days often gives some relief from the discomfort of arthritis. It may take eight to twelve weeks to gain the peak response. Long-term use (months to years) requires physician supervision and periodic evaluation. It's not unusual to change or combine medicines in RA.

Typical Treatment Goals and Measurements (Outcomes and Markers)
Pain: Most clinicians treating pain use a device called an algometer to check your pain. This looks like a small ruler, but lets the clinician better understand your pain. The goals of treatment then relate to where the level of pain started (for example, a rating of 7 on a zero-to-ten scale) and what the cause of the pain was. Pain medicines may also be used together (in combination) in order to get the best result or outcome. If your pain control is not acceptable to YOU, be sure to call your doctor as you may need a different medicine or combination.
Arthritis: Control of arthritis symptoms (pain, loss of mobility, decreased ability to accomplish activities of daily living) is paramount in returning

patient quality of life and to checking the results (beneficial outcomes) from this medicine. CRP and RA titer may decrease. See WOMAC in Glossary for rheumatoid arthritis. ACR 20 and higher (see Glossary) refers to the number of signs and symptoms relieved by this medicine.

Possible Advantages of This Drug
Fewer side effects than many other nonselective NSAIDS. Once-daily dosing helps adherence.

▷ **This Drug Should Not Be Taken If**
- you have had an allergic reaction to it previously.
- you are subject to asthma or nasal polyps caused by aspirin.
- you have active peptic ulcer disease or any form of gastrointestinal bleeding.
- you have a bleeding disorder or a blood cell disorder.
- you have active liver disease or severe impairment of kidney function.

▷ **Inform Your Physician Before Taking This Drug If**
- you are allergic to aspirin or to other aspirin substitutes.
- you have a history of peptic ulcer disease, regional enteritis, or ulcerative colitis.
- you have a history of any type of bleeding disorder.
- you have impaired liver or kidney function.
- you develop signs or symptoms of pancreatitis while taking this medicine (talk with your doctor).
- you have high blood pressure or a history of heart failure.
- you take acetaminophen, aspirin or other aspirin substitutes, anticoagulants, or oral antidiabetic drugs.
- you have an infection.
- you plan to have surgery of any type in the near future.

Possible Side Effects (natural, expected, and unavoidable drug actions)
Fluid retention (weight gain, edema), prolongation of bleeding time.

▷ **Possible Adverse Effects** (unusual, unexpected, and infrequent reactions)
If any of the following develop, consult your physician promptly for guidance.
Mild Adverse Effects
Allergic reactions: skin rash, itching, spontaneous bruising.
Headache, dizziness, hair loss (alopecia), altered vision, ringing in ears (tinnitus), drowsiness, fatigue, paresthesias, inability to concentrate—rare to infrequent.
Indigestion, nausea, vomiting, abdominal pain, diarrhea—infrequent to frequent.
Serious Adverse Effects
Esophagitis or active peptic ulcer, stomach or intestinal bleeding—possible and more likely in elderly.
Drug-induced liver or kidney damage—rare to infrequent.
Serious skin damage (toxic epidermal necrolysis)—case reports.
Worsening of congestive heart failure—possible.
Pancreatitis—rare.
Enteropathy—possible.
Bone marrow depression (see Glossary): abnormal bleeding or bruising—case reports.
Blood-clotting problems—related to dose and half-life.
Increased blood potassium or decreased sodium—case reports.

▷ **Possible Effects on Sexual Function:** None reported.

Possible Delayed Adverse Effects: Mild anemia due to "silent" blood loss from the stomach.

▷ **Adverse Effects That May Mimic Natural Diseases or Disorders**
   Liver reaction may suggest viral hepatitis.

Natural Diseases or Disorders That May Be Activated by This Drug
   Peptic ulcer disease, ulcerative colitis. This drug may hide symptoms of gout.

Possible Effects on Laboratory Tests
   Red blood cell count and hemoglobin level or sodium: decreased.
   Bleeding time: increased.
   Blood uric acid level or potassium: increased.
   Liver function tests: increased liver enzymes (ALT/GPT, AST/GOT, and alkaline phosphatase), increased bilirubin.
   Kidney function tests: blood creatinine and urea nitrogen (BUN) levels increased; urine analysis positive for red blood cells, casts, and increased protein content (kidney damage).
   Fecal occult blood test: positive.

CAUTION
   1. The smallest effective dose should always be used.
   2. This drug may hide early signs of infection. Tell your doctor if you think you are getting one.
   3. Congestive heart failure in elderly patients may be unmasked or worsened. Risk appears to increase with use of higher doses.
   4. This medicine helps treat the signs and symptoms and may help prevent structural damage in rheumatoid arthritis (RA), does not work like the Disease Modifying AntiRheumatic Drugs (DMARDs) to help stop the damage/progression of RA itself.

Precautions for Use
   By Infants and Children: Indications and dose recommendations for those under 12 years of age are not established.
   By Those Over 60 Years of Age: Small doses are advisable until tolerance is determined. Watch for any indications of liver or kidney toxicity, fluid retention, dizziness, confusion, impaired memory, stomach bleeding, or constipation. People in this age group are often more likely to have stomach problems from the medicine itself. Existing congestive heart failure may be worsened.

▷ **Advisability of Use During Pregnancy**
   Pregnancy Category: B. D in the final 3 months of pregnancy. See Pregnancy Risk Categories at the back of this book.
   Animal Studies: No birth defects reported due to this drug.
   Human Studies: Adequate studies of pregnant women are not available.
   The manufacturer does not recommend the use of this drug during pregnancy.

Advisability of Use If Breast-Feeding
   Presence of this drug in breast milk: Yes.
   Talk to your doctor about this decision. The American Academy of Pediatrics considers this medicine to be usually compatible with breast-feeding.

Habit-Forming Potential: None.

Effects of Overdose: Possible drowsiness, dizziness, ringing in the ears, nausea, vomiting, indigestion.

Possible Effects of Long-Term Use: Development of anemia due to "silent" bleeding from the gastrointestinal tract.

Suggested Periodic Examinations While Taking This Drug (at physician's discretion)
> Complete blood cell counts.
> Liver and kidney function tests.
> Complete eye examinations if vision is altered in any way.
> Sedimentation rate (ESR) and C-reactive Protein (CRP) checks.
> ACR progress.
> Hearing examinations if ringing in the ears or hearing loss develops.

▷ **While Taking This Drug, Observe the Following**

Foods: No restrictions. No data from objective studies are available for combination use of this medicine and glucosamine. Talk to your doctor about possible combination.

Herbal Medicines or Minerals: Since St. John's wort and this drug may cause increased sun sensitivity, caution is advised. Feverfew, ginseng, ginkgo, alfalfa, clove oil, cinchona bark, white willow bark, and garlic may also change clotting, so combining those herbals with these medicines is not recommended. Talk to your doctor BEFORE combining any medicines. NSAIDs may decrease feverfew effects. Hay flower, mistletoe herb, and white mustard seed carry German Commission E monograph indications for arthritis but have not been tested in combination with this medicine. Herbals such as eucalyptus, kava, and valerian that can have toxic effects on the liver should be avoided while taking piroxicam. Talk to your doctor BEFORE adding any herbal to piroxicam.

Beverages: No restrictions. May be taken with milk.

▷ *Alcohol:* Use with caution. Both alcohol and piroxicam can irritate the stomach lining and can increase the risk of stomach ulceration and/or bleeding.

Tobacco Smoking: No interactions expected. I advise everyone to quit smoking.

▷ *Other Drugs*

Piroxicam may ***increase*** the effects of
- adrenocortical steroids (see Drug Classes) and may result in additive stomach irritation.
- anticoagulants (Coumadin, etc.) and increase the risk of bleeding; more frequent INR (prothrombin time or protime) testing is needed, and dosing should then be adjusted accordingly. Low-molecular-weight heparins (see Drug Classes) combined with this medicine increase risk of hematoma.
- beta blockers (atenolol and others)—can decrease the effectiveness of the beta blocker.
- cyclosporine (Sandimmune) may increase seizure risk.
- enoxaparin (Lovenox) and may increase bleeding risk.
- lithium (Lithobid, others) and can lead to lithium toxicity.
- methotrexate (Mexate) and may lead to methotrexate toxicity.

Piroxicam ***taken concurrently*** with
- alendronate (Fosamax) may increase risk of stomach and intestinal irritation, and use at the same time will decrease the amount of alendronate that gets into your body. Separate doses by 2 hours.
- antihypertensives such as thiazides (see Drug Classes), loop diuretics and others (ACE inhibitors) will blunt their therapeutic benefits.
- cholestyramine (Questran) may blunt piroxicam effectiveness.
- diuretics (see Drug Classes) may blunt diuretic benefits.
- eptifibatide (Integrilin) may increase bleeding risk.

- ofloxacin (Floxin) and other quinolones such as levofloxacin (Levaquin) may increase seizure risk.
- oral hypoglycemics (see sulfonylureas) may increase risk of low blood sugar.
- ritonavir (Norvir) and perhaps other protease inhibitors (see Drug Classes) can lead to toxicity.
- tacrolimus (Prograf) may increase risk of kidney failure.

Piroxicam *taken concurrently* with the following drugs may increase bleeding risk. Avoid these:

- aspirin or other NSAIDs.
- clopidogrel (Plavix). Follow patients closely and check for early signs or symptoms of bleeding.
- dipyridamole (Persantine).
- indomethacin (Indocin).
- sulfinpyrazone (Anturane).
- valproic acid (Depakene).

▷ *Driving, Hazardous Activities:* This drug may cause drowsiness or dizziness. Restrict activities as necessary.

Aviation Note: The use of this drug *may be a disqualification* for piloting. Consult a designated Aviation Medical Examiner.

Exposure to Sun: This drug may cause photosensitivity (see Glossary). Use caution.

OXTRIPHYLLINE (ox TRY fi lin)

Other Names: Choline theophyllinate, theophylline cholinate

Introduced: 1965   **Class:**   Antiasthmatic, bronchodilator, xanthines   **Prescription:**   USA: Yes

Controlled Drug: USA: No; Canada: No   **Available as Generic:**   Yes

Brand Names: ✤Apo-Oxtriphylline, Choledyl, Choledyl Delayed-Release, Choledyl SA, ✤Novotriphyl

Author's Note: This medicine is converted to 64% theophylline by the body. See the theophylline profile for further information.

OXYCODONE (ox ee KOH dohn)

Introduced: 1950   **Class:**   Analgesic, strong; opioids   **Prescription:** USA: Yes   **Controlled Drug:** USA: C-II*; Canada: No   **Available as Generic:**   USA: Yes; Canada: No

Brand Names: ✤Endocet [CD], ✤Endodan [CD], ✤Oxycocet [CD], ✤Oxycodan [CD], OxyContin, Percocet [CD], ✤Percocet-Demi [CD], Percodan [CD], Percodan-Demi [CD], Roxicet, Roxicodone, Roxilox, Roxiprin [CD], SK-Oxycodone, ✤Supeudol, Tylox [CD]

*See Schedules of Controlled Drugs at the back of this book.

BENEFITS versus RISKS

Possible Benefits	*Possible Risks*
EFFECTIVE RELIEF OF MODERATE-TO-SEVERE AND ONGOING PAIN	POTENTIAL FOR HABIT FORMATION (ADDICTION, DEPENDENCE)
	Sedative effects
	Mild allergic reactions—infrequent
	Nausea, constipation

▷ **Principal Uses**

As a Single Drug Product: Uses currently included in FDA-approved labeling: (1) Used in tablet and suppository form (Canada) to relieve moderate to severe pain; (2) OxyContin form is approved for use appropriate to a schedule II narcotic to treat people in moderate to severe pain who are expected to require continuous PAIN medicines (opioids) for an extended time. An important factor to be considered for OxyContin use is the severity and persistent nature of the pain that a patient is facing.

Other (unlabeled) generally accepted uses: None.

As a Combination Drug Product [CD]: Oxycodone is available in combinations with acetaminophen and with aspirin. These milder pain relievers are added to enhance the analgesic effect and reduce fever when present.

Author's Note: The FDA and Purdue Pharmaceuticals have worked together to strengthen warnings for OxyContin because of continuing reports of abuse and diversion of this medicine. A "Dear Healthcare Professional" letter was sent out that explains the strengthening of the labeling including proper prescribing information and also highlights the problems associated with abuse and diversion of OxyContin. An important factor that MUST be considered when OxyContin is prescribed is the severity of the pain that is being treated and the ongoing persistent nature of the pain that results, not simply the disease that is the root cause of the painful symptoms. The company has also responsibly undertaken a "Profiles in Pain Management" series in the *Pharmacy Today* journal of the American Pharmaceutical Association to increase awareness of prescription medication abuse. Because ALL opioids are subject to abuse, the FDA is also encouraging all makers of opioids sold in the US to voluntarily review and revise product labeling as needed to help ensure adequate warnings and precautions regarding risks of abuse, misuse and diversion are presented and that responsible prescribing practices are promoted. A MedWatch safety summary is available at *www.fda.gov/medwatch/safety/2001/safety01.htm#oxycon.*

How This Drug Works: Acting primarily as a depressant of certain brain functions (by attaching to specific receptors—Mu receptors), this drug suppresses pain perception and calms the emotional response to pain.

▷ **Widely Used Guidelines That Involve This Medicine (representative sample):** Please look at the section at the very beginning of this profile called "Class." Next, turn to Table 22 and you will find guidelines listed by the class involved!

Available Dosage Forms and Strengths

Solution — 5 mg/5 mL

Suppositories — 10 mg, 20 mg (Canada)

Tablets — 5 mg, 10 mg (Canada)

Tablets — 2.44 mg, 4.88 mg (in combination drugs)

Tablets, combination (newer Percocet forms) — 7.5 mg oxycodone/325mg acetaminophen and 10 mg/325 mg

Tablets, controlled-release — 10 mg, 20 mg, 40 mg, 80 mg, 160 mg

▷ **Usual Adult Dosage Ranges:** Percodan is taken as one tablet (5 mg) every 6 hours. Current pain theory says that pain medicines should be scheduled—for example, given every 6 hours. The outdated "wait until it hurts" or PRN method tended to result in suffering. May be increased to 10 mg every 4 hours if needed for severe pain. The total daily dose should not exceed 60 mg.

Percocet (oxycodone and acetaminophen combination) tablets are available in more strengths that minimize the amount of acetaminophen [previously 2.5/325, 5/325, 7.5/500, and 10/650] and now 7.5 mg oxycodone with 325 mg acetaminophen and 10 mg/325 mg have been added. These strengths represent the amount of oxycodone followed by the amount of acetaminophen and give pain management specialists more flexibility in treating pain. Make sure you understand how much and how often to take this medicine. The "lower acetaminophen" forms make it less likely that too much acetaminophen will be taken and will lower the risk of damage to the liver (hepatotoxicity).

OxyContin is taken every 12 hours and is a controlled-release formulation. This product has an 80-mg and 120-mg strength that is used for increasing (escalating) pain in people who have been taking opioids and have become tolerant. Some clinicians use a rescue dose of the immediate-release forms of oxycodone to manage (rescue) breakthrough pain (usually dosed as 10 to 30 mg every 4 hours as needed for pain in people who are already taking opioid pain medicines) and then add a percentage of the total daily rescue dosage used back to the extended-release formulation. The amount of medicine given every 12 hours should be increased if needed, rather than changing the time between doses. Taking this medicine more often than every 12 hours has not been studied. Increases in total daily OxyContin doses can usually be made in steps of 25% of the existing dose excepting the change from 10 mg to 20 mg. Current labeling for this form of oxycodone is meant to decrease the chance that OxyContin could be prescribed inappropriately for pain of lesser severity than the approved use or for other disorders or conditions inappropriate for a schedule II narcotic.

Note: Actual dose and schedule must be determined for each patient individually.

Conditions Requiring Dosing Adjustments

Liver Function: Dose adjustments should be empirically made in liver failure.

Kidney Function: Dose adjustment does not appear to be needed. Some combination products contain aspirin, which may be contraindicated in kidney failure.

▷ **Dosing Instructions:** The immediate-release tablets may be crushed and taken with or following food to reduce stomach upset or nausea. Controlled-release forms such as OxyContin should never be broken, chewed, crushed, or injected. Taking altered controlled-release forms can lead to excessively fast drug release and death. As with other medicines for pain management, dosing is provided around the clock. If you forget a dose: For immediate-release forms: Take the missed dose as soon as you remember it, unless it's nearly time for your next dose—if that is the case, skip the missed dose and take the next dose right on schedule. For sustained-release forms: Call your doctor. DO NOT double doses. Talk with your doctor if you find yourself missing doses.

    Author's Note: Current pain treatment theory calls for timed or scheduled dosing. This tends to prevent pain, rather than allowing pain to recur and then having to be treated. Some clinicians will use timed dosing immediately after surgery and then revert to as-needed dosing once the most severe period of pain has passed. Pain is the fifth vital sign.

Usual Duration of Use: As long as significant pain is present and as required to control pain. Continual use of the immediate-release form should not exceed 5 to 7 days without interruption and reassessment of need (excepting use as a "rescue medicine.") Use of the OxyContin form (consistent with newer labeling) will be for painful conditions requiring longer-term treatment with a potent opioid. Ongoing use frequently requires use of bowel medicines (such as Senokot) to address constipation.

Typical Treatment Goals and Measurements (Outcomes and Markers)

Pain: Most clinicians treating pain use a device called an algometer to check your pain. This looks like a small ruler, but lets the clinician better understand your pain. The goals of treatment then relate to where the level of pain started (for example, a rating of 7 on a 0–10 scale) and what the cause of the pain was. I use the PQRSTBG (see Glossary) system. Pain medicines may also be used together (in combination) in order to get the best result or outcome. If your pain control is not acceptable to YOU and if after a reasonable attempt with good adherence, results are not acceptable, be sure to call your doctor. You may need a different dose, different medicine or combination. Specific clinical practice guidelines from the American Geriatrics Society (AGS) for pain management in older people should be used to help guide treatments in people over 60.

▷ **This Drug Should Not Be Taken If**
- you had an allergic reaction to it previously.
- you are having an acute attack of asthma, severe asthma, or excessive carbon dioxide (CO_2).
- you are having significant depression of breathing (respiratory depression).
- you have a blockage in your bowel (paralytic ileus).
- patients allergic to aspirin should not be given Percodan.

▷ **Inform Your Physician Before Taking This Drug If**
- you had an unfavorable reaction to any narcotic drug or are prone to constipation.
- you have had a head injury with increased pressure (intracranial) in the head.
- you have a history of drug abuse, misuse, or alcoholism (benefit-to-risk decision).
- you have chronic lung disease with impaired breathing or another condition that would make it likely that you have a lowered lung or respiratory reserve.

- you are dehydrated or are in circulatory shock.
- you have impaired liver or kidney function.
- you have gallbladder disease, a seizure disorder, or an underactive thyroid gland.
- you have difficulty emptying the urinary bladder.
- you are taking any other drugs that have a sedative effect.
- you plan to have surgery under general anesthesia in the near future.

Possible Side Effects (natural, expected, and unavoidable drug actions)
Drowsiness, light-headedness, dry mouth, urinary retention, constipation.

▷ **Possible Adverse Effects** (unusual, unexpected, and infrequent reactions)
If any of the following develop, consult your physician promptly for guidance.
Mild Adverse Effects
Allergic reactions: skin rash, hives, itching.
Idiosyncratic reactions: skin rash and itching when combined with dairy products (milk or cheese).
Dizziness, sensation of drunkenness, depression, blurred or double vision—dose-related.
Nausea, vomiting—may be dose related.
Serious Adverse Effects
Impaired breathing: use with caution in chronic lung disease—variable and can be dose related.
Abnormal body movements, if the drug is abruptly stopped.

▷ **Possible Effects on Sexual Function:** Blunted sexual responses—case reports.

Possible Effects on Laboratory Tests
Urine screening tests for drug abuse: test result may be falsely **positive;** confirmatory test result may be **negative.** (Test results depend upon amount of drug taken and testing method used.)

CAUTION
1. If you have been prescribed Percocet, please be aware that there are now more strengths. Make certain that you understand how much to take. The strengths (oxycodone/acetaminophen) may be confusing. For example, it may be tempting for some prescribers to shorten Percocet 5/325 to Percocet-5. This kind of name change could lead to an impression that five tablets are to be taken instead of a correct one-tablet dose. Talk to your doctor and make sure you understand how much and how often you are to take this medicine.
2. If you have asthma, chronic bronchitis or emphysema, excessive use of this drug may cause significant respiratory difficulty, thickening of bronchial secretions, and suppression of coughing.
3. If you have been taking an oxycodone form on an ongoing basis, slow tapering rather than sudden discontinuation is prudent.
4. The concurrent use of this drug with atropinelike drugs can increase the risk of urinary retention and reduced intestinal function.
5. Constipation can be a serious problem, particularly in older patients (as bowel function tends to slow down). Many clinicians prescribe a medicine (such as Senokot-S) to promote bowel movements at the same time that oxycodone is prescribed.
6. The FDA and the maker of OxyContin have worked together to strengthen the warnings and precautions section of the OxyContin labeling. It would

be prudent to discuss these changes with your doctor. The fact that this drug has been misused, altered, and used inappropriately by addicts does not mean that it lost an important place in pain management.

7. Do not take this drug following acute head injury.
8. Females will generally have a 25% higher oxycodone blood (plasma) level than males when weight is considered (on a body weight adjusted basis).
9. Physical dependence and tolerance can happen with repeated use (see Glossary).
10. If you are taking a large dose of OxyContin (such as 160 mg) make sure you understand that a high-fat meal can increase drug levels by 25%—and could impact breathing.

Precautions for Use

By Infants and Children: Do not use this drug in children under 2 years of age because of their vulnerability to life-threatening respiratory depression.

By Those Over 60 Years of Age: Small starting doses and short-term therapy are indicated. There may be increased susceptibility to the development of drowsiness, dizziness, unsteadiness, falling, urinary retention, and constipation (may lead to fecal impaction).

▷ **Advisability of Use During Pregnancy**

Pregnancy Category: B. D when taken for an extended amount of time or if used at high doses when the baby is born. See Pregnancy Risk Categories at the back of this book.

Animal Studies: No information available.

Human Studies: Adequate studies of pregnant women are not available. Oxycodone taken repeatedly during the final few weeks before delivery may cause withdrawal symptoms in the newborn.

Use only if clearly needed and in small, infrequent doses.

Advisability of Use If Breast-Feeding

Presence of this drug in breast milk: Yes.

Avoid drug or refrain from nursing.

Habit-Forming Potential: Psychological and/or physical dependence can develop. The FDA and the maker of OxyContin have taken expanded steps to enhance prescriber awareness of possible diversion and abuse of OxyContin. Newer labeling also helps more clearly define patients who will benefit from this medicine.

Effects of Overdose: Drowsiness, restlessness, agitation, nausea, vomiting, dry mouth, vertigo, weakness, lethargy, stupor, coma, seizures.

Possible Effects of Long-Term Use: Psychological and physical dependence, chronic constipation.

Suggested Periodic Examinations While Taking This Drug (at physician's discretion)

Check for constipation. Balance of pain relief versus alertness. Assessment of pain relief. For example, as diseases such as cancer progress, it is not unusual for pain management needs to change.

▷ **While Taking This Drug, Observe the Following**

Foods: Generally, no restrictions—however, the 160 mg OxyContin form should NOT be taken with a high fat meal. Higher dose is closer to level that can lead to breathing problems, and a high-fat meal can increase oxycodone levels from OxyContin by 25%.

Herbal Medicines or Minerals: Caution is advised in combining any medicine that leads to drowsiness. St. John's wort can change (inducing or increasing)

P450 enzymes, blunting the effects of oxycodone. Talk to your doctor BEFORE you combine any herbal medicines with oxycodone.

Beverages: No restrictions. May be taken with milk.

▷   *Alcohol:* Oxycodone can intensify the intoxicating effects of alcohol, and alcohol can intensify the depressant effects of oxycodone on brain function, breathing, and circulation. Combined use is best avoided.

Tobacco Smoking: No interactions expected. I advise everyone to quit smoking.

Marijuana Smoking: Increase in drowsiness and pain relief; impairment of mental and physical performance.

▷   *Other Drugs*

Oxycodone may ***increase*** the effects of

• atropinelike drugs and increase the risk of constipation and urinary retention.

• other drugs with sedative effects (see Drug Classes for benzodiazepines, tricyclic antidepressants, antihistamines, MAO inhibitors, phenothiazines, and opioid drugs [narcotics]).

Oxycodone ***taken concurrently*** with

• naltrexone (ReVia) may lead to withdrawal symptoms.

• rifabutin (Rifater, others) may blunt oxycodone benefits.

• ritonavir (Norvir) and perhaps other protease inhibitors (see Drug Classes) may lead to toxicity.

• sertraline (Zoloft) resulted in a serotonin syndrome in one case report. Caution is advised.

• tramadol (Ultram) may increase risk of adverse effects.

▷   *Driving, Hazardous Activities:* This drug can impair mental alertness, judgment, reaction time and physical coordination. Avoid hazardous activities accordingly.

Aviation Note: The use of this drug ***is a disqualification*** for piloting. Consult a designated Aviation Medical Examiner.

Exposure to Sun: No restrictions.

Discontinuation: It is best to limit this drug to short-term use. If extended use is needed, discontinuation should be gradual to minimize possible effects of withdrawal.

PANTOPRAZOLE (pan TOE prah sole)

Introduced: 2000   **Class:**   Antiulcer, proton pump inhibitor   **Prescription:**   USA: Yes   **Controlled Drug:**   USA: No; Canada: No   **Available as Generic:**   USA: No; Canada: No

Brand Name: Protonix

Author's Note: Information in this profile will be broadened if further data on this medicine warrants inclusion.

PAROXETINE (pa ROCKS a teen)

Introduced: 1993   **Class:**   Antidepressant, other   **Prescription:** USA: Yes   **Controlled Drug:**   USA: No; Canada: No   **Available as Generic:**   USA: No; Canada: No

Brand Names: Paxil, Paxil CD

BENEFITS versus RISKS

Possible Benefits	Possible Risks
EFFECTIVE CONTROL OF DEPRESSION	Abnormal ejaculation in males
CONTROL OF SOCIAL ANXIETY DISORDER	POSSIBLE ASSOCIATION WITH INCREASED RISK OF SUICIDAL THINKING OR ATTEMPTS IF USED IN CHILDREN LESS THAN 18 TO TREAT MAJOR DEPRESSION
EFFECTIVE USE IN PANIC ATTACKS IN CHILDREN	
HELPS CONTROL OBSESSIVE-COMPULSIVE DISORDER	
TREATS POST-TRAUMATIC STRESS DISORDER	
Fewer adverse effects than tricyclic antidepressants	
May help premature ejaculation	
Useful in some pain syndromes	

▷ **Principal Uses**

As a Single Drug Product: Uses currently included in FDA-approved labeling: (1) Treatment of depression; (2) helps control obsessive-compulsive disorder; (3) helps control panic attacks (panic disorder) in adults; (4) control of social anxiety disorder (SAD); (5) eases social phobia; (6) relatively new approval to treat post-traumatic stress disorder (PTSD); (7) eases generalized anxiety disorder (GAD).

Other (unlabeled) generally accepted uses: (1) Can have a role in diabetic nerve pain (neuropathy); (2) helps long-standing (chronic) daily headaches; (3) can help premature ejaculation; (4) has previously been used to help prevent panic attacks in children (however, newer data regarding use in children and increased suicidal behavior may change this—see controversies in medicine note below).

How This Drug Works: Inhibits uptake of serotonin. When more of this chemical is available in the brain, a positive impact on thinking results. Because the specific cause of panic attacks is not known, how this medicine works to prevent panic attacks has not been identified.

▷ **Widely Used Guidelines That Involve This Medicine (representative sample):** Please look at the section at the very beginning of this profile called "Class." Next, turn to Table 22 and you will find guidelines listed by the class involved!

Available Dosage Forms and Strengths

Tablets, controlled-release — 12.5 mg, 25 mg
Tablets, immediate-release — 10 mg, 20 mg, 30 mg, 40 mg
Oral suspension — 10 mg/5 mL

▷ **Recommended Dose Ranges** (Actual dose and schedule must be determined for each patient individually.)

Infants and Children: Some clinicians have used 5 to 10 mg per day in children with panic disorder (or 0.25 to 0.5 mg per kg per day). The British Medicine and Healthcare Products Regulatory Agency ordered British doctors to stop using this medicine in patients less than 18 years old due to their contention that it is linked to suicidal behavior. The FDA issued a statement about paroxetine saying that it is reviewing POSSIBLE increased risk of suicidal thinking and/or suicide attempts in children less than 18 who are treated for major depression (major depressive disorder (MDD). The FDA is NOT recommending use of paroxetine in children or adolescents with MDD (currently is NOT approved for that use). Parents should talk to their doctor about what actions to take or not take and how to take them with appropriate medical supervision. See *www.fda.gov/ceder/drug/infopage/paxil/default.htm*.

18 to 60 Years of Age: Depression: Immediate-release form: The usual starting dose is 20 mg, taken in the morning. Dose can then be increased as needed and tolerated in 10-mg intervals to a maximum of 50 mg daily.

Depression: Controlled-release form: Started with 25 milligrams (mg) daily. If patient response does not meet physician goals, the dose may be increased by 12.5 mg daily (at intervals of 7 days or more). The maximum recommended dose is 62.5 mg daily.

Obsessive-compulsive disorder (immediate-release form): Started with 20 mg daily with increases as in depression to a usual benefit at 40 mg per day. Maximum dose is 60 mg daily.

Panic disorder: Dosing is started with 10 mg per day, and doses are increased (at weekly intervals) as needed and tolerated to the usual dose of 40 mg a day. Daily maximum is 60 mg.

Social anxiety disorder: 20 mg daily.

PTSD: The starting dose is 20 mg, which is given in the morning. Dosing is adjusted in 10 mg steps. Typical doses are 20-40 mg daily.

Over 60 Years of Age: The starting dose in this population is 10 mg daily. The maximum dose is 40 mg daily.

Conditions Requiring Dosing Adjustments

Liver Function: Starting dose is 10 mg, and the maximum dose is 40 mg daily. Drug levels may be needed.

Kidney Function: Same starting dose and maximum dose as in liver compromise.

▷ **Dosing Instructions:** The absorption of this medicine is not changed by food. The geomatrix form (CR) should not be altered before taking it. If you have trouble swallowing, the liquid form is a clear benefit. People using the suspension form (liquid) should shake the bottle just before they use it, and use a medicine cup or measuring spoon to get just the right dose. If you forget a dose: Take the missed dose as soon as you remember it, unless it's nearly time for your next dose—if that is the case, skip the missed dose and take the next dose right on schedule. DO NOT double doses. Talk with your doctor if you find yourself missing doses.

Usual Duration of Use: Continual use on a regular schedule for 14 days is usually necessary to determine this drug's effectiveness in treating depression. It may be 4 weeks before you get the full benefit of this medicine. Long-term use (months to years) requires periodic evaluation of response and dose adjustment by your doctor. Controversy about how long to continue a medicine for depression exists and must be individualized. Some clinicians advocate 4–9 months after depression eases, while others advocate longer or ongoing preventive use.

Typical Treatment Goals and Measurements (Outcomes and Markers)

Depression: The general goal: to at least help lessen the degree and severity of depression, letting patients return to their daily lives. Specific measures of depression involve testing or inventories and can be valuable in helping check benefits from this medicine. The Hamilton Depression Scale is widely used to assess depression. In any case the ability of the patient to return to normal activities or not have them interrupted is a hallmark of successful treatment.

Panic: Goals for panic tend to be more vague and subjective than hypertension or cholesterol. Frequently, the patient (in conjunction with physician assessment) will largely decide if panic has been successfully controlled. Decreased number of trips to the hospital or Emergency Room (ER) visits may also be a useful measure. The Liebowitz Social Anxiety Scale (LSAS) is a tool as well as the Clinical Global Impressions–Global Improvement Scale, which can be used to help figure out benefits in patients with anxiety and panic. The Hamilton Rating Scale for Anxiety anxious mood section is also helpful. The ability of the patient to return to normal activities is a hallmark of successful treatment.

Social Phobia: The Liebowitz Social Anxiety Scale (LSAS) is also used to check benefits in social anxiety disorder. Undertaking or returning to social activities is a practical gauge.

Possible Advantages of This Drug

Fewer side effects than tricyclic antidepressants. May be a drug of choice in people with heart disease who are also depressed. Since a large National Cancer Institute study found that those who suffer depression for 6 years or more have a generally increased risk of cancer, one benefit of effective treatment of depression with this drug may be a generally reduced risk of cancer. This was the first medicine approved to treat social anxiety disorder. The controlled-release form offers a geomatrix technology that may help minimize adverse events and improve how well patients take this medicine (adherence).

▷ This Drug Should Not Be Taken If

- you had an allergic reaction to it previously.
- you have taken a MAO inhibitor (see Drug Classes) in the last 14 days.

▷ Inform Your Physician Before Taking This Drug If

- you are pregnant or breast-feeding.
- you have a history of mania or seizures.
- you take diuretics or typically drink little water.
- you have a history of liver or kidney disease.
- you take prescription or nonprescription medicines not discussed with your doctor when paroxetine was prescribed.

Possible Side Effects (natural, expected, and unavoidable drug actions)

Lowered blood pressure and fainting upon standing (postural hypotension). Sedation. Nausea (up to 27%). Often decreases in 3 weeks. May require ondansetron or a lower paroxetine dose. Withdrawal syndrome possible if this medicine is stopped abruptly. Best to slowly decrease (taper) this medicine over 2–4 weeks.

▷ Possible Adverse Effects (unusual, unexpected, and infrequent reactions)

If any of the following develop, consult your physician promptly for guidance.

Mild Adverse Effects

Allergic reactions: skin rash and itching.

Headache, nervousness, or insomnia—infrequent to frequent.

Palpitations—infrequent.

Teeth grinding (bruxism)—case report.

Sense of inner restlessness (akathisia)—infrequent.

Loss of appetite, nausea, taste disorders, or constipation—infrequent to frequent.

Tingling of the hands (paresthesias)—infrequent.

Sweating—frequent.

Dizziness, blurred vision—infrequent to frequent.

Serious Adverse Effects

Allergic reactions: anaphylaxis—reported.

Idiosyncratic reactions: bruising and excessive menstrual bleeding—case report (reversed with vitamin C).

Increased risk of suicidal thinking or behavior in patients being treated with this and several other antidepressants (see controversies in medicine note). Any patient taking this or any medicine who begins to have thoughts about suicide or aggressive mood changes should call their doctor and get additional help and guidance immediately.

Abnormal movements or positioning of the mouth or face—infrequent.

Abnormal urination (SIADH)—case report.

Seizures—rare.

Liver toxicity—rare.

▷ **Possible Effects on Sexual Function:** Galactorrhea. USED TO TREAT premature ejaculation.

Abnormal ejaculation—infrequent to frequent.

Inability to achieve orgasm, impotence, or sexual dysfunction—infrequent.

Prolonged and painful erection (priapism)—rare.

Possible Delayed Adverse Effects: None reported.

▷ **Adverse Effects That May Mimic Natural Diseases or Disorders**

Increased liver enzymes may mimic early hepatitis.

Natural Diseases or Disorders That May Be Activated by This Drug

None reported.

Possible Effects on Laboratory Tests

Liver function tests: increased.

CAUTION

1. Take this medicine as prescribed, and do not stop taking it without talking with your doctor.
2. A withdrawal syndrome is possible if this medicine is abruptly stopped. Best to slowly decrease (taper) the dose over 2–4 weeks if this medicine needs to be stopped.
3. An FDA Public Health Advisory was released in March 2004 recommending pediatric and adult patients treated with this medicine should be closely watched for worsening depression or suicidal thinking. The FDA has required makers of antidepressants such as this one to alert health-care professionals to the fact that children and adults with major depression may develop worsening depression or suicidal thoughts and behavior whether they take medicine for depression or do not take it. Patients should be carefully followed for such clinical worsening (particularly when treatment is started or doses are increased or decreased).

Precautions for Use

By Infants and Children: Safety and effectiveness for use by those under 18 years of age have not been established (see controversies in medicines note below).

Current Controversies in Medicine: The British Medicines and Health-care Products Regulatory Agency reviewed paroxetine (known as Seroxat in the UK). Their conclusion was to order physicians to stop prescribing this medicine to children 18 and younger. The reason was a government study that in their opinion, established the link between paroxetine and suicidal behavior when the medicine was taken by children.

By Those Over 60 Years of Age: Lower starting and maximum doses are indicated.

▷ **Advisability of Use During Pregnancy**
Pregnancy Category: C. See Pregnancy Risk Categories at the back of this book.
Animal Studies: Reproduction studies in rabbits or rats using doses of up to 10 times the typical human dose have not revealed any fetal changes.
Human Studies: Information from adequate studies of pregnant women is not available.
Ask your doctor for guidance.

Advisability of Use If Breast-Feeding
Presence of this drug in breast milk: Yes, in small amounts (up to roughly 2.9% of the mother's dose in one study).
Some clinicians use a guideline that says that if less than 10% of the dose that a mother takes goes into the breast milk, then breast-feeding is safe. Ask your doctor for help.

Habit-Forming Potential: None, but a withdrawal syndrome characterized by dizziness, confusion, sweating, and tremor has been described.

Effects of Overdose: Confusion, heart rhythm changes, seizures.

Possible Effects of Long-Term Use: Not defined.

Suggested Periodic Examinations While Taking This Drug (at physician's discretion)
Liver function tests.

▷ **While Taking This Drug, Observe the Following**
Foods: No restrictions. Vitamin C reversed abnormal bruising and increased menstrual bleeding in one patient.
Herbal Medicines or Minerals: Since paroxetine and St. John's wort may act to increase serotonin, the combination is not advised. Since part of the way ginseng and ginkgo work may be as a MAO inhibitor, it may be ill advised to combine ginseng and ginkgo with paroxetine. Ma huang, guarana, yohimbe, Indian snakeroot, and kava kava (no longer recommended in Canada) are also best avoided while taking this medicine. One case report of dehydroepiandrosterone (DHEA) leading to acute mania when combined with sertraline precludes use of paroxetine with DHEA as well (same SSRI family).
Beverages: No restrictions.
▷ *Alcohol:* The manufacturer recommends avoiding alcohol while taking this medicine.
Tobacco Smoking: No interactions expected. I advise everyone to quit smoking.
Marijuana Smoking: Additive sedation, possible signs and symptoms of mania—DO NOT COMBINE.
▷ *Other Drugs*
Paroxetine may *increase* the effects of
• benzodiazepines (see Drug Classes).
• buspirone (Buspar).
• desipramine (and potentially other tricyclic antidepressants: see Drug Classes).
• dofetilide (Tikosyn) by increasing blood levels. Checks of patient clinical status and dosing changes are appropriate.
• encainide (Enkaid) and flecainide (Tambocor) because paroxetine inhibits an enzyme system needed to remove flecainide. More frequent encainide or flecainide blood levels are prudent.

- galantamine (Reminyl) because paroxetine inhibits an enzyme system needed to remove galantamine. Caution: careful patient monitoring and possible dose decreases of galantamine may be prudent.
- haloperidol (Haldol), because paroxetine blocks an enzyme system needed to remove haloperidol.
- labetalol (Normodyne), metoprolol (Toprol XL), and perhaps other beta blockers (see Drug Classes), because paroxetine inhibits an enzyme system needed to remove them (P450 2D6).

Paroxetine *taken concurrently* with

- activated charcoal will reduce absorption of paroxetine.
- astemizole (Hismanal) now removed from the U.S. market may lead to heart toxicity—DO NOT COMBINE.
- dextromethorphan (the DM ingredient in many cough suppressants) may lead to serotonin syndrome—DO NOT COMBINE.
- digoxin (Lanoxin) may lead to lowered digoxin levels. More frequent digoxin levels are prudent.
- fenfluramine (Pondimin) may cause toxicity (serotonin syndrome).
- lithium (Lithobid, others) may lead to increased adverse effects.
- MAO inhibitors (see Drug Classes) may result in a fatal serotonin syndrome. Do not combine these medicines.
- phenytoin (Dilantin) or fosphenytoin (Cerebyx) may result in decreased paroxetine blood levels and lessening of therapeutic benefits. Dose increases may be needed.
- propafenone (Rythmol, others) may result in increased propafenone levels and toxicity, careful patient follow-up and more frequent propafenone levels are prudent.
- quinidine (Quinaglute, others) may result in increased paroxetine levels and toxicity; decreased paroxetine doses may be needed.
- risperidone (Risperdal) may lead to serotonin syndrome.
- ritonavir (Norvir) may lead to paroxetine toxicity.
- sibutramine (Meridia) increases risk of serotonin syndrome.
- sumatriptan (Imitrex) and other triptan-type medicines (see Drug Classes) can lead to hyperreflexia and poor coordination—the combination may not be advisable and if combination is required, careful patient follow-up is very important.
- tramadol (Ultram) may lead to increased risk of seizures—DO NOT combine.
- tryptophan may result in sweating, nausea and dizziness.
- venlafaxine (Effexor) can increase risk of serious serotonin syndrome.
- warfarin (Coumadin) may result in bleeding; more frequent INR (prothrombin time or protime) testing is recommended. Warfarin doses should be adjusted based on laboratory results.

The following drug may *increase* the effects of paroxetine:

- cimetidine (Tagamet).
- bupropion (Zyban, Wellbutrin). Low paroxetine doses and close patient follow-up are needed if these medicines must be combined. Bupropion inhibits P450 2D6—a liver enzyme that helps remove paroxetine from the body.

Driving, Hazardous Activities: This drug may frequently cause sedation. Restrict activities as necessary.

Aviation Note: The use of this drug *is a disqualification* for piloting. Consult a designated Aviation Medical Examiner.

Exposure to Sun: No specific restrictions.

Exposure to Heat: This medicine can cause excessive sweating. If you work or are frequently in a hot environment, be careful to replace enough fluids to avoid dehydration.

Heavy Exercise or Exertion: Since this medicine may cause excessive sweating, be careful to replace lost fluids.

Occurrence of Unrelated Illness: Fevers may cause more severe dehydration.

Discontinuation: Do not stop this medicine without talking with your doctor. For patients taking this medicine for an extended period of time, gradual dosing decreases (tapering) over several weeks or longer is recommended.

PEGINTERFERON ALPHA-2A (PEG in tur fear on)

Introduced: 2002   **Class:** Antiviral, pegylated interferon alpha-2a
Prescription: USA: Yes   **Controlled Drug:** USA: No; Canada: No
Available as Generic: USA: No; Canada: No
Brand Name: Pegasys

Author's Note: Used in hepatitis C in combination with ribavirin (Copegus–see ribavirin profile later in this book). Specific genotypes help drive dosing of this medicine and the ribavirin combination (see below).

BENEFITS versus RISKS	
Possible Benefits	*Possible Risks*
SINGLE AGENT TREATMENT OF HEPATITIS C (DRUG NAIVE)	HEADACHE
COMBINATION TREATMENT OF HEPATITIS C WITH RIBAVIRIN	FATIGUE
	NAUSEA OR DIARRHEA
MORE EFFECTIVE THAN UNMODIFIED INTERFERON AGAINST HEPATITIS C	MUSCLE CHANGES
	INSOMNIA
	DEPRESSION
	BLOOD CELL CHANGES
Improved quality of life versus some other Hepatitis C treatments	

▷ **Principal Uses**

As a Single Drug Product: Uses currently included in FDA-approved labeling: (1) Treats hepatitis C in people who were not previously given interferon alpha; (2) combination treatment of hepatitis C with ribavirin in those not previously given interferon alpha.

Other (unlabeled) generally accepted uses: (1) Not defined at present, possible emerging use in kidney (renal cell) carcinoma.

How This Drug Works: This specific form of interferon alpha-2a is a modified form of the original molecule. A branched methoxy-polyethlene glycol compound is attached (covalently) to the original interferon molecule. The effect of attaching this additional substance to the interferon is to keep it in the body longer (reduces clearance) by the kidney, protects against compounds in the body (enzymes) which might break the interferon alpha-2a down, and allows once-a-week dosing. The attachment also appears to attack the hepatitis C virus more forcefully since the drug stays at a higher level than other interferon alpha-2a formulations which are given three times a week (allowing peaks and valleys in concentration and giving the virus more time to recover).

▷ **Widely Used Guidelines That Involve This Medicine (representative sample):** Please look at the section at the very beginning of this profile called "Class." Next, turn to Table 22 and you will find guidelines listed by the class involved!

Available Dosage Forms and Strengths
Injectable solution—180 mcg per vial

▷ **Usual Adult Dosage Ranges**

Ongoing Hepatitis C in Adults: 180 mcg (micrograms) is given ONCE A WEEK for 48 weeks. This is given to patients who have or do not have cirrhosis. The company package insert notes that if a viral response (antiviral effect) is NOT seen in 12 weeks, stopping the treatment should be considered.

Combination Hepatitis C Treatment in Adults (with Copegus-ribavirin): The same dose of 180 mcg once weekly of the peginterferon alpha-2a is given, however, the ribavirin dose changes. Here, genetics are considered: Patients who have genotypes 1 or 4 and who weigh more than 75 kilograms are given 1,200 mg a day. For those less than 75 kg, 1,000 mg a day is given, and combination is continued for 48 weeks. People with genotypes 2 or 3 are given 800 mg of ribavirin (divided into two 400-mg doses given twice a day) coupled with 180 mcg once a week of peginterferon alpha-2a and the combination is only continued for 24 weeks. If an antiviral effect is not seen 12 weeks into therapy, consideration is given to stopping the medicine.

Note: Actual dose and schedule must be determined for each patient individually.

Conditions Requiring Dosing Adjustments

Liver Function: Patients who have a liver function test called ALT progressively increase should have their dose lowered to 135 micrograms a week. If ALT continues to rise, after the dose is reduced coupled with evidence of liver decline (hepatic decompensation) or increases in a compound called bilirubin, the medicine should be stopped.

Kidney Function: People with creatinine clearance (a measure of how well the kidneys work) of less than 50 mL/minute should NOT be given peginterferon alpha-2a.

Anemia: For people with a history of stable heart disease who have a decrease in hemoglobin of 2 gram per deciliter noted as g/dL (for example, a drop in the hemoglobin lab test result from 12g/dL to 10 g/dL during any four-week period of therapy) or for patients who do not have heart disease, but have a hemoglobin laboratory test result of 10 grams/deciliter, the ribavirin dose should be lowered to 600 mg a day. If people with a history of stable heart disease are given the lower ribavirin dose for 4 weeks and the hemoglobin stays lower than 12 g/dL or in people without heart disease who have a hemoglobin less than 8.5 g/dL, peginterferon alpha- 2a should be stopped.

Depression: People who become *mildly depressed:* (your doctor may use signs and symptoms or one of the inventories of depression such as Ham D to check this), doses can remain constant, but weekly visits to the doctor's office or weekly phone calls to the patient are needed. For *moderate depression:* the dose of peginterferon alpha-2a should be decreased to 90–135 micrograms, and the patient should be evaluated at a weekly visit at the doctor's office. If signs and symptoms of depression improve and remain the same for more than 4 weeks, patients can go back to the previous schedule of office visits. The dose of peginterferon alpha-2a can then be kept at the lower amount or increased to the prior dose based on clinician judgment. If a patient becomes *severely depressed:* Peginterferon alpha-2a should be stopped and the patient referred to a psychiatrist immediately.

Low White Blood Cells (Neutropenia): If a specific kind of white blood cell count (absolute neutrophil count or ANC) decreases to an ANC of less than 750 per cubic millimeter (/mm3), peginterferon alpha-2a dose is decreased to 135 mcg a week. If ANC drops to less than 500/mm3, the medicine should be stopped until the ANC goes back up to more than 1,000/mm3. Once ANC is more than 1,000/mm3, peginterferon alpha-2a can be restarted at a dose of 90 mcg a week.

Low Blood Platelets (Thrombocytopenia): If a blood element involved in clotting called a platelet (thrombocyte) falls to less than 50,000 per cubic millimeter (/mm3), the Pegasys dose is lowered to 90 mcg a week. If the platelet count falls to less than 25,000/mm3, Pegasys should be stopped.

▷ **Dosing Instructions:** May be taken alone or combined with a form of ribavirin called (Copegus). While the benefit-to-risk decision favors use of these/this medicine for some patients, care must be taken to carefully follow possible undesirable effects such as anemia, depression and changes in red blood cells and platelets. Dosing should be carefully decided by a qualified specialist, and is given as a single injection once a week. This/these medicines are best taken/given on the same day and time each week. Very specific instructions are present in a Med Guide that comes with Pegasys. It is important NOT to use Pegasys if some things about the medicine change. A simple way to remember this is CEPC: Don't use it if it is Cloudy, has Expired, has Particles floating in it, or if it is any other Color than a light yellow or is colorless. Call your doctor or prescriber if you are unsure how much to inject. If you know the correct dose, clean off the area of skin where you have decided to inject, then gently roll the medicine vial in your hands to warm it, and then pull the syringe back to the correct mark on the barrel. After removing (flipping off the plastic top on the vial) and cleaning it with an alcohol pad, push the needle into the rubber stopper on the vial and push the air in the syringe inside of the vial. Follow the instructions your doctor or nurse has given you to draw up the correct dose and to remove air bubbles. Finally, inject the medicine slowly under the skin using the technique that your nurse or doctor explained to you. Make sure you dispose of the syringe and needle the way you were instructed. Each syringe and medicine vial is to be used only once. If you are also going to use Copegus in combination with Pegasys, read the Med Guide that came with that medicine and follow the instructions carefully.

Usual Duration of Use: Use on a regular schedule for up to 12 weeks may be needed to see best effects from this medicine or from the combination of medicines already discussed. Ongoing use for more than 48 weeks does not have efficacy or safety data. Ongoing use requires periodic check of response (such as viral load), check for side effects, laboratory monitoring and possibly dose changes. Make sure you keep follow-up appointments with your doctor and for laboratory or other testing.

Typical Treatment Goals and Measurements (Outcomes and Markers)
The general goal is to lower the amount of virus in the body and ideally to kill all of it. Viral load or burden tests help guide therapy. A test for viral genetic material in the serum called HCV-RNA is taken. The goal is to achieve undetectable amounts. The technical term for this is an undetectable HCV-RNA by PCR. Because the usual limit of the test is 100 copies per milliliter, the goal is to achieve "undetectable." When and if lower detection tests become available (as has happened with HIV testing), a lower goal will

become the standard. Additional beneficial effects will be quality of life, halting of progression, or cessation of liver damage.

Possible Advantages of This Medicine/These Drugs: The combination of peginterferon alpha-2a with ribavirin gives a more prolonged (durable) lowering of the amount of virus (viral load or viral burden) and in general viral response. For people who have been infected with the hepatitis C virus (HCV) with the genotype 1 form, pegylated forms of interferon (2a or 2b) are drugs of choice.

▷ **This Drug Should Not Be Taken If**
- you have had an allergic reaction to it previously.
- you have autoimmune hepatitis or unstable liver disease or have had a liver transplant.
- you have previously taken and did not respond to other alpha interferon treatment.
- you are taking this medicine and your hemoglobin drops below acceptable levels (see anemia above).
- you are taking this medicine and your neutrophils (ANC) or your platelet count drops below acceptable level (see above).
- you have sickle-cell anemia, thalassemia major, or some other form of abnormal red blood cells.
- you become seriously depressed while taking this medicine.
- you become pregnant while taking this medicine.
- you are a woman of childbearing age and have not had a negative pregnancy test before starting this medicine.

▷ **Inform Your Physician Before Taking This Drug If**
- you have a history of bone marrow depression or cancer.
- you have a history of a serious emotional or mental disorder, particularly depression.
- you have a history of alcohol or drug abuse.
- you have a history of heart disease, a prior heart attack, or poor heart circulation (ischemic heart disease).
- you have impaired liver function from hepatitis B (no data) or impaired kidney function.
- you have a history of lung problems (pulmonary dysfunction) or chronic obstructive pulmonary disease (this medicine may worsen them).
- you have a history of diabetes or low thyroid function (hypothyroidism).
- you develop a fever, which gets higher or does not go away.
- you have psoriasis and it gets worse while taking this medicine.
- you are taking any drugs for emotional or mental disorders.
- you have a history of eye problems (such as blood clots in the retinal artery, edema of the macula, or optic neuritis)—talk to your doctor.
- you have a history of low white blood cell counts or cancer.
- you have a history of autoimmune disease (such as lupus erythematosus or rheumatoid arthritis) or are HIV positive.
- you have a history of colon inflammation (colitis).
- you ask the person prescribing this medicine about HCV genotyping of the virus causing your hepatitis C infection, and learn that this testing has not yet been performed (genotype of the virus is very important).
- you are unsure how much or how often to take this medicine.

Possible Side Effects (natural, expected, and unavoidable drug actions)
Injection site reactions (frequent).

▷ **Possible Adverse Effects** (unusual, unexpected, and infrequent reactions)
   If any of the following develop, consult your physician promptly for guidance.
   Mild Adverse Effects
   Allergic reaction: skin rash, itching (pruritis)—may be frequent.
   Headache, fatigue or fever—frequent.
   Insomnia—frequent (may be prudent to anticipate this effect and ask your doctor for help when this medicine is prescribed).
   Depression (see depression note above)—frequent.
   Blurred vision—possible.
   Dizziness, nausea or abdominal pain—frequent.
   Sweating—infrequent.
   Loss of appetite (anorexia), diarrhea, abdominal pain—frequent.
   Muscle aches or joint pain—frequent.
   Blood sugar changes—possible.
   Hair loss—alopecia—may be frequent.
   Dry mouth—infrequent.
   Serious Adverse Effects
   Allergic reaction: Not clearly defined.
   Depression—see note above (may be serious enough to require stopping the medicine).
   Decrease or loss of vision (optic neuritis, macular edema, retinal artery blood clots—reported (see vision check below).
   Muscle stiffness (rigors)—may be frequent.
   Abnormal heart rhythms (supraventricular arrhythmia) or heart attack—case reports.
   Low white blood cell counts: fever, sore throat, infection—possible (see note above regarding dosing).
   Aggravation of excessively low or high thyroid function (hypo- or hyperthyroidism).
   Blood sugar changes—possible.
   Pancreatitis—possible with alpha interferon and ribavirin treatment.
   Decreased hemoglobin—possible (see note above regarding dosing).
   Decreased platelets—possible (see note above regarding dosing).
   Bloody diarrhea—possible.
   Lung problems (pneumonia, interstitial pneumonitis, others)—reported as aggravated or caused by this medicine.
   Aggravation of or development of autoimmune problems (muscle inflammation (myositis), rheumatoid arthritis, systemic lupus erythematosus, others)—possible.
▷ **Possible Effects on Sexual Function:** May impair fertility in some women. Female cynomolgus monkeys experience amenorrhea or prolonged menstrual cycles.
Adverse Effects That May Mimic Natural Diseases or Disorders
   Mood changes, depression may suggest a psychotic disorder.
   Dropping neutrophils (ANC) may mimic other hematologic problems, yet actually be an adverse drug reaction.
Natural Diseases or Disorders That May Be Activated by This Drug
   Latent or subclinical depression, epilepsy, incipient congestive heart failure.
Possible Effects on Laboratory Tests
   Development of neutralizing antibodies—rare.
   Development of binding antibodies—infrequent.

Liver function tests: increased (ALT, bilirubin, others).
White blood cells (neutrophils): lowered ANC.
Hemoglobin: may be decreased.
Triglycerides: increased (frequent).
Platelets: may be decreased.
Blood sugar changes.
Amylase and/or lipase: increased.

CAUTION

1. Talk to your doctor if you or your significant other or a family member notices that you are starting to become depressed (see note on depression in dosing), or think about suicide. This medicine can be a cause of severe depression.
2. While this medicine can successfully attack the hepatitis C virus (particularly in combination with ribavirin), serious possible adverse effects require follow-up and laboratory testing while taking this medicine.
3. Call your doctor if you have trouble breathing, a change in vision or unusual bleeding or bruising.
4. Call 911 if you start to have severe chest pain (some cardiovascular problems have been associated with this medicine).
5. Call your doctor immediately if you become pregnant (see pregnancy note).
6. You develop an ongoing or increasing temperature, sore throat, or other signs of an infection.
7. Triglycerides may be increased. Talk to your doctor about this.

Precautions for Use

By Infants and Children: Safety and effectiveness for those under 18 not established.

By Those Over 60 Years of Age: Some of the measures of how the medicine is distributed in the body (area under the curve-AUC and half life) were increased or prolonged in people more than 60. Adverse effects from this medicine may be more pronounced in this patient population. Prudent to follow the patient more carefully, and adjust dosing based on undesirable signs and symptoms.

▷ ### Advisability of Use During Pregnancy

Pregnancy Category: C. See Pregnancy Risk Categories at the back of this book.

Animal Studies: High doses were not associated with birth defects (teratogenicity) in animals, but have been listed as a potential cause of fetal birth defects in the Med Guide. Abortion HAS been reported with high dose, nonpegylated forms in animals.

Human Studies: Adequate studies of pregnant women are not available.

A negative pregnancy test BEFORE starting this medicine and TWO forms of birth control while taking this medicine and for at least six months AFTER STOPPING it are needed. Male partners of women taking this medicine are advised to use a condom. Talk to your doctor about how to address the issue of pregnancy and the possible transmission of hepatitis C. If you DO become pregnant, YOU or YOUR DOCTOR should call 1-800-526-6367.

Advisability of Use If Breast-Feeding

Presence of this drug in breast milk: Not defined.

Blood and body fluids may transfer the hepatitis C virus. Breast-feeding is NOT advisable.

Habit-Forming Potential: None.

Effects of Overdose: Management of the symptoms that a patient has at the time that they are seen by a doctor (symptomatic management).

Possible Effects of Long-Term Use: See anemia, white blood cell, and platelet notes above.

Suggested Periodic Examinations While Taking This Drug (at physician's discretion)

Hepatitis C RNA testing (PCR) before and periodically during treatment
Vision testing/eye exam before (baseline) treatment.
Complete blood counts, ANC (baseline, two weeks, four weeks).
Liver biopsy may be needed for some patients, possibly before and during treatment.
Thyroid stimulating hormone (TSH).
Liver (ALT, AST and bilirubin) before treatment (baseline) and usually every two months.
Kidney function tests.
Amylase and lipase.
Blood sugar, A1C.
Evaluation of heart function at baseline (before therapy) and periodically.
Baseline pregnancy test in females of child bearing age.
Checks for signs and symptoms of depression such as appetite, change in pleasure gained from usually pleasurable activities, or administration of typical depression inventories such as the Hamilton Depression Scale (Ham-D).

Author's Note: Baseline blood and biochemical tests and pregnancy tests for females are needed. Once treatment is started, blood (hematological) tests are checked at 2 and 4 weeks, and repeat biochemical testing done at 4 weeks. In clinical trials, CBC and chemistries (including liver function tests and uric acid) were checked at weeks 1 and 2, 4, 6 and 8. For ongoing treatment, testing was done every four weeks. Testing was obtained more frequently if abnormal results were obtained. TSH was checked every twelve weeks. Pregnancy testing was checked before therapy was started, during combination therapy was checked monthly and for six months after the medicine was stopped.

▷ **While Taking This Drug, Observe the Following**

Foods: Taking this medicine with a high-fat meal increases the amount that gets into your body. Talk to your doctor about how he or she would like you to take this medicine. Use of smaller, more nutrient dense meals may help provide nutrition while acting as a coping mechanism for nausea.

Herbal Medicines or Minerals: Some herbal medicines such as eucalyptus, kava, and valerian have possible toxic effects on the liver. These herbals should NOT be taken, both because of the viral presence in the liver and because of possible additive undesirable effects on the liver.

Beverages: No restrictions. May be taken with milk.

▷ *Alcohol:* Since alcohol can add to liver problems, any use should be discussed with your doctor.

Tobacco Smoking: No interactions expected. I advise everyone to quit smoking.

Marijuana Smoking: Added dizziness.

▷ *Other Drugs*

Peginterferon alpha-2A *taken concurrently* with
- didanosine (Videx) is NOT recommended. Increased risk of fatal liver failure, pancreatitis, lactic acidosis, and/or peripheral neuropathy preclude this.
- medicines known to have toxic effects on the liver would be best avoided if

possible due to overlapping undesirable effects on the liver. Some combinations may represent a benefit-to-risk decision.

- medicines removed by a liver enzyme called CYP 450 1A2 may be increased to toxic levels because peginterferon inhibits this enzyme. Checking blood levels of the medicines combined with peginterferon that undergo such removal is prudent, with dosing adjustments based on blood levels.
- theophylline (Theo Dur, others) can lead to an increased (roughly 25%) blood level of theophylline. More frequent checks of blood levels and dosing changes are needed.

Peginterferon alpha-2a and ribavirin *taken concurrently* with

- stavudine (Zerit) or zidovudine (AZT) may blunt the antiviral benefits of these two HIV medicines.

▷ *Driving, Hazardous Activities:* May cause dizziness, blurred vision, or fatigue. Use caution and assess the extent of these possible undesirable effects BEFORE undertaking such activities.

Aviation Note: The use of this drug *may be a disqualification* for piloting. Consult a designated Aviation Medical Examiner.

Exposure to Sun: No restrictions.

Special Storage Instructions: Care must be taken for proper disposal of needles and avoidance of possible needle sticks by caregivers. The medicine itself should be stored in a refrigerator with a temperature of 36–46 degrees F. (2–8 degrees Centigrade) because lack of refrigeration can break down the medicine. DO NOT SHAKE the bottle as this can also inactivate the medicine. Protect the medicine from light and also make certain that the medicine is not frozen. It is important NOT to leave the medicine out of the refrigerator for more than a day. Once you have drawn up a dose from a given vial of medicine, throw the rest of the medicine in the vial away. Please note the CEPC characteristics of the medicine in dosing instructions above.

Discontinuation: See notes on white blood cell, platelet counts, liver function tests, and time that the medicine should be given to work in the profile above. Talk to your doctor BEFORE making any changes in dosing or making any decision to stop this medicine.

PENBUTOLOL (pen BYU toh lohl)

Introduced: 1976 **Class:** Antihypertensive, beta-adrenergic blocker
Prescription: USA: Yes **Controlled Drug:** USA: No; Canada: No
Available as Generic: Yes

Brand Name: Levatol

Author's Note: Information in this profile has been truncated to make room for more widely used medicines.

PENICILLAMINE (pen i SIL a meen)

Introduced: 1963 **Class:** Antiarthritic **Prescription:** USA: Yes
Controlled Drug: USA: No; Canada: No **Available as Generic:** USA: No; Canada: No

Brand Names: Cuprimine, Depen

BENEFITS versus RISKS

Possible Benefits	*Possible Risks*
EFFECTIVE TREATMENT OF WILSON'S DISEASE (COPPER TOXICITY)	SEVERE ALLERGIC REACTIONS BONE MARROW DEPRESSION
Effective treatment of cystinuria and cystine kidney stones	Drug-induced damage of lungs, liver, pancreas, and kidneys
Partially effective treatment of rheumatoid arthritis and poisoning due to heavy metals: iron, lead, mercury, and zinc	

Author's Note: Due to proliferation of new medicines, this profile has been abbreviated in order to make room for more widely used medicines.

PENICILLIN ANTIBIOTIC FAMILY

Amoxicillin (a mox i SIL in)   **Amoxicillin/Clavulanate** (a mox i SIL in/KLAV yu lan ayt)   **Ampicillin** (am pi SIL in)   **Bacampicillin** (bak am pi SIL in)   **Cloxacillin** (klox a SIL in)   **Penicillin VK** (pen i SIL in VEE KAY)

Introduced: 1969, 1982 (2002 for Augmentin XR form), 1961, 1979, 1962, 1953, respectively   **Class:** Antibiotics, penicillins   **Prescription:** USA: Yes   **Controlled Drug:** USA: No; Canada: No   **Available as Generic:** USA: Yes (all but amoxicillin/clavulanate); Canada: Yes

Brand Names: Amoxicillin: A-Cillin, Amoxil, ✤Apo-Amoxi, ✤Clavulin, Larotid, ✤Novamoxin, ✤Nu-Amoxi, Polymox, Prevpac [CD], Trimox, Wymox, Amoxicillin/Clavulanate: Augmentin, Augmentin XR, Ampicillin: Amcill, ✤Ampicin, ✤Ampicin PRB [CD], ✤Ampilean, ✤Apo-Ampi, Augmentin, ✤Clavulin, D-Amp, Faspak Ampicillin, 500 Kit [CD], ✤Novo-Ampicillin, Nu-Ampi, Omnipen, Omnipen Pediatric Drops, Pardec Capsules [CD], ✤Penbritin, Polycillin, Polycillin Pediatric Drops, Polycillin-PRB [CD], ✤Pondocillin, Principen, SK-Ampicillin, Totacillin, Bacampicillin: ✤Penglobe, Spectrobid, Cloxacillin: ✤Apo-Cloxi, ✤Bactopen, Cloxapen, ✤Novo-Cloxin, ✤Nu-Cloxi, ✤Orbenin, Tegopen, Penicillin VK: ✤Apo-Pen-VK, Beepen VK, Betapen-VK, Ledercillin VK, ✤Nadopen-V, ✤Novopen-VK, ✤Nu-Pen-VK, Penapar VK, Pen-V, ✤Pen-Vee, Pen-Vee K, Pfizerpen VK, ✤PVF, ✤PVF K, Robicillin VK, SK-Penicillin VK, Uticillin VK, V-Cillin K, ✤VC-K 500, Veetids, Win-Cillin

---

BENEFITS versus RISKS

Possible Benefits	*Possible Risks*
EFFECTIVE TREATMENT OF INFECTIONS DUE TO SUSCEPTIBLE MICROORGANISMS	ALLERGIC REACTIONS, MILD TO SEVERE Superinfections (yeast) Drug-induced colitis—possible Lowering of white blood cells (amoxicillin/clavulanate, ampicillin, cloxacillin) Decreased kidney function

---

▷ **Principal Uses**

As a Single Drug Product: Uses currently included in FDA-approved labeling: (1) Used to treat responsive infections of the upper and lower respiratory tract, the middle ear (acute otitis media). Amoxicillin resistance has prompted dosing changes. Approved to treat susceptible skin infections; (2) helps prevent rheumatic fever and bacterial endocarditis in people with valvular heart disease; (3) treats some *Haemophilus influenzae* infections (amoxicillin); (4) treats some genitourinary tract infections (amoxicillin/clavulanate, ampicillin, penicillin VK); (5) treats some cases of sinusitis; (6) ampicillin is used in combination to treat some kinds of septicemia and meningitis; (7) amoxicillin is approved in combination with other medicines (such as omeprazole) to treat some *Helicobacter pylori* infections; (8) some forms treat anthrax; (9) Augmentin XR form approved for community acquired pneumonia or sudden (acute) sinusitis caused by streptococcus pneumoniae with reduced susceptibility (MIC of 2 micrograms per mL).

Other (unlabeled) generally accepted uses: (1) Combined therapy of animal bite wounds; (2) treats stage one Lyme disease in children (amoxicillin or penicillin VK); (3) therapy of Lyme disease in the central nervous system (penicillin VK); (4) can treat some dental abscesses (penicillin VK); (5) treats typhoid fever (amoxicillin); (6) prevention of bacterial endocarditis (amoxicillin); (7) treats biliary tract infections or chancroid (amoxicillin/clavulanate); (8) cloxacillin treats some bone infections if intravenous (IV) drugs are not tolerated.

As a Combination Drug Product [CD]: Amoxicillin and clavulanate are combined (Augmentin) to give the benefits of amoxicillin combined with the ability to treat more resistant bacteria (clavulanate). Amoxicillin is available combined with two drugs: clarithromycin and lansoprazole. Since resistant (refractory) ulcers are often actually *Helicobacter pylori* infections, the combination works to kill the bacteria and lower acid production.

How These Drugs Work: Destroy susceptible infecting bacteria by damaging ability to make protective cell walls as they multiply and grow. Amoxicillin/clavulanate uses clavulanate blockage of enzymes to enable treatment of resistant bacteria. Bacampicillin is converted to ampicillin, giving peak blood levels three times higher than ampicillin. This allows bacampicillin dosing every 12 hours.

▷ **Widely Used Guidelines That Involve This Medicine (representative sample):** Please look at the section at the very beginning of this profile called "Class." Next, turn to Table 22 and you will find guidelines listed by the class involved!

Available Dosage Forms and Strengths

Amoxicillin:

Capsules — 250 mg, 500 mg
Oral liquid — 3 g
Oral suspension — 50 mg/mL, 125 mg/mL, 250 mg/5 mL
Pediatric drops — 50 mg/mL
Tablets, chewable — 125 mg, 250 mg

Amoxicillin/clavulanate:

Oral suspension — 125 mg (amoxicillin) and 31.25 mg (clavulanate) per 5 mL; 250 mg (amoxicillin) and 62.5 mg (clavulanate) per 5 mL; 250 mg (amoxicillin) and 125 mg (clavulanate); 500 mg (amoxicillin) and 125 mg (clavulanate)
Pediatric formulation, twice daily — 200 mg (amoxicillin) and 28.6 mg (clavulanate) per 5 mL; 400 mg (amoxicillin) and 57.1 (clavulanate) per 5 mL
Tablets — 500 mg (amoxicillin) and 125 mg (clavulanate); 875 mg (amoxicillin) and 125 mg (clavulanate)
Tablets, chewable — 125 mg (amoxicillin) and 31.25 mg (clavulanate); 250 mg (amoxicillin) and 62.5 mg (clavulanate)
Tablets, chewable twice-daily formulation — 200 mg (amoxicillin) and 28.6 mg (clavulanate); 400 mg (amoxicillin) and 57.1 mg (clavulanate)

Ampicillin:

Capsules — 250 mg, 500 mg
Oral suspension — 100 mg/mL, 125 mg/mL, 250 mg/mL, 500 mg/5 mL
Pediatric drops — 100 mg/mL

Bacampicillin:

Oral suspension — 125 mg/5 mL
Tablets — 400 mg, 800 mg (800 mg in Canada only)

Cloxacillin:

Capsules — 250 mg, 500 mg
Oral suspension — 125 mg/5 mL
Oral liquid — 125 mg/5 mL

Penicillin VK:

Oral solution — 125 mg/5 mL, 250 mg/5 mL
Tablets — 125 mg, 250 mg, 500 mg

▷ **Recommended Dosage Ranges** (Actual dose and schedule must be determined for each patient individually for all of these medicines.)
Dose is based on how sensitive the infection-causing bacteria are, infection severity, and patient response.

Penicillin VK: Dose range is 125 to 500 mg every 6 to 8 hours. For prevention of bacterial endocarditis: 2 g (2,000 mg) taken 1 hour before the procedure, followed by 1 g 6 hours later. Daily maximum is 7 g (7,000 mg).

Infants and Children:

Amoxicillin: For susceptible infections: Up to 6 kg of body mass—25 to 50 mg every 8 hours. 6 to 8 kg of body mass—50 to 100 mg every 8 hours. 8 to 20 kg of body mass—6.7 to 13.3 mg per kg of body mass every 8 hours. 20 kg of body mass and over—same as 12 to 60 years of age. Note: See higher dosing in ear infection (otitis media) below.

Amoxicillin/clavulanate: Up to 40 kg of body mass—6.7 to 13.3 mg (amoxicillin) per kg of body mass, every 8 hours. 40 kg of body mass and over—same as 12 to 60 years of age. 12-hour formula: For severe infections—45 mg amoxicillin per kg of body mass **per day** (divided into two doses given every 12 hours). For less severe infections (as in skin infections)—25 mg per kg of body mass **per day** (divided into two doses given every 12 hours).

Bacampicillin: 25 mg per kg of body mass per day is given, divided into two equal doses every 12 hours, for respiratory infections.

Cloxacillin: Children weighing less than 44 lb (20 kg) receive 50 to 100 mg per kg of body mass per day, divided into four doses. Children greater than 20 kg get the adult dose. Intravenous dosing may be required for severe infections.

12 to 60 Years of Age:

Amoxicillin: Usual dose—250 to 500 mg every 8 hours. Daily maximum is 4.5 g. For gonorrhea—3 g, with 1 g of probenecid, taken as a single dose. For Lyme disease—250 to 500 mg, three or four times a day, for 10 to 30 days; dose and duration depends on severity of infection and response to treatment.

Author's Note: American Heart Association (AHA) guidelines for prevention of bacterial endocarditis in patients at risk suggest amoxicillin in an initial dose of 2 g BEFORE (check current guidelines for timing and best choices) oral or dental procedures. There is no recommendation for follow-up doses of antibiotics.

Because of limits on how well amoxicillin gets into the middle ear and prevalence of penicillin-resistant *Strep pneumoniae* causing middle ear infections, some clinicians are using 80–90 mg per kg per day, divided into two or three equal doses (12 or 8 hours apart) in children with sudden onset (acute) otitis media with *S. pneumoniae*. Resistance patterns of bacteria are changing in many areas making other antibiotics medicines of choice depending on the specific resistance patterns and bacteria being treated.

Amoxicillin/clavulanate: Usual dose—250 to 500 mg (amoxicillin) every 8 hours. In some severe infections, 875/125 mg tablets are taken twice a day. Daily maximum (of amoxicillin) is 4.5 g. Augmentin XR form: two tablets every 12 hours.

Ampicillin: 50 to 100 mg per kg of body mass per day divided into four doses or 500 to 1,000 mg every 6 hours. Usual daily maximum is 6,000 mg daily.

Bacampicillin: For those with a body mass of 25 kg or more—400 to 800 mg every 12 hours.

Cloxacillin: 250 to 500 mg every 6 hours. The maximum dose is 6,000 mg (6 g) every 24 hours.

Over 60 Years of Age: Amoxicillin: Same as 12 to 60 years of age.

Amoxicillin/clavulanate: Same as 12 to 60 years of age. Note: The above doses refer to the amoxicillin component of amoxicillin/clavulanate. The 250-mg regular tablet and the 250-mg chewable tablet contain different amounts of clavulanate and are NOT interchangeable.

Ampicillin: Drug is removed more slowly by patients in this age group, but specific dose decreases are not defined.

Bacampicillin: Tests of kidney function should be obtained. Doses of 400 mg per day have been used in moderate kidney disease or decline (age-related decline in kidney function may be moderate).

Cloxacillin: No specific dosing changes are available.

Conditions Requiring Dosing Adjustments

Liver Function: Dose adjustments do not appear to be needed (amoxicillin, amoxicillin/clavulanate, ampicillin, and penicillin VK). Caution is advised for bacampicillin use by these patients. The dose is decreased or time between doses increased for cloxacillin.

Kidney Function:

Amoxicillin, amoxicillin/clavulanate, ampicillin: Dosing interval **must** be adjusted in renal compromise.

Bacampicillin: The dose must be decreased to 400 mg per day in moderate kidney failure. In severe kidney failure, a dose of 400 mg every 36 hours is used.

Cloxacillin: Patients should be watched closely for adverse effects in severe kidney compromise.

Penicillin VK: For patients with severe kidney compromise, the usual dose is taken every 8 hours.

▷ **Dosing Instructions:** The tablet (amoxicillin, bacampicillin, penicillin VK) may be crushed (or amoxicillin and amoxicillin/clavulanate chew-tabs chewed) or the capsule (amoxicillin) opened and taken on an empty stomach or with food or milk (amoxicillin). Augmentin XR or other extended-release forms should NOT be crushed or altered. Absorption may be slightly faster if taken when stomach is empty (penicillin VK). Ampicillin, bacampicillin, and cloxacillin are best taken on an empty stomach. Oral suspension forms should be shaken well before measuring each dose. Use a measuring cup or calibrated measuring spoon to make sure you get just the right dose. If you forget a dose: Take the missed dose as soon as you remember it, unless it's nearly time for your next dose—if that is the case, skip the missed dose and take the next dose right on schedule. If the dose missed was the first dose of the day, separate the remaining doses into evenly spaced intervals. DO NOT double doses. Talk with your doctor if you find yourself missing doses.

Usual Duration of Use: For all streptococcal infections—not less than 10 consecutive uninterrupted days to reduce risk of rheumatic fever or glomerulonephritis. For all other infections—as long as needed to eradicate the infection. Incomplete treatment may lead to serious resistance and dangerous infections.

Typical Treatment Goals and Measurements (Outcomes and Markers)

Infections: The most commonly used measures of serious infections are white blood cell counts and differentials (the kind of blood cells that occur most often in your blood), and temperature. Many clinicians look for positive changes in 24–48 hours. NEVER stop an antibiotic because you start to feel better. For many infections, a full 14 days is REQUIRED to kill the bacteria. The goals and time frame (see peak benefits above) should be discussed with you when the prescription is written, as well as how soon to expect a decline in temperature or other signs and symptoms and what to do if symptoms worsen.

Possible Advantages of These Drugs: The Augmentin XR form requires less frequent dosing (better adherence) and kills more resistant (high MIC) forms of streptococcus.

▷ **These Drugs Should Not Be Taken If**
- you had an allergic reaction to them previously.
- you are certain you are allergic to any form of penicillin.

▷ **Inform Your Physician Before Taking These Drugs If**
- you suspect you may be allergic to penicillin or have a history of a previous "reaction."
- you are allergic to any cephalosporin antibiotic (Ancef, Ceclor, etc.—see Drug Classes).
- you are allergic by nature (hay fever, asthma, hives, eczema).
- you are unsure how much to take or how often.
- you have a history of liver or kidney disease.
- you have a history of low blood counts (amoxicillin/clavulanate, ampicillin, cloxacillin).

Possible Side Effects (natural, expected, and unavoidable drug actions)
Superinfections (see Glossary), often due to yeast organisms or for some penicillins due to Clostridium difficile.

▷ **Possible Adverse Effects** (unusual, unexpected, and infrequent reactions)
If any of the following develop, consult your physician promptly for guidance.
Mild Adverse Effects
Allergic reactions: skin rashes, hives, itching.
Irritations of mouth or tongue, "black tongue," nausea, vomiting, diarrhea, dizziness—rare to infrequent.
Serious Adverse Effects
Allergic reactions: anaphylactic reaction (see Glossary), severe skin reactions, drug fever, swollen painful joints, sore throat, abnormal bleeding or bruising.
Severe skin reactions (Stevens-Johnson syndrome, bullous pemphigoid)—case reports.
Drug-induced colitis—rare.
Hemolytic anemia—case reports (penicillin VK).
Drug-induced periarteritis nodosa, meningitis, or porphyria—case reports (penicillin VK).
Abnormal liver or kidney changes—rare.
Drug-induced abnormal lowering of white blood cells—rare (amoxicillin/clavulanate, ampicillin, cloxacillin, penicillin VK).

▷ **Possible Effects on Sexual Function:** None reported except for case reports of a small decrease in sperm counts for ampicillin.

Possible Effects on Laboratory Tests
Complete blood counts: decreased red cells, hemoglobin, white cells (therapeutic effects of each antibiotic) and platelets (penicillin VK); increased eosinophils (allergic reactions).
INR (prothrombin time): occasionally increased (ampicillin, cloxacillin, and penicillin VK).

Liver function tests: increased aspartate aminotransferase (AST/GOT) and bilirubin (cloxacillin and penicillin VK).

Coombs test: may be positive with ampicillin or penicillin VK therapy.

CAUTION

1. If your infection does not respond in 24–48 hours (reduced symptoms, temperature, etc.), CALL YOUR DOCTOR.
2. Take the exact dose and the full course prescribed (even if you feel better).
3. These medicines DO NOT treat viral infections. Considerable controversy has erupted regarding inappropriate prescribing of antibiotics to treat viral infections. Some intelligent clinicians are writing contingency antibiotics where the differential diagnosis of a bacterial infection versus a viral infection is unclear. Demanding an antibiotic or expecting an antibiotic to treat a viral infection (except in the case of a secondary bacterial infection) is an inappropriate patient action in most cases and only serves to lead to emergence of bacterial resistance.
4. If these drugs must be used concurrently with antibiotics, such as erythromycin or tetracycline, take the penicillin first.

Precautions for Use

By Infants and Children: Watch children with allergies closely for evidence of a developing allergy to penicillin. These drugs (amoxicillin, penicillin VK) may cause diarrhea, which sometimes necessitates discontinuation. Up to 90% of patients with mononucleosis who take amoxicillin, amoxicillin/clavulanate, or ampicillin get a rash.

By Those Over 60 Years of Age: Natural skin changes may predispose to prolonged itching in the genital and anal regions. Report such reactions promptly.

▷ **Advisability of Use During Pregnancy**

Pregnancy Category: B. See Pregnancy Risk Categories at the back of this book.

Animal Studies: Birth defects of the limbs reported in mice (penicillin VK only). (Not confirmed in other studies.)

Human Studies: Adequate studies of pregnant women indicate no increased risk of birth defects.

Ask your doctor for guidance, but these drugs are generally considered safe for use during any period of pregnancy.

Advisability of Use If Breast-Feeding

Presence of these drugs in breast milk: Yes.

The nursing infant may be sensitized to penicillin and be at risk for developing diarrhea or yeast infections. Talk with your doctor. Penicillins may be drugs of choice versus chloramphenicol or tetracyclines.

Habit-Forming Potential: None.

Effects of Overdose: Possible nausea, vomiting, and/or diarrhea.

Possible Effects of Long-Term Use: Superinfections, often due to yeast organisms or Clostridium difficile.

Suggested Periodic Examinations While Taking These Drugs (at physician's discretion)

Complete blood cell counts.

Kidney function tests.

▷ **While Taking These Drugs, Observe the Following**

Foods: No restrictions, except ampicillin, bacampicillin, and cloxacillin, which are best taken on an empty stomach.

Herbal Medicines or Minerals: Some patients use echinacea to attempt to boost their immune systems. Unfortunately, use of echinacea is not recommended in people with damaged immune systems. This herb may also actually weaken any immune system if it is used too often or for too long a time. Do NOT take mistletoe herb, oak bark or F.C. of marshmallow root and licorice. Guar gum decreased how much of one kind of penicillin got in the body. Avoid that combination.

Since St. John's wort and ampicillin may cause increased sun sensitivity, caution is advised.

Beverages: No restrictions (except as above). May be taken with milk.

▷   *Alcohol:* No interactions expected, but alcohol can blunt the immune response. It is best NOT to drink while you have an infection severe enough to require antibiotics.

Tobacco Smoking: No interactions expected. I advise everyone to quit smoking.

▷   *Other Drugs*

Penicillins *taken concurrently* with

- disulfiram (Antabuse) can cause a disulfiramlike reaction (see Glossary) (bacampicillin only); avoid the combination of these drugs.
- entacapone (Comtan) (and other medicines) are removed by the bile tract (biliary elimination), and medicines such as ampicillin that have been found to change removal by the bile. These and similar medicines may also alter blood levels by interfering with a process known as glucuronidation and/or intestinal beta glucuronidase may lead to an increased entacapone effect or adverse effects (such as movement disorders or diarrhea) in some patients. Closer patient follow-up and caution are prudent.
- live typhoid vaccine may blunt the vaccine response and benefits (amoxicillin and amoxicillin/clavulanate).
- methotrexate (Mexate) may increase risk of methotrexate toxicity (especially amoxicillin and oral penicillin).
- omeprazole (Prilosec) and other proton pump inhibitors (see Drug Classes) will decrease the amount of ampicillin that gets into the body because ampicillin requires an acid environment to optimally be absorbed.
- probenecid (Benemid) will increase and sustain blood levels. This interaction is often used to therapeutic advantage.

Ampicillin *taken concurrently* with

- allopurinol may increase the risk of rashes.
- atenolol can blunt the therapeutic benefits of atenolol.

Ampicillin, cloxacillin or penicillin VK *taken concurrently* with

- warfarin (Coumadin) may intensify the anticoagulant effect and increase risk of bleeding; more frequent INR (prothrombin time or protime) testing is needed.

Penicillins may *decrease* the effects of

- birth control pills (oral contraceptives) and impair their effectiveness in preventing pregnancy.

The following drugs may *decrease* the effects of penicillins:

- antacids, histamine (H2) blockers or proton pump inhibitors (see Drug Classes)—may reduce the absorption of penicillins.
- chloramphenicol (Chloromycetin).
- cholestyramine (Questran, etc.) can delay penicillins such as penicillin G. If these medicines must be used together, the penicillin should be taken (or given) an hour before the cholestyramine or alternatively, the penicillin should be taken four to six hours AFTER the cholestyramine.
- erythromycin (Erythrocin, E-Mycin, etc.).
- tetracyclines (Achromycin, Declomycin, doxycycline, Minocin, etc.: see Drug Classes).

▷ *Driving, Hazardous Activities:* Usually no restrictions. Be alert to the rare occurrence of dizziness and/or nausea and restrict activities accordingly.

Aviation Note: The use of these drugs **may be a disqualification** for piloting. Consult a designated Aviation Medical Examiner.

Exposure to Sun: Ampicillin may increase sensitivity to the sun. Use caution.

Special Storage Instructions: Oral solutions and pediatric drops (amoxicillin) should be refrigerated.

Observe the Following Expiration Times: Do not take the oral solution of these drugs if older than 7 days (cloxacillin is good for only 3 days) if kept at room temperature or 14 days when kept refrigerated.

PENTAZOCINE (pen TAZ oh seen)

Introduced: 1967   **Class:**   Analgesic, strong   **Prescription:** USA: Yes   **Controlled Drug:**   USA: C-IV*; Canada: No   **Available as Generic:**   USA: No; Canada: No

Brand Names: Talacen [CD], Talwin, Talwin Compound [CD], ♣Talwin Compound-50 [CD], Talwin Nx [CD]

BENEFITS versus RISKS	
Possible Benefits	*Possible Risks*
RELIEF OF MODERATE TO SEVERE PAIN	POTENTIAL FOR HABIT FORMATION (DEPENDENCE)
	Respiratory depression
	Sedative effects
	Mental and behavioral disturbances
	Low blood pressure, fainting
	Nausea, constipation

Author's Note: The information in this profile has been shortened to make room for more widely used medicines.

PENTOXIFYLLINE (pen tox I fi leen)

Other Name: Oxpentifylline

Introduced: 1972   **Class:**   Blood flow agent, xanthines   **Prescription:**   USA: Yes   **Controlled Drug:**   USA: No; Canada: No   **Available as Generic:**   No

Brand Name: Trental

*See Schedules of Controlled Drugs at the back of this book.

BENEFITS versus RISKS	
Possible Benefits	**Possible Risks**
IMPROVED BLOOD FLOW IN PERIPHERAL ARTERIAL DISEASE	Reduced blood pressure, angina, abnormal heart rhythms
REDUCTION OF INTERMITTENT CLAUDICATION PAIN	Rare low blood counts and aplastic anemia
May help in some AIDS-related pain	Indigestion, nausea, vomiting
	Dizziness, flushing

Author's Note: A medicine called cilostazol (Pletal) was approved by the FDA to treat intermittent claudication. Information in this profile has been shortened to make room for more widely used medicines.

PERGOLIDE (PER go lide)

Introduced: 1980 **Class:** Anti-Parkinsonism, ergot derivative **Prescription:** USA: Yes **Controlled Drug:** USA: No; Canada: No **Available as Generic:** USA: No

Brand Names: ✦Drax-Pergolide, Permax

BENEFITS versus RISKS	
Possible Benefits	**Possible Risks**
ADDITIVE RELIEF OF SYMPTOMS OF PARKINSON'S DISEASE WHEN USED CONCURRENTLY WITH LEVODOPA/CARBIDOPA PERMITS A REDUCTION IN SINEMET DOSE	ABNORMAL INVOLUNTARY MOVEMENTS HALLUCINATIONS INITIAL FALL IN BLOOD PRESSURE/ORTHOSTATIC HYPOTENSION
Reduces tics in some children with Tourette's and/or chronic tics	Premature heart contractions (ventricular)

▷ **Principal Uses**

As a Single Drug Product: Uses currently included in FDA-approved labeling: As an adjunct to levodopa/carbidopa treatment of Parkinson's disease for people who experience intolerable abnormal movements (dyskinesia) and/or increasing "on-off" episodes due to levodopa. The addition of pergolide (1) permits reduction of the daily dose of levodopa with consequent lessening of dyskinesia and erratic drug response and (2) provides additional relief of Parkinsonian symptoms.

Other (unlabeled) generally accepted uses: (1) helps in some conditions where excess prolactin is made; (2) may be of use in acromegaly; (3) works to lower increased prolactin levels (as in some pituitary tumors); (4) lowered tic occurrence significantly in one study of patients with chronic tics and/or Tourette's syndrome.

How This Drug Works: By directly stimulating part of the brain (dopamine receptor sites in the corpus striatum), this drug helps to compensate for the deficiency of dopamine that is responsible for the rigidity, tremor and sluggish movement characteristic of Parkinson's disease.

▷ **Widely Used Guidelines That Involve This Medicine (representative sample):** Please look at the section at the very beginning of this profile called "Class." Next, turn to Table 22 and you will find guidelines listed by the class involved!

Available Dosage Forms and Strengths
Tablets — 0.05 mg, 0.25 mg, 1 mg

▷ **Usual Adult Dosage Ranges:** *Parkinson's (in conjunction with levodopa plus carbidopa)*: Starts at 0.05 mg daily (first 2 days); slowly increased by 0.1 mg daily or 0.15 mg every third day over the next 12 days. If needed and tolerated, daily dose may be increased by 0.25 mg every third day until best response. Total daily dose, 0.4 mg, should be divided into three equal portions taken at 6- to 8-hour intervals. Usual ongoing dose is 3 mg every 24 hours; do not exceed 5 mg every 24 hours.

During gradual start of pergolide, dose of levodopa/carbidopa (Sinemet) may be lowered by your doctor.

Note: Actual dose and schedule must be determined for each patient individually.

Typical Treatment Goals and Measurements (Outcomes and Markers)
Parkinson's disease: The general goal is to minimize symptoms (tremor, sluggish movements, analysis of walking or gait, etc.) to the fullest extent possible. Additionally, many neurologists use Hahn-Yahr scores and the time it takes to maximum amount of finger tapping as indicators of the benefits of this drug.
Tic Reduction: The goal is to minimize the frequency of tics. The Yale Global Tic Severity Scale (YGTSS) is widely used to check results.

Conditions Requiring Dosing Adjustments
Liver Function: Used with caution in liver disease.
Kidney Function: Consideration should be given to empirical decreases in dose.

▷ **Dosing Instructions:** The tablet may be crushed and taken with food or milk to reduce stomach irritation. If you forget a dose: Take the missed dose as soon as you remember it, unless it's nearly time for your next dose—if that is the case, skip the missed dose and take the next dose right on schedule. DO NOT double doses. Talk with your doctor if you find yourself missing doses.

Usual Duration of Use: Regular use for 4 to 6 weeks reveals benefits controlling Parkinson's symptoms and permitting lower levodopa/carbidopa dose. Onset time for conditions involving excessive prolactin (hyperprolactinemia) will require a similar length of time to work. Long-term use requires follow-up with your doctor.

Possible Advantages of This Drug: May give more effective and uniform control of Parkinsonian symptoms and fewer adverse effects from levodopa therapy. More powerful (potent) and longer lasting than bromocriptine.

▷ **This Drug Should Not Be Taken If**
• you have had an allergic reaction to this medicine or to the components previously.
• you have had a serious adverse effect from any ergot preparation.
• you have severe coronary artery disease or peripheral vascular disease.

▷ **Inform Your Physician Before Taking This Drug If**
• you have constitutionally low blood pressure.
• you are pregnant or breast-feeding your infant.
• you are taking any antihypertensive drugs or antipsychotic drugs (see Drug Classes).

- you have any degree of coronary artery disease, especially angina, or a history of heart attack.
- you have any type of heart rhythm disorder.
- you have impaired liver or kidney function.
- you have a seizure disorder.

Possible Side Effects (natural, expected, and unavoidable drug actions)
Weakness; chest pain (possibly heart-related or anginal); peripheral edema; orthostatic hypotension (see Glossary)—infrequent.

▷ **Possible Adverse Effects** (unusual, unexpected, and infrequent reactions)
If any of the following develop, consult your physician promptly for guidance.
Mild Adverse Effects
Allergic reactions: skin rash, facial swelling—rare.
Headache, dizziness, confusion, drowsiness, insomnia, anxiety, double vision—rare to infrequent.
Nasal congestion, shortness of breath, palpitation, fainting—rare to infrequent.
Altered taste, dry mouth, indigestion, nausea, vomiting, constipation, diarrhea—infrequent.
Serious Adverse Effects
Allergic reactions: none reported.
Idiosyncratic reactions: flu-like symptoms.
Abnormal involuntary movements (dyskinesia)—frequent.
Psychotic behavior—case reports.
Hallucinations (accounted for 7.8% of patient withdrawals from therapy; 13.8% occurrence in clinical trials).
Abnormal heartbeat (ventricular arrhythmias)—infrequent to frequent.
Heart valve changes—case reports.
Anemia—rare.

▷ **Possible Effects on Sexual Function:** Infrequent reports of altered libido (increased or decreased), impotence, breast pain, priapism (see Glossary).

▷ **Adverse Effects That May Mimic Natural Diseases or Disorders**
Effects on mental function and behavior may resemble psychotic disorders.

Natural Diseases or Disorders That May Be Activated by This Drug
Coronary artery disease with anginal syndrome, heart rhythm disorders, Raynaud's phenomenon (see Glossary), seizure disorders.

Possible Effects on Laboratory Tests
Blood prolactin level: decreased (marked reduction).

CAUTION
1. May cause abnormal movements (dyskinesias), or intensify existing dyskinesias. Watch for tremors, twitching or abnormal involuntary movements of any kind. Report these promptly.
2. Low starting doses help prevent possibility of excessive drop in blood pressure. See dose routine outlined above.
3. Tell your doctor promptly if you become pregnant or plan pregnancy. This drug has been reported (rarely) to cause abortion and birth defects.
4. May lead to abnormal heart rhythms in people prone to arrhythmia.

Precautions for Use
By Infants and Children: One study in children 7–17 years old started with 25 mcg a day, then increased in seven days by 25 mcg to 50 mcg three times a

day. A study in children with chronic tics and/or Tourette's used 0.15 to
0.45 mg a day.

By Those Over 60 Years of Age: Small initial doses are mandatory. Watch closely
for any tendency to light-headedness or faintness, especially on arising
from a lying or sitting position. You may be more susceptible to the development of impaired thinking, confusion, agitation, nightmares, or hallucinations.

▷ **Advisability of Use During Pregnancy**

Pregnancy Category: B. See Pregnancy Risk Categories at the back of this book.

Animal Studies: No birth defects due to this drug were found in mouse or rabbit studies.

Human Studies: Adequate studies of pregnant women are not available. However, there are four reports of birth defects associated with the use of this
drug and infrequent reports of abortion. Causal relationships have not
been established, but prudence advises against the use of this drug during
pregnancy.

Consult your physician for guidance.

Advisability of Use If Breast-Feeding

Presence of this drug in breast milk: Unknown.

Avoid drug or refrain from nursing.

Habit-Forming Potential: None.

Effects of Overdose: Nausea, vomiting, palpitations, low blood pressure, agitation, severe involuntary movements, hallucinations, seizures.

Possible Effects of Long-Term Use: Increased risk of developing dyskinesias.

Suggested Periodic Examinations While Taking This Drug (at physician's discretion)

Regular evaluation of drug response.

Heart function and blood pressure status.

▷ **While Taking This Drug, Observe the Following**

Foods: No restrictions.

Herbal Medicines or Minerals: Calcium and garlic may lower blood pressure.
Since this medicine may also lower blood pressure, talk to your doctor
BEFORE you add garlic or additional amounts of calcium to your diet.
Calabar bean (chop nut, Fabia, ordeal nut, others) is unsafe when taken by
mouth (physostigmine is the active ingredient) and should never be taken
by people with Parkinson's disease. Some theory to suggest that kava (no
longer advised in Canada due to liver toxicity questions) may blunt pergolide effectiveness. Octacosanol (a cousin of vitamin E) can worsen
movement problems and should also be avoided.

Beverages: No restrictions. May be taken with milk.

▷ *Alcohol:* Alcohol can exaggerate the blood pressure–lowering and sedative
effects of this drug.

Tobacco Smoking: No interactions expected. I advise everyone to quit smoking.

▷ *Other Drugs*

Pergolide *taken concurrently* with
• antihypertensive drugs (and other drugs that can lower blood pressure)
requires careful monitoring for excessive drops in pressure (lisinopril case
report); dose changes may be needed.

The following drugs may *decrease* the effects of pergolide and diminish its
effectiveness:
• chlorprothixene (Taractan).
• haloperidol (Haldol).

- metoclopramide (Reglan).
- phenothiazines (see Drug Classes).
- thiothixene (Navane).

▷ *Driving, Hazardous Activities:* This drug may cause dizziness, drowsiness, impaired coordination, or fainting. Restrict activities as necessary.

Aviation Note: The use of this drug *is a disqualification* for piloting. Consult a designated Aviation Medical Examiner.

Exposure to Sun: No restrictions.

Exposure to Heat: Use caution until the combined effects have been determined. Hot environments can cause lowering of blood pressure.

Discontinuation: **Do not stop this drug abruptly.** Sudden withdrawal can cause confusion, paranoid thinking, and severe hallucinations. Consult your physician regarding a schedule for gradual withdrawal.

PERPHENAZINE (per FEN a zeen)

Introduced: 1957   **Class:**   Tranquilizer,   major;   phenothiazines
Prescription: USA: Yes   **Controlled Drug:**   USA: No; Canada: No
Available as Generic: USA: Yes; Canada: Yes

Brand Names: ✤Apo-Perphenazine, ✤Elavil Plus [CD], ✤Etrafon, Etrafon [CD], Etrafon-A [CD], Etrafon Forte [CD], ✤Phenazine, ✤PMS-Levazine, ✤PMS-Perphenazine, Triavil [CD], Trilafon

BENEFITS versus RISKS	
Possible Benefits	*Possible Risks*
EFFECTIVE CONTROL OF ACUTE MENTAL DISORDERS	SERIOUS TOXIC EFFECTS ON BRAIN WITH LONG-TERM USE
Beneficial effects on thinking, mood, and behavior	Liver damage with jaundice
Relief of anxiety and tension	Blood cell disorders: hemolytic anemia, abnormally low white
Moderately effective control of nausea and vomiting	blood cell and platelet counts

▷ **Principal Uses**

As a Single Drug Product: Uses currently included in FDA-approved labeling: (1) Treats acute and chronic psychotic disorders: agitated depression, schizophrenia, and similar mental dysfunction; (2) used as a tranquilizer to help agitated and disruptive behavior; (3) severe nausea and vomiting treatment; (4) used to prevent vomiting from cisplatin; (5) eases vertigo.

Other (unlabeled) generally accepted uses: (1) Can ease tremors caused by tricyclic antidepressants.

As a Combination Drug Product [CD]: Available combined with amitriptyline. In some severe agitated depression, combining an antipsychotic drug and an antidepressant will be more effective than either drug used alone.

Author's Note: Information in this profile has been shortened to make room for more widely used medicines.

PHENELZINE (FEN el zeen)

Introduced: 1961   **Class:** Antidepressant, MAO type A inhibitor
Prescription: USA: Yes   **Controlled Drug:** USA: No; Canada: No
Available as Generic: No
Brand Name: Nardil

BENEFITS versus RISKS

Possible Benefits	*Possible Risks*
EFFECTIVE RELIEF OF REACTIVE, NEUROTIC, ATYPICAL DEPRESSIONS WITH ASSOCIATED ANXIETY OR PHOBIA	DANGEROUS INTERACTIONS WITH MANY DRUGS AND FOODS CONDUCIVE TO HYPERTENSIVE CRISIS
Beneficial in some depressions that are not responsive to other treatments	DISORDERED HEART RATE AND RHYTHM
	Drug-induced hepatitis—rare
	Mental changes: agitation, confusion, impaired memory, hypomania

---

Author's Note: Since other medicines are more widely used, the information in this profile has been shortened.

PHENOBARBITAL (fee noh BAR bi tawl)

Other Name: Phenobarbitone

Introduced: 1912   **Class:** Sedative, anticonvulsant, barbiturates
Prescription: USA: Yes   **Controlled Drug:** USA: C-IV*; Canada: Yes
Available as Generic: Yes

Brand Names: Aasquel, Alised, Alubelap [CD], Aminodrox-Forte, Antispasmodic [CD], Azpan, Barbidonna [CD], Barbidonna Elixir [CD], Barbita, Belap, Belladenal [CD], Belladenal-S [CD], ✤Belladenal Spacetabs [CD], ✤Bellergal [CD], Bellergal-S [CD], ✤Bellergal Spacetabs [CD], Bronchotabs [CD], Bronkolixir [CD], ✤Cafergot-PB, Chardonna-2 [CD], Daricon PB, ✤Diclophen [CD], Dilantin w/Phenobarbital [CD], Donna-Sed, Donnatal [CD], Donphen, Ergobel [CD], Eskabarb, Eskaphen B [CD], Floramine, ✤Gardenal, Hybephen [CD], Hypnaldyne [CD], Isuprel Compound [CD], Kinesed [CD], Luminal, Mudrane GG Elixir and Tablets [CD], Mudrane Tablets [CD], Neospect, ✤Neuro-Spasex [CD], ✤Neuro-Trasentin [CD], ✤Neuro-Trasentin Forte [CD], Novalene, Phedral [CD], ✤Phenaphen Capsules [CD], ✤Phenaphen No. 2, 3, 4 [CD], Phenergan w/Codeine [CD], Phyldrox, Quadrinal [CD], Relaxadron, SBP [CD], Scodonnar [CD], Sedacord [CD], SK-Phenobarbital, Solfoton, Spasquid [CD], Spazcaps, Tedral Preparations [CD], T.E.P. [CD], Thalfed [CD], Theocardone, Theocord [CD], Theolixer, Vitaphen

---

*See Schedules of Controlled Drugs at the back of this book.

BENEFITS versus RISKS

Possible Benefits	*Possible Risks*
EFFECTIVE CONTROL OF TONIC-CLONIC SEIZURES AND ALL TYPES OF PARTIAL SEIZURES	POTENTIAL FOR DEPENDENCE LIFE-THREATENING TOXICITY WITH OVERDOSE
EFFECTIVE CONTROL OF FEBRILE SEIZURES OF CHILDHOOD	Drug-induced hepatitis or decreased kidney function
Effective relief of anxiety and nervous tension	Blood cell disorders: abnormally low red cell, white cell, and platelet counts

▷ **Principal Uses**

As a Single Drug Product: Uses currently included in FDA-approved labeling: (1) Used as a mild sedative; (2) used as an anticonvulsant to control grand mal epilepsy and all types of partial seizures, including febrile seizures of childhood; (3) used as a sedative, yet newer agents carry fewer drug interactions or effects on sleep cycles.

Other (unlabeled) generally accepted uses: (1) May be helpful in detoxification of sedative-hypnotic addiction; (2) can help control seizures found in cerebral malaria; (3) eases neonatal seizures; (4) may have a role in treating pain syndromes.

As a Combination Drug Product [CD]: This drug is available in many combinations with derivatives of belladonna, an antispasmodic commonly used to treat functional disorders of the gastrointestinal tract. It is also available in combination with bronchodilators for the treatment of asthma and with ergotamine for the treatment of headaches.

How This Drug Works: Impedes transfer of sodium and potassium across cells and selectively blocks nerve impulses. This can give a sedative effect or suppress nerve impulses that cause seizures.

Author's Note: Information in this profile has been shortened to make room for more widely used medicines.

PHENYTOIN (FEN i toh in)

Other Name: Diphenylhydantoin

Introduced: 1938   **Class:**   Anticonvulsant, hydantoins, pain syndrome modifier   **Prescription:**   USA: Yes   **Controlled Drug:**   USA: No; Canada: No   **Available as Generic:**   USA: Yes; Canada: Yes

Brand Names: Dilantin, Dilantin Infatabs, Dilantin w/Phenobarbital [CD], Di-Phen, Diphenylan, Ekko JR, Ekko SR, Ekko Three, ✿Mebroin [CD], ✿Phelantin

---

BENEFITS versus RISKS

Possible Benefits	Possible Risks
EFFECTIVE CONTROL OF TONIC-CLONIC (GRAND MAL), PSYCHOMOTOR (TEMPORAL LOBE), MYOCLONIC and FOCAL SEIZURE	VERY NARROW TREATMENT MARGIN
	POSSIBLE BIRTH DEFECTS
	Overgrowth of gums
May have a role used as a powder helping heal wounds (diabetic wounds and pressure or bed sores)	Excessive hair growth
	Blood cell disorders: impaired production of all blood cells
	Drug-induced hepatitis or nephritis

▷ **Principal Uses**

As a Single Drug Product: Uses currently included in FDA-approved labeling: As an antiepileptic drug to control grand mal, psychomotor, myoclonic and focal seizures. It can also be used to control seizures following brain surgery (neurosurgery).

Other (unlabeled) generally accepted uses: (1) Used to initiate treatment of trigeminal neuralgia—it is sometimes effective in relieving the severe facial pain of this disorder; (2) used in chronic pain syndromes; (3) may have a role (as an applied powder) in helping heal wounds (such as bed sores and diabetic wounds); (4) effective in eclampsia or pre-eclampsia.

As a Combination Drug Product [CD]: This drug is available in combination with phenobarbital, another effective anticonvulsant. Some seizure disorders require the combined actions of these two drugs for effective control.

How This Drug Works: By promoting the loss of sodium from nerve fibers, this drug lowers and stabilizes their excitability and thereby inhibits the repetitious spread of electrical impulses along nerve pathways. This action may prevent seizures altogether or it may reduce their frequency and severity. In helping wound healing it probably works in a similar way as the adverse effect of causing excessive gum growth. Phenytoin appears to promote fibroblast growth leading to collagen, etc.

▷ **Widely Used Guidelines That Involve This Medicine (representative sample):** Please look at the section at the very beginning of this profile called "Class." Next, turn to Table 22 and you will find guidelines listed by the class involved!

Available Dosage Forms and Strengths

Capsules, extended — 30 mg, 100 mg

Capsules, prompt — 30 mg, 100 mg

Injection — 50 mg/mL

Kapseals — 30 mg, 100 mg

Oral suspension — 30 mg/5 mL, 125 mg/5 mL

Tablets, chewable — 50 mg

▷ **Usual Adult Dosage Ranges:** *Seizures:* Initially (prompt or extended form) 100 mg three times a day. Dose may be increased cautiously by 100 mg/week as needed and tolerated. Once the optimal maintenance dose has been identified, the total daily dose may be taken as a single dose every 24 hours if Dilantin capsules are used. No other formulation is approved for once-a-day use. The total daily dose should not exceed 600 mg. In wound healing, some clinicians have used a phenytoin capsule content mixed with sterile saline using sterile technique. A sterile gauze pad is then soaked in the mixture and the gauze applied to the wound. Others have applied phenytoin powder USP directly to the wound once a day and then covered the wound with a sterile dressing. This is not an FDA-approved use and standardized protocols and research are needed.

Note: Actual dose and schedule must be determined for each patient individually.

Conditions Requiring Dosing Adjustments

Liver Function: The ongoing dose should be decreased based on blood levels.

Kidney Function: The dose or dosing interval must be decreased in moderate kidney failure.

Obesity: The way this medicine is distributed (volume of distribution) changes with increasing body fat. Loading doses must be calculated based on ideal body weight. The product of 1.33 times actual weight divided by the ideal weight is then added to the original number to decide the final loading dose.

▷ **Dosing Instructions:** May be taken with or after food to reduce stomach irritation. The capsule may be opened, and the tablet may be crushed. Chew tabs or liquid forms can help if you have problems swallowing. If liquid suspension form is used, shake the medicine well, then use a measuring spoon or calibrated medicine dose cup to get exactly the right dose. If you forget a dose: Take the missed dose as soon as you remember it, unless it's nearly time for your next dose—if that is the case, skip the missed dose and take the next dose right on schedule. DO NOT double doses unless your doctor tells you to do that. If you miss two doses or more in a row, call your doctor.

Usual Duration of Use: Use on a regular schedule for 2 to 3 weeks usually determines benefit in reducing frequency and severity of seizures. Optimal control will require careful dose adjustments over a period of several months. Long-term use (months to years) requires ongoing physician supervision.

Typical Treatment Goals and Measurements (Outcomes and Markers)

Seizures: The general goal for this medicine is effective seizure control. Neurologists tend to define "effective" on a case-by-case basis depending on the seizure type and patient factors. If seizure control is not effective, it's not unusual to use combination treatment. For this medicine, a balance must be struck between too little medicine and too much medicine. Blood levels are used to make certain that the blood level is in the right range.

▷ **This Drug Should Not Be Taken If**
• you have had an allergic reaction to this drug or other hydantoin drugs previously.
• you have sinus bradycardia or serious heart block.

▷ **Inform Your Physician Before Taking This Drug If**
• you are taking any other drugs at this time.
• you have a history of liver disease or impaired liver function.
• you have a history of alcohol abuse. Alcohol can change blood levels of this medicine.
• you have low blood pressure, diabetes, or any type of heart disease.
• you are pregnant or planning pregnancy.
• you plan to have surgery under general anesthesia in the near future.

Possible Side Effects (natural, expected, and unavoidable drug actions)
Mild fatigue, sluggishness and drowsiness (in sensitive individuals).
Pink to red to brown coloration of urine (of no significance).

▷ **Possible Adverse Effects** (unusual, unexpected, and infrequent reactions)
If any of the following develop, consult your physician promptly for guidance.

Mild Adverse Effects

Allergic reactions: skin rashes, hives, drug fever (see Glossary).

Headache, dizziness, nervousness, insomnia, muscle twitching—infrequent.

Nausea, vomiting, constipation—infrequent.

Bedwetting—case reports.

Abnormal eye movements—dose-related.

Low blood calcium (and potential osteoporosis) and elevated blood sugar— possible.

Overgrowth of gum tissues—most common in children.

Excessive growth of body hair—most common in young girls.

Serious Adverse Effects

Allergic reactions: drug-induced hepatitis, with or without jaundice (see Glossary).

Drug-induced nephritis, with acute kidney failure.

Severe skin reactions (toxic epidermal necrolysis, Stevens-Johnson syndrome or erythema multiforme).

Myocarditis, generalized enlargement of lymph glands (pseudolymphoma)— case reports.

Idiosyncratic reactions: hemolytic anemia (see Glossary).

Acute psychotic episodes—case reports.

Mental confusion, unsteadiness, double vision, jerky eye movements, slurred speech—possible.

Drug-induced seizures—possible.

Blood-clotting disorders in infants of mothers maintained on phenytoin— rare.

Bone marrow depression (see Glossary): weakness, fever, sore throat, bleeding, or bruising—case reports.

Lupus erythematosus—case report.

Drug-induced periarteritis nodosa, low thyroid function, or myasthenia gravis—case reports.

Tardive dyskinesia or porphyria—case reports.

Abnormal IgA (increased risk of respiratory infections)—possible.

Peripheral nerve damage (neuropathy) or muscle damage (myopathy)—case reports.

Serious heart rhythm problems (such as ventricular fibrillation)—with rapid intravenous use.

Elevated blood sugar, due to inhibition of insulin release—possible.

▷ **Possible Effects on Sexual Function:** Decreased libido and/or impotence— infrequent.

Swelling and tenderness of male breast tissue (gynecomastia) or Peyronie's disease (see Glossary)—rare.

Decreased effectiveness of oral contraceptives.

▷ **Adverse Effects That May Mimic Natural Diseases or Disorders**

Drug-induced hepatitis may suggest viral hepatitis. Skin reactions may resemble lupus erythematosus.

Natural Diseases or Disorders That May Be Activated by This Drug

Latent diabetes, porphyria, systemic lupus erythematosus, low bone mineral density predisposing to osteoporosis.

Possible Effects on Laboratory Tests

Complete blood cell counts: decreased red cells, hemoglobin, white cells, and platelets; increased eosinophils (allergic reaction).

Blood lupus erythematosus (LE) cells: positive.

Prothrombin time: increased (when phenytoin is taken concurrently with warfarin).

Blood calcium level: decreased.

Blood total cholesterol, LDL and VLDL cholesterol levels: no effects.

Blood HDL cholesterol level: increased.

Blood triglyceride levels: no effect.

Blood glucose level: increased.

Blood thyroid hormone levels: T3, T4, and free T4: increased.

Liver function tests: increased liver enzymes (ALT/GPT, AST/GOT, alkaline phosphatase) and bilirubin.

CAUTION

1. Some brand-name capsules of this drug have a significantly longer duration of action than generic-name capsules of the same strength. To assure a correct dosing schedule, it is necessary to distinguish between "prompt"-action and "extended"-action capsules. Do not substitute one for the other without your physician's knowledge and guidance.
2. When used for the treatment of epilepsy, *this drug must not be stopped abruptly.*
3. Periodic blood levels of this drug are essential to get the right dose (see "Therapeutic Drug Monitoring" in Section One).
4. Use of phenytoin in wound healing has some early data, but requires further research and standardization of protocols.
5. Take this medicine EXACTLY as prescribed and at the same time each day.
6. Shake the suspension form of this drug thoroughly before measuring the dose. Use a standard measuring device to assure that the dose is accurate.
7. Side effects and mild adverse effects are usually most apparent during the first several days of treatment and often subside with continued use.
8. It may be necessary to take folic acid to prevent anemia. Talk with your doctor about this.
9. Case reports have been made about atypical allergy (cross-sensitivity) between phenytoin and carbamazepine (Tegretol, others). Talk to your doctor if you are allergic to phenytoin.
10. This medicine has an unusual pathway for removal that can fill up (become saturated) and stop working. This means that a small change in dose may give a huge change in blood levels. Make certain you know exactly how much phenytoin your doctor wants you to take.
11. Carry personal identification card that says you are taking this drug.

Precautions for Use

By Infants and Children: Elimination of this drug varies widely with age. Periodic measurement of blood levels is essential for all ages. Some children will require more than one dose daily for good control.

Observe for early indications of drug toxicity: jerky eye movements, unsteadiness in stance and gait, slurred speech, abnormal involuntary movements of the extremities, and odd behavior.

By Those Over 60 Years of Age: You may be more sensitive to all of the actions of this drug and require smaller doses. Observe closely for any indications of early toxicity: drowsiness, fatigue, confusion, unsteadiness, disturbances of vision, slurred speech, muscle twitching.

▷ **Advisability of Use During Pregnancy**

Pregnancy Category: D. See Pregnancy Risk Categories at the back of this book.

Animal Studies: Cleft lip and palate, skeletal and visceral defects in mice and rats.

Human Studies: Available information is conflicting. Some studies suggest a small but significant increase in birth defects. The incidence of birth defects in children of epileptics not taking anticonvulsant drugs is 3.2%; incidence increases to 6.4% with anticonvulsant use in pregnancy. The "fetal hydantoin syndrome" in infants exposed to phenytoin during pregnancy shows birth defects of skull, face, and limbs; deficient growth and development; and subnormal intelligence. Other effects on the infant include reduction in blood-clotting factors that predispose it to severe bruising and hemorrhage.

Discuss the benefits and risks of using this drug during pregnancy with your doctor. It is advisable to use the smallest maintenance dose that will control seizures. In addition, you should take vitamin K during the final month of pregnancy to prevent a deficiency of fetal blood-clotting factors.

Advisability of Use If Breast-Feeding

Presence of this drug in breast milk: Yes, in trace amounts.

Monitor nursing infant closely, and discontinue drug or nursing if adverse effects develop.

Habit-Forming Potential: None.

Effects of Overdose: Drowsiness, jerky eye movements, hand tremor, unsteadiness, slurred speech, hallucinations, delusions, nausea, vomiting, stupor progressing to coma.

Possible Effects of Long-Term Use: Low blood calcium resulting in rickets or osteomalacia; megaloblastic anemia; peripheral neuropathy (see Glossary); schizophreniclike psychosis. Lymphosarcoma, malignant lymphoma, and leukemia have been associated with long-term use; a cause-and-effect relationship (see Glossary) has not been established.

Suggested Periodic Examinations While Taking This Drug (at physician's discretion)

Monitoring of blood phenytoin levels to guide dose. Time to sample blood for phenytoin level: just before next dose. Recommended therapeutic range: 10 to 20 mg/mL.

Complete blood cell counts.

Liver function tests.

Measurements of the following blood levels: glucose, calcium, phosphorus, folic acid, vitamin B_{12}.

Bone mineral density testing (DEXA) to check risk for osteoporosis and fracture.

▷ **While Taking This Drug, Observe the Following**

Foods: No restrictions.

Herbal Medicines or Minerals: Using kola, guarana, or ma huang may result in unacceptable central nervous system stimulation. Evening primrose oil may increase seizure risk. Some ginkgo products have a contaminant in them called 4-O-methylpyridoxine, which may increase seizure risk. Combination is not advisable. Valerian and kava kava (use questionable due to possible liver toxicity) may interact to increase drowsiness. St. John's wort may also cause increased sun sensitivity—caution is advised. Increased calcium and vitamin D are prudent.

Nutritional Support: Supplements of folic acid, calcium, vitamin D, and vitamin K may be necessary.

Beverages: No restrictions. May be taken with milk.

▷   *Alcohol:* Use extreme caution. Alcohol (in large quantities or with continual use) may reduce this drug's effectiveness in preventing seizures.

Tobacco Smoking: No interactions expected. I advise everyone to quit smoking.

▷   *Other Drugs*

Phenytoin may ***decrease*** the effects of

- acetaminophen (Tylenol, others).
- acyclovir (Zovirax).
- amprenavir (Agenerase), atazanavir (Reyataz), indinavir (Crixivan), ritonavir (Norvir) and perhaps other protease inhibitors.
- atorvastatin (Lipitor) and simvastatin (Zocor) probably by increasing liver enzymes (cytochrome P450 3A4), which are partly involved in removing atorvastatin. More frequent checks of progress toward cholesterol goals are prudent if these medicines must be combined.
- bupropion (Wellbutrin).
- cholecalciferol (vitamin D).
- clofibrate (Atromid-S).
- clozapine (Clozaril).
- conjugated estrogens (Premarin).
- cortisonelike drugs (see Drug Classes).
- cyclosporine (Sandimmune).
- disopyramide (Norpace).
- donepezil (Aricept).
- doxycycline (Vibramycin, etc.).
- imatinib (Gleevec). Checks of imatinib levels used to guide dosing are prudent.
- itraconazole (Sporanox), voriconazole (Vfend), and other antifungals using the same liver removal system.
- lamotrigine (Lamictal). Blood levels of lamotrigine and dosing adjustments as indicated are needed.
- levodopa (Larodopa, Sinemet).
- levothyroxine (Synthroid, others).
- meperidine (Demerol).
- methadone (Dolophine).
- mexiletine (Mexitil).
- miconazole (Monistat, Micatin, others).
- neuromuscular blocking agents (such as pancuronium-Pavulon or vecuronium-Norcuron).
- oral antidiabetic drugs (see Drug Classes).
- oral contraceptives (birth control pills).
- paclitaxel (Taxol).
- paroxetine (Paxil).
- quetiapine (Seroquel).
- quinidine (Quinaglute, etc.).
- sirolimus (Rapamune) and tacrolimus (Prograf).
- tiagabine (Gabitril).
- triamcinolone.

Phenytoin ***taken concurrently*** with

- acetazolamide (Diamox) may lead to bone problems (osteomalacia).
- aprepitant (Emend) may result in decreased benefits of phenytoin OR aprepitant.

- carbamazepine (Tegretol) may result in increased or decreased levels of phenytoin.
- chlordiazepoxide (Librium, and perhaps other benzodiazepines) may increase or decrease phenytoin levels; levels should be obtained more frequently if these drugs are combined.
- ciprofloxacin (Cipro) may increase or decrease phenytoin levels. Check phenytoin levels more frequently.
- dopamine will result in very low blood pressure.
- flu shots (influenza vaccine) may change phenytoin levels.
- ketorolac (Toradol) may result in seizures—DO NOT COMBINE these medicines.
- oral anticoagulants (Coumadin, etc.) can either increase or decrease the anticoagulant effect; monitor this combination very closely with INR (serial prothrombin) testing.
- primidone (Mysoline) may alter primidone actions and enhance its toxicity.
- theophyllines (Aminophyllin, Theo-Dur, etc.) may cause a decrease in the effectiveness of both drugs.
- valproic acid (Depakene) may result in altered phenytoin or valproic acid levels; increased blood level testing of both medicines is needed if these medicines are to be combined.
- warfarin (Coumadin) may lead to initial increased bleeding risk and subsequent decrease in anticoagulation; more frequent INR (prothrombin time or protime) testing is needed. Warfarin doses should be adjusted to results.

The following drugs may ***increase*** the effects of phenytoin:
- amiodarone (Cordarone).
- chloramphenicol (Chloromycetin).
- chlorpheniramine.
- cimetidine (Tagamet).
- clopidogrel (Plavix)—extent unknown—yet clopidogrel inhibits cytochrome P450 2C9 which helps remove phenytoin from the body. More frequent checks of phenytoin levels are prudent if these medicines are combined.
- cotrimoxazole (Bactrim).
- diltiazem (Cardizem).
- disulfiram (Antabuse).
- felbamate (Felbatol).
- fluconazole (Diflucan).
- fluoxetine (Prozac).
- fluvoxamine (Luvox).
- gabapentin (Neurontin).
- ibuprofen and perhaps other NSAIDs.
- isoniazid (INH, Niconyl, etc.).
- metronidazole (Flagyl).
- nefazodone (Serzone).
- nifedipine (Adalat).
- omeprazole (Prilosec).
- phenacemide (Phenurone).
- S-Liposomal doxorubicin.
- sertraline (Zoloft).
- sulfonamides (see Drug Classes).
- topiramate (Topamax).
- trazodone (Desyrel).

- tricyclic antidepressants (see Drug Classes).
- trimethoprim (Proloprim, Trimpex).
- valproic acid (Depakene).
- venlafaxine (Effexor).
- zotepine (Nipolept).

The following drugs may ***decrease*** the effects of phenytoin:

- antacids (various)—separate doses by two hours.
- aspirin (high dose, various brands)—more frequent checks of total and free phenytoin levels.
- bleomycin (Blenoxane).
- carmustine (BiCNU).
- cisplatin (Platinol).
- diazoxide (Proglycem, Hyperstat).
- folic acid (various).
- methotrexate (Mexate).
- rifampin (Rifadin).
- vinblastine (Velban).

▷ *Driving, Hazardous Activities:* This drug may impair mental alertness, vision and coordination. Restrict activities as necessary.

Aviation Note: The use of this drug ***is a disqualification*** for piloting. Consult a designated Aviation Medical Examiner.

Exposure to Sun: Use caution—this drug may cause photosensitivity (see Glossary).

Occurrence of Unrelated Illness: Intercurrent infections may slow the elimination of this drug and increase the risk of toxicity, due to higher blood levels.

Discontinuation: ***This drug must not be discontinued abruptly.*** Sudden withdrawal can precipitate severe and repeated seizures. If this drug is to be discontinued, gradual reduction in dose should be made over a period of 3 months. Total drug withdrawal may be attempted after a period of 3 to 4 years without a seizure. However, seizures are likely to recur in 40% of adults and in 20–30% of children.

PILOCARPINE (pi loh KAR peen)

Introduced: **1875** Class: Antiglaucoma **Prescription:** USA: Yes **Controlled Drug:** USA: No; Canada: No **Available as Generic:** Yes

Brand Names: Adsorbocarpine, Akarpine, Almocarpine, Betoptic Pilo [CD], E-PiloPreparations[CD], I-Pilopine, IsoptoCarpine, ✤Minims, ✤Miocarpine, Ocusert Pilo-20, Ocusert Pilo-40, PE Preparations [CD], Pilagan, Pilocar, Pilopine HS, Piloptic-1, Piloptic-2, Pilosyst 20/40, Salagen, ✤Spersacarpine

BENEFITS versus RISKS

Possible Benefits	***Possible Risks***
EFFECTIVE REDUCTION OF INTERNAL EYE PRESSURE FOR CONTROL OF ACUTE AND CHRONIC GLAUCOMA	Mild side effects with systemic absorption Minor eye discomfort Altered vision

▷ **Principal Uses**

As a Single Drug Product: Uses currently included in FDA-approved labeling: (1) Used to manage all types of glaucoma (selection of the appropriate dose form and strength must be carefully individualized); (2) can help in dry mouth (xerostomia) even after radiation therapy; (3) eases symptoms in Sjögren's syndrome.

Other (unlabeled) generally accepted uses: (1) Treatment of Adie syndrome; (2) can help before laser surgery in order to prevent excessive increases in eye (intraocular) pressure after surgery.

As a Combination Drug Product [CD]: This drug is combined with epinephrine (in eyedrop solutions) to utilize the actions of both drugs in lowering internal eye pressure. The opposite effects of these two drugs on the size of the pupil (pilocarpine constricts, epinephrine dilates) provides a balance that prevents excessive constriction or dilation. The Betopic Pilo form offers the combination benefits of a beta blocker (betaxolol).

How This Drug Works: By directly stimulating constriction of the pupil, this drug enlarges the outflow canal in the anterior chamber of the eye and promotes the drainage of excess fluid (aqueous humor), thus lowering the internal eye pressure.

▷ **Widely Used Guidelines That Involve This Medicine (representative sample):** Please look at the section at the very beginning of this profile called "Class." Next, turn to Table 22 and you will find guidelines listed by the class involved!

Available Dosage Forms and Strengths

Combination solution — 1.75% pilocarpine and 0.25% betaxolol

Eyedrop solutions — 0.25%, 0.5%, 1%, 2%, 3%, 4%, 5%, 6%

Gel — 4%

Ocuserts — 20 mcg, 40 mcg

Tablets — 5 mg

▷ **Usual Adult Dosage Ranges:** *For open-angle glaucoma*: Eyedrop solutions—one drop of a 1% to 2% solution three to four times daily (every 6–8 hours). Dosing is adjusted to keep the eye pressure (intraocular pressure) at the goal decided upon. See betaxolol profile for combination form dosing. Eye gel—apply 0.5-inch strip of gel into the eye once daily at bedtime. Ocusert—insert one into affected eye and replace every 7 days with a new one.

Note: Actual dose and dosing schedule must be determined for each patient individually.

Conditions Requiring Dosing Adjustments

Liver Function: Decreased removal from the body (roughly 30% slower in one small study). Empiric small steps in dosing and possible increased effects with "normal doses" are to be watched for in patients with moderate liver compromise.

Kidney Function: The elimination of this drug has yet to be defined.

▷ **Dosing Instructions:** To avoid excessive absorption into the body, press finger against inner corner of the eye (to close off the tear duct) during and for 2 minutes following instillation of the eyedrop. Place the gel and the Ocusert in the eye at bedtime. If you forget a dose: Use the missed dose as soon as you remember it, unless it's nearly time for your next dose—if that is the case, skip the missed dose and take the next dose right on schedule. DO NOT double doses. Talk with your doctor and pharmacist if you find yourself missing doses. Taking the medicine is crucial to getting results.

Usual Duration of Use: Use on a regular schedule for 1 to 2 weeks usually determines this drug's effectiveness in controlling internal eye pressure. Long-term use (months to years) requires physician supervision and follow-up to make sure pressure stays in the desired range.

Typical Treatment Goals and Measurements (Outcomes and Markers)
Glaucoma: Ophthalmologists measure eye pressure (intraocular pressure [IOP]), and then check IOP lowering once this medicine is started, adjusting (titrating) the medicine(s) to get and keep eye pressure in the desired range. The chamber angle can be checked prior to treatment.

Currently a "Drug of Choice"
For primary open-angle glaucoma (along with timolol and dipivefrin) especially in people over 50 years old.

▷ **This Drug Should Not Be Taken If**
- you have had an allergic reaction to it previously.
- you have sudden (acute) iritis or other eye problems where a key effect of this medicine (miosis) is not acceptable.
- you have active bronchial asthma and are using the tablet form.

▷ **Inform Your Physician Before Taking This Drug If**
- you have a history of bronchial asthma.
- you have a history of acute iritis.
- you have significant heart, kidney, or liver disease.
- your thyroid is overactive (hyperthyroidism).
- you have chronic obstructive pulmonary disease.
- you have gallstones.
- you are trying to have a baby.

Possible Side Effects (natural, expected, and unavoidable drug actions)
Temporary impairment of vision, usually lasting 2 to 3 hours following instillation of drops. Burning of the eyes, sensitivity to light and trouble seeing at night—frequent.

▷ **Possible Adverse Effects** (unusual, unexpected, and infrequent reactions)
If any of the following develop, consult your physician promptly for guidance.
Mild Adverse Effects
Allergic reactions: itching of the eyes, eyelid itching and/or swelling.
Headache, heart palpitation, tremors—infrequent.
Sweating—frequent.
Nausea—case reports.
Serious Adverse Effects
Provocation of acute asthma in susceptible patients.
Mental status changes (memory loss, confusion, or hallucinations)—case reports.
Atrioventricular block (abnormal heart conduction), slow heartbeats (bradycardia) and blood pressure changes (hypo or hypertension)—case reports.
Retinal detachment—possible.

▷ **Possible Effects on Sexual Function:** Possible impaired fertility.

Possible Effects on Laboratory Tests
Red blood cell and white blood cell counts: increased.

Precautions for Use
By Those Over 60 Years of Age: Maintain personal cleanliness to prevent eye infections. Report promptly any indication of eye infection.

▷ **Advisability of Use During Pregnancy**

Pregnancy Category: C. See Pregnancy Risk Categories at the back of this book.

Animal Studies: Significant birth defects due to this drug reported in rats.

Human Studies: Adequate studies of pregnant women are not available. Limit use to the smallest effective dose. Minimize systemic absorption (see "Dosing Instructions" above).

Advisability of Use If Breast-Feeding

Presence of this drug in breast milk: May be present in small amounts. Monitor nursing infant closely, and discontinue drug or nursing if adverse effects develop.

Habit-Forming Potential: None.

Effects of Overdose: Flushing of face, increased flow of saliva, sweating. If solution is swallowed: nausea, vomiting, diarrhea, profuse sweating, rapid pulse, difficult breathing, loss of consciousness.

Possible Effects of Long-Term Use: Development of tolerance (see Glossary), temporary loss of effectiveness.

Suggested Periodic Examinations While Taking This Drug (at physician's discretion)

Measurement of internal eye pressure on a regular basis.

Examination of eyes for development of cataracts.

▷ **While Taking This Drug, Observe the Following**

Foods: No restrictions.

Herbal Medicines or Minerals: St. John's wort may also cause increased sun sensitivity—caution is advised. Scopolia root has glaucoma as a possible side effect. DO NOT COMBINE. Henbane, ephedra–ma huang (now removed from the market for weight loss), and belladonna should also be avoided.

Beverages: No restrictions.

▷   *Alcohol:* Use caution. If this drug is absorbed, it may prolong the effect of alcohol on the brain.

Tobacco Smoking: No interactions expected. I advise everyone to quit smoking.

Marijuana Smoking: Sustained additional decrease in internal eye pressure.

▷   *Other Drugs*

The following drugs may **decrease** the effects of pilocarpine:

• atropine and drugs with atropinelike actions (see Drug Classes).

Pilocarpine **taken concurrently** with

• dipivefrin (Propine) may result in increased myopia and blurred vision.

• epinephrine (various) will result in increased myopia.

• latanoprost (Xalatan) may decrease latanoprost effectiveness. The bedtime dose of pilocarpine should be given an hour after the latanoprost dose.

• sulfacetamide (Sulamyd) may lead to pilocarpine precipitation. Separate these drugs by 20 minutes.

• timolol can produce additive effects in treating glaucoma.

▷   *Driving, Hazardous Activities:* This drug may impair your ability to focus your vision properly. Restrict activities as necessary.

Aviation Note: The use of this drug **may be a disqualification** for piloting. Consult a designated Aviation Medical Examiner.

Exposure to Sun: This medicine may make you very sensitive to the sun. Wear sunglasses.

Discontinuation: Do not stop regular use of this drug without consulting your physician. Periodic discontinuation and temporary substitution of another drug may be necessary to preserve its effectiveness in treating glaucoma.

PINDOLOL (PIN doh lohl)

Introduced: 1972   **Class:**   Antihypertensive, beta-adrenergic blocker
Prescription: USA: Yes   **Controlled Drug:**   USA: No; Canada: No
Available as Generic: Yes

Brand Names: ✤Alti-Pindol, ✤Apo-Pindol, ✤Dom-Pindolol, ✤Novo-Pindol, ✤Nu-Pindol, ✤Syn-Pindolol, ✤Viskazide [CD], Visken

---

BENEFITS versus RISKS

Possible Benefits	*Possible Risks*
EFFECTIVE, WELL-TOLERATED ANTIHYPERTENSIVE IN MILD TO MODERATE HIGH BLOOD PRESSURE	CONGESTIVE HEART FAILURE IN ADVANCED HEART DISEASE
EFFECTIVE PREVENTION OF ANGINA	Worsening of angina in coronary heart disease (abrupt withdrawal)
PROBABLY HELPS PREVENT (LIKE OTHER BETA BLOCKERS) REPEAT HEART ATTACKS	Masking of low blood sugar (hypoglycemia) in drug-treated diabetes
	Provocation of asthma (with high doses in asthmatics)

▷ **Principal Uses**

As a *Single Drug Product:* Uses currently included in FDA-approved labeling: Treats mild to moderate high blood pressure, alone or with other drugs.

Other (unlabeled) generally accepted uses: (1) May be of benefit in helping control aggressive behavior; (2) can help prevent migraine headaches; (3) combination therapy with digoxin may be effective in limiting some abnormal heart rhythms (atrial fibrillation); (4) can be of benefit in some kinds of anxiety; (5) decreases sympathetic output in hyperthyroidism; (5) helps prevent angina.

As a *Combination Drug Product [CD]:* This drug is available in combination with hydrochlorothiazide (in Canada). The addition of a thiazide diuretic to this beta-blocker drug enhances its effectiveness as an antihypertensive.

How This Drug Works: Blocks certain actions of the sympathetic nervous system:

• reducing rate and contraction force of the heart, thus lowering ejection pressure of blood leaving the heart
• reducing degree of contraction of blood vessel walls, lowering blood pressure.

▷ **Widely Used Guidelines That Involve This Medicine (representative sample):** Please look at the section at the very beginning of this profile called "Class." Next, turn to Table 22 and you will find guidelines listed by the class involved!

Available Dosage Forms and Strengths
Tablets — 5 mg, 10 mg
Tablets (Canada) — 15 mg

▷ **Usual Adult Dosage Ranges:** *Hypertension*: Starts with 5 mg twice a day (12 hours apart). The dose may be increased gradually by 10 mg/day at intervals of 3 to 4 weeks as needed and tolerated, up to 60 mg/day. For ongoing use (maintenance), 5 to 10 mg two or three times daily is often effective. The total daily dose should not exceed 60 mg. *Angina prevention*: Starting dose is 2.5 to 5 mg. This starting dose can then be increased as needed and tolerated over several weeks.

Note: Actual dose and schedule must be determined for each patient individually.

Conditions Requiring Dosing Adjustments

Liver Function: See comment below. Lower starting doses are prudent, coupled with careful patient follow-up. People with combined liver and kidney disease should be given lower starting doses and vigilant follow-up.

Kidney Function: This medicine had two ways that it is removed from the body (kidney and liver). While some sources advocate no adjustment in kidney failure, lower starting doses and careful patient monitoring of blood pressure is prudent and doses lowered if blood pressure becomes unacceptably low.

▷ **Dosing Instructions:** The tablet may be crushed and taken without regard to eating. Do not stop this drug abruptly. If you forget a dose: Take the missed dose as soon as you remember it, unless it's 4 hours or less until your next scheduled dose—if that is the case, skip the missed dose and take the next dose right on schedule. DO NOT double doses. Talk with your doctor if you find yourself missing doses.

Usual Duration of Use: Use on a regular schedule for 2 to 3 weeks usually determines effectiveness in lowering blood pressure. The long-term use of this drug (months to years) will be determined by the course of your blood pressure over time and your response to an overall treatment program (weight reduction, salt restriction, smoking cessation, etc.). See your doctor on a regular basis. Reaching and maintaining goal blood pressure is critical to long-term health.

Typical Treatment Goals and Measurements (Outcomes and Markers)

Blood Pressure: Guidelines (JNC VII) define normal blood pressure (BP) as **less than** 120/80 and **pre-hypertension** as 120/80 to 139/89. This new range is intended to help doctors encourage lifestyle changes (or in the case of people with a risk factor for high blood pressure, start treatment) much earlier—so that damage to blood vessels, heart, kidneys, sexual potency, or eyes might be minimized or avoided altogether. Stage 1 hypertension is 140/90 to 159/99 and stage 2 hypertension equal to or greater than 160/100 mm Hg. These guidelines also recommend that clinicians work with their patients to agree on the goals and a plan of treatment. The first-ever guidelines for blood pressure (hypertension) in African Americans recommends that MOST black patients be started on TWO antihypertensive medicines with the goal of lowering blood pressure to 130/80 for those with high risk for heart and blood vessel disease or with diabetes. The American Diabetes Association also recommends 130/80 as the target for diabetics and less than 125/75 for those who spill more than one gram of protein into their urine. Most clinicians try to achieve a BP that confers the best balance of lower cardiovascular risk and avoids the problem of too low a blood pressure. Blood pressure duration is generally increased with beneficial restriction of sodium. If goals are not met, it is not unusual to intensify doses or add on medicines.

Possible Advantages of This Drug

Causes less slowing of the heart rate than most other beta-blocker drugs. Is one of the most potent (weight to weight, mg to mg) beta blockers. Two routes of removal from the body make this medicine safer to use than some of the other beta blockers (such as atenolol, nadolol, or sotolol) in patients with compromised kidneys.

Currently a "Drug of Choice"

For starting treatment of hypertension (diuretics such as hydrochloro-thiazide are the other class) with a single drug.

▷ **This Drug Should Not Be Taken If**
- you have bronchial asthma.
- you have had an allergic reaction to it previously.
- you have an abnormally slow heart rate or a serious form of heart block.
- you are taking, or have taken within the past 14 days, any monoamine oxi-dase (MAO) type A inhibitor (see Drug Classes).

▷ **Inform Your Physician Before Taking This Drug If**
- you had an adverse reaction to any beta blocker (see Drug Classes).
- you have a history of serious heart disease, or congestive heart failure.
- you have a history of hay fever (allergic rhinitis), asthma, chronic bronchi-tis, or emphysema.
- you have a history of overactive thyroid function (hyperthyroidism).
- you have a history of low blood sugar (hypoglycemia) or diabetes.
- you have impaired liver or kidney function.
- you have diabetes or myasthenia gravis.
- you take digitalis, quinidine, or reserpine, or any calcium-channel-blocker drug (see Drug Classes).
- you have bad circulation to your legs or arms (peripheral vascular disease).
- you plan to have surgery under general anesthesia in the near future.

Possible Side Effects (natural, expected, and unavoidable drug actions)

Lethargy and fatigability, cold extremities, slow heart rate, light-headedness in upright position (see orthostatic hypotension in Glossary). May (like other beta blockers) make patients somewhat resistant to epinephrine used in serious allergic reactions (anaphylaxis).

▷ **Possible Adverse Effects** (unusual, unexpected, and infrequent reactions)

If any of the following develop, consult your physician promptly for guidance.

Mild Adverse Effects

Allergic reactions: skin rash, itching.

Headache, dizziness, insomnia, abnormal dreams, fainting—infrequent.

Indigestion, nausea, vomiting, constipation, diarrhea—infrequent.

Joint and muscle discomfort, tremor, fluid retention (edema)—infrequent.

Serious Adverse Effects

Allergic reactions: typical reactions to known allergens (such as bee stings) may be exaggerated.

Mental depression, anxiety—infrequent.

Chest pain, shortness of breath—possible.

Induction of bronchial asthma—in asthmatic individuals.

Abnormally slow heartbeat or congestive heart failure—possible to infrequent.

Drug-induced systemic lupus erythematosus or myasthenia gravis—case reports.

Worsening of poor circulation to the arms or legs (intermittent claudica-tion)—possible. May be prudent to check for hidden Peripheral Artery Dis-ease (PAD) by checking ankle brachial index (ABI). ABI check (see Glossary) can help find PAD early, and avoid claudication that may result if this medication is taken by someone who has PAD but does not know it.

Carpal tunnel syndrome—reported with other beta blockers.

▷ **Possible Effects on Sexual Function:** Decreased libido or impaired erection—infrequent.

Possible Effects on Laboratory Tests
Blood lupus erythematosus (LE) cells: possibly positive (one case of drug-induced LE).
Blood total cholesterol level: decreased (with long-term use).
Blood HDL cholesterol level: increased.
Blood LDL and VLDL cholesterol levels: no effects.
Blood triglyceride levels: no effects.
Glucose tolerance test (GTT): decreased or increased.
Liver function tests: slightly increased liver enzymes (ALT/GPT and AST/GOT): possible.

CAUTION
1. **Do not stop this drug suddenly** without the knowledge and help of your doctor. Carry a card that says you are taking this drug.
2. Ask your doctor or pharmacist before using nasal decongestants, which are usually present in over-the-counter cold preparations and nose drops. These can cause sudden increases in blood pressure when taken concurrently with beta blocker drugs.
3. Report the development of any tendency to emotional depression.

Precautions for Use
By Infants and Children: Safety and effectiveness for those under 12 years of age are not established. If this drug is used, however, observe for the development of low blood sugar (hypoglycemia) during periods of reduced food intake.

By Those Over 60 Years of Age: Unacceptably high blood pressure should be reduced without creating the risks associated with excessively low blood pressure. Small starting doses and frequent blood pressure checks are indicated. Sudden, rapid, and excessive reduction of blood pressure can predispose to stroke or heart attack. Watch for dizziness, unsteadiness, tendency to fall, confusion, hallucinations, depression, or urinary frequency.

▷ ## Advisability of Use During Pregnancy
Pregnancy Category: B. See Pregnancy Risk Categories at the back of this book.
Animal Studies: No significant increase in birth defects due to this drug.
Human Studies: Adequate studies of pregnant women not available, but there are some reports of lower growth and fetal problems. Ask your physician for guidance.

Advisability of Use If Breast-Feeding
Presence of this drug in breast milk: Yes.
Avoid drug or refrain from nursing.

Habit-Forming Potential: None.

Effects of Overdose: Weakness, slow pulse, low blood pressure, fainting, cold and sweaty skin, congestive heart failure, possible coma, and convulsions.

Possible Effects of Long-Term Use: Reduced heart reserve and eventual heart failure in susceptible individuals with advanced heart disease.

Suggested Periodic Examinations While Taking This Drug (at physician's discretion)
Measurements of blood pressure.
Evaluation of heart function.
May be prudent to check for hidden Peripheral Artery Disease (PAD) by checking ankle brachial index (ABI). ABI check (see Glossary) can help find PAD early, and avoid claudication that may result if this medication is taken by someone who has PAD but does not know it.
LE prep, ANA.

▷ **While Taking This Drug, Observe the Following**

Foods: No restrictions. Avoid excessive salt intake.

Herbal Medicines or Minerals: Ginseng, hawthorn, saw palmetto, bitter orange, country mallow, ma huang (no longer on the US market for weight loss), guarana and mate (caffeine), goldenseal, yohimbe, and licorice may also cause increased blood pressure. Dong quai may block one route of removal of this medicine from the body leading to toxic effects with "normal" doses. St. John's wort may increase removal of this medicine from the body leading to loss of benefits despite appropriate doses. Calcium and garlic may help lower blood pressure. Ginkgo benefits in helping peripheral artery disease are as yet unproven. Indian snakeroot has a German Commission E monograph indication for hypertension. Eleuthero root and ephedra (ma huang) should be avoided by people living with hypertension. Talk to your doctor BEFORE combining any herbal with any prescription drug or herbal product.

Beverages: No restrictions. May be taken with milk.

▷ *Alcohol:* Use with caution. Alcohol may exaggerate lowering of blood pressure or increase mild sedative effect.

Tobacco Smoking: Nicotine may reduce this drug's effectiveness. I advise everyone to quit smoking.

▷ *Other Drugs*

Pindolol may ***increase*** the effects of

- other antihypertensive drugs and cause excessive lowering of blood pressure; dose adjustments may be necessary.
- digoxin (Lanoxin) on the heart conduction system, leading to AV block and possible digoxin toxicity as well.
- reserpine (Ser-Ap-Es, etc.) and cause sedation, depression, slowing of the heart rate, and lowering of blood pressure.
- verapamil (Calan, Isoptin) and cause excessive depression of heart function; monitor this combination closely.

Pindolol ***taken concurrently*** with

- amiodarone (Cordarone) may cause extremely slow heartbeats and risk of sinus arrest.
- clonidine (Catapres) requires close monitoring for rebound high blood pressure if clonidine is withdrawn while pindolol is still being taken.
- epinephrine (various) will result in a large increase in blood pressure and reflex increase in heart rate (tachycardia).
- fentanyl (various) can lead to severe decreases in blood pressure. Extreme caution and dose adjustments are warranted if these medicines must be combined.
- fluoxetine (Prozac) may result in increased risk of pindolol toxicity.
- fluvoxamine (Luvox) may result in increased risk of pindolol toxicity.
- insulin requires close monitoring to avoid undetected hypoglycemia (see Glossary).
- oral antidiabetic drugs (see Drug Classes) can result in slowed recovery from low blood sugar.
- phenylpropanolamine (various—now removed from US products) may result in severe increases in blood pressure—avoid this combination.
- ritodrine (Yutopar) will blunt the effects (tocolytic). Dose changes may be needed.
- venlafaxine (Effexor) may result in beta-blocker or venlafaxine toxicity—avoid this combination if possible or use decreased doses of both medicines.

The following drugs may *increase* the effects of pindolol:
- cimetidine (Tagamet).
- methimazole (Tapazole).
- oral contraceptives.
- propylthiouracil (Propacil).
- ritonavir (Norvir) and perhaps other protease inhibitors (see Drug Classes).
- zileuton (Zyflo), close patient monitoring is prudent and dose adjustments may be required.

The following drugs may *decrease* the effects of pindolol:
- barbiturates (phenobarbital, etc.).
- indomethacin (Indocin) and possibly other NSAIDs—may impair pindolol's antihypertensive effect.
- rifampin (Rifadin, Rimactane).
- theophylline (Theo-Dur, others).

▷ *Driving, Hazardous Activities:* Use caution until the full extent of fatigue, dizziness and blood pressure change has been determined.

Aviation Note: The use of this drug *is a disqualification* for piloting. Consult a designated Aviation Medical Examiner.

Exposure to Sun: No restrictions.

Exposure to Heat: Caution is advised. Hot environments can lower blood pressure and exaggerate the effects of this drug.

Exposure to Cold: Caution is advised. Cold environments can enhance the circulatory deficiency in the extremities that may occur with this drug. The elderly should take precautions to prevent hypothermia (see Glossary).

Heavy Exercise or Exertion: It is advisable to avoid exertion that produces light-headedness, excessive fatigue or muscle cramping. The use of this drug may intensify the hypertensive response to isometric exercise.

Occurrence of Unrelated Illness: Fever can lower blood pressure and require adjustment of dose. Nausea or vomiting may interrupt regular doses. Ask your doctor for help.

Discontinuation: It is advisable to avoid sudden discontinuation of this drug in all situations. If possible, gradual reduction of dose over a period of 2 to 3 weeks is recommended. Ask your physician for specific guidance.

PIRBUTEROL (peer BYU ter ohl)

Introduced: 1983 **Class:** Antiasthmatic, bronchodilator **Prescription:** Yes **Controlled Drug:** USA: No; Canada: No **Available as Generic:** No

Brand Name: Maxair

BENEFITS versus RISKS	
Possible Benefits	*Possible Risks*
VERY EFFECTIVE RELIEF OF BRONCHOSPASM	Increased blood pressure
	Nervousness
	Fine hand tremor
	Irregular heart rhythm (with excessive use)

▷ **Principal Uses**

As a Single Drug Product: Uses currently included in FDA-approved labeling: (1) Relieves acute attacks of bronchial asthma; (2) reduces the frequency and severity of chronic, recurrent asthmatic attacks (prevention); (3) relieves reversible bronchospasm seen in chronic bronchitis, bronchiectasis, and emphysema.

Other (unlabeled) generally accepted uses: None at present.

How This Drug Works: By increasing the production of cyclic AMP, this drug relaxes constricted bronchial muscles to relieve asthmatic wheezing.

▷ **Widely Used Guidelines That Involve This Medicine (representative sample):** Please look at the section at the very beginning of this profile called "Class." Next, turn to Table 22 and you will find guidelines listed by the class involved!

Available Dosage Forms and Strengths

Aerosol (in canisters of 300 inhalations) — 200 mcg per actuation

▷ **Usual Adult Dosage Range (or children over 12):** Inhaler: Two puffs (inhalations) (400 mcg) every 4 to 6 hours. **Do not exceed** 12 inhalations (2,400 mcg) every 24 hours. Some patients may get benefits from one puff every 4 to 6 hours.

Note: Actual dose and schedule must be determined for each patient individually.

Conditions Requiring Dosing Adjustments

Liver Function: Used with caution by patients with liver disease who use it often.

Kidney Function: No dose adjustments thought to be needed.

▷ **Dosing Instructions:** Carefully follow the "Patient's Instructions for Use" provided with the inhaler as the amount of medicine that goes to work for you depends on your technique. Gently shake the inhaler before each use. Do not overuse. If you forget a dose: Use the missed dose as soon as you remember it, unless it's nearly time for your next dose—if that is the case, skip the missed dose and take the next dose right on schedule. DO NOT double doses. Talk with your doctor if you find yourself missing doses.

Usual Duration of Use: According to individual requirements. Do not use beyond the time necessary to stop (terminate) episodes of asthma.

Typical Treatment Goals and Measurements (Outcomes and Markers)

Asthma: Short-acting beta agonists like albuterol are used to prevent or treat reversible spasms of the bronchial tubes. The peak effect happens 1 to 2 hours after dosing. Some pulmonologists use arterial blood gases in extreme cases. FEV-1 in mild to moderate cases is important for checking response. Clinical symptoms such as chest tightening and wheezing should also ease. If the usual benefit is not realized, call your doctor.

Possible Advantages of This Drug

Has a more rapid onset of action and a longer duration of effect than most other drugs of this class.

▷ **This Drug Should Not Be Taken If**

• you have had an allergic reaction to it previously.
• you are taking, or have taken within the past 2 weeks, any monoamine oxidase (MAO) type A inhibitor (see Drug Classes).

▷ **Inform Your Physician Before Taking This Drug If**

• you have any type of heart or circulatory disorder, especially high blood pressure, coronary heart disease or heart rhythm abnormality.

- you have diabetes or an excessively active thyroid gland (hyperthyroidism).
- you have any type of seizure disorder.
- you are taking any form of digitalis or any stimulant drug.

Possible Side Effects (natural, expected, and unavoidable drug actions)
Aerosol—dryness or irritation of mouth or throat, altered taste. Cough.

▷ **Possible Adverse Effects** (unusual, unexpected, and infrequent reactions)
If any of the following develop, consult your physician promptly for guidance.
Mild Adverse Effects
Allergic reactions: skin rash, itching—rare.
Headache, dizziness, nervousness, fine tremor of hands—infrequent.
Palpitations, rapid heart rate, chest pain, cough—rare to infrequent.
Nausea, diarrhea, taste disorders—rare.
Serious Adverse Effects
Irregular heart rhythm, increased blood pressure—possible.
Paradoxical spasm of the bronchi—possible.

▷ **Possible Effects on Sexual Function:** None reported.

Natural Diseases or Disorders That May Be Activated by This Drug
Latent coronary artery disease, diabetes, epilepsy, or high blood pressure.

Possible Effects on Laboratory Tests
None reported.

CAUTION
1. Combined use of this drug by inhalation with beclomethasone aerosol (Beclovent, Vanceril) may increase the risk of toxicity due to fluorocarbon propellants (fluorocarbons are being phased out). It is advisable to use pirbuterol aerosol 20 to 30 minutes before beclomethasone aerosol. This will reduce the risk of toxicity and help beclomethasone reach the lung.
2. Excessive or prolonged use of this drug by inhalation can reduce its effectiveness (tolerance) and cause serious heart rhythm, disturbances, including cardiac arrest.

Precautions for Use
By Infants and Children: Safety and effectiveness of use in children under 12 years of age have not been established.
By Those Over 60 Years of Age: Avoid excessive and continual use. If acute asthma is not relieved promptly, other drugs may be needed. Watch for nervousness, palpitations, irregular heart rhythm, and muscle tremors.

▷ **Advisability of Use During Pregnancy**
Pregnancy Category: C. See Pregnancy Risk Categories at the back of this book.
Animal Studies: High-dose studies in rabbits revealed abortion and increased fetal deaths. Studies in rats and rabbits found no drug-associated birth defects.
Human Studies: Adequate studies of pregnant women are not available.
Avoid use during first 3 months if possible.

Advisability of Use If Breast-Feeding
Presence of this drug in breast milk: Unknown.
Avoid drug or refrain from nursing.

Habit-Forming Potential: None. Tolerance to beneficial effects has been reported.

Effects of Overdose: Nervousness, palpitation, rapid heart rate, sweating, headache, tremor, vomiting, chest pain.

Possible Effects of Long-Term Use: Loss of effectiveness (tolerance).

Suggested Periodic Examinations While Taking This Drug (at physician's discretion)
Blood pressure measurements.
Evaluation of heart status.

▷ **While Taking This Drug, Observe the Following**
Foods: No restrictions.
Herbal Medicines or Minerals: Using St. John's wort, ma huang, bitter orange, country mallow, ephedrine-like compounds, mate or kola while taking this medicine may result in unacceptable central nervous system stimulation. Fir or pine needle oil should NOT be used by asthmatics. Ephedra alone does carry a German Commission E monograph indication for asthma treatment. If you are allergic to plants in the Asteraceae family (aster, chrysanthemum, daisy, or ragweed), you may also be allergic to echinacea, chamomile, feverfew, and St. John's wort. Since part of the way that ginseng works may be as a MAO inhibitor, DO NOT combine with pirbuterol.
Beverages: Avoid excessive use of caffeine-containing beverages—coffee, tea, cola, chocolate.
▷ *Alcohol:* No interactions expected.
Tobacco Smoking: No interactions expected. I advise everyone to quit smoking.
▷ *Other Drugs*
Pirbuterol **taken concurrently** with
• albuterol (Proventil, Ventolin) may result in adverse effects on the heart.
• monoamine oxidase (MAO) type A inhibitors may cause excessive increase in blood pressure and undesirable heart stimulation.
• phenothiazines (see Drug Classes) may result in blunting of the therapeutic effects of pirbuterol.
▷ *Driving, Hazardous Activities:* Use caution if excessive nervousness or dizziness occurs.
Aviation Note: The use of this drug **is a disqualification** for piloting. Consult a designated Aviation Medical Examiner.
Exposure to Sun: No restrictions.
Heavy Exercise or Exertion: Use caution—excessive exercise can induce asthma in sensitive individuals.

PIROXICAM (peer OX i kam)

Please see the oxicam (nonsteroidal anti-inflammatory drug) family profile.

PNEUMOCOCCAL CONJUGATE VACCINE (NEW mo kok uhl)

Other Name: Pneumonia vaccine

Introduced: Presently this is a specific formulation to help confer immunity to seven kinds (4, 6B, 9V, 14, 18C, 19F and 23F) of bacteria called pneumococcus **Class:**   Antibacterial vaccine   **Prescription:**   USA: Yes   **Controlled Drug:**   USA: No; Canada: No   **Available as Generic:**   USA: No; Canada: No

Brand Name: Prevnar

Author's Note: The American Diabetes Association (*www.diabetes.org* **or 1-877-CDC-DIAB for more information) recommends that people living with diabetes get both a flu and pneumococcal shot (vaccine). If you would like a copy of the ACIP recommendations, call 1-888-232-3228. Information on current recommendations for shots (vaccines) can be found at** *www.cdc.gov/nip/recs/child-schedule.htm*. **Don't become a statistic (23-valent forms only). This profile will be broadened to include data on Pnu-Immune-23 and Pneumovax 23 in subsequent editions. The focus for this profile will be on Prevnar (7 valent form) as it is now part of the recommendations (ACIP) for vaccinations in children (not recommended for use in adults).**

BENEFITS versus RISKS

Possible Benefits	*Possible Risks*
PREVENTION OF DISEASE CAUSED BY THE MOST SERIOUS OR PREVALENT STRAINS OF STREPTOCOCCUS PNEUMONIA	Lowered platelets Hypersensitivity Fever
PREVENTION OF PNEUMOCOCCAL MENINGITIS	
PREVENTION OF BACTEREMIC PNEUMONIA CAUSED BY STREPTOCOCCUS	
PREVENTION OF EAR INFECTION (OTITIS MEDIA) IN INFANTS AND TODDLERS CAUSED BY THE SEVEN STRAINS IN THE VACCINE	
Possible cross-protection from other similar bacterial strains	

▷ **Principal Uses**

As a Single Drug Product: Uses currently included in FDA-approved labeling: Prevention of pneumococcal infection (Prevnar only).

Other (unlabeled) generally accepted uses: (1) Used in patients with compromised immune systems such as HIV-positive, cancer and bone marrow transplant patients (23-valent forms only); (2) can be of use in isolated outbreaks such as in nursing homes or military camps (23-valent forms only).

How This Drug Works: Surprisingly, there are more than 90 kinds of pneumococcus, but disease is actually caused by a few kinds of this bacteria. While we usually think of this bacteria as a cause of lung infection (pneumonia), it is actually the cause of some 20–40% of middle ear infections in children (Strep pneumoniae). Additionally, there has been a trend toward bacteria that can outsmart (resist) widely used antibiotics. What this shot (vaccine) does is to take part (capsular antigen saccharides) of the seven most likely bacteria types that cause middle ear infections and place them in a sterile solution. These components are purified, then inactivated and used to form a shot (vaccine), which is a suspension. When injected, it stimulates the immune system to make antibodies. The antibodies (present to all vaccine serotypes after four doses of the vaccine) act to prevent middle ear infections or reduce infection severity if infection does occur.

▷ **Widely Used Guidelines That Involve This Medicine (representative sample):** Please look at the section at the very beginning of this profile called "Class." Next, turn to Table 22 and you will find guidelines listed by the class involved!

Available Dosage Forms and Strengths

Prevnar form: (2 micrograms each of 4, 9v, 14, 18 C, 19F and 23F. Four mcg of 6B) for a total of 16 mcg/0.5 mL of the seven selected strains.

▷ **Recommended Dosage Ranges** (Actual dose and schedule must be determined for each patient and each flu season individually.)

Infants and Children: Current ACIP recommendations include this vaccine as part of routine pediatric care. After the vial is resuspended, 0.5 mL is injected. Shots are given into the muscle (intramuscular) on a schedule at two, four, six and between 12-15 months of age. While the first dose is usually given at 2 months, it can be given as early as 6 weeks. Subsequent doses in that case are given every 4-8 weeks, and the last dose (fourth) is given two months after the third dose.

The Prevnar form is NOT to be used in adults.

Conditions Requiring Dosing Adjustments

Liver Function: Not involved.

Kidney Function: Not involved.

▷ **Dosing Instructions:** The vial should be gently, but well shaken before the shot is given. The fluid in the vial should appear white when resuspended. This vaccine should be given into a muscle. Appropriate sites are the anterolateral part of the thigh in infants and the upper arm (deltoid muscle) in toddlers and young children. Care should be taken NOT to inject into a vein. Once the injection site is cleaned, this is often accomplished by inserting the needle, pulling back on the syringe (aspiration), and making sure that blood does not appear. If blood does appear, this indicates a blood vessel, and the needle should be withdrawn without injecting and the steps for injection taken once again. Some tenderness at the injection site is possible. Fever and muscular aches or pains are also possible and may be treated with acetaminophen (Tylenol, others). Prudent to give the acetaminophen (pre-treat) BEFORE the injection is given.

Usual Duration of Use: Four doses are given as outlined previously.

Typical Treatment Goals and Measurements (Outcomes and Markers)

Prevention of Strep Pneumoniae Infection: Prevention of infection from the seven serotypes of strep is the goal of vaccination. Because strep can cause pneumonia, middle ear and other infections, it is logical that these infections from the seven serotypes would be prevented or would be much milder in nature than they otherwise would have been. Antibody checks can be performed at some laboratories.

Possible Advantages of This Drug

Confers immunity in children to a prevalent bacteria, which is becoming more resistant to antibiotics.

Currently a Drug of Choice

For preventing S. Pneumoniae infections due to the seven serotypes present in the vaccine for children starting at 2 months of age (with four shot course completion).

▷ **This Vaccine Should Not Be Given If**

- you have had an allergic reaction to any dose form of it previously (any other pneumococcal shot or to a diphtheria shot).

- you are giving the shot and are in a blood vessel (shot should be given into a muscle).

▷ **Inform Your Physician Before Taking/Giving This Vaccine If**
- you are HIV positive.
- you have a history of blood clotting disorders.
- you have clinical reasons against getting a shot in the muscle (such as low platelets or a blood clotting disorder, where a benefit-to-risk decision should be made).
- you have a history of allergy to latex (packaging does have dry natural rubber in it).
- you are the person giving the shot and you are unsure if you are in a vein or not (best to go to another injection site).

Possible Side Effects (natural, expected, and unavoidable drug actions)
Pain at the vaccination site—frequent. Muscle aches, fever, or bothersome tiredness (malaise). These symptoms are a reaction to the components of the vaccine.

▷ **Possible Adverse Effects** (unusual, unexpected, and infrequent reactions)
If any of the following develop, consult your physician promptly for guidance.
Mild Adverse Effects
Allergic reactions: swelling and redness—possible.
Muscle aches or fever—rare.
Fatigue, nausea and headache—infrequent.
Serious Adverse Effects
Allergic reactions: anaphylactic reactions.
Febrile seizures—case reports.
Low blood platelets—case reports for the earlier 23-valent forms.
Guillain-Barré syndrome or paresthesias—rare for the Pneumovax form.

▷ **Possible Effects on Sexual Function:** None reported.

Possible Delayed Adverse Effects: None reported.

▷ **Adverse Effects That May Mimic Natural Diseases or Disorders**
Reaction to vaccine contents may mimic the flu.

Natural Diseases or Disorders That May Be Activated by This Drug
None reported.

Possible Effects on Laboratory Tests
Antibodies to the seven pneumococcal strains in the shot: positive (beneficial effect).

CAUTION
1. Prevnar form not approved for HIV positive or patients without a spleen (asplenics). The 23-valent form is approved for such use (also in transplant patients).
2. Prevnar will NOT protect against S. pneumoniae infection caused by strains not in the shot.
3. If muscle aches or fever occurs after vaccination, acetaminophen (Tylenol, others) is recommended. **Do not** take aspirin, and especially do not give aspirin to children. Prudent to take acetaminophen BEFORE vaccination to prevent such reactions.
4. Call your doctor immediately if you develop hives, swelling of the face, unexplained high fever, unexplained bleeding or bruising, seizures or difficulty breathing after the vaccination.

5. People with allergy to latex should be given this shot as a benefit-to-risk decision as the packaging contains dry natural rubber.
6. Safety and efficacy have not been defined for people less than 6 weeks old.
7. Patients with impaired immunity (HIV, chemotherapy, steroid use, etc.) may have a blunted response to the vaccine.
8. This vaccine has an aluminum adjuvant and should be well shaken prior to injection.
9. A benefit-to-risk decision should be made for patients who are taking blood thinners (anticoagulants).

Precautions for Use
By Infants and Children: Safety and effectiveness for use by those under 6 WEEKS of age have not been established.
By Those Over 60 Years of Age: Prevnar form is not indicated.

▷ Advisability of Use During Pregnancy
Pregnancy Category: C. See Pregnancy Risk Categories at the back of this book.
Animal Studies: Animal studies have not been conducted.
Human Studies: Information from adequate studies of pregnant women is not available.
Ask your doctor for guidance.

Advisability of Use If Breast-Feeding
Presence of this drug in breast milk: Not defined.
This vaccine is NOT recommended for use in adults, but is also NOT recommended in nursing mothers.

Habit-Forming Potential: None.

Effects of Overdose: No specific cases reported. Treatment would be consistent with any symptoms of the patient.

Possible Effects of Long-Term Use: Not indicated for long-term use.

Suggested Periodic Examinations After Giving This Vaccine (at physician's discretion)
None indicated, other than possible check for antibody formation to the seven strains in the shot.

▷ While Taking This Drug, Observe the Following
Foods: No restrictions.
Herbal Medicines or Minerals: Some patients use echinacea to attempt to boost their immune systems. Unfortunately, use of echinacea is not recommended in people with damaged immune systems. This herb may also actually weaken any immune system if it is used too often or for too long a time.
Beverages: No restrictions.
▷   *Alcohol:* No restrictions.
Tobacco Smoking: No interactions expected. I advise everyone to quit smoking.
▷   *Other Drugs*
Prevnar pneumococcal vaccine may ***increase*** the effects of
• specific interactions where effects have been increased are not yet identified.
Influenza vaccine ***taken concurrently*** with
• anticoagulants (such as warfarin, low molecular weight heparins, etc.) may lead to increased risk of complications when Prevnar is given as an intramuscular shot.
• chemotherapy (see Drug Classes) can result in blunting of the immune response to this vaccine. Some clinicians will still give the shot in the hope of conferring some immunity.

- cyclosporine (Sandimmune) can cause blunting of the immune response to the vaccine.
- immunosuppressive agents (chemotherapy, corticosteroids, perhaps some DMARDs, etc.) may impair or blunt immune response to the vaccine.
- methotrexate (Rheumatrex) can result in blunting of the immune response to this vaccine.

▷ *Driving, Hazardous Activities:* This drug may cause excessive tiredness and muscle aches. Restrict activities as necessary.

Aviation Note: The use of this drug *may be a short-term disqualification* for piloting. Consult a designated Aviation Medical Examiner.

Exposure to Sun: No restrictions.

Exposure to Heat: Since this vaccine may cause short-duration fevers, it is wise to avoid hot environments for a day after vaccination.

Heavy Exercise or Exertion: A fever may result, and it is wise to avoid strenuous exercise for a day after vaccination.

Special Storage Instructions: This vaccine is ideally stored in the refrigerator. If this is how storage is accomplished, the outdate specified by the manufacturer is valid. If the vaccine is stored at room temperature, it is stable for up to 7 days.

Observe the Following Expiration Times: If the vaccine is stored at room temperature, it is stable for up to 7 days.

Author's Note: There is a Vaccine Adverse Event Reporting System (VAERS). The toll-free number is 1-800-822-7967.

PRAMIPEXOLE (PRAM ih pex ohl)

Other Name: None

Introduced: 1997   **Class:**   Anti-Parkinsonian, dopamine receptor agonist   **Prescription:**   USA: Yes   **Controlled Drug:**   USA: No; Canada: No   **Available as Generic:**   MSA: No; Canada: No

Brand Name: Mirapex

BENEFITS versus RISKS

Possible Benefits	*Possible Risks*
EFFECTIVE SYMPTOM RELIEF IN IDIOPATHIC PARKINSON'S DISEASE	Movement disorders
	Hallucinations
	Somnolence
BINDS SEVEN TIMES MORE AGGRESSIVELY TO D3 RECEPTORS THAN TO D2 RECEPTORS	Postural hypotension
SOME EARLY DATA FROM CELLS OUTSIDE THE BODY FOUND THAT PRAMIPEXOLE MAY PROTECT AGAINST DISEASE PROGRESSION	
May be an alternative therapy for restless leg syndrome when other medicines like carbidopa/levodopa have not worked	

▷ **Principal Uses**

As a Single Drug Product: Uses currently included in FDA-approved labeling: Treats major types of Parkinson's disease: paralysis agitans ("shaking palsy" of unknown cause), the type that follows encephalitis and Parkinsonism that develops with aging (associated with hardening of the brain arteries).

Other (unlabeled) generally accepted uses: (1) May have a limited role in restless leg syndrome; (2) can improve depression.

As a Combination Drug Product [CD]: Not available.

How This Drug Works: This drug acts as a dopamine receptor activator (agonist). This drug is also unique in that it has a strong affinity for a specific receptor (D3).

▷ **Widely Used Guidelines That Involve This Medicine (representative sample):** Please look at the section at the very beginning of this profile called "Class." Next, turn to Table 22 and you will find guidelines listed by the class involved!

Available Dosage Forms and Strengths

Tablets—0.125 mg, 0.25 mg, 0.5 mg, 1 mg, 1.5 mg

Author's Note: Information in this profile will be broadened once further information is available and if clinical use supports it.

PRAVASTATIN (pra vah STA tin)

Introduced: 1986 **Class:** Cholesterol-lowering agent, HMG-CoA reductase inhibitor **Prescription:** USA: Yes **Controlled Drug:** USA: No; Canada: No **Available as Generic:** USA: No; Canada: No

Brand Names: ✦Lin-Pravastatin, Pravachol, Pravigard Pac

Author's Note: At present, applications for pravastatin (Pravachol) and lovastatin (Mevacor) have been made to the FDA to change low doses of these medicines to nonprescription (OTC) status. At the time of this writing, the OTC issue has not been resolved (see Sources—Cohen, J.D. and Larouche, S.J.).

BENEFITS versus RISKS

Possible Benefits	*Possible Risks*
REDUCES RISK OF STROKES	Drug-induced increase in liver enzymes
EFFECTIVE REDUCTION OF TOTAL BLOOD CHOLESTEROL AND LDL CHOLESTEROL	Drug-induced myositis (muscle inflammation)
EFFECTIVE REDUCTION IN THE NUMBER OF FIRST-TIME AND REPEAT HEART ATTACKS (PRIMARY AND SECONDARY PREVENTION)	Decreased co-enzyme Q10 Rhabodmyolysis
REDUCTION IN THE NUMBER OF PATIENT DEATHS	
SLOWS PROGRESSION OF ATHEROSCLEROSIS	
REDUCES RISK OF TRANSIENT ISCHEMIC ATTACKS (TIAs)	
LOWERS APOLIPOPROTEIN B and TRIGLYCERIDES	
INCREASES HDL-C IN PEOPLE WITH HETEROZYGOUS FAMILIAL AND NONFAMILIAL PRIMARY HYPERCHOLESTEROLEMIA AND MIXED DYSLIPIDEMIA (FREDERICKSON TYPES 2a AND 2b)	
NEUTRALIZES INFLAMMATORY RISK (SUCH AS C REACTIVE PROTEIN)	
PACKAGED WITH ASPIRIN IN THE PRAVIGARD FORM HELPS PATIENTS REMEMBER THIS VALUABLE COMBINATION	
May have a role in preventing development of type 2 diabetes in men	
May have a role in preventing osteoporosis	

▷ **Principal Uses**

As a Single Drug Product: Uses currently included in FDA-approved labeling: (1) Treats abnormally high total blood cholesterol levels (in people with types IIa and IIb hypercholesterolemia) due to increased low-density lipoprotein (LDL) cholesterol (used with a cholesterol-lowering diet after an adequate trial of nondrug methods has failed); (2) helps prevent a first heart attack or stroke and reduces death from cardiovascular disease in people with increased blood cholesterol levels at risk of a first heart attack. Also serves to help prevent a repeat heart attack; (3) slows progression and in some cases makes small reversals in coronary artery disease (atherosclerosis); (4) used to decrease triglycerides in mixed lipidemias; (5) reduces risk of strokes or transient ischemic attacks (TIAs)—the CARE trial of 4,159 patients found that strokes were lowered by 32%; (6) approved to increase HDL-C in patients with heterozygous familial and nonfamilial primary hypercholesterolemia and mixed dyslipidemia; (7) lowers apolipoprotein B.

Other (unlabeled) generally accepted uses: (1) Reduces temporary blood flow (to the heart) problems (myocardial ischemia) when combined with other therapies; (2) may have a role in decreasing development of type 2 diabetes in men (WOSCOPS); (3) may have a role in reducing development of osteoporosis (emerging data).

As a Combination Drug Product [CD]: This drug is available packaged with aspirin, giving the advantage of convenient and clinically valuable combination therapy.

How This Drug Works: This drug blocks the liver enzyme that starts production of cholesterol. Its principal action is the reduction of low-density lipoproteins (LDL), the fraction of total blood cholesterol that is thought to increase the risk of coronary heart disease. This drug also increases the level of high-density lipoproteins (HDL), the cholesterol fraction that is thought to reduce the risk of heart disease. There is an increasing evidence base that tells us that this drug has strong beneficial effects on blood flow, the blood vessel walls and what is in the blood itself. Specific compounds or effects of platelet derived growth factor (PDGF), undesirable blood clotting via thrombin-antithrombin III, thrombomodulin and other chemicals may be beneficially lowered or effects mitigated by statins. Pravastatin lowered the likelihood of blood to clot (thrombogenicity) caused by both platelets and endothelial cells. This medicine also leads to improvement in opening (vasodilation) of the brachial artery that required the lining or endothelium. Combination with aspirin gives the added benefit of making platelets less likely to form undesirable blood clots (an antiplatelet effect which lowers risk of heart attack and stroke).

▷ **Widely Used Guidelines That Involve This Medicine (representative sample):** Please look at the section at the very beginning of this profile called "Class." Next, turn to Table 22 and you will find guidelines listed by the class involved!

Available Dosage Forms and Strengths
Tablets — 10 mg, 20 mg, 40 mg, 80 mg

▷ **Recommended Dose Ranges** (Actual dose and schedule must be determined for each patient individually.)

Infants and Children: Under 2 years of age—do not use this drug. 2 to 18 years of age—dose not established.

18 to 60 Years of Age: Hypercholesterolemia: Patients are put on a standard cholesterol lowering diet (see *www.americanheart.org*). Patients remain on this diet once the medicine is started, and dosing is begun with 40 mg once a day at bedtime. Because the peak benefit is seen in 4 weeks, lipid tests should be obtained periodically, and dosing adjusted depending on reaching goals and on treatment guidelines (such as NCEP ATP 3). If goals are not reached after 4 weeks, add on therapy of a different medicine (such as ezetimibe) or the 80 mg dose is appropriate. Some newer data found a related medicine in higher dose gave better results when used in the higher dose after a heart attack.

Over 60 Years of Age: Starting dose for those with kidney or liver compromise is 10 mg daily. A geriatric use subsection has been added to the Precautions of FDA-sanctioned labeling. The results of the CARE and LIPID studies had

6,593 people who used 40 mg for up to 6 years. In those studies, 36.1% were 65 or older. Adverse events and responses were similar to those seen in younger people. A measure called area under the curve (AUC) was 25–50% higher than in younger patients, but peak level and half life were similar. Dosing changes are not thought to be needed.

Conditions Requiring Dosing Adjustments

Liver Function: Used with caution by patients with liver disease. Starting dose is decreased to 10 mg per day. Pravastatin should not be used in sudden (acute) liver disease.

Kidney Function: Those with significant kidney disease take a starting dose of 10 mg per day. Used with caution in kidney compromise.

▷ **Dosing Instructions:** The tablet may be crushed and can be taken without regard to eating. Labeling says that it can be taken at any time. Previously, it was preferably taken at bedtime. (Highest rates of cholesterol production occur between midnight and 5 A.M.) If you forget a dose: Take the missed dose as soon as you remember it, unless it's nearly time for your next dose—if that is the case, skip the missed dose and take the next dose right on schedule. DO NOT double doses. Talk with your doctor if you find yourself missing doses.

Usual Duration of Use: Use on a regular schedule for 4 to 6 weeks usually determines effectiveness in reducing blood levels of total and LDL-C cholesterol. Long-term use (months to years) requires periodic physician evaluation. It is critical to take this medicine as directed to take control of an ongoing condition such as increased cholesterol, stroke risk, or heart attack risk.

Typical Treatment Goals and Measurements (Outcomes and Markers)

Cholesterol: Current guidelines (National Cholesterol Education Program or NCEP) acknowledge diabetes as one of the conditions that increases risk of heart disease, modifying risk factors, therapeutic lifestyle changes (TLC), and recommending routine testing for all of the cholesterol fractions (lipoprotein profile) versus total cholesterol alone. Goals are: a total cholesterol of 200 mg/dL, and optimal bad cholesterol (LDL) of less than 100 mg/dL. Less than 70 mg/dL (see Grundy, S.M. in Sources) is a reasonable optional goal for very high risk patients (such as diabetics with acute coronary syndromes, etc.). 130–159 mg/dL as borderline high, 160 mg/dL as high and 190 mg/dL as very high. Did you know that there are at least five different kinds of "good cholesterol" or HDL? The "too low" measure for HDL is still 40mg/dL, but in order to learn more about cholesterol types some doctors are starting to order lipid panels. There are at least seven different kinds of "bad cholesterol." The new panels tell doctors about the kinds of cholesterol that your body makes. This is important because some kinds (small dense particles) tend to stick to blood vessels (are highly atherogenic). Take your medicine to reach your goals! Two additional tests you will hear about will be electron beam computed tomography (EBCT) and CRP. EBCT is an important tool used in conjunction with laboratory studies. Findings show that even patients who meet cholesterol goals (particularly females over 55) can still be at significant cardiovascular risk. EBCT then defines risk by giving a calcium score and a "virtual tour" of the coronary arteries. C Reactive Protein, or CRP, is a relatively new and apparently independent predictor of heart disease risk. A large study (see Ridker, P.M. in Sources) found that CRP predicted heart disease risk independently of bad cholesterol (low density lipoprotein). Talk to your doctor about this laboratory test and ask about current guidelines for who should be tested (see Pearson, T.A. in Sources).

Possible Advantages of This Drug

Several studies show that drugs of this class (HMG-CoA reductase inhibitors) are more effective and better tolerated than other drugs currently available for reducing total and LDL-C cholesterol. This medicine is proven to increase HDL, has emerging bone health and diabetes data, works in primary and secondary heart (coronary) events, and also helps prevent stroke. Uses less common ways (liver enzymes) for removal from the body and thus avoids many drug interactions possible with other medicines in this same family.

▷ **This Drug Should Not Be Taken If**
- you have had an allergic reaction to it or to similar medicines previously.
- you have an unexplained and ongoing increase in liver function tests.
- you have active liver disease.
- you are pregnant or breast-feeding your infant.

▷ **Inform Your Physician Before Taking This Drug If**
- you have previously taken and have not tolerated any other drugs in this class: lovastatin (Mevacor), simvastatin (Zocor), others.
- you have a history of liver disease or impaired liver function.
- you are not using any method of birth control or you are planning pregnancy.
- you regularly consume substantial amounts of alcohol.
- you have kidney disease.
- you have cataracts or impaired vision.
- you get unexplained muscle weakness, pain, or tenderness (call your doctor).
- you have any type of chronic muscular disorder.
- you have an increase in certain liver enzymes (transaminases), which increase to three times the upper normal limit (pravastatin should be stopped immediately).

Possible Side Effects (natural, expected, and unavoidable drug actions)

Decreased co-enzyme Q10 (co-Q10 or ubiquinone) levels.

▷ **Possible Adverse Effects** (unusual, unexpected, and infrequent reactions)

If any of the following develop, consult your physician promptly for guidance.

Mild Adverse Effects

Allergic reactions: skin rash, itching—rare.

Headache, dizziness, depression—case reports to rare.

Flu-like syndrome, cough—case reports.

Indigestion, stomach pain, nausea, excessive gas, constipation, diarrhea—rare to infrequent.

Muscle cramps and/or pain—rare.

Serious Adverse Effects

Allergic reactions: rash (lichenoid dermatitis).

Porphyria cutanea tarda (PCT)—case reports.

Marked and persistent abnormal liver function tests with focal hepatitis (without jaundice)—rare.

Acute myositis (muscle pain and tenderness) during long-term use—case reports.

Rhabdomyolysis—rare and more likely if combined with fibrates.

Low white blood cells (leukopenia)—rare and questionable causation.

Roughly sixty cases of short-term memory loss (pravastatin [1], atorvastatin [23], and simvastatin [36] have been made.

Neuropathy—case report.

▷ **Possible Effects on Sexual Function:** Impotence—questionable causation with medicines that lower cholesterol.

Possible Delayed Adverse Effects: Increased liver enzymes, decreased co-Q10.

Natural Diseases or Disorders That May Be Activated by This Drug
Latent liver disease.

Possible Effects on Laboratory Tests
Blood alanine aminotransferase (ALT) enzyme level: possible increase (with higher doses of drug).
Blood total cholesterol, LDL cholesterol, and triglyceride levels: decreased.
Blood HDL cholesterol level: increased.

CAUTION
1. If pregnancy occurs while taking this drug, discontinue the drug immediately and consult your physician.
2. Report promptly any development of unexplained muscle pain or tenderness, especially if accompanied by fever or malaise.
3. Report promptly the development of altered or impaired vision so that appropriate evaluation can be made (reported with lovastatin in high doses, but not this medicine).
4. If transaminase levels increase to three times the upper limit of normal values, this medicine should be stopped.

Precautions for Use
By Infants and Children: Safety and effectiveness for those less than 18 years of age are not established.
By Those Over 60 Years of Age: Tell your doctor about any personal or family history of cataracts. Comply with all recommendations regarding periodic eye examinations. Report promptly any alterations in vision. 10 mg starting dose is prudent.

▷ **Advisability of Use During Pregnancy**
Pregnancy Category: X. See Pregnancy Risk Categories at the back of this book.
Animal Studies: Mouse and rat studies reveal skeletal birth defects due to a closely related drug of this class.
Human Studies: Adequate studies of pregnant women are not available.
This drug should be avoided during entire pregnancy.

Advisability of Use If Breast-Feeding
Presence of this drug in breast milk: Yes, in small amounts.
Avoid drug or refrain from nursing.

Habit-Forming Potential: None.

Effects of Overdose: Increased indigestion, stomach distress, nausea, and diarrhea.

Possible Effects of Long-Term Use: Beneficial effects on cholesterol, blood vessels, the bones, and inflammation.

Suggested Periodic Examinations While Taking This Drug (at physician's discretion)
Blood cholesterol studies: total cholesterol, HDL and LDL fractions (Berkeley Heart Lab), LP (a), homocysteine. Other markers of atherogenic fats and CRP are prudent—not because of the medicine, but because they help further define needed treatment.
Liver function tests before treatment, before increasing the dose and when clinically indicated thereafter. **Pravastatin was the first HMG-CoA reductase inhibitor to receive labeling from the FDA for less-frequent liver**

testing. Complete eye examination at beginning of treatment and at any time that significant change in vision occurs. Ask your doctor for guidance. Bone mineral density tests (DEXA, PDEXA, or ultrasound) will help show retention of bone mineral density (a newer possible beneficial effect). Electron beam computed tomography (EBCT) can help predict silent ischemia and other problems with blood vessels that supply the heart itself. This also may help define the results (outcomes) you are getting from this medicine.

▷ **While Taking This Drug, Observe the Following**

Foods: Follow a standard low-cholesterol diet. Your doctor may also recommend some specific foods such as increased vegetables or functional foods such as Benecol. Three well-designed studies found that both in women and men and before and after a heart attack, people who ate more fish (2–4 servings a week) appeared to avoid heart disease. Additionally putting supplements containing Omega 3 polyunsaturated fatty acids (PUFA) into the diet also appeared to protect against abnormal heart rhythms and sudden death from heart attack. Increasing oat bran in the diet may be of additional help in lowering cholesterol, but can decrease the amount of medicine that gets into your body. Take oat bran 2 hours before pravastatin or 4–6 hours after. Your doctor may also recommend increasing B vitamins. See Tables 19 and 20 about lifestyle changes and risk factors you can fix.

Herbal Medicines or Minerals: No data exist from well-designed clinical studies about garlic and pravastatin combinations and they cannot presently be recommended. Additionally, garlic may inhibit blood-clotting (platelet) aggregation—something to consider if you are already taking a platelet inhibitor. The FDA has allowed one dietary supplement called Cholestin to continue to be sold. This preparation actually contains lovastatin. Since use of two HMG-CoA inhibitors may increase risk of rhabdomyolysis or myopathy, the combination is NOT advised. Medicines such as eucalyptus, kava, valerian, or other herbals that can cause liver damage are not advisable.

Soy (milk, tofu, etc.) contains phytoestrogens, which has led to an FDA-approved health claim for reducing risk of heart disease (if there is at least 6.25 g of soy protein per serving). Substituting soy for some of the meat in your diet can also help lower cholesterol. Policosanol may have added benefits in lowering cholesterol but no data using it in combination. Because pravastatin like other medicines in this drug class can deplete co-Q10, supplementation may be needed. One report of type 2 diabetics with low co-Q10 found beneficial effects from supplementation.

Beverages: No restrictions. May be taken with milk.

▷ *Alcohol:* No interactions expected. Use sparingly.

Tobacco Smoking: No interactions expected. I advise everyone to quit smoking.

▷ *Other Drugs*

Pravastatin **taken concurrently** with

- amprenavir (Agenerase) and ritonavir (Norvir) and perhaps other protease inhibitors may increase pravastatin levels and the risk of muscle damage (myopathy); however, the risk of such combination is not as great as with other medicines in the same family as pravastatin relies less on CYP 3A4 for removal from the body.
- clofibrate (Atromid-S) has been associated with muscle damage (rhabdomyolysis).
- cyclosporine (Sandimmune) increases the risk for myopathy. Dosing of 10 mg is used with a maximum of 20 mg.
- erythromycin (various) may increase muscle damage risk. Do not combine.

- itraconazole (Sporanox—24% increase in serum concentration in one study). May increase risk of muscle problems. Decreased doses are prudent if these medicines must be combined.
- gemfibrozil (Lopid) may alter the absorption and excretion of pravastatin and may also increase risk of muscle damage (rhabdomyolysis); these drugs should not be taken concurrently.
- niacin (various) may increase muscle damage risk.
- quinupristin/dalfopristin (Synercid) may increase the risk for myopathy by increasing cerivastatin blood levels.
- warfarin (Coumadin) can increase the risk of bleeding; more frequent INR (prothrombin time or protime) testing is indicated. Ongoing warfarin doses should be based on laboratory results.

The following drug may *decrease* the effects of pravastatin:

- cholestyramine (Questran)—may reduce absorption of pravastatin; take pravastatin 1 hour before or 4 hours after cholestyramine.

▷ *Driving, Hazardous Activities:* This drug may cause dizziness. Restrict activities as necessary.

Aviation Note: The use of this drug *may be a disqualification* for piloting. Consult a designated Aviation Medical Examiner.

Exposure to Sun: No restrictions.

Discontinuation: Do not stop this drug without your doctor's knowledge and help. There may be a significant increase in blood cholesterol levels if this medicine is stopped. Patients who have acute coronary syndromes or ACS (such as unstable angina, heart attack [non-p; Q-wave myocardial infarction], and Q-wave myocardial infarction) were reviewed as part of the Platelet Receptor Inhibitor in Ischemic Syndrome Management (PRISM) study. It was found that pretreatment with statin type medicines (HMG-CoA reductase inhibitors such as the medicine in this profile) significantly lowered risk during the first 30 days after ACS symptoms started. Talk with your doctor BEFORE stopping any statin type medicine.

PRAZOSIN (PRA zoh sin)

Introduced: 1970 **Class:** Antihypertensive **Prescription:** USA: Yes **Controlled Drug:** USA: No; Canada: No **Available as Generic:** USA: Yes; Canada: Yes

Brand Names: ✤Apo-Prazo, Minipres, Minizide [CD], ✤Novo-Prazin, ✤Nu-Prazo

```
┌──────────────────────────────────────────────────────────────────────┐
│                      BENEFITS versus RISKS                             │
│        Possible Benefits                    Possible Risks             │
│  EFFECTIVE INITIAL THERAPY FOR     "First-dose" drop in blood pressure │
│    MILD TO MODERATE                  with fainting                     │
│    HYPERTENSION                    May cause increased heart rate      │
│  EFFECTIVE ANTIHYPERTENSIVE          (paroxysmal tachycardia)          │
│    IN MODERATE TO SEVERE                                               │
│    HYPERTENSION                                                        │
│  EFFECTIVE CONTROL OF                                                  │
│    HYPERTENSION IN                                                     │
│    PHEOCHROMOCYTOMA                                                    │
│  HELPS URINE FLOW IN BENIGN                                            │
│    PROSTATIC HYPERPLASIA                                               │
│  Effective in presence of impaired                                    │
│    kidney function                                                     │
└──────────────────────────────────────────────────────────────────────┘
```

Author's Note: Data from the ALLHAT trial found that alpha blockers such as this medicine are not drugs of first choice in high blood pressure. Information in this profile has been shortened for more widely used medicines.

PREDNISOLONE (pred NIS oh lohn)

Introduced: 1955 **Class:** Cortisonelike drugs **Prescription:** USA: Yes **Controlled Drug:** USA: No; Canada: No **Available as Generic:** USA: Yes; Canada: Yes

Brand Names: A&D w/Prednisolone [CD], ✿Ak-Cide [CD], ✿Ak-Pred, ✿Ak-Tate, Blephamide, Cortalone, Delta-Cortef, Duapred, Econopred Ophthalmic, Fernisolone-P, Hydelta-TBA, Hydeltrasol, ✿Inflamase, ✿Inflamase Forte, Isopto Cetapred [CD], Key-Pred, Meticortelone, Meti-Derm, Metimyd [CD], Metreton, ✿Minims Prednisolone, Mydrapred, Niscort, Nor-Pred, ✿Nova-Pred, ✿Novoprednisolone, Ophtho-Tate, Optimyd [CD], Otobione [CD], Pediaject, Pediapred, Polypred, Predcor, ✿Pred Forte, Pred-G [CD], ✿Pred Mild, Prelone, PSP-IV, Savacort, Sterane, TBA Pred, ✿Vasocidin [CD]

BENEFITS versus RISKS

Possible Benefits	*Possible Risks*
EFFECTIVE RELIEF OF SYMPTOMS IN A WIDE VARIETY OF INFLAMMATORY AND ALLERGIC DISORDERS	Ongoing systemic use (variable onset) can be associated with increased possible emergence of effects such as:
EFFECTIVE IMMUNOSUPPRESSION IN SELECTED BENIGN AND MALIGNANT DISORDERS	ALTERED MOOD AND PERSONALITY
	CATARACTS, GLAUCOMA
Prevention of rejection in organ transplantation	HYPERTENSION, ARRHYTHMIA
	OSTEOPOROSIS, INCREASED SUSCEPTIBILITY TO INFECTIONS
	ASEPTIC BONE NECROSIS (OSTEONECROSIS) IS AN AREA OF CONTROVERSY, UNCLEAR ONSET, PATIENT RISK FACTORS AND CORRELATION VERSUS CAUSATION (SEE CONTROVERSY IN MEDICINES)

Author's Note: Adverse effects from ophthalmic use are much more limited and more rare than those from systemic use.

▷ **Principal Uses**

As a Single Drug Product: Uses currently included in FDA-approved labeling: (1) Used in the treatment of a wide variety of allergic and inflammatory conditions—it is used most commonly in the management of serious skin disorders, asthma, regional enteritis, ulcerative colitis and all types of major rheumatic disorders including bursitis, tendonitis, most forms of arthritis, and inflammatory eye conditions; (2) used as part of combination therapy in lymphoma; (3) used in some kinds of adrenal insufficiencies; (4) used to help tuberculosis patients who also have inflammation around the heart without fluid buildup; (5) eases symptoms in ulcerative colitis.

Other (unlabeled) generally accepted uses: (1) Used as part of combination therapy in acute leukemias (lymphoblastic, lymphocytic, and myelogenous); (2) may have a role in combination therapy of breast cancer; (3) can help relieve the muscle pain of familial Mediterranean fever; (4) part of a combination therapy in treating abnormal liver tumors (hemangiomas); (5) can help subfertile men decrease seminal antibodies and become fertile; (6) helps people who have drug-induced lowering of white blood cells recover; (7) treats anaphylactic reactions of unknown cause; (8) treats thrombocytopenic purpura of unknown cause; (9) eases symptoms in myasthenia gravis; (10) can help reflex sympathetic dystrophy.

How This Drug Works: It is thought that this drug's anti-inflammatory effect is due to its ability to inhibit the normal defensive functions of certain white blood cells. Its immunosuppressant effect is attributed to a reduced production of lymphocytes and antibodies and increase of a protein called lipocortin.

▷ **Widely Used Guidelines That Involve This Medicine (representative sample):** Please look at the section at the very beginning of this profile called

"Class." Next, turn to Table 22 and you will find guidelines listed by the class involved!

Available Dosage Forms and Strengths
Eye ointment — 0.6%
Eye suspension — 0.5%, 1%
Oral liquid — 6.7 mg/5 mL
Syrup — 15 mg/5 mL
Tablets — 5 mg

▷ **Usual Adult Dosage Ranges:** 5 to 60 mg daily as a single dose or in divided doses (some patients are put on alternate-day schedules). Once an adequate response is achieved, the dose should be decreased to the lowest effective dose. Ophthalmic drops—one to two drops is instilled into the eye sac (conjunctival sac) every 3 to 12 hours. Dosing may be increased to every hour in severe cases.

Note: Actual dose and schedule must be determined for each patient individually.

Typical Treatment Goals and Measurements (Outcomes and Markers)
Inflammation: The general goal is to relieve the swelling and the inflammatory response. Use in asthma should help decrease the frequency and severity of acute attacks. Some clinicians use decreased frequency of rescue inhaler use as a measure of success. Improvement in lung (pulmonary function) testing also helps define results in asthma. Lastly, clinical signs and symptoms such as wheezing, tightness in the chest, and exercise tolerance should all move in favorable directions.

Conditions Requiring Dosing Adjustments
Liver Function: Dosing adjustments do not appear to be needed in liver compromise.
Kidney Function: Dosing adjustments in renal compromise do not appear to be needed. This drug can cause proteinuria. It is a benefit-to-risk decision for kidney compromise (nephropathy) patients who tend to lose protein.

▷ **Dosing Instructions:** The tablet may be crushed and taken with or following food to prevent stomach irritation, preferably in the morning. Suspensions should be gently mixed before using. If you forget a dose: Call your doctor for instructions.

Usual Duration of Use: For acute disorders: 4 to 10 days generally, depending on patient reaction, disease flare and the condition being treated. For chronic disorders: according to individual requirements. Use only for time needed to relieve symptoms in acute self-limiting conditions or the time required to stabilize a chronic condition and permit gradual withdrawal. Because of its intermediate duration of action, this drug is appropriate for alternate-day dosing for many forms. See your doctor regularly.

Author's Note: The information categories provided in this profile are appropriate for prednisolone. For specific information that is normally found in those categories that have been omitted from this profile, see the following profile of prednisone. Prednisolone is a derivative of prednisone; both drugs share all significant actions and effects.

PREDNISONE (PRED ni sohn)

Introduced: 1955 **Class:** Cortisonelike drugs **Prescription:**
USA: Yes **Controlled Drug:** USA: No; Canada: No **Available as**
Generic: USA: Yes; Canada: Yes

Brand Names: ✸Apo-Prednisone, Aspred-C [CD], Deltasone, Liquid Pred, Meticorten, ✸Metreton [CD], ✸Novoprednisone, Orasone, Panasol-S, Paracort, Prednicen-M, Prednisone Intensol, SK-Prednisone, Sterapred, Sterapred-DS, ✸Winpred

---

BENEFITS versus RISKS

Possible Benefits	*Possible Risks*
EFFECTIVE RELIEF OF SYMPTOMS IN A WIDE VARIETY OF INFLAMMATORY AND ALLERGIC DISORDERS	Ongoing systemic use (variable onset) can be associated with increased possible emergence of effects such as:
EFFECTIVE IMMUNOSUPPRESSION IN SELECTED BENIGN AND MALIGNANT DISORDERS	ALTERED MOOD AND PERSONALITY
Prevention of rejection in organ transplantation	CATARACTS, GLAUCOMA
	HYPERTENSION, ABNORMAL HEARTBEATS
	OSTEOPOROSIS, INCREASED SUSCEPTIBILITY TO INFECTIONS AND OTHERS
	ASEPTIC BONE NECROSIS (OSTEONECROSIS) IS AN AREA OF CONTROVERSY, UNCLEAR ONSET, PATIENT RISK FACTORS AND CORRELATION VERSUS CAUSATION (SEE CONTROVERSY IN MEDICINES)

▷ **Principal Uses**

As a Single Drug Product: Uses currently included in FDA-approved labeling: (1) Treats a wide variety of allergic and inflammatory conditions—it is used most commonly in the management of serious skin disorders (such as severe psoriasis, contact dermatitis and drug hypersensitivity reactions, etc.), asthma, gout, lupus erythematosus, regional enteritis, ulcerative colitis, nephrotic syndrome and all types of major rheumatic disorders including bursitis, tendonitis, most forms of arthritis and severe allergic conjunctivitis of the eye; (2) used as part of combination therapy of lymphoma; (3) helps address adrenal insufficiency; (4) used as part of combination therapy of several kinds of leukemia; (5) used in kidney transplant patients; (6) helps patients recover from symptoms of multiple sclerosis.

Other (unlabeled) generally accepted uses: (1) Used in combination therapy of acute (lymphoblastic, lymphocytic and myelogenous) leukemias; (2) combination therapy of breast cancer; (3) may be helpful in therapy of familial Mediterranean fever; (4) used with other medications to treat liver tumors (hemangiomas); (5) may help subfertile men decrease seminal antibodies and become fertile; (6) helps prevent early lung deterioration in children with AIDS; (7) eases symptoms in alcoholics who have hepatitis and encephalopathy; (8) used in some chronic pain syndromes.

How This Drug Works: Anti-inflammatory effect is due to its ability to inhibit normal defensive functions of certain white blood cells. Its immunosuppressant effect is due to a reduced production of lymphocytes and antibodies.

▷ **Widely Used Guidelines That Involve This Medicine (representative sample):** Please look at the section at the very beginning of this profile called "Class." Next, turn to Table 22 and you will find guidelines listed by the class involved!

Available Dosage Forms and Strengths
Oral solution — 5 mg/5 mL
    Syrup — 5 mg/5 mL (5% alcohol)
    Tablets — 1 mg, 2.5 mg, 5 mg, 10 mg, 20 mg, 25 mg, 50 mg

▷ **Usual Adult Dosage Ranges:** Five to 60 mg daily as a single dose or in divided doses depending on the condition being treated. With myasthenia gravis, patients not responding to 100 mg will not respond to higher doses. Once initial inflammation has eased, the dose should be gradually lowered to the lowest effective dose for the condition being treated. Some clinicians use alternate day therapy once response is judged to be clinically adequate. This may help minimize cushingoid side effects of long-term therapy.
Note: Actual dose and schedule must be determined for each patient individually.

Conditions Requiring Dosing Adjustments
Liver Function: No dosing changes thought to be needed.
Kidney Function: Dosing adjustments in kidney disease do not appear to be needed.

▷ **Dosing Instructions:** The tablet may be crushed and taken with food or milk to help prevent stomach irritation, preferably in the morning. Liquid form doses should be measured with a dosing cup or a calibrated measuring spoon. If you forget a dose: Call your doctor for instructions. Be sure to check with your doctor BEFORE getting any vaccines (blunting of vaccine response may occur).

Usual Duration of Use: For acute disorders: 4 to 10 days generally with additional considerations of patient reaction, disease flare and tapering. For chronic disorders: according to individual requirements. Use should not exceed time needed for symptomatic relief in acute self-limiting conditions or time required to stabilize a chronic condition and permit gradual withdrawal. Intermediate duration of action allows alternate-day dosing. See your doctor regularly.

Typical Treatment Goals and Measurements (Outcomes and Markers)
Inflammation: The general goal is to relieve the swelling and the inflammatory response. Markers such as erythrocyte sedimentation rate (ESR), increased joint mobility and decreased time that joints are stiff in the morning can be used. Use in asthma should help decrease the frequency and severity of acute attacks. Some clinicians use decreased frequency of rescue inhaler use as a measure of success. Improvement in lung (pulmonary function) testing such as PEFR and FEV1 also help define results in asthma. Lastly, clinical signs and symptoms such as wheezing, tightness in the chest, and exercise tolerance should all move in favorable directions if asthma is being treated. If signs and symptoms worsen or do not ease or if new signs or symptoms occur, call your doctor.

▷ **This Drug Should Not Be Taken If**
- you had an allergic reaction to it previously.
- you have active peptic ulcer disease.
- you have an active herpes simplex virus eye infection.
- you have active tuberculosis.
- you have a fungal infection in a large area inside your body (systemic fungal infection).

▷ **Inform Your Physician Before Taking This Drug If**
- you have had an adverse reaction to any cortisonelike drug.
- you have a history of peptic ulcer disease, thrombophlebitis, or tuberculosis.
- you have diabetes, kidney failure, glaucoma, high blood pressure, deficient thyroid function, or myasthenia gravis.
- you have osteoporosis.
- you develop unexplained joint pain (such as in the knees, hip, or shoulder) while taking this medicine, or after you've taken it. These may be early signs of aseptic necrosis (osteonecrosis). Call your doctor right away.
- you have been exposed to any viral illness, such as measles or chicken pox. (Cases may be severe if you are taking this medicine.)
- you are prone to depression.
- you have diverticulitis.
- you plan to have surgery of any kind in the near future or have had some kinds of intestinal surgery.

Possible Side Effects (natural, expected, and unavoidable drug actions)

Increased appetite, weight gain, retention of salt and water leading to increased blood pressure, excretion of potassium, increased susceptibility to infection because of immune suppression. Increased white blood cell count (granulocytes)—not a symptom of infection, but a drug effect. Decreased white blood cell count (monocytes and lymphocytes). Growth changes in children. Mild depression or euphoria (may be common). Impaired wound healing. Easy bruising (ecchymosis). Adrenal gland suppression.

▷ **Possible Adverse Effects** (unusual, unexpected, and infrequent reactions)
If any of the following develop, consult your physician promptly for guidance.

Mild Adverse Effects

Allergic reaction: skin rash.

Headache, dizziness, insomnia—infrequent.

Acid indigestion, abdominal distention—infrequent.

Patchy blue areas on the great toe (blue toe syndrome)—case reports.

Muscle cramping and weakness—possible.

Elevated intracranial pressure (pseudotumor cerebri)—infrequent.

Acne, excessive growth of facial hair—frequent.

Serious Adverse Effects

Serious mental or emotional disturbances—case reports.

Reactivation of latent tuberculosis—possible in those with past tuberculosis.

Development of peptic ulcer—possible and more likely in those with previous ulcers.

Development of inflammation of the pancreas—rare (pancreatitis more likely with prolonged treatment or high doses).

Thrombophlebitis (inflammation of a vein with the formation of blood clot): pain or tenderness in thigh or leg, with or without swelling of the foot, ankle, or leg—rare.

Increased intraocular (inner eye) pressure, glaucoma, or cataracts—infrequent.

Kaposi's sarcoma—case reports.

Growth retardation—possible in children with long-term use.

Cushing's syndrome—possible with long-term use (central obesity, "buffalo hump," and moon-shaped face).

Necrosis of bone (osteonecrosis, avascular necrosis, or aseptic necrosis)—Questions remain as to correlation versus causation, but may be more likely with high initial corticosteroid doses, long-term treatment, and cumulative doses of 4.32 grams. May also happen with short-term, modest doses. Individual patient risk factors and/or diseases or conditions appear to be important. Call your doctor if unexplained joint pain happens.

Osteoporosis—possible with long-term use.

Superinfections—possible.

Inflammation or wasting of muscle (myositis or myopathy)—infrequent.

Increased blood sugar—possible and may be dose-related.

Drug-induced porphyria or seizures—case reports.

Pulmonary embolism (movement of a blood clot to the lung): may show as sudden shortness of breath, pain in the chest, coughing, bloody sputum—increased risk.

▷ **Possible Effects on Sexual Function:** Altered timing and pattern of menstruation. Correction of male infertility when due to autoantibodies that suppress sperm activity.

▷ **Adverse Effects That May Mimic Natural Diseases or Disorders**
Pattern of symptoms and signs resembling Cushing's syndrome, osteoporosis may resemble bone loss occurring after menopause.

Natural Diseases or Disorders That May Be Activated by This Drug
Latent diabetes, glaucoma, peptic ulcer disease, tuberculosis.

Possible Effects on Laboratory Tests
Complete blood cell counts: decreased eosinophils, lymphocytes, and platelets.

Blood amylase level: increased (possible pancreatitis).

Blood total cholesterol and HDL cholesterol levels: increased.

Blood LDL cholesterol level: no effect.

Blood digoxin (Lanoxin, others): FALSE increase with Abbott TDx method.

Blood triglyceride levels: no significant effect.

Blood glucose level: increased.

Glucose tolerance test (GTT): decreased.

Blood potassium or testosterone level: decreased.

Blood thyroid hormone (T3): decreased.

Blood uric acid level: increased.

Urine sugar tests: no effect with Tes-Tape; false low result with Clinistix and Diastix.

Fecal occult blood test: positive (if gastrointestinal bleeding).

CAUTION
1. If therapy exceeds 1 week, carry an identification card noting that you are taking this drug.
2. Do not stop this drug abruptly after long-term use.
3. If vaccination against measles, rabies, smallpox, or yellow fever is required, discontinue this drug 72 hours before vaccination and do not resume it for at least 14 days after vaccination.

4. Because of the way that this medicine works on the immune system, you will have an increased risk of infections while you are taking it. It is prudent to avoid patients with flu or other viral illnesses such as chicken pox. Call your doctor if exposure happens.

5. A variety of patient risk factors appear to be important in possible development of osteonecrosis. Talk to your doctor about the current list. Call your doctor if unexplained joint pain occurs.

Controversies in Medicine: Medicines in this class have had conflicting reports regarding correlation with or causation of aseptic bone necrosis (osteonecrosis-ON). There appear to be patient risk factors, possible delayed onset with occurrence even after the medicine is stopped, and some diseases or conditions where corticosteroids are often used and ON is more frequent than the general population. It is unclear if this is because of the disease or condition or the use of corticosteroids. Previous data regarding cumulative dosing (4.32 grams) appears controversial, with more recent case reports of 6 days of treatment with some doses being associated with ON. Some existing and emerging patient risk factors include alcohol use versus abuse, initial high doses, HIV positive patients who weight trained, Systemic Lupus Erythematosus, some clotting disorders, and high homocysteine levels amongst others appear to increase risk. Early research regarding use of alendronate (Fosamax) to treat ON appears to show that it is important for patients to quickly return to their doctors if unexplained joint pain (such as in the hip or knee) happens. Some centers note that ON has been poorly studied, and while the weight of data is growing, it is yet too early to say more than ON is correlated with corticosteroid use.

Precautions for Use

By Infants and Children: Avoid prolonged use if possible. During long-term use, observe for suppression of normal growth and the possibility of increased intracranial pressure. Following long-term use, the child may be at risk for adrenal gland deficiency during stress for as long as 18 months after cessation of this drug.

By Those Over 60 Years of Age: Cortisonelike drugs should only be used when the disorder under treatment is unresponsive to adequate trials of unrelated drugs. Avoid the prolonged use of this drug if possible. Continual use (even in small doses) can increase severity of diabetes, enhance fluid retention, raise blood pressure, weaken resistance to infection, induce stomach ulcer, and accelerate development of cataract and osteoporosis or other bone problems.

▷ Advisability of Use During Pregnancy

Pregnancy Category: B. See Pregnancy Risk Categories at the back of this book.
Animal Studies: Birth defects reported in mice, rats, and rabbits.
Human Studies: Adequate studies of pregnant women are not available.

Avoid completely during the first 3 months. Limit use during the final 6 months as much as possible. If used, examine infant for possible deficiency of adrenal gland function.

Advisability of Use If Breast-Feeding

Presence of this drug in breast milk: Yes, but amounts received via breast milk are generally less than 0.1% of a therapeutic dose. Talk to your doctor. Prednisolone or prednisone may be drugs of choice in women who wish to breast-feed while taking one of those medicines for one of its indicated uses.

Habit-Forming Potential: Long-term use of this drug may produce a state of functional dependence (see Glossary). In therapy of asthma and rheumatoid arthritis, it is advisable to keep the dose as small as possible and attempt drug withdrawal after periods of reasonable improvement. Such procedures may reduce the degree of "steroid rebound"—the return of symptoms as the drug is withdrawn.

Effects of Overdose: Fatigue, muscle weakness, stomach irritation, acid indigestion, excessive sweating, facial flushing, fluid retention, swelling of extremities, increased blood pressure.

Possible Effects of Long-Term Use: Increased blood sugar (possible diabetes), increased fat deposits on the trunk of the body ("buffalo hump"), rounding of the face ("moon face"), thinning and fragility of skin, loss of texture and strength of bones (osteoporosis, aseptic necrosis), cataracts, glaucoma, retarded growth and development in children.

Suggested Periodic Examinations While Taking This Drug (at physician's discretion)

Measurements of blood pressure, blood sugar, and potassium levels.

Complete eye examinations at regular intervals.

Chest X ray if history of tuberculosis.

Bone mineral density testing (DEXA) to check for osteoporosis. Check of bone status relative to osteonecrosis (such as unexplained joint pain). Such pain may need MRI follow-up.

Determination of the rate of development of the growing child to detect retardation of normal growth.

▷ **While Taking This Drug, Observe the Following**

Foods: Alfalfa may negate benefits of prednisone in SLE patients (possible L-canavanine effect). Otherwise, no drug lowering by food reported. Ask your doctor about restricting salt or eating potassium-rich foods. Higher protein diet may be prudent in long-term use. Taking drug with food can help avoid stomach upset.

Herbal Medicines or Minerals: Hawthorn, ginger, garlic, ma huang, ginseng, guar gum, fenugreek, and nettle may change blood sugar. Since prednisone may also change blood sugar control, caution is advised. Ma huang has ephedra in it and may also decrease prednisone benefits.

Fir or pine needle oil should NOT be used by asthmatics. Ephedra alone does carry a German Commission E monograph indication for asthma treatment. If you are allergic to plants in the Asteraceae family (aster, chrysanthemum, daisy, or ragweed), you may also be allergic to echinacea, chamomile, feverfew, and St. John's wort. During long-term use, take a vitamin D supplement and increase calcium. During wound repair, take a zinc supplement. Potassium loss may need to be replaced. Ask your doctor if glucosamine makes sense for you. Ginseng and echinacea may blunt prednisone benefits. Licorice (glycyrrhizine in it) may increase risk of adverse effects. Talk to your doctor BEFORE adding any herbal to any other medicines that you already take.

Beverages: No restrictions. Drink all forms of milk liberally.

▷ *Alcohol:* Use caution if you are prone to peptic ulcers. Talk to your doctor to get his or her approval of drinking beer, wine, or other liquor while taking this medicine. Controversy exists as to any alcohol use versus abuse as a risk factor for osteonecrosis.

Tobacco Smoking: Nicotine increases the blood levels of naturally produced cortisone. I advise everyone to quit smoking.

Marijuana Smoking: May cause additional impairment of immunity.

▷ *Other Drugs*

Prednisone may ***decrease*** the effects of

- insulin (various), or oral hypoglycemic drugs, requiring dosing changes of insulin or hypoglycemic.
- isoniazid (INH, Niconyl, etc.).
- quetiapine (Seroquel).
- salicylates (aspirin, sodium salicylate, etc.) and also increases the risk of stomach irritation.
- vaccines (such as flu vaccine), by blunting the immune response to them.

Prednisone ***taken concurrently*** with

- amphotericin B (Abelcet, Fungizone) may result in additive potassium loss.
- asparaginase (Elspar) may result in increased risk of toxicity if given with or before prednisone. Asparaginase dosing should be accomplished after prednisone dosing.
- birth control pills (oral contraceptives) will prolong the prednisone effect.
- clarithromycin (Biaxin) may lead to psychotic symptoms (one case report). Patients must be closely watched if these medicines are combined.
- cyclosporine (Sandimmune) can cause increased cyclosporine levels and increased prednisone levels. Dose decreases may be needed for both drugs.
- foscarnet (Foscavir) may result in additive potassium loss.
- ketoconazole (Nizoral) has increased a metabolite of prednisone in some studies (prednisolone), but not in other studies. Increased patient follow-up and check for increased prednisone side effects are prudent if combined treatment continues for 5–7 days.
- levofloxacin (Levaquin) and perhaps other fluoroquinolone antibiotics may increase the risk of tendon rupture. Caution in exercise is needed.
- loop diuretics (furosemide [Lasix], bumetanide [Bumex]) may blunt their effects.
- macrolide antibiotics (erythromycin, troleandomycin, and perhaps others) can lead to prednisone toxicity.
- montelukast (Singulair) resulted in severe edema (peripheral) in one case report. Caution and close patient monitoring are prudent if these medicines must be combined.
- neuromuscular blocking agents (such as pancuronium-Pavulon, vecuronium-Norcuron, others) can result in increased risk and or severity of muscle problems (myopathy and flaccid paralysis) and can also antagonize blockade from these medicines. Caution and unparalyzed periods are prudent.
- NSAIDs may result in additive stomach and intestinal irritation.
- oral anticoagulants may either increase or decrease their effectiveness; consult your physician regarding the need for prothrombin time testing and dose adjustment.
- oral antidiabetic drugs (see Drug Classes) or insulin may result in loss of glucose control.
- ritonavir (Norvir) and perhaps other protease inhibitors (see Drug Classes) may lead to toxicity.
- theophylline (Theo-Dur, others) may result in variable responses to this medicine. Increased frequency of theophylline level testing is recommended.
- thiazide diuretics (see Drug Classes) or loop diuretics may result in additive potassium loss.
- vaccines (flu, pneumococcal, varicella, and others) may result in blunted response to the vaccine and decreased preventive benefits.

The following drugs may *decrease* the effects of prednisone:
- antacids—may reduce its absorption.
- barbiturates (Amytal, Butisol, phenobarbital, etc.).
- carbamazepine (Tegretol).
- phenytoin (Dilantin, etc.) and fosphenytoin (Cerebyx).
- primidone (Mysoline).
- rifampin (Rifadin, Rimactane, etc.).

▷ *Driving, Hazardous Activities:* Usually no restrictions. Be alert to the rare occurrence of dizziness.

Aviation Note: The use of this drug **may be a disqualification** for piloting. Consult a designated Aviation Medical Examiner.

Exposure to Sun: No restrictions.

Occurrence of Unrelated Illness: This drug may decrease resistance to infection. Tell your doctor if you develop an infection of any kind. It may also reduce your ability to respond to the stress of acute illness, injury, or surgery. Keep your doctor informed of any changes in health.

Discontinuation: Do not stop this drug abruptly after chronic use. Ask your doctor for help about gradual, individualized withdrawal. Some clinicians change from daily to every other day therapy for four weeks BEFORE starting to lower the dose in a stepwise fashion. Many patients tolerate dose reductions of 2.5 mg of prednisone (other steroids are calculated on the basis of prednisone equivalents) with those decreases made every 3–7 days. If a disease flare occurs (worsening of symptoms), the dose should be increased to the last dose before the disease flare and should be tapered more slowly down to 5–10 mg or lower. Some clinicians use 8 A.M. predose plasma cortisol to guide tapering. If this lab test is less than 10 mcg/deciliter, tapering is continued until the daily prednisone equivalent is 2–5 mg. In general, if long-term treatment or high doses were used, prednisone equivalents should be tapered over 9–12 months. For up to 2 years after stopping this drug, you may require it again if you have an injury, surgery, or an illness.

PRIMIDONE (PRI mi dohn)

Introduced: 1953   **Class:** Anticonvulsant   **Prescription:** USA: Yes   **Controlled Drug:** USA: No; Canada: No   **Available as Generic:** USA: Yes; Canada: Yes

Brand Names: ❧Apo-Primidone, Myidone, Mysoline, ❧PMS-Primidone and ❧Sertan

Author's Note: **Information in this profile has been shortened to make room for more widely used medicines.**

PROBENECID (proh BEN e sid)

Introduced: 1951   **Class:** Antigout   **Prescription:** USA: Yes   **Controlled Drug:** USA: No; Canada: No   **Available as Generic:** USA: Yes; Canada: No

Brand Names: Ampicillin-Probenecid, ❧Ampicin PRB [CD], Benemid, ❧Benuryl, Colabid [CD], ColBenemid [CD], Polycillin-PRB [CD], Probalan, Probampacin [CD], Proben-C [CD], Probenecid with Colchicine, ❧Pro-Biosan 500 Kit [CD], SK-Probenecid

---

BENEFITS versus RISKS

Possible Benefits	*Possible Risks*
EFFECTIVE LONG-TERM PREVENTION OF ACUTE ATTACKS OF GOUT	Formation of uric acid kidney stones
Useful adjunct to penicillin therapy (to achieve high blood and tissue levels of penicillin)	Bone marrow depression (aplastic anemia)
Used with cidofovir (Vistide) to ease kidney toxicity	Drug-induced liver and kidney damage

---

▷ **Principal Uses**

As a Single Drug Product: Uses currently included in FDA-approved labeling: (1) Used in helping maintain penicillin levels in therapy of gonorrhea; (2) helps prevent gout.

Other (unlabeled) generally accepted uses: (1) May have a role in preventing kidney toxicity in cisplatin chemotherapy; (2) adjunctive use in maintaining effective antibiotic levels in treatment of syphilis; (3) may prevent kidney damage from some kinds of kidney toxic (nephrotoxic) drugs (such as cidofovir-Vistide for CMV in HIV patients); (4) helps lower increased uric acid levels that can be caused by medicines such as thiazide diuretics.

As a Combination Drug Product [CD]: This drug is available in combination with colchicine, a drug often used for the treatment of acute gout. Each drug works in a different way; when used in combination they provide both relief of the acute gout and some measure of protection from recurrence of acute attacks. Also available combined with penicillin so that the penicillin stays in the body longer than usual to fight the infection.

How This Drug Works: Works in the kidney (tubular systems) to increase uric acid excretion in the urine; this drug reduces the levels of uric acid in the blood and body tissues. It also works in the kidney to decrease the amount of penicillin excreted in the urine, prolongs the presence of penicillin in the blood and helps achieve higher concentrations in body tissues.

▷ **Widely Used Guidelines That Involve This Medicine (representative sample):**
Please look at the section at the very beginning of this profile called "Class." Next, turn to Table 22 and you will find guidelines listed by the class involved!

Available Dosage Forms and Strengths
Tablets — 500 mg
Tablets (combination) — 0.5 mg colchicine and 500 mg of probenecid

▷ **Usual Adult Dosage Ranges:** *Antigout (non-combination tablet)*: Initially 250 mg twice a day for 1 week and then 500 mg twice a day. When there have been no sudden gout attacks for six months, the dose can usually be decreased by 500 mg a day every six months until uric acid levels start to rise again. *Adjunct to penicillin therapy (non-combination tablet)*: 500 mg four times a day.
Note: Actual dose and schedule must be determined for each patient individually.

Conditions Requiring Dosing Adjustments
Liver Function: Specific guidelines for dose adjustment in liver compromise are not available. This drug should be used with caution.
Kidney Function: Patients with kidney failure (creatinine clearance less than 30 mL/min) should not use this drug, as the effectiveness is questionable. Those with moderate kidney failure may still benefit from this medicine,

and dose increases (as needed and tolerated) in 500-mg steps up to 2,000 mg a day in equally divided doses may be required.

▷ **Dosing Instructions:** The tablet may be crushed and taken with or following food to reduce stomach irritation. Drink 2.5 to 3 quarts of liquids (10 to 12 full glasses) daily unless your doctor tells you it is not a good idea in your case. If you forget a dose: Take the missed dose as soon as you remember it, unless it's nearly time for your next dose—if that is the case, skip the missed dose and take the next dose right on schedule. DO NOT double doses. Talk with your doctor and pharmacist if you find yourself missing doses as there are many strategies to help.

Usual Duration of Use: Use on a regular schedule for several months usually determines effectiveness in preventing acute attacks of gout. If six months pass without a sudden (acute) gout attack, the dose can usually be decreased. Long-term use (months to years) requires supervision and periodic evaluation by your physician.

Typical Treatment Goals and Measurements (Outcomes and Markers)
Uric Acid: Blood uric acid levels often decrease in 48 to 72 hours and may reach normal range in 1 to 3 weeks. Attacks of gout should become shorter and lessen in severity over time.

▷ **This Drug Should Not Be Taken If**
- you have had an allergic reaction to it previously.
- you have active liver disease.
- you have acute kidney failure or kidney stones made of uric acid.
- you are less than 2 years old.
- you have an active blood cell or bone marrow disorder.
- you are taking any drug product that contains aspirin or aspirinlike drugs.
- you are having an attack of acute gout at the present time.

▷ **Inform Your Physician Before Taking This Drug If**
- you have a history of kidney disease or kidney stones.
- you have a history of liver disease or impaired liver function.
- you have a history of peptic ulcer disease.
- you have a history of a blood cell or bone marrow disorder.

Possible Side Effects (natural, expected, and unavoidable drug actions)
Development of kidney stones (composed of uric acid)—this is preventable. Consult your physician regarding the use of sodium bicarbonate (or other urine alkalinizer) to prevent stone formation.

▷ **Possible Adverse Effects** (unusual, unexpected, and infrequent reactions)
If any of the following develop, consult your physician promptly for guidance.
Mild Adverse Effects
Allergic reactions: skin rash, itching, drug fever (see Glossary).
Headache, dizziness, flushing of face—infrequent.
Hair loss (alopecia): possible.
Reduced appetite, sore gums, nausea, vomiting—possible to infrequent.
Serious Adverse Effects
Allergic reactions: anaphylactic reaction (see Glossary).
Idiosyncratic reactions: hemolytic anemia (see Glossary).
Bone marrow depression (see Glossary): fatigue, sore throat, bleeding/bruising—case reports.
Drug-induced liver damage with jaundice (see Glossary—also includes hepatic necrosis) or porphyria—case reports.

Fluid in the retina (retinal edema)—case reports.

Drug-induced kidney damage: marked fluid retention, reduced urine formation—case reports.

▷ **Possible Effects on Sexual Function:** None reported.

▷ **Adverse Effects That May Mimic Natural Diseases or Disorders**

Liver reactions may suggest viral hepatitis. Kidney reactions may suggest nephrosis.

Possible Effects on Laboratory Tests

Complete blood cell counts: decreased red cells, hemoglobin, white cells, and platelets.

INR (prothrombin time): increased (when taken concurrently with warfarin).

Blood glucose level and uric acid level: decreased.

Blood urea nitrogen (BUN) level: increased (kidney damage).

Liver function tests: increased enzymes (ALT/GPT, AST/GOT, alkaline phosphatase) or bilirubin.

Urine sugar tests: false positive with Benedict's solution and Clinitest.

CAUTION

1. This drug should not be started until 2 to 3 weeks after an acute attack of gout has subsided.
2. This drug may increase the frequency of acute attacks of gout during the first few months of treatment. Concurrent use of colchicine is advised to prevent acute attacks (see combination forms).
3. Aspirin (and aspirin-containing drug products) can reduce the effectiveness of this drug. Use acetaminophen or a nonaspirin analgesic for pain relief as needed.

Precautions for Use

By Infants and Children: Safety and effectiveness for those less than 2 years of age are not established.

By Those Over 60 Years of Age: The natural decline in kidney function that occurs after 60 may require adjustment of your dose. You may be more susceptible to the serious adverse effects of this drug. Report any unusual symptoms promptly for evaluation.

▷ **Advisability of Use During Pregnancy**

Pregnancy Category: B. See Pregnancy Risk Categories at the back of this book.

Animal Studies: No information available.

Human Studies: Adequate studies of pregnant women are not available.

This drug has been used during pregnancy with no reports of birth defects or adverse effects on the fetus. Ask your physician for guidance.

Advisability of Use If Breast-Feeding

Presence of this drug in breast milk: Unknown.

Avoid drug or refrain from nursing.

Habit-Forming Potential: None.

Effects of Overdose: Stomach irritation, nausea, vomiting, nervous agitation, delirium, seizures, coma.

Possible Effects of Long-Term Use: Formation of kidney stones. Kidney damage in sensitive patients.

Suggested Periodic Examinations While Taking This Drug (at physician's discretion)

Complete blood cell counts.

Blood uric acid.

Liver and kidney function tests.

▷ **While Taking This Drug, Observe the Following**

Foods: Follow your physician's advice regarding the need for a low-purine diet.

Herbal Medicines or Minerals: Acerola is high in vitamin C. Inosine, like acerola, may increase uric acid levels. Aspen should be avoided in gout. Lipase may worsen gout. Goutweed (aegopodium podagraria) does not have enough data to assess effectiveness in treating gout.

Beverages: A large intake of coffee, tea, or cola beverages may reduce the effectiveness of treatment.

▷ *Alcohol:* No interactions expected, but large amounts of alcohol can raise the blood uric acid level and reduce the effectiveness of treatment.

Tobacco Smoking: No interactions expected. I advise everyone to quit smoking.

▷ *Other Drugs*

Probenecid may ***increase*** the effects of

- acetaminophen (Tylenol), increasing risk of toxicity.
- acyclovir (Zovirax) and result in toxicity unless doses are reduced.
- ciprofloxacin (Cipro) and gatifloxacin (Tequin), increasing toxicity risk.
- clofibrate (Atromid-S).
- dyphylline (Neothylline).
- entacapone (Comtan).
- ganciclovir (Cytovene).
- ketoprofen and perhaps other NSAIDs (see Drug Classes).
- ketorolac (Toradol) and increase toxicity risk.
- methotrexate (Mexate) and increase its toxicity.
- midazolam (Versed) and increase CNS depression.
- oral antidiabetic agents (see Drug Classes—sulfonlyureas).
- oseltamivir (Tamiflu).
- thiazide diuretics (see Drug Classes).
- thiopental (Pentothal) and prolong its anesthetic effect.
- valacyclovir (Valtrex) and result in toxicity unless doses are reduced.
- valgancyclovir (Valcyte) and result in toxicity unless doses are reduced.
- zalcitabine (Hivid).
- zidovudine (Retrovir) and increase toxicity risk.

Probenecid ***taken concurrently*** with

- allopurinol (Zyloprim) may result in extended allopurinol half-life.
- cephalosporins (see Drug Classes) may cause a doubling of antibiotic levels. Caution must be used to avoid toxicity.
- dapsone may cause up to a 50% increased dapsone level and result in toxicity unless dapsone doses are decreased.
- penicillins (see Drug Classes) may cause a threefold to fivefold increase in penicillin blood levels, greatly increasing the effectiveness of each penicillin dose.
- rifampin (Rifadin, others) may result in increased blood levels of rifampin.
- ritonavir (Norvir) may lead to changes in probenecid blood levels.

The following drugs may ***decrease*** the effects of probenecid:

- aspirin and other salicylates—may reduce its effectiveness in promoting the excretion of uric acid.
- bismuth subsalicylate (Pepto-Bismol, others).

▷ *Driving, Hazardous Activities:* This drug may cause dizziness. Restrict activities as necessary.

Aviation Note: The use of this drug ***may be a disqualification*** for piloting. Consult a designated Aviation Medical Examiner.

Exposure to Sun: No restrictions.
Discontinuation: Do not stop this drug without consulting your physician.

PROCAINAMIDE (proh KAYN a mide)

Introduced: 1950 **Class:** Antiarrhythmic **Prescription:** USA: Yes **Controlled Drug:** USA: No; Canada: No **Available as Generic:** USA: Yes; Canada: No

Brand Names: ✤Apo-Procainamide, Procamide SR, Procanbid, Procan SR (no longer manufactured), Promine, Pronestyl, Pronestyl-SR, Rhythmin

Author's Note: Information in this profile has been shortened to make room for more widely used medicines.

PROCHLORPERAZINE (proh klor PER a zeen)

Introduced: 1956 **Class:** Antipsychotic, antiemetic, phenothiazines **Prescription:** USA: Yes **Controlled Drug:** USA: No; Canada: No **Available as Generic:** USA: Yes; Canada: Yes

Brand Names: ✤Combid [CD], Compazine, Eskatrol, Isopro, ✤Nu-Prochlor, ✤PMS-Prochlorperazine, Regal-BID, ✤Stemetil, Ultrazine [CD]

BENEFITS versus RISKS	
Possible Benefits	*Possible Risks*
EFFECTIVE CONTROL OF ACUTE MENTAL DISORDERS, NAUSEA, AND VOMITING	SERIOUS TOXIC EFFECTS ON BRAIN WITH LONG-TERM USE
Relief of anxiety and nervous tension	Liver damage with jaundice
	Blood cell disorders: abnormally low white cell and platelet counts

▷ **Principal Uses**
As a Single Drug Product: Uses currently included in FDA-approved labeling: (1) Relieves severe nausea and vomiting (such as from chemotherapy); (2) may be used to treat schizophrenia; (3) helps prevent motion sickness; (4) eases anxiety.
Other (unlabeled) generally accepted uses: (1) Sometimes used to increase the effects of anesthesia; (2) may be of use in treating Ménière's disease (for nausea and vomiting); (3) may have a role in migraine.
As a Combination Drug Product [CD]: This drug is available in combination with isopropamide for use in treating stomach (peptic) ulcers.

How This Drug Works: By inhibiting the action of dopamine, this drug acts to correct an imbalance of nerve impulse transmissions that is thought to be responsible for certain mental disorders. By blocking dopamine in the brain's chemoreceptor trigger zone, this drug prevents stimulation of this vomiting center.

▷ **Widely Used Guidelines That Involve This Medicine (representative sample):** Please look at the section at the very beginning of this profile called "Class." Next, turn to Table 22 and you will find guidelines listed by the class involved!

Available Dosage Forms and Strengths
Capsules, prolonged action — 10 mg, 15 mg, 30 mg
Injection — 5 mg/mL
Suppositories — 2.5 mg, 5 mg, 25 mg
Syrup — 5 mg/5 mL
Tablets — 5 mg, 10 mg, 25 mg

▷ **Usual Adult Dosage Ranges:** *For Nausea and Vomiting*: 5 to 10 mg three or four times daily. The sustained-release capsule can be taken as 15 mg when you wake up in the morning or 10 mg of the sustained-release form every 12 hours. Doses above 40 mg should be reserved only for resistant cases.

For Moderate to Severe Psychotic Problems: Initially 10 mg of the immediate-release form every 6 to 8 hours. If needed and tolerated, dose may be increased by 5 mg at intervals of 3 to 4 days. Usual range is 50 to 75 mg daily.

Note: Actual dose and dosing schedule must be determined for each patient individually.

Conditions Requiring Dosing Adjustments
Liver Function: This drug should be used with caution by patients with liver compromise. Specific guidelines for dose adjustment are not available.

Kidney Function: Specific guidelines for adjustment of doses are not available.

▷ **Dosing Instructions:** Immediate release tablets may be crushed and taken with or following food to reduce stomach irritation. Prolonged-action capsules should be swallowed whole without alteration. For the syrup form, make certain to use a dosing cup or a calibrated measuring spoon. If you forget a dose and you take several doses a day, take the missed dose as soon as you remember it, unless your next dose is due in about an hour—if that is the case, skip the missed dose and take the next dose right on schedule. If you only take one dose a day, take the missed dose as soon as you remember it, unless it's almost time for your next dose—then skip the dose you forgot and take the next dose on schedule. Talk with your doctor and pharmacist if you find yourself missing doses.

Usual Duration of Use: Use on a regular schedule for 12 to 24 hours usually determines effectiveness in controlling nausea and vomiting. If used for severe anxiety-tension states or acute psychotic behavior, a trial of several weeks is usually necessary to determine effectiveness. If not significantly beneficial within 6 weeks, it should be stopped. Consult your physician on a regular basis.

Typical Treatment Goals and Measurements (Outcomes and Markers)
Vomiting: The goal is to prevent or at least to decrease vomiting (emesis) frequency, amount, or severity. If goals are NOT met, call your doctor—there are a number of other medicines that can be tried.

▷ **This Drug Should Not Be Taken If**
- you have had an allergic reaction to it previously.
- you have active liver disease.
- you have signs that are indicative of Reye's syndrome.
- you have extremely low blood pressure.
- this drug was prescribed for a child who is less than 2 years old or who weighs less than 20 lb.
- you have a current blood cell or bone marrow disorder.

▷ **Inform Your Physician Before Taking This Drug If**
- you are allergic or abnormally sensitive to any phenothiazine drug (see Drug Classes).

- you have impaired liver or kidney function.
- you have any type of seizure disorder.
- you have bone marrow depression or a history of blood diseases or ulcers.
- you have diabetes, glaucoma or heart disease.
- you have prostate trouble (prostatic hypertrophy).
- you are pregnant.
- you have had neuroleptic malignant syndrome or lupus erythematosus.
- you are taking any drug with sedative effects.
- you plan to have surgery under general or spinal anesthesia in the near future.

Possible Side Effects (natural, expected, and unavoidable drug actions)
Drowsiness (usually during the first 2 weeks), orthostatic hypotension (see Glossary), blurred vision, dry mouth, nasal congestion, constipation, impaired urination. Pink or purple coloration of urine—of no significance.

▷ **Possible Adverse Effects** (unusual, unexpected, and infrequent reactions)
If any of the following develop, consult your physician promptly for guidance.
Mild Adverse Effects
Allergic reactions: skin rash, hives, low-grade fever.
Lowering of body temperature, especially in the elderly (see hypothermia in Glossary)—possible.
Increased appetite and weight gain—possible.
Increased blood pressure—infrequent.
Dizziness, weakness—frequent.
Agitation, insomnia, impaired day and night vision—infrequent.
Chronic constipation, fecal impaction, incontinence—infrequent.
Serious Adverse Effects
Allergic reactions: hepatitis with jaundice (see Glossary), usually between second and fourth week; high fever; asthma; anaphylactic reaction (see Glossary).
Idiosyncratic reactions: toxic dermatitis, Stevens-Johnson Syndrome.
Neuroleptic malignant syndrome (see Glossary).
Liver toxicity or porphyria—case reports.
Abnormal eye positioning (oculogyric crisis)—case reports.
Depression, disorientation, seizures—case reports.
Abnormally high blood pressure—rare.
Disturbances of heart rhythm, rapid heart rate—rare.
Bone marrow depression (see Glossary)—case reports (call your doctor if you get a sore throat or infection).
Parkinson-like disorders (see Glossary); muscle spasms of face, jaw, neck, back, extremities; slowed movements, muscle rigidity, tremors; tardive dyskinesias (see Glossary)—case reports.

▷ **Possible Effects on Sexual Function:** Altered timing and pattern of menstruation.
Female breast enlargement with milk production—case reports.
Causes false-positive pregnancy test result.
Male breast enlargement and tenderness (gynecomastia), inhibited ejaculation or priapism (see Glossary)—case reports.

▷ **Adverse Effects That May Mimic Natural Diseases or Disorders**
Nervous system reactions may suggest Parkinson's disease. Liver reactions may suggest viral hepatitis. Reactions resembling systemic lupus erythematosus can occur.

Natural Diseases or Disorders That May Be Activated by This Drug
Latent epilepsy, glaucoma, diabetes mellitus, prostatism (see Glossary).

Possible Effects on Laboratory Tests
White blood cell count: decreased.
Liver function tests: increased enzymes (ALT/GPT, AST/GOT, alkaline phosphatase) or bilirubin.

CAUTION
1. Many over-the-counter medications (see Glossary) for allergies, colds and coughs contain drugs that can interact unfavorably with this drug. Ask your doctor or pharmacist for help before using any such medications.
2. Aluminum- or magnesium-containing antacids can limit absorption of this drug and reduce its effectiveness.
3. Obtain prompt evaluation of any change or disturbance of vision.

Precautions for Use
By Infants and Children: Do not use this drug in infants under 2 years of age (or less than 20 pounds) or in children of any age with symptoms suggestive of Reye's syndrome (see Glossary). Children with acute illnesses ("flu-like" infections, measles, chicken pox, etc.) are very susceptible to adverse effects when this drug is given to control nausea and vomiting.
By Those Over 60 Years of Age: Small starting doses are advisable. You may be more susceptible to drowsiness, lethargy, constipation, lowering of body temperature (hypothermia), and orthostatic hypotension (see Glossary). This drug can worsen existing prostatism (see Glossary). You may also be more susceptible to the development of Parkinson-like reactions and/or tardive dyskinesia (see discussion of these terms in Glossary). These reactions must be recognized early, because they may become unresponsive to treatment and irreversible.

▷ **Advisability of Use During Pregnancy**
Pregnancy Category: C. See Pregnancy Risk Categories at the back of this book.
Animal Studies: Cleft palate reported in mouse and rat studies.
Human Studies: Case reports of congenital problems (atrophy of a hand and amputation) with use of this medicine during the first three months (trimester) of pregnancy have been reported, but cause and effect not proven. Information from adequate studies of pregnant women is not available.
Talk to your doctor about this benefit-to-risk decision. Avoid drug during the first three months and the final month because of possible effects on the newborn infant. Limit use to small and infrequent doses.

Advisability of Use If Breast-Feeding
Presence of this drug in breast milk: Yes, in small amounts.
Stop nursing or change to a different medicine. Talk to your doctor before making any medicine changes.

Habit-Forming Potential: None, but it has been used in combination with pentazocine as a heroin substitute by some drug abusers.

Effects of Overdose: Marked drowsiness, weakness, tremor, agitation, unsteadiness, deep sleep, coma, convulsions.

Possible Effects of Long-Term Use: Tardive dyskinesia. Eye changes—opacities in cornea or lens, retinal pigmentation.

Suggested Periodic Examinations While Taking This Drug (at physician's discretion)
Complete blood cell counts, especially between the 4th and 10th weeks of treatment.

Liver function tests.

Electrocardiograms.

Complete eye examinations—eye structures and vision.

Careful inspection of the tongue for early evidence of fine, involuntary, wavelike movements that could indicate the beginning of tardive dyskinesia.

▷ **While Taking This Drug, Observe the Following**

Foods: No restrictions. Vitamin C in high doses may lower therapeutic benefits.

Herbal Medicines or Minerals: Since part of the way that ginkgo and ginseng works may be as a MAO inhibitor, the combination is NOT advisable. Eucalyptus, kava, valerian, and other herbal products, which may have toxic effects on the liver, are not advisable. Combination is also not advisable for betel nut as movement disorders have been reported with combined use of medicines from the same family. Both prochlorperazine and St. John's wort may lead to increased sun sensitivity—CAUTION IS ADVISED. Evening primrose oil may increase seizure risk if combined with medicines in this family and is not advisable.

Nutritional Support: A riboflavin (vitamin B_2) supplement should be taken with long-term use.

Beverages: No restrictions. May be taken with milk.

▷ *Alcohol:* Avoid completely. Alcohol can increase phenothiazine sedation and accentuate depressant effects on brain function and blood pressure. Phenothiazines can increase intoxicating effects of alcohol.

Tobacco Smoking: Possible reduction of drowsiness from drug. I advise everyone to quit smoking.

Marijuana Smoking: Moderate increase in drowsiness; accentuation of orthostatic hypotension; increased risk of precipitating latent psychoses, confusing the interpretation of mental status and drug responses.

▷ *Other Drugs*

Prochlorperazine may *increase* the effects of

- all atropinelike drugs and cause nervous system toxicity.
- cisapride (Propulsid), increasing risk of dangerous heart rhythms.
- gatifloxacin (Tequin), grepafloxacin (Raxar), moxifloxacin (Avelox), or sparfloxacin (Zagam), increasing risk of abnormal heartbeats.
- all sedative drugs, especially meperidine (Demerol), and cause excessive sedation.

Prochlorperazine may *decrease* the effects of

- guanethidine (Ismelin, Esimil) and reduce its effectiveness in lowering blood pressure.

Prochlorperazine *taken concurrently* with

- dofetilide (Tikosyn), increases risk of abnormal heartbeats.
- lithium (Lithobid, others) may lead to movement disorders and brain damage.
- MAO inhibitors (see Drug Classes) may result in increased risk of abnormal body movements (extrapyramidal reactions).
- medicines such as amiodarone (Cordarone), dofetilide (Tikosyn) and other medicines such as class I, IA, or III antiarrhythmics, clarithromycin, cotrimoxazole, ondansetron, ziprazidone, and others may lead to prolongation of the QTc interval and undesirable effects. Combination is not recommended.
- oral antidiabetic drugs (see Drug Classes) may blunt their therapeutic benefits.

- phenytoin (Dilantin, others) or fosphenytoin (Cerebyx) may have variable effects on phenytoin blood levels; more frequent blood levels are prudent if these drugs are combined.
- propranolol (Inderal) may cause increased effects of both drugs; monitor drug effects closely and adjust doses as necessary.
- ritonavir (Norvir) may lead to prochlorperazine toxicity.
- tramadol (Ultram) may increase seizure risk.
- zotepine (Nipolept) may increase seizure risk.

The following drugs may decrease the effects of prochlorperazine:
- antacids containing aluminum and/or magnesium.
- benztropine (Cogentin).
- trihexyphenidyl (Artane).

▷ *Driving, Hazardous Activities:* This drug can impair mental alertness, judgment, and physical coordination. Avoid hazardous activities.

Aviation Note: The use of this drug *is a disqualification* for piloting. Consult a designated Aviation Medical Examiner.

Exposure to Sun: Use caution until sensitivity has been determined. Some phenothiazines can cause photosensitivity (see Glossary).

Exposure to Heat: Use caution and avoid excessive heat as much as possible. This drug may impair the regulation of body temperature and increase the risk of heatstroke.

Exposure to Cold: Use caution and dress warmly. This drug can increase the risk of hypothermia in the elderly.

Discontinuation: After long-term use, do not stop this drug suddenly. Gradual withdrawal over 2 to 3 weeks under physician supervision is recommended.

PROPAFENONE (pro PAAF in own)

Introduced: 1998   **Class:** Antiarrhythmic (1C)   **Prescription:**
USA: Yes   **Controlled Drug:** USA: No; Canada: No   **Available as**
Generic: Yes

Brand Names: ✦Apo-Propafenone, ✦Gen-Propafenone, Rythmol, Rythmol SR

BENEFITS versus RISKS	
Possible Benefits	*Possible Risks*
EFFECTIVE TREATMENT IN SELECTED HEART RHYTHM DISORDERS BENEFICIAL IN LIFE-THREATENING VENTRICULAR ARRHYTHMIAS	NARROW TREATMENT RANGE May worsen some arrhythmias Rare liver injury, reduced white blood cell count or positive ANA

▷ **Principal Uses**

As a Single Drug Product: Uses currently included in FDA-approved labeling: (1) Helps correct abnormal heartbeats (symptomatic paroxysmal atrial fibrillation or PAF or symptomatic paroxysmal supraventricular tachycardia or PSVT) in people who do not have structural heart disease; (2) treats life-threatening ventricular arrhythmias (such as sustained ventricular tachycardia); (3) PREVENTS abnormal heartbeats arising in the ventricles (ventricular arrhythmias) that are caused (induced) by exercise.

Other (unlabeled) generally accepted uses: (1) Treats a variety of abnormal heartbeats not arising from the ventricles (such as supraventricular tachycardia, Wolff-Parkinson-White syndrome, and atrial flutter or fibrillation); (2) helps correct or prevent ventricular arrhythmias that are started (induced) by exercise.

How This Drug Works: Slows transmission of electrical impulses in the heart, restoring normal heart rate and rhythm in selected types of arrhythmia. (Class 1C agent that blocks the fast sodium current in Purkinje fibers and heart muscle and slows the rate of increase of Phase 0 of the action potential.) Because this medicine is chemically (structurally) close to propranolol (Inderal) a beta blocker, it does have some action as a beta blocker.

▷ **Widely Used Guidelines That Involve This Medicine (representative sample):** Please look at the section at the very beginning of this profile called "Class." Next, turn to Table 22 and you will find guidelines listed by the class involved!

Available Dosage Forms and Strengths
Capsules (sustained release)—225 mg, 325 mg and 425 mg
Tablets, coated—150 mg, 225 mg, 300 mg

▷ **Usual Adult Dosage Ranges:** *Arrhythmia (immediate release)*: Dosing is started with 150 mg every 8 hours (450 mg daily). Dosing can then be increased (every 3 to 4 days), as needed and tolerated to 225 mg every eight hours or 300 mg every eight hours (900 mg daily). If the heartbeat changes (QRS widens) or if there is second- or third-degree heart (atrioventricular) block, consideration should be given to lowering the dose. Testing blood levels is advised even though they have not related well to clinical effects.

Recently Started (Onset) Atrial Fibrillation: One loading dose by mouth of 600 mg often works, but intravenous treatment gets better results in the first two hours. Some clinicians have used 150 mg every 4 hours to convert this kind of atrial fibrillation to normal sinus rhythm in 48 hours (for patients who do not have cardiovascular decompensation). Sustained release for paroxysmal atrial fibrillation: Sustained release capsules in a dose of 325 mg twice daily.

Note: Actual dose and schedule must be determined for each patient individually.

Conditions Requiring Dosing Adjustments
Liver Function: The dose should be decreased by 20 to 30 percent, and blood levels should be checked more frequently.
Kidney Function: The kidneys remove only one percent of this drug. More frequent check of blood levels is prudent.

▷ **Dosing Instructions:** The immediate release tablet may be crushed and taken with food or milk to reduce stomach upset. Take at the same times each day to obtain uniform results (even blood levels). If you forget a dose: Take the missed dose as soon as you remember it, unless you are more than four hours late—if that is the case, skip the missed dose and take the next dose right on schedule. DO NOT double doses. The sustained release capsule should NOT be altered. Talk with your doctor and pharmacist if you find yourself missing doses.

Usual Duration of Use: Use on a regular schedule determines effectiveness in correcting or preventing responsive rhythm disorders. If effective, use will often be ongoing. The time it takes to reach its peak effect can vary from patient to patient and may require dosing adjustments. Long-term use requires physician supervision. Use in stopping (aborting) recent onset atrial fibrillation may produce immediate results.

Typical Treatment Goals and Measurements (Outcomes and Markers)

Abnormal Heartbeats: The general goal is to return the heart to a normal rhythm or at least to markedly reduce the occurrence of abnormal heartbeats. In life-threatening arrhythmias, the goal is to abort the abnormal beats and return the pattern to normal. Success at ongoing suppression may involve ambulatory checks of heart rate and rhythm for a day (such as in Holter monitoring). This kind of testing involves placement of adhesive-backed temporary electrodes on the skin in several positions around the heart. A small heart rate and rhythm (EKG or ECG) recording device is carried around via a shoulder strap and records what the heart is doing over 24 hours. Once the recording is made, a scanning machine reviews the record, tallies abnormal heartbeats or rhythms and gives a close and extended look at how the heart is reacting or benefiting from the medicines that the patient is taking. Repeat measurements can be made if doses are changed to check the success at keeping the heart in normal sinus rhythm.

▷ **This Drug Should Not Be Taken If**
- you have had an allergic reaction to it previously.
- your electrolytes are out of balance (talk to your doctor).
- you have second- or third-degree heart block (determined by electrocardiogram), uncorrected by a pacemaker.
- you have congestive heart failure that is not controlled.
- your bronchi are subject to spasm (bronchospasm).
- you have an excessively slow heartbeat (bradycardia).

▷ **Inform Your Physician Before Taking This Drug If**
- you had adverse reactions to other antiarrhythmic drugs.
- you have a seizure disorder.
- you have a history of heart disease of any kind, especially "heart block" or heart failure AND YOU DO NOT HAVE A PACEMAKER.
- you have impaired liver function.
- you have had an antinuclear antibody (ANA) test and the result (titer) was elevated.
- you have difficulty making sperm (spermatogenesis).
- you are prone to low blood pressure.
- you take digitalis, a potassium supplement or any diuretic drug that can cause potassium loss (ask your doctor).

Possible Side Effects (natural, expected, and unavoidable drug actions)

Dizziness (may be frequent), unpleasant taste (bitter).

▷ **Possible Adverse Effects** (unusual, unexpected, and infrequent reactions)
If any of the following develop, consult your physician promptly for guidance.

Mild Adverse Effects
Allergic reaction: skin rash.
Fatigue, sleep problems, headache, tremor—rare to infrequent.
Drug-induced fever—case report.
Cough or wheezing—case report.
Hair loss (alopecia)—rare.
Loss of appetite, nausea, vomiting, constipation, diarrhea, abdominal pain—rare to infrequent.

Serious Adverse Effects
Allergic reactions: anaphylaxis—case report.
Idiosyncratic reactions: not reported.

Peripheral neuropathy—case report.

Seizure—case report.

Drug-induced heart rhythm disorders: shortness of breath, palpitations, chest pain, swelling, ventricular fibrillation—infrequent.

Congestive heart failure—rare.

Lowered sodium and increased urination (SIADH)—case reports.

Systemic lupus erythematosus—case report.

Kidney (renal) failure—case reports.

Liver damage with jaundice (see Glossary)—case reports (may happen after 2–4 weeks or after prolonged therapy).

Low white blood cell or platelet counts: fever, sore throat, abnormal bleeding/bruising—case reports.

▷ **Possible Effects on Sexual Function:**

Decreased sperm formation—possible.

Impotence—rare.

▷ **Adverse Effects That May Mimic Natural Diseases or Disorders**

Liver toxicity may suggest viral hepatitis.

Natural Diseases or Disorders That May Be Activated by This Drug

Latent epilepsy.

Possible Effects on Laboratory Tests

Blood white cell and platelet counts: decreased.

Liver function tests: increased liver enzymes (ALT/GPT, AST/GOT)—rare.

ANA titer: possibly increasing.

CAUTION

1. Thorough evaluation of your heart function (including electrocardiograms) is necessary prior to using this drug.

2. Periodic evaluation of your heart function is needed to determine your response to this drug. Some individuals may experience worsening of their heart rhythm disorder and/or deterioration of heart function. Close monitoring of heart rate, rhythm, and overall performance is essential.

3. Dose must be adjusted carefully for each person. Do not change your dose without talking to your doctor.

4. Do not take any other antiarrhythmic drug while taking this drug unless you are directed to do so by your physician.

5. Carry a card in your purse or wallet saying that you take this drug. Tell health care providers that you take it.

6. In roughly 10% of patients and in people who also take quinidine, propafenone removal (metabolism) is slower than in other patients. Lower doses and more frequent blood level checks are prudent.

7. Removal of this drug from the body happens in a way that can become filled up (saturable biotransformation). This means that a small dose change may result in a larger than normally expected increase in blood level. If dosing is changed, a recheck of blood levels is prudent.

8. In a study called CAST (Cardiac Arrhythmia Suppression Trial), medicines similar to propafenone (Class 1C) used in patients who had a heart attack (MI) more than 6 days after the heart attack in treating non-life-threatening ventricular arrhythmias were found to actually lead to an increased risk of reversed cardiac arrest or death.

9. If an Antinuclear Antibody (ANA) titer is checked and persists or worsens, consideration must be given to stopping this medicine.

Precautions for Use

By Infants and Children: Safety and effectiveness have not been established.

By Those Over 60 Years of Age: Reduced liver function may require reduction in dose. Lower doses and slower increases (if required) in doses are prudent, and are needed in those with previous heart (myocardial) damage. Watch carefully for light-headedness, dizziness, unsteadiness, and tendency to fall. One study reported use of one 600-mg loading dose of propafenone as effective for treating atrial fibrillation that has recently started.

▷ **Advisability of Use During Pregnancy**

Pregnancy Category: C. See Pregnancy Risk Categories at the back of this book.

Animal Studies: No birth defects reported in mice, rats, or rabbits, but an increased rate of fetal resorption was found.

Human Studies: Adequate studies of pregnant women are not available.

Avoid during first 3 months. Use this drug only if clearly needed. Ask your physician for guidance.

Advisability of Use If Breast-Feeding

Presence of this drug in breast milk: Yes.

This is a benefit-to-risk decision to be discussed with your doctor.

Habit-Forming Potential: None.

Effects of Overdose: Marked drop in blood pressure, abnormal heart rhythms, slow heartbeat, seizures.

Possible Effects of Long-Term Use: Liver function tests may increase.

Suggested Periodic Examinations While Taking This Drug (at physician's discretion)

Electrocardiograms.

Complete blood cell counts.

Liver function tests.

Blood levels.

ANA titer.

▷ **While Taking This Drug, Observe the Following**

Foods: No restrictions. Ask your physician about the need for salt restriction.

Herbal Medicines or Minerals: Kola, mate, guarana, St. John's wort, ma huang, bitter orange, country mallow and yohimbe may cause additive heart rate or rhythm problems. These are not advisable if you have heart rhythm difficulties. Using St. John's wort, ma huang, ephedra (no longer on the US market for weight loss) while taking this medicine may result in unacceptable heart stimulation. Belladonna, henbane, scopolia, pheasant's eye extract or lily of the valley, or squill powdered extracts should NOT be taken if you have abnormal heart rhythms. Licorice may increase risk of abnormal heartbeats.

Beverages: Caffeine may have an effect on heart rate and may not be desirable. Talk to your doctor about caffeine. Can be taken with milk.

▷ *Alcohol:* Use caution. Alcohol can increase the blood pressure–lowering effects of this drug.

Tobacco Smoking: Nicotine may irritate the heart, reducing drug effectiveness. I advise everyone to quit smoking.

▷ *Other Drugs*

Propafenone may ***increase*** the effects of

- amitriptyline (Elavil, others) and perhaps other tricyclic antidepressants.
- antihypertensive drugs and cause excessive lowering of blood pressure.
- beta blockers (such as metoprolol or propranolol: see Drug Classes).

- clozapine (Clozaril), leading to toxicity. Downward dose adjustments and blood levels are prudent.
- cyclosporine (Sandimmune), leading to toxicity.
- quinidine (Quinaglute, various).
- theophylline (Theo-Dur, others), leading to theophylline toxicity and seizures.
- warfarin (Coumadin, others); more frequent INR tests and dose adjustments are needed.

Propafenone *taken concurrently* with

- amiodarone (Cordarone) may lead to excessive propafenone levels and toxicity, and because of possible undesirable effects on heart rhythm, combination not recommended.
- bupropion (Zyban, Wellbutrin) increases propafenone levels and can cause toxicity.
- digoxin (Lanoxin, others) increases digoxin levels and can cause toxicity.
- drugs that inhibit or are removed by CYP 2D6 (talk to your doctor) may increase propafenone effects.
- fluoxetine (Prozac) may lead to increased propafenone blood levels and toxicity if doses are not adjusted.
- medicines such as amiodarone (Cordarone), dofetilide (Tikosyn) and other medicines such as class I, IA, or III antiarrhythmics, clarithromycin, cotrimoxazole, ondansetron, ziprazidone, zolmitriptan and others may lead to prolongation of the QTc interval and undesirable effects. Combination is not recommended.
- paroxetine (Paxil) may lead to increased propafenone blood levels and toxicity if doses are not adjusted.
- quinidine (Quinaglute) may increase propafenone levels and lead to toxicity if doses are not adjusted.
- ritonavir (Norvir) and perhaps other protease inhibitors (see Drug Classes) may lead to propafenone toxicity.
- sertraline (Zoloft) may lead to propafenone toxicity.

The following drugs may *decrease* the effects of propafenone:

- carbamazepine (Tegretol).
- phenobarbital (various).
- rifampin (Rifadin, Rimactane).

▷ *Driving, Hazardous Activities:* This drug may cause weakness, dizziness, or blurred vision. Restrict activities as necessary.

Aviation Note: The use of this drug *may be a disqualification* for piloting. Consult a designated Aviation Medical Examiner.

Exposure to Sun: No restrictions.

Occurrence of Unrelated Illness: Vomiting, diarrhea, or dehydration can affect this drug's action adversely. Report such developments promptly.

Discontinuation: Should not be stopped abruptly after long-term use. Ask your doctor about slowly reducing the dose.

PROPIONIC ACID (NONSTEROIDAL ANTI-INFLAMMATORY DRUG) FAMILY

Fenoprofen   (FEN oh proh fen)   **Flurbiprofen**   (flur BI proh fen)
Ibuprofen   (common: I byu PROH fen; correct: i BYU proh fen)   **Ketoprofen**   (kee toh PROH fen)   **Naproxen**   (na PROX in)   **Oxaprozin** (OX a proh zin)

Introduced: 1976, 1977, 1974, 1973, 1974, 1992, respectively   **Class:** Analgesic, mild; NSAIDs   **Prescription:**   USA: Varies   **Controlled Drug:**   USA: No; Canada: No   **Available as Generic:**   Yes

Brand Names: *Fenoprofen*: Nalfon, *Flurbiprofen*: Ansaid, ✤Apo-Flurbiprofen, ✤Froben, ✤Froben-SR, Novo-Flurbiprofen, Ocufen, *Ibuprofen*: Aches-N-Pain, Actiprofen, Advil, Advil Migraine, ✤Amersol, ✤Apo-Ibuprofen, Arthritis Foundation Pain Reliever/Fever Reducer, Bayer Select, Children's Advil, Children's Motrin, Children's Motrin Drops (nonprescription), Children's Motrin Suspension (nonprescription), CoAdvil [CD], Dimetapp Sinus [CD], Dologesic, Dristan Sinus, Excedrin IB, Genpril, Guildprofen, Haltran, Ibu, Ibuprohm, Junior Strength Motrin Caplets (nonprescription), Medipren, Medi-Profen, Midol IB, Motrin, Motrin IB, ✤Novo-Profen, Nuprin, PediaProfen, Profen-IB, Rufen, Superior Pain Medicine, Supreme Pain Medicine, Tab-Profen, *Ketoprofen*: Actron (12.5 mg nonprescription), ✤Apo-Keto, ✤Apo-Keto E, Orudis, Orudis E-50, Orudis E-100, Orudis KT (nonprescription), Orudis SR, Oruvail, Oruvail ER, ✤Oruvail SR, ✤Rhodis, ✤Rhodis EC, ✤Rhodis EC Suppository, *Naproxen*: Aleve (220 mg nonprescription), Anaprox, Anaprox DS, ✤Apo-Naproxen, Naprelan, Naprelan Once Daily, Naprosyn, ✤Naxen, Neo-Prox, ✤Novo-Naprox, ✤Nu-Naprox, ✤Synflex, *Oxaprozin*: Daypro

Author's Note: Ibuprofen has been shown to interfere with the beneficial effects of aspirin on the heart (MI prophylaxis). At the time of this writing, the combination is NOT advisable. Talk to your doctor about the state of this data and his or her impression.

BENEFITS versus RISKS

Possible Benefits	*Possible Risks*
EFFECTIVE RELIEF OF MILD TO MODERATE PAIN AND INFLAMMATION	Gastrointestinal pain, ulceration, bleeding
EFFECTIVE RELIEF OF FEVER	Kidney damage
ADVIL MIGRAINE WORKS TO TREAT MIGRAINE HEADACHES	Fluid retention
	Bone marrow depression (except oxaprozin)
	Liver toxicity (all rare)
	Combination with ibuprofen may blunt heart protective effects of aspirin

---

▷ **Principal Uses**

As a Single Drug Product: Uses currently included in FDA-approved labeling: (1) All six agents in this class treat rheumatoid and osteoarthritis; (2) naproxen is useful in treating bursitis, gout, dysmenorrhea (ketoprofen and ibuprofen are also approved for use in primary dysmenorrhea), pain, juvenile rheumatoid arthritis, and tendonitis; (3) fenoprofen is the only agent approved to treat tennis elbow; (4) flurbiprofen ophthalmic is used to prevent intraoperative miosis; (5) Advil Migraine form treats migraine headaches.

Other (unlabeled) generally accepted uses: (1) Naproxen has been used to treat migraine and colds caused by rhinoviruses; (2) oxaprozin is useful in gout and tendonitis; (3) ketoprofen may have a role in temporal arteritis; (4) flurbiprofen has some support for therapy of periodontal disease; (5) fenoprofen has been used successfully in therapy of migraine; (6) ibuprofen treats interleukin-2 toxicity and chronic urticaria and can decrease IUD-associated bleeding; (7) all of the agents have been used for a variety of pains and fever; (8) ibuprofen has data from a study of 148 infants with patent ductus arteriosus comparing it to indomethacin. The research concluded that benefits were similar, and ibuprofen caused less decreased urine (oliguria).

How These Drugs Work: They reduce levels of prostaglandins (and related compounds), chemicals involved in inflammation and pain.

▷ **Widely Used Guidelines That Involve This Medicine (representative sample):** Please look at the section at the very beginning of this profile called "Class." Next, turn to Table 22 and you will find guidelines listed by the class involved!

Available Dosage Forms and Strengths

Fenoprofen:

Capsules — 200 mg, 300 mg, 600 mg
Tablets — 600 mg

Flurbiprofen:

Ophthalmic drops — 0.03%
Tablets — 50 mg, 100 mg

Ibuprofen:

Caplets — 200 mg
Oral suspension — 50 mg/1.25 mg, 100 mg/5 mL
Tablets — 40 mg, 200 mg, 300 mg, 400 mg, 600 mg, 800 mg
Tablets, chewable — 50 mg, 100 mg

Ketoprofen:

Capsules — 50 mg, 75 mg, 100 mg, 150 mg
Suppositories (Canada) — 100 mg
Tablets, enteric (Canada) — 50 mg
Tablets (nonprescription) — 12.5 mg

Naproxen:

Caplets — 220 mg
Naprelan Once Daily — 375 mg, 500 mg
Oral suspension — 125 mg/5 mL
Rectal suppository (Canada) — 500 mg
Tablets — 125 mg, 250 mg, 275 mg, 375 mg, 500 mg, 550 mg
Tablets, controlled-release — 375 mg, 500 mg

Oxaprozin:

Caplets — 600 mg
Tablets — 600 mg

▷ **Usual Adult Dosage Ranges:**

Fenoprofen: 300 to 600 mg three or four times daily. Daily maximum is 3,200 mg.

Flurbiprofen: 100 to 300 mg daily in two to four divided doses. The lowest effective dose should be used. Daily maximum is 300 mg.

Ibuprofen: 200 to 800 mg three or four times daily. Total daily dose should not exceed 3,200 mg.

Ketoprofen: 75 mg three times daily or 50 mg four times daily. Usual daily dose is 100 to 300 mg, divided into three or four doses. Daily maximum is 300 mg.

Naproxen: Gout—750 mg initially and then 250 mg every 8 hours until attack is relieved. Arthritis—250 mg, 375 mg or 500 mg twice daily, 12 hours apart.

The sustained-release form (Naprelan) offers an intestinal-protective drug absorption system (IPDAS) and once-daily (two tablets once a day) dosing. Menstrual pain—500 mg initially and then 250 mg every 6 to 8 hours as needed. Maximum dose for pain is 1,375 mg.

Oxaprozin: 1,200 mg as a single daily dose in the morning. Daily maximum is 1,800 mg (or 26 mg per kg of body mass for patients with normal liver and kidney function).

Author's Note: Medicines in this class with available nonprescription forms usually have lower daily maximum doses. For example, Children's Motrin is approved for nonprescription use as temporary relief of minor aches and pains or reduction of fever in children 2 years of age and older. Adverse effects are also less common and fewer in number. Less than 11 kg of body mass and under 2 years old—consult your doctor; 2 to 3 years old and 11–15.9 kg of body mass—100 mg every 6 to 8 hours. Up to four doses may be given a day. Use should NOT go on for longer than 3 days. Please look carefully at individual package labels or ask your pharmacist or doctor for dosing advice.

Note: Actual dose and dosing schedule must be determined for each patient individually.

Conditions Requiring Dosing Adjustments

Liver Function: All of these drugs are metabolized in the liver and therefore should be used with caution and consideration given to lower doses, by patients with liver compromise.

Kidney Function: These drugs share the risks common to most nonsteroidal anti-inflammatory drugs (NSAIDs). Some patients with kidney compromise are dependent on prostaglandins for kidney function. A benefit-to-risk decision must be made regarding the use of NSAIDs by these patients.

▷ **Dosing Instructions:** Take with food or milk and a full glass of water to prevent stomach irritation and remain upright (do not lie down) for 30 minutes. The tablets may be crushed and the capsules opened, except for ketoprofen tablets (should not be crushed or altered). Sustained-release forms available in other countries should NOT be altered. Be sure to use a calibrated medication spoon or a calibrated medicine dosing cup for liquid forms. If you forget a dose: Take the missed dose as soon as you remember it, unless it's nearly time for your next dose—if that is the case, skip the missed dose and take the next dose right on schedule. DO NOT double doses. Talk with your doctor if you find yourself missing doses.

Usual Duration of Use: Use on a regular schedule for 1 to 2 weeks usually determines effectiveness for some conditions. Peak oxaprozin effect may take 6 weeks in arthritis. Long-term use requires supervision and periodic physician evaluation. If you feel that you require a nonprescription form for more than occasional use, please talk to your doctor about an evaluation of the problem you are taking the nonprescription form for.

Typical Treatment Goals and Measurements (Outcomes and Markers)

Pain: Most clinicians treating pain use a device called an algometer to check your pain. This looks like a small ruler, but lets the clinician better understand your pain. The goals of treatment then relate to where the level of pain started (for example, a rating of seven on a zero to ten scale) and what the cause of the pain was. I use the PQRSTBG method (see Glossary). Pain medicines may also be used together (in combination) in order to get the best result or outcome. If your pain control is not acceptable to YOU (remember, in hospitals and outpatient settings, etc., pain control is a patient right) and if after a week of arthritis pain treatment, results are not acceptable, be sure to call your doctor—you may need a different medicine or combination.

Arthritis: Control of arthritis symptoms (pain, loss of mobility, decreased ability to accomplish activities of daily living, range of motion, etc.) is paramount in returning patient quality of life and to checking the results (beneficial outcomes) from these medicines. Clinicians use the WOMAC osteoarthritis index (see Glossary) to globally assess the health status of people living with osteoarthritis. Many arthritis management or pain centers use interdisciplinary teams (physicians from several specialties, nurses, physician's assistants, physical and occupational therapists, pharmacotherapists, psychotherapists, social workers and others) to get the best results. Laboratory measures of results for rheumatoid arthritis include decreases in chemicals released by the body (acute phase reactants) such as C-reactive protein. A more general test to roughly measure inflammation is a sed rate (erythrocyte sedimentation rate). ACR improvements in characteristic signs and symptoms of RA, such as ACR 20 are widely used.

▷ **These Drugs Should Not Be Taken If**
- you have had an allergic reaction to them previously.
- you are subject to asthma or nasal polyps caused by aspirin.
- you have a bleeding disorder or a blood cell disorder.
- flurbiprofen ophthalmic drops should NOT be used by people with herpes simplex keratitis.
- you have severe impairment of kidney function (some cases).

▷ **Inform Your Physician Before Taking These Drugs If**
- you are allergic to aspirin or other aspirin substitutes.
- you have active peptic ulcer disease or any form of gastrointestinal bleeding.
- you have a history of peptic ulcer disease or any type of bleeding disorder.
- you have impaired liver or kidney function or any active infection.
- you start to have signs and symptoms of meningitis and are taking ibuprofen (call your doctor as the medicine should be stopped and additional tests run).
- you have high blood pressure or a history of heart failure.
- you are taking acetaminophen, aspirin or other aspirin substitutes, or anticoagulants.

Possible Side Effects (natural, expected, and unavoidable drug actions)
Fluid retention (weight gain); ringing in the ears. Pink, red, purple, or rust coloration of urine (ibuprofen only).

▷ **Possible Adverse Effects** (unusual, unexpected, and infrequent reactions)
If any of the following develop, consult your physician promptly for guidance.

Mild Adverse Effects
Allergic reactions: skin rash, hives, itching.
Headache, dizziness, altered or blurred vision, ringing in the ears, depression—infrequent.
Stinging or burning of the eyes with ophthalmic flurbiprofen drops—possible.
Sleep disturbances—infrequent (oxaprozin).
Mouth sores, indigestion, nausea, vomiting, constipation, diarrhea—infrequent.
Palpitations—rare (fenoprofen).

Serious Adverse Effects

Allergic reactions: anaphylactic reaction (see Glossary), severe skin reactions—rare.

Lung inflammation (naproxen—pneumonitis)—rare.

Idiosyncratic reactions: drug-induced meningitis (aseptic meningitis) with fever and coma—rare (ibuprofen and naproxen).

Active peptic ulcer, with or without bleeding—rare with 6 months of use, infrequent after 1 year of use.

Inflammation of the colon—rare.

Porphyria—case reports (some drugs in this class).

Pancreatitis or lupus erythematosus—two case reports with naproxen.

Some medicines in this class may cause Parkinson-like symptoms in susceptible patients—case reports.

Worsening of congestive heart failure—possible.

Inflammation of the esophagus—probable if patients lie down soon after taking these medicines.

Liver damage with jaundice (see Glossary)—case reports.

Kidney damage with or without painful urination, bloody urine, reduced urine formation—possible.

Bone marrow depression (see Glossary): fatigue, sore throat, abnormal bleeding/bruising—case reports.

▷ **Possible Effects on Sexual Function:** Altered timing and pattern of menstruation (ibuprofen, ketoprofen, and naproxen) and excessive menstrual bleeding (ibuprofen and ketoprofen)—case reports.

Male breast enlargement and tenderness—rare (ibuprofen).

Naproxen may rarely inhibit ejaculation.

Ketoprofen may rarely decrease libido.

Possible Delayed Adverse Effects: Mild anemia due to "silent" blood loss from the stomach.

▷ **Adverse Effects That May Mimic Natural Diseases or Disorders**

Liver reaction may suggest viral hepatitis.

Natural Diseases or Disorders That May Be Activated by These Drugs

Peptic ulcer disease, ulcerative colitis.

Possible Effects on Laboratory Tests

Erythrocyte sedimentation rate: decreased (a desired effect).

Complete blood cell counts: decreased red cells, hemoglobin, white cells, and platelets.

Blood cholesterol or uric acid levels: increased.

Blood lithium level: increased.

Liver function tests: increased enzymes (ALT/GPT, AST/GOT, alkaline phosphatase), or bilirubin.

Kidney function tests: increased blood creatinine and urea nitrogen (BUN) levels.

Fecal occult blood test: positive.

CAUTION

1. Dose should always be limited to the smallest amount that produces reasonable improvement.

2. These drugs may hide (mask) early signs (indications) of infection. Tell your doctor if you think you are developing an infection of any kind.

3. Congestive heart failure in elderly patients may be unmasked or worsened. Risk appears to increase with use of higher doses.

4. Controversy erupted when ibuprofen was found to have the potential to interfere with the beneficial effects of aspirin. At the time of this writing the two medicines should NOT be combined. Talk to your doctor to get the latest information on this interaction.

Precautions for Use

By Infants and Children: Safety and effectiveness for some uses for those under 12 not well established. For children with fever, ibuprofen dosing is accomplished like other medicines on a weight basis. In fever in children 6 months to 12 years, the ibuprofen prescription dose is 5 mg per kg of body weight if the fever is less than 102.5, and 10 mg per kg if the temperature is 102.5 degrees or higher. The dose can be repeated every 6-8 hours, and the maximum dose is 40 mg/kg per day. Naproxen and some other medicines in this class are limited to children 12 and over for use in fighting fevers. Call your doctor if temperature continues.

By Those Over 60 Years of Age: Small doses are prudent until tolerance is determined. Watch for signs of liver or kidney toxicity, fluid retention, dizziness, confusion, impaired memory, stomach bleeding, or constipation.

▷ **Advisability of Use During Pregnancy**

Pregnancy Category: B for ibuprofen, fenoprofen, flurbiprofen, ketoprofen, and naproxen. C for oxaprozin. Ibuprofen, and fenoprofen are FDA category D if used in the final 3 months (trimester) of pregnancy. The manufacturers of ketoprofen and flurbiprofen say that both medicines should be avoided in late pregnancy. See Pregnancy Risk Categories at the back of this book.

Animal Studies: No birth defects reported in rats or rabbits.

Human Studies: Adequate studies of pregnant women are not available.

Avoid these drugs during the final 3 months. Use during the first 6 months only if clearly needed. Ask your physician for guidance.

Advisability of Use If Breast-Feeding

Presence of these drugs in breast milk: Yes or expected.

Avoid drugs or refrain from nursing for others. Ibuprofen is generally considered compatible with breast-feeding (American Academy of Pediatrics).

Habit-Forming Potential: None.

Effects of Overdose: Drowsiness, dizziness, ringing in the ears, nausea, vomiting, diarrhea, confusion, unsteadiness, stupor progressing to coma.

Possible Effects of Long-Term Use: Fluid retention.

Suggested Periodic Examinations While Taking These Drugs (at physician's discretion)

Complete blood cell counts.

Liver and kidney function tests.

Complete eye examinations if vision is altered in any way.

▷ **While Taking These Drugs, Observe the Following**

Foods: Spicy foods may add to stomach irritation potential. Please remember that herbals are regulated as foods and see below.

Herbal Medicines or Minerals: Ginseng, ginkgo, alfalfa, clove oil, feverfew, cinchona bark, white willow bark, and garlic may also change clotting, so combining those herbals with these medicines is not recommended. Eucalyptus, kava, valerian, and other herbals may have undesirable toxic effects on the liver and should be avoided while taking these medicines on an ongoing basis. Talk to your doctor BEFORE combining any medicines. NSAIDs may decrease feverfew effects. Since St. John's wort and some of these medicines may increase sensitivity to the sun, CAUTION IS ADVISED.

Hay flower, mistletoe herb, and white mustard seed carry German Commission E monograph indications for arthritis.

Beverages: No restrictions. May be taken with milk.

▷ *Alcohol:* Use with caution. The irritant action of alcohol on the stomach lining, added to the irritant action of these drugs, can increase the risk of stomach ulceration and/or bleeding.

Tobacco Smoking: No interactions expected. I advise everyone to quit smoking.

▷ *Other Drugs*

These medicines may ***increase*** the effects of

- anticoagulants (Coumadin, etc.) and increase the risk of bleeding; more frequent INR (prothrombin time or protime) tests are needed, and ongoing doses should be adjusted to the laboratory test results.
- cyclosporine (Sandimmune), leading to toxicity.
- fosphenytoin (Cerebyx) or phenytoin (Dilantin) and may lead to increased risk of antiepileptic toxicity.
- lithium (Lithobid, others), by causing toxic lithium levels.
- methotrexate (Mexate, others) and result in major methotrexate toxicity with possible anemia, hemorrhage and blood infections.
- oral hypoglycemic agents (Sulfonylureas).

These medicines may ***decrease*** the effects of

- beta blockers (see Drug Classes), such as carteolol (Cartrol).
- diuretics (see Drug Classes—Thiazides, etc.), such as hydrochlorothiazide (Esidrix) and furosemide (Lasix).

These medicines ***taken concurrently*** with the following drugs may increase the risk of bleeding; avoid these combinations if possible and closely monitor patients for bleeding (PTT or PT may not fully estimate bleeding risk):

- aspirin.
- dipyridamole (Persantine).
- eptifibatide (Integrilin).
- indomethacin (Indocin).
- ketorolac (Toradol).
- low molecular weight heparins (Lovenox, others see Drug Classes).
- sulfinpyrazone (Anturane).
- valproic acid (Depakene).
- warfarin (Coumadin).

These medicines ***taken concurrently*** with

- ACE inhibitors (see Drug Classes) can worsen kidney diseases and blunt benefits.
- alendronate (Fosamax) can worsen stomach irritation. Caution is advised.
- histamine (H2) blockers (see Drug Classes) may increase toxicity from NSAIDs.
- ofloxacin (and perhaps other fluoroquinolones; see Drug Classes) may increase risk of seizures.
- ritonavir (Norvir) may lead to toxic propionic acid NSAID levels.
- tacrine (Cognex) led to delirium in a patient taking ibuprofen.
- tacrolimus (Prograf) poses a serious risk for kidney failure. This combination is not advisable.

▷ *Driving, Hazardous Activities:* These drugs may cause drowsiness or dizziness. Restrict activities as necessary.

Aviation Note: The use of these drugs ***may be a disqualification*** for piloting. Consult a designated Aviation Medical Examiner.

Exposure to Sun: Use caution until sensitivity is determined. Ibuprofen, ketoprofen, flurbiprofen, and naproxen cause photosensitivity (see Glossary).

PROPRANOLOL (proh PRAN oh lohl)

Introduced: 1966 **Class:** Anti-anginal, antiarrhythmic, antihypertensive, antimigraine, beta blocker **Prescription:** USA: Yes **Controlled Drug:** USA: No; Canada: No **Available as Generic:** Yes

Brand Names: ❧Apo-Propranolol, Betachron, ❧Detensol, Inderal, Inderal-LA, Inderide [CD], Inderide LA [CD], Innopran XL, Ipran, ❧Novo-Pranol, ❧PMS Propranolol

---

BENEFITS versus RISKS

Possible Benefits	*Possible Risks*
EFFECTIVE, WELL-TOLERATED AS ANTIANGINAL DRUG EFFORT-INDUCED ANGINA; ANTIARRHYTHMIC DRUG IN CERTAIN HEART RHYTHM DISORDERS; ANTIHYPERTENSIVE DRUG IN MILD TO MODERATE HYPERTENSION	Worsening of angina in coronary heart disease (if drug is abruptly withdrawn)
	Masking of low blood sugar (hypoglycemia) in drug-treated diabetes
PREVENTION OF MIGRAINE HEADACHES	Provocation of asthma (in asthmatics)
REDUCES DEATH AND LOSS OF FUNCTION AFTER A HEART ATTACK	Depression
EASES ESSENTIAL TREMOR IN ADULTS (FAMILIAL)	Blood cell disorders: low white cell and platelet counts
Effective adjunct in the management of pheochromocytoma	

▷ **Principal Uses**

    As a Single Drug Product: Uses currently included in FDA-approved labeling: (1) Treats several cardiovascular disorders: classical effort-induced angina, certain types of heart rhythm disturbance and high blood pressure; (2) also helps prevent repeat heart attacks (myocardial infarction); (3) reduces frequency and severity of migraine headaches; (4) decreases tremors in essential and action tremor.

    Other (unlabeled) generally accepted uses: (1) Helps control physical signs of anxiety and nervous tension (as in stage fright); (2) helps control familial tremors and symptoms seen with markedly overactive thyroid function (thyrotoxicosis); (3) decreases abnormal abdominal fluid accumulation (ascites) in people with cirrhosis of the liver; (4) may have a role in combination therapy with metronidazole in resistant Giardia infections; (5) helps control headaches caused by cyclosporine (Sandimmune); (6) may be useful in certain kinds of pain, especially after amputations; (7) can help control panic attacks; (8) helps fight symptoms in narcotic withdrawal cases.

    As a Combination Drug Product [CD]: This drug is available in combination with hydrochlorothiazide for the treatment of hypertension. This combination product includes two drugs with different mechanisms of action; it is intended to provide greater effectiveness and convenience for long-term use.

How This Drug Works: Blocks certain actions of the sympathetic nervous system:
- reducing rate and contraction force of the heart, lowering the ejection pressure of the blood leaving the heart and reducing the oxygen requirement for heart function.
- reduces degree of contraction of blood vessel walls, lowering blood pressure.
- prolongs conduction time of nerve impulses through the heart, helping manage certain heart rhythm disorders.

▷ **Widely Used Guidelines That Involve This Medicine (representative sample):** Please look at the section at the very beginning of this profile called "Class." Next, turn to Table 22 and you will find guidelines listed by the class involved!

Available Dosage Forms and Strengths

Capsules, nighttime, prolonged-action — 80 mg, 120 mg
Capsules, prolonged-action — 60 mg, 80 mg, 120 mg, 160 mg
Concentrate — 80 mg/mL
Injection — 1 mg/mL
Oral solution — 4 mg/mL, 8 mg/mL
Tablets — 10 mg, 20 mg, 40 mg, 60 mg, 80 mg, 90 mg, 120 mg

▷ **Usual Adult Dosage Ranges:**

Anti-anginal: Initially 20 mg three or four times a day; increase dose gradually based on patient response (slowly) as needed and tolerated. The total daily dose should not exceed 320 mg. Long-acting forms are started at 80-160 mg once a day.

Antiarrhythmic: 10 to 30 mg three or four times a day as needed and tolerated.

Antihypertensive: Initially 40 mg twice a day; increase dose gradually as needed and tolerated. The total daily dose should not exceed 640 mg. The sustained-release form is started at 80 mg as single drug therapy or as combination treatment with a diuretic. Doses are slowly increased because several days to several weeks may be needed to see peak benefit from any given dose. The Inderide LA form is used after patient needs are determined individually, but is given in a starting dose of one capsule daily. The Innopran XL form is specifically formulated to be taken at bedtime (roughly 10 P.M.). The usual starting dose is 80 mg. Some patients may require 120 mg daily.

Essential Tremor: Dosing is usually started at 40 mg twice a day. Dosing is increased as needed and tolerated to 60 to 320 mg a day. Many patients respond to 120 mg a day.

Migraine Headache Prevention: Initially 20 mg four times a day; increase dose gradually as needed and tolerated. The total daily dose should not exceed 480 mg. Long-acting formulations offer the advantage of once-daily dosing.

Note: Actual dose and schedule must be determined for each patient individually.

Conditions Requiring Dosing Adjustments

Liver Function: Used with caution by patients with liver disease. In general, lower starting doses and slower dose increases are indicated.

Kidney Function: This drug should be used with caution by people with combined kidney and liver compromise. Dose adjustments are not needed for people with compromised kidneys.

▷ **Dosing Instructions:** This drug is preferably taken 1 hour before eating to max-imize absorption. The regular-release tablets may be crushed; to prevent harmless numbing effect, mix with soft food and swallow promptly. The prolonged-action (extended-release) forms should be swallowed whole (do NOT crush or chew). The Innopran XL form is specifically made as a chronotherapeutic form to be taken at night. Do not stop any form of this drug abruptly. If you forget a dose: Take the missed dose as soon as you remember it, unless it's WITHIN 8 hours of your next dose for an extended-release form or if your next dose is DUE in 4 hours for the immediate-release forms—if that is the case, skip the missed dose and take the next dose right on schedule. DO NOT double doses. Talk with your doctor and phar-macist if you find yourself missing doses. There are some pager-based and phone-based and other reminder systems for medicines that can be of great help.

Usual Duration of Use: Use on a regular schedule for 10 to 14 days usually determines effectiveness in preventing angina, controlling heart rhythm disorders and lowering blood pressure. Peak benefits may take as long as 6 to 8 weeks. Long-term use is determined by your symptoms over time and response to the overall treatment program (weight reduction, salt restric-tion, smoking cessation, etc.). See your physician on a regular basis.

Typical Treatment Goals and Measurements (Outcomes and Markers)

Blood Pressure: Guidelines (JNC VII) define normal blood pressure (BP) as **less than** 120/80 and **pre-hypertension** as 120/80 to 139/89. This new range is intended to help doctors encourage lifestyle changes (or in the case of people with a risk factor for high blood pressure, start treatment) much earlier—so that damage to blood vessels, heart, kidneys, sexual potency, or eyes might be minimized or avoided altogether. Stage 1 hypertension is 140/90 to 159/99 and stage 2 hypertension equal to or greater than: 160/100 mm Hg. These guidelines also recommend that clinicians work with their patients to agree on the goals and a plan of treatment. The first-ever guidelines for blood pressure (hypertension) in African Americans recommends that MOST black patients be started on TWO antihypertensive medicines with the goal of lowering blood pressure to 130/80 for those with high risk for heart and blood vessel disease or with diabetes. The American Diabetes Association also recommends 130/80 as the target for diabetics and less than 125/75 for those who spill more than one gram of protein into their urine. Most clinicians try to achieve a BP that confers the best balance of lower cardiovascular risk and avoids the problem of too low a blood pres-sure. Blood pressure duration is generally increased with beneficial restric-tion of sodium. If goals are not met, it is not unusual to intensify doses or add on medicines.

Abnormal Heartbeats: The general goal is to return the heart to a normal rhythm or at least to markedly reduce the occurrence of abnormal heartbeats. In life-threatening arrhythmias, the goal is to abort the abnormal beats and return the pattern to normal. Success at ongoing suppression may involve ambulatory checks of heart rate and rhythm for a day (such as in Holter monitoring). This kind of testing involves placement of adhesive-backed temporary electrodes on the skin in several positions around the heart. A small heart rate and rhythm (EKG or ECG) recording device is carried around via a shoulder strap and records what the heart is doing over 24 hours. Once the recording is made, a scanning machine reviews the record, tallies abnormal heartbeats or rhythms and gives a close and extended look at how the heart is reacting or benefiting from the medicines that the patient is taking. Repeat measurements can be made if doses are changed to check the success at keeping the heart in normal sinus rhythm.

Possible Advantage of This Drug

Has a clear benefit in reducing the chance of a second heart attack once a first heart attack has been diagnosed. Data from one large research project showed that early morning blood pressure surges are an independent risk factor for strokes. The Innopran XL form may be the ideal (optimal) dosage form to address this phenomenon.

▷ **This Drug Should Not Be Taken If**
- you have bronchial asthma.
- you have had an allergic reaction to it previously.
- you have Prinzmetal's variant angina (coronary artery spasm).
- you have heart failure (overt).
- you have Raynaud's phenomenon.
- you have an abnormally slow heart rate (bradycardia) or a serious form of heart block (second or third degree AV block).
- you are taking, or have taken within the past 14 days, any monoamine oxidase (MAO) type A inhibitor (see Drug Classes).

▷ **Inform Your Physician Before Taking This Drug If**
- you had an adverse reaction to a beta blocker (see Drug Classes).
- you have a history of serious heart disease.
- you have a history of hay fever (allergic rhinitis), asthma, chronic bronchitis or emphysema.
- you have a history of overactive thyroid function (hyperthyroidism).
- you have a history of low blood sugar (hypoglycemia).
- you have impaired liver or kidney function.
- you are allergic to bee stings.
- you have diabetes or myasthenia gravis.
- you take digitalis, quinidine or reserpine or any calcium-channel-blocker drug (see Drug Classes).
- you plan to have surgery under general anesthesia in the near future.

Possible Side Effects (natural, expected, and unavoidable drug actions)

Lethargy and fatigability, cold extremities, slow heart rate, light-headedness in upright position (see orthostatic hypotension in Glossary). Increased bowel movements.

▷ **Possible Adverse Effects** (unusual, unexpected, and infrequent reactions)

If any of the following develop, consult your physician promptly for guidance.

Mild Adverse Effects

Allergic reactions: skin rash, temporary loss of hair, drug fever (see Glossary).
Joint pain—case reports.
Headache, dizziness, insomnia, vivid dreams—infrequent.
Decreased tear production, hyperemia of the conjunctiva—rare.
Indigestion, taste disorder, nausea, vomiting, diarrhea—infrequent.
Weight gain—possible.

Serious Adverse Effects

Allergic reactions: anaphylaxis. Reactions may be exaggerated if a patient is taking this medicine and is exposed to the allergen. For example, epinephrine use can result in epinephrine resistance and severe increases in blood pressure and a reactionary (reflex) slowing of the heart rate.

Idiosyncratic reactions: acute behavioral disturbances (agitation, disorientation, confusion, hallucinations, amnesia)—case reports.

Paradoxical hypertension—case reports.

Mental depression, anxiety—case reports and dose-related.

Chest pain, shortness of breath, precipitation of congestive heart failure—possible.

Peripheral neuropathy or hyperthyroidism—rare.

Drug-induced systemic lupus erythematosus, myasthenia gravis or porphyria—case reports.

Kidney problems (interstitial nephritis)—rare.

Induction of bronchial asthma—in asthmatics.

May precipitate problems walking (intermittent claudication)—possible. May be prudent to check for hidden Peripheral Artery Disease (PAD) by checking ankle brachial index (ABI). ABI check (see Glossary) can help find PAD early, and avoid claudication that may result if this medication is taken by someone who has PAD but does not know it.

Blood cell disorders: abnormally low white blood cell or platelet counts—case reports.

Carpal tunnel syndrome—case reports.

▷ **Possible Effects on Sexual Function:** Decreased libido; impaired erection; impotence—infrequent (has the highest incidence of libido reduction and erectile impairment of all beta-blocker drugs).

Male infertility (inhibited sperm motility); Peyronie's disease (see Glossary)—possible.

▷ **Adverse Effects That May Mimic Natural Diseases or Disorders**

Reduced blood flow to extremities may resemble Raynaud's phenomenon (see Glossary).

Natural Diseases or Disorders That May Be Activated by This Drug

Prinzmetal's variant angina, Raynaud's phenomenon, intermittent claudication, myasthenia gravis (questionable).

Possible Effects on Laboratory Tests

White blood cell count: occasionally decreased.

Blood platelet count: increased or decreased.

Bleeding time: increased.

Blood total cholesterol, triglycerides or VLDL level: no effect in some; increased in others.

Blood HDL cholesterol level: no effect in some; decreased in others.

Blood LDL cholesterol level: no effect in some; increased and decreased in others.

Blood glucose level: no effect in some; increased or decreased in others (hypoglycemia more likely in type 1 diabetics).

Blood thyroid hormone levels: T3—no effect in some, decreased in others; T4—increased; free T4—increased.

Blood uric acid level: no effect in some; increased in others.

Liver function tests: increased liver enzymes (ALT/GPT, AST/GOT, and alkaline phosphatase); effects probably not due to liver damage.

CAUTION

1. ***Do not stop this drug suddenly*** without the knowledge and help of your doctor. Carry a card in your purse or wallet that says you are taking this drug.

2. Ask your physician or pharmacist before using nasal decongestants, which are usually present in over-the-counter cold preparations and nose

drops. These can cause sudden increases in blood pressure when taken concurrently with beta-blocker drugs.
3. Report the development of any tendency to emotional depression.

Precautions for Use
By Infants and Children: Safety and effectiveness for those less than 12 years of age are not established, but if this drug is used, watch for low blood sugar (hypoglycemia) during periods of reduced food intake.
By Those Over 60 Years of Age: Unacceptably high blood pressure should be reduced without creating the risks associated with excessively low blood pressure. Therapy is started with small doses and blood pressure checked frequently. Sudden, rapid, and excessive reduction of blood pressure can predispose to stroke or heart attack. Observe for dizziness, unsteadiness, tendency to fall, confusion, hallucinations, depression, or urinary frequency.

▷ **Advisability of Use During Pregnancy**
Pregnancy Category: C. See Pregnancy Risk Categories at the back of this book.
Animal Studies: No significant increase in birth defects due to this drug. Some toxic effects on embryo reported.
Human Studies: Adequate studies of pregnant women are not available.
Avoid use of drug during the first 3 months if possible. Ask your physician for guidance.

Advisability of Use If Breast-Feeding
Presence of this drug in breast milk: Yes.
Monitor nursing infant closely, and discontinue drug or nursing if adverse effects develop.

Habit-Forming Potential: None.

Effects of Overdose: Weakness, slow pulse, low blood pressure, fainting, cold and sweaty skin, congestive heart failure, possible coma, and convulsions.

Possible Effects of Long-Term Use: Reduced heart reserve and eventual heart failure in susceptible patients with advanced heart disease.

Suggested Periodic Examinations While Taking This Drug (at physician's discretion)
Complete blood cell counts.
Measurements of blood pressure.
Evaluation of heart function.
Liver function tests.
ABI check for Peripheral Artery Disease (PAD).

▷ **While Taking This Drug, Observe the Following**
Foods: Avoid excessive salt intake. Excessive fat intake can worsen existing cardiovascular disease. Talk to your doctor about a sensible diet. Some of the therapeutic lifestyle changes (Table 20) apply here.
Herbal Medicines or Minerals: Ginseng, hawthorn, saw palmetto, ma huang, bitter orange, country mallow, goldenseal, yohimbe, and licorice may also cause increased blood pressure. Dong quai may block the removal of this medicine from the body leading to toxic effects with "normal" doses. St. John's wort may increase removal of this medicine from the body leading to loss of benefits despite appropriate doses. Calcium and garlic may help lower blood pressure. Indian snakeroot has a German Commission E monograph indication for hypertension—talk to your doctor. Eleuthero root and ephedra–ma huang (no longer on the US market) should be avoided by people living with hypertension. Ginger, vanadium, and nettle

may also change blood sugar. Talk to your doctor and pharmacist BEFORE combining any herbals with this drug.

Beverages: No restrictions. May be taken with milk.

▷ *Alcohol:* Use with caution. Alcohol may exaggerate this drug's ability to lower blood pressure and may increase its mild sedative effect.

Tobacco Smoking: Nicotine may reduce this drug's effectiveness in treating angina, heart rhythm disorders, and high blood pressure. Smoking increases the rate of elimination of this drug. I advise everyone to quit smoking.

▷ *Other Drugs*

Propranolol may *increase* the effects of

• other antihypertensive drugs and cause excessive lowering of blood pressure; dose adjustments may be necessary.
• lidocaine (Xylocaine, etc.).
• quinidine (Quinaglute). Careful patient monitoring for heart failure, excessively low blood pressure, and very slow heart rate is required.
• reserpine (Ser-Ap-Es, etc.) and cause sedation, depression, slowing of the heart rate, and lowering of blood pressure.
• rizatriptan (Maxalt); a 5-mg starting dose and a maximum of 15 mg of rizatriptan should be used if these medicines are combined.
• verapamil (Calan, Isoptin) and cause excessive depression of heart function; monitor this combination closely.
• warfarin (Coumadin) and increase bleeding risk; more frequent INR (prothrombin time or protime) testing is needed. Warfarin dosing should be adjusted to laboratory results.

Propranolol may *decrease* the effects of

• albuterol (Proventil).
• theophyllines (Aminophyllin, Theo-Dur, etc.) and reduce their antiasthmatic effectiveness and blunt the benefits of propranolol.

Propranolol *taken concurrently* with

• amiodarone (Cordarone) may result in abnormal heart rhythms and low pulse—these agents should not be combined.
• clonidine (Catapres) requires close monitoring for rebound high blood pressure if clonidine is withdrawn while propranolol is still being taken.
• cocaine may lead to heart attack.
• colestipol (Colestid) may decrease propranolol benefits.
• digoxin (Lanoxin) can result in severe slowing of the heart (bradycardia).
• epinephrine (Adrenalin, etc.) may cause marked rise in blood pressure and slowing of the heart rate.
• ergot derivatives (see Drug Classes) may lead to excessive blood vessel constriction and cold extremities (peripheral ischemia).
• fluoxetine (Prozac) may increase the risk of slow heartbeat and sedation.
• fluvoxamine (Luvox) may increase the risk of slow heartbeat and sedation.
• insulin requires close monitoring to avoid undetected hypoglycemia (see Glossary).
• methyldopa (various) can lead to an excessive blood pressure increase during stress.
• nefazodone (Serzone) may decrease propranolol benefits and lead to nefazodone toxicity.
• oral antidiabetic drugs (see Drug Classes) and cause slow recovery from any low blood sugar that may occur.
• quinidine (Quinaglute) can increase adverse effects without increased therapeutic benefits.

- sertraline (Zoloft) may lead to sudden chest pain.
- venlafaxine (Effexor) may result in increased risk of propranolol toxicity.
- X-ray contrast media such as diatrizoate results in up to an eightfold increase in risk of severe allergic (anaphylactic) drug reactions.
- zolmitriptan (Zomig) or rizatriptan (Maxalt) may increase risk of rizatriptan or zolmitriptan adverse effects.
- zotepine (Nipolept) may increase risk of toxicity from both drugs.

The following drugs may *increase* the effects of propranolol:
- chlorpromazine (Thorazine, etc.)—may also lead to seizures. Close patient follow-up is required.
- cimetidine (Tagamet).
- ciprofloxacin (Cipro).
- diltiazem (Cardizem).
- disopyramide (Norpace).
- furosemide or other diuretics.
- methimazole (Tapazole).
- metoclopramide (Reglan) (conventional immediate-release forms of propranolol).
- nicardipine (Cardene).
- propafenone (Rythmol) especially if doses of 150 mg a day or more of propafenone are used.
- propoxyphene (various).
- propylthiouracil (Propacil).
- ritonavir (Norvir) and perhaps other protease inhibitors (see Drug Classes).
- zileuton (Zyflo).

The following drugs may *decrease* the effects of propranolol:
- antacids.
- barbiturates (phenobarbital, etc.).
- indomethacin (Indocin) and possibly other "aspirin substitutes," or NSAIDs—may impair propranolol's antihypertensive effect.
- rifampin (Rifadin, Rimactane).
- sertraline (Zoloft) may increase risk of chest pain.
- simvastatin (Zocor) by decreasing the peak blood concentration.

▷ *Driving, Hazardous Activities:* Use caution until the full extent of drowsiness, lethargy, and blood pressure change have been determined.

Aviation Note: The use of this drug *may be a disqualification* for piloting. Consult a designated Aviation Medical Examiner.

Exposure to Sun: No restrictions.

Exposure to Heat: Caution is advised. Hot environments can lower blood pressure and exaggerate the effects of this drug.

Exposure to Cold: Caution is advised. Cold environments can enhance the circulatory deficiency in the extremities that may occur with this drug. The elderly should take precautions to prevent hypothermia (see Glossary).

Heavy Exercise or Exertion: It is advisable to avoid exertion that produces light-headedness, excessive fatigue, or muscle cramping. The use of this drug may intensify the hypertensive response to isometric exercise.

Occurrence of Unrelated Illness: Fever can lower blood pressure and require adjustment of dose. Nausea or vomiting may interrupt the regular dose schedule. Ask your physician for guidance.

Discontinuation: Best to avoid sudden stopping of this drug, especially in coronary artery disease. If possible, a gradual reduction of dose over a period of 2 to 3 weeks is recommended. Ask your physician for specific guidance.

PROTEASE INHIBITOR FAMILY

Atazanavir   (Aht ah zan ah veer),   **Lopinavir and Ritonavir**   (Loh PIN a veer and ri TOHN a veer)   **Amprenavir**   (am PREN a veer)   **Indinavir** (in DIN a veer)   **Nelfinavir**   (nel FIN a veer)   **Ritonavir**   (ri TOHN a veer)   **Saquinavir**   (sa KWIN a veer) **Tenofovir**   (ten OH fo Veer) **Investigational: Mozenavir and Tipranavir**

Introduced: 2003, 2000, 1999, 1996, 1997, 1996, 1995, and 2001, respectively **Class:**   Protease inhibitor, antiviral, anti-AIDS   **Prescription:**   USA: Yes **Controlled Drug:**   USA: No; Canada: Yes   **Available as Generic:**   USA: No; Canada: No

Author's Note: Information on atazanavir will be broadened as additional information becomes available.

Brand Names: *Atazanavir:* Reyataz, *Lopinavir and Ritonavir*: Kaletra, *Amprenavir*: Agenerase, *Indinavir*: Crixivan, *Nelfinavir*: Viracept, *Ritonavir*: Kaletra [CD], Norvir, *Saquinavir*: Fortovase, Invirase, *Tenofovir*: Viread

---

BENEFITS versus RISKS

Possible Benefits	*Possible Risks*
INCREASED CD4 COUNTS	SERIOUS CHANGES IN INSULIN
DECREASED OPPORTUNISTIC	LEVELS TO KETOACIDOSIS
INFECTIONS	SERIOUS INCREASES IN
EFFECTIVE COMBINATION	CHOLESTEROL
THERAPY OF HIV	Increased liver function tests (not
MAY DECREASE HIV TO	reported for amprenavir)
UNDETECTABLE LEVELS WITH	Kidney stones (indinavir)
EARLY THERAPY	May have SERIOUS drug interactions
ATAZANAVIR OFFERS ONCE DAILY	(see below)
DOSING	

▷ **Principal Uses**

As a Single Drug Product: Uses currently included in FDA-approved labeling: Treatment of HIV infection when antiretroviral therapy is indicated, in combination with other antiretroviral agents.

Author's Note: Combination therapy has become a standard of care. NIAID antiretroviral therapy guidelines take into account how easily HIV therapy can fit into a patient's life. The NIH AIDS information site at *WWW.AIDSINFO.NIH.GOV* is excellent. Adherence or taking medicines for HIV exactly on time and in the right amount is ABSOLUTELY CRITICAL to getting the best possible results or outcomes. Most experts recommend supervision of treatment decisions by an infectious disease specialist. Structured therapy interruptions (STI) or structured interruptions of therapy (SIT) are controversial and can't be recommended.

Other (unlabeled) generally accepted uses: Used in making HIV infection undetectable with combination therapy.

As a Combination Drug Product [CD]: Ritonavir is available combined with lopinavir (Kaletra). This combination works to use the blood level–sustaining role of ritonavir and the mechanism of action of lopinavir. While we usually think of drug interactions as undesirable, low-dose ritonavir in this combination inhibits the cytochrome P450 3A4 leading to increased and sustained lopinavir blood levels.

How These Drugs Work: They inhibit HIV reproduction (replication) by inhibiting an HIV enzyme (protease), which blocks the ability of the virus to make mature, infectious virus particles.

▷ **Widely Used Guidelines That Involve This Medicine (representative sample):** Please look at the section at the very beginning of this profile called "Class." Next, turn to Table 22 and you will find guidelines listed by the class involved!

Available Dosage Forms and Strengths
Amprenavir:
> Capsules — 50 mg, 150 mg
> Oral solution — 15 mg/mL

Indinavir:
> Capsules — 200 mg, 400 mg

Nelfinavir:
> Oral powder — 50 mg/g
> Tablet — 250 mg

Ritonavir:
> Capsule — 100 mg
> Oral solution — 80 mg/mL
> Soft gel capsule — 100 mg

Ritonavir/lopinavir (Kaletra):
> Capsule — 33.3 mg ritonavir and 133.3 mg lopinavir
> Oral solution — 20 mg/mL ritonavir and 80 mg/mL lopinavir

Saquinavir:
> Gelcap (Fortovase) — 200 mg
> Gelcap (Invirase) — 200 mg

Author's Note: This profile gives Fortovase data.

▷ **Recommended Dose Ranges** (Actual dose and schedule must be determined for each patient individually.)

18 to 60 Years of Age:
Amprenavir: 1,200 mg twice a day (in combination with other antiretrovirals).
Indinavir: 800 mg by mouth every 8 hours.
Nelfinavir: 750 mg every 8 hours.
Ritonavir: In order to help minimize adverse effects, ritonavir is started at 300 mg twice daily and then is increased by 100 mg twice daily at two- to three-day intervals. The desired "goal dose" is 600 mg twice daily. If ritonavir is taken with saquinavir, dose is reduced to 400 mg twice daily.
Ritonavir/lopinavir: Three capsules or 5 mL of the oral solution twice a day with food.
Saquinavir: 1,200 mg three times daily.

Over 65 Years of Age: These drugs have not been specifically studied in those over 65.

Conditions Requiring Dosing Adjustments
Liver Function:
Amprenavir: People with impaired liver function (Child-Pugh score of 5–8) require dosing adjustments. Those with this degree of compromise are given 450 mg twice daily and should be closely followed for possible adverse effects.
Indinavir: The dose should be decreased to 600 mg by mouth every 8 hours in mild to moderate liver failure.

Nelfinavir, ritonavir and saquinavir: Have not been studied in liver disease, but caution is advised as much of these drugs are removed by the liver.

Kidney Function: Amprenavir, indinavir, nelfinavir, ritonavir, and saquinavir: Dosing changes are not thought to be needed.

▷ **Dosing Instructions:** Indinavir is best taken on an empty stomach, but may be taken with a light snack, such as dry toast with jelly, apple juice or coffee. Nelfinavir, ritonavir and saquinavir should be taken with a meal or light snack. Ritonavir oral solution SHOULD NOT be refrigerated and should be shaken well BEFORE you take your dose. Amprenavir can be taken with or without food but SHOULD NOT be taken with a high-fat meal. IT IS CRITICAL THAT PROTEASE INHIBITOR DOSES NOT BE MISSED, as resistance to the medicine may develop. Since reports of altered blood sugar have been made, knowledge of signs and symptoms of high blood sugar or ketoacidosis and periodic checks of blood sugar appear prudent. If you forget a dose: Take the missed dose as soon as you remember it, unless it's nearly time for your next dose—if that is the case, skip the missed dose and take the next dose right on schedule. DO NOT double doses. Talk with your doctor if you find yourself missing doses. There are several excellent timers and even beeper-based systems to help you remember your medicine.

Usual Duration of Use: Use on a regular schedule for several months usually determines effectiveness in lowering the viral burden. The lowest level of viral burden, the 12-week level of viral burden, and how consistently you take these medicines (adherence) are key factors in long-term results. Long-term use (months to years) requires periodic physician evaluation of response (viral burden and CD4).

Typical Treatment Goals and Measurements (Outcomes and Markers)

HIV: Goals for HIV treatment presently are maximum suppression of viral replication, maximum lowering of the amount of virus in your body (viral load or burden), and maximum patient survival. Markers of successful therapy include undetectable viral load, increased CD4 cells, absence of indicator or opportunistic infections (OIs), and in the case of the HIV-positive patient, failure of the infection to progress to AIDS. If goals are not achieved in the time your doctor has set, typical strategies include intensification as well as phenotypic resistance testing of the virus itself. If goals are achieved and the viral load later rebounds despite excellent compliance, medication change (salvage therapy) is indicated.

Possible Advantages of These Drugs

These medicines are part of combination regimens (termed cocktails by television news) that can lower the amount of HIV in the body to nondetectable levels in many patients. Resistance to these medicines still occurs in a variety of ways. Amprenavir appeared to have a novel resistance pattern (codon 50V mutation that confers resistance), however, overlapping secondary resistance locations have become problematic. Newer dosing strategies and even the once-a-day protease inhibitor (see Reyataz or atazanavir) has been approved. Regardless of the patient, it is not unusual for HIV treatment to have to be changed. PI-containing regimens tend to offer reasonably durable virus suppression. The newest PI, **atazanavir (Reyataz),** is also the first once-a-day protease inhibitor—something that I believe will greatly improve how well patients take this medicine (lower pill burden than the other available PIs).

▷ **These Drugs Should Not Be Taken If**
- you had an allergic reaction to any dose form.
- you are taking cisapride, ergotamine, or triazolam (see Other Drugs section).

▷ **Inform Your Physician Before Taking These Drugs If**
- you have diabetes or a history of blood sugar regulation problems.
- you are taking amprenavir and develop a rash.
- you are allergic to sulfonamide-type medicines (amprenavir).
- you have elevated cholesterol or lipids.
- you have had kidney stones previously (indinavir especially).
- you have kidney or liver compromise.
- you have phenylketonuria (nelfinavir powder has 11.2 mg of phenylalanine in each gram).
- you are taking one of the medicines that interacts with a protease inhibitor and have not had a blood level check.
- you have had adverse reactions to other protease inhibitors.
- you are unsure how much to take or how often to take them.

Possible Side Effects (natural, expected, and unavoidable drug actions)
Rare kidney stones (indinavir). Increased liver function tests.

▷ **Possible Adverse Effects** (unusual, unexpected, and infrequent reactions)
If any of the following develop, consult your physician promptly for guidance.

Mild Adverse Effects
Allergic reaction: skin rash.
Headache (frequent with amprenavir) or dizziness—rare to infrequent.
Weakness—infrequent.
Toenail changes (ingrown)—possible.
Blurred vision—rare.
Chills, fever, or sweating—rare to infrequent.
Nausea and vomiting or abdominal pain—infrequent to frequent.
Palpitations—rare.
Joint pain—rare.
Tingling around the mouth (paresthesias)—frequent for ritonavir and agenerase.
Lipodystrophy—possible.
Author's Note: Current controversy as to possible lipid changes (lipodystrophy or LD) from protease inhibitors and/or nucleoside reverse transcriptase inhibitors involves presence of mild changes versus moderate to severe problems. The HOPS data found that risk of LD increases with increasing time on antiretrovirals and that LD increases with an increasing number of nondrug factors (age 40 or older, HIV infection 7 or more years, AIDS 2 or more years, hemophiliacs, nadir CD4 count less than 100 or less than 15 and time since nadir 3 or more years).
Diarrhea—infrequent to frequent (frequent with nelfinavir).

Serious Adverse Effects
Allergic reactions: life-threatening rash (Stevens-Johnson syndrome)—rare for amprenavir.
Anemia or spleen disorder—rare (indinavir, ritonavir, and saquinavir).
Hemolytic anemia—case report for agenerase.
Kidney stones—infrequent (indinavir).
Changes in insulin levels (increased blood sugar [hyperglycemia]) or ketoacidosis—many case reports for the protease inhibitors.

Increased cholesterol—many case reports.

Fat redistribution (lipodystrophy)—possible (starts from 4–61 weeks and greatest risk appears to be with indinavir).

Increased risk of blood clots (thrombosis)—possible (indinavir only).

Increased bleeding risk in people with hemophilia (nelfinavir).

▷ **Possible Effects on Sexual Function:** Rare reports of premenstrual syndrome in some early studies with indinavir. Four cases of extended and excessive menstruation (hypermenorrhea) have been reported with ritonavir.

Possible Delayed Adverse Effects: Kidney stones (indinavir). Blood sugar problems (low blood sugar or ketoacidosis) or cholesterol changes. Fat redistribution. Ingrown toenails.

▷ **Adverse Effects That May Mimic Natural Diseases or Disorders**

Increased liver function tests may mimic hepatitis (not reported for amprenavir). Changes in insulin levels may mimic diabetes.

Possible Effects on Laboratory Tests

Liver function tests: increased (not reported for amprenavir).
Complete blood counts: decreased red blood cells and hematocrit.
Insulin levels: lowered.
Blood sugar (glucose): increased.
Cholesterol—may be significantly increased.

CAUTION

1. Serious increases in cholesterol (lipids) have been reported.
2. Serious increases in blood sugar have been reported in many case reports to date for protease inhibitors. This effect has been seen in early reports on average after 76 days of therapy, but has also been reported after as little as 4 days of treatment with protease inhibitors.
3. Make certain you know high blood sugar (hyperglycemia) and ketoacidosis signs and symptoms if you are taking this medicine. Blood sugar problems have been reported for protease inhibitors.
4. These medicines may decrease the amount of virus in your body, but the virus can still be spread to others through sexual contact or blood contamination.
5. Promptly report flank pain or blood in the urine; this could indicate a kidney stone.
6. Periodic measures of viral load and CD4 are critical to make certain that therapy is still working.
7. IT IS CRITICAL to take these medicines exactly as directed to get the best results.
8. Ritonavir (Norvir) has MANY drug interactions. Ask your pharmacist to check the most current list. Amprenavir also has some serious drug interactions. Doses of the protease inhibitor may need to be increased or decreased.
9. Fat redistribution should be reported to your doctor (one patient responded to ketoconazole treatment).
10. Amprenavir contains a significant amount of vitamin E. DO NOT USE vitamin E supplements while taking this medicine.

Precautions for Use

By Infants and Children:

Amprenavir: Capsules: 4–12 years old or if 13–16 and weight is less than 50 kg—20 mg per kg twice daily or 15 mg per kg three times daily up to

2,400 mg. 13–16 years of age and weighing more than 50 kg—same as adult dose. Oral solution (NOT INTERCHANGEABLE WITH CAPSULES): 4–12 years old or if 13–16 and weight is less than 50 kg: 22.5 mg per kg twice daily or 17 mg per kg three times daily up to 2,800 mg.

Indinavir: Dosing in children is not clearly defined.

Nelfinavir: 2–13 years old—One open-label study used 20–30 mg per kg per dose, which was taken three times daily with a meal or light snack.

Ritonavir: Started at 250 mg per square meter and increased at 2- to 3-day intervals by 30 mg per square meter. The goal dose is 400 mg per square meter twice daily in combination with other antiretroviral agents (up to 600 mg twice daily).

Saquinavir: Dosing in those less than 16 years old has not been defined.

By Those Over 65 Years of Age: Have not been studied in this age group.

▷ **Advisability of Use During Pregnancy**

Pregnancy Category: Nelfinavir, ritonavir and saquinavir: B; Amprenavir, indinavir: C. See Pregnancy Risk Categories at the back of this book.

Animal Studies: Clinical doses in rats and rabbits have not revealed teratogenicity.

Human Studies: Adequate studies of pregnant women are not available. Ask your doctor for help.

Advisability of Use If Breast-Feeding

Presence of this drug in breast milk: Yes in rats (amprenavir, indinavir); unknown (nelfinavir, ritonavir, saquinavir).

Refrain from nursing if you are HIV-positive or are taking this drug. Breast milk may also transfer the AIDS virus from mother to infant.

Habit-Forming Potential: None.

Effects of Overdose:

Amprenavir: No known antidote exists. If overdose occurs, the manufacturer suggests the patients should be treated according to the signs and symptoms they develop.

Indinavir: No human data are available. Doses of 20 times the human dose in rats and 10 times the human dose in mice were not lethal for indinavir.

Ritonavir: Limited experience, with one case reporting paresthesias and another showed sudden kidney failure with eosinophilia.

Possible Effects of Long-Term Use: Resistance may develop. Lipodystrophy and blood sugar problems may occur.

Suggested Periodic Examinations While Taking These Drugs (at physician's discretion)

Liver function tests.

Complete blood counts.

CD4 or viral load measurement.

Measurement of blood sugar (glucose), especially for those with prior blood sugar problems or patients who show signs or symptoms of hyperglycemia or ketoacidosis.

Measurement of cholesterol and fractions before starting therapy and periodically while taking these medicines.

▷ **While Taking These Drugs, Observe the Following**

Foods: If indinavir is taken with a meal high in fat, calories, or protein, a 77% to 91% decrease in the total amount of drug absorbed has been reported.

Amprenavir absorption is decreased if it is taken with a high-fat meal. The other medicines in this class are better absorbed if taken with food.

Herbal Medicines or Minerals: Some patients use echinacea to attempt to boost their immune systems. Unfortunately, use of echinacea is not recommended in people with damaged immune systems. This herb may also actually weaken any immune system if it is used too often or for too long (more than 8 weeks). Garlic is often used to help lower cholesterol, but dropped blood levels by 50% in one study—do not combine with saquinavir and talk to your doctor before combining garlic with any HIV medicine. St. John's wort significantly decreased indinavir levels in one study. Because protease inhibitors as well as nonnucleoside reverse transcriptase inhibitors (see Drug Classes), use the P450 3A4 pathway—use of this herbal is NOT recommended for people taking those medicines.

Nutritional Support: Since amprenavir contains a significant amount of vitamin E, supplements or multivitamins high in vitamin E should be avoided.

Beverages: No restrictions.

▷ *Alcohol:* No interactions expected.

Tobacco Smoking: May blunt therapeutic benefits of ritonavir. I advise everyone to quit smoking.

Marijuana Smoking: Ritonavir and other PIs removed by the same liver enzymes can increase blood levels leading to toxicity (see dronabinol interaction).

▷ *Other Drugs*

These medicines *taken concurrently* with

- amiodarone (Cordarone) increase heart toxicity risk—DO NOT COMBINE with ritonavir; if combined with indinavir, blood levels are required.
- antacids (various, didanosine also) may lead to lower blood levels of these medicines and poor antiviral effects; separate antacid dosing by at least an hour.
- astemizole (Hismanal) may cause serious toxicity—DO NOT COMBINE (astemizole now removed from the US market).
- azole antifungals (itraconazole, ketoconazole, others) may lead to increased protease inhibitor levels and toxicity.
- bepridil (Vascor) may lead to serious toxicity—DO NOT COMBINE with these medicines.
- birth control pills (oral contraceptives) may lead to low birth control levels and pregnancy (ritonavir, saquinavir, and amprenavir).
- bupropion (Wellbutrin) increase seizure risk with ritonavir—DO NOT COMBINE.
- carbamazepine (Tegretol) decrease protease inhibitor levels.
- cimetidine (Tagamet) may lead to cimetidine toxicity (ritonavir only).
- cisapride (Propulsid) may cause serious toxicity—DO NOT COMBINE.
- cyclosporine (Sandimmune) may lead to cyclosporine toxicity. Blood levels and dosing changes are prudent.
- delavirdine (Rescriptor) may lead to delavirdine toxicity.
- diazepam (Valium, others) may be increased by protease inhibitors to toxic levels—DO NOT COMBINE.
- didanosine (Videx) may blunt therapeutic benefits; separate doses by 1 hour.
- digoxin (Lanoxin, others) may increase digoxin levels; lower doses of digoxin and digoxin blood levels are needed.

- diltiazem (Cardizem) may lead to diltiazem toxicity (ritonavir and saquinavir, perhaps others).
- dofetilide (Tikosyn) may lead to dofetilide toxicity.
- dronabinol (Marinol) may increase dronabinol levels, lower doses of dronabinol, and close patient follow-up are needed.
- efavirez (Sustiva) combined with ritonavir can increase levels of both medicines. Careful patient follow-up and close monitoring of liver enzymes are needed.
- ergot derivatives (see Drug Classes) may lead to toxicity—DO NOT COMBINE.
- felodipine (Plendil) may lead to felodipine toxicity.
- flecainide (Tambocor) SHOULD NOT be taken with ritonavir.
- fluticasone (Flonase) may lead to flonase toxicity when combined with ritonavir (perhaps other PIs).
- fluvastatin (Lescol) and other HMG-CoA reductase inhibitors (see Drug Classes) removed by liver CYP3A4 (atorvastatin, lovastatin, pravastatin, and simvastatin) may lead to HMG-CoA toxicity. Cerivastatin (Baycol) is also removed by CYP3A4, but it is equally removed by CYP2C8 and may be a safer alternative.
- fluvoxamine (Luvox) may lead to fluvoxamine toxicity (ritonavir, perhaps others).
- gemfibrozil (Lopid) may increase gemfibrozil levels (ritonavir); patients who show signs of gemfibrozil toxicity should have gemfibrozil doses lowered.
- glimepiride (Amaryl), glipizide (Glucotrol) or glyburide (Glynase) may have blood levels changed (ritonavir); caution and possible oral hypoglycemic dosing changes are prudent.
- ibuprofen (Motrin, others) and other NSAIDs may lead to ibuprofen or other NSAID toxicity (ritonavir only)—caution is advised.
- isradipine (DynaCirc) may lead to isradipine toxicity.
- itraconazole (Sporanox) or ketoconazole (Nizoral) may cause protease inhibitor toxicity and doses of the protease inhibitor may need to be reduced. Combination with ritonavir may lead to itraconazole or ketoconazole toxicity.
- macrolide antibiotics (clarithromycin, erythromycin) may increase antibiotic levels; macrolide doses may need to be lowered (based on increased nausea/vomiting). Azithromycin may be the best macrolide to use if one is needed.
- medicines removed (metabolized) by CYP3A4 may increase blood levels greater than expected and increase risk of toxicity.
- methylenedioxymethamphetamine (MDMA or ecstasy) led to a serotonin reaction and death in one case report for ritonavir—DO NOT COMBINE.
- midazolam (Versed) may cause serious toxicity—DO NOT COMBINE.
- narcotics such as morphine (MS Contin) or methadone (Dolophine) may lead to toxic narcotic levels.
- nevirapine (Viramune) may blunt therapeutic effects of indinavir—Caution and dosing changes are prudent.
- oral hypoglycemics (see Drug Classes) may lead to excessive lowering of blood sugar (ritonavir only).
- other antiretrovirals may reduce viral load to nondetectable levels but may also interact (ritonavir lowers nelfinavir levels, while indinavir increases nelfinavir or saquinavir levels).

- other drugs that are toxic to the liver may result in additive toxicity (except amprenavir).
- other drugs that can lead to kidney stones may result in additive risk with indinavir.
- paclitaxel (Taxol) may lead to paclitaxel toxicity (ritonavir).
- phenytoin (Dilantin) or fosphenytoin (Cerebyx) may lower protease benefits.
- propafenone (Rythmol) should NOT be taken with ritonavir and may be contraindicated with other protease inhibitors.
- quinidine (Quinaglute, others) should NOT be taken with ritonavir, nelfinavir. Other protease inhibitors may increase quinidine blood levels, and more frequent quinidine levels are prudent. Indinavir is considered to be safe to give with quinidine.
- quinupristin/dalfopristin (Synercid) should be combined with ritonavir or ritonavir combinations only after careful consideration and caution. Levels of ritonavir may need to be checked and doses reduced.
- rifabutin (Mycobutin) may increase rifabutin and decrease indinavir levels; half the usual dose of rifabutin is used if these drugs are combined.
- rifampin (Rifater, others) may cause loss of indinavir and amprenavir benefits—DO NOT COMBINE.
- risperidone (Risperdol) may lead to toxicity if combined with ritonavir or ritonavir combinations. Careful patient follow-up and checks for risperidone toxicity are needed.
- saquinavir (Fortovase) and ritonavir may lead to increased saquinavir levels and possible toxicity unless doses are reduced.
- sirolimus (Rapamune) may cause sirolimus or tacrolimus (Prograf) with ritonavir may lead to toxicity.
- sildenafil (Viagra), vardenafil (Levitra) and tadalafil (Cialis) may lead to excessive blood levels of the erectile dysfunction medicine and possible toxicity (amprenavir, atazanavir, ritonavir, and saquinavir).
- tramadol (Ultram) may lead to tramadol toxicity; reduced tramadol doses are mandatory if these medicines are combined.
- triazolam (Halcion) and perhaps other benzodiazepines may cause serious toxicity.
- tricyclic antidepressants (see Drug Classes) should have blood levels checked.
- venlafaxine (Effexor) may increase risk of venlafaxine toxicity when combined with some PIs.
- warfarin (Coumadin) may increase risk of bleeding (amprenavir, ritonavir, and nelfinavir only); frequent INR checks are prudent.
- zolpidem (Ambien) may produce toxic zolpidem levels (if combined with ritonavir)—DO NOT COMBINE.

▷ *Driving, Hazardous Activities:* Some of these drugs may rarely cause sleepiness. Restrict activities as necessary.

Aviation Note: The use of these drugs **may be a disqualification** for piloting. Consult a designated Aviation Medical Examiner.

Exposure to Sun: No restrictions.

Special Storage Instructions: The ritonavir soft gelatin capsules DO NOT require refrigeration if they are stored below 77° F.

Discontinuation: Do not stop these drugs without your doctor's knowledge and guidance.

PROTRIPTYLINE (proh TRIP ti lin)

Introduced: 1966 **Class:** Antidepressant **Prescription:** USA: Yes **Controlled Drug:** USA: No; Canada: No **Available as Generic:** USA: Yes; Canada: No

Author's Note: The information in this profile has been shortened to make room for more widely used medicines.

PYRAZINAMIDE (peer a ZIN a mide)

Introduced: 1968 **Class:** Anti-infective, antituberculosis **Prescription:** USA: Yes **Controlled Drug:** USA:No; Canada: No **Available as Generic:** USA: Yes; Canada: No

Brand Names: ♣PMS Pyrazinamide, Rifater [CD], ♣Tebrazid

BENEFITS versus RISKS	
Possible Benefits	*Possible Risks*
EFFECTIVE ADJUNCTIVE TREATMENT OF TUBERCULOSIS	DRUG-INDUCED HEPATITIS—rare
Adjunctive treatment of atypical mycobacterial infections	Activation of gouty arthritis and porphyria
	Decreased platelets and hemoglobin

▷ **Principal Uses**

As a Single Drug Product: Uses currently included in FDA-approved labeling: Treatment of active tuberculosis, in combination with other antitubercular drugs.

Other (unlabeled) generally accepted uses: (1) Combination therapy of Mycobacterium xenopi infections; (2) combination therapy of resistant tuberculosis; (3) combination therapy of tuberculosis in AIDS.

As a Combination Drug Product [CD]: This medicine is combined with other antituberculosis medicines (isoniazid and rifampin) in order to attack tuberculosis with combination treatment in a single-dose form. This undoubtedly helps adherence.

How This Drug Works: This drug is ideal for killing tuberculosis organisms that are in acid environments, such as in some kinds of white blood (macrophages) cells.

▷ **Widely Used Guidelines That Involve This Medicine (representative sample):** Please look at the section at the very beginning of this profile called "Class." Next, turn to Table 22 and you will find guidelines listed by the class involved!

Available Dosage Forms and Strengths

Tablets — 500 mg

Tablets — 300 mg pyrazinamide, 50 mg isoniazid and 120 mg of rifampin (Rifater brand)

▷ **Recommended Dosage Ranges** (Actual dose and schedule must be determined for each patient individually.)

Children: 15–30 mg per kg of body mass, once a day. Total daily dose should not exceed 2,000 mg.

12 to 60 Years of Age: For tuberculosis—using lean body weight in kilograms (kg): 40–55 kg are given 1,000 mg daily, 56–75 kg are given 1,500 mg daily and those 76–90 kg are given 2,000 mg daily. Some patients do better with twice-weekly dosing with those of lean body weight in kilograms 40–55 kg are given 2,000 mg twice a week, 56–75 kg are given 3,000 mg and those 76–90 kg are given 4,000 mg twice a week.

Author's Note: Because of the current resistant tuberculosis problem, most clinicians start all patients on a four-drug regimen for 8 weeks (until laboratory culture results are available). Treatment of this widespread resistant organism should be based on local resistance trends and individual patient organisms and typically continues for about 6 (range of 4-7) months.

Over 60 Years of Age: Same as 12 to 60 years of age.

Conditions Requiring Dosing Adjustments

Liver Function: This drug should be used with caution and in decreased doses by patients with liver compromise. Should not be used (contraindicated) in patients with severe liver dysfunction.

Kidney Function: Not used in patients with creatinine clearance less than 50 mL/minute. One researcher recommends 60 mg per kg of body mass, twice weekly. The dose of pyrazinamide should be given at least 24 hours before any given dialysis session. Other sources say to avoid in dialysis patients. Patients should be closely monitored.

▷ **Dosing Instructions:** The tablet may be crushed and taken with or following food to reduce stomach irritation. Take the full course prescribed. This drug should be taken concurrently with other antitubercular drugs to prevent the development of drug-resistant strains of tuberculosis bacteria. The Rifater product accomplishes triple therapy in a single pill. If you forget a dose: Take the missed dose as soon as you remember it, unless it's nearly time for your next dose—if that is the case, skip the missed dose and take the next dose right on schedule. DO NOT take two doses at the same time. Talk with your doctor if you find yourself missing doses. IT IS CRITICAL to take this medicine exactly as prescribed and for as long as prescribed.

Usual Duration of Use: Use on a regular schedule for 2 months usually determines effectiveness in controlling active tuberculosis. Long-term use of antitubercular drugs requires periodic physician evaluation. (Bone infections may require a year of therapy).

Typical Treatment Goals and Measurements (Outcomes and Markers)

Infections: The most commonly used measures of serious infections are white blood cell counts and differentials (the kind of blood cells that occur most often in your blood), and temperature. While clinicians look for positive changes in 24–48 hours in typical infections, this kind of infection REQUIRES long-term treatment to kill it. NEVER stop a treatment for an infection because you start to feel better. The goals and time frame (see peak benefits above) should be discussed with you when the prescription is written. Months of treatment are usually required to kill this very tough (resistant) organism.

Possible Advantages of This Drug

May reduce the period of drug treatment from 9 months down to 6 months in responsive infections.

▷ **This Drug Should Not Be Taken If**
- you have had an allergic reaction to it previously.
- you have permanent liver damage with impaired function.
- you have active gout, sudden (acute).

▷ **Inform Your Physician Before Taking This Drug If**
- you have had an allergic reaction to ethionamide, isoniazid, or niacin (nicotinic acid).
- you have a history of liver disease.
- you have a history of peptic ulcer or porphyria.
- you tried to take medicines for tuberculosis before, but did not complete the prescribed therapy.
- you have gout or diabetes.
- you have impaired kidney function.

Possible Side Effects (natural, expected, and unavoidable drug actions)
Increased blood uric acid levels. Fever.

▷ **Possible Adverse Effects** (unusual, unexpected, and infrequent reactions)
If any of the following develop, consult your physician promptly for guidance.

Mild Adverse Effects
Allergic reactions: skin rash, itching, fever.
Loss of appetite, mild nausea, vomiting—frequent.
Joint pain—frequent.
Acne—rare.

Serious Adverse Effects
Idiosyncratic reactions: Rare sideroblastic anemia.
Decreased blood platelets—rare.
Seizures—rare.
Drug-induced porphyria or pellagra—case reports.
Loss of blood sugar control in diabetics—reported.
Kidney problems (interstitial nephritis)—case reports.
Drug-induced hepatitis, with and without jaundice (see Glossary)—more likely with higher doses.
Gouty arthritis, due to increased blood uric acid levels—possible.

▷ **Possible Effects on Sexual Function:** None reported other than rare reports of painful urination.

▷ **Adverse Effects That May Mimic Natural Diseases or Disorders**
Drug-induced hepatitis may suggest viral hepatitis.

Natural Diseases or Disorders That May Be Activated by This Drug
Gout, peptic ulcer, porphyria.

Possible Effects on Laboratory Tests
Complete blood cell counts: decreased red cells, hemoglobin, and platelets.
INR (prothrombin time): increased.
Blood sugar: tight control may become more difficult.
Blood uric acid level: increased.
Liver function tests: increased enzymes (ALT/GPT, AST/GOT, alkaline phosphatase) or bilirubin.
Urine ketone tests: false-positive test result with Acetest and Ketostix.

CAUTION
1. When this drug is used alone, tuberculosis bacteria rapidly develop resistance to it. To be effective, this drug must be used in combination with

other effective antitubercular drugs, such as isoniazid and rifampin. The CDC states that the rifampin combination requires frequent liver tests.
2. This drug may interfere with control of diabetes.

Precautions for Use

By Infants and Children: Safety and effectiveness for those under 12 years of age are not established. The rare occurrence of drug-related seizure has been reported in a 2-year-old child.

By Those Over 60 Years of Age: No specific information available.

▷ **Advisability of Use During Pregnancy**

Pregnancy Category: C. See Pregnancy Risk Categories at the back of this book.
Animal Studies: No information available.
Human Studies: Adequate studies of pregnant women are not available.
Use this drug only if clearly needed. Ask your physician for guidance.

Advisability of Use If Breast-Feeding

Presence of this drug in breast milk: Yes.
Avoid drug or refrain from nursing.

Habit-Forming Potential: None.

Effects of Overdose: Nausea, vomiting, malaise.

Possible Effects of Long-Term Use: Liver damage.

Suggested Periodic Examinations While Taking This Drug (at physician's discretion)

Complete blood cell counts.
Liver function tests.
Uric acid blood levels.

▷ **While Taking This Drug, Observe the Following**

Foods: No restrictions.

Herbal Medicines or Minerals: Some patients use echinacea to attempt to boost their immune systems. Unfortunately, use of echinacea is not recommended in people with damaged immune systems. This herb may also actually weaken any immune system if it is used too often or for too long a time. Do NOT take mistletoe herb, oak bark or F.C. of marshmallow root, woody nightshade stem, or licorice. Since St. John's wort and pyrazinamide may cause increased sun sensitivity, caution is advised.

Beverages: No restrictions. May be taken with milk.

▷ *Alcohol:* Use sparingly to minimize liver toxicity.

Tobacco Smoking: No interactions expected. I advise everyone to quit smoking.

▷ *Other Drugs*

Pyrazinamide may ***decrease*** the effects of
• allopurinol (Zyloprim).
• BCG vaccine.
• cyclosporine (Sandimmune).
• probenecid (Benemid).
• sulfinpyrazone (Anturane).

Pyrazinamide ***taken concurrently*** with
• phenytoin (Dilantin) or fosphenytoin (Cerebyx) may lead to phenytoin or fosphenytoin toxicity.
• zidovudine (AZT) may lead to low pyrazinamide levels. Dosing changes may be needed.

▷ *Driving, Hazardous Activities:* No restrictions.

Aviation Note: The use of this drug is probably not a disqualification for piloting. Consult a designated Aviation Medical Examiner.

Exposure to Sun: Use caution—this drug may cause photosensitivity (see Glossary).

Discontinuation: If tolerated, this drug is usually taken for a minimum of 2 months. Do not stop it without your physician's knowledge and guidance.

PYRIDOSTIGMINE (peer id oh STIG meen)

Introduced: 1962   **Class:**   Antimyasthenic   **Prescription:**   USA: Yes   **Controlled Drug:**   USA: No; Canada: No   **Available as Generic:** USA: No; Canada: No

Brand Names: ✤Anaplex SR, Mestinon, Mestinon-SR, Mestinon Timespan, Regonol

---

BENEFITS versus RISKS

Possible Benefits	*Possible Risks*
MODERATELY EFFECTIVE TREATMENT OF OCULAR AND MILD FORMS OF MYASTHENIA GRAVIS (symptomatic relief of muscle weakness) PRETREATMENT MEDICINE WHEN NERVE AGENT EXPOSURE IS POSSIBLE	Cholinergic crisis (overdose): excessive salivation, nausea, vomiting, stomach cramps, diarrhea, shortness of breath (asthmalike wheezing), excessive weakness

---

▷ **Principal Uses**

As a Single Drug Product: Uses currently included in FDA-approved labeling: (1) Used to treat the ocular and milder forms of myasthenia gravis by providing temporary relief of muscle weakness and fatigability (most useful in long-term treatment when there is little or no swallowing difficulty); (2) used to reverse skeletal muscle relaxants; (3) used to pretreat the effects of nerve gas.

Other (unlabeled) generally accepted uses: (1) Combination therapy in chronic pain; (2) may help in combination therapy of Huntington's chorea and Lambert-Eaton syndrome; (3) adjunctive use with scopolamine to prevent side effects of scopolamine in treating motion sickness; (4) may have a role in treating nonepidemic parotitis; (5) used in pediatrics to treat myasthenia gravis.

How This Drug Works: This drug inhibits cholinesterase, the enzyme that destroys acetylcholine. This results in higher levels of acetylcholine, the nerve transmitter that facilitates the stimulation of muscular activity. The net effects are increased muscle strength and endurance.

▷ **Widely Used Guidelines That Involve This Medicine (representative sample):** Please look at the section at the very beginning of this profile called "Class." Next, turn to Table 22 and you will find guidelines listed by the class involved!

Available Dosage Forms and Strengths

Solution for injection — 5 mg/mL

Syrup — 60 mg/5 mL (5% alcohol)

Tablets — 30 mg, 60 mg

Tablets, prolonged-action — 180 mg

▷ **Usual Adult Dosage Ranges:** *Myasthenia Gravis:* Initially 1 to 6 normal-release tablets, spaced throughout the day when maximum strength is needed (or ten of the 5 mL liquid dose). Maintenance varies with the severity of the disease—1 to 3 extended-release tablets once or twice a day. If twice-daily extended-release doses are needed, they should be separated by 6 hours. Some patients may need to supplement the extended-release tablets with the 30-mg, immediate-release tablets or the syrup in order to best control symptoms (some patients require up to 1,500 mg a day).

Nerve Gas or Agent Protection: 30 mg every 8 hours when the threat of a nerve agent attack is present. PRETREATMENT IS CRITICAL. Pralidoxime (600 mg) and atropine citrate (2 mg) are also given injected into a muscle if there actually is nerve gas exposure. If exposure is confirmed, the pyridostigmine is stopped.

Note: Actual dose and schedule must be determined for each patient individually.

Conditions Requiring Dosing Adjustments

Liver Function: No dosing changes are defined in liver compromise.

Kidney Function: This drug is primarily eliminated in the urine, but specific guidelines for dose adjustments in renal compromise are not available.

▷ **Dosing Instructions:** Take with food or milk to reduce the intensity of side effects. Larger portions of the daily maintenance dose should be timed according to the pattern of fatigue and weakness. The syrup will permit a finer adjustment of dose. Dosing should be accomplished using a dose cup or calibrated measuring spoon. The regular tablet may be crushed. Mestinon sustained-release tablets can be cut in half. These tablets may NOT be crushed or cut into four pieces, as that would change the way that the drug is released. If you forget a dose: Take the missed dose as soon as you remember it, unless it's nearly time for your next dose—if that is the case, skip the missed dose and take the next dose right on schedule. DO NOT double doses. Talk with your doctor if you find yourself missing doses.

Usual Duration of Use: Use on a regular schedule (with dose adjustment) for 10 to 14 days usually determines effectiveness in relieving myasthenia symptoms. Long-term use (months to years) requires periodic physician evaluation. Nerve agent prophylaxis should also be followed by a physician.

Typical Treatment Goals and Measurements (Outcomes and Markers)

Myasthenia Gravis: The general goal is to increase muscle strength while avoiding nicotinic or muscarinic effects (diarrhea, salivation, nausea and vomiting). Immediate-release-form dosing is timed to correspond to fatigue or weakness.

▷ **This Drug Should Not Be Taken If**
- you are known to be allergic to bromide compounds.
- you have a urinary obstruction or mechanical intestinal obstruction.

▷ **Inform Your Physician Before Taking This Drug If**
- you have heart rhythm disorders or bronchial asthma.
- you are sensitive to bromides.
- you have recurrent urinary tract infections.
- you have prostatism (see Glossary).
- you will have surgery with general anesthesia.

Possible Side Effects (natural, expected, and unavoidable drug actions)

Small pupils (miosis), watering of eyes, slow pulse, excessive salivation, nausea, vomiting, stomach cramps, diarrhea, urge to urinate, increased sweating, increased bronchial secretions (muscarinic/nicotinic side effects).

▷ **Possible Adverse Effects** (unusual, unexpected, and infrequent reactions)
If any of the following develop, consult your physician promptly for guidance.

Mild Adverse Effects

Allergic reaction: skin rash.

Nervousness, anxiety, unsteadiness, muscle cramps or twitching—infrequent.

Loss of scalp hair (alopecia)—case report.

Serious Adverse Effects

Confusion, slurred speech, seizures, difficult breathing (asthmatic wheezing).

Increased muscle weakness or paralysis—case report.

Psychosis—rare.

Excessive vomiting or diarrhea may cause low potassium levels (hypokalemia). This accentuates muscle weakness.

▷ **Possible Effects on Sexual Function:** None reported.

▷ **Adverse Effects That May Mimic Natural Diseases or Disorders**

Seizures may suggest the possibility of epilepsy.

Natural Diseases or Disorders That May Be Activated by This Drug

Latent bronchial asthma.

Possible Effects on Laboratory Tests: None reported.

CAUTION

1. Some drugs block this drug, reducing effectiveness in treating myasthenia gravis. Ask your doctor before starting any other medicine.
2. Variations in response may occur from time to time. Because generalized muscle weakness is a major symptom of both myasthenia crisis (underdose) and cholinergic crisis (overdose), it may be difficult to recognize the correct cause. As a rule, weakness that starts an hour after taking this drug probably represents overdose; weakness that begins 3 or more hours after taking this drug is probably due to underdose. Watch these relationships and tell your doctor.
3. During long-term use, watch for development of resistance to the therapeutic action (loss of effect). Ask your doctor if the drug should be stopped for a few days to see if response can be restored.

Precautions for Use

By Infants and Children: The syrup form of this drug permits greater precision of dose adjustment and ease of administration in this age group. Neonates have received 5 mg every 4 to 6 hours. Since this is often self-limiting in neonates, the medicine can frequently be tapered and stopped.

By Those Over 60 Years of Age: The natural decline of kidney function with aging may require smaller doses to prevent accumulation of this drug to toxic levels.

▷ **Advisability of Use During Pregnancy**

Pregnancy Category: C. See Pregnancy Risk Categories at the back of this book.

Animal Studies: No information available.

Human Studies: Adequate studies of pregnant women are not available.

There are no reports of birth defects due to the use of this drug during pregnancy. However, there are reports of significant muscular weakness in newborn infants whose mothers had taken this drug during pregnancy.

Ask your physician for guidance.

Advisability of Use If Breast-Feeding

Presence of this drug in breast milk: Yes, as roughly 0.01% of the mother's dose.

Monitor nursing infant closely, and discontinue drug or nursing if adverse effects develop.

Habit-Forming Potential: None.

Effects of Overdose: Generalized muscular weakness, blurred vision, very small pupils, slow heart rate, difficult breathing (wheezing), excessive salivation, nausea, vomiting, stomach cramps, diarrhea, muscle cramps or twitching. This syndrome constitutes the cholinergic crisis.

Possible Effects of Long-Term Use: Development of tolerance (see Glossary) with loss of therapeutic effectiveness.

Suggested Periodic Examinations While Taking This Drug (at physician's discretion)

Assessment of drug effectiveness and dose schedule for optimal therapeutic results.

▷ **While Taking This Drug, Observe the Following**

Foods: No restrictions.

Herbal Medicines or Minerals: Echinacea pallida root or purpurea herb as well as woody nightshade stem or belladonna should be avoided.

Beverages: No restrictions. May be taken with milk.

▷ *Alcohol:* Use caution until the combined effects are determined. Weakness and unsteadiness may be accentuated.

Tobacco Smoking: No interactions expected. I advise everyone to quit smoking.

▷ *Other Drugs*

Pyridostigmine *taken concurrently* with

* disopyramide (Norpace) may ease undesirable anticholinergic effects (problems urinating, decreased sweating, etc.).
* succinylcholine (various) may increase muscular problems (neuromuscular blockade). This combination should usually be avoided in patients taking pyridostigmine.

The following drugs may *decrease* the effects of pyridostigmine:

* adrenocortical steroids (corticosteroids-such as prednisone and others—see Drug Classes).
* atropine (belladonna).
* clindamycin (Cleocin).
* guanadrel (Hylorel).
* guanethidine (Esimil, Ismelin).
* procainamide (Procan SR, Pronestyl).
* quinidine (Cardioquin, Duraquin, etc.).
* quinine (Quinamm).

▷ *Driving, Hazardous Activities:* This drug may cause blurred vision, confusion, or generalized weakness. Restrict activities as necessary.

Aviation Note: The use of this drug *is a disqualification* for piloting. Consult a designated Aviation Medical Examiner.

Exposure to Sun: No restrictions.

Exposure to Heat: Use caution—this drug may cause excessive sweating and increased weakness.

Exposure to Environmental Chemicals: Avoid excessive exposure (inhalation, skin contamination) to the insecticides Baygon, Diazinon, and Sevin. These can worsen potential drug toxicity.

Discontinuation: Do not stop this drug abruptly without your doctor's knowledge and guidance.

QUAZEPAM (KWAH zee pam)

Introduced: 1982 **Class:** Hypnotic, benzodiazepines **Prescription:** USA: Yes **Controlled Drug:** USA: C-IV* **Available as Generic:** USA: No

Brand Names: Doral, Dormalin

Author's Note: The National Institute of Mental Health has an information page on anxiety. It can be found on the World Wide Web (*www.nimh.nih.gov/anxiety*). The information in this profile has been abbreviated to make room for more widely used medicines.

QUINAPRIL (KWIN a pril)

Introduced: 1984 **Class:** Antihypertensive, ACE inhibitor

Please see the angiotensin converting enzyme (ACE) inhibitor family profile.

QUINIDINE (KWIN i deen)

Introduced: 1918 **Class:** Antiarrhythmic **Prescription:** USA: Yes **Controlled Drug:** USA: No; Canada: No **Available as Generic:** Yes

Brand Names: ❧Apo-Quinidine, ❧Biquin Durules, Cardioquin, Cin-Quin, Duraquin, ❧Natisedine, ❧Novo-Quinidin, Quinaglute Dura-Tabs, Quinate, Quinatime, Quinidex Extentabs, ❧Quinobarb [CD], Quinora, Quin-Release, SK-Quinidine Sulfate

BENEFITS versus RISKS	
Possible Benefits	*Possible Risks*
EFFECTIVE TREATMENT OF SELECTED HEART RHYTHM DISORDERS IDIOSYNCRATIC REACTIONS	NARROW TREATMENT RANGE FREQUENT ADVERSE EFFECTS NUMEROUS ALLERGIC AND DOSE-RELATED TOXICITIES Provocation of abnormal heart rhythms Abnormally low blood platelet count Hemolytic anemia Kidney or liver toxicity

▷ **Principal Uses**

As a Single Drug Product: Uses currently included in FDA-approved labeling: (1) Helps control the following types of abnormal heart rhythm: atrial fibrillation and flutter, paroxysmal atrial tachycardia, paroxysmal ventricular

*See Schedules of Controlled Drugs at the back of this book.

tachycardia, premature atrial, and ventricular contractions; (2) intravenous treatment of malaria in people who cannot take medicine by mouth.

Other (unlabeled) generally accepted uses: Not defined at present.

As a Combination Drug Product [CD]: This drug is available (in Canada) in combination with a barbiturate, a mild sedative that is added to allay the anxiety and nervous tension that may accompany heart rhythm disorders.

How This Drug Works: Slows activity of the heart pacemaker and delays electrical impulses through the heart conduction system, restoring normal heart rate and rhythm.

▷ **Widely Used Guidelines That Involve This Medicine (representative sample):** Please look at the section at the very beginning of this profile called "Class." Next, turn to Table 22 and you will find guidelines listed by the class involved!

Available Dosage Forms and Strengths

> Capsules — 200 mg, 300 mg
> Injections — 80 mg/mL, 200 mg/mL
> Tablets — 100 mg, 200 mg, 275 mg, 300 mg
> Tablets, prolonged-action — 250 mg, 300 mg, 324 mg, 330 mg

▷ **Usual Adult Dosage Ranges:** *Premature Atrial or Ventricular Contractions*: Quinidine sulfate immediate-release—200 to 400 mg every 4 to 6 hours. Quinidine sulfate extended-release (Quinidex Extentabs)—300 to 600 mg every 8–12 hours. Quinidine gluconate—324 mg to 648 mg or 1–2 tablets every 8–12 hours. Dosing is adjusted to patient response and blood levels (2–8 mcg/mL).

Paroxysmal Atrial Tachycardia: 400 to 600 mg every 2 to 3 hours until paroxysm is terminated.

Atrial Flutter: Digoxin is given first (digitalize); then individualize dose schedule as appropriate.

Atrial Fibrillation: Digoxin is given first (digitalize); then try 200 mg every 2 to 3 hours for five to eight doses; increase dose daily until normal rhythm is restored or toxic effects develop.

Ongoing (Maintenance) Schedule: Generally 200 to 300 mg three or four times daily.

Note: Actual dose and schedule must be determined for each patient individually.

Conditions Requiring Dosing Adjustments

Liver Function: This drug is extensively metabolized in the liver. Blood levels should be obtained to guide dosing. A larger loading dose and a 50% decreased ongoing (maintenance) dose may be required.

Kidney Function: Blood levels should be obtained and used to guide dosing. Quinidine should be used with **CAUTION** in renal compromise.

▷ **Dosing Instructions:** This drug is preferably taken on an empty stomach to achieve high blood levels rapidly. However, it may be taken with or following food to reduce stomach irritation. The regular tablets may be crushed and the capsules opened. Prolonged-action forms should be swallowed whole without alteration. If you forget a dose: Take the missed dose as soon as you remember it, unless you've missed your dose by 2 hours for immediate-release forms or 4 hours for sustained-release forms—if that is the case, skip the missed dose and take the next dose right on schedule. Call your doctor if you've missed more than two doses. Talk with your doctor and pharmacist if you find yourself missing doses. There are a variety of reminder pill boxes or even phone call systems to help.

Usual Duration of Use: Use on a regular schedule for 2 to 4 days usually determines effectiveness in correcting or preventing responsive abnormal rhythms. Long-term use (months to years) requires physician supervision and periodic evaluation and blood levels.

Typical Treatment Goals and Measurements (Outcomes and Markers)

Abnormal Heartbeats: The general goal is to return the heart to a normal rhythm or at least to markedly reduce the occurrence of abnormal heartbeats. In life-threatening arrhythmias, the goal is to abort the abnormal beats and return the pattern to normal. Success at ongoing suppression may involve ambulatory checks of heart rate and rhythm for a day (such as in Holter monitoring). This kind of testing involves placement of adhesive-backed temporary electrodes on the skin in several positions around the heart. A small heart rate and rhythm (EKG or ECG) recording device is carried around via a shoulder strap and records what the heart is doing over 24 hours. Once the recording is made, a scanning machine reviews the record, tallies abnormal heartbeats or rhythms, and gives a close and extended look at how the heart is reacting or benefiting from the medicines that the patient is taking. Repeat measurements can be made if doses are changed to check the success at keeping the heart at normal sinus rhythm.

▷ **This Drug Should Not Be Taken If**
- you have had an allergic or idiosyncratic reaction to it or to quinine previously.
- you currently have an acute infection of any kind.
- you have taken too much digoxin (digoxin toxicity).
- you have myasthenia gravis or kidney disease.
- you have an AV block (complete) and do not have an artificial pacemaker or you have conduction problems in the ventricles (intraventricular conduction defects).
- you have abnormal heart rhythms caused by an escape mechanism (ask your specialist).

▷ **Inform Your Physician Before Taking This Drug If**
- you have coronary artery disease or sick sinus syndrome.
- you have a history of excessive thyroid function (hyperthyroidism).
- you usually have very low blood pressure.
- you have had a deficiency of blood platelets in the past from any cause.
- your blood chemistry (electrolyte content) is not in balance.
- you are now taking, or have taken recently, any digitalis preparation (digitoxin, digoxin, etc.).
- you will have surgery with general anesthesia.
- you have a history of passing out (syncopal episodes).
- you have acute rheumatic fever or subacute bacterial endocarditis (SBE).

Possible Side Effects (natural, expected, and unavoidable drug actions)

Drop in blood pressure, may be marked in some patients and cause passing out (syncope). Drug fever—reported.

▷ **Possible Adverse Effects** (unusual, unexpected, and infrequent reactions)

If any of the following develop, consult your physician promptly for guidance.

Mild Adverse Effects

Allergic reactions: skin rash, hives, itching, drug fever—rare.
Irritation of the esophagus (esophagitis)—possible.
Nausea, vomiting, diarrhea—infrequent.

Serious Adverse Effects

Allergic reactions: severe skin reactions, hemolytic anemia (see Glossary), joint and muscle pains, anaphylactic reaction (see Glossary), reduced blood platelet count, drug-induced hepatitis (see Glossary).

Idiosyncratic reactions: skin rash, fast heart rate, delirium, difficult breathing.

Dose-related toxicity (cinchonism): blurred vision, ringing ears, hearing loss, coma, heart (cardiac) arrest.

Mental status changes: paranoia, memory loss, depression, psychosis—reported.

Drug-induced myasthenia gravis, systemic lupus erythematosus (SLE) or carpal tunnel syndrome—case reports.

Swelling of the lymph glands in the inguinal area (lymphadenopathy)—case report.

Kidney toxicity—case reports.

Heart conduction abnormalities (Torsade de Pointes, others)—case reports.

Optic neuritis, impaired vision—case report.

Abnormally low white blood cell count: fever, sore throat, infections—case reports.

Abnormally low platelet count—case reports.

▷ **Possible Effects on Sexual Function:** None reported.

▷ **Adverse Effects That May Mimic Natural Diseases or Disorders**

Drug-induced hepatitis may suggest viral hepatitis.

Natural Diseases or Disorders That May Be Activated by This Drug

Systemic lupus erythematosus, myasthenia gravis, psoriasis (in sensitive people).

Possible Effects on Laboratory Tests

Complete blood cell counts: decreased red cells, hemoglobin, white cells, and platelets; increased eosinophils (allergic reaction); marked increase of white blood cells in association with "quinidine fever"—very rare.

Antinuclear antibodies (ANA): positive.

INR (protime): increased (when *taken concurrently* with warfarin).

Liver function tests: increased enzymes (ALT/GPT, AST/GOT, alkaline phosphatase) or bilirubin.

CAUTION

1. Dose adjustments must be based upon individual reaction.
2. Dosing schedules differ for the various salt forms (the second part of the generic name). For example, quinidine sulfate (83% anhydrous quinidine) is not the same as quinidine gluconate (62% anhydrous quinidine) or quinidine polygalacturonate (60% anhydrous quinidine). MAKE CERTAIN that any refill prescriptions contain the correct medicine.
3. It is prudent to carry a card saying that you take this drug in case of an accident.

Precautions for Use

By Infants and Children: A test for drug idiosyncrasy should be made before starting treatment with this drug. Dosing is made on weight and is an unlabeled use of this medicine. If there is no beneficial response after 3 days of adequate dose, this drug should be discontinued.

By Those Over 60 Years of Age: Small doses are mandatory until your individual response has been determined. Observe for the development of light-headedness, dizziness, weakness, or sense of impending faint. Use *CAUTION* to prevent falls.

▷ **Advisability of Use During Pregnancy**
  Pregnancy Category: C. See Pregnancy Risk Categories at the back of this book.
  Animal Studies: No information available.
  Human Studies: Adequate studies of pregnant women are not available. No birth
    defects have been reported following use of this drug during pregnancy.
    Use this drug only if clearly needed.

Advisability of Use If Breast-Feeding
  Presence of this drug in breast milk: Yes.
  Avoid drug or refrain from nursing.

Habit-Forming Potential: None.

Effects of Overdose: Nausea, vomiting, ringing in the ears, headache, jerky eye
  movements, double vision, altered color vision, confusion, delirium, hot
  skin, seizures, coma.

Possible Effects of Long-Term Use: None reported.

Suggested Periodic Examinations While Taking This Drug (at physician's dis-
  cretion)
  Complete blood cell counts.
  Electrocardiograms.
  Blood levels.

▷ **While Taking This Drug, Observe the Following**
  Foods: Restrict or eliminate grapefruit (delays absorption and slows the speed
    at which the body changes this medicine to the active form).
  Herbal Medicines or Minerals: Kola, St. John's wort, ma huang (no longer avail-
    able for weight loss), bitter orange, country mallow, guarana, and yohimbe
    may cause additive heart rate or rhythm problems. These are not advisable
    if you have heart rhythm difficulties. Using St. John's wort, ma huang,
    ephedra, or kola while taking this medicine may result in unacceptable
    heart stimulation. Belladonna, henbane, scopolia, pheasant's eye extract or
    lily of the valley, or squill powdered extracts should NOT be taken if you
    have abnormal heart rhythms. Since St. John's wort and quinidine may
    increase sun sensitivity, the combination is NOT advised.
  Beverages: Ask your doctor about caffeine intake. Avoid grapefruit juice (delays
    absorption and slows the speed at which the body changes this medicine
    to the active form).
  May be taken with milk.

▷ *Alcohol:* Use caution—alcohol may enhance the blood pressure–lowering effects
    of this drug.
  Tobacco Smoking: Nicotine can increase irritability of the heart and aggravate
    rhythm disorders. Avoid all forms of tobacco.

▷ *Other Drugs*
  Quinidine *taken concurrently* with
  • aspirin may prolong the bleeding time.
  • beta blockers (see Drug Classes) may result in additive and undesirable
    beta-blockade; lower starting doses may be needed for both medicines.
  • cisapride (Propulsid) may lead to serious heart rhythm problems—DO
    NOT COMBINE.
  • clomipramine (Anafranil) may lead to dry mouth, sedation, or abnormal
    heartbeats. Careful patient follow-up is needed if these two medicines
    must be combined.
  • codeine may blunt the effectiveness of codeine.
  • dextromethorphan (the DM in many cough preparations) can lead to dex-
    tromethorphan toxicity—DO NOT COMBINE.

- dofetilide (Tikosyn) may lead to serious heart rhythm problems—DO NOT COMBINE. Prudent to wait roughly five (4.32 half-lives) after stopping a prior class-one antiarrhythmic or other QTc prolonging drug before starting dofetilide.
- fluoxetine (Prozac) may lead to quinidine or fluoxetine toxicity.
- gatifloxacin (Tequin), grepafloxacin (Raxar), moxifloxacin (Avelox), or sparfloxacin (Zagam) may lead to abnormal heartbeats.
- magnesium-containing antacids (various) may lead to excessive accumulation of quinidine and quinidine toxicity. More frequent checks of blood levels are prudent if these medicines must be combined.
- medicines such as class I, IA, or III antiarrhythmics (dofetilide [Tikosyn], clarithromycin, cotrimoxazole, ondansetron, ziprazidone, zolmitriptan and others) may lead to prolongation of the QTc interval and undesirable effects. Combination is not recommended (see amiodarone note above regarding extreme caution if these two medicines are combined or if transition is made from quinidine to amiodarone).
- metformin (Glucophage) may increase risk of lactic acidosis.
- neuromuscular blocking agents (such as pancuronium-Pavulon, vecuronium-Norcuron, others) can result in increased severity of muscle blockade. Use of lower neuromuscular blocker doses is prudent.
- nisoldipine (Sular) may blunt nisoldipine benefits.
- tramadol (Ultram) may lead to tramadol toxicity.
- tricyclic antidepressants (see Drug Classes) may result in antidepressant toxicity.
- venlafaxine (Effexor) may result in venlafaxine toxicity.

Quinidine may *increase* the effects of
- anticoagulants (Coumadin, etc.) and increase the risk of bleeding; more frequent INR (prothrombin time or protime) testing is needed.
- aripiprazole (Abilify) and cause aripiprazole toxicity. The Abilify dose should be lowered by 50% while the combination is made and increased if quinidine is stopped.
- digitoxin and digoxin (Lanoxin) and cause digitalis toxicity.
- disopyramide (Norpace).
- metformin (Glucophage).
- propafenone (Rythmol) may lead to propafenone toxicity. Careful patient follow-up is critical as propafenone dosing adjustments may be required.
- tricyclic antidepressants (amitriptyline, doxepin).
- warfarin (Coumadin) and may result in coagulation changes (inconsistent effect). More frequent INR checks are prudent.

The following drugs may *increase* the effects of quinidine:
- amiodarone (Cordarone). The quinidine dose should be about half the usually recommended dose for patients who are already taking amiodarone and a decision has been made to switch from amiodarone to quinidine. If combination treatment is thought to be required, careful checks of dosing and cautious checks of blood levels are critical to avoid development of atypical quick heart rates in the ventricles (such as Torsade de Pointes).
- amprenavir (Agenerase), atazanavir (Reyataz), ritonavir (Norvir), nelfinavir (Viracept), saquinavir (Viracept), and perhaps other protease inhibitors (see Drug Classes)—If the combination must be made, aggressive follow-up of blood levels and checks for signs and symptoms of quinidine toxicity (low blood pressure, dizziness, arrhythmias) are required.
- cimetidine (Tagamet).

- delavirdine (Rescriptor).
- diclofenac (Voltaren).
- diltiazem (Cardizem).
- erythromycin (various).
- itraconazole (Sporanox), ketoconazole (Nizoral), or voriconazole (Vfend).
- quinupristin/dalfopristin (Synercid) may lead to serious heart rhythm problems—extremely careful quinidine level follow-up and careful patient monitoring are critical if these medicines must be combined.
- sertraline (Zoloft).
- verapamil (Verelan).

The following drugs may *decrease* the effects of quinidine:
- barbiturates (phenobarbital, etc.).
- phenytoin (Dilantin) or fosphenytoin (Cerebyx).
- rifabutin (Mycobutin).
- rifampin (Rifadin, Rimactane).
- sucralfate (Carafate).

▷ *Driving, Hazardous Activities:* This drug may cause dizziness and alter vision. Restrict activities as necessary.

Aviation Note: The use of this drug *may be a disqualification* for piloting. Consult a designated Aviation Medical Examiner.

Exposure to Sun: Use caution—this drug may cause photosensitivity (see Glossary).

RABEPRAZOLE (rah BEP rah zohl)

Introduced: 2001   **Class:**   Proton pump inhibitor, Antiulcer, GERD treatment   **Prescription:**   USA: Yes   **Controlled Drug:**   USA: No; Canada: No   **Available as Generic:**   No

Brand Name: Aciphex

Author's Note: Like lansoprazole, this medicine may offer faster onset and quicker sign and symptom relief in heartburn (GERD). In a recent study in *Helicobacter pylori* (see Mario, FD in Sources), a 20 mg dose twice daily of rabeprazole in combination with clarithromycin (Biaxin) used for seven days was 91.4 percent successful in eliminating *Helicobacter pylori*. Further head-to-head research is needed to define the place of rabeprazole. Information in this profile will be broadened in future editions if clinical data warrant.

RALOXIFENE (rah LOX i feen)

Introduced: 1997   **Class:**   Antiestrogen, selective estrogen receptor inhibitor (SERM), anti-osteoporosis   **Prescription:**   USA: Yes   **Controlled Drug:**   USA: No; Canada: No   **Available as Generic:**   No

Brand Name: Evista

BENEFITS versus RISKS

Possible Benefits	*Possible Risks*
EFFECTIVE PREVENTION OF POSTMENOPAUSAL OSTEOPOROSIS	Changes in blood clotting
EFFECTIVE TREATMENT OF POSTMENOPAUSAL OSTEOPOROSIS	Hot flashes (flushes)
DECREASES RISK OF NEW VERTEBRAL FRACTURES	Weight gain
REDUCED LDL CHOLESTEROL	
Possible benefits on heart health in women at increased risk of cardiovascular disease	
Possible benefits in preventing breast cancer (being studied in the STAR trial)	
Avoids the risk of endometrial cancer possible with hormones	

▷ **Principal Uses**

As a Single Drug Product: Uses currently included in FDA-approved labeling: (1) Helps prevent osteoporosis in women after menopause; (2) treats osteoporosis after menopause.

Other (unlabeled) generally accepted uses: (1) Because of LDL and homocysteine lowering, may have a role in maintaining heart (cardiovascular) health; (2) may have a role in preventing breast cancer (one study found a 76% lower risk of breast cancer in a group of women who took this drug for 3 years [MORE trial], and is now being studied in the STAR trial); (3) Based on the MORE trial, data accumulated on cardiovascular benefits of this drug. The RUTH trial is under way to further define the benefits of raloxifene on the heart. Appears likely to have a significant role in preventing cardiovascular disease.

Author's Note: Tamoxifen reduced breast cancer rates by almost half in a very large (13,388 patients) cancer prevention study performed by the National Cancer Institute over 6 years. The FDA has launched a new oncology tools website. Visit this at *www.fda.gov/cder/cancer.* **There is a listing of cancer medicine trials on the World Wide Web at** *http://cancertrials.nci.nih.gov.* **The STAR (Study of Tamoxifen and Raloxifene) trial is under way. This is a National Cancer Institute study evaluating 19,000 women who are at risk for breast cancer and now is fully enrolled at the time of this writing. They will be given either 20 mg per day of tamoxifen or 60 mg of raloxifene each day for five years. For more information, you can reach the National Cancer Institute at 1-800-422-6237. An analysis done after the Multiple Outcomes of Raloxifene Evaluation (MORE) trial (secondary analysis— see Barrett-Connor in references) showed that raloxifene use in 1,035 women with high heart (cardiovascular) risk, the rate of cardiovascular events was much lower than with placebo (40% decrease when cardiovascular events are defined as coronary plus cerebrovascular events). The Raloxifene Use for The Heart (RUTH) trial is ongoing**

(started in 1998, is a seven-year trial) and is studying raloxifene in women with known heart (coronary) risk factors or coronary disease.

How This Drug Works: Works similar to estrogen itself on the bone (increasing bone density) and on LDL cholesterol (lowering it). Because of this, some people in the news media call raloxifene a designer estrogen. May block use (uptake) of estrogen (estradiol) and remove one stimulus for breast cancer. Benefits in preventing cardiovascular disease may involve decreases in fibrinogen, positive changes in endothelial function, decreased LDL and homocysteine. It also decreases a specific measure of the carotid arteries (carotid artery pulsatility index). More data are needed.

▷ **Widely Used Guidelines That Involve This Medicine (representative sample):** Please look at the section at the very beginning of this profile called "Class." Next, turn to Table 22 and you will find guidelines listed by the class involved!

Available Dosage Forms and Strengths
Tablets — 60 mg

▷ **Usual Adult Dosage Ranges:**
Prevention of Postmenopausal Osteoporosis: 60 mg once daily. Supplemental calcium and vitamin D are prudent.
Treatment of Postmenopausal Osteoporosis: 60 mg once daily. Supplemental calcium and vitamin D are prudent.
Note: Actual dose and schedule must be determined for each patient individually.

Conditions Requiring Dosing Adjustments
Liver Function: Extensively changed (metabolized) in the liver. Dose decreases appear prudent, but drug use not studied in this population. Most of the drug removal from the body is via feces.
Kidney Function: Not studied in people with kidney disease or compromise.

▷ **Dosing Instructions:** The tablet may be crushed and taken without regard to food. If you forget a dose: Take the missed dose as soon as you remember it, unless it's nearly time for your next dose—if that is the case, skip the missed dose and take the next dose right on schedule. Talk with your doctor if you find yourself missing doses. There are beeper-based systems to help you. If a switch is being made from estrogen to raloxifene, some clinicians taper estrogen over at least a month to help decrease the chance of sudden menopause symptoms. It may also be best to have stopped taking estrogen for a month before starting raloxifene—this approach will allow any raloxifene-related problems to be clearly identified.

Usual Duration of Use: Use in clinical trials compared two years of raloxifene use to calcium use alone. The RUTH trial is ongoing. Some trials used measures of bone mineral density (BMD) to check the benefits of this drug. It appears prudent to check BMD before starting this medicine and then to recheck markers of bone turnover (such as N-telopeptides) and BMD once the medicine has been started to make sure that it is working. Long-term use requires physician supervision.

Typical Treatment Goals and Measurements (Outcomes and Markers)
Bone Mineral Density: The general goal is to at least prevent further bone loss, and ideally, increase bone mineral density or BMD. Results can be checked by a lab test (N-telopeptide) and repeat DEXA, PDEXA, or ultrasound. The overall goal is to decrease fracture risk.

Possible Advantages of This Drug

Effective treatment of osteoporosis. Appears to confer heart (cardioprotective) benefits as well as possible prevention of breast cancer with a single medicine. Large studies are under way.

▷ **This Drug Should Not Be Taken If**
- you had a serious allergic or adverse reaction to it before.
- you have a history of blood clots (clot in the retinal vein, DVT, or pulmonary embolism [PE]).
- you are pregnant or are breast-feeding your infant.

▷ **Inform Your Physician Before Taking This Drug If**
- you are taking estrogen (not studied with this drug).
- you have a history of thrombophlebitis or pulmonary embolism.
- you have impaired liver function.
- you plan to have surgery or will be immobilized (prolonged rest in bed) in the near future.
- you have an active malignancy (benefit-to-risk decision).
- your diet is low in calcium or vitamin D (smart to take a supplement if your diet is deficient).

Possible Side Effects (natural, expected, and unavoidable drug actions)

Hot flashes—may be frequent.

▷ **Possible Adverse Effects** (unusual, unexpected, and infrequent reactions)
If any of the following develop, consult your physician promptly for guidance.

Mild Adverse Effects

Allergic reaction: skin rash.
Insomnia, migraine, nerve pain, or depression—infrequent.
Weight gain—infrequent.
Sweating—infrequent.
Indigestion (dyspepsia), nausea, or vomiting—infrequent.
Cough, sinusitis, or pharyngitis—infrequent.
Joint pain (may be frequent) or leg cramps or muscle pain—infrequent.
Varicose veins—rare.
Swelling of the ankles or wrists (edema)—infrequent.

Serious Adverse Effects

Increased uterine cancer risk was found in mice and rats. How this applies to humans is not known, but not associated with increased risk in one analysis of trials involving more than 9,837 patients.
Chest pain—infrequent.
Liver toxicity—case report.
Blood clots (thromboembolism)—twofold increased risk of lung (PE) and 3.4-fold increased risk of clots (relative to sugar pill or placebo) in veins (venous thromboembolism).

▷ **Possible Effects on Sexual Function:** Vaginitis (up to 4.3 %).

Possible Effects on Laboratory Tests

Markers of bone turnover (bone specific alkaline phosphatase): decreased.
Bone mineral density: increased (beneficial).
Liver function tests: may be increased (questionable cause).

CAUTION

1. Calcium supplements should be added to your diet if your diet does not include enough calcium. Talk to your doctor about the need for vitamin D.
2. Research has not been done combining this medicine with estrogen.

3. Ask your doctor about how to decrease risk factors for osteoporosis. Also ask about an exercise program appropriate to your degree of bone loss.
4. One researcher questioned mouse and rat data that showed raloxifene causing cancer of the ovaries in those animals. The manufacturer said that cancer in rodents did not correspond to risk of cancer in humans.
5. This drug has not been studied for use in men.
6. A head-to-head trial of tamoxifen and raloxifene has started to look at benefits and risks of use in preventing breast cancer (STAR trial).
7. Data are available (MORE trial) that show that this medicine can help prevent fractures in the spine (vertebral fractures) as well as fractures of the hip.
8. This medicine may increase risk of blood clots, and therefore use is a benefit-to-risk decision in patients with active malignancies (which may also increase blood clots).
9. Ask your doctor about how prudent it would be for sitting for extended periods (such as on a long flight or a long trip in the car).

▷ **Advisability of Use During Pregnancy**
Pregnancy Category: X. See Pregnancy Risk Categories at the back of this book.
Human Studies: Studies of pregnant women will not be done. This drug should NOT be used during pregnancy.

Advisability of Use If Breast-Feeding
Presence of this drug in breast milk: Unknown.
Avoid drug or refrain from nursing.

Habit-Forming Potential: None.

Effects of Overdose: An accidental dose of 600 mg was tolerated in clinical trials.

Possible Effects of Long-Term Use: Increased bone mineral density, prevention of spine fractures.

Suggested Periodic Examinations While Taking This Drug (at physician's discretion)
Bone mineral density testing.
Laboratory tests of bone turnover.
Periodic liver function tests.
Check for blood clots.
Regular gynecological examinations.

▷ **While Taking This Drug, Observe the Following**
Foods: No restrictions.
Herbal Medicines or Minerals: Make certain that you are getting adequate calcium in your diet if you have osteoporosis or thin bones (osteopenia). The average American diet has about 200–400 mg. Most people need 1,000 to 1,500 mg per day. Effervescent calcium (resulting in a solution) may be absorbed more rapidly than other forms of calcium and can help prevent osteoporosis. Vitamin D and adequate sunlight are also needed. Soy or other plant-derived phytoestrogens may work to complement raloxifene, but have not been studied together with raloxifene. Some breast cancer patients are taking mistletoe (Iscador, others). This herbal is available by prescription in Europe and may work to stimulate the immune system, but there are no combined raloxifene trials.
Beverages: Smart to lower intake of soda (phosphorous decreases calcium). May be taken with milk.

▷ *Alcohol:* No interactions with the medicine expected, but clinicians count alcohol as something that slows the cells that make bone, potentially worsening osteopenia or osteoporosis.

Tobacco Smoking: No interactions expected. I advise everyone to quit smoking.

▷ *Other Drugs*

The following drugs may ***decrease*** the effects of raloxifene:

- ampicillin (Polycillin, Principen).
- ampicillin/sulbactam (Unasyn).
- cholestyramine (Questran).
- corticosteroids such as prednisone (Deltasone, others), as long-term use of those medicines can lead to osteoporosis.

Raloxifene ***taken concurrently*** with

- other highly protein bound medicines, such as diazepam (Valium), indomethacin (Indocin), naproxen (Naprosyn), or others, should be done only with great caution.
- warfarin (Coumadin) may lower benefits of warfarin; increased frequency of INR (prothrombin time or protime) testing is needed.

▷ *Driving, Hazardous Activities:* No restrictions thought to be needed.

Aviation Note: The use of this drug ***is probably not a disqualification*** for piloting. Consult a designated Aviation Medical Examiner.

Exposure to Sun: No restrictions.

RAMIPRIL (ra MI pril)

Introduced: 1985   **Class:**   Antihypertensive, ACE inhibitor

Please see the angiotensin converting enzyme (ACE) inhibitor family profile.

RANITIDINE (ra NI te deen)

Author's Note: ALL of the four available histamine (H2) receptor blocking drugs are now available without prescription. See the histamine (H2) blocking drug family profile.

REPAGLINIDE (ra PAG lyn ide)

Author's Note: Information in this profile has been truncated in order to make room for nateglinide, which has a more favorable benefit-to-risk profile.

Introduced: 1998   **Class:**   Antidiabetic, meglitinides   **Prescription:** USA: Yes   **Controlled Drug:**   USA: No; Canada: No   **Available as Generic:**   No

Brand Names: ✤Gluconorm, Prandin

RIBAVIRIN (RHI bah vye ron)

Author's Note: This medicine is used in conjunction with peginterferon alpha-2A (see profile previously detailed) to treat hepatitis C, and this

profile will focus on that combined use and on Copegus form. Specific genotypes drive ribavirin dosing (see below).

Introduced: 2003 (Copegus form)   **Class:** Antiviral   **Prescription:** USA: Yes   **Controlled Drug:** USA: No; Canada: No   **Available as Generic:** No

Brand Names: Copegus, Rebetrol, Virazole

BENEFITS versus RISKS	
Possible Benefits	*Possible Risks (Combination)*
COMBINATION TREATMENT OF HEPATITIS C (DRUG NAIVE) COMBINATION TREATMENT OF HEPATITIS C WITH INTERFERON MORE EFFECTIVE THAN UNMODIFIED INTERFERON COMBINATION FOR HEPATITIS C WHEN USED WITH PEGASYS Improved quality of life versus some other Hepatitis C treatments	HEADACHE FATIGUE NAUSEA OR DIARRHEA MUSCLE CHANGES INSOMNIA DEPRESSION BLOOD CELL CHANGES

▷ **Principal Uses**

As a Single Drug Product: Uses currently included in FDA-approved labeling: (1) Treats hepatitis C in combination with interferon alpha-2a (Pegasys), in people who were not previously given interferon alpha, who have compensated liver disease and have evidence of cirrhosis (histological basis and Child-Pugh class A).

Other (unlabeled) generally accepted uses: (1) Some interest in use in SARS.

How This Drug Works: For the combination use: The specific form of interferon alpha-2a (Pegasys) is a modified form of the original molecule. A branched methoxy-polyethylene glycol compound is attached (covalently) to the original interferon molecule. The effect of attaching this additional substance to the interferon is to keep it in the body longer (reduces clearance) by the kidney, protects against compounds in the body (enzymes) which might break the interferon alpha-2a down, and allows once-a-week dosing. The attachment also appears to attack the Hepatitis C Virus more forcefully since the drug stays at a higher level than other interferon alpha-2a formulations which are given three times a week (allowing peaks and valleys in concentration and giving the virus more time to recover). The antiviral action of ribavirin is not fully defined.

▷ **Widely Used Guidelines That Involve This Medicine (representative sample):** Please look at the section at the very beginning of this profile called "Class." Next, turn to Table 22 and you will find guidelines listed by the class involved!

Available Dosage Forms and Strengths

Tablets (Copegus) — 200 mg

▷ **Usual Adult Dosage Ranges**

Combination Hepatitis C Treatment in Adults (with Pegasys-interferon Alpha-2a): The same dose of 180 mcg once weekly of the peginterferon alpha-2a is given, however, the ribavirin dose changes. Here, genetics of the virus are considered: Patients who have genotypes 1 or 4 and who weigh more than 75 kilograms are given 1,200 mg a day. For those less than 75 kg, 1,000 mg a day is given, and combination is continued for 48 weeks. People with genotypes 2 or 3 are given 800 mg of ribavirin (divided into two-400 mg doses given twice a day) coupled with 180 mcg once a week of peginterferon alpha-2a and the combination is only continued for 24 weeks. If an antiviral effect is not seen 12–24 weeks into therapy, consideration is given to stopping the medicine. **DOSING IS ADJUSTED FOR HEMOGLOBIN AND HEART (cardiac) HISTORY—SEE BELOW.**

Note: **Actual dose and schedule must be determined for each patient individually.**

Conditions Requiring Dosing Adjustments

Liver Function: Patients who have a liver function compromise (Child-Pugh Class A) may be given ribavirin. Other patients with more severe compromise have not been studied and SHOULD NOT be given ribavirin.

Kidney Function: People with creatinine clearance (a measure of how well the kidneys work) of less than 50 mL/minute should NOT be given ribavirin.

Hemoglobin adjustment without a heart (cardiac) history: People who have their hemoglobin decrease to less than 10 g/dL have the ribavirin decreased to 600 mg daily (given as 200 mg in the morning and 400 mg in the evening). People who have their hemoglobin decrease to less than 8.5 g/dL have the ribavirin permanently stopped.

Hemoglobin adjustment WITH a heart (cardiac) history: People who have their hemoglobin decrease by 2 g/dL or more during any four-week treatment period have the dose decreased to 600 mg daily (given as 200 mg in the morning and 400 mg in the evening). If the hemoglobin drops to less than 12 g/dL following four weeks of this lower dose, the ribavirin is permanently stopped.

▷ **Dosing Instructions:** Used in combination with a form of interferon alpha-2a (Pegasys). A qualified specialist should carefully decide dosing, and dosing depends on the genotype of the virus. Pegasys is best taken/given on the same day and time each week. Very specific instructions are present in a Med Guide that comes with Pegasys. If you are going to use Copegus in combination with Pegasys, read the Med Guide that came with that medicine and follow the instructions carefully. It is best to take Copegus twice a day, with food.

Usual Duration of Use: Use on a regular schedule for up to 12-24 weeks may be needed to see best effects from the combination of medicines already discussed. Ongoing use for more than 48 weeks does not have efficacy or safety data. Ongoing use requires periodic check of response (such as viral load), check for side effects, laboratory monitoring and possibly dose changes. Make sure you keep follow-up appointments with your doctor and for laboratory or other testing.

Typical Treatment Goals and Measurements (Outcomes and Markers)

The general goal is to lower the amount of virus in the body and ideally to kill all of it. Viral load or burden tests help guide therapy. A test for viral genetic material in the serum called HCV-RNA is taken. The goal is to achieve undetectable amounts. The technical term for this is an undetectable HCV-RNA by PCR. Because the usual limit of the test is 100 copies per milliliter, the goal is to achieve "undetectable." When and if lower detection tests become available (as has happened with HIV testing), a new lower goal will become the standard. Additional beneficial effects will be quality of life, halting of progression or cessation of liver damage.

Possible Advantages of This Medicine/These Drugs: The combination of peginterferon alpha-2a with ribavirin gives a more prolonged (durable) lowering of the amount of virus (viral load or viral burden) and in general viral response. For people who have been infected with the Hepatitis C Virus (HCV) with the genotype 1 form, pegylated forms of interferon (2a or 2b) are drugs of choice.

▷ **This Drug or Combination Should Not Be Taken If**
- you have had an allergic reaction to it previously.
- you have autoimmune hepatitis or unstable liver disease or have had a liver transplant.
- you have previously taken and did not respond to other alpha interferon treatment.
- you are taking this medicine and your hemoglobin drops below acceptable levels (see dosing).
- you are taking this medicine and your neutrophils (Absolute Neutrophil Count), or your platelet count drops below acceptable level (see ANC in Pegasys profile).
- you have sickle cell anemia, thalassemia major or some other form of abnormal red blood cells (Pegasys).
- you become seriously depressed while taking this medicine (Pegasys).
- you are pregnant or become pregnant while taking this medicine.
- you are a man who has a female partner who is pregnant.
- you are a woman of childbearing age and have not had a negative pregnancy test before starting this medicine.

▷ **Inform Your Physician Before Taking These Drugs If**
- you have a history of bone marrow depression or cancer.
- you have a history of a serious emotional or mental disorder, particularly depression.
- you have a history of alcohol or drug abuse.
- you have a history of heart disease, a prior heart attack, or poor heart circulation (ischemic heart disease).
- you have impaired liver function from hepatitis B (no data) or impaired kidney function.
- you have a history of lung problems (pulmonary dysfunction) or chronic obstructive pulmonary disease (this medicine may worsen them).
- you have a history of diabetes or low thyroid function (hypothyroidism).
- you develop a fever, which gets higher or does not go away.
- you have psoriasis and it gets worse while taking this medicine.
- you are taking any drugs for emotional or mental disorders.
- you have a history of eye problems (such as blood clots in the retinal artery, edema of the macula, or optic neuritis)—talk to your doctor.
- you have a history of low white blood cell counts or cancer.
- you have a history of autoimmune disease (such as lupus erythematosus or rheumatoid arthritis) or are HIV positive
- you have a history of colon inflammation (colitis).
- you ask the person prescribing this medicine about HCV genotyping of the virus causing your hepatitis C infection, and learn that this testing has not yet been performed (genotype of the virus is very important).
- you are unsure how much or how often to take this medicine.

Possible Side Effects (natural, expected, and unavoidable drug actions)
Injection site reactions (frequent for Pegasys).

▷ **Possible Adverse Effects** (unusual, unexpected, and infrequent reactions)

If any of the following develop, consult your physician promptly for guidance.

Mild Adverse Effects

Allergic reaction: skin rash, itching (pruritis)—may be frequent.

Headache, fatigue, or fever—frequent.

Insomnia—frequent (may be prudent to anticipate this effect and ask your doctor for help when this medicine is prescribed).

Depression (see depression note above)—frequent.

Blurred vision—possible.

Dizziness, nausea, or abdominal pain—frequent.

Sweating—infrequent.

Loss of appetite (anorexia), diarrhea, abdominal pain—frequent.

Muscle aches or joint pain—frequent.

Blood sugar changes—possible.

Hair loss—alopecia.

Dry mouth—infrequent.

Serious Adverse Effects

Allergic reaction: Copegus form must be stopped IMMEDIATELY and 911 called if hives (urticaria), swelling (angioedema), difficulty breathing (bronchospasm/bronchoconstriction) or anaphylactic signs and symptoms start.

Depression—see note in Pegasys (may be serious enough to require stopping the medicine).

Decrease or loss of vision (optic neuritis, macular edema, retinal artery blood clots—reported (see vision check below with combination).

Muscle stiffness (rigors)—may be frequent with combination.

Heart attack—case reports for people who became anemic while taking ribavirin.

Low white blood cell counts: fever, sore throat, infection—possible (see Pegasys note regarding dosing).

Aggravation of excessively low or high thyroid function (hypo- or hyperthyroidism with combination).

Blood sugar changes—possible with combination.

Pancreatitis—possible with alfa interferon and ribavirin treatment.

Hemolytic anemia (Copegus)—may be frequent (see CBC note below for baseline, etc.).

Decreased platelets—possible (see note in Pegasys profile).

Bloody diarrhea—possible with combination.

Lung problems (pneumonia, interstitial pneumonitis, others)—reported as aggravated or caused by combination.

Aggravation of or development of autoimmune problems (muscle inflammation (myositis), rheumatoid arthritis, systemic lupus erythematosus, others)—possible with combination.

▷ **Possible Effects on Sexual Function:** Animals treated with ribavirin had lowered sperm counts, but no apparent change in fertility. Pegasys may impair fertility in some women. Female cynomolgus monkeys experience amenorrhea or prolonged menstrual cycles.

Adverse Effects That May Mimic Natural Diseases or Disorders

Mood changes, depression may suggest a psychotic disorder from combined use.

Dropping neutrophils (ANC) may mimic other hematologic problems, yet actually be an adverse drug reaction from the Pegasys form during combined use.

Natural Diseases or Disorders That May Be Activated by This Drug
Latent or subclinical depression, epilepsy, incipient congestive heart failure (combined use).

Possible Effects on Laboratory Tests (combined use)
Development of neutralizing antibodies—rare.
Development of binding antibodies—infrequent.
Liver function tests: increased (ALT, bilirubin, others)
White blood cells (neutrophils): lowered ANC.
Hemoglobin: may be decreased.
Triglycerides: increased (frequent).
Platelets: may be decreased.
Blood sugar changes.
Amylase and/or lipase: increased.

CAUTION
1. Talk to your doctor if you or your significant other or a family member notices that you are starting to become depressed (see note on depression in dosing), or think about suicide. This medicine can be a cause of severe depression.
2. While this medicine can successfully attack the hepatitis C virus (particularly in combination with ribavirin), serious possible adverse effects require follow-up and laboratory testing while taking this medicine.
3. Call your doctor if you have trouble breathing, a change in vision or unusual bleeding or bruising.
4. Call 911 if you start to have severe chest pain (some cardiovascular problems have been associated with Pegasys).
5. Negative pregnancy test before starting treatment, two forms of birth control for females and use of a condom for males required while taking this combination. Call your doctor immediately if you become pregnant (see pregnancy note).
6. You develop an ongoing or increasing temperature, sore throat, or other signs of an infection.
7. Triglycerides may be increased. Talk to your doctor about this.

Precautions for Use
By Infants and Children: Safety and effectiveness for those under 18 not established.
By Those Over 60 Years of Age: Some of the measures of how Pegasys is distributed in the body (area under the curve—AUC and half life) were increased or prolonged in people more than 60. Adverse effects from this medicine may be more pronounced in this patient population. Prudent to follow the patient more carefully, and adjust dosing based on undesirable signs and symptoms. Patients over 65 were NOT included in Copegus clinical studies. Because of age-related kidney compromise, risk of adverse effects may be greater in this population if given ribavirin.

▷ **Advisability of Use During Pregnancy**
Pregnancy Category: X for Copegus, C for Pegasys. See Pregnancy Risk Categories at the back of this book.
Animal Studies: Significant teratogenic effects in all animal species where tested as well as embryocidal effects.
Human Studies: Adequate studies of pregnant women are not available.
A negative pregnancy test BEFORE starting this medicine and TWO forms of birth control while taking this medicine and for at least six months AFTER STOPPING it are needed. Male partners of women taking this medicine

are advised to use a condom. Not to be taken in pregnancy. Talk to your doctor about how to address the issue of pregnancy and the possible transmission of hepatitis C. If you DO become pregnant, YOU or YOUR DOCTOR should call 1-800-526-6367.

Advisability of Use If Breast-Feeding

Presence of this drug in breast milk: Not defined.

Blood and body fluids may transfer the hepatitis C virus. Breast-feeding is NOT advisable.

Habit-Forming Potential: None.

Effects of Overdose: Management of the symptoms that a patient has at the time that they are seen by a doctor (symptomatic management).

Possible Effects of Long-Term Use: See anemia, white blood cell, and platelet notes for Pegasys.

Suggested Periodic Examinations While Taking This Drug (at physician's discretion—combination use)

Hepatitis C RNA testing (PCR) before (baseline) and periodically during treatment

Vision testing/eye exam before (baseline) treatment.

Complete blood counts, ANC (baseline, two weeks, four weeks).

Liver biopsy may be needed for some patients, possibly before and during treatment.

Thyroid stimulating hormone (TSH).

Liver (ALT, AST, and bilirubin) before treatment (baseline) and usually every two months.

Kidney function tests.

Amylase and lipase.

Blood sugar, A1C.

Evaluation of heart function at baseline (before therapy) and periodically.

Baseline pregnancy test in females of childbearing age.

Checks for signs and symptoms of depression such as appetite, change in pleasure gained from usually pleasurable activities, or administration of typical depression inventories such as the Hamilton Depression Scale (Ham-D).

Author's Note: Baseline blood and biochemical tests and pregnancy tests for females are needed. Once treatment is started, blood (hematological) tests are checked at 2 and 4 weeks, and repeat biochemical testing done at 4 weeks. In clinical trials, CBC and chemistries (including liver function tests and uric acid) were checked at weeks 1 and 2, 4, 6 and 8. For ongoing treatment, testing was done every four weeks. Testing was obtained more frequently if abnormal results were obtained. TSH was checked every twelve weeks. Pregnancy testing was checked before therapy was started, during combination therapy was checked monthly and for six months after the medicine was stopped.

▷ **While Taking This Drug, Observe the Following**

Foods: Taking Pegasys with a high-fat meal increases the amount that gets into your body. Talk to your doctor about how he or she would like you to take this medicine. Use of smaller, more nutrient dense meals may help provide nutrition while acting as a coping mechanism for nausea. Ribavirin should be taken with food.

Herbal Medicines or Minerals: Some herbal medicines such as eucalyptus, kava, and valerian have possible toxic effects on the liver. These herbals should

NOT be taken, both because of the viral presence in the liver and because of possible additive undesirable effects on the liver.

Beverages: No restrictions. May be taken with milk.

▷ *Alcohol:* Since alcohol can add to liver problems, any use should be discussed with your doctor for Pegasys. DO NOT drink while taking the combination.

Tobacco Smoking: No interactions expected. I advise everyone to quit smoking.

Marijuana Smoking: Added dizziness.

▷ *Other Drugs*

Peginterferon alpha-2a *taken concurrently* with

- didanosine (Videx) is NOT recommended for the combination or for Pegasys alone. Increased risk of fatal liver failure, pancreatitis, lactic acidosis, and/or peripheral neuropathy preclude this.
- medicines known to have toxic effects on the liver would be best avoided if possible due to overlapping undesirable effects on the liver. Some combinations may represent a benefit-to-risk decision.
- medicines removed by a liver enzyme called CYP 450 1A2 may be increased to toxic levels because peginterferon inhibits this enzyme. Checking blood levels of the medicines combined with peginterferon that undergo such removal is prudent, with dosing adjustments based on blood levels.

Peginterferon alpha-2a and ribavirin *taken concurrently* with

- stavudine (Zerit) or zidovudine (AZT) may blunt the antiviral benefits of these two HIV medicines. The stavudine combination may lead to a serious and sometimes fatal metabolic complication (lactic acidosis).

▷ *Driving, Hazardous Activities:* May cause dizziness, blurred vision, or fatigue. Use caution and assess the extent of these possible undesirable effects BEFORE undertaking such activities.

Aviation Note: The use of this drug *may be a disqualification* for piloting. Consult a designated Aviation Medical Examiner.

Exposure to Sun: No restrictions.

Special Storage Instructions: For Pegasys: care must be taken for proper disposal of needles and avoidance of possible needle sticks by caregivers. The medicine itself should be stored in a refrigerator with a temperature of 36–46°F., (2–8°C.) because lack of refrigeration can break down the medicine. DO NOT SHAKE the bottle as this can also inactivate the medicine. Protect the medicine from light and also make certain that the medicine is not frozen. It is important NOT to leave the medicine out of the refrigerator for more than a day. Once you have drawn up a dose from a given vial of medicine, throw the rest of the medicine in the vial away. Please note the CEPC characteristics of the medicine in dosing instructions for Pegasys. For ribavirin tablets, storage at room temperature is fine.

Discontinuation: See notes on white blood cell, platelet counts, liver function tests, and time that the medicine should be given to work in the Pegasys profile above. Talk to your doctor BEFORE making any changes in dosing or stopping this medicine or the combination.

RIFABUTIN (RIF a byu tin)

Introduced: 1993   **Class:**   Antimycobacterial agent (antitubercular)
Prescription: USA: Yes   **Controlled Drug:**   USA: No; Canada: No
Available as Generic: USA: No; Canada: No
Brand Name: Mycobutin

Warning: Rifabutin prophylaxis must not be taken by people with active tuberculosis.

BENEFITS versus RISKS

Possible Benefits	*Possible Risks*
PREVENTION OF DISSEMINATED MYCOBACTERIUM AVIUM-INTRACELLULARE COMPLEX IN PEOPLE WITH ADVANCED HIV INFECTION	NEUTROPENIA Low platelet counts

---

▷ **Principal Uses**

As a Single Drug Product: Uses currently included in FDA-approved labeling: (1) Prevention of disseminated *Mycobacterium avium-intracellulare* complex in patients with advanced HIV infection; (2) combination treatment of *Mycobacterium avium-intracellulare* complex infection.

Other (unlabeled) generally accepted uses: (1) Some clinicians are using rifabutin in cases of resistant *H. Pylori* that can cause stomach ulcers; (2) early data for use as part of combination treatment of Crohn's disease.

How This Drug Works: Rifabutin inhibits DNA-dependent RNA polymerase (an enzyme critical to cells that are dividing) in *E. coli*. The exact mechanism of action of rifabutin in *Mycobacterium avium* or *Mycobacterium avium-intracellulare* complex is not known.

▷ **Widely Used Guidelines That Involve This Medicine (representative sample):** Please look at the section at the very beginning of this profile called "Class." Next, turn to Table 22 and you will find guidelines listed by the class involved!

Available Dosage Forms and Strengths

Capsules (Mycobutin) — 150 mg

How to Store: Keep at room temperature, and avoid exposure to excessive humidity.

▷ **Recommended Dose Ranges** (Actual dose and schedule must be determined for each patient individually.)

Infants and Children: Safety and effectiveness of rifabutin in *Mycobacterium avium-intracellulare* complex prophylaxis has not been clearly established. Safety data comes from a trial of 22 children who were HIV positive.

Infants 1 Year of Age: 18.5 mg per kg of body mass per day.

Children 2–10 Years: 8.6 mg per kg of body mass per day.

Adolescents up to 14 years: 4.0 mg per kg of body mass per day.

14 to 60 Years of Age: 300 mg once a day. Those prone to nausea and vomiting may take 150 mg two times a day with food.

Over 60 Years of Age: Same as 14 to 60 years of age.

Conditions Requiring Dosing Adjustments

Liver Function: At present, clear adjustments of dose in hepatic compromise are not defined, but the drug should be used with caution.

Kidney Function: Elimination of rifabutin may actually be increased in people with compromised kidneys, although the clinical effect is as yet unknown.

Author's Note: The information in this profile has been shortened to make room for more widely used medicines.

RIFAMPIN (ri FAM pin)

Other Name: Rifampicin

Introduced: 1967   **Class:**   Antibiotic,   rifamycins   **Prescription:**
USA: Yes   **Controlled Drug:**   USA: No; Canada: No   **Available as**
Generic: Yes

Brand Names: Rifadin, Rifadin IV, Rifamate [CD], Rifater [CD], Rimactane,
Rimactane/INH Dual Pack [CD], ✚Rofact

```
┌─────────────────────────────────────────────────────────────────┐
│                       BENEFITS versus RISKS                        │
│        Possible Benefits              Possible Risks               │
│  EFFECTIVE TREATMENT OF          DRUG-INDUCED KIDNEY OR            │
│    TUBERCULOSIS IN                 LIVER DAMAGE                     │
│    COMBINATION WITH OTHER        Blood cell or coagulation disorders│
│    DRUGS                         Colitis (pseudomembranous)        │
│  EFFECTIVE PREVENTION OF                                           │
│    MENINGITIS                                                      │
│  COMBINATION TREATMENT OF                                          │
│    SOME STAPH INFECTIONS                                           │
└─────────────────────────────────────────────────────────────────┘
```

▷ **Principal Uses**

As a Single Drug Product: Uses currently included in FDA-approved labeling:
(1) Treats active tuberculosis—usually given concurrently with other antitubercular drugs to enhance its effectiveness; (2) also used to eliminate the
meningitis germ (meningococcus) from the throats of healthy carriers so
that it cannot be spread to others; (3) treats tuberculosis in coal workers
(good results combined with other antitubercular drugs); (4) used to prevent tuberculosis in people exposed to patients with active disease; (5)
helps prevent meningitis in patients exposed to Neisseria meningitides
(best if used within 24 hours of diagnosis of the case from which the person was exposed).

Other (unlabeled) generally accepted uses: (1) Second-line agent in combination with doxycycline in treatment of brucellosis; (2) has a place in preventing *Haemophilus influenzae* infections in people exposed to patients
with active disease; (3) combination therapy of lepromatous leprosy; (4)
used with cotrimoxazole to eliminate methicillin-resistant Staphylococcus
aureus (MRSA) from people who have the bacteria; (5) used with other
drugs to treat Staph endocarditis; (6) can be an additional antibiotic in a
multiple drug regimen for treating anthrax; (7) part of combination therapy (with ofloxacin) in diabetic bone infection (osteomyelitis) in the foot.

As a Combination Drug Product [CD]: This drug is available in combination
with isoniazid and pyrazinamide, additional drugs that delay development
of drug-resistant strains of the tuberculosis germ (Rifater). It is also combined with isoniazid in a double combination form for the same reason
(Rifamate).

In the Pipeline: The Health and Human Services secretary has identified a group
of medicines to be tested for use in children. Rifampin was on that list of
the 12 highest priority medicines to be studied in children (find out more
at *www.hhs.gov/news/press/2003pres/20030121.html*).

How This Drug Works: This drug prevents the growth and multiplication of susceptible tuberculosis organisms by blocking specific enzyme systems that are involved in the formation of essential proteins.

▷ **Widely Used Guidelines That Involve This Medicine (representative sample):** Please look at the section at the very beginning of this profile called "Class." Next, turn to Table 22 and you will find guidelines listed by the class involved!

Available Dosage Forms and Strengths
Capsules — 150 mg, 300 mg

▷ **Usual Adult Dosage Ranges**
For Tuberculosis: 10 mg per kg of body mass per day, up to 600 mg once daily. Initial (empiric) therapy involves combination treatment until the sensitivity pattern of the tuberculosis mycobacteria that is causing the infection is known. After this, rifampin is combined with isoniazid and pyrazinamide for the first 2 months and isoniazid and rifampin are then continued in the subsequent 4 months (longer depending on the site of the infection such as in bone).

For Meningococcus carriers: 600 mg every 12 hours for two days or 600 mg once daily for 4 days. The total daily dose should not exceed 600 mg.

Note: Actual dose and schedule must be determined for each patient individually.

Conditions Requiring Dosing Adjustments
Liver Function: This drug can cause liver damage, and patients should be followed closely. In severe failure, the dose should be limited to 6 to 8 mg per kg of body mass twice a week.

Kidney Function: For patients with a creatinine clearance (see Glossary) of 10 to 50 mL/min, one researcher suggests that 50% to 100% of the usual dose should be given.

▷ **Dosing Instructions:** This drug is preferably taken with 8 ounces of water on an empty stomach (1 hour before or 2 hours after eating). However, it may be taken with food if necessary to reduce stomach irritation. The capsule may be opened and the contents mixed with applesauce or jelly to take it. Solution form (Australia) should be dosed using a dosing cup or calibrated measuring spoon. If you forget a dose: Take the missed dose as soon as you remember it, unless it's nearly time for your next dose—if that is the case, skip the missed dose and take the next dose right on schedule. DO NOT double doses. Talk with your doctor if you find yourself missing doses.

Usual Duration of Use: Use on a regular schedule for several months usually determines effectiveness in promoting recovery from tuberculosis. Long-term use requires ongoing physician supervision and periodic evaluation.

Typical Treatment Goals and Measurements (Outcomes and Markers)
Infections: The most commonly used measures of serious infections are white blood cell counts and differentials (the kind of blood cells that occur most often in your blood), and temperature. In tuberculosis, clinicians start four medicines for the 8 weeks it typically takes for sputum specimens containing this organism to grow to reveal their sensitivity patterns. While clinicians look for positive changes in 24–48 hours in typical infections, tuberculosis REQUIRES long-term treatment to kill it. NEVER stop an antibiotic because you start to feel better. The goals and time frame (see peak benefits above) should be discussed with you when the prescription is written.

▷ **This Drug Should Not Be Taken If**
   • you have had an allergic reaction to it previously.

▷ **Inform Your Physician Before Taking This Drug If**
   • you are pregnant.
   • you have a history of liver disease or impaired liver function.
   • you have active liver disease.
   • you consume alcohol daily.
   • you are taking an oral contraceptive—an alternate method of contraception is advised.
   • you are taking an anticoagulant.

Possible Side Effects (natural, expected, and unavoidable drug actions)
   Red, orange, or brown discoloration of tears, sweat, saliva, sputum, urine, or stool. Yellow coloring of the skin (not jaundice). **Note:** In the absence of illness symptoms, any discoloration is a harmless drug effect and does not mean toxicity. Possible fungal superinfections (see Glossary).

▷ **Possible Adverse Effects** (unusual, unexpected, and infrequent reactions)
   If any of the following develop, consult your physician promptly for guidance.
   Mild Adverse Effects
   Allergic reactions: skin rash syndrome, hives, itching, drug fever (see Glossary).
   Headache, dizziness, blurred vision, impaired hearing, vague numbness, and tingling—infrequent.
   Joint and muscle pain—infrequent and often subsides after a few weeks.
   Loss of appetite, heartburn, nausea, vomiting, abdominal cramps, diarrhea—infrequent.
   Serious Adverse Effects
   Serious skin problems (Stevens-Johnson syndrome or toxic epidermal necrolysis)—case reports.
   Flu-like syndrome: fever, headache, dizziness, musculoskeletal pain, difficult breathing—case reports.
   Drug-induced liver damage, with or without jaundice—frequent.
   Kidney damage—infrequent.
   Drug-induced porphyria, pancreatitis, gallstones, or pseudomembranous colitis—case reports.
   Excessively low blood platelet count: abnormal bleeding or bruising—rare.
   Blood-clotting problems (disseminated intravascular coagulopathy)—case report.
   Hemolytic anemia—case reports.
   Suppression of the adrenal gland—possible.
   Some case reports have been made regarding lung tumors (pulmonary malignancies). Cause-and-effect relationship not defined.

▷ **Possible Effects on Sexual Function:** Altered timing and pattern of menstruation—case reports.
   Decreased effectiveness of oral contraceptives.

▷ **Adverse Effects That May Mimic Natural Diseases or Disorders**
   Liver reactions may suggest viral hepatitis. Kidney reactions may suggest an infectious nephritis.

Possible Effects on Laboratory Tests
   Complete blood cell counts: decreased red cells, hemoglobin, white cells, and platelets; increased eosinophils (allergic reaction).
   INR (protime): increased (when taken with warfarin).

Liver function tests: increased liver enzymes (ALT/GPT, AST/GOT, and alkaline phosphatase), increased bilirubin.

CAUTION

1. This drug may permanently discolor soft contact lenses.
2. This drug may reduce the effects of oral contraceptives—pregnancy could occur. An alternate method of contraception is advised.
3. Resistance may develop rapidly if this drug is used alone to treat tuberculosis. Only use with other antitubercular drugs.
4. TAKE THE FULL course prescribed; this may be many months.

Precautions for Use

By Infants and Children: Monitor closely for possible liver toxicity or deficiency of blood platelets.

By Those Over 60 Years of Age: Natural changes in body composition and function make you more susceptible to the adverse effects of this drug. Report promptly any indications of possible drug toxicity.

▷ **Advisability of Use During Pregnancy**

Pregnancy Category: C. See Pregnancy Risk Categories at the back of this book.
Animal Studies: Cleft palate and spinal defects reported in rodent studies.
Human Studies: Adequate studies of pregnant women are not available.
   If possible, avoid use of drug during the first 3 months.

Advisability of Use If Breast-Feeding

Presence of this drug in breast milk: Yes, but to a small extent (0.05% of the mother's dose goes to the breast milk in 24 hours in one study).
   Talk to your doctor about this decision.

Habit-Forming Potential: None.

Effects of Overdose: Nausea, vomiting, drowsiness, unconsciousness, severe liver damage, jaundice.

Possible Effects of Long-Term Use: Superinfections, fungal overgrowth of mouth or tongue.

Suggested Periodic Examinations While Taking This Drug (at physician's discretion)

Complete blood cell counts.
Liver and kidney function tests (frequent liver tests if used with pyrazinamide). Chest X-ray, sputum culture.
Hearing acuity tests if hearing loss is suspected.

▷ **While Taking This Drug, Observe the Following**

Foods: No restrictions.

Herbal Medicines or Minerals: Some patients use echinacea to attempt to boost their immune systems. Unfortunately, use of echinacea is not recommended in people with damaged immune systems. This herb may also actually weaken any immune system if it is used too often or for too long a time. DO NOT take mistletoe herb, oak bark, or F.C. of marshmallow root, woody nightshade stem, or licorice.

Beverages: No restrictions.

▷ *Alcohol:* It is best to avoid alcohol completely to reduce the risk of liver toxicity.

Tobacco Smoking: No specific drug interactions expected, but adding smoke to lungs already compromised by a serious infection is not prudent. I advise everyone to quit smoking.

▷ *Other Drugs*

Rifampin *taken concurrently* with
   • halothane anesthesia may result in serious liver damage.

Rifampin may *decrease* the effects of
- amiodarone (Cordarone).
- amprenavir (Agenerase), atazanavir (Reyataz), indinavir (Crixivan), and nelfinavir (Viracept).
- antianxiety agents such as diazepam and perhaps other benzodiazepines (see Drug Classes).
- anticoagulants such as warfarin (Coumadin).
- anticonvulsant drugs such as phenytoin (Dilantin).
- barbiturates (see Drug Classes).
- BCG live-attenuated vaccine.
- beta blockers such as metoprolol or propranolol (see Drug Classes).
- birth control pills (oral contraceptives).
- buspirone (Buspar).
- some calcium channel blockers (see Drug Classes).
- carbamazepine (Tegretol)—may lead to carbamazepine toxicity.
- carvedilol (Coreg).
- caspofungin (Cancidas).
- chloramphenicol (Chloromycetin).
- clofibrate (Atromid-S).
- clozapine (Clozaril).
- cortisonelike drugs (see Drug Classes).
- cyclosporine (Sandimmune).
- dapsone.
- delavirdine (Rescriptor).
- digitalis preparations (Lanoxin, others).
- disopyramide (Norpace).
- donepezil (Aricept).
- doxycycline (various).
- enalapril (Vasotec).
- fluconazole (Diflucan), itraconazole (Sporanox), ketoconazole (Nizoral), or voriconazole (Vfend).
- fluvastatin (Lescol).
- fosphenytoin (Cerebyx).
- some HMG-CoA reductase inhibitors (fluvastatin).
- imatinib (Gleevec).
- leflunomide (Arava).
- losartan (Cozaar).
- methadone (Dolophine).
- metoprolol (Lopressor).
- mexiletine (Mexitil).
- montelukast (Singulair).
- narcotics such as methadone (see Opioids in Drug Classes).
- nelfinavir (Viracept).
- nevirapine (Viramune).
- nicardipine (Cardene).
- nifedipine (Adalat).
- olanzapine (Zyprexa).
- oral hypoglycemic agents (sulfonylureas such as tolbutamide: see Drug Classes).
- phenytoin (Dilantin).
- progestins.
- propafenone (Rythmol).
- quinidine (Quinaglute, others).

- repaglinide (Prandin).
- ritonavir (Norvir)—this combination may also lead to rifampin toxicity.
- rofecoxib (Vioxx).
- sertraline (Zoloft).
- sildenafil (Viagra), vardenafil (Levitra), and tadalafil (Cialis).
- sirolimus (Rapamune) or tacrolimus (Prograf).
- theophylline (Theo-Dur, others).
- tocainide (Tonocard).
- tretinoin (Vesanoid).
- tricyclic antidepressants (see Drug Classes).
- trimexate (Neutrexin).
- verapamil (Verelan).
- warfarin (Coumadin); increased INR testing is needed.
- zaleplon (Sonata).
- zidovudine (AZT); the therapeutic effect will be lessened by a decreased drug level.
- zolpidem (Ambien).

The following drug may *decrease* the effects of rifampin:

- para-aminosalicylic acid (PAS) may reduce its antitubercular effectiveness.

▷ *Driving, Hazardous Activities:* This drug may cause dizziness, drowsiness, impaired vision, and impaired hearing. Restrict activities as necessary.

Aviation Note: The use of this drug *may be a disqualification* for piloting. Consult a designated Aviation Medical Examiner.

Exposure to Sun: No restrictions.

Discontinuation: It is advisable not to interrupt or stop this drug without consulting your physician. Intermittent use can increase risk of developing allergic reactions.

RISEDRONATE (RIH seh druh nate)

Introduced: 1999 **Class:** Third-generation bisphosphonate **Prescription:** USA: Yes **Controlled Drug:** USA: No **Available as Generic:** No

Brand Name: Actonel

BENEFITS versus RISKS	
Possible Benefits	*Possible Risks*
TREATMENT OF POST-MENOPAUSAL OSTEOPOROSIS	DIARRHEA
TREATS AND PREVENTS CORTICOSTEROID-CAUSED OSTEOPOROSIS	Irritation of the esophagus
SYMPTOM RELIEF IN PAGET'S DISEASE	Minor flu-like symptoms
MORE POTENT THAN PREVIOUSLY AVAILABLE BISPHOSPHONATES	

▷ **Principal Uses**

As a Single Drug Product: Uses currently included in FDA-approved labeling: (1) Treatment of postmenopausal osteoporosis; (2) treatment of Paget's disease; (3) prevention and treatment of corticosteroid-induced osteoporosis.

Other (unlabeled) generally accepted uses: None at present.

How This Drug Works: This medicine works at the brush border of the osteoclast cell. This prevents this cell from resorbing (gobbling up) bone while the osteoblast (bone-building cell) continues to work. This results in bone building and decreased fracture risk.

▷ **Widely Used Guidelines That Involve This Medicine (representative sample):** Please look at the section at the very beginning of this profile called "Class." Next, turn to Table 22 and you will find guidelines listed by the class involved!

Available Dosage Forms and Strengths

Tablets — 30 mg

Author's Note: Information in this profile will be broadened as more data are available and clinical studies are completed. A head-to-head clinical trial of risedronate and alendronate is underway.

RISPERIDONE (RIS peer i dohn)

Introduced: 1993, 2003, 2003 for M-tab form **Class:** Antipsychotic agent **Prescription:** USA: Yes **Controlled Drug:** USA: No; Canada: No **Available as Generic:** USA: No; Canada: No

Brand Names: Risperdal, Risperdal CONSTA, Risperdal M-tab

BENEFITS versus RISKS	
Possible Benefits	*Possible Risks*
TREATMENT OF SCHIZOPHRENIA REFRACTORY TO OTHER AGENTS	INCREASED RISK OF CEREBROVASCULAR PROBLEMS (including stroke) in elderly, dementia patients
DECREASED SIDE EFFECTS COMPARED TO OTHER AVAILABLE DRUGS	BLOOD SUGAR CHANGES (HYPERGLYCEMIA)
EFFECTIVE TREATMENT OF CERTAIN PSYCHOTIC DISORDERS	Involuntary movement disorder Neuroleptic malignant syndrome Change in heart function (in the elderly)
M-TAB FORM OFFERS THE ABILITY TO TAKE THE MEDICINE WITHOUT NEEDING WATER	
RISPERDAL CONSTA FORM IS THE FIRST ATYPICAL ANTIPSYCHOTIC AVAILABLE IN A LONG-ACTING FORMULATION	
May have a role in easing agitation in dementia patients	

▷ **Principal Uses**

As a Single Drug Product: Uses currently included in FDA-approved labeling: (1) Manages psychotic disorders such as chronic schizophrenia; (2) treats AIDS-related psychosis.

Other (unlabeled) generally accepted uses: (1) Eases behavioral difficulties associated with autism; (2) treatment of aggression; (3) treatment of Tourette's syndrome; (4) can have a role in helping behavioral problems in people with mental retardation; (5) helps treatment-resistant obsessive-compulsive disorder and catatonia; (6) eased psychiatric problems associated with levodopa in one small study of Parkinson's patients.

How This Drug Works: Balances two nerve transmitters (dopamine and serotonin), helping restore more normal thinking and mood.

▷ **Widely Used Guidelines That Involve This Medicine (representative sample):** Please look at the section at the very beginning of this profile called "Class." Next, turn to Table 22 and you will find guidelines listed by the class involved!

Available Dosage Forms and Strengths

Oral solution — 1 mg/mL

Tablets, orally disintegrating — 0.5 mg, 1 mg, 2 mg

Tablets — 0.25 mg, 0.5 mg, 1 mg, 2 mg, 3 mg, 4 mg, 5 mg

▷ **Recommended Dose Ranges** (Actual dose and schedule must be determined for each patient individually.)

Infants and Children: Safety and efficacy for those less than 18 years of age are not established.

18 to 60 Years of Age: Past starting dose was 1 mg taken twice daily (to avoid first-dose problems seen with alpha adrenoceptor antagonists). Approved dosing has shown doses up to 8 mg taken once a day to be effective. Doses in the twice-daily (BID) approach may be started as 1 mg twice daily and increased as needed and tolerated by 1 mg on the second and third day, for a total of 3 mg twice daily by the third day. If further dose changes are needed, they should be made at 1-week intervals. Doses greater than 8 mg per day are not recommended. Doses more than 16 mg a day have not been studied. If the once-a-day or twice-a-day approach is used, it is prudent (given other medical conditions) for some patients to be started on lower doses and more slowly increased than others.

Over 60 Years of Age: Therapy is started with 0.5 mg twice daily. The dose is increased if needed and tolerated by 0.5 mg twice daily. Doses greater than 1.5 mg daily are achieved by small increases made at 1-week intervals. Careful attention must be paid to blood pressure and development of adverse effects.

Conditions Requiring Dosing Adjustments

Liver Function: The starting dose must be decreased and adjusted as for those over 60 years old. Additionally, there may be an increased amount of the active drug that results from each dose (increased free fraction), and, as such, a greater than expected effect may be seen.

Kidney Function: The starting dose must be decreased and adjusted as for those over 60 years old.

▷ **Dosing Instructions:** The original tablet may be crushed, and the medication's effect is not changed by food. Water is the best liquid to take this medicine with. M-tab form dissolves without water. Measuring pipettes (calibrated) are provided with the liquid form. Cola or tea is NOT compatible with the liquid (solution) form (coffee, orange juice, low-fat milk, or water is okay). If you forget a dose: Take the missed dose as soon as you remember it, unless it's nearly time for your next dose—if that is the case, skip the missed dose and take the next dose right on schedule. DO

NOT double doses. Talk with your doctor if you find yourself missing doses as there are a lot of timers and even beeper-based systems to help you.

Usual Duration of Use: Use on a regular schedule for 1 to 2 weeks usually determines effectiveness in helping control chronic schizophrenia. Ongoing use must be individualized. If the need for ongoing use is established, the lowest effective dose should be used. Periodic physician evaluation of response and dose is required.

Typical Treatment Goals and Measurements (Outcomes and Markers)

Psychosis: The general goal: to lessen the degree and severity of abnormal thinking, letting patients return to their daily lives. Specific measures of psychosis may involve testing or inventories (and can be valuable in helping check benefits from this medicine).

Possible Advantages of This Drug

Treatment of schizophrenia resistant (refractory) to other therapy. Probably a drug of choice in older adults. The M-tab form offers convenience, ease of swallowing for patients with swallowing problems, and dosing flexibility. This form also helps in some psychiatric settings where patients may be trying to avoid taking their medicine by "cheeking" their pills. Risperdal consta form is the first atypical antipsychotic to be formulated in a long-acting form.

▷ **This Drug Should Not Be Taken If**
- you had an allergic reaction to it previously.
- you had neuroleptic malignant syndrome (ask your doctor).
- you have excessive prolactin in your blood (hyperprolactinemia—talk to your doctor).

▷ **Inform Your Physician Before Taking This Drug If**
- you have a history of breast cancer.
- you have liver or kidney compromise.
- you have a history of prediabetes or diabetes.
- you are pregnant or plan to become pregnant or are breast-feeding your infant.
- you have had tardive dyskinesia in the past.
- you have a history of Parkinson's disease or seizures.
- you have a history of heart rhythm disturbances (especially QTc prolongation).
- you are unsure how much to take or how often to take it.

Possible Side Effects (natural, expected, and unavoidable drug actions)

Increased prolactin levels may result in male and female breast tenderness and swelling.

Sleepiness.

Orthostatic hypotension (see Glossary)—rare.

Weight gain—may be frequent (18% in one source).

▷ **Possible Adverse Effects** (unusual, unexpected, and infrequent reactions)

If any of the following develop, consult your physician promptly for guidance.

Mild Adverse Effects

Allergic reaction: skin rash.

Difficulty in concentrating—rare.

Headache or increased dreaming—rare to infrequent.

Constipation, diarrhea, or nausea—infrequent.

Palpitations, edema—rare.

Increased urination—rare.

Serious Adverse Effects

Allergic reactions: anaphylactic reactions.

Abnormal heart function (prolonged QTc interval, PACs, others)—rare.

Tardive dyskinesia (see Glossary) or neuroleptic malignant syndrome—case reports.

Chest pain/myocarditis—rare.

Parkinsonian tremor—case report.

Low sodium—rare.

Opioid withdrawal—case reports in two patients taking opioid (narcotics).

Paresthesia—case reports.

Seizures—rare.

Cerebrovascular problems (stroke, TIA, etc.)—increased risk in elderly, dementia patients (not an approved use).

Lowered white blood cells or platelets—case reports.

Like all atypical antipsychotic medicines—risk of increased blood sugar and diabetes has been reported—incidence unknown.

Abnormal liver function—rare.

Pancreatitis—case reports.

▷ **Possible Effects on Sexual Function:** Diminished sexual desire; delayed or absent orgasm; erectile dysfunction including priapism; male (gynecomastia) breast tenderness or swelling; dry vagina or menstrual changes (hypermenorrhea)—rare. Ejaculation failure—case reports and may be dose-related. Female breast (galactorrhea) milk excretion in the absence of pregnancy—infrequent.

Possible Delayed Adverse Effects: Swelling and tenderness of male and female breast tissue.

Natural Diseases or Disorders That May Be Activated by This Drug: Some human cancers depend on prolactin for growth, and since risperidone increases prolactin, it should be used with *CAUTION* by people with previously diagnosed breast cancer.

Possible Effects on Laboratory Tests

Liver Function Tests: increased SGPT, SGOT, and LDH.

Complete Blood Counts: decreased platelets, white blood cells, and hemoglobin.

Prolactin: increased.

Blood sugar: may be increased.

CAUTION

1. This drug should be used with great caution in patients with diabetes and in patients with breast cancer.
2. Call your doctor promptly if you have an increased tendency to infection or abnormal bleeding or bruising while taking this drug.
3. This drug should be used with great caution, if at all, by patients with a history of seizures.
4. Increased risk of cerebrovascular problems (such as stroke, TIAs) in elderly patients with dementia.

Precautions for Use

By Infants and Children: Safety and effectiveness for those under 18 years of age are not established.

By Those Over 60 Years of Age: The starting dose of 0.5 mg twice daily is used for patients who are elderly or debilitated, and slower increases in dose as needed and tolerated are indicated. Great care should be taken in patients with heart disease. You may be more likely to experience postural hypotension (see Glossary) and problems with motor skills. Those with prostate problems may have increased risk of urine retention.

▷ **Advisability of Use During Pregnancy**

Pregnancy Category: C. See Pregnancy Risk Categories at the back of this book.

Animal Studies: Increased rat pup death during the first few days of lactation.

Human Studies: Adequate studies of pregnant women are not available. One case report of lack of formation of the corpus callosum of the brain in a fetus exposed to this drug while in the uterus.

Ask your doctor for guidance.

Advisability of Use If Breast-Feeding

Presence of this drug in breast milk: Yes.

Avoid drug or refrain from nursing.

Habit-Forming Potential: None, but a withdrawal syndrome associated with mania has been reported.

Effects of Overdose: Drowsiness, hypotension, tachycardia, low sodium and potassium, ECG changes (prolonged QT interval), and seizure.

Suggested Periodic Examinations While Taking This Drug (at physician's discretion)

Liver function tests.

Electrolytes (sodium and potassium).

ECG.

Prolactin levels.

▷ **While Taking This Drug, Observe the Following**

Foods: No restrictions.

Herbal Medicines or Minerals: Data from a small study of forty patients (see Emsley, R. in Sources) found that add-on therapy with one of the components of fish oil (eicosapentanoic acid or EPA) helped schizophrenic patients (Positive and Negative Syndrome Scale scores) and was well-tolerated (also has a heart benefit).

Since risperidone and St. John's wort may act to increase serotonin, the combination is not advised. St. John's wort may also worsen sensitivity to the sun. Ma huang and yohimbe are also best avoided while taking this medicine. Because part of the way that ginkgo and ginseng work is as an MAO inhibitor, DO NOT combine with risperidone. Evening primrose oil can increase risk of seizures. Combination is NOT recommended.

Beverages: No restrictions.

▷ *Alcohol:* Patients should avoid alcohol while taking risperidone.

Tobacco Smoking: No interactions expected. I advise everyone to quit smoking.

Marijuana Smoking: Increased somnolence.

▷ *Other Drugs*

Risperidone may *decrease* the effects of

• levodopa (Sinemet, others).

Risperidone *taken concurrently* with

• bupropion (Zyban, Wellbutrin) can lead to increased blood levels and toxicity from "normal" doses of risperidone. Caution, careful patient monitoring, and possible dose reductions are prudent if these medicines must be combined.

• carbamazepine (Tegretol) will decrease the drug level and perhaps the therapeutic effects of risperidone.

- other centrally acting medicines may result in increased central effects.
- clozapine (Clozaril) may decrease the therapeutic effects of risperidone.
- lithium (Lithobid, others) may lead to increased adverse effects.
- medicines that inhibit the liver enzyme Cytochrome P450 2D6 will increase risperidone levels and may lead to toxicity with "normal" doses. Medicines that increase cytochrome P450 2D6 will blunt the benefits of risperidone.
- medicines such as class I, IA, or III antiarrhythmics such as amiodarone (Cordarone), clarithromycin, cotrimoxazole, dofetilide (Tikosyn), erythromycin, ondansetron, ziprazidone, zolmitriptan, and others may lead to prolongation of the QTc interval and undesirable heart rhythm effects such as Torsades de Pointes. Combination is not recommended.
- methadone (various) may decrease methadone levels and lead to withdrawal symptoms.
- paroxetine (Paxil) and perhaps other SSRIs may lead to serotonin syndrome.
- phenytoin (Dilantin) or fosphenytoin (Cerebyx) may decrease risperidone blood levels and blunt risperidone therapeutic benefits.
- propafenone (Rythmol) may lead to propafenone toxicity.
- ritonavir (Norvir) and perhaps other protease inhibitors (see Drug Classes) may lead to toxicity.
- tramadol (Ultram) may increase seizure risk.
- valproic acid (Depakene, Depakote) may increase valproic acid toxicity risk. Careful patient follow-up and more frequent blood levels are needed.
- venlafaxine (Effexor) may increase risperidone toxicity risk.
- zotepine (Nipolept) may increase seizure risk.

▷ *Driving, Hazardous Activities:* This drug may cause drowsiness and difficulty in concentrating. Restrict activities as necessary.

Aviation Note: The use of this drug **is a disqualification** for piloting. Consult a designated Aviation Medical Examiner.

Exposure to Sun: Use caution—this drug may cause photosensitivity.

Discontinuation: Consult your doctor before stopping this medication.

RIZATRIPTAN (rye zah TRIP tan)

Introduced: 1998 **Class:** Antimigraine, serotonin-1-receptor agonist
Prescription: USA: Yes **Controlled Drug:** USA: No; Canada: No
Available as Generic: USA: No; Canada: No
Brand Names: Maxalt, Maxalt-MLT, ✣Maxalt RPD

```
BENEFITS versus RISKS
        Possible Benefits                    Possible Risks
RAPID AND EFFECTIVE RELIEF OR   Fainting
  PREVENTION OF MIGRAINE        Small increases in blood pressure
GENERALLY WELL TOLERATED        Exacerbation of ischemic heart
Relieves photophobia (light       disease (should not be given to
  sensitivity)                    those patients)
Relieves phonophobia (sound     Not to be used in hemiplegic or
  sensitivity)                    basilar migraine
Relieves nausea and vomiting    Not to be used in significant
More potent than some of the other  cardiovascular disease
  "triptans" currently available
```

▷ **Principal Uses**

As a Single Drug Product: Uses currently included in FDA-approved labeling: Acute treatment of migraine with or without aura in adults.

Other (unlabeled) generally accepted uses: None at present.

How This Drug Works: Rizatriptan acts on blood vessels (by acting as a serotonin-1D agonist) to cause vasoconstriction (shrinking of the blood vessels). This relieves swelling, thought to be the cause of migraine. It is more potent dose-to-dose than sumatriptan (Imitrex).

Available Dosage Forms and Strengths

Tablets — 5 mg, 10 mg

Tablets, orally disintegrating (MLT) — 5 mg, 10 mg

Wafer, orally disintegrating (RPD) — 5 mg, 10 mg

Possible Advantages of This Drug: Offers a novel dosage form that is an orally disintegrating tablet. The convenience of this form makes it unobtrusive and easy to take. This medicine is more potent than sumatriptan (mg-to-mg) and may lead to better effects in stopping a migraine headache. Head-to-head trials are needed.

ROSUVASTATIN (Rah SUE vah statin)

Introduced: 2003   **Class:**   Cholesterol-lowering agent, HMG-CoA reductase inhibitor   **Prescription:**   USA: Yes   **Controlled Drug:**   USA: No; Canada: Not available   **Available as Generic:**   USA: No

Brand Name: Crestor

Author's Note: Due to availability of other agents and questions from one group regarding data on this medicine, this profile will not be broadened in this edition.

SALMETEROL (Sal ME Ter Ohl)

Introduced: 1994   **Class:**   Bronchodilator   **Prescription:**   USA: Yes   **Controlled Drug:**   USA: No; Canada: Not available   **Available as Generic:** USA: No

Brand Names: ❦Advair [CD], Advair Diskus, Aeromax, Serevent, Serevent Diskus

+--+
| **BENEFITS versus RISKS** |
| |
| *Possible Benefits*   *Possible Risks* |
| LONG-ACTING RELIEF OF   Rapid heart rate (tachycardia) |
| BRONCHIAL ASTHMA |
| PREVENTION OF NIGHTTIME |
| (NOCTURNAL) ASTHMA |
| SYMPTOMS |
+--+

▷ **Principal Uses**

   As a Single Drug Product: Uses currently included in FDA-approved labeling:
   (1) Treatment and prevention of bronchospasm in asthma; (2) prevention
   of nocturnal asthma; (3) prevention of exercise-induced bronchospasm;
   (4) ongoing treatment of chronic obstructive pulmonary disease (COPD).
   Helps avoid spasm of the bronchi of the lungs (bronchospasm).

   Other (unlabeled) generally accepted uses: (1) Could have a role in treating
   cystic fibrosis.

   As a Combination Drug Product [CD]: This drug has been available in combination with fluticasone. Fluticasone is a corticosteroid that fights inflammation and asthma in a different way than salmeterol (a long-acting beta-2
   agonist). This profile will focus on the single medicine form.

How This Drug Works: Acts at specific sites (beta-2) in the lung and opens the
   airways (bronchodilation), decreasing airway reactivity and increasing
   movement of mucus. It also blocks release of chemicals from cells
   (basophils, eosinophils, macrophages, and mast) that worsen asthma.

▷ **Widely Used Guidelines That Involve This Medicine (representative sample):** Please look at the section at the very beginning of this profile called
   "Class." Next, turn to Table 22 and you will find guidelines listed by the
   class involved!

Available Dosage Forms and Strengths

   Advair Diskus form — 100/50, 250/50, and 500 mcg fluticasone and 50 mcg
                        of salmeterol per use.
              Inhaler — 13-g canister that gives 21 mcg of salmeterol per use.
   Serevent Diskus — 50 mcg of salmeterol per use.

▷ **Recommended Dose Ranges** (Actual dose and schedule must be determined for
   each patient individually.)

   Infants and Children: Safety and efficacy in those less than 12 years of age not
   established.

   Combination form: Salmeterol/fluticasone (50 micrograms/100 micrograms)
   newly approved for use in those 4 to 11 years old who have asthma and
   continue to have symptoms while taking inhaled corticosteroid therapy by
   itself.

   12 to 60 Years of Age: For Prevention of Asthma:

   Inhalation Aerosol Form (Serevent): Two inhalations (42 mcg) twice daily in
   the morning and evening. Doses are taken 12 hours apart.

   Salmeterol Powder for Inhalation (Diskus Form): One disc (contains 50 mcg
   of salmeterol) 12 hours apart.

   Combination form: For asthma: *Fluticasone/salmeterol combination:* the starting dose is 100 mcg fluticasone and 50 mcg of salmeterol in people who are
   not presently taking an inhaled steroid (corticosteroid). If they are taking
   an inhaled corticosteroid such as budesonide and the steroid dose is less

than or equal to 400 mcg a day, then the combination inhaler containing 100 mcg of fluticasone and 50 mcg of salmeterol is substituted and is taken twice a day. Other doses of budesonide or other corticosteroids require different combinations of fluticasone/salmeterol to get the best results.

For Prevention of Exercised-Induced Asthma:
    Inhalation Aerosol Form (Serevent): Two inhalations at least 30 to 60 minutes before exercise. Additional doses of salmeterol should not be taken for 12 hours.
    Salmeterol powder for inhalation (Diskus form): One disc (has 50 mcg of salmeterol) given or taken at least 30 minutes before exercise.
Over 60 Years of Age: Same as 12 to 60 years of age.

Conditions Requiring Dosing Adjustments
Liver Function: Use with caution, as the drug may accumulate in liver failure.
Kidney Function: Salmeterol has not been studied in kidney failure patients.

▷ **Dosing Instructions:** Follow written instructions closely. Shake well before using. You may need to use a spacer with the metered-dose inhaler form. If you forget a dose: Take the missed dose as soon as you remember it, unless it's nearly time for your next dose—if that is the case, skip the missed dose and Take the next dose right on schedule. Talk with your doctor if you find yourself missing doses. Like other medicines, benefits come from using the medicine correctly.

Usual Duration of Use: Use on a regular schedule for 4 to 6 weeks usually determines effectiveness in preventing asthma attacks. Long-term use (months to years) requires periodic physician evaluation of response and dose adjustment.

Typical Treatment Goals and Measurements (Outcomes and Markers)
Asthma: Signs and symptoms of asthma such as difficulty breathing (dyspnea), cough, light-headedness, and wheezing should lessen. Forced expiratory volume at one second (FEV1) and/or peak expiratory flow rate (PEF) are checked by most pulmonologists as indicators of successful treatment. If the usual benefit is not realized, call your doctor.

Possible Advantages of This Drug
Longer-acting beta-2 agent than previously available. Combination form offers two mechanisms of action and may last 12 hours or longer in some patients.

▷ **This Drug Should Not Be Taken If**
- you had an allergic reaction to it previously.
- you currently have an irregular heart rhythm.
- you are taking, or have taken within the past 2 weeks, any monoamine oxidase (MAO) type A inhibitor.
- you have sudden onset asthma or status asthmaticus. (Fluticasone or fluticasone/salmeterol WON'T WORK.)

▷ **Inform Your Physician Before Taking This Drug If**
- your breathing does not improve after taking this drug.
- you have an overactive thyroid (hyperthyroidism).
- you have diabetes.
- you have a history of heart problems (such as arrhythmias, coronary insufficiency).
- you have abnormally high blood pressure.
- you are unsure how much to take or how often to take it.

Possible Side Effects (natural, expected, and unavoidable drug actions)
Dryness or irritation of the mouth or throat, altered taste. Nervousness, tremor, or palpitations.

▷ **Possible Adverse Effects** (unusual, unexpected, and infrequent reactions)
If any of the following develop, consult your physician promptly for guidance.
Mild Adverse Effects
Allergic reactions: skin rash and urticaria.
Rhinitis and laryngitis—possible.
Rapid heart rate (tachycardia)—case reports.
Tachyphylaxis—conflicting data and reports.
Sleep disturbances—rare to infrequent.
Blood sugar changes—possible.
Headache, tremor, dizziness, and nervousness—infrequent.
Serious Adverse Effects
Allergic reactions: anaphylactic reactions.
Paradoxical bronchospasm—possible.
Respiratory arrest—case reports.
Prolonged QTc interval of the heart—reported, but appears to diminish over time (tachyphylaxis).

▷ **Possible Effects on Sexual Function:** Not defined.

Possible Delayed Adverse Effects: None defined at present.

▷ **Adverse Effects That May Mimic Natural Diseases or Disorders**
Rapid heart rate may mimic heart disease. Bronchospasm may mimic asthma.

Natural Diseases or Disorders That May Be Activated by This Drug
Latent coronary artery disease. Diabetes or high blood pressure.

Possible Effects on Laboratory Tests
Blood cholesterol profile: may be increased.
Blood glucose level: increased.

CAUTION
1. A small yet significant increased risk of asthma-related death was found in one large study comparing Serevent to usual asthma treatment. A follow-up analysis suggested that this risk may be larger in African American patients.
2. Use of this drug by inhalation with beclomethasone aerosol (Beclovent, Vanceril) may increase the risk of fluorocarbon propellant (fluorocarbons being eliminated from these products), but those still containing fluorocarbon propellants may lead to toxicity. Use salmeterol aerosol 20 to 30 minutes **before** beclomethasone aerosol to reduce toxicity and enhance penetration of beclomethasone into the lungs.
3. Serious heart rhythm problems or cardiac arrest can result from excessive and prolonged use.
4. Call your doctor if asthma symptoms appear more often than usual, or if you begin to increase use of the immediate bronchodilator.
5. *Guidelines for the Diagnosis and Management of Asthma* from the National Institutes of Health states that salmeterol should NOT be used for acute symptoms or asthma exacerbations.
6. Combination form works primarily locally in the lung. Because of this, blood (plasma) levels don't predict the benefit (therapeutic effect). Additionally, Advair Diskus form should NOT be used to transfer people who have required systemic steroids due to possible adrenal insufficiency.

Precautions for Use

> *By Infants and Children:* Safety and effectiveness for those under 12 not established for the aerosol form (Serevent). Safety and effectiveness for those under 4 not established for the inhalation powder form (Serevent Diskus).

> *By Those Over 60 Years of Age:* Avoid increased use. If asthma is not controlled as it has been in the past, call your doctor.

▷ Advisability of Use During Pregnancy

Pregnancy Category: C. See Pregnancy Risk Categories at the back of this book.

Animal Studies: Rabbit studies have revealed cleft palate, limb and paw flexures and delayed bone formation.

Human Studies: Adequate studies of pregnant women are not available. Ask your doctor for guidance.

Advisability of Use If Breast-Feeding

Presence of this drug in breast milk: not defined.
Avoid drug or refrain from nursing.

Habit-Forming Potential: None.

Effects of Overdose: Exaggeration of pharmacological effects: tachycardia and/or arrhythmia, muscle cramps, cardiac arrest, and death.

Suggested Periodic Examinations While Taking This Drug (at physician's discretion)

Blood pressure checks.
Evaluations of heart (cardiac) status.
PFTs.

▷ While Taking This Drug, Observe the Following

Foods: No restrictions.

Herbal Medicines or Minerals: Using St. John's wort, ma huang, bitter orange, country mallow, ephedrine-like compounds, mate, guarana, or kola while taking this medicine may result in unacceptable central nervous system stimulation. Fir or pine needle oil should NOT be used by asthmatics. Ephedra alone does carry a German Commission E monograph indication for asthma treatment. If you are allergic to plants in the Asteraceae family (aster, chrysanthemum, daisy, or ragweed), you may also be allergic to echinacea, chamomile, feverfew, and St. John's wort. Since part of the way ginseng works may be as an MAO inhibitor, do not combine ginseng with salmeterol.

Beverages: Avoid excessive caffeine as in coffee, tea, cola, and chocolate.

▷   *Alcohol:* No interactions expected.

Tobacco Smoking: No interactions expected. Asthma may be worsened by irritation from smoking. I advise everyone to quit smoking.

▷   *Other Drugs*

Salmeterol ***taken concurrently*** with

- monoamine oxidase (MAO) type A inhibitors can cause extreme increases in blood pressure and heart stimulation.

The following drugs may ***increase*** the effects of salmeterol:

- methylxanthines such as caffeine or theophylline (Theodur, others).
- tricyclic antidepressants.

▷   *Driving, Hazardous Activities:* This drug may cause nervousness or dizziness. Restrict activities as necessary.

Aviation Note: The use of this drug ***is a disqualification*** for piloting. Consult a designated Aviation Medical Examiner.

Exposure to Sun: No restrictions.

Heavy Exercise or Exertion: Use caution—this may stress the protective effects of this drug.

SELEGILINE (se LEDGE i leen)

Other Name: Deprenyl

Introduced: 1981   **Class:**   Anti-Parkinsonism, monoamine oxidase (MAO) type B inhibitor   **Prescription:**   USA: Yes   **Controlled Drug:** USA: No; Canada: No   **Available as Generic:**.   USA: Yes

Brand Names: ❧Apo-Selegiline, Carbex, ❧Dom-Selegiline, Eldepryl, ❧Med-Selegiline, ❧Novo-Selegiline, ❧PMS-Selegiline

---

BENEFITS versus RISKS

Possible Benefits	*Possible Risks*
EFFECTIVE INITIAL TREATMENT OF PARKINSON'S DISEASE WHEN STARTED AT THE ONSET OF SYMPTOMS	ABNORMAL INVOLUNTARY MOVEMENTS
	HALLUCINATIONS
ADDITIVE RELIEF OF SYMPTOMS OF PARKINSON'S DISEASE WHEN USED CONCURRENTLY WITH LEVODOPA/CARBIDOPA	INITIAL FALL IN BLOOD PRESSURE/ORTHOSTATIC HYPOTENSION
PERMITS REDUCTION IN SINEMET DOSE	
May have a role in Alzheimer's disease	

▷ **Principal Uses**

As a Single Drug Product: Uses currently included in FDA-approved labeling: (1) Used to start drug treatment of very early Parkinson's disease (soon after onset of symptoms), thus delaying the use of levodopa/carbidopa; (2) also used as an adjunct to levodopa/carbidopa treatment of Parkinson's disease if intolerable abnormal movements (dyskinesia) and/or increasing "on-off" episodes occur—addition of selegiline (a) permits reduction of the daily dose of levodopa with consequent lessening of dyskinesia and erratic drug response and (b) provides additional relief of Parkinsonian symptoms.

Other (unlabeled) generally accepted uses: (1) Some improvement achieved in Alzheimer's disease (some trials also used high-dose vitamin E) in patients treated with this drug; (2) narcolepsy; (3) may have a role in attention deficit hyperactivity disorder (ADHD) where methylphenidate is not tolerated; (4) may work as adjunctive treatment in some schizophrenia cases (in combination with risperidone in one study); (5) has some benefit in depression and bipolar disorder, but not for routine use.

How This Drug Works: By inhibiting monoamine oxidase type B (the enzyme that inactivates dopamine in the brain) and by slowing how quickly dopamine is stored back into nerves once it's been released (restorage of released dopamine at nerve terminals), this drug helps correct dopamine deficiency responsible for rigidity, tremor, and sluggish movement characteristic of Parkinson's disease. Selegiline is changed (metabolized) to amphetamine and methamphetamine in the body, but how these compounds work in the beneficial effect of the drug is unclear.

▷ **Widely Used Guidelines That Involve This Medicine (representative sample):** Please look at the section at the very beginning of this profile called "Class." Next, turn to Table 22 and you will find guidelines listed by the class involved!

Available Dosage Forms and Strengths
Capsules — 5 mg
Tablets — 5 mg
Author's Note: The capsule form of this medicine may eventually replace the tablet form and is an astute attempt by the company to help avoid confusion with other white tablets or counterfeit copies of Eldepryl.

▷ **Usual Adult Dosage Ranges:** *Parkinsonism*: 5 mg once or twice daily. The usual maintenance dose is 5 mg after breakfast and 5 mg after lunch. Daily dose of 10 mg is adequate to achieve optimal benefit. Higher doses do not result in further improvement and are not advised. During gradual introduction of selegiline, dose of levodopa/carbidopa (Sinemet) may be cautiously decreased. Sinemet dose should be reduced by 10% to 20% when selegiline is started.
Note: Actual dose and schedule must be determined for each patient individually.

Conditions Requiring Dosing Adjustments
Liver Function: This drug is extensively metabolized in the liver. Patients with liver compromise should be followed closely.
Kidney Function: No dosing changes thought to be needed. It can cause prostatic enlargement (hypertrophy) and should be used with caution in patients with urine outflow problems.

▷ **Dosing Instructions:** The tablet may be crushed and taken with food or milk to reduce stomach irritation. Talk to your doctor about foods high in tyramine (such as soy sauce, red [such as Chianti] and white wines, beer, aged cheese, and figs, etc.). If you forget a dose: Take the missed dose as soon as you remember it, unless it's nearly time for your next dose—if that is the case, skip the missed dose and take the next dose right on schedule. DO NOT double doses. Taking this medicine with breakfast and/or lunch is usually best because taking it with dinner can disrupt your sleep. Talk with your doctor if you find yourself missing doses or having difficulty sleeping.

Usual Duration of Use: Use on a regular schedule for 4 to 6 weeks usually determines effectiveness in controlling the symptoms of Parkinson's disease and permitting reduction of levodopa/carbidopa dose. Long-term use (months to years) requires periodic physician evaluation and goal assessment.

Typical Treatment Goals and Measurements (Outcomes and Markers)
Parkinson's Disease: The general goal is to minimize symptoms (tremor, sluggish movements, analysis of walking or gait, etc.) to the fullest extent possible. Additionally, many neurologists use Hàhn-Yahr scores and the time it takes to maximum amount of finger tapping as indicators of the benefits of this drug.

Possible Advantages of This Drug
It may provide a more effective and uniform control of Parkinsonian symptoms and a significant reduction of some adverse effects associated with long-term levodopa therapy.

▷ **This Drug Should Not Be Taken If**
• you have had an allergic reaction to it previously.
• you have Huntington's disease, hereditary (essential) tremor, or tardive dyskinesia (see Glossary).

- you are pregnant or breast-feeding.
- you take meperidine (Demerol).

▷ **Inform Your Physician Before Taking This Drug If**
- you have constitutionally low blood pressure.
- you have peptic ulcer disease.
- you are taking levodopa.
- you have a history of heart rhythm disorder.
- you are taking any antihypertensive drugs, antidepressants, or antipsychotic drugs (see Drug Classes).

Possible Side Effects (natural, expected, and unavoidable drug actions)
Weakness, orthostatic hypotension (see Glossary), dry mouth, insomnia—all rare.

▷ **Possible Adverse Effects** (unusual, unexpected, and infrequent reactions)
If any of the following develop, consult your physician promptly for guidance.
Mild Adverse Effects
Headache, dizziness, blurred vision, agitation—rare.
Change in sleep patterns—reported with conflicting effects of insomnia or improved sleep.
Palpitations, fainting—rare.
Altered taste—rare.
Nausea and vomiting, stomach pain, anorexia—rare to frequent.
Serious Adverse Effects
Dyskinesias: abnormal involuntary movements—infrequent.
Confusion and hallucinations, depression, psychosis, vivid dreams—rare.
Angina and fast heart rate (tachycardia)—infrequent.
Aggravation of peptic ulcer, gastrointestinal bleeding—rare.
Growth of the prostate—rare.

▷ **Possible Effects on Sexual Function:** Transient decreases in penile sensation and anorgasmia have rarely been reported if doses exceed 10 mg per day. Increased libido may occur.

▷ **Adverse Effects That May Mimic Natural Diseases or Disorders**
Effects on mental function and behavior may resemble psychotic disorders.

Natural Diseases or Disorders That May Be Activated by This Drug
Peptic ulcer disease.

Possible Effects on Laboratory Tests
Vanillylmandelic acid (VMA) test will be falsely low.

CAUTION
1. This drug can start dyskinesias and intensify existing dyskinesias. Watch carefully for tremors, twitching, or abnormal, involuntary movements of any kind. Report these promptly.
2. This drug potentiates the effects of levodopa. When added to current levodopa treatment, adverse effects of levodopa may develop or be intensified. Levodopa dose must be reduced by 10% to 20% when treatment with selegiline begins.
3. Tell your doctor promptly if you become pregnant or plan pregnancy. The manufacturer does not recommend the use of this drug during pregnancy.
4. Some foods (tyramine-containing—see Glossary) have led to rare increases in blood pressure with selegiline doses greater than 10 mg. Talk to your doctor.

Precautions for Use

By Infants and Children: This drug is not utilized by this age group.

By Those Over 60 Years of Age: This drug is usually well tolerated by the elderly. Observe closely for any tendency to light-headedness or faintness, especially on arising from a lying or sitting position.

▷ **Advisability of Use During Pregnancy**

Pregnancy Category: C. See Pregnancy Risk Categories at the back of this book.

Animal Studies: No birth defects due to this drug were found in rat studies.

Human Studies: Adequate studies of pregnant women are not available.

The manufacturer advises that this drug should not be taken during pregnancy.

Advisability of Use If Breast-Feeding

Presence of this drug in breast milk: Unknown.

Avoid drug or refrain from nursing.

Habit-Forming Potential: None.

Effects of Overdose: Nausea, vomiting, palpitations, low blood pressure, agitation, severe involuntary movements, hallucinations.

Possible Effects of Long-Term Use: None reported.

Suggested Periodic Examinations While Taking This Drug (at physician's discretion)

Regular evaluation of drug response, heart function, and blood pressure status.

▷ **While Taking This Drug, Observe the Following**

Foods: **CAUTION** should be used regarding foods containing tyramine (see Glossary for a list), although the reaction with this drug may not be as severe as that seen with other MAO inhibitors (avocado, others).

Herbal Medicines or Minerals: St. John's wort: **CAUTION** is advised because of possible serotonin syndrome. St. John's wort may also worsen sensitivity to the sun. The principle active ingredient of guarana and mate is caffeine—and use should be avoided. Since part of the way ginkgo and ginseng work may be as MAO inhibitors, do not combine with selegiline. Ma huang (contains ephedra), nutmeg, bitter orange, country mallow, kava, mate, and yohimbe are also best avoided while taking this medicine. Calabar bean (chop nut, fabia, ordeal nut, others) is unsafe when taken by mouth (physostigmine is the active ingredient) and should never be taken by people with Parkinson's disease. Octacosanol (a cousin of vitamin E) can worsen movement problems and should also be avoided.

Beverages: Caffeine-containing beverages may have more of an effect than previously. Limit caffeine consumption. May be taken with milk.

▷ *Alcohol:* Use **CAUTION** until the combined effects have been determined. Alcohol may exaggerate the blood pressure–lowering and sedative effects of this drug. Aged wines, etc., containing tyramine may cause a reaction of varying severity.

Tobacco Smoking: No interactions expected. I advise everyone to quit smoking.

Marijuana Smoking: Additive drowsiness may occur.

▷ *Other Drugs*

Selegiline *taken concurrently* with

- albuterol (Ventolin, others) may result in increased adverse vascular effects.
- amphetamine (Dexedrine, others) can cause a severe increase in blood pressure.

- antidepressants (see Drug Classes) such as amitriptyline (Elavil) may cause neurotoxic reactions such as seizures.
- antihypertensive drugs (and other drugs that can lower blood pressure) require careful monitoring for excessive drops in pressure; dose adjustments may be necessary.
- benzodiazepines (see Drug Classes) may result in increased central nervous system depression.
- beta 2 type agonist medicines may increase risk of rapid heart rate, hypomania, or agitation.
- birth control pills (oral contraceptives) may increase risk of selegiline toxicity.
- bupropion (Wellbutrin) may cause seizures.
- buspirone (Buspar) may result in increases in blood pressure.
- carbamazepine (Tegretol) may result in high fevers and seizures—still, some studies found benefits in resistant depression.
- citalopram (Celexa) may lead to toxicity—DO NOT COMBINE.
- cyclobenzaprine (Flexeril) may lead to toxicity—DO NOT COMBINE.
- dextromethorphan (various), a cough suppressant used in many nonprescription cough medicines, has been reported to cause toxicity with low blood pressure, spasms, high fevers, and some deaths—these medicines should not be combined.
- ephedrine (various) can result in severe increases in temperature.
- fluoxetine (Prozac) may cause serotonin toxicity syndrome.
- fluvoxamine (Luvox) may result in extreme agitation, rigidity, excessive temperatures, and coma—DO NOT combine these medicines.
- lithium (Lithobid) may increase risk of the serotonin toxicity syndrome.
- meperidine (Demerol) may cause a life-threatening reaction of unknown cause; avoid this combination.
- methyldopa (Aldomet) MAY LEAD TO HYPERTENSIVE CRISIS—DO NOT COMBINE.
- methylphenidate (Concerta, others) MAY LEAD TO HYPERTENSIVE CRISIS—DO NOT COMBINE.
- mirtazapine (Remeron) may lead to adverse seizures.
- morphine (MS Contin, various) may lead to excessive CNS and lowered blood pressure effects—DO NOT COMBINE.
- nefazodone (Serzone) may lead to serotonin syndrome—DO NOT COMBINE.
- opioid medicines (oxycodone, morphine, others) may lead to excessive CNS depression. Manufacturer does NOT recommend combining.
- oral hypoglycemic agents (see Oral Antidiabetic Drugs in Drug Classes) may cause very low blood sugars.
- paroxetine (Paxil) may result in central nervous system toxicity.
- phenothiazines (see Drug Classes) may result in increased occurrence of movement disorders.
- phentermine (Fastin) may lead to hypertensive crisis—DO NOT COMBINE.
- phenylpropanolamine (now removed from the U.S. market—various) or phenylephrine (various) can cause severe increases in temperature and blood pressure—DO NOT combine.
- pseudoephedrine (various) can cause severe increases in temperature and blood pressure—DO NOT combine (this includes combination forms of pseudoephedrine such as loratadine/pseudoephedrine [Claritin-D]).
- sertraline (Zoloft) may result in central nervous system toxicity.

- sibutramine (Meridia) may lead to toxicity.
- sumatriptan (Imitrex) or zolmitriptan (Zomig) may lead to toxicity.
- tramadol (Ultram) may lead to seizures.
- tryptophan may cause a fatal serotonin syndrome.
- venlafaxine (Effexor) can result in central and autonomic nervous system toxicity.

The following drugs may **decrease** the effects of selegiline and diminish its effectiveness:

- chlorprothixene (Taractan).
- haloperidol (Haldol).
- metoclopramide (Reglan).
- phenothiazines (see Drug Classes).
- reserpine (Ser-Ap-Es, etc.), in high doses.
- thiothixene (Navane).

▷ *Driving, Hazardous Activities:* This drug may cause dizziness, drowsiness, impaired coordination, or fainting. Restrict activities as necessary.

Aviation Note: The use of this drug *is a disqualification* for piloting. Consult a designated Aviation Medical Examiner.

Exposure to Sun: Use caution—photosensitivity has been reported.

Exposure to Heat: Use caution until the combined effects have been determined. Hot environments can cause lowering of blood pressure.

Discontinuation: **Do not stop this drug abruptly.** Sudden withdrawal can cause prompt increase in Parkinsonian symptoms and deterioration of control. Consult your physician regarding a schedule for gradual withdrawal and concurrent adjustment of Sinemet or other appropriate drugs.

SERTRALINE (SER tra leen)

Introduced: 1986 **Class:**   Antidepressant   **Prescription:**   USA: Yes
Controlled Drug: USA: No; Canada: No **Available as Generic:** USA: No
Brand Names: ✿Apo-sertraline, ✿Dom-sertraline, ✿Gen-sertraline, ✿Novo-sertraline, ✿Ratio-sertraline, ✿Rhoxal-sertraline, ✿Riva-sertraline, Zoloft

BENEFITS versus RISKS	
Possible Benefits	*Possible Risks*
EFFECTIVE TREATMENT OF DEPRESSION	Male sexual dysfunction
TREATS PANIC DISORDER	Seizures
TREATMENT OF OBSESSIVE-COMPULSIVE DISORDER	
TREATS POST-TRAUMATIC STRESS DISORDER (PTSD)	
TREATS PREMENSTRUAL DYSPHORIC DISORDER (PMDD)	
May be of particular use after a heart attack or stroke	

▷ **Principal Uses**

As a Single Drug Product: Uses currently included in FDA-approved labeling: Treats (1) major depression; (2) obsessive-compulsive disorder; (3) panic disorder; (4) post-traumatic stress disorder; (5) premenstrual dysphoric disorder; (6) social anxiety disorder and social phobia.

Other (unlabeled) generally accepted uses: (1) May have a role in treating obesity—rat studies have shown a decrease in eating that depends on the dose that is taken, and studies in humans are being conducted; (2) may help some kinds of sexual problems (premature ejaculation); (3) helps clozapine-caused (induced) obsessive-compulsive disorder; (4) can ease the feeling of loss of breath in mild to severe obstructive lung disease; (5) may have a role in depression after a heart attack, both in treating the depression and in heart rate variability.

How This Drug Works: This drug relieves depression by slowly restoring to normal levels a specific constituent of brain tissue (serotonin) that transmits nerve impulses.

▷ **Widely Used Guidelines That Involve This Medicine (representative sample):** Please look at the section at the very beginning of this profile called "Class." Next, turn to Table 22 and you will find guidelines listed by the class involved!

Available Dosage Forms and Strengths
Solution — 20 mg per mL
Tablets — 25 mg, 50 mg, 100 mg

▷ **Recommended Dose Ranges** (Actual dose and schedule must be determined for each patient individually.)

Infants and Children: In children 6 to 12 years old: 25 mg once daily has been approved to treat obsessive-compulsive disorder.

12 to 60 Years of Age: Depression: Initially 50 mg once daily, taken in the morning or evening. The dose is then slowly increased, as needed and tolerated, in increments of 50 mg at intervals of 1 week. The total daily dose should not exceed 200 mg.

Panic disorder: Dosing is started at 25 mg a day (morning or evening). After 7 days, the dose can be increased to 50 mg once daily. If needed and tolerated, the dose can then be increased (at 7-day intervals) to a 200 mg per day maximum.

PTSD: Similar to dosing for depression.

Obsessive-compulsive disorder: Same as dosing in depression.

Over 60 Years of Age: Dose amounts are the same as 12 to 60 years of age, unless liver function is compromised. Because the drug is removed some 40% more slowly than in younger patients, any changes in dose should be made at 2–3-week intervals.

Conditions Requiring Dosing Adjustments
Liver Function: Drug is a rare cause of liver damage. Patients with liver disease should be watched closely and lower doses used.
Kidney Function: The role of the kidneys is minimal and dosing adjustments are not thought to be needed.

▷ **Dosing Instructions:** The tablet may be crushed and is best taken with food to enhance absorption, but it may be taken at any time with or without food. The oral liquid form (concentrate) has 20 mg in each mL. Use the calibrated dropper to get the right dose. Just before you are going to take it, the dose can be mixed with 4 ounces of water, orange juice, ginger ale, lemonade, or other suitable liquid (talk to your pharmacist). It is okay if a haze appears once the concentrate has been added to the liquid. Taking this medicine regularly is important. If you forget a dose: Skip the missed dose and take the next dose right on schedule. DO NOT double doses. Talk with your doctor if you find yourself missing doses.

Usual Duration of Use: Use on a regular schedule for 4 to 8 weeks usually determines effectiveness in relieving depression and pattern of both favorable and unfavorable drug effects. Clinical studies suggest that people who respond during the first 8 weeks of treatment will benefit from another 8 weeks of sertraline therapy. Benefits of use in obsessive-compulsive disorder (OCD) have not been shown longer than 12 weeks in clinical trials. Since OCD tends to be ongoing, patients who benefit from this medicine should discuss the benefits and risks of continued sertraline. Long-term use requires periodic physician evaluation. The lowest effective dose should be used.

Typical Treatment Goals and Measurements (Outcomes and Markers)

Depression: The general goal: to lessen the degree and severity of depression, letting patients return to their daily lives. Specific measures of depression involve testing or inventories (such as Hamilton Depression or HAM-D) and can be valuable in helping check benefits from this medicine.

Panic Disorder: Goals for panic tend to be more vague and subjective than hypertension or cholesterol. Frequently, the patient (in conjunction with physician assessment) will largely decide if panic has been modified to a successful extent. Additionally, decreased number of trips to the hospital or ER visits may be a useful measure. The Liebowitz Social Anxiety Scale (LSAS) is a tool as well as the Clinical Global Impressions–Global Improvement Scale, which can be used to help figure out benefits in patients with anxiety and panic. The Hamilton Rating Scale for Anxiety anxious mood section is also helpful. The ability of the patient to return to normal activities is a hallmark of successful treatment.

Possible Advantages of This Drug

Does not cause weight gain, a common side effect of tricyclic antidepressants. Less likely to cause dry mouth, constipation, urinary retention, orthostatic hypotension (see Glossary), and heart rhythm disturbances than tricyclic antidepressants. May have fewer drug interactions than other medicines in this same class. Has data from the SADHART trial (see Glassman, AH in Sources) that shows that this medicine is safe and effective in people with recent heart attack and unstable angina.

▷ **This Drug Should Not Be Taken If**
- you have had an allergic reaction to it previously or you have a latex allergy and were prescribed the solution form (the dropper bulb is made of natural rubber).
- you took a monoamine oxidase (MAO) type A inhibitor (see Drug Classes) in the last 14 days.
- you take disulfiram and were prescribed the oral solution form (has 12% alcohol).

▷ **Inform Your Physician Before Taking This Drug If**
- you had any adverse effects from antidepressant drugs.
- you have impaired liver or kidney function.
- you have Parkinson's disease.
- you or a loved one does not understand or want to face the risk of possible suicide; careful follow-up by caregivers and your physician is prudent.
- you have had a recent heart attack.
- you have a seizure disorder.
- you have a bleeding problem or take a diuretic.
- you are pregnant or plan pregnancy while taking this drug.

Possible Side Effects (natural, expected, and unavoidable drug actions)
>   Decreased appetite, weight loss (average 1 to 2 lb). Withdrawal syndrome possible if this medicine is abruptly stopped.

▷ **Possible Adverse Effects** (unusual, unexpected, and infrequent reactions)
   If any of the following develop, consult your physician promptly for guidance.

Mild Adverse Effects
>   Allergic reactions: skin rash, itching—rare.
>   Headache, nervousness, insomnia, fatigue, tremor, dizziness, impaired concentration—rare.
>   Sleepwalking—case reports.
>   Abnormal vision, numbness, and tingling—rare.
>   Confusion—rare.
>   Alopecia—infrequent.
>   Easy bruising (ecchymoses) or nosebleeds (epistaxis)—reported.
>   Night sweats—case report.
>   Chest pain and increased blood pressure—rare.
>   Paresthesias—rare.
>   Muscle aches (myalgia)—may be frequent.
>   Dry mouth, altered taste, nausea, vomiting, diarrhea, tongue ulceration—rare to frequent.

Serious Adverse Effects
>   Allergic reactions: dermatitis (various forms such as Stevens-Johnson Syndrome)—rare.
>   Drug-induced seizures—rare.
>   Hemorrhage into the anterior chamber of the eye or anemia—rare.
>   Hallucinations—case reports.
>   Low blood platelets (thrombocytopenia), changes in bleeding time—case reports.
>   Increased blood cholesterol (hypercholesterolemia)—infrequent.
>   Low blood sugar—case reports.
>   Pancreatitis—associated in time (temporal association) with use of this medicine.
>   Bronchospasm—infrequent.
>   QT interval changes, Torsade de Pointes—case reports.
>   Movement disorders (extrapyramidal reactions)—case reports.
>   Neuroleptic malignant syndrome—case reports with other SSRIs.
>   Serotonin syndrome (hyperreflexia, tachycardia, palpitations, etc.)—possible as with other SSRIs
>   Low blood sodium—rare.
>   SIADH—case reports (may also occur with other selective serotonin reuptake inhibitors).

▷ **Possible Effects on Sexual Function:** Male sexual dysfunction: delayed ejaculation—may be frequent.
>   Female sexual dysfunction: inhibited orgasm—rare.
>   Swelling and tenderness of male (gynecomastia) and female breast tissue with milk production (galactorrhea)—case reports.
>   Infrequent dysmenorrhea, intermenstrual bleeding, atrophic vaginitis, painful erections (priapism)—possible, case reports.
>   May help some kinds of sexual disorders.

Natural Diseases or Disorders That May Be Activated by This Drug
>   Latent epilepsy.

Possible Effects on Laboratory Tests
Blood total cholesterol and triglyceride levels: increased—infrequent.
Blood uric acid levels: decreased.
Hemoglobin or hematocrit: decreased—rare.
Liver function tests: increased liver enzymes (ALT/GPT, AST/GOT, and alkaline phosphatase).
Blood sodium: decreased (with rare SIADH).

CAUTION
1. If any type of skin reaction develops (rash, hives, etc.), stop this drug and call your doctor promptly.
2. If dryness of the mouth develops and persists for more than 2 weeks, consult your dentist for guidance.
3. Ask your doctor or pharmacist before taking any other prescription or over-the-counter drug while taking sertraline.
4. If you are advised to take any monoamine oxidase (MAO) type A inhibitor (see Drug Classes), allow an interval of 5 weeks after discontinuing this drug before starting the MAO inhibitor.
5. It is advisable to withhold this drug if electroconvulsive therapy (ECT, "shock" treatment) is to be used to treat your depression.
6. Movement reactions if they happen usually occur in the first month of treatment, and close patient follow-up is advisable.
7. A withdrawal syndrome is possible if this medicine is abruptly stopped. Best to slowly (taper) this medicine over 2–4 weeks or longer.
8. If you are taking disulfiram (Antabuse), avoid taking the oral liquid form because it has 12% alcohol.
9. Pediatric and adult patients treated with this medicine should be closely watched for worsening depression or suicidal thinking. The FDA has required makers of antidepressants such as this one to alert healthcare professionals to the fact that children and adults with major depression may develop worsening depression or suicidal thoughts and behavior whether they take medicine for depression or do not take it. Patients should be carefully followed for such clinical worsening (particularly when treatment is started or doses are increased or decreased).

Precautions for Use
By Infants and Children: Safety and effectiveness for those less than 12 years of age are not established.
By Those Over 60 Years of Age: The lowest effective dose should be used for maintenance treatment and adjusted as needed for reduced kidney function.

▷ **Advisability of Use During Pregnancy**
Pregnancy Category: C. See Pregnancy Risk Categories at the back of this book.
Animal Studies: Delayed bone development due to this drug found in rat and rabbit studies.
Human Studies: Adequate studies of pregnant women are not available.
Use this drug only if clearly needed. Ask your physician for guidance.

Advisability of Use If Breast-Feeding
Presence of this drug in breast milk: Yes, variable amounts.
One small study found undetectable blood levels in infants who were breast-fed while their mothers were taking sertraline. Another found detectable levels. May be a drug of choice for mothers who breast-feed their infants. Discuss breast-feeding with your doctor.

Habit-Forming Potential: None.

Effects of Overdose: Agitation, restlessness, excitement, nausea, vomiting, seizures.

Possible Effects of Long-Term Use: None reported.

Suggested Periodic Examinations While Taking This Drug (at physician's discretion)

▷ **While Taking This Drug, Observe the Following**

Foods: May increase peak blood level. Grapefruit juice can block removal of this medicine from the body and lead to toxicity. DO NOT COMBINE.

Herbal Medicines or Minerals: Since sertraline and St. John's wort may act to increase serotonin, the combination is not advised. Because part of the way ginseng and ginkgo work may be as MAO inhibitors, the combination is not advisable. Ma huang, yohimbe, Indian snakeroot, and kava kava (not recommended by Health Canada due to liver concerns) are also best avoided while taking this medicine. DHEA led to a manic episode in one patient who combined the two medicines.

Calcium now has excellent data (1,200–1,600 mg per day unless contraindicated) in helping prevent premenstrual dysphoric syndrome (PMDS). This may be an intelligent first-line therapy or valuable adjunctive use. Talk to your doctor to see if this makes sense for you.

Beverages: Do not drink grapefruit juice while taking this medicine. May be taken with milk.

▷ *Alcohol:* Avoid completely.

Tobacco Smoking: No interactions expected. I advise everyone to quit smoking.

Marijuana Smoking: The active ingredient (cannabinoids) found in marijuana combined with a similar medicine (fluoxetine) led to sudden mania in one patient. COMBINATION IS NOT ADVISABLE.

▷ *Other Drugs*

Sertraline may ***increase*** the effects of

- almotriptan (Axert), naratriptan (Amerge), sumatriptan (Imitrex), rizatriptan (Maxalt), zolmitriptan (Zomig), and any triptan-type medicine, leading to loss of coordination and weakness.
- astemizole (Hismanal—see medicines removed from the market), leading to Torsade de Pointes or other heart rhythm problems—DO NOT COMBINE.
- carbamazepine (Tegretol, others), leading to toxicity. Careful patient monitoring and more frequent carbamazepine-level checks are prudent.
- clozapine (Clozaril), leading to clozapine toxicity.
- dextromethorphan (in many cough "DM" suppressants).
- diazepam (Valium) and perhaps other benzodiazepines (see Drug Classes).
- diltiazem (Cardizem).
- dofetilide (Tikosyn), leading to toxicity. CAUTION and more frequent blood-level checks are prudent.
- fosphenytoin (Cerebyx) or phenytoin (Dilantin). Blood-level checks are prudent if these medicines must be combined.
- lamotrigine (Lamictal).
- propafenone (Rythmol), leading to toxicity. Blood levels and clinical monitoring are prudent.
- sibutramine (Meridia), which may lead to toxicity (serotonin syndrome)—DO NOT COMBINE.
- theophylline (Theo-Dur, others) may lead to theophylline toxicity.
- tolbutamide (Orinase).

- warfarin (Coumadin) and related oral anticoagulants; more frequent INR (prothrombin time or protime) testing is needed. Ongoing warfarin doses should be based on INR results.

Sertraline *taken concurrently* with

- antidiabetic drugs (insulin, oral hypoglycemics: see Oral Antidiabetic Drugs in Drug Classes) may increase the risk of hypoglycemic reactions; monitor blood and urine sugar levels carefully.
- benzodiazepines removed by the CYP 3A4 family of liver enzymes (such as triazolam or alprazolam) may lead to benzodiazepine toxicity.
- bupropion (Wellbutrin, Zyban) may lead to sertraline toxicity. Caution and dosing in the lower end of the dose range are prudent.
- cimetidine (Tagamet, Tagamet HB 200) may lead to sertraline toxicity. Careful patient monitoring and lower sertraline doses are prudent.
- erythromycin (various) led to a serotonin syndrome in one patient; other macrolide antibiotics such as clarithromycin may also lead to this effect. Doses of sertraline should be lowered if these medicines must be combined.
- flecainide (Tambocor) may lead to flecainide toxicity.
- lithium (Lithobid, others) may lead to changes. Lithium blood levels are prudent.
- metoclopramide (Reglan) may lead to sertraline toxicity.
- monoamine oxidase (MAO) type A inhibitors may cause confusion, agitation, high fever, seizures, and dangerous elevations of blood pressure—avoid the concurrent use of these drugs.
- quinidine (Quinaglute, others) may lead to quinidine toxicity—CAUTION is advised.
- ritonavir (Norvir) and perhaps other protease inhibitors (see Drug Classes) may lead to toxicity.
- terfenadine (Seldane) may lead to toxicity.
- tramadol (Ultram) may lead to seizures.
- zolpidem (Ambien) may lead to hallucinations—DO NOT COMBINE.

▷ *Driving, Hazardous Activities:* This drug may cause drowsiness, dizziness, impaired judgment, and altered vision. Restrict activities as necessary.

Aviation Note: The use of this drug *is a disqualification* for piloting. Consult a designated Aviation Medical Examiner.

Exposure to Sun: Use caution—this drug may (rarely) cause photosensitivity (see Glossary).

Discontinuation: Best to slowly decrease (taper) the dose over 2–4 weeks or longer. Call your doctor if you plan to stop this drug for any reason.

SIBUTRAMINE (si BYOU trah meen)

Introduced: 1998 **Class:** Serotonin reuptake inhibitor, anorexiant, weight loss agent **Prescription:** USA: Yes **Controlled Drug:** USA: C-IV*; Canada: Yes **Available as Generic:** USA: No

Brand Name: Meridia

Author's Note: A U.S. consumer group has petitioned the FDA to remove sibutramine. Italy suspended sales of sibutramine last year, then reinstated the

*See Schedules of Controlled Drugs at the back of this book.

medicine. Canada reviewed the medicine, and subsequently decided that the benefits outweighed the risks. Controversy arose because of serious heart effects such as stroke, heart attack, abnormal heartbeats (arrhythmias), and more than 28 deaths. The question yet to be resolved is if this is a cause-and-effect relationship (see Glossary). Does the fact that the medicine was taken by patients with significant risk factors for heart disease mean that the medicine caused the problem or that the risk of the problem would have happened anyway? People who are obese or overweight are certainly subject to increased risk of heart problems. Based on current concerns, patients and clinicians must remember that sibutramine is contraindicated in people with coronary artery disease, arrhythmias, heart failure, and uncontrolled high blood pressure. Careful patient selection and close consideration of this benefit-to-risk decision are needed.

BENEFITS versus RISKS

Possible Benefits	*Possible Risks*
EFFECTIVE WEIGHT LOSS	SIGNIFICANT INCREASES IN
ASSOCIATED DECREASES IN	BLOOD PRESSURE AND HEART
TRIGLYCERIDE AND DESIRABLE	RATE (DIASTOLIC)
HDL CHANGES WITH WEIGHT	Increased premature (asymptomatic)
LOSS	heart contractions
	Possible increased risk of serious
	cardiovascular problems

▷ **Principal Uses**

As a Single Drug Product: Uses currently included in FDA-approved labeling: Used to manage obesity, including weight loss and maintaining weight loss in people on a reduced-calorie diet. Used in those with an initial body mass index (BMI: see Glossary) greater than or equal to 30 kg per square meter or 27 kg per square meter if there are other risk factors (such as diabetes, hyperlipidemia, or hypertension).

Other (unlabeled) generally accepted uses: (1) Could help some cases of peripheral neuropathy. Further research is needed.

How This Drug Works: This medicine helps treat obesity by decreasing the desire to eat by blocking reuptake of nerve transmitters (norepinephrine serotonin and dopamine) in brain synapses. People who took the drug in clinical studies were satisfied more quickly when they ate. Since metabolism is also increased, they used more of the food that they did eat than patients not receiving the medicine. Most of this effect comes from two active compounds (metabolites) that the body changes sibutramine into (M1 and M2). May also have some action as an antidepressant.

▷ **Widely Used Guidelines That Involve This Medicine (representative sample):** Please look at the section at the very beginning of this profile called "Class." Next, turn to Table 22 and you will find guidelines listed by the class involved!

Available Dosage Forms and Strengths

Capsules — 5 mg, 10 mg, 15 mg

▷ **Recommended Dosage Ranges** (Actual dose and schedule must be determined for each patient individually.)

Dosing is started at 10 mg once a day in the morning. Status of heart rate and blood pressure should be checked before any dose increases. If the clinician feels that those and other parameters are acceptable, and if weight loss goals have not been met, the dose may be increased after 4 weeks to a daily dose of 15 mg. Conversely, the dose should be decreased to 5 mg daily if not tolerated (using blood pressure and heart rate as guides). The daily maximum is 15 mg.

Conditions Requiring Dosing Adjustments

Liver Function: This drug is changed in the liver; however, dose changes are not thought to be needed in mild to moderate liver failure. Drug should NOT be used in severe liver failure.

Kidney Function: No changes needed in mild to moderate kidney failure. Drug should NOT be used in severe kidney failure.

▷ **Dosing Instructions:** Capsule may be taken before or following food. It was usually taken in the morning in clinical trials because nighttime dosing can lead to sleep problems. If the starting dose of 10 mg isn't tolerated (using heart rate and blood pressure as a guide), discuss this with your doctor. The dose is usually then lowered to 5 mg daily in those cases. If you forget a dose: Take the missed dose as soon as you remember it, unless it's nearly time for your next dose—if that is the case, skip the missed dose and take the next dose right on schedule. DO NOT double up on doses. Talk with your doctor and pharmacist if you find yourself missing doses.

Usual Duration of Use: This medicine has been used up to 2 years. Longer-term use should be discussed with your doctor. One study found that 77% of those who took the medicine as part of a program not only lowered cholesterol but also helped achieve and maintain significant weight loss. Ongoing use requires periodic physician follow-up.

Typical Treatment Goals and Measurements (Outcomes and Markers)

Weight Loss: The goal is to lower body weight or maintain weight loss. Body weight (body mass index, or BMI), percent body fat, and laboratory tests such as triglycerides, VLDL, LDL, and HDL can be checked to assess successful combination treatment. Be sure to talk to your doctor about the benefits of losing some weight and keeping it off versus crash or fad diets and weight yo-yoing.

Possible Advantages of This Drug

Use has not been associated with heart valve problems seen with dexfenfluramine (Redux). The STORM study (Sibutramine Trial in Obesity Reduction and Maintenance) showed that 67% of people who took sibutramine maintained their 6-month weight loss for up to 2 years. In a more recent European study, 77% of people who took the medicine as part of an organized program lowered cholesterol and maintained significant weight loss.

▷ **This Drug Should Not Be Taken If**

- you had an allergic reaction to any form of it previously.
- you've had a stroke.
- you are anorexic.
- you have a history of abnormal heart rhythms, irregular heartbeat, or heart disease.
- you have pulmonary hypertension.
- you have poorly controlled or uncontrolled high blood pressure.
- you have congestive heart failure or disease of the coronary arteries.
- other causes of obesity such as untreated low thyroid function (hypothyroidism) were not ruled out.
- you have glaucoma (narrow angle).

- you take, or have taken within the last 14 days, a monoamine oxidase (MAO) inhibitor (see Drug Classes).
- you have severe kidney or liver disease.

▷ **Inform Your Physician Before Taking This Drug If**
- you have heart (cardiovascular) disease or have had an unfavorable reaction to any serotonin reuptake inhibitor.
- you have glaucoma.
- your work requires balance or operation of hazardous machinery (this medicine can cause dizziness).
- you have a history of high blood pressure.
- you have a history of kidney or liver compromise.
- you have a history of gallstones.
- you have a history of psychiatric disorders or drug abuse.
- you have taken other weight loss medicines (anorexiants) in the last year.
- you have a seizure disorder.
- you develop unexplained difficulty in breathing, fainting, chest pain, fast or irregular heartbeat, or swelling of the ankles. Call if you have any kind of seizure or blackout. These signs and symptoms can be early warnings of problems, or some of them could be part of pulmonary hypertension.

Possible Side Effects (natural, expected, and unavoidable drug actions)
Since some weight-loss agents that cause increased levels of serotonin have been associated with development of a fatal lung problem (primary pulmonary hypertension, or PPH), it is prudent to talk about this with your doctor. It is unknown if sibutramine can cause this problem. Serotonin syndrome may result with combined use with MAO inhibitors or other medicines that increase serotonin.

▷ **Possible Adverse Effects** (unusual, unexpected, and infrequent reactions)
If any of the following develop, consult your physician promptly for guidance.
Mild Adverse Effects
Allergic reaction: skin rash.
Headache and anorexia—frequent.
Sleep disturbances—infrequent.
Anxiety—reported.
Dry mouth or constipation—frequent (but may ease over time).
Palpitations or tachycardia—rare.
Fast heart rate (tachycardia)—infrequent.
Increased liver enzymes—frequent (questionable cause).
Serious Adverse Effects
High blood pressure (increased up to 30% of the level present before starting the medicine) as well as some cases of increased diastolic pressure—infrequent.
Abnormal heartbeats—case reports.
Heart attack—case reports.
Stroke—case reports.
Psychosis—case report.
Seizures—case reports.
Abnormal liver enzymes (ALT)—rare.
Low blood platelets—case reports.

▷ **Possible Effects on Sexual Function:** Painful menstruation—infrequent.

Natural Diseases or Disorders That May Be Activated by This Drug
High blood pressure controlled by other medicines may return. Untreated

high blood pressure may worsen. See "This Drug Should Not Be Taken If" section above.

Possible Effects on Laboratory Tests

Drug testing: may cause false positive tests for amphetamines.

CAUTION

1. It is best to carry a card saying you are taking this drug. A medicine alert bracelet is also a good idea.
2. This medicine may cause false positive urine drug tests for amphetamines.
3. Other conditions (organic causes) leading to obesity (such as low activity of the thyroid gland—hypothyroidism) should be ruled out prior to starting this medicine.
4. Safety and efficacy of use of sibutramine with other weight-loss agents have NOT been established. Combination therapy is NOT recommended.
5. This medicine has NOT been found to cause lung problems (primary pulmonary hypertension, or PPH); however, other drugs that increase serotonin were subsequently found to do this. If you develop unexplained difficulty in breathing, fainting, chest pain, or swelling of the ankles, call your doctor. These may be early symptoms of pulmonary hypertension.
6. Because of the increased risk of increased blood pressure, periodic checks of blood pressure are prudent.
7. Nonprescription medicines such as pseudoephedrine, ephedrine, or phenylpropanolamine can increase heart rate or blood pressure. Talk with your pharmacist or doctor BEFORE you combine any type of decongestant, cough, allergy, or cold medicine.
8. Serotonin syndrome is possible with medicines that increase brain serotonin. Call your doctor if disorientation, hyperreflexia, or palpitations happen while taking this medicine.

Precautions for Use

By Infants and Children: Safety and effectiveness have not been established in those less than 16 years old.

By Those Over 60 Years of Age: The drug levels this medicine achieves and the places in the body where this medicine goes are no different for those over 60 than those under 60. *CAUTION* should be used (as with all medicines active in the central nervous system) in treating elderly patients with sibutramine. Since there is also a higher occurrence of high blood pressure and heart disease, caution and lower doses appear prudent.

▷ **Advisability of Use During Pregnancy**

Pregnancy Category: C. See Pregnancy Risk Categories at the back of this book.
Human Studies: Adequate studies of pregnant women are not available.
NOT recommended for pregnant women.

Advisability of Use If Breast-Feeding

Presence of this drug in breast milk: unknown in humans.
Avoid drug or refrain from nursing.

Habit-Forming Potential: The possibility of physical dependence is low, but this medicine is a schedule 4 drug (see Controlled Drug Schedules in the back of this edition). Further study is needed to confirm an accurate probability of dependence risk. There was no evidence of addictive or drug-seeking behavior in premarketing studies.

Effects of Overdose: Few cases of overdose have been reported. Rapid heart rate was seen in one overdose.

Possible Effects of Long-Term Use: Weight loss (the desired effect). Increased blood pressure.

Suggested Periodic Examinations While Taking This Drug
   Periodic weigh-ins.
   Liver function tests.
   Checks for early signs of primary pulmonary hypertension and hypertension in general are prudent.
   Periodic blood pressure checks are prudent.

▷ **While Taking This Drug, Observe the Following**
   Foods: Follow prescribed portion control and menu choices. Tryptophan (found in some health food stores) increases risk of serotonin syndrome.
   Herbal Medicines or Minerals: Combining this medicine with St. John's wort IS NOT advised because of possible serotonin syndrome. Since part of the way ginseng works may be as an MAO inhibitor, do not combine ginseng with sibutramine. Ma huang, kola, bitter orange, country mallow, guarana, mate, ephedra (no longer available in the U.S. for weight loss), and yohimbe are also best avoided while taking this medicine.
   Nutritional Support: Dietary counseling and physician- or dietitian-directed menus and portion control are suggested. Make a rational plan to take the undesirable weight off and keep it off.
   Beverages: No restrictions except as described in your dietary guidelines.
▷ *Alcohol:* The manufacturer does not recommend use of excessive alcohol and sibutramine.
   Tobacco Smoking: No interactions are described in current literature. I advise everyone to quit smoking.
▷ *Other Drugs*
   Sibutramine *taken concurrently* with
   • antimigraine agents (such as sumatriptan-Imitrex) and dihydroergotamine may rarely result in a serotonin syndrome—DO NOT COMBINE.
   • central nervous system active medicines (see Drug Classes of benzodiazepines, opioids [fentanyl, etc.], phenothiazines, and others) may have additive effects—CAUTION is advised.
   • dextromethorphan (various brands of cough medicine) may increase risk of serotonin syndrome—DO NOT COMBINE.
   • fentanyl (Duragesic, others) increases risk of serotonin syndrome—DO NOT COMBINE.
   • lithium (Lithobid, others) increases risk of serotonin syndrome—DO NOT COMBINE.
   • meperidine (Demerol, others) increases risk of serotonin syndrome—DO NOT COMBINE.
   • monoamine oxidase (MAO) inhibitors (see Drug Classes) may result in serious, even fatal, reactions. Fourteen days should pass between stopping an MAO inhibitor and starting sibutramine.
   • pentazocine (Talwin, others) increases risk of serotonin syndrome—DO NOT COMBINE.
   • selective serotonin reuptake inhibitors (SSRIs: see Drug Classes) increases risk of serotonin syndrome—DO NOT COMBINE.
   • tricyclic antidepressants (some, such as desipramine [Norpramin] and amitriptyline [Elavil]) increase serotonin syndrome risk.
   • tryptophan (various) increases risk of serotonin syndrome—DO NOT COMBINE.
   Sibutramine *taken concurrently* with the following may result in increased sibutramine levels:

- erythromycins (see Drug Classes).
- itraconazole (Sporanox), ketoconazole (Nizoral), and voriconazole (Vfend).
- mibefradil (Posicor) (removed from the U.S. market).
- nelfinavir (Viracept) and perhaps other protease inhibitors (see Drug Classes)—may increase blood levels.
- any medicine that interferes with cytochrome CYP3A4 or is removed from the body by those enzymes will potentially increase sibutramine blood levels. For example, if sildenafil (Viagra) and sibutramine are combined, I expect that doses of one or both drugs may need to be adjusted.

The following drugs may **decrease** the effects of sibutramine:
- rifabutin (Mycobutin).
- rifampin (Rifadin, Rimactane).

▷ *Driving, Hazardous Activities:* Use caution.

Aviation Note: The use of this drug **may be a disqualification** for piloting. Consult a designated Aviation Medical Examiner.

Exposure to Sun: No restrictions at present.

Occurrence of Unrelated Illness: Since weight loss may modify the need for medicines used to control blood pressure and lipids, the medicines used in these conditions may need to be adjusted.

Discontinuation: Ask your doctor for help if you are considering stopping this medicine.

SILDENAFIL CITRATE (sill DEN ah fill)

Introduced: 1998   **Class:** Anti-impotence, phosphodiesterase inhibitor
Prescription: USA: Yes   **Controlled Drug:** USA: No; Canada: No
Available as Generic: USA: No; Canada: No
Brand Name: Viagra

BENEFITS versus RISKS	
Possible Benefits	*Possible Risks*
SUCCESSFUL ACHIEVEMENT OF AN ERECTION	SERIOUS DRUG INTERACTIONS
SUFFICIENT ERECTION TO ACHIEVE INTERCOURSE	Drug-induced vision changes
May work in female orgasm problems (Italian data)	Headache

▷ **Principal Uses**

As a Single Drug Product: Uses currently included in FDA-approved labeling: (1) Treats difficulties getting or maintaining an erection (erectile dysfunction).

Other (unlabeled) generally accepted uses: (1) Many anecdotal and/or conflicting reports of improvement in sexuality (enhancement) and benefits in females have been made; (2) may have a role in premature ejaculation problems; (3) helps reverse sexual problems caused by antidepressant medicines.

▷ **How This Drug Works:** Causes smooth muscle in the penis to relax, increasing blood flow into the penis, resulting in erection. Sildenafil causes release of nitric oxide (NO) in part of the penis called the corpus cavernosum. This then increases an enzyme called guanylate cyclase. This enzyme increases cyclic guanosine monophosphate (CGMP). The CGMP causes the smooth muscle in the penis to relax. Once the smooth muscle relaxes, blood flows into the penis, resulting in erection.

▷ **Widely Used Guidelines That Involve This Medicine (representative sample):** Please look at the section at the very beginning of this profile called "Class." Next, turn to Table 22 and you will find guidelines listed by the class involved!

Available Dosage Forms and Strengths
Tablets — 25 mg, 50 mg, 100 mg

▷ **Recommended Dose Ranges** (Actual dose and schedule must be determined for each patient individually.)

Infants and Children: Not used in this age group.

18 to 65 Years of Age: Doses typically range from 25–100 mg used once daily. The dose that your doctor chooses is taken from half an hour up to four hours before sexual activity. This medicine has worked in more than 70% of patients who took the 50–100 mg daily dose. For people who are taking medicines that inhibit a liver enzyme called cytochrome P450 3A4 (such as itraconazole, ketoconazole, or some macrolide antibiotics such as erythromycin), the 25 mg dose is used by clinicians who have patients who take one of those medicines at the same time as sildenafil. Further caution is required, and it would be a benefit-to-risk decision if multiple 3A4 inhibitors are being taken and sildenafil is being considered. Additionally, some medicines used in combination therapy of HIV/AIDS may interact, and caution and lower doses are prudent; use is a benefit-to-risk decision for your doctor. (See additional medicine combination comments in the drug interactions section below.)

Over 65 Years of Age: Because plasma levels of sildenafil may be increased in this age group, doses should be reduced to 25 mg once daily. If kidney function has decreased to less than 30 mL/min further in a patient in this age group, further benefit-to-risk decision should be given.

Conditions Requiring Dosing Adjustments
Liver Function: A starting dose of 25 mg is prudent in liver disease.
Kidney Function: Caution is advised, as one measure of drug levels is doubled in those with compromised kidneys. A starting dose of 25 mg is prudent.

▷ **Dosing Instructions:** The tablet may be crushed and taken without regard to eating (high-fat meals decreased absorption time and may make the medicine take longer to work). It can be taken an hour before sexual activity, and the manufacturer mentions an acceptable range of half an hour to 4 hours before sexual activity. If you forget a dose: There is a 4-hour to as little as 30-minute time frame to work with. DO NOT take the medicine more than once a day.

Usual Duration of Use: Use is only recommended ONCE a day. If use is to be ongoing on a daily basis, this should be discussed with your doctor.

Typical Treatment Goals and Measurements (Outcomes and Markers)
Erectile dysfunction: The general goal is to help you attain an erection that will help you have sex. Typical desired results are stiffness or tone of the penis and how often you have an erection in response to this medicine.

Possible Advantages of This Drug: Avoids direct injections into the penis (such as Caverject). Avoids surgical placement of an implant. Excellent response rate.

▷ **This Drug Should Not Be Taken If**
  • you have had an allergic reaction to it previously.
  • you have a disease or condition that would result in serious health hazard if lowering of the blood pressure or sexual activity occurred.

- you are taking any nitrate (see Drug Classes). NEVER combine these nitrates with sildenafil (see also "Other Drug" interactions).
- you have preexisting cardiovascular disease of a severity that precludes sexual activity.
- you have not fully discussed this medicine or all of the other medicines you take with your doctor, or have obtained it from an alternative source.

▷ **Inform Your Physician Before Taking This Drug If**
- you have liver or kidney disease.
- the drug was prescribed for you without a complete medical history or physical examination.
- you have a history of heart disease (such as congestive heart failure, past heart attack, unstable angina, arrhythmias, or coronary ischemia).
- you have multiple myeloma, leukemia, or sickle-cell syndrome (may predispose you to painful and sustained erections called priapism).
- you are over 65 and a 50 mg dose has been prescribed.
- you have vision changes while taking this medicine.
- you have cataracts or impaired vision (such as retinitis pigmentosa).
- you have had structural damage to the penis (Peyronie's disease: see Glossary).
- you are taking a medicine that blocks or enhances the liver cytochrome system (CYP3A4 or 2C9) (talk to your doctor or pharmacist about this).
- you are prone to heartburn or have other stomach conditions or a bleeding disorder.
- you do not have any improvement in erections or sexual performance while taking this medicine.
- you are unsure how much to take or how often to take this medicine.

Possible Side Effects (natural, expected, and unavoidable drug actions)
Changes in vision (blue tint) or dry eyes—up to 3% in clinical trials. Nasal congestion—possible.

▷ **Possible Adverse Effects** (unusual, unexpected, and infrequent reactions)
If any of the following develop, consult your physician promptly for guidance.
Mild Adverse Effects
Allergic reaction: rash.
Headache—infrequent to frequent.
Flushing—infrequent to frequent.
Indigestion—infrequent.
Sensitivity to light or blurred vision—possible to infrequent (more likely with the 100 mg dose).
Inability to distinguish between blue and green—possible and may be dose-related.
Serious Adverse Effects
DEATH RESULTING FROM DRUG INTERACTIONS—possible with nitrates.
Temporary vision loss—case reports.
Stroke—case report.
Decrease in blood supplied to the heart muscle (myocardial ischemia)—rare.
Heart attack—case reports with preexisting heart conditions and rare reports in people without preexisting heart conditions.
Decreased preload and afterload—possible (in patients with cardiomyopathy).
Arrhythmias (ventricular tachycardia) or atrial fibrillation—case reports.

▷ **Possible Effects on Sexual Function:**
   Abnormal ejaculation—case reports.
   Sustained and painful erection (priapism)—case reports.

Possible Delayed Adverse Effects: None reported to date.

Natural Diseases or Disorders That May Be Activated by This Drug
   Patient perception of any preexisting retinal disease may be worsened if
   sildenafil haze or bluish vision tinting happens. Some cardiovascular conditions may be worsened by this drug.

Possible Effects on Laboratory Tests
   None reported.

CAUTION
   **Author's Note: Early case reports of 6 deaths were reviewed by the FDA
   in May 1998. A total of 30 deaths were reviewed as of June 1998.
   Based on the review, Viagra itself was NOT found to be the cause of
   the deaths and NO CHANGES were made to the package insert. Subsequently, expanded safety information was added to required FDA
   labeling including drug interaction data. During this controversial
   and rapidly changing period, conflicting reports, possible interactions
   as absolute contraindications, and unclear benefit-to-risk decisions
   were reported and evolved or failed to evolve. Talk to your doctor or
   pharmacist about the most current combinations of medicines that
   are thought to be inappropriate versus those requiring lower doses
   and those that should never be undertaken. Because a medicine has
   serious possible interactions does not mean that it is an undesirable
   medicine, only that some combinations are never to be made.**

   1. Because of the possibility of SERIOUS drug interactions, keep a card in
      your purse or wallet or get a medicine alert bracelet to wear that says you
      are taking sildenafil.
   2. If this medicine does not help you get or maintain an erection, it is
      important that you follow up with your doctor.
   3. Safety and efficacy of sildenafil combined with other treatments for erec-
      tile problems (dysfunction) have not been established and may not be
      recommended by your doctor.
   4. Some people use illegal "poppers," which are actually ampules of alkyl
      nitrites, to enhance sexual activity. These should NEVER be combined
      with Viagra.
   5. The American Academy of Ophthalmology recommended further studies
      of sildenafil's long-term effects on the eyes and also warned that those
      with conditions of the retina should take the drug in the lowest effective
      dose and with caution. Promptly report altered or impaired vision so that
      appropriate evaluation can be made.
   6. The manufacturer notes that it is important to have a physical exam and
      medical history taken to properly diagnose problems with erections (erec-
      tile dysfunction) and to identify (where possible) any underlying disease or
      condition that may actually be the cause of the problem (such as diabetes).
   7. If your erection lasts more than 4 hours, go to the nearest emergency
      room. Such persistent erections may lead to damage of the penis that is
      not reversible.

Precautions for Use
   By Infants and Children: Safety and effectiveness for those under 18 not estab-
      lished.
   By Those Over 60 Years of Age: Because this medicine is more slowly removed

from the body in this age group, drug levels may be higher. The recommended starting dose is 25 mg.

▷ **Advisability of Use During Pregnancy**
Pregnancy Category: B. See Pregnancy Risk Categories at the back of this book.
Animal Studies: No evidence of embryotoxicity, fetotoxicity, or teratogenicity in rats and rabbits.
Human Studies: Adequate studies of pregnant women are not available.
NOT indicated for use in women, children, or newborns.

Advisability of Use If Breast-Feeding
Presence of this drug in breast milk: Unknown.
Avoid drug or refrain from nursing.

Habit-Forming Potential: None.

Effects of Overdose: Adverse effects were similar to accepted dosing adverse effects, but increased in frequency with clinical trials of 800 mg doses. Supportive care is indicated with the caveat of extremely careful cardiac monitoring in those with existing heart disease.

Possible Effects of Long-Term Use: Not defined.

Suggested Periodic Examinations While Taking This Drug (at physician's discretion)
Follow-up on success in achieving an erection and having intercourse.
Complete eye examination at beginning of treatment and at any time that significant change in vision occurs. Ask your doctor for help.

▷ **While Taking This Drug, Observe the Following**
Foods: Grapefruit juice can be an inhibitor of CYP3A4. DO NOT combine. Water is the safest liquid to take this medicine with.
Herbal Medicines or Minerals: Using St. John's wort, ma huang (no longer available for weight loss), mate, bitter orange, country mallow, or kola while taking this medicine may result in unacceptable heart stimulation. Since St. John's wort and sildenafil may increase sun sensitivity, the combination is NOT advised. There are no data regarding combining yohimbe (Pausinystala yohimbe) with sildenafil, and yohimbe can lead to serious heart complications. The combination is NOT advised. Numan has had some small cohort studies, but has also not been studied and cannot be recommended in combination with sildenafil. A product from Health Nutrition labs called Viga or Viga for Women was the subject of an FDA MedWatch safety alert. The warning noted that this dietary supplement contained sildenafil as an unlabeled ingredient. See *www.fda.gov/medwatch/SAFETY/2003/safety/safety02.htm#vigarma*.
Beverages: Grapefruit juice can be an inhibitor of the enzyme that removes sildenafil from the body (CYP3A4). DO NOT combine as toxicity may result. Drug may be taken with milk or water.
▷ *Alcohol:* Excess alcohol intake may blunt the benefits of this medicine.
Tobacco Smoking: No interactions expected. I advise everyone to quit smoking.
Marijuana Smoking: The active ingredient (cannabinoids) found in marijuana can act as an inhibitor of the principal enzyme (CYP3A4) that removes sildenafil from the body. COMBINATION IS NOT RECOMMENDED.
▷ *Other Drugs*
Sildenafil may increase the effects of
• nitrates (see Drug Classes)—NEVER COMBINE.
The following drugs may *increase* the effects of sildenafil:
• cimetidine (Tagamet).

- delavirdine (Rescriptor).
- diltiazem (Cardizem).
- erythromycins (erythromycin and clarithromycin: see Drug Classes).
- indinavir (Crixivan), nelfinavir (Viracept), saquinavir (Invirase, Fortovase), and perhaps other protease inhibitors (see Drug Classes).
- itraconazole (Sporanox), ketoconazole (Nizoral), and perhaps similar anti-fungals.
- metronidazole (Flagyl).
- mibefradil (Posicor) (removed from the U.S. market).
- nitroprusside (Nitropress).
- ritonavir (Norvir) can increase sildenafil blood levels by up to 1,000%. A maximum dose of 25 mg every 48 hours is suggested along with careful patient monitoring.
- saquinavir (Fortovase). Starting dose should be 25 mg.
- sertraline (Zoloft).
- any medicine that interferes with cytochrome (CYP3A4-major or 2C9-minor, such as sibutramine [Meridia], which uses CYP3A4) will potentially increase (or decrease) sildenafil blood levels. In some cases, I expect that sildenafil dosing will need to be adjusted, and in others, the combination should be avoided.

Sildenafil **taken concurrently** with

- amprenavir (Agenerase) and atazanavir (Reyataz) may lead to excessive sildenafil levels. Lower doses are prudent.
- amyl nitrite will result in serious decreases in blood pressure—DO NOT COMBINE.
- medicines that cause vision changes (see Table 4) may result in additive vision problems.
- oral hypoglycemic agents tolbutamide (Orinase an inhibitor of 2C9) and glipizide (Glucotrol)—one early case report of a serious interaction are representative of medicines that may lead to problems and in the case of glipizide had one reported problem. Talk to your doctor about the latest information on possible interactions of these medicines with sildenafil.

The following drugs may **decrease** the effects of sildenafil:

- carbamazepine (Tegretol).
- phenytoin (Dilantin).
- rifabutin (Mycobutin).
- rifampin (Rifadin, Rimactane).

▷ *Driving, Hazardous Activities:* No restrictions.

Aviation Note: The use of this drug **may be a disqualification** for piloting. Consult a designated Aviation Medical Examiner.

Exposure to Sun: May increase sensitivity of your eyes to sunlight. Talk to your doctor about sunglasses or other protective measures.

Discontinuation: Talk to your doctor about your results from taking this drug.

SIMVASTATIN (sim vah STA tin)

Introduced: 1986 **Class:** Anticholesterol **Prescription:** USA: Yes **Controlled Drug:** USA: No; Canada: No **Available as Generic:** USA: No; Canada: No

Brand Names: ✤Apo-Simvastatin, ✤Gen-Simvastatin, ✤Nu-Simvastatin, ✤Ratio-Simvastatin, Vytorin, Zocor, Zocor Heart-Pro (OTC in UK)

BENEFITS versus RISKS

Possible Benefits	*Possible Risks*
EFFECTIVE REDUCTION OF TOTAL BLOOD CHOLESTEROL AND LDL CHOLESTEROL	Drug-induced liver problems (hepatitis)—rare
INCREASES HDL-C (GOOD CHOLESTEROL) IN PATIENTS WITH PRIMARY HYPER-CHOLESTEROLEMIA AND MIXED DYSLIPIDEMIA	Drug-induced muscle damage (myositis)—rare
TREATS ISOLATED HYPER-TRIGLYCERIDEMIA AND TYPE THREE HYPER-LIPOPROTEINEMIA	Decreased coenzyme Q10
REDUCES RISK FROM CORONARY DISEASE	
REDUCES DEATH FROM CORONARY REVASCULARIZATION	
REDUCES NONFATAL MYOCARDIAL INFARCTIONS AND THE NEED FOR BYPASS SURGERY AND ANGIOPLASTY	
REDUCES RISK OF STROKES	
May help prevent or preserve mental status in Alzheimer's	
May help maintain bone health	

▷ **Principal Uses**

As a Single Drug Product: Uses currently included in FDA-approved labeling: (1) Used by patients with elevated cholesterol to reduce death from heart disease and decrease the number of nonfatal heart attacks; (2) treats high total blood cholesterol levels (in people with types IIa and IIb hypercholesterolemia)—used in conjunction with a cholesterol-lowering diet (it should not be used until an adequate trial of nondrug methods for lowering cholesterol has proved to be ineffective); (3) stops progression and decreases number of deaths of patients with coronary artery disease as well as the need for bypass surgery and angioplasty; (4) decreases risk of strokes; (5) treats isolated hypertriglyceridemia and type three hyperlipoproteinemia; (6) increases HDL-C in people with primary hypercholesterolemia and mixed dyslipidemia.

Other (unlabeled) generally accepted uses: (1) Used in combination with estrogen (in one study of women averaging 57 years old) lowered LDL, increased HDL, and reduced undesirable blood-clotting factors and inflammation; (2) may help reduce lipid disorders that occur in kidney problems (nephrotic syndrome); (3) combination therapy in preventing gallstones; (4) may have a role after heart transplants to decrease death and lower LDL-C levels; (5) a small study of 32 patients with multiple sclerosis (MS) is under way looking at the benefits of high dose simvastatin in easing MS symptoms; (5) may help preserve bone health; (6) could have a role in Alzheimer's patients helping prevent it or preserve function.

How This Drug Works: Blocks the liver enzyme starting production of cholesterol. Reduces low-density lipoproteins (LDL), the fraction of cholesterol thought to increase risk of coronary heart disease. Also increases, high-density lipoproteins (HDL), the cholesterol fraction that reduces the risk of heart disease. There is a growing body of evidence that "statins" also have beneficial changes on what is in the blood, blood flow, and even the blood vessel walls themselves (some of this may account for benefits in decreasing Alzheimer's risk). Specific compounds or effects of platelet derived growth factor (PDGF), undesirable blood clotting via thrombin-antithrombin III, thrombomodulin, and other chemicals may be beneficially lowered or effects mitigated by statins.

▷ **Widely Used Guidelines That Involve This Medicine (representative sample):** Please look at the section at the very beginning of this profile called "Class." Next, turn to Table 22 and you will find guidelines listed by the class involved!

Available Dosage Forms and Strengths
   Tablets — 5 mg, 10 mg, 20 mg, 40 mg, 80 mg

▷ **Recommended Dosage Ranges** (Actual dose and schedule must be determined for each patient individually.)
   Infants and Children: Under 2 years of age—do not use this drug.
   2 to 20 years of Age: Dose not established for children or adolescents.
   20 to 60 Years of Age: Initially 20 mg daily, taken at bedtime. Dose is increased as needed to reach desired goals (such as decreased LDL-C percent). The drug is then increased as needed and tolerated by increments of 5 to 10 mg at intervals of 4 weeks. The total daily dose should not exceed 80 mg. For patients who require more than a 45% decrease in bad cholesterol (LDL), the starting dose is 40 mg per day. Some clinicians add on therapy, which lowers cholesterol by a different mechanism. One study of related medicines found that the higher dose after a heart attack gave better results than lower doses (ask your doctor about this). **See dosing based on drug interactions in the Other Drugs section below in order to give your medicines a checkup.**
   Over 60 Years of Age: Initially 5 mg daily. Increase dose as needed and tolerated by increments of 5 mg at intervals of 4 weeks. The total daily dose should not exceed 40 mg.

Conditions Requiring Dosing Adjustments
   Liver Function: This drug achieves a high concentration in the liver and is subsequently eliminated in the bile. It can be a rare cause of liver damage, and patients should be followed closely.
   Kidney Function: In severe kidney failure, the dose should be started at 5 mg and the patient closely followed.
   Heart Transplants: People who are getting immunosuppressive therapy should be started on 5 mg of simvastatin. The maximum dose in these patients should be 10 mg.

▷ **Dosing Instructions:** The tablet may be crushed and taken without regard to eating, preferably at bedtime (the highest rates of cholesterol production occur between midnight and 5 A.M.). If you forget a dose: Take the missed dose as soon as you remember it, unless it's nearly time for your next dose—if that is the case, skip the missed dose and take the next dose right on schedule. DO NOT double doses. Talk with your doctor and pharmacist if you find yourself missing doses, as there are many effective reminder systems available.

Usual Duration of Use: Use on a regular schedule for 4 to 6 weeks usually determines effectiveness in reducing blood levels of total and LDL cholesterol. Long-term use (months to years) requires periodic physician evaluation of response and dose adjustment, as cholesterol tends to increase as we age. See your doctor on a regular basis to make certain you are on track.

Typical Treatment Goals and Measurements (Outcomes and Markers)

Cholesterol: Current guidelines (National Cholesterol Education Program, or NCEP) acknowledge diabetes as one of the conditions that increases risk of heart disease, modifying risk factors, therapeutic lifestyle changes (TLC), and recommending routine testing for all of the cholesterol fractions (lipoprotein profile) versus total cholesterol alone. Goals are: a total cholesterol of 200 mg/dL, and optimal bad cholesterol (LDL) of less than 100 mg/dL. Less than 70 mg/dL (see Grundy, S.M. in Sources) is a reasonable optional goal for very high risk patients (such as diabetics with acute coronary syndromes, etc.). 130–159 mg/dL as borderline high, 160 mg/dL as high and 190 mg/dL as very high. Did you know that there are at least five different kinds of "good cholesterol" or HDL? The "too low" measure for HDL is still 40mg/dL, but in order to learn more about cholesterol types some doctors are starting to order lipid panels. There are at least seven different kinds of "bad cholesterol." The new panels tell doctors about the kinds of cholesterol that your body makes. This is important because some kinds (small dense particles) tend to stick to blood vessels (are highly atherogenic). Take your medicine to reach your goals! Two additional tests you will hear about will be electron beam computed tomography (EBCT) and CRP. EBCT is an important tool used in conjunction with laboratory studies. Findings show that even patients who meet cholesterol goals (particularly females over 55) can still be at significant cardiovascular risk. EBCT then defines risk by giving a calcium score and a "virtual tour" of the coronary arteries. C Reactive Protein, or CRP, is a relatively new and apparently independent predictor of heart disease risk. A large study (see Ridker, P.M. in Sources) found that CRP predicted heart disease risk independently of bad cholesterol (low density lipoprotein). Talk to your doctor about this laboratory test and ask about current guidelines for who should be tested (see Pearson, T.A. in Sources).

Possible Advantages of This Drug: Several studies indicate that HMG-CoA reductase inhibitors are more effective and better tolerated than other drugs currently available for reducing total and LDL cholesterol. Additional benefits in preventing other problems are emerging.

▷ **This Drug Should Not Be Taken If**
- you have had an allergic reaction to it previously.
- you have active liver disease.
- your liver enzyme levels (serum transaminases) have increased without explanation.
- you are pregnant or breast-feeding your infant.

▷ **Inform Your Physician Before Taking This Drug If**
- you have previously taken any other drugs in this class: lovastatin (Mevacor) or pravastatin (Pravachol).
- you have a history of liver disease or impaired liver function.
- you are taking any of the medicines listed in the Other Drugs section of this profile.
- you are not using any method of birth control or you are planning pregnancy.
- you regularly consume substantial amounts of alcohol.
- you have cataracts or impaired vision.
- you have any type of chronic muscular disorder.

- you develop muscle pain, weakness, or soreness that is unexplained while taking this medicine.
- you plan to have major surgery in the near future.

Possible Side Effects (natural, expected, and unavoidable drug actions)
Development of abnormal liver function tests without associated symptoms.
Decreased co-enzyme Q10 (co-Q10 or ubiquinone).

▷ **Possible Adverse Effects** (unusual, unexpected, and infrequent reactions)
If any of the following develop, consult your physician promptly for guidance.
Mild Adverse Effects
Allergic reaction: rash.
Headache, dizziness, or fatigue—infrequent.
Nausea, excessive gas, constipation, or diarrhea—rare to infrequent.
Lowering of blood pressure—possible.
Serious Adverse Effects
Marked and persistent abnormal liver function tests with focal hepatitis—rare.
Acute myositis (muscle pain and tenderness)—infrequent.
Rhabdomyolysis—rare (may be more likely with higher doses).
Potential for cataracts—based on animal data, not reported in humans.
Lowered blood platelets (thrombocytopenia)—rare.
Neuropathy—case report.
Depression—rare.
Protein in the urine—rare.
Lichen planus skin rash—rare.
Roughly 60 cases of short-term memory loss (simvastatin [36], atorvastatin [23], pravastatin [1]) have been made.

▷ **Possible Effects on Sexual Function:** Impotence—case reports.

Possible Delayed Adverse Effects: Increased liver enzymes. Lowered levels of co-enzyme Q10.

Natural Diseases or Disorders That May Be Activated by This Drug
Latent liver disease.

Possible Effects on Laboratory Tests
Blood alanine aminotransferase (ALT) enzyme level: increased (with higher doses of drug).
Blood total cholesterol, LDL cholesterol, and triglyceride levels: decreased.
Blood HDL cholesterol level: increased.
Bone mineral density tests (DEXA, PDEXA, and quantitative ultrasound) will remain the same or increase in many cases (beneficial effect).

CAUTION
1. If pregnancy occurs while taking this drug, stop the drug immediately and call your physician.
2. Call your doctor to report promptly any development of muscle pain or tenderness, especially if accompanied by fever or weakness (malaise).
3. Promptly report altered or impaired vision so that appropriate evaluation can be made.

Precautions for Use
By Infants and Children: Safety and effectiveness for those less than 17 years of age are not established.
By Those Over 60 Years of Age: Inform your physician regarding any personal or family history of cataracts. Comply with all recommendations regarding periodic eye examinations. Report promptly any alterations in vision.

▷ **Advisability of Use During Pregnancy**

Pregnancy Category: X. See Pregnancy Risk Categories at the back of this book.

Animal Studies: Mouse and rat studies reveal skeletal birth defects due to a closely related drug of this class.

Human Studies: Adequate studies of pregnant women are not available.

This drug should be avoided during entire pregnancy.

Advisability of Use If Breast-Feeding

Presence of this drug in breast milk: Unknown, but expected since a similar drug from this class does go into breast milk.

Avoid drug or refrain from nursing.

Habit-Forming Potential: None.

Effects of Overdose: Increased indigestion, stomach distress, nausea, and diarrhea.

Possible Effects of Long-Term Use: Abnormal liver function with focal hepatitis.

Suggested Periodic Examinations While Taking This Drug (at physician's discretion)

Blood cholesterol studies: total cholesterol, HDL, and LDL fractions. CRP, homocysteine, and LP(a).

Liver function tests before treatment and every 6 months for the first year of treatment—or until 1 year has passed after the last dose increase. People who require the 80 mg dose should get another test at 3 months after the increase to 80 mg. In patients who have had an increase in liver enzymes, repeat testing should be done to confirm the first finding. After this, testing should continue frequently until the enzymes return to normal. IF THE ENZYMES INCREASE TO THREE TIMES THE UPPER LIMIT OF NORMAL, SIMVASTATIN SHOULD BE STOPPED.

A complete eye examination may be prudent at beginning of treatment and at any time that significant change in vision occurs (based on animal data). Ask your doctor for help.

EBCT can help define blood vessel damage (calcium score) and track results from this medicine.

▷ **While Taking This Drug, Observe the Following**

Foods: Combination use of B vitamin supplements may help lower additional heart disease risk factors such as homocysteine. Follow a standard low-cholesterol diet. Your doctor may recommend specific foods such as increased vegetables or functional foods such as Benecol. Three well-designed studies found that both in women and men before or after a heart attack, people who ate more fish (2–4 servings a week) appeared to avoid heart disease. Additionally, supplements containing Omega 3 polyunsaturated fatty acids (PUFA) also appeared to protect against abnormal heart rhythms and sudden death from heart attack. Your doctor may also recommend increasing B vitamins. See Tables 19 and 20 about lifestyle changes and risk factors you can fix.

Herbal Medicines or Minerals: No data exist from well-designed clinical studies about garlic and simvastatin combinations, and the combination cannot presently be recommended. Additionally, garlic may inhibit blood-clotting (platelet) aggregation—something to consider if you are already taking a platelet inhibitor. The FDA has allowed one dietary supplement called Cholestin to continue to be sold. This preparation actually contains lovastatin. Since use of two HMG-CoA inhibitors may increase risk of rhabdomyolysis or myopathy, the combination is NOT advised. Because St. John's wort and this medicine can increase sun sensitivity, the combination is not advised. Herbal medicines such as eucalyptus, kava, valerian, and others, which can have a toxic effect on the liver, should be avoided while taking simvastatin.

Using plant stanol ester products (Benecol) with this medicine can help further lower total and LDL cholesterol. Soy products (milk, tofu, etc.) contain phytoestrogens that have led to an FDA-approved health claim for reducing risk of heart disease (if they have at least 6.25 g of soy protein per serving). Substituting soy for some of the meat in your diet can also help further lower cholesterol. Policosanol also appears to have benefits. Because simvastatin can deplete co-enzyme Q10, supplementation may be needed.

Beverages: DO NOT take this medicine with grapefruit juice. Blood levels may be markedly increased, increasing risk of muscle damage. May be taken with milk or water.

▷ *Alcohol:* No interactions expected. Use sparingly.

Tobacco Smoking: No interactions expected. I advise everyone to quit smoking.

▷ *Other Drugs*

Author's Note: The company has strengthened myopathy/rhabdomyolysis risk language with some drug combinations versus earlier package inserts.

Simvastatin may *increase* the effects of
- digoxin (Lanoxin).
- imatinib (Gleevec); blood levels of imatinib are needed and should be used to guide lower dosing.
- warfarin (Coumadin); more frequent testing of INR (prothrombin time or protime) will be needed. (Possible increased risk of muscle damage, so any unexplained muscle stiffness or weakness should lead to a call to your doctor.)

Simvastatin *taken concurrently* with
- amiodarone (Cordarone) may increase risk of muscle damage. DOSE REDUCTION TO 20 MG MAXIMUM AND CAREFUL PATIENT MONITORING ARE REQUIRED IF THESE MEDICINES MUST BE COMBINED.
- amprenavir (Agenerase), indinavir (Crixivan), atazanavir (Reyataz), ritonavir (Norvir), and perhaps other protease inhibitors INCREASE THE RISK OF MUSCLE DAMAGE. DOSING OF SIMVASTATIN SHOULD BE SUSPENDED.
- clarithromycin (Biaxin) and erythromycin (various) INCREASES THE RISK OF MUSCLE DAMAGE. IF THESE MEDICINES MUST BE USED, DOSING OF SIMVASTATIN SHOULD BE SUSPENDED.
- clofibrate (Atromid-S) or other fibrates may result in increased risk of serious muscle toxicity. AVOID IF POSSIBLE—IF NOT—DOSE REDUCTION TO 10 mg MAXIMUM AND CAREFUL PATIENT MONITORING ARE REQUIRED IF THESE MEDICINES MUST BE COMBINED.
- colesevelam (Welchol) results in better lowering of LDL-C (desirable effect).
- cyclosporine (Sandimmune) 10 mg DAILY DOSE MAXIMUM. Careful follow-up for effects on the kidney and muscles (kidney failure and myopathy) is needed.
- gemfibrozil (Lopid) may alter absorption and excretion of simvastatin and may also increase risk of muscle damage (rhabdomyolysis)—10 mg MAXIMUM AND CAREFUL PATIENT FOLLOW-UP ARE NEEDED.
- itraconazole (Sporanox), voriconazole (Vfend), or ketoconazole (Nizoral)

seriously increases risk of muscle damage—DO NOT COMBINE. DOSING OF SIMVASTATIN SHOULD BE SUSPENDED WHILE ITRACONAZOLE OR KETOCONAZOLE ARE BEING TAKEN.

- medicines that change cytochrome P450 3A4 (inhibitors will increase simvastatin levels, and inducers will blunt simvastatin therapeutic effects).
- nefazodone (Serzone) may increase risk of muscle damage. IF NEFAZODONE IS REQUIRED, RISK OF MYOPATHY IS INCREASED. CAREFUL PATIENT MONITORING IS MANDATORY.
- niacin may cause an increased frequency of muscle problems (myopathy) when combined with a related medicine (lovastatin). DOSE REDUCTION TO 10 MG MAXIMUM AND CAREFUL PATIENT MONITORING ARE REQUIRED IF THESE MEDICINES MUST BE COMBINED (niacin doses of 1g a day or more). THIS IS A BENEFIT-TO-RISK DECISION.
- quinupristin/dalfopristin (Synercid) may increase the risk for myopathy by increasing simvastatin blood levels.
- verapamil (Verelan) may increase risk of muscle damage. DOSE REDUCTION TO 20 MG MAXIMUM AND CAREFUL PATIENT MONITORING ARE REQUIRED IF THESE MEDICINES MUST BE COMBINED.

The following drug may *decrease* the effects of simvastatin:

- cholestyramine (Questran) may reduce absorption of simvastatin; take simvastatin 1 hour before or 4 hours after cholestyramine.
- fosphenytoin (Cerebyx) or phenytoin (Dilantin) may increase the body chemicals (enzymes) that remove simvastatin and blunt simvastatin benefits. Careful patient monitoring and dose increases may be needed.

▷ *Driving, Hazardous Activities:* No restrictions.

Aviation Note: The use of this drug *may be a disqualification* for piloting. Consult a designated Aviation Medical Examiner.

Exposure to Sun: One case of skin reaction to the sun (photosensitivity/photodermatitis) has been reported.

Discontinuation: **Do not stop this drug without your doctor's knowledge and help.** There may be a significant increase in blood cholesterol levels if this medicine is stopped. Patients who have acute coronary syndromes or ACS (such as unstable angina, heart attack [non-p; Q-wave myocardial infarction], and Q-wave myocardial infarction) were reviewed as part of the Platelet Receptor Inhibitor in Ischemic Syndrome Management (PRISM) study. It was found that pretreatment with statin type medicines (HMG-CoA reductase inhibitors such as the medicine in this profile) significantly lowered risk during the first 30 days after ACS symptoms started. Talk with your doctor BEFORE stopping any statin-type medicine.

SPIRONOLACTONE (speer oh noh LAK tohn)

Introduced: 1959　**Class:** Diuretic, aldosterone receptor antagonist　**Prescription:** USA: Yes　**Controlled Drug:** USA: No; Canada: No　**Available as Generic:** USA: Yes

Author's Note: A medicine called eplerenone (Inspra) may have a more favorable profile, but further research is needed.

Brand Names: Alatone, Aldactazide [CD], Aldactone, ✚Apo-Spirozide, ✚Novo-Spiroton, ✚Novo-Spirozine [CD], ✚Sincomen, Spironazide

```
┌─────────────────────────────────────────────────────────────────────┐
│                     BENEFITS versus RISKS                             │
│    Possible Benefits                     Possible Risks               │
│ REDUCES RISK OF DEATH AND         ABNORMALLY HIGH BLOOD               │
│   HOSPITALIZATION BY 30%            POTASSIUM LEVEL WITH              │
│   WHEN USED AS PART OF              EXCESSIVE USE                      │
│   COMBINATION THERAPY FOR         Enlargement of male breast tissue   │
│   SEVERE HEART FAILURE            Masculinization effects in women:   │
│ EFFECTIVE PREVENTION OF             excessive hair growth, deepening of│
│   POTASSIUM LOSS WHEN USED          the voice                         │
│   ADJUNCTIVELY WITH OTHER         Liver damage (case reports)         │
│   DIURETICS                                                           │
│ EFFECTIVE DIURETIC IN                                                 │
│   REFRACTORY CASES OF FLUID                                           │
│   RETENTION WHEN USED                                                 │
│   ADJUNCTIVELY WITH OTHER                                             │
│   DIURETICS                                                           │
│ HELPS LESSEN ABNORMAL                                                 │
│   HEART CHANGES                                                       │
│   (REMODELING) AFTER A HEART                                          │
│   ATTACK (WHEN COMBINED                                               │
│   WITH AN ACE INHIBITOR)                                              │
└─────────────────────────────────────────────────────────────────────┘
```

▷ **Principal Uses**

As a Single Drug Product: Uses currently included in FDA-approved labeling: (1) Manages congestive heart failure and disorders of the liver and kidney that are accompanied by excessive fluid retention (edema); (2) also used with other measures to treat high blood pressure where prevention of potassium loss is needed; (3) used to decrease fluid in patients who have failed gluco-corticoid treatment and have nephrotic syndrome; (4) works to restore blood potassium to normal in drug caused (induced) low potassium (hypokalemia); (5) used in congestive heart failure (CHF) to reduce frequency of hospitalizations and death in patients with moderate to severe (NYHA class III when the principal study began and up to class IV) heart failure when used in combination with standard CHF treatment (usually a loop diuretic and ACE inhibitor [if tolerated] and in some cases digoxin).

Other (unlabeled) generally accepted uses: (1) May have an adjunctive role in treating acne; (2) can help treat lung problems (bronchopulmonary dysplasia) and slow the disease process; (3) can help precocious puberty in females; (4) eases fluid buildup in premenstrual syndrome; (5) may help women with excessive facial hair growth (hirsutism); (6) may protect against mountain sickness; (7) may help prevent bone loss in women who have polycystic ovary syndrome (PCOS) and are given a gonadotropin releasing hormone agonist; (8) used in combination with an ACE inhibitor (see Drug Classes) after a heart attack to help prevent abnormal heart changes (remodeling) and decreased heart function.

As a Combination Drug Product [CD]: This drug is available in combination with hydrochlorothiazide, a different kind of diuretic that promotes the loss of potassium from the body. Spironolactone is used in this combination to counteract the potassium-wasting effect of the thiazide diuretic.

In the Pipeline: The Health and Human Services secretary has identified a group of medicines to be tested for use in children. Spironolactone was on that list of the 12 highest priority medicines to be studied in children (find out more at *www.hhs.gov/news/press/2003pres/20030121.html*).

How This Drug Works: By inhibiting the action of aldosterone (an adrenal gland hormone), this drug prevents the reabsorption of sodium and the excretion of potassium by the kidney. Thus the drug promotes the excretion of sodium (and water with it) and the retention of potassium. In heart failure, spironolactone works to protect the heart from too much aldosterone (a hormone that can lower the ability of the heart to pump).

▷ **Widely Used Guidelines That Involve This Medicine (representative sample):** Please look at the section at the very beginning of this profile called "Class." Next, turn to Table 22 and you will find guidelines listed by the class involved!

Available Dosage Forms and Strengths
Tablets — 25 mg, 50 mg, 100 mg
Combination Tablets — 25 mg spironolactone/25 mg HCTZ, 50 mg spironolactone/50 mg HCTZ

▷ **Usual Adult Dosage Ranges:** For *edema:* Initially 100 mg per day in one dose or divided into several doses. The dose is then adjusted according to individual response. The usual maintenance dose is 50 to 200 mg daily, divided into two to four doses. If response is not adequate after 5 days, a second fluid medicine (diuretic) is added.

For hypertension: Spironolactone alone: 50–100 mg a day in one dose or divided into equal doses. The ongoing dose is adjusted as needed and tolerated 14 days after the drug is started. For the Aldactazide form: 50–100 mg of each medicine in one dose or separated into several equal doses.

In moderate to severe heart failure: Many clinicians are recommending use of 25 mg per day in combination with an ACE inhibitor, a loop diuretic, and possibly digoxin.

Acne: 50 mg a day has lead to clearing of acne.

Note: Actual dosage and administration schedule must be determined for each patient individually.

Conditions Requiring Dosing Adjustments
Liver Function: This drug can be a rare cause of liver damage, and patients should be followed closely.

Kidney Function: For patients with mild kidney failure, the drug can be taken every 12 hours in the usual dose. In moderate kidney failure (GFR 10–50 mL/min), spironolactone can be taken every 12 to 24 hours in the usual dose. In severe kidney failure (GFR less than 10 mL/min or creatinine greater than 2.5 mg/dL), this drug should not be taken. Spironolactone is contraindicated in acute renal failure and severe chronic renal compromise.

▷ **Dosing Instructions:** The tablet may be crushed and taken with or following meals to promote absorption of the drug and reduce stomach irritation. If you forget a dose: Take the missed dose as soon as you remember it, unless it's nearly time for your next dose—if that is the case, skip the missed dose and take the next dose right on schedule. DO NOT double doses. Talk with your doctor if you find yourself missing doses.

Usual Duration of Use: Use on a regular schedule for 5 to 10 days usually determines effectiveness in clearing edema, and for 2 to 3 weeks to determine its effect on hypertension. Because patient response may vary in congestive heart failure (CHF) and the aldosterone antagonism data are relatively new, talk over goals of CHF use individually. Long-term use (months to years) requires physician supervision and periodic evaluation.

Typical Treatment Goals and Measurements (Outcomes and Markers)

Congestive Heart Failure: The goal is to help remove excess fluid (edema) and hence decrease blood pressure while helping ease the amount of work the heart has to do. Additionally, when this medicine is combined with standard CHF treatment, death and adverse consequences of CHF as well as the number of times a given patient will generally have to be hospitalized are reduced. Clinical signs and symptoms such as ankle swelling, difficulty breathing and walking, or exercise tolerance may also improve. Surrogate end points (a marker that offers vital information about how well a patient is responding to a treatment) are useful to clinicians. Two possible surrogate markers for CHF are left ventricular end diastolic volume (LVEDV) and b-type natriuretic peptide (BNP). These will be updated as more information becomes available.

Blood Pressure: Guidelines (JNC VII) define normal blood pressure (BP) as **less than** 120/80 and **pre-hypertension** as 120/80 to 139/89. This new range is intended to help doctors encourage lifestyle changes (or, in the case of people with a risk factor for high blood pressure, start treatment) much earlier—so that damage to blood vessels, heart, kidneys, sexual potency, or eyes might be minimized or avoided altogether. Stage 1 hypertension is 140/90 to 159/99, and stage 2 hypertension equal to or greater than 160/100 mm Hg. These guidelines also recommend that clinicians work with their patients to agree on the goals and a plan of treatment. The first-ever guidelines for blood pressure (hypertension) in African Americans recommend that MOST black patients be started on TWO antihypertensive medicines with the goal of lowering blood pressure to 130/80 for those with high risk for heart and blood vessel disease or with diabetes. The American Diabetes Association also recommends 130/80 as the target for diabetics and less than 125/75 for those who spill more than 1 g of protein into their urine. Most clinicians try to achieve a BP that confers the best balance of lower cardiovascular risk and avoids the problem of too low a blood pressure. Blood pressure duration is generally increased with beneficial restriction of sodium. If goals are not met, it is not unusual to intensify doses or add on medicines.

This Drug Should Not Be Taken If
- you have had an allergic reaction to it previously.
- you have severely impaired liver or kidney function.
- your kidneys are not making any urine.
- your blood potassium is excessively high (hyperkalemia).

Inform Your Physician Before Taking This Drug If
- you have a history of liver or kidney disease.
- you have diabetes.
- you take an anticoagulant, antihypertensives, a digitalis preparation, another diuretic, lithium, or a potassium preparation.
- your blood chemistry (electrolytes) are out of balance.
- you plan to have surgery under general anesthesia in the near future.
- you have a potassium-rich diet. Talk to your doctor and see Table 13.

Possible Side Effects (natural, expected, and unavoidable drug actions)
Abnormally high blood potassium levels—possible and may be frequent; abnormally low blood sodium levels or dehydration—infrequent.

Possible Adverse Effects (unusual, unexpected, and infrequent reactions)
If any of the following develop, consult your physician promptly for guidance.

Mild Adverse Effects

Allergic Reactions: Skin rash, hives, itching, drug fever (see Glossary).

Headache, dizziness, unsteadiness, weakness, drowsiness, lethargy, confusion—infrequent.

Dry mouth, nausea, vomiting, diarrhea—infrequent.

Masculine pattern of hair growth and deepening of the voice in women—case reports.

Taste disturbances—possible.

Serious Adverse Effects

Allergic reactions: Abnormally low blood platelet count—rare.

Systemic-lupus-erythematosus-like syndrome—case reports.

Symptomatic potassium excess: confusion, numbness and tingling in lips and extremities, fatigue, weakness, shortness of breath, slow heart rate, low blood pressure—possible.

Stomach ulceration with bleeding—case reports.

Disruption in the acid base balance of body (hyperchloremic or hyperkalemic acidosis)—possible.

Liver toxicity (hepatitis) or kidney toxicity (nephrotoxicity)—case reports.

Porphyria or systemic-lupus-erythematosus-like syndrome—case reports.

Excessively low white blood cells (granulocytes) or platelets—case reports.

Thinning of the bones—case report.

This medicine is a tumorigen in chronic rat toxicity studies. Current labeling notes that unnecessary use of this medicine should be avoided.

▷ **Possible Effects on Sexual Function**

Decreased libido or impaired erection or impotence—possible.

Male breast enlargement and tenderness (gynecomastia) (increases with higher doses). Some gynecomastia reports were associated with impotence. Female breast enlargement; altered timing and pattern of menstruation; postmenopausal bleeding.

Decreased vaginal secretion—case reports.

Possible Effects on Laboratory Tests

White blood cell count: possibly decreased.

Blood platelet count: possibly decreased.

Blood potassium level: increased.

Blood uric acid level: no effect in some; increased and decreased in others.

CAUTION

1. Do not take potassium supplements or increase intake of potassium-rich foods (see Table 13) while taking this drug.
2. Do not stop this drug abruptly unless abnormally high blood levels of potassium develop.
3. Ordinary doses of aspirin (more than 650 mg) may reverse the diuretic effect of this drug. Discuss aspirin or NSAID use with your doctor.
4. Avoid excessive use of salt substitutes containing potassium; these are potential causes of potassium excess.
5. Spironolactone may interfere with laboratory checks (falsely LOW) levels of digoxin and changes in cortisol results.

Precautions for Use

By Infants and Children: Limit the continual use of this drug in children to 1 month.

Watch closely for indications of potassium accumulation. Dosing is accomplished based on weight using 1–3 mg/kilogram per day, up to 200 mg/24 hours (given in a single dose or in 2–4 equal doses).

By Those Over 60 Years of Age: The natural decline in kidney function may predispose to potassium retention in the body. Watch for indications of potassium excess: slow heart rate, irregular heart rhythms, low blood pressure, confusion, or drowsiness. The excessive use of diuretics can cause harmful loss of body water (dehydration), increased viscosity of the blood, and an increased tendency of the blood to clot, predisposing to stroke, heart attack, or thrombophlebitis.

▷ **Advisability of Use During Pregnancy**

Pregnancy Category: C in the package insert, D by one researcher. See Pregnancy Risk Categories at the back of this book.

Animal Studies: This drug causes feminization of male rat fetuses.

Human Studies: Adequate studies of pregnant women are not available.

This drug should not be used during pregnancy unless a very serious complication of pregnancy occurs for which this drug is significantly beneficial.

Advisability of Use If Breast-Feeding

Presence of this drug in breast milk: A metabolic end product (canrenone) is present.

Avoid drug or refrain from nursing.

Habit-Forming Potential: None.

Effects of Overdosage: Thirst, drowsiness, fatigue, weakness, nausea, vomiting, confusion, irregular heart rhythm, low blood pressure.

Possible Effects of Long-Term Use: Potassium accumulation to abnormally high blood levels. Male breast enlargement

Suggested Periodic Examinations While Taking This Drug (at physician's discretion)

Measurements of blood sodium, potassium, magnesium, and chloride levels. Kidney and liver function tests.

▷ **While Taking This Drug, Observe the Following**

Foods: Talk to your doctor about possible need to avoid high-potassium foods (see Table 13). Avoid excessive restriction of salt.

Herbal Medicines or Minerals: Hawthorn (Crataegus variety) and co-enzyme Q10 (co-Q10) can affect the way the heart works. BE CERTAIN to tell your doctor that you are taking or are considering taking these herbs if you are taking spironolactone or if a spironolactone prescription is being considered for you or a loved one. Issues remain regarding optimum doses, monitoring strategies, and possible interactions for co-Q10. One objective review recognized co-Q10 as adjunctive therapy for congestive heart failure. Co-Q10 may also interact badly with aspirin. Soy products (milk, tofu, etc.) contain phytoestrogens that have led to an FDA-approved health claim for reducing risk of heart disease (if they have at least 6.25 g of soy protein per serving). It is important that potassium and magnesium levels be kept in the normal range while you are taking spironolactone. Licorice may increase risk of excessively low potassium and should be avoided. Couch grass or nettle should NOT be taken by patients who have increased fluid (edema) caused by heart weakness. Ginseng, guarana, bitter orange, country mallow, mate, eleuthero root, hawthorn, saw palmetto, ma huang (no longer on the U.S. market for weight loss—not to be combined), goldenseal, and licorice may cause increased blood pressure. Couch grass may worsen edema due to heart or kidney problems. Indian snakeroot, calcium, and garlic may help lower blood pressure. Talk to your doctor BEFORE combining any herbal medicine with spironolactone.

Beverages: No restrictions. May be taken with milk.

▷ *Alcohol:* Use with caution. Alcohol may enhance the drowsiness and the blood-pressure-lowering effect of this drug.

Tobacco Smoking: No interactions expected, but I advise everyone to quit smoking.

▷ *Other Drugs*

Spironolactone may ***increase*** the effects of
- digoxin (Lanoxin). Cautious and increased checks of digoxin levels are prudent.

Spironolactone may ***decrease*** the effects of
- anticoagulants (Coumadin, etc.). Increased frequency of INR (prothrombin time or protime) testing is needed.
- digoxin (Lanoxin). Falsely lowering the laboratory test results on some test kits. Cautious checks and increased checks of digoxin levels are prudent.

Spironolactone ***taken concurrently*** with
- arginine (various) may lead to excessive potassium levels.
- captopril (Capoten) or other ACE inhibitors (see Drug Classes) may cause further increases in blood potassium levels. More frequent laboratory tests are prudent.
- cortisone-like drugs (fludrocortisone, others) may lead to excessive potassium loss.
- cyclosporine (Sandimmune) may result in very elevated potassium levels.
- digitoxin (Crystodigin) may cause either increased or decreased digitoxin effects (unpredictable).
- lithium (Lithobid, others) may cause accumulation of lithium to toxic levels.
- norepinephrine (various) may blunt norepinephrine effects.
- potassium preparations may cause excessively high blood potassium levels.
- tacrolimus (Prograf) may lead to excessive potassium levels. USE IS NOT ADVISED.
- valsartan (Diovan) may lead to increased potassium levels. More frequent potassium checks are prudent.
- warfarin (Coumadin) may blunt effectiveness of warfarin. More frequent INR checks are prudent. Dose adjustments may be needed.

The following drugs may ***decrease*** the effects of spironolactone:
- aspirin (higher doses) or other NSAIDs (see Drug Classes)—may reduce its diuretic effectiveness.

▷ *Driving, Hazardous Activities:* This drug may cause dizziness and drowsiness. Restrict activities as necessary.

Aviation Note: The use of this drug ***may be a disqualification*** for piloting. Consult a designated Aviation Medical Examiner.

Exposure to Sun: No restrictions.

Discontinuation: With high dosage or prolonged use, it is advisable to withdraw this drug gradually. Ask your physician for guidance.

STAVUDINE (STAV u dine)

Other Name: D4T **Introduced:** 1994 **Class:** Antiretroviral, Anti-HIV, Anti-AIDS **Prescription:** USA: Yes **Controlled Drug:** USA: No; Canada: No **Available as Generic:** USA: No; Canada: No
Brand Name: Zerit

BENEFITS versus RISKS	
Possible Benefits	*Possible Risks*
INCREASED CD4 COUNTS IN ADULTS WITH ADVANCED HIV	PERIPHERAL NEUROPATHY
	Pancreatitis
LESS LIKELY THAN OTHER AGENTS TO DEVELOP RESISTANCE	Hyperlactatemia
	Lactic acidosis syndrome (LAS)
AVOIDS BONE MARROW TOXICITY OF ZIDOVUDINE	
EFFECTIVE COMBINATION THERAPY OF HIV	
EXTENDED-RELEASE FORM GIVES BENEFIT OF ONCE-A-DAY DOSING	

▷ **Principal Uses**

As a Single Drug Product: Uses currently included in FDA-approved labeling: Treatment of HIV in adults and children as part of combination therapy (a study of stavudine plus didanosine plus nevirapine is an effective triple medicine combination).

Author's Note: Adherence—taking medicines for HIV exactly on time and in the right amount—is ABSOLUTELY critical to getting the best possible results or outcomes. The antiretroviral therapy guidelines from NIAID take into account how easily the medicine treating HIV can fit into a patient's life (once-daily dosing is a distinct advantage). Structured therapy interruptions (STI) or structured interruptions of therapy (SIT) are controversial.

Other (unlabeled) generally accepted uses: (1) postoccupational exposure to HIV.

How This Drug Works: This drug inhibits HIV reproduction (replication) by (1) inhibiting an HIV enzyme (reverse transcriptase), which blocks the ability of the virus to make nuclear material; and (2) inhibiting an enzyme (DNA polymerase-gamma and -beta), which blocks the ability to make DNA in the mitochondria.

▷ **Widely Used Guidelines That Involve This Medicine (representative sample):** Please look at the section at the very beginning of this profile called "Class." Next, turn to Table 22 and you will find guidelines listed by the class involved!

Available Dosage Forms and Strengths

Capsules — 15 mg, 20 mg, 30 mg, 40 mg

Capsules, extended release — 37.5 mg, 50 mg, 75 mg, 100 mg

Powder — 1 mg/mL

▷ **Recommended Dose Ranges** (Actual dose and schedule must be determined for each patient individually.)

Infants and Children: Children weighing less than 30 kg are given 2 mg per kg per day separated into two equal doses 12 hours apart. Those weighing greater than 30 kg are given the adult dose.

18 to 60 Years of Age: Regular release form: Patients with a body mass of 60 kg (132 lb) or more should take 40 mg every 12 hours. Patients with a body mass of less than 60 kg should take 30 mg twice daily. For those who have had to stop because of peripheral neuropathy (after complete resolution of symptoms)—20 mg twice daily for patients with a body mass of 60 kg or more; 15 mg twice daily for those with a body mass less than 60 kg. Some suggestion has been made that doses greater than 1 mg per kg per day carry a greater risk of peripheral neuropathy. If peripheral neuropathy does happen, most clinicians will interrupt stavudine treatment. For patients in whom symptoms (tingling and numbness or pain in the hands or feet) resolve completely, stavudine can be restarted at 20 mg twice daily for people who weigh 60 kg or more or at 15 mg twice a day for those less than 60 mg. Some clinicians separate the total daily dose into three equal doses given three times a day. *Extended release form:* 100 mg once a day for people who weigh more than 60 kg and 75 mg once a day for those less than 60 kg.

Over 65 Years of Age: This drug has not been studied in those over 65.

Conditions Requiring Dosing Adjustments

Liver Function: If liver enzymes increase significantly, therapy may need to be stopped and then reintroduced with 20 mg daily for those weighing more than 60 kg and 15 mg daily if less than 60 kg.

Kidney Function: Patients with mild kidney compromise (creatinine clearance greater than 50 mL/min) take the usual weight-adjusted dose for adults. Mild to moderate kidney compromise (creatinine clearance 26 to 50 mL/min) should take one-half of the usual weight-adjusted dose every 12 hours. In severe kidney compromise (creatinine clearance 10 to 25 mL/ min), one-half the usual weight-adjusted dose should be taken every 24 hours.

▷ **Dosing Instructions:** This drug may be taken without regard to food. Not missing doses (adherence) is critical, as missed doses will make resistance more likely. The oral solution should be mixed (reconstituted) with water by your pharmacist by adding 202 mL of purified water to the dry powder. SHAKE THE CONTAINER VIGOROUSLY BEFORE you give or take a dose. The reconstituted medicine should be refrigerated and expires 30 days after it is mixed. If signs and symptoms of peripheral neuropathy (pain in the feet or hands, numbness, or tingling sensations) start—treatment with stavudine should be interrupted. When symptoms resolve completely, stavudine is restarted at 20 mg twice a day for people 60 kg or more and 15 mg twice daily for those less than 60 kg. If you forget a dose: Take the missed dose as soon as you remember it, unless it's nearly time for your next dose—if that is the case, skip the missed dose and take the next dose right on schedule. DO NOT double doses. The once-daily formulation allows less frequent dosing, and should not be modified. IT IS ABSOLUTELY CRITICAL to take HIV medicines exactly as prescribed. Talk with your doctor if you find yourself missing doses. There are beeper-based systems that can be a great help.

Usual Duration of Use: Use on a regular schedule for several months usually determines effectiveness in shutting down HIV replication and increasing CD4 counts. Long-term use (months to years) requires periodic physician evaluation of response (viral burden and CD4).

Typical Treatment Goals and Measurements (Outcomes and Markers)

HIV: Goals for HIV treatment presently are maximum suppression of viral replication, maximum lowering of the amount of virus in your body (viral load or burden), and maximum patient survival. Markers of successful therapy include undetectable viral load, increased CD4 cells, absence of indicator or opportunistic infections (OIs), and, in the case of the HIV-positive patient, failure of the infection to progress to AIDS.

Possible Advantages of This Drug
More favorable side-effect profile than other nucleoside analogs. Favorable profile for combination therapy. Favorable once-daily dosing, decreasing pill burden.

▷ **This Drug Should Not Be Taken If**
- you had an allergic reaction to it previously.

▷ **Inform Your Physician Before Taking This Drug If**
- you have had peripheral neuropathy caused by other drugs before.
- you have kidney or liver compromise.
- you have had pancreatitis.
- your bone marrow is depressed.
- you are pregnant.
- you have vitamin B_{12} deficiency or folic acid deficiency.
- you are unsure how much to take or how often to take it.

Possible Side Effects (natural, expected, and unavoidable drug actions)
Chills or fever—infrequent.
Peripheral neuropathy—infrequent to frequent.
Pancreatitis—infrequent.

▷ **Possible Adverse Effects** (unusual, unexpected, and infrequent reactions)
If any of the following develop, consult your physician promptly for guidance.
Mild Adverse Effects
Allergic reaction: skin rash.
Rapidly ascending neuromuscular weakness (mimics Guillain-Barré)—case reports.
Sleep disorder (early awakening and anxiety)—reported, but questionable causation.
Nausea and vomiting or abdominal pain—infrequent.
Increased liver enzymes—frequent.
Lipodystrophy—possible (incidence undetermined).
Author's Note: Possible lipid changes (lipodystrophy or LD) from protease inhibitors and/or nucleoside reverse transcriptase inhibitors involve presence of mild changes versus moderate to severe problems. The HOPS data found that risk of LD increases with increasing time on antiretrovirals and that LD increases with an increasing number of nondrug factors (age 40 or older, HIV infection 7 or more years, AIDS 2 or more years, hemophiliacs, nadir CD4 count less than 100 or less than 15, and time since nadir 3 or more years). Patients who did not have these risk factors DID NOT develop significant LD in the HOPS data.
Serious Adverse Effects
Allergic reactions: anaphylactic reactions—rare.
Anemia—case reports.
Low white blood cell or platelet counts—rare to infrequent in phase three data, not found in later data.
Lactic acidosis syndrome (LAS)—case reports.
Respiratory failure as part of a Guillain-Barré type syndrome—case reports.
Severe liver problems (hepatomegaly with statuses)—case reports with nucleoside analogs.

▷ **Possible Effects on Sexual Function:** Impotence—rare in phase three data. One case report of swelling of male breast tissue (gynecomastia).

Possible Delayed Adverse Effects: Peripheral neuropathy—up to 24%.

▷ **Adverse Effects That May Mimic Natural Diseases or Disorders**

Increased liver function tests may mimic hepatitis. Rapidly ascending neuro-muscular weakness may mimic Guillain-Barré syndrome.

Possible Effects on Laboratory Tests

Liver function tests: increased.

Amylase: increased.

Complete blood counts: decreased platelets and white blood cells—possible.

CAUTION

1. Taking stavudine and even an undetectable viral burden **does not** remove risk of giving (transmission) HIV to others through sexual contact or blood contamination.
2. Promptly report the development of stomach pain and vomiting; this could indicate pancreatitis.
3. Report development of pain, numbness, tingling, or burning in the hands or feet, as this may be peripheral neuropathy.

Precautions for Use

By Infants and Children: Watch carefully for adverse effects.

By Those Over 65 Years of Age: Age-related decline in kidney function may require dosing changes.

▷ **Advisability of Use During Pregnancy**

Pregnancy Category: C. See Pregnancy Risk Categories at the back of this book.

Animal Studies: Clinical doses in rats have not revealed teratogenicity, but doses of 399 times those used in humans have resulted in skeletal problems. Increased early rat death has also occurred at 399 times the human dose.

Human Studies: Adequate studies of pregnant women are not available.

Ask your doctor for guidance.

Advisability of Use If Breast-Feeding

Presence of this drug in breast milk: Yes.

Refrain from nursing if you are HIV positive or are taking this drug. HIV can be transmitted through breast milk.

Habit-Forming Potential: None.

Effects of Overdose: Adults treated with 12 to 24 times the recommended daily dose revealed no acute toxicity.

Possible Effects of Long-Term Use: Peripheral neuropathy and hepatic toxicity.

Suggested Periodic Examinations While Taking This Drug (at physician's discretion)

Liver function tests.

Amylase and complete blood counts.

CD4 or viral load measurement.

▷ **While Taking This Drug, Observe the Following**

Foods: No restrictions.

Herbal Medicines or Minerals: Some patients use echinacea to attempt to boost their immune systems. Unfortunately, use of echinacea is not recommended in people with damaged immune systems. This herb may also actually weaken any immune system if it is used too often or for too long a time. St. John's wort can blunt the blood levels and benefits of stavudine. DO NOT combine.

Beverages: No restrictions.

▷ *Alcohol:* No interactions expected.

Tobacco Smoking: No interactions expected. I advise everyone to quit smoking.

▷ *Other Drugs*
Stavudine *taken concurrently* with
- hydroxyurea (Droxia, Hydrea) may lead to fatal pancreatitis and liver toxicity. DO NOT COMBINE.
- other drugs such as metronidazole (Flagyl) that can cause peripheral neuropathy should be avoided if possible.

Stavudine may *increase* the effects of
- didanosine (Videx) at specific drug concentration ratios. Careful monitoring for liver toxicity should be undertaken.

Stavudine may *decrease* the effects of
- didanosine (Videx) at specific drug concentration ratios.
- zidovudine (AZT) at specific drug concentration ratios. The combination is NOT recommended.

▷ *Driving, Hazardous Activities:* This drug may cause dizziness. Restrict activities as necessary.

Aviation Note: The use of this drug *may be a disqualification* for piloting. Consult a designated Aviation Medical Examiner.

Exposure to Sun: No restrictions.

Discontinuation: Do not stop this drug without your doctor's knowledge and guidance.

STRONTIUM-89 (STRON tee um)

Introduced: 1993   **Class:**   Systemic radionuclide, pain syndrome modifier   **Prescription:**   USA: Yes   **Controlled Drug:**   USA: No; Canada: No   **Available as Generic:**   USA: No; Canada: No

Brand Name: Metastron

BENEFITS versus RISKS	
Possible Benefits	*Possible Risks*
EFFECTIVE RELIEF OF PRIMARY OR METASTATIC (SUCH AS FROM PROSTATE OR BREAST CANCER) CANCER OF THE BONE PAIN	BONE MARROW TOXICITY (DECREASED WHITE BLOOD CELLS AND PLATELETS) Transient increase in bone pain

▷ **Principal Uses**
As a Single Drug Product: Uses currently included in FDA-approved labeling: Used to treat metastatic bone cancer pain.
Other (unlabeled) generally accepted uses: None at present.

How This Drug Works: This radiopharmaceutical is selectively taken up by areas of bone cancer. Once it accumulates in cancerous areas, it emits radiation directly at the site of the cancer.

▷ **Widely Used Guidelines That Involve This Medicine (representative sample):** Please look at the section at the very beginning of this profile called "Class." Next, turn to Table 22 and you will find guidelines listed by the class involved!

Available Dosage Forms and Strengths
Injection — 10.9 to 22.6 mg of strontium in a total of 1 mL of water

▷ **Recommended Dose Ranges** (Actual dose and schedule must be determined for each patient individually.)

Infants and Children: Safety and efficacy for those less than 18 years old are not established.

18 to 60 Years of Age: A dose of 1.5–2.2 megabecquerels/kg or 40–60 microcuries/kg of body weight is given intravenously over 1 to 2 minutes. The dose may be repeated at 90-day intervals, if needed, and is based on how well the patient responds to the original dosing as well as to how acceptable the blood cell counts are (hematological status).

Over 60 Years of Age: Same as 18 to 60 years of age.

Conditions Requiring Dosing Adjustments

Liver Function: Dosing changes in liver compromise do not appear to be needed.

Kidney Function: This agent is primarily removed by the kidneys, but decreases in doses are not presently defined.

▷ **Dosing Instructions:** You may eat and drink as you normally would. During the first week after injection, strontium-89 will be present in the blood and the urine. A normal toilet should be used in preference to a urinal. The radiation in this medicine is NOT considered a hazard to family members or to staff in the hospital or cancer center. If you forget a dose: CALL your doctor for instructions. This medicine must be taken on a regular basis.

Usual Duration of Use: Use of previously prescribed pain medicine will be expected for 7 to 21 days after the injection, and there may be a flare in pain (prudent to anticipate this). A maximum of 42 days after injection has been needed to determine peak effectiveness in controlling bone cancer pain. The dose may be repeated (if blood tests are acceptable) 90 days after the prior dose was given. See your physician on a regular basis.

Typical Treatment Goals and Measurements (Outcomes and Markers)

Pain: Most clinicians treating pain use a device called an algometer to check your pain. This looks like a small ruler, but lets the clinician better understand your pain. The goals of treatment then relate to where the level of pain started (for example, a rating of seven on a zero to ten scale) and what the cause of the pain was. I use the PQRSTBG method (see Glossary). Pain medicines may also be used together (in combination) in order to get the best result or outcome. Relief of bone pain is a hallmark of successful treatment with this medicine. Decreasing use of primary pain medicine as well as rescue doses can be used to track response. It is important to note that little progress may be made in the first 3 weeks. Sleep patterns should also improve. If your pain control is not acceptable to YOU (remember, in hospitals, outpatient settings, etc., pain control is a patient right), call your doctor.

Possible Advantages of This Drug

Effective control of bone cancer pain without the risks or compromise of narcotics. This medicine may also allow lower doses of medicines such as morphine with excellent pain control, thereby reducing the risk of adverse effects from the opioid (such as morphine).

▷ **This Drug Should Not Be Taken If**
- you had an allergic reaction to it previously.
- you have cancer that does not involve the bone.

▷ **Inform Your Physician Before Taking This Drug If**
- you have a history of low platelets (less than 60,000) or white blood cell counts (less than 2,400).
- you take other drugs that may lower white cells or platelets.
- you have an increased calcium.
- you do not understand how to appropriately dispose of your urine.

Possible Side Effects (natural, expected, and unavoidable drug actions)
May cause a calcium-like flushing when injected. May cause transient (up to 72 hours) increase in bone pain. Drug fever may result.

▷ **Possible Adverse Effects** (unusual, unexpected, and infrequent reactions)
If any of the following develop, consult your physician promptly for guidance.
Mild Adverse Effects
Allergic reactions: not defined.
Chills and fever—possible.
Serious Adverse Effects
Allergic reactions: none defined.
Bone marrow toxicity: 20–30% decrease in white cell or platelet counts—may be dose-related. Lowest point (nadir) happens 5–16 weeks after a dose.
Bacterial infection of blood (septicemia) following drug-induced decreases in white blood cells—possible.
Animal data shows that this drug is a possible carcinogen—case reports of two patients given this drug for refractory prostate cancer and subsequently developed sudden (acute) myelogenous leukemia (still of questionable cause due to multiple treatments).

▷ **Possible Effects on Sexual Function:** None reported.

Possible Delayed Adverse Effects: Lowering of white blood cells (recovery in up to 6 months) and blood platelets (lowest count 5 to 16 weeks after therapy).

Natural Diseases or Disorders That May Be Activated by This Drug
Aplastic anemia.

Possible Effects on Laboratory Tests
White blood cell counts: decreased.
Platelet counts: decreased.

CAUTION
1. Promptly report any signs of infection (lethargy, temperature, sore throat) to your doctor.
2. It may take up to 21 days for this agent to work. Narcotics will need to be continued.
3. Your blood and urine will contain radioactive strontium for 7 days after injection. Ask your doctor for help on appropriate disposal.
4. This drug is a potential carcinogen.
5. Promptly report any abnormal bleeding or bruising.

Precautions for Use
By Infants and Children: Safety and effectiveness for those less than 18 years of age are not established.
By Those Over 60 Years of Age: Specific changes are not presently needed.

▷ **Advisability of Use During Pregnancy**
Pregnancy Category: D. See Pregnancy Risk Categories at the back of this book.

Animal Studies: Adequate studies evaluating potential to cause birth defects have not been performed.

Human Studies: Adequate studies of pregnant women are not available. This drug may cause fetal harm. Ask your doctor for advice.

Advisability of Use If Breast-Feeding
Presence of this drug in breast milk: This drug acts like calcium and is expected to be present in breast milk.
Avoid drug or refrain from nursing.

Habit-Forming Potential: None.

Effects of Overdose: May result in acute radiation syndrome with initial nausea and vomiting followed by depressed white cells and platelets and tendency to infections. Careful dose calculations are indicated, as this drug emits beta-radiation.

Possible Effects of Long-Term Use: Not indicated for long-term use.

Suggested Periodic Examinations While Taking This Drug (at physician's discretion)
Complete blood counts should be tested once every other week during therapy.

▷ **While Taking This Drug, Observe the Following**
Foods: No restrictions.
Herbal Medicines or Minerals: Some patients use echinacea to attempt to boost their immune systems. Unfortunately, use of echinacea is not recommended in people with damaged immune systems. This herb may also actually weaken any immune system if it is used too often or for too long a time.
Beverages: No restrictions.
▷ *Alcohol:* No interactions expected.
Tobacco Smoking: No interactions expected. I advise everyone to quit smoking.
Marijuana Smoking: No interactions expected.
▷ *Other Drugs*
Strontium-89 **taken concurrently** with
• medications that lower white blood cells or platelets may result in severe decreases in white blood cells or platelets.
▷ *Driving, Hazardous Activities:* This drug may cause a transient increase in bone pain. Restrict activities as necessary.
Aviation Note: The use of this drug **may be a disqualification** for piloting. Consult a designated Aviation Medical Examiner.
Exposure to Sun: No restrictions.
Discontinuation: Dosing may be repeated if blood counts are acceptable.

SUCRALFATE (soo KRAL fayt)

Introduced: 1978 **Class:** Antiulcer, gastrointestinal drug **Prescription:** USA: Yes **Controlled Drug:** USA: No; Canada: No **Available as Generic:** Yes

Brand Names: ✽Apo-Sucralfate, Carafate, ✽Dom-Sucralfate, ✽Novo-Sucralfate, ✽Sulcrate

---

BENEFITS versus RISKS

Possible Benefits	*Possible Risks*
EFFECTIVE TREATMENT IN DUODENAL ULCER DISEASE	Constipation
	Skin rash, hives, itching
No serious adverse effects	Aluminum toxicity in kidney compromise

---

▷ **Principal Uses**

As a Single Drug Product: Uses currently included in FDA-approved labeling: Treats and prevents recurrence of duodenal ulcer disease in adults and children. Effective when used alone, but may be used with antacids for pain relief.

Other (unlabeled) generally accepted uses: (1) May be useful in treating stomach (gastric ulcers) if other therapy isn't tolerated; (2) can reduce the frequency of diarrhea caused by radiation therapy; (3) may have a role as a douche in promoting healing of vaginal ulcerations that are resistant to other measures; (4) can ease the pain and spasms associated with tonsillectomy; (5) appears to increase healing in burn patients.

Author's Note: Information in this profile has been shortened to make room for more widely used medicines.

SULFAMETHOXAZOLE (sul fa meth OX a zohl)

Please see the sulfonamide antibiotic family profile.

SULFASALAZINE (sul fa SAL a zeen)

Introduced: 1949   **Class:**   Bowel anti-inflammatory, sulfonamides
Prescription: USA: Yes   **Controlled Drug:**   USA: No; Canada: No
Available as Generic: USA: Yes; Canada: No

Brand Names: ❦Alti-Sulfasalazine, Azaline, Azulfidine, Azulfidine EN-Tabs, ❦PMS Sulfasalazine, ❦PMS Sulfasalazine E.C., ❦Salazopyrin, ❦Salazopyrin EN, ❦SAS-Enema, ❦SAS Enteric-500, SAS-500, Sulfazine EC

BENEFITS versus RISKS

Possible Benefits	*Possible Risks*
EFFECTIVE SUPPRESSION OF INFLAMMATORY BOWEL DISEASE	Allergic reactions: mild to severe skin reactions
SYMPTOMATIC RELIEF OF REGIONAL ENTERITIS AND ULCERATIVE COLITIS	Blood cell disorders: aplastic anemia, hemolytic anemia, abnormally low white cell or platelet counts
HELPFUL IN REFRACTORY RHEUMATOID ARTHRITIS	Drug-induced liver damage
	Drug-induced kidney damage
	Seizures

▷ **Principal Uses**

As a Single Drug Product: Uses currently included in FDA-approved labeling: (1) Treats inflammatory disease of the lower intestinal tract and then helps

retain remissions: regional enteritis (Crohn's disease) and ulcerative colitis—
it is usually taken by mouth, but may also be used in retention enemas; (2)
helps rheumatoid arthritis.

Other (unlabeled) generally accepted uses: (1) Short-term use in therapy of
ankylosing spondylitis; (2) treatment of mild to moderate psoriasis; (3)
may have a role in juvenile arthritis; (4) may decrease risk of colorectal
cancer in ulcerative colitis patients.

How This Drug Works: Suppresses the formation of prostaglandins and related
tissue substances that cause inflammation, diarrhea, and tissue destruction.

▷ **Widely Used Guidelines That Involve This Medicine (representative sample):** Please look at the section at the very beginning of this profile called
"Class." Next, turn to Table 22 and you will find guidelines listed by the
class involved!

Available Dosage Forms and Strengths
Oral suspension — 250 mg/5 mL
Tablets — 500 mg
Tablets, enteric coated — 500 mg

▷ **Usual Adult Dosage Ranges:** *Ulcerative colitis:* Some clinicians start with 3 to
4 g per day of this medicine, separated into equal doses given every 6 to 8
hours until symptoms are adequately controlled. For maintenance, 500 mg
every 6 hours. Other clinicians use a starting dose of 1–2 g a day in order to
decrease stomach and intestinal adverse effects (consistent with product
labeling). Some patients tolerate up to 6 g a day, but doses of 4 g a day or
greater bring increased risk of adverse effects. If diarrhea occurs, the dose
is often decreased to the earlier dose that worked and did not cause diarrhea. Some patients do not remove this medicine well (slow acetylators)
and are given 2.5 to 3 g a day.

Rheumatoid arthritis (when salicylates or NSAIDs have not worked): 2 grams
daily is taken in equally divided doses. If the delayed-release form (Azulfidine EN-Tabs) is used, 500 mg is taken for 1 week in the evening, then
500 mg twice daily for a week, then 500 mg in the morning and 1 g in the
evening for a week and continuing with 1 g twice a day. Maximum dose is
3 grams.

Note: Actual dose and schedule must be individually determined.

Conditions Requiring Dosing Adjustments
Liver Function: This drug can be a cause of liver damage, and patients should
be followed closely.
Kidney Function: Empiric decreases in doses should be considered. This drug
should be used with *CAUTION* in kidney compromise.

▷ **Dosing Instructions:** This drug is preferably taken with 8 ounces of water on an
empty stomach, 1 hour before or 2 hours after eating. However, it may be
taken with or following food to reduce stomach irritation. Intervals
between doses (day and night) should be no longer than 8 hours. The regular tablet may be crushed; the enteric-coated tablet should be swallowed
whole without changing it. Suspension form should be shaken well and
measured using a dose cup or calibrated dosing spoon. If you forget a dose:
Take the missed dose as soon as you remember it, unless it's nearly time for
your next dose—if that is the case, skip the missed dose and take the next
dose right on schedule. DO NOT double doses. Talk with your doctor and
pharmacist if you find yourself missing doses. There are many effective
medicine reminder systems to help you.

Usual Duration of Use: Use on a regular schedule for 1 to 3 weeks usually determines effectiveness in controlling the symptoms of regional enteritis or ulcerative colitis. Benefits in rheumatoid arthritis (RA) may be seen in 4 to 12 weeks. Long-term use (months to years) requires physician supervision. It is not unusual to change therapies in RA.

Typical Treatment Goals and Measurements (Outcomes and Markers)
Inflammatory Bowel Disease: The goal is to cause (induce) a remission and maintain it. Symptoms that will resolve include rectal bleeding and diarrhea. More involved exams will reveal an absence of bowel ulceration and easing of friability or granularity of the bowel itself.

▷ **This Drug Should Not Be Taken If**
   • you are allergic to any sulfonamide drug (see Drug Classes) or aspirin (or other salicylates).
   • you are in the final month of pregnancy (near term).
   • it has been prescribed for an infant less than 2 years old.
   • you have a urinary or intestinal obstruction or porphyria.
   • you are breast-feeding.

▷ **Inform Your Physician Before Taking This Drug If**
   • you are allergic by nature: history of hay fever, asthma, hives, and eczema.
   • you have asthma.
   • you have impaired liver or kidney function.
   • you have a glucose-6-phosphate dehydrogenase (G6PD) deficiency or are known to be a slow acetylator.
   • you have a personal or family history of porphyria.
   • you have juvenile rheumatoid arthritis that is in the systemic course because there is a high rate of a serum sickness–like reaction.
   • you have had a drug-induced blood cell or bone marrow disorder.
   • you currently take any oral anticoagulant, antidiabetic drug, or phenytoin.
   • you plan to have surgery under pentothal anesthesia soon.

Possible Side Effects (natural, expected, and unavoidable drug actions)
Brownish coloration of the urine—of no significance. Skin pigmentation. Superinfections, bacterial or fungal (see Glossary).

▷ **Possible Adverse Effects** (unusual, unexpected, and infrequent reactions)
   If any of the following develop, consult your physician promptly for guidance.
   Mild Adverse Effects
   Allergic reactions: skin rashes, hives, itching.
   Headache—frequent.
   Dizziness—infrequent.
   Discoloration (yellow stains) on contact lenses—possible.
   Ringing in the ears—case reports.
   Loss of appetite, irritation of mouth or tongue, nausea, vomiting, diarrhea—infrequent to frequent.
   Taste disorders—rare.
   Serious Adverse Effects
   Allergic reactions: drug fever (see Glossary), swollen glands, painful joints, anaphylaxis (see Glossary).
   Allergic pneumonitis, allergic liver damage (hepatitis).
   Severe skin reactions (Stevens-Johnson syndrome or toxic epidermal necrolysis).
   Idiosyncratic reactions: hemolytic anemia (see Glossary).

Bone marrow depression (see Glossary): fever, sore throat, abnormal bleed-ing/bruising—rare to infrequent.

Serum sickness (increased bilirubin, fever, red rash, hepatitis)—case reports.

Pancreatitis, myopathy, or drug-induced lupus erythematosus—case reports.

Hearing loss—case reports.

Folic acid deficiency—possible.

Kidney damage—case reports.

Peripheral neuropathy (see Glossary)—case reports.

Inflammation of tissue around the heart (pericarditis)—case reports.

▷ **Possible Effects on Sexual Function:** Decreased production of sperm, reversible infertility—case reports.

▷ **Adverse Effects That May Mimic Natural Diseases or Disorders**

Liver reactions may suggest viral hepatitis. Lung reactions may suggest an infectious pneumonia.

Natural Diseases or Disorders That May Be Activated by This Drug

Goiter, acute intermittent porphyria.

Possible Effects on Laboratory Tests

Complete blood cell counts: decreased red cells, hemoglobin, white cells, and platelets; increased eosinophils (allergic reaction).

Liver function tests: increased enzymes (ALT/GPT, AST/GOT, alkaline phos-phatase) or bilirubin.

Sperm count: decreased; abnormal sperm common; effects reversible on dis-continuation of drug.

CAUTION

1. A large intake of water (up to 2 quarts daily) is necessary to ensure an adequate volume of urine to help prevent kidney (renal) problems.
2. Shake liquid dose forms well before measuring each dose.

Precautions for Use

By Infants and Children: Safety and effectiveness for those less than 2 years of age are not established.

By Those Over 60 Years of Age: Watch for development of reduced urine volume, fever, sore throat, abnormal bleeding or bruising, or skin irritation with itching, particularly in the anal or genital regions.

▷ **Advisability of Use During Pregnancy**

Pregnancy Category: B; however, this drug should not be used near the time of the birth of the baby. See Pregnancy Risk Categories at the back of this book.

Animal Studies: Cleft palate and skeletal birth defects due to sulfonamides reported in mice and rats.

Human Studies: No increase in birth defects reported in 4,584 exposures to var-ious sulfonamides during pregnancy.

Avoid use of drug during the final month of pregnancy because of possible adverse effects on the newborn infant.

Advisability of Use If Breast-Feeding

Presence of this drug in breast milk: Yes.

Avoid drug or refrain from nursing.

Habit-Forming Potential: None.

Effects of Overdose: Headache, dizziness, nausea, vomiting, abdominal cramp-ing, toxic fever, coma, jaundice, kidney failure.

Possible Effects of Long-Term Use: Development of goiter, with or without hypothyroidism. An orange-yellow discoloration of the skin has been reported. This is not jaundice.

Suggested Periodic Examinations While Taking This Drug (at physician's discretion)

Complete blood cell counts, weekly for the first 8 weeks.

Urine analysis weekly.

Check of sulfapyridine levels (less than 50 mcg/mL may be associated with fewer problems).

Liver and kidney function tests.

▷ **While Taking This Drug, Observe the Following**

Foods: Follow prescribed diet. See iron salt interaction below.

Herbal Medicines or Minerals: Since St. John's wort and sulfasalazine may increase sun sensitivity, the combination is NOT advised. Flaxseed, peppermint oil, and psyllium husk have Commission E monograph indications for irritable bowel syndrome. This is NOT the same as ulcerative colitis, and those products have not been studied in ulcerative colitis. Aloe, buckhorn berry or bark, cascara sagrada bark, rhubarb root, and senna should not be taken by people living with ulcerative colitis.

Beverages: No restrictions. May be taken with milk.

▷ *Alcohol:* Use caution. Sulfonamide drugs can increase the intoxicating effects of alcohol.

Tobacco Smoking: No interactions expected. I advise everyone to quit smoking.

▷ *Other Drugs*

Sulfasalazine may ***increase*** the effects of

• anticoagulants (warfarin-Coumadin, etc.) and increase bleeding risk; more frequent INR (prothrombin time) testing is needed.

• sulfonylureas or other oral hypoglycemic agents (see Sulfonylureas and Oral Antidiabetic Drugs in Drug Classes) and increase the risk of hypoglycemia.

Sulfasalazine may ***decrease*** the effects of

• digoxin (Lanoxin).

• live typhoid vaccine (Vivotif).

Sulfasalazine ***taken concurrently*** with

• ampicillin and perhaps other penicillins may lower therapeutic benefits from sulfasalazine.

• some barbiturates (see Drug Classes) may result in decreased sulfasalazine therapeutic benefits.

• calcium supplements (calcium gluconate) may result in decreased therapeutic benefits from sulfasalazine.

• folic acid (various) may decrease folate absorption.

• iron salts or calcium may decrease sulfasalazine's benefits.

• mercaptopurine (Purinethol) may increase risk of bone marrow depression.

• riluzole (Rilutek) increases risk of liver toxicity.

• varicella vaccine (Varivax) may result in Reye's syndrome; avoid taking this medicine for 6 weeks following varicella vaccine.

▷ *Driving, Hazardous Activities:* This drug may cause dizziness. Restrict activities as necessary.

Aviation Note: The use of this drug ***may be a disqualification*** for piloting. Consult a designated Aviation Medical Examiner.

Exposure to Sun: Use caution—some sulfonamide drugs can cause photosensitivity (see Glossary).

SULFONAMIDE ANTIBIOTIC FAMILY

Sulfamethoxazole   (sul fa meth OX a zohl)   **Sulfisoxazole**   (sul fi SOX a zohl)

Introduced: 1961, 1949, respectively   **Class:**   Anti-infective, sulfonamides   **Prescription:**   USA: Yes   **Controlled Drug:**   USA: No; Canada: No   **Available as Generic:**   Yes

Brand Names: Sulfamethoxazole: ✢Apo-Sulfamethoxazole, ✢Apo-Sulfatrim [CD], ✢Apo-Sulfatrim DS [CD], Azo Gantanol [CD], Bactrim [CD], Bactrim DS [CD], Bethaprim [CD], Comoxol [CD], Cotrim [CD], Gantanol, ✢Novo-Trimel [CD], ✢Novo-Trimel DS [CD], ✢Nu-Cotrimox, ✢Protrin [CD], ✢Protrin DF [CD], ✢Roubac [CD], Septra [CD], Septra DS [CD], Sulfatrim [CD], ✢Uro Gantanol [CD], Uroplus DS [CD], Uroplus SS [CD], Vagitrol; Sulfisoxazole: Azo Gantrisin [CD], Azo-Sulfisoxazole, Eryzole [CD], Gantrisin, Gulfasin, Lipo Gantrisin, ✢Novosoxazole, Pediazole [CD], SK-Soxazole, Sulfalar, Vagila

---

BENEFITS versus RISKS

Possible Benefits	*Possible Risks*
EFFECTIVE ANTIMICROBIAL ACTION AGAINST SUSCEPTIBLE BACTERIA AND PROTOZOA	Allergic reactions: mild to severe skin reactions, anaphylaxis, myocarditis
Effective adjunctive prevention and treatment of *Pneumocystis carinii* pneumonia (AIDS-related sulfamethoxazole)	Blood cell disorders: aplastic anemia, hemolytic anemia, abnormally low white cell or platelet counts
	Drug-induced liver or kidney damage
	Cotrimoxazole form may prolong the QT interval of the heart

▷ **Principal Uses**

As a Single Drug Product: Uses currently included in FDA-approved labeling: (1) Sulfamethoxazole is used to treat some bacterial or protozoan infections: chancroid, cystitis, and other infections of the urinary tract. **Sulfamethoxazole should not be used to treat group A streptococcal infections.** (2) Sulfisoxazole is used in treating ear infections (otitis media), chloroquine-resistant malaria, and toxoplasmosis.

Other (unlabeled) generally accepted uses: (1) Treats *Chlamydia* infections; (2) combination therapy of resistant *Mycobacterium kansasii* infections; (3) sulfisoxazole may work in long-term prevention of ear infections; (4) some patients with rheumatoid arthritis have shown benefit from sulfamethoxazole.

As a Combination Drug Product [CD]: These medicines are available in combination with phenazopyridine, an analgesic to ease discomfort associated with acute urethral infections. Sulfamethoxazole is also available in combination with another antibacterial drug, trimethoprim; in some countries this combination is given the generic name cotrimoxazole. This combination is quite effective in the treatment of certain types of middle ear infection, bronchitis, and pneumonia, and certain infections of the intestinal tract and urinary tract. It is now used as primary prevention and treatment for *Pneumocystis carinii* pneumonia associated with AIDS.

Author's Note: This medicine in the combination form (Bactrim, Septra) has assumed a major role in helping prevent a prevalent opportunistic infection in HIV-positive people (PCP pneumonia).

How These Drugs Work: Prevent the growth and multiplication of susceptible bacteria or protozoa by interfering with their formation of folic acid, an essential nutrient.

▷ Widely Used Guidelines That Involve This Medicine (representative sample): Please look at the section at the very beginning of this profile called "Class." Next, turn to Table 22 and you will find guidelines listed by the class involved!

Available Dosage Forms and Strengths

Sulfamethoxazole:

Oral suspension — 500 mg/5 mL

Tablets — 500 mg, 1 g

Tablets, combination — 400 mg sulfa/80 mg trimethoprim and 800 mg sulfa/160 mg of trimethoprim (DS form)

Sulfisoxazole:

Emulsion, prolonged action — 1 g/5 mL

Eyedrops — 4%

Eye ointment — 4%

Injection — 400 mg/mL

Pediatric suspension — 500 mg/5 mL

Syrup — 500 mg/5 mL

Tablets — 500 mg

▷ Recommended Dosage Ranges (Actual dose and schedule must be determined for each patient individually.)

Infants and Children:

Sulfamethoxazole: Children over 2 months—50 to 60 mg per kg of body mass to start and then 25 to 30 mg per kg of body mass every 12 hours, up to a maximum of 75 mg per kg of body mass daily.

Sulfisoxazole: Children over 2 months—50 mg per kg of body mass to start and then 100 mg per kg of body mass per day, divided into equal doses given two to four times daily.

Recommended Dosage Range:

Sulfamethoxazole: Initially 2 g and then 1 g every 8 to 12 hours, depending upon the severity of the infection. The total daily dose should not exceed 3 g.

Combination form: For prevention of PCP pneumonia: one DS tablet a day.

Sulfisoxazole: Initially 2 to 4 g (may not be required in urinary tract infections) and then 750 to 1,500 mg (1.5 g) every 4 hours or 1 to 2 g every 6 hours, depending upon the severity of the infection. The total daily dose should not exceed 8 g.

Conditions Requiring Dosing Adjustments

Liver Function: Patients with compromised livers should be followed closely, but specific guidelines for decreasing doses are not defined. Sulfisoxazole may cause liver damage.

Kidney Function: Doses should be decreased for patients with compromised kidneys. For patients with mild to moderate kidney failure, sulfisoxazole can be taken every 6 hours in the usual dose. In moderate to severe kidney failure, it can be taken every 12 to 24 hours in the usual dose. In severe kidney failure, it can be taken once a day. It should be used with **CAUTION** in renal compromise. Increased elimination of this drug may be seen in patients with alkaline urine. For sulfamethoxazole: Specific dosing changes have not been made for the single agent. For cotrimoxazole, it has been recommended that the dosing interval be increased for patients with impaired kidneys.

▷ **Dosing Instructions:** The tablet may be crushed and is preferably taken on an empty stomach, 1 hour before or 2 hours after eating. However, both drugs may be taken with or following food to reduce stomach irritation. Be certain to drink liberal amounts of water while taking this medicine if you are not restricted from doing so. Suspension forms should be shaken well and dosed using a measuring cup or calibrated dosing spoon. If you forget a dose: Take the missed dose as soon as you remember it, unless it's nearly time for your next dose—if that is the case, skip the missed dose and take the next dose right on schedule. DO NOT double doses. Talk with your doctor if you find yourself missing doses, as compliance ensures treatment or best possible prevention of infection.

Usual Duration of Use: Use on a regular schedule for 4 to 7 days usually determines effectiveness in controlling responsive infections. Treatment should be continued until the patient is free of symptoms for 48 hours. Limit treatment to no more than 14 days if possible. Preventive use of trimethoprim/sulfamethoxazole will be ongoing, based on CD4 recovery/reconstitution.

Typical Treatment Goals and Measurements (Outcomes and Markers)
Infections: The most commonly used measures of serious infections are white blood cell counts and differentials (the kind of blood cells that occur most often in your blood), and temperature. Many clinicians look for positive changes in 24–48 hours. NEVER stop an antibiotic because you start to feel better. For treating infections, the full course is REQUIRED to kill the bacteria. Prophylaxis (for example of PCP) often requires ongoing use. The goals and time frame (see possible benefits above) should be discussed with you when the prescription is written.

Currently a "Drug of Choice"
Sulfamethoxazole (when combined with trimethoprim) is the drug of choice for preventing pneumonia (due to *Pneumocystis carinii*) in HIV-positive patients or those with AIDS.

▷ **These Drugs Should Not Be Taken If**
- you are allergic to any sulfonamide drug (see Drug Classes).
- you are in the final month of pregnancy.
- you are breast-feeding your infant.
- it has been prescribed for an infant less than 2 months old (unless congenital toxoplasmosis is being treated—sulfisoxazole).

▷ **Inform Your Physician Before Taking These Drugs If**
- you are allergic to any sulfonamide derivative: acetazolamide, thiazide diuretics, sulfonylurea antidiabetics (see Drug Classes).
- you are allergic by nature: history of hay fever, asthma, hives, and eczema.
- you have impaired liver or kidney function.
- you have a personal or family history of porphyria.
- you have had a drug-induced blood cell or bone marrow disorder.
- you have a glucose-6-phosphate dehydrogenase (G6PD) deficiency in your red blood cells (ask your doctor).

- you currently take any oral anticoagulant, antidiabetic drug, or phenytoin.
- you plan to have surgery under pentothal anesthesia while taking this drug.

Possible Side Effects (natural, expected, and unavoidable drug actions)

Brownish coloration of the urine—of no significance. Superinfections, bacterial or fungal (see Glossary).

▷ ## Possible Adverse Effects (unusual, unexpected, and infrequent reactions)

If any of the following develop, consult your physician promptly for guidance.

Mild Adverse Effects

Allergic reactions: skin rashes, hives, itching, localized swellings, reddened eyes, temporary myopia.

Myopia—infrequent.

Headache, dizziness, unsteadiness, ringing in the ears (tinnitus)—possible.

Loss of appetite, irritation of mouth or tongue, nausea, vomiting, abdominal pain, diarrhea—infrequent.

Serious Adverse Effects

Allergic reactions: drug fever (see Glossary), swollen glands, painful joints, anaphylaxis (see Glossary).

Allergic reaction in the heart muscle (myocarditis), allergic pneumonitis, allergic hepatitis.

Severe skin reactions (Stevens-Johnson syndrome, TEN, Jarisch-Herxheimer)—rare.

Idiosyncratic reactions: hemolytic anemia (see Glossary)—possible.

Bone marrow depression (see Glossary): fatigue, weakness, fever, sore throat, abnormal bleeding or bruising—case reports.

Liver damage—rare.

Pancreatitis—case reports.

Kidney damage: bloody or cloudy urine, reduced urine volume—possible.

Psychotic reactions, hallucinations, seizures, hearing changes (loss or vestibular symptoms), peripheral neuropathy (see Glossary)—case reports.

Severe hypoglycemia—case report (sulfamethoxazole).

Methemoglobinemia—rare.

Drug-induced lupus erythematosus or blood-clotting problems (hypoprothrombinemia)—rare.

Drug-induced disulfiramlike reaction (sulfisoxazole)—possible.

▷ ## Possible Effects on Sexual Function: None reported.

▷ ## Adverse Effects That May Mimic Natural Diseases or Disorders

Liver reactions may suggest viral hepatitis. Lung reactions may suggest an infectious pneumonia.

Natural Diseases or Disorders That May Be Activated by These Drugs

Goiter, acute intermittent porphyria, polyarteritis nodosa, systemic lupus erythematosus (questionable).

Possible Effects on Laboratory Tests

Complete blood cell counts: decreased red cells, hemoglobin, white cells, and platelets; increased eosinophils (allergic reaction).

INR (prothrombin time): increased (when taken concurrently with warfarin).

Liver function tests: increased enzymes (ALT/GPT, AST/GOT, alkaline phosphatase) or bilirubin.

CAUTION
1. A large intake of water (up to 2 quarts daily) is necessary to ensure an adequate volume of urine.
2. Shake liquid dose forms well before measuring each dose.

Precautions for Use
By Infants and Children: These drugs should not be used in infants under 2 months of age.
By Those Over 60 Years of Age: Small doses taken at longer intervals often achieve adequate blood and tissue drug levels. Observe for the development of reduced urine volume, fever, sore throat, abnormal bleeding or bruising, or skin irritation with itching, particularly in the anal or genital regions.

▷ **Advisability of Use During Pregnancy**
Pregnancy Category: C; however, these drugs **SHOULD NOT BE TAKEN** (are contraindicated) near the time of the birth of the baby. See Pregnancy Risk Categories at the back of this book.
Animal Studies: Cleft palate and skeletal birth defects reported in mice and rats.
Human Studies: No increase in birth defects reported in 4,584 exposures to various sulfonamides during pregnancy.
Avoid use of drug during the final 3 months of pregnancy because of possible adverse effects on the newborn infant.

Advisability of Use If Breast-Feeding
Presence of these drugs in breast milk: Yes.
Avoid drug or refrain from nursing.

Habit-Forming Potential: None.

Effects of Overdose: Headache, dizziness, nausea, vomiting, abdominal cramping, toxic fever, coma, jaundice, kidney failure.

Possible Effects of Long-Term Use
Superinfections, bacterial or fungal. Development of goiter, with or without hypothyroidism. Excessive loss of vitamin C via urine.

Suggested Periodic Examinations While Taking These Drugs (at physician's discretion)
Complete blood cell counts, weekly for the first 8 weeks.
Urine analysis weekly.
ANA or LE prep.
Liver and kidney function tests.

▷ **While Taking These Drugs, Observe the Following**
Foods: No restrictions.
Herbal Medicines or Minerals: Since St. John's wort and these medicines may increase sun sensitivity, the combination is NOT advised. Some patients use echinacea to attempt to boost their immune systems. Unfortunately, use of echinacea is not recommended in people with damaged immune systems. This herb may also actually weaken any immune system if it is used too often or for too long a time. DO NOT take mistletoe herb, oak bark, or F.C. of marshmallow root and licorice extracts. Pure cranberry juice may help keep harmful bacteria from attaching to the bladder wall and may be useful in helping to prevent urinary tract infections.
Beverages: No restrictions. May be taken with milk. Note recommendations for increased fluid intake.
▷ *Alcohol:* Use caution. Sulfonamide drugs can increase the intoxicating effects of alcohol and may also lead to a disulfiram (see Glossary) reaction.
Tobacco Smoking: No interactions expected. I advise everyone to quit smoking.

▷   *Other Drugs*

These medicines may ***increase*** the effects of

- abacavir/lamivudine/zidovudine (Trizivir) and result in zidovudine or lamivudine toxicity in the combination product.
- amantadine (Symmetrel) and cause abnormal heart rhythms and CNS stimulation (confusion, disorientation).
- anticoagulants (Coumadin, etc.) and increase the risk of bleeding; more frequent INR testing (prothrombin time or protime) is needed. Ongoing warfarin doses should be decided based on laboratory results.
- metformin (Glucophage) and lead to increased risk of lowered blood sugar or lactic acidosis.
- methotrexate (Mexate) and cause severe blood toxicity.
- sulfonylureas (see Drug Classes) or other oral hypoglycemic agents and increase the risk of excessively low blood sugar (hypoglycemia).
- zidovudine (AZT) and lamivudine and result in zidovudine or lamivudine toxicity in the single product or in their combination forms.

These medicines may ***decrease*** the effects of

- birth control pills (oral contraceptives).
- cyclosporine (Sandimmune) and reduce its immunosuppressive effect.
- live typhoid vaccine (Vivotif).
- penicillins (see Drug Classes).

These medicines ***taken concurrently*** with

- metronidazole (Flagyl) may lead to a disulfiram reaction.
- ritonavir (Norvir) may lead to changes in cotrimoxazole amounts that get into the body (bioavailability). Close patient follow-up is prudent.
- warfarin (Coumadin) may lead to increased risk of bleeding. More frequent INR checks are prudent.

Sulfamethoxazole ***taken concurrently*** with

- medicines such as class I, IA, or III antiarrhythmics (dofetilide [Tikosyn], clarithromycin, cotrimoxazole, erythromycin, ondansetron, ziprazidone, zolmitriptan, and others) may lead to prolongation of the QTc interval and undesirable effects. Combination is not recommended.

▷   *Driving, Hazardous Activities:* These drugs may cause dizziness. Restrict activities as necessary.

Aviation Note: The use of these drugs ***may be a disqualification*** for piloting. Consult a designated Aviation Medical Examiner.

Exposure to Sun: Use caution. Some sulfonamide drugs can cause photosensitivity (see Glossary).

SULINDAC (sul IN dak)

Please see the acetic acid (nonsteroidal anti-inflammatory drug) family profile.

SUMATRIPTAN (soo ma TRIP tan)

Introduced: 1993   **Class:**   Antimigraine drug, serotonin-1-receptor agonist   **Prescription:**   USA: Yes   **Controlled Drug:**   USA: No; Canada: No   **Available as Generic:**   USA: No; Canada: No

Brand Names: Imitrex, Imitrex Nasal Spray

```
┌─────────────────────────────────────────────────────────────┐
│                    BENEFITS versus RISKS                      │
│        Possible Benefits              Possible Risks          │
│                                                               │
│  RAPID AND EFFECTIVE RELIEF OR   Fainting                     │
│    PREVENTION OF MIGRAINE        Myocardial infarction (probably │
│  GENERALLY WELL-TOLERATED          secondary to coronary vasospasm) │
│    NASAL SPRAY FORM              Serious atrial and ventricular │
│  Relieves photophobia (light       arrhythmias                │
│    sensitivity)                  Exacerbation of ischemic heart │
│  Relieves phonophobia (sound       disease (should not be given to │
│    sensitivity)                    those patients)            │
│  Relieves nausea and vomiting    Not to be used in hemiplegic or │
│                                    basilar migraine           │
│                                  Not to be used in significant │
│                                    cardiovascular disease     │
│                                  Not compatible with patients with │
│                                    seizure disorders (see This Drug │
│                                    Should Not Be Taken If)    │
└─────────────────────────────────────────────────────────────┘
```

▷ **Principal Uses**

As a Single Drug Product: Uses currently included in FDA-approved labeling: (1) Acute treatment of migraine with or without aura in adults; (2) treatment of cluster headache in adults.

Other (unlabeled) generally accepted uses: Treatment of post-traumatic headaches.

How This Drug Works: Sumatriptan acts on blood vessels to cause vasoconstriction (shrinking of the blood vessels). This relieves swelling, thought to be the cause of migraine. The drug binds to receptor arteries such as the basilar artery and in vasculature (blood vessels) associated with the dura mater (part of the lining of the brain).

▷ **Widely Used Guidelines That Involve This Medicine (representative sample):** Please look at the section at the very beginning of this profile called "Class." Next, turn to Table 22 and you will find guidelines listed by the class involved!

Available Dosage Forms and Strengths

Nasal spray — 5 mg/100 mcL, 20 mg/100 mcL

Sumatriptan succinate (Imitrex) — 2 syringes with 6 mg in 0.5 mL of liquid

Injection self-dose system kit — in each 1 mL size syringe, a dosing device and instructions

Unit-of-use syringes — 6 mg in 0.5 mL of liquid in a 1 mL syringe in a carton of two syringes.

6 mg single-dose vials — 0.5 mL of liquid in a 2 mL vial.

All the liquid should be a colorless to pale yellow clear solution. Particles or precipitates should NEVER appear.

Tablets — 25 mg, 50 mg, 100 mg

How to Store

Keep out of reach of children. Store at room temperature in a room where the temperature will not exceed 86 degrees F (30 degrees C). Keep away from heat and light.

▷ **Recommended Dosage Ranges** (Actual dose and schedule must be determined for each patient individually.)

Infants and Children: The safety and effectiveness in pediatrics have not been determined.

18 to 60 Years of Age:

Subcutaneous: Maximum adult dose is 6 mg. The dose should be taken as soon as possible after the symptoms of acute migraine are recognized. Controlled clinical trials have failed to demonstrate a benefit of repeated injections if the initial injection is unsuccessful. If symptoms return, a second 6 mg injection may be taken 12 hours after the first injection. If side effects occur, use the lowest dose in the approved dose range that is effective for you. Maximum is 12 mg per 24 hours.

Oral: 25 mg taken with water or other acceptable liquids as soon as possible after a headache starts. The dose chosen must balance possible benefit of the higher dose with increased risk of adverse effects of higher doses. Take the dose your doctor prescribes as soon as headache pain starts. If the headache returns or if there is a partial response, single tablets can be taken at least 2 hours after the first dose (up to 200 mg a day). If symptoms come back, subsequent doses can be taken (talk this over with your doctor first) separated by 2 hours after the last dose and taken up to a total of 200 mg in 24 hours.

Author's Note: The tablet form of this medicine has been reformulated to dissolve more quickly.

Nasal: 5 to 20 mg as a one-time dose. Labeled dosing says that more patients taking the 20 mg dose had headache relief. The dose chosen must balance possible benefit of the higher dose with increased risk of adverse effects of higher doses. Take the dose prescribed as soon as headache pain starts. For example, 10 mg may be taken by spraying 5 mg in each nostril. A 20 mg dose can be taken as 10 mg in each nostril. Data exist that show that single doses more than 20 mg do not give additional benefit. If symptoms return, the dose can be taken once again (2 hours after the first dose was taken), but the daily maximum of 40 mg must not be exceeded. Safety in treating more than 4 headaches in 30 days is unknown with any dosage form.

Over 65 Years of Age: NOT recommended in this age group since declines in kidney (renal) and liver (hepatic) function and coronary artery disease are more common in those over 65, and side effects (such as blood pressure increase) may be more severe.

Conditions Requiring Dosing Adjustments

Liver Function: Oral tablets will give unpredictable variations in blood levels if used in liver disease. Maximum dose is 50 mg per dose and 100 mg per 24 hours.

Kidney Function: No changes in dose thought to be needed in kidney disease.

Dosing Instructions: The injection form must be given subcutaneously, not intravenously. Intravenous injection must be avoided because of potential to cause coronary vasospasm (constriction of the blood vessels that supply the heart). This medicine should be colorless to pale yellow and clear. Particles should never be present. There is extensive information on self-injection available from your doctor or pharmacist. The first dose is usually given in the doctor's office. The tablet form may take more than an hour to work. The tablet form may be taken with food. Follow directions for the nasal form closely. The nasal form should be used in only one nostril each time (unless your doctor tells you to use it differently). Close the bottle tightly after each nasal use. If you forget a dose: This medicine is used when you get a migraine headache, NOT on an ongoing basis.

Usual Duration of Use: The maximum dose is two 6 mg doses (injections) in 24 hours. This medication relieves existing migraines and will not change the frequency or number of attacks (ask your doctor about preventive or prophylactic medicines). Recurring use of this medicine will be needed. If your migraines increase in frequency or severity, call your doctor. If this medicine is not effective in helping your migraine, call your doctor.

Typical Treatment Goals and Measurements (Outcomes and Markers)

Migraine Pain: Most clinicians treating pain use a device called an algometer to check your pain. This looks like a small ruler, but lets the clinician better understand your pain. The goals of treatment then relate to where the level of pain started (for example, a rating of seven on a zero to ten scale) and what the cause of the pain was. I use the PQRSTBG system (see Glossary). Pain medicines may also be used together (in combination) in order to get the best result or outcome. Specific results to migraine relate to stopping (aborting) an attack or easing the severity of an attack. Once again, the role of prophylactic medicines is clear in helping some patients avoid attacks altogether. A migraine diary can help you figure out which foods may lead to migraines (trigger foods) as well as medication response.

▷ **This Drug Should Not Be Taken If**
- you had an allergic reaction to it previously.
- you are unfamiliar with the subcutaneous route. Particular care must be taken to avoid intravenous use because this may lead to coronary vasospasm (constriction of the blood vessels that supply the heart).
- you have ischemic heart disease with symptoms such as angina pectoris or silent ischemia, or history of MI (myocardial infarction).
- you have peripheral vascular disease (including ischemic bowel disease).
- you have a seizure disorder, transient ischemic attack (TIA), stroke, or other cerebrovascular syndrome.
- you have Prinzmetal's angina (a specific kind of chest pain).
- you have uncontrolled hypertension (high blood pressure).
- you have basilar or hemiplegic migraine.
- you have taken an MAO inhibitor within the last 2 weeks.
- you have (within 24 hours) taken an ergotamine preparation.

▷ **Inform Your Physician Before Taking This Drug If**
- you are pregnant or plan to become pregnant.
- you are breast-feeding your infant.
- you have high blood pressure, high cholesterol, or a strong family history of coronary artery disease.
- you have chest pain, heart disease, or irregular heartbeats.
- you smoke.
- you have taken or have prescriptions for other migraine medications.
- you have allergies or trouble taking other medications, whether prescription or over the counter.
- you are a woman after menopause or are a man over 40.
- you have liver or kidney disease.
- you are uncertain of how much to take or when to take this medicine.
- you do not understand the subcutaneous injection technique.
- you have Raynaud's phenomenon.

Possible Side Effects (natural, expected, and unavoidable drug actions)
Excessive thirst and frequent urination. Transient rises in blood pressure. Vision changes—rare. Taste changes—frequent.

▷ **Possible Adverse Effects** (unusual, unexpected, and infrequent reactions)
If any of the following develop, consult your physician promptly for guidance.

Mild Adverse Effects
Allergic reactions: red, itching skin; skin rash and tenderness.
Atypical sensations such as tingling (rare with injection, infrequent with tablet form).
Confusion and other mental changes or dizziness—rare.
Flushing—rare.
Tightness in the chest or jaw—infrequent.
Gastroesophageal reflux and diarrhea—case report.
Pain at the injection site; joint pain, weakness, and stiffness—rare.

Serious Adverse Effects
Allergic reactions: anaphylactic reactions.
Syncope (fainting), CVA, dysphasia, seizure—rare.
Serious changes in heart rate and rhythm—rare.
Raynaud's phenomenon, dyspnea (difficulty breathing)—rare.
Kidney stones (renal calculi)—rare.
Prinzmetal's angina—rare.
Heart attack (myocardial infarction)—rare.

▷ **Possible Effects on Sexual Function:** Dysmenorrhea, erection problems—case reports.

Possible Delayed Adverse Effects: None identified.

▷ **Adverse Effects That May Mimic Natural Diseases or Disorders**
Changes in heart rate and rhythm may mimic a number of cardiac conditions. Drug-induced hypertension may mimic hypertension from other causes. Urological symptoms may mimic benign prostatic hypertrophy. Sumatriptan can mimic Raynaud's phenomenon.

Natural Diseases or Disorders That May Be Activated by This Drug
Hypertension.

Possible Effects on Laboratory Tests
Liver function tests: rare increases in SGOT and SGPT.

CAUTION
1. Do not use sumatriptan if you are pregnant.
2. Call your doctor if you have any pain or tightness in the chest or throat when you use this medicine.
3. Do not use sumatriptan if you have used an ergotamine preparation within the last 24 hours.
4. This medication is **not** to be used intravenously.
5. If you are diagnosed as having ischemic heart disease after sumatriptan has been prescribed for you, do not use the medicine again.

Precautions for Use
By Infants and Children: Safety and effectiveness for those less than 18 years of age are not established.
By Those Over 65 Years of Age: Not recommended in this population.

▷ **Advisability of Use During Pregnancy**
Pregnancy Category: C. See Pregnancy Risk Categories at the back of this book.
Animal Studies: Sumatriptan has been lethal to rabbit embryos when given in doses that were threefold higher than those produced by a 6 mg dose. Term fetuses from rabbits treated with sumatriptan exhibited an increase in cervicothoracic vascular defects and minor skeletal abnormalities.

Human Studies: Adequate studies of pregnant women are not available. Ask your physician for guidance.

Advisability of Use If Breast-Feeding
Presence of this drug in breast milk: Yes.
Use of this medication by nursing mothers is a benefit-to-risk decision to be made by a physician.

Habit-Forming Potential: Not clearly defined, but seems to have a low potential for abuse.

Effects of Overdose: Patients have received doses of 8 to 12 mg without adverse effects. This DOES NOT mean this is advisable. Healthy volunteers have taken up to 16 mg subcutaneously without serious adverse events. Coronary vasospasm has resulted from intravenous doses. Animal data present convulsions, tremor, flushing, decreased breathing and activity, cyanosis, ataxia, and paralysis.

Possible Effects of Long-Term Use: Not defined.

Suggested Periodic Examinations While Taking This Drug (at physician's discretion)
Liver function tests.
Electrocardiogram.

▷ **While Taking This Drug, Observe the Following**
Foods: No restrictions; however, some foods or additives such as monosodium glutamate or chocolate may be a risk factor for migraines. Skipping meals can also be a risk factor for migraines. Keeping a migraine diary can help identify triggers.
Herbal Medicines or Minerals: Using St. John's wort, ma huang, guarana, or kola while taking this medicine may trigger a migraine. Trigger compounds must be individually identified. Since part of the way that ginseng works (mechanism of action) may involve MAO inhibition, combination with sumatriptan is NOT recommended. Using ma huang or ephedra (ephedra—removed from the U.S. market for weight loss) or ephedrine-like compounds such as bitter orange or country mallow may result in additive and undesirable vasoconstriction. If you are allergic to plants in the Asteraceae family (aster, chrysanthemum, daisy, or ragweed), you may also be allergic to echinacea, chamomile, feverfew, and St. John's wort. St. John's wort can cause changes in the liver enzymes that help remove this medicine—talk to your doctor before combining any herbal medicine or mineral with sumatriptan.
Beverages: An individual trigger beverage list should be identified.
▷ *Alcohol:* May cause additive sedation. Alcohol may also be a precipitating factor for migraine.
Tobacco Smoking: No interactions expected. I advise everyone to quit smoking.
Marijuana Smoking: May cause additive dizziness, drowsiness, and lethargy; may cause additive increases in blood pressure.
▷ *Other Drugs*
Sumatriptan *taken concurrently* with
• citalopram (Celexa) or the related escitalopram (Lexapro) may lead to loss of coordination and excessive reflex response—NOT RECOMMENDED. Close monitoring is appropriate if they must be combined.
• ergotamine-containing preparations (see Drug Classes) may result in additive vasospasm (prolonged constriction of the blood vessels)—these medicines SHOULD NOT be taken within 24 hours of any sumatriptan dose.

There is a case report of heart attack after sumatriptan was combined with methysergide.

- fluoxetine (Prozac) may result in coordination problems.
- fluvoxamine (Luvox) and other SSRIs may result in coordination problems.
- monoamine oxidase (MAO) inhibitors (see Drug Classes) may result in toxic levels of sumatriptan—MAO inhibitors and sumatriptan should never be combined. It is important that 14 days go by after your last dose of an MAO inhibitor before you take any form of sumatriptan.
- naratriptan (Amerge), zolmitriptan (Zomig), or other "triptans" (5HT1 agonists) may lead to prolonged spasm of the blood vessels—DO NOT COMBINE.
- paroxetine (Paxil) may result in coordination problems.
- sertraline (Zoloft) may result in coordination problems.
- sibutramine (Meridia) may increase risk of serotonin syndrome—DO NOT COMBINE.
- venlafaxine (Effexor) may result in coordination problems.

▷ *Driving, Hazardous Activities:* This drug may cause dizziness and drowsiness. Restrict activities as necessary.

Aviation Note: The use of this drug *may be a disqualification* for piloting. Consult a designated Aviation Medical Examiner.

Exposure to Sun: No restrictions.

Exposure to Cold: Use *CAUTION* until tolerance is determined. Cold may enhance sumatriptan vasoconstriction.

Heavy Exercise or Exertion: Strenuous exercise can be a risk factor for migraines in some patients.

Special Storage Instructions: Keep this medicine out of reach of children. Store at room temperature in a room where the temperature will not exceed 86°F (30°C). Keep away from heat and light.

Observe the Following Expiration Times: There is an expiration date printed on the treatment package. Throw the medication away if it has expired. The autoinjector may be used again.

SYNTHETIC CONJUGATED ESTROGENS, A
(CHEMICALLY DERIVED FROM PLANTS [YAMS AND SOY])

Other Names: Sodium estrone sulfate, sodium equilin sulfate, sodium 17 alpha-dihydroequilin sulfate, sodium 17 alpha estradiol sulfate, sodium 17 beta dihydroequilin sulfate, sodium 17 beta estradiol sulfate, sodium equilin sulfate (higher molecular weight), sodium 17 alpha dihydroequilin sulfate, and sodium 17 beta dihydroequilin sulfate (higher molecular weight). All of these nine compounds are present in Cenestin.

Author's Note: Since this medicine contains compounds that work like the estrogen that the body makes before menopause (estrogenic substances), and because these came from plants (versus horse urine for many other estrogen replacement medicines), the FDA approved Cenestin as an entirely new class. Many of the warnings, etc., in this profile are those for estrogens in general. Reports from phase four prescribing will determine further uses (indications) as well as the full scope of specific possible side effects and benefits. Alternative synthetic conjugated estrogen combinations such as Cenestin are further detailed below. A new plant-derived

synthetic conjugated estrogen called synthetic conjugated estrogens, B (brand name Enjuvia), has been approved and will be detailed in subsequent editions if clinical results and research warrants.

The estrogen-alone part of the Women's Health Initiative (WHI) was stopped in February 2004 because there was no lowering of risk of coronary heart disease and there was found to be an increased risk of stroke. (Visit *www.nhlbi.nih.gov* for more information. At the time of this writing, there is a press release at *www.nhlbi.nih.gov/new/press/04-04-13.htm*). Controversy about estrogen therapy (ERT) and use of combination hormone replacement therapy (HRT) started with the HERS (Heart and Estrogen/Progestin Replacement Study). HERS negated the role of estrogen/progestin in preventing a second heart attack. The Women's Health Initiative (WHI) combination arm was stopped early (see *www.whi.org;* July 17, 2002, *JAMA* article, especially Table 4; *www.acog.org;* and *www.menopause.org*). Importantly, the WHI data showed that if 10,000 women took the 0.626 mg conjugated estrogens and 2.5 mg medroxyprogesterone daily (as in Prempro), versus not taking it, 8 more women would develop invasive breast cancer, 7 more would have a heart attack or other coronary, and 8 more would have blood clots in the lungs or a stroke. Five fewer would have hip fracture and 6 fewer would have colorectal cancers. The WHIMS group (Women's Health Initiative Memory Study) of the WHI (May 27, 2003—see FDA talk paper T03-39 in Sources) found that this medicine should NOT be used to help prevent dementia or Alzheimer's, and for the data analyzed, showed an increased risk of undesirable mental status change (dementia) in women over 65 who used the combination for longer periods. A two-month time frame of use was recommended by the WHI panel (shortest period and in the lowest dose to meet treatment goals).

A continued analysis of the 16,608 women from the Women's Health Initiative (WHI), published in the July 25, 2003, issue of *JAMA* reported that in women who used the combination of estrogen plus progesterone and who developed breast cancer, the tumors tended to be larger than women who did not take the combination. Additionally, 25.4% of the combined product users who developed breast cancer had tumors that had begun to spread. In general, women who took the combination formulation had a 24% increased breast cancer risk. Increased risk did not become apparent in the first 2 years of those studied. Some question regarding difficulty of discovering tumors because of increased breast density caused by the hormone progestin has been postulated.

The low-dose Prempro form contains 0.45 mg of conjugated estrogens and 1.5 mg of medroxyprogesterone acetate. This combination form is indicated for use by women who have a uterus and is used to treat moderate to severe vasomotor symptoms (night sweats and hot flashes) as well as moderate to severe vulvar and vaginal changes (atrophy) that may show as vaginal dryness. Topical forms should be considered if the combination is only being used for vulvar and vaginal atrophy. Alternatives for patients who can't take estrogen currently include clonidine, fluoxetine (Prozac), gabapentin (Neurontin), and venlafaxine (Effexor).

Introduced: 1999   **Class:**   Female sex hormones   **Prescription:** USA: Yes   **Controlled Drug:**   USA: No; Canada: No   **Available as Generic:**   USA: No; Canada: No
Brand Names: Cenestin, ♣C.E.S.

BENEFITS versus RISKS

Possible Benefits	*Possible Risks*
RELIEF OF MENOPAUSAL HOT FLASHES AND NIGHT SWEATS	INCREASED RISK OF CANCER OF THE UTERUS (endometrium— possible and risk increases with longer use)
DECREASED RISK OF HIP FRACTURE	
DECREASED RISK OF COLORECTAL CANCER	INCREASED RISK OF BREAST CANCER (possible and expected to be more probable with longer use)
Possible prevention or relief of atrophic vaginitis or atrophy of the vulva and urethra	INCREASED RISK OF HEART ATTACK
Works to help prevent postmenopausal osteoporosis	INCREASED RISK OF STROKE
Works to increase bone mineral density	INCREASED RISK OF LONG OR DEEP VEIN CLOTS (THROMBOSIS)
	INCREASED RISK OF CANCER OF THE OVARY
	Accelerated growth of preexisting fibroid tumors of the uterus
	Fluid retention
	Lowered tolerance for blood sugar
	Postmenopausal bleeding
	Increased gall stone risk

▷ **Principal Uses**

As a *Single Drug Product:* Uses currently included in FDA-approved labeling: (1) Treatment of moderate to severe menopausal symptoms (vasomotor symptoms) in menopause; (2) treats severe or moderate vaginal and vulvar atrophy symptoms that can be seen with menopause.

Other (unlabeled) generally accepted uses: None at present.

How This Drug Works: When used to correct hormonal deficiency states, estrogens restore normal cellular activity by increasing nuclear material and protein synthesis. Frequency and intensity of menopausal symptoms are reduced when normal levels of estrogen are restored.

▷ **Widely Used Guidelines That Involve This Medicine (representative sample):** Please look at the section at the very beginning of this profile called "Class." Next, turn to Table 22 and you will find guidelines listed by the class involved!

Available Dosage Forms and Strengths

Tablets — 0.3 mg, 0.625 mg, 0.9 mg, 1.25 mg

▷ **Usual Adult Dosage Ranges:** *For moderate to severe symptoms associated with menopause:* Dosing is started at 0.625 mg a day. The dose may be increased to a maximum of 1.25 mg daily if needed and tolerated. The lowest effective dose should be used and attempts to stop and taper medicine made at 3- to 6-month intervals. *For vaginal atrophy:* 0.3 mg is taken once daily. Once again, the medicine should be used in the lowest effective dose for the shortest possible time with attempts to taper at 3–6-month intervals.

Note: Actual dose and schedule must be determined for each patient individually.

Conditions Requiring Dosing Adjustments

Liver Function: Since this medicine is metabolized in the liver, blood levels should be checked and the dose adjusted as needed in liver compromise. Estrogens should not be used in acute or severe liver compromise. This drug can be lithogenic (capable of causing stones) in bile.

Kidney Function: No expected dosing changes in kidney compromise.

▷ **Dosing Instructions:** The effect of food on this medicine is not known. At present, it is best to take this medicine on an empty stomach. If you forget a dose: Take the missed dose as soon as you remember it, unless it's nearly time for your next dose—if that is the case, skip the missed dose and take the next dose right on schedule. DO NOT double doses. Talk with your doctor if you find yourself missing doses.

Usual Duration of Use: Regular use for 10 to 20 days needed to see effectiveness in easing menopausal symptoms. Attempts to stop or lower the dose (taper) this medicine should be made at 3- to 6-month intervals. Follow-up with your doctor is required.

Typical Treatment Goals and Measurements (Outcomes and Markers)

Menopause: Most clinicians treating menopause seek goals of reduction or cessation of hot flashes, greater sense of well-being, and avoidance of rapid bone loss (which can also be measured by some lab tests and DEXA testing). The WHI study and substudies changed treatment to the smallest effective dose for the shortest possible time that is appropriate to the goals and benefit-to-risk profile of the individual patient.

Possible Advantages of This Drug

THIS DRUG IS NOT derived from horse urine and avoids the possible allergic potential of products that are. Effective with once-a-day dose.

▷ **This Drug Should Not Be Taken If**
- you have had an allergic reaction to it or to the ingredients in the tablet previously.
- you have a history of thrombophlebitis, embolism, heart attack, or stroke.
- you have seriously impaired liver function or recent onset of liver disease.
- you have abnormal and unexplained vaginal bleeding.
- you are pregnant.
- you have or are suspected to have breast cancer.
- you have known or suspected estrogen-dependent cancer (your doctor will determine this).

▷ **Inform Your Physician Before Taking This Drug If**
- you have had an unfavorable reaction to estrogen therapy previously.
- you have a history of breast, endometrial, or reproductive organ cancer.
- you have fibrocystic breast changes, fibroid tumors of the uterus, endometriosis, migraine headaches, epilepsy, asthma, heart disease, high blood pressure, gallbladder disease, diabetes, or porphyria.
- you have retention of fluid.
- you have elevated calcium and kidney disease.
- you've used this medicine for 3 or 6 months and have not tried to stop using it.
- you smoke tobacco on a regular basis.
- you have a history of blood-clotting disorders.
- you plan to have surgery in the near future.

Possible Side Effects (natural, expected, and unavoidable drug actions)

Fluid retention, weight gain, "breakthrough" bleeding (spotting), altered menstrual pattern, resumption of menstrual flow ("periods") after natural cessation (postmenopausal bleeding).

▷ **Possible Adverse Effects** (unusual, unexpected, and infrequent reactions)

If any of the following develop, consult your physician promptly for guidance.

Mild Adverse Effects

Allergic reaction: skin rash—reported with other estrogens.

Headache, nervous tension, depression, accentuation of migraine headaches—infrequent.

Vision change (steepening of the curve of the cornea)—possible.

Nausea, vomiting, bloating, diarrhea—infrequent to frequent.

Tannish pigmentation of the face—possible.

Serious Adverse Effects

Allergic reactions: anaphylaxis—case reports with other estrogens.

Idiosyncratic reaction: not reported with this product.

Can produce or worsen high blood pressure—more likely with higher doses.

Gallbladder disease—two- to four fold increased risk.

Intolerance to sugar—possible.

Thrombophlebitis (inflammation of a vein with formation of blood clot): pain or tenderness in thigh or leg, with or without swelling of foot or leg—low dose has minimal increased risk; higher doses may carry more risk.

Pulmonary embolism (movement of blood clot to lung): sudden shortness of breath, pain in chest, coughing, bloody sputum—possible.

Systemic lupus erythematosus or worsening of porphyria—rare.

Stroke (blood clot in brain): headaches, blackout, sudden weakness, or paralysis of any part of the body, severe dizziness, altered vision, slurred speech, inability to speak—case reports with other estrogens.

Endometrial cancer—increased risk from using estrogens alone (unopposed estrogen) may be 2–12 times more than people who do not use estrogens. Many studies do not show increased cancer risk if estrogens are used for less than a year. Risk with longer term use may persist for 8–15 years after the drug is stopped. There is no evidence that natural estrogens are more or less likely than other estrogens to increase risk.

Nonfatal heart attack (blood clot in coronary artery): sudden pain in chest, neck, jaw, or arm; weakness; sweating; nausea. Has been associated with women taking higher doses and with men using estrogen to treat prostate cancer; however, this is not clearly decided as yet with this product.

Breast cancer—increased risk with the combination form use in WHI found 26% increased risk of invasive breast cancer in women with a uterus who took the combination treatment. A re-analysis of the WHI data found that tumor risk did not appear in the first 2 years that the combination form was used (see Chlebowski, R.T. in Sources). A subset analysis (see Li, C.I. in Sources) found that the greatest risk was seen in combination use for at least 5 years. Those using estrogen alone who had undergone a hysterectomy had use for as long as 25 years and did not appear to show any appreciable increased risk of breast cancer.

Ovarian cancer—use of estrogens alone for more than 10 years increased risk in some studies, not in others.

Benign liver adenomas or blood clots in the liver—reported with oral contraceptives.

▷ **Possible Effects on Sexual Function:** Swelling and tenderness of breasts, milk production. Increased vaginal secretions.

Possible Delayed Adverse Effects: Estrogens taken during pregnancy may predispose a female child to the later development of cancer of the vagina or cervix following puberty.

▷ **Adverse Effects That May Mimic Natural Diseases or Disorders**
Blood clots may mimic clots forming for other reasons.

Natural Diseases or Disorders That May Be Activated by This Drug
Latent hypertension, diabetes mellitus, acute intermittent porphyria.

Possible Effects on Laboratory Tests
Serum folate: may be decreased (the effect of possible lowering of folate by Cenestin on red blood cells is not yet defined).
Accelerated prothrombin time (reported as INR).
Glucose tolerance test (GTT): decreased tolerance.
Liver function tests: increased with other estrogens if a rare liver clot forms.

CAUTION
1. Yearly mammography is needed for ALL women who take this medicine who are more than 50 years old.
2. Bone mineral density tests (DEXA or PDEXA) are prudent to see whether this medicine is helping bone mass.
3. While this product is derived from plants (yam and soy), it was approved by the FDA as an estrogen and as such may carry the benefits and risks of existing estrogens. Many consumers think that because something is derived from a natural source, it is somehow safer. This tablet is a blend of nine estrogenic compounds derived from soy and yams, and may or may not carry similar risks and benefits of existing estrogens. Ongoing use will define how possible side effects or benefits of prior estrogens apply to Cenestin. Any unusual vaginal bleeding should be immediately reported your doctor.
4. See WHI note above regarding benefit to risk and individualization, etc. Best to take this medicine for the shortest amount of time in the smallest dose that is consistent with the benefit-to-risk profile of the patient and the goals of therapy.

Precautions for Use
By Those Over 60 Years of Age: May help women who are at increased risk for osteoporosis. In this age group, it may be advisable to attempt relief of hot flashes with nonestrogenic medicines. During use, report promptly any indications of impaired circulation: speech disturbances, altered vision, sudden hearing loss, vertigo, sudden weakness or paralysis, angina, leg pains.

▷ **Advisability of Use During Pregnancy**
Pregnancy Category: X. See Pregnancy Risk Categories at the back of this book.
Animal Studies: Genital defects reported in mice and guinea pigs; cleft palate reported in rodents from other estrogens.
Human Studies: Information from studies of pregnant women indicates that estrogens can masculinize the female fetus. In addition, limb defects and heart malformations have been reported. It is now known that estrogens taken during pregnancy can predispose the female child to the development of cancer of the vagina or cervix following puberty.

Avoid estrogens completely during entire pregnancy.

Advisability of Use If Breast-Feeding
Presence of this drug in breast milk: Yes, in minute amounts.

Estrogens in large doses can suppress milk formation. Breast-feeding is considered to be safe during the use of estrogens. Malnourished mothers may have unacceptable decreases in protein and nitrogen in their breast milk if this drug is used while breast-feeding. Estrogens should NOT be used to try to stop breast milk formation after giving birth, as this may increase risk of blood clots.

Habit-Forming Potential: There has been some suggestion of estrogens having potential for psychological dependence and tolerance because of their mood-elevating properties, but clinical reports have not been presented.

Effects of Overdose: Nausea, vomiting, fluid retention, abnormal vaginal bleeding, breast enlargement and discomfort.

Possible Effects of Long-Term Use: Long-term use of combination form no longer recommended. Ongoing study of WHI is for the estrogen only "arm" of the study. Prudence dictates that women with intact uteri should use estrogens only if the benefits outweigh the risks, with proper supervision and in the lowest effect dose for the shortest possible time consistent with the goals, benefit-to-risk profile, etc.

Suggested Periodic Examinations While Taking This Drug (at physician's discretion)

Checks every 3–6 months for benefits and continued need. Regular evaluation of the breasts (self-exam). Yearly mammography for ALL women who take this medicine.

Regular (every 6 months) evaluation of the breasts and pelvic organs, including Pap smears.

Liver function tests as indicated.

▷ **While Taking This Drug, Observe the Following**

Foods: Avoid excessive use of salt if fluid retention occurs. Combined use of calcium and vitamin D can be a further step to help avoid osteoporosis. Combining DHEA with estrogen can lead to signs and symptoms (such as nausea, colitis, or breakthrough bleeding) of excess estrogen.

Herbal Medicines or Minerals: Black cohosh appears to work by (1) suppressing luteinizing hormone, (2) binding to estrogen receptors in the pituitary and inhibiting luteinizing hormone release, and (3) binding to estrogen receptors in the pituitary. The net effect is that this herb eases symptoms of menopause, but little is known about long-term use or heart and bone protective effects. This herb may interfere with the benefits of estrogen replacement therapy. Talk to your doctor before starting black cohosh if you are currently taking any form of estrogen. Use of St. John's wort, echinacea, or ginkgo completely stopped or lowered the ability of sperm to penetrate eggs in one study. DO NOT use these herbs if you are using a conjugated estrogen product to augment mucous quality and help infertility. St. John's wort may also increase sun sensitivity.

Beverages: No restrictions. May be taken with milk.

▷ *Alcohol:* No interactions expected.

Tobacco Smoking: Studies show that smoking, especially heavy smoking (15 or more cigarettes daily) in association with use of estrogen-containing oral contraceptives, significantly increases risk of heart attack (coronary thrombosis). I advise everyone to stop smoking.

▷ *Other Drugs*

Estrogens **taken concurrently** with

• alendronate (Fosamax) have not been specifically studied but had beneficial effects in one part of a larger study using a different medicine. The combination of a different kind of estrogen used with alendronate is now approved in Canada.

- amprenavir (Agenerase) may blunt benefits of amprenavir in fighting HIV, and may also result in loss of contraceptive benefits (efficacy). Other protease inhibitors such as nelfinavir (Viracept) may lead to contraceptive failure also.
- aprepitant (Emend) may lower estrogen levels (in the case of birth control pills lead to pregnancy).
- atazanavir (Reyataz) may lead to increased estrogen levels.
- atorvastatin (Lipitor) may lead to increased birth control pill medicine levels.
- fluconazole (Diflucan) may increase contraceptive medicine blood levels (ethinyl estradiol).
- lamotrigene (Lamictal) may increase or decrease lamotrigene levels. More frequent blood level checks are needed with doses adjusted accordingly.
- naratriptan (Amerge) may increase naratriptan as well as zolmitriptan (Zomig) blood levels. Patients should be closely followed for increased naratriptan or zolmitriptan adverse effects.
- oral antidiabetic drugs (see Drug Classes) or oral blood-sugar-lowering medicines may cause loss of glucose control and high blood sugars.
- progestins (various) may increase risk of breast cancer versus estrogen use by itself.
- tacrine (Cognex) increases the risk of tacrine adverse effects.
- thyroid hormones may increase the bound (inactive) drug and require an increase in thyroid dose.
- tricyclic antidepressants (Elavil, Sinequan, etc.) may enhance their adverse effects and reduce their antidepressant effectiveness.
- vitamin C (ascorbic acid, various brands) in higher doses may result in increased estrogen effects—a lower dose of estrogens may be indicated if higher-dose vitamin C will be taken on an ongoing basis.
- warfarin (Coumadin) may cause alterations of prothrombin activity; increased doses may be needed, and more frequent INR testing is indicated.
- zolmitriptan (Zomig) may increase risk of zolmitriptan adverse effects.

The following drugs may decrease the effects of estrogens:

- carbamazepine (Tegretol).
- penicillin (various) may blunt contraceptive benefits.
- phenobarbital (various).
- phenytoin (Dilantin) or fosphenytoin (Cerebyx).
- primidone (Mysoline).
- rifampin (Rifadin, Rimactane).

Author's Note: The possible drug interactions above are those detailed for existing estrogens in the estrogen profile earlier in this book.

▷ *Driving, Hazardous Activities:* Usually no restrictions. Talk to your doctor for assessment of individual risk and for guidance regarding specific restrictions.

Aviation Note: Usually no restrictions, but watch for the rare occurrence of disturbed vision (curvature changes) and restrict activities accordingly. Consult a designated Aviation Medical Examiner.

Exposure to Sun: Caution—existing estrogens may cause photosensitivity (see Glossary).

Discontinuation: Best to use estrogens in the smallest effective dose for the shortest amount of time consistent with the benefit-to-risk profile of the patient and the goals of treatment. If used to control menopausal symptoms, the dose is reduced gradually to prevent acute withdrawal hot flashes. Avoid continual, uninterrupted use of large doses. Ask your doctor for help.

TACRINE (TA kreen)

Please see the anti-Alzheimer's drug family profile.

TADALAFIL (Tah DAHL ah fill)

Introduced: 2003   **Class:** Anti-impotence,   phosphodiesterase inhibitor (PDE5)   **Prescription:**   USA: Yes   **Controlled Drug:**   USA: No; Canada: No   **Available as Generic:**   USA: No; Canada: No
Brand Name: Cialis

```
┌─────────────────────────────────────────────────────────────────┐
│                    BENEFITS versus RISKS                          │
│     Possible Benefits                  Possible Risks             │
│ SUCCESSFUL ACHIEVEMENT OF      SERIOUS DRUG INTERACTIONS          │
│   AN ERECTION                  Drug-induced vision changes        │
│ SUFFICIENT ERECTION TO         Headache                          │
│   ACHIEVE INTERCOURSE                                             │
│ BENEFICIAL EFFECT MAY LAST                                        │
│   FOR UP TO 36 HOURS                                             │
└─────────────────────────────────────────────────────────────────┘
```

▷ **Principal Uses**
  As a Single Drug Product: Uses currently included in FDA-approved labeling: (1) Treats difficulties getting or maintaining an erection (erectile dysfunction). Other (unlabeled) generally accepted uses: None at present.
▷ **How This Drug Works:** Causes smooth muscle in the penis to relax, increasing blood flow into the penis, resulting in erection. Sildenafil causes release of nitric oxide (NO) in part of the penis called the corpus cavernosum. This then increases an enzyme called guanylate cyclase. This enzyme increases cyclic guanosine monophosphate (CGMP). The CGMP causes the smooth muscle in the penis to relax. Once the smooth muscle relaxes, blood flows into the penis, resulting in erection.
▷ **Widely Used Guidelines That Involve This Medicine (representative sample):** Please look at the section at the very beginning of this profile called "Class." Next, turn to Table 22 and you will find guidelines listed by the class involved!
Available Dosage Forms and Strengths
  Tablets — 5 mg, 10 mg, 20 mg
▷ **Recommended Dose Ranges** (Actual dose and schedule must be determined for each patient individually.)
  Infants and Children: Not used in this age group.
  18 to 65 Years of Age: The usual starting dose is 10 mg taken before sexual activity (some people get a benefit half an hour after taking it). This medicine should only be used once a day. Depending on individual response or how

well the medicine is tolerated, the dose can be increased to 20 mg or decreased to 5 mg once a day. For people who are taking medicines that inhibit a liver enzyme called cytochrome P450 3A4 (such as itraconazole, ketoconazole, and some macrolide antibiotics such as erythromycin), the 10 mg dose is the maximum recommended and should only be taken once every 3 days (72 hours). Further caution is required and it would be a benefit-to-risk decision if multiple 3A4 inhibitors are being taken and tadalafil is being considered. Additionally, some medicines used in combination therapy of HIV/AIDS may interact; caution and lower doses are prudent, and use is a benefit-to-risk decision for your doctor. (See additional medicine combination comments in the drug interactions section below.)

Over 65 Years of Age: Current labeling says that dosing does not need to be decreased based on age, but dosing SHOULD BE DECREASED based on kidney function (e.g., starting dose of only 5 mg if creatinine clearance [CrCl] is 31–50 mL/Min and a maximum dose of 10 mg every two days). Because our kidneys don't work as well as we age, talk to your doctor about your dose being adjusted for the age-related decline in kidney function.

Conditions Requiring Dosing Adjustments

Liver Function: For mild to moderately impaired liver function (Child-Pugh Class A or B), the dose of tadalafil should NOT be more than 10 mg once a day. If the liver is severely impaired (Child-Pugh Class C), this medicine SHOULD NOT be used.

Kidney Function: Dosing SHOULD BE DECREASED based on kidney function (e.g. starting dose of only 5 mg if creatinine clearance [CrCl] is 31–50 mL/Min and a maximum dose of 10 mg every two days). Because our kidneys don't work as well as we age, (yes—even 65 WITHOUT a diagnosis of kidney disease), talk to your doctor about your dose being adjusted for the age-related decline in kidney function. You'll need a laboratory test and have to get some blood taken—but it's smart to check.

▷ **Dosing Instructions:** The tablet may be crushed and taken without regard to eating (high-fat meals decreased absorption time for a different medicine for Erectile Dysfunction [ED] which may be an advantage). It goes to work in 30 minutes for many people and can last for 36 hours. If you forget a dose: There is as little as a 30-minute wait. DO NOT take the medicine more than once a day.

Usual Duration of Use: Use is only recommended ONCE a day. If use is to be ongoing on a daily basis, this should be discussed with your doctor.

Typical Treatment Goals and Measurements (Outcomes and Markers)

Erectile dysfunction: The general goal is to help you attain an erection that will stay firm enough to let you have sex. Typical desired results are stiffness or tone of the penis and how often you have an erection in response to this medicine.

Possible Advantages of This Drug: Avoids direct injections into the penis (such as Caverject). Avoids surgical placement of an implant. Excellent response rate that may last for up to 36 hours.

▷ **This Drug Should Not Be Taken If**
- you have had an allergic reaction to it previously.
- you have a disease or condition that would result in serious health hazard if lowering of the blood pressure or sexual activity occurred.
- you are taking any nitrate (see Drug Classes). NEVER combine these nitrates with tadalafil (see also Other Drug interactions).

- you have preexisting cardiovascular disease of a severity that precludes sexual activity.
- you have not fully discussed this medicine or all of the other medicines you take with your doctor, or have obtained it from an alternative source.

▷ **Inform Your Physician Before Taking This Drug If**
- you have a decline in liver or kidney function.
- the drug was prescribed for you without a complete medical history or physical examination.
- you have a history of heart disease (such as congestive heart failure, past heart attack, unstable angina, arrhythmias, or coronary ischemia). This medicine has not been studied well in those patients.
- you have multiple myeloma, leukemia, or sickle-cell syndrome (may predispose you to painful and sustained erections called priapism).
- you are over 65, kidney function has not been checked, and more than a 10-mg dose has been prescribed.
- you have vision changes while taking this medicine.
- you have cataracts or impaired vision (such as retinitis pigmentosa).
- you have had structural damage to the penis (Peyronie's disease: see Glossary).
- you are taking a medicine that blocks or enhances the liver cytochrome system (CYP3A4) (talk to your doctor or pharmacist about this).
- you are prone to heartburn or have other stomach conditions or a bleeding disorder.
- you do not have any improvement in erections or sexual performance while taking this medicine.
- you are unsure how much to take or how often to take this medicine.

Possible Side Effects (natural, expected, and unavoidable drug actions)
Changes in vision (blue/green) or dry eyes—possible.

▷ **Possible Adverse Effects** (unusual, unexpected, and infrequent reactions)
If any of the following develop, consult your physician promptly for guidance.
Mild Adverse Effects
Allergic reaction: rash.
Headache—infrequent to frequent.
Congestion of the nose (nasal)—infrequent.
Indigestion—infrequent.
Sensitivity to light or blurred vision—possible to infrequent.
Inability to distinguish between blue and green—possible.
Flushing—infrequent.
Serious Adverse Effects
Serious DRUG INTERACTIONS—possible (see below).
Chest pain, fast heart rate, low blood pressure, heart attack—case reports infrequent to rare—and of uncertain cause-and-effect relationship.
Abnormal liver function tests—rare—and of uncertain cause-and-effect relationship.

▷ **Possible Effects on Sexual Function:**
Sustained and painful erection (priapism)—case reports.

Possible Delayed Adverse Effects: None reported to date.

Natural Diseases or Disorders That May Be Activated by This Drug
Patient perception of any preexisting retinal disease may be worsened if tadalafil haze or blue/green vision change happens. Cardiovascular changes

seen in clinical trials were rare and of uncertain cause-and-effect relationship. Heart condition caution relative to sexual activity being safe for patients is in the present patient information.

Possible Effects on Laboratory Tests
None reported.

CAUTION
1. Because of the possibility of SERIOUS drug interactions, keep a card in your purse or wallet or get a medicine alert bracelet to wear that says you are taking tadalafil.
2. If this medicine does not help you get or maintain an erection, it is important that you follow up with your doctor.
3. Safety and efficacy of tadalafil combined with other treatments for erectile problems (dysfunction) have not been established and may not be recommended by your doctor.
4. Some people use illegal "poppers," which are actually ampules of alkyl nitrites, to enhance sexual activity. These should NEVER be combined with tadalafil.
5. If your erection lasts more than 4 hours, go to the nearest emergency room. Such persistent erections may lead to damage of the penis that is not reversible.

Precautions for Use
By Infants and Children: Safety and effectiveness for those under 18 not established.
By Those Over 65 Years of Age: Check of kidney function is prudent.

▷ ## Advisability of Use During Pregnancy
Pregnancy Category: B. See Pregnancy Risk Categories at the back of this book.
Animal Studies: no evidence of embryotoxicity, fetotoxicity, or teratogenicity in rats and rabbits.
Human Studies: Adequate studies of pregnant women are not available.
NOT indicated for use in women, children, or newborns.

Advisability of Use If Breast-Feeding
Presence of this drug in breast milk: Unknown.
Use in nursing mothers is NOT recommended.

Habit-Forming Potential: None.

Effects of Overdose: Supportive care is indicated with the caveat of extremely careful cardiac monitoring in those with existing heart disease.

Possible Effects of Long-Term Use: Not defined.

Suggested Periodic Examinations While Taking This Drug (at physician's discretion)
Follow-up on success in achieving an erection and having intercourse.
Complete eye examination at beginning of treatment may be prudent. Ask your doctor for help.

▷ ## While Taking This Drug, Observe the Following
Foods: Grapefruit juice can be an inhibitor of CYP3A4. DO NOT combine. Water is the safest liquid to take this medicine with.
Herbal Medicines or Minerals: Using St. John's wort, ma huang (no longer available for weight loss), mate, bitter orange, country mallow, or kola while taking this medicine may result in unacceptable heart stimulation. There are no data regarding combining yohimbe (Pausinystala yohimbe) with

tadalafil, and yohimbe can lead to serious heart complications. The combination is NOT advised. Numan has had some small cohort studies, but has also not been studied and cannot be recommended in combination with tadalafil. A product from Health Nutrition labs called Viga or Viga for Women was the subject of an FDA MedWatch safety alert. The warning noted that this dietary supplement contained sildenafil as an unlabeled ingredient. See *www.fda.gov/medwatch/SAFETY/2003/safety/safety02.htm#vigarma*. Combining two medicines from the same medicine family would not make sense.

Beverages: Grapefruit juice can be an inhibitor of the enzyme that removes tadalafil from the body (CYP3A4). DO NOT combine as toxicity may result. Drug may be taken with milk or water.

▷ *Alcohol:* Excess alcohol intake (such as 0.7 gms per kilogram of weight—as in 5 shots of whiskey or 5 glasses of wine) may excessively lower blood pressure. Do not drink large amounts of alcohol. Talk to your doctor about alcohol and how much is acceptable for you.

Tobacco Smoking: No interactions expected. I advise everyone to quit smoking.

Marijuana Smoking: The active ingredient (cannabinoids) found in marijuana can act as an inhibitor of the principal enzyme (CYP3A4) that removes tadalafil from the body. COMBINATION IS NOT RECOMMENDED.

▷ *Other Drugs*

Tadalafil may increase the effects of
- nitrates (see Drug Classes)—NEVER COMBINE.

The following drugs may ***increase*** the effects of tadalafil:
- erythromycins (erythromycin and clarithromycin: see Drug Classes).
- indinavir (Crixivan), nelfinavir (Viracept), saquinavir (Invirase, Fortovase), amprenavir (Agenerase), and atazanavir (Reyataz).
- itraconazole (Sporanox), ketoconazole (Nizoral), and perhaps similar antifungals.
- metronidazole (Flagyl).
- mibefradil (Posicor) (removed from the U.S. market).
- nitroprusside (Nitropress).
- sertraline (Zoloft).
- any medicine that interferes with cytochrome (CYP3A4), or even those such as sibutramine [Meridia], which use (CYP3A4), will potentially increase (or decrease) tadalafil blood levels. In some cases, I expect that tadalafil dosing will need to be adjusted, and in others, the combination should be avoided.

Tadalafil ***taken concurrently*** with
- alpha-1 adrenergic blockers (such as terazocin, tamsulosin, doxazosin, prazocin, and alfuzosin; see Drug Classes), with the exception of tamsulosin in a dose of 0.4 mg once a day, should NOT be combined with tadalafil as they can severely lower blood pressure.
- amyl nitrite will result in serious decreases in blood pressure—DO NOT COMBINE.
- medicines that cause vision changes (see Table 4) may result in additive vision problems.

The following drugs may ***decrease*** the effects of tadalafil:
- carbamazepine (Tegretol).
- phenytoin (Dilantin).

- rifabutin (Mycobutin).
- rifampin (Rifadin, Rimactane).
▷ *Driving, Hazardous Activities:* No restrictions.
Aviation Note: The use of this drug **may be a disqualification** for piloting. Consult a designated Aviation Medical Examiner.
Exposure to Sun: May increase sensitivity of your eyes to sunlight. Talk to your doctor about sunglasses or other protective measures.
Discontinuation: Talk to your doctor about your results from taking this drug.

TAMOXIFEN (ta MOX i fen)

Introduced: 1973 **Class:** Anticancer, chemotherapy, selective estrogen receptor modulator (SERM) **Prescription:** USA: Yes **Controlled Drug:** USA: No; Canada: No **Available as Generic:** Yes

BrandNames: ✤Alpha-Tamoxifen, ✤Apo-Tamox,✤Dom-Tamoxifen, Nolvadex, ✤Nolvadex-D, ✤Novo-Tamoxifen, ✤PMS-Tamoxifen, ✤Tamofen, ✤Tamone

Author's Note: A medicine called anastrozole (Arimidex) has shown extremely promising results in early results from the one of the largest cancer studies ever undertaken (more than 9,000 women). This trial is unusual in that it is very very large and compares tamoxifen to anastrozole and also looks at the combination of the two drugs.

BENEFITS versus RISKS	
Possible Benefits	*Possible Risks*
DECREASED RISK OF BREAST CANCER	UTERINE CANCER
PREVENTION OF BREAST CANCER IN HIGH-RISK FEMALES	Severe increase in tumor or bone pain, transient thrombophlebitis, pulmonary embolism
EFFECTIVE ADJUNCTIVE TREATMENT IN ADVANCED BREAST CANCER	Abnormally high blood calcium levels
MAY INCREASE THE CHANCES OF BREAST CONSERVATION	Eye changes: corneal opacities, retinal injury
ADDITION OF TAMOXIFEN TO LUMPECTOMY AND RADIATION TREATMENT REDUCES OCCURRENCE OF INVASIVE BREAST CANCER IN WOMEN WITH DUCTAL CARCINOMA IN SITU	

▷ **Principal Uses**
As a Single Drug Product: Uses currently included in FDA-approved labeling: (1) An alternative to estrogens and androgens (male sex hormones) to treat advanced breast cancer in postmenopausal women; (2) treats advanced breast cancer in women that has spread (metastasized) from a prior site; (3) used to delay or prevent the recurrence of breast cancer in high-risk females (5-year predicted risk greater than or equal to 1.67% by the Gail

Model). Reduced breast cancer in the National Surgical Adjuvant Breast and Bowel Project (NSABP-P1) by 62% in healthy BRCA2 carriers, but did not reduce risk in healthy women 35 or older who were BRCA1 carriers; (4) approved for use in advanced metastatic breast cancer in men; (5) addition of tamoxifen to radiation therapy and surgery (may be a lumpectomy) in women with ductal carcinoma *in situ* led to a 43% decrease in invasive breast cancer in the same breast or in the opposite breast versus a dummy pill or placebo.

Other (unlabeled) generally accepted uses: (1) May have a role in treating cancer of the liver or lung; (2) used to stimulate ovulation in premenopausal women with infertility; (3) used to treat rare desmoid tumors; (4) helps prevent osteoporosis in women in whom the drug is being used to prevent the recurrence of cancer; (5) can help retroperitoneal fibrosis; (6) could have a role in treating tenderness and swelling of male breast tissue (gynecomastia) of unknown cause (idiopathic).

Author's Note: Tamoxifen reduced breast cancer rates by almost half in a very large (13,388 patients) cancer prevention study performed by the National Cancer Institute over a period of 6 years. The FDA has launched a new oncology tools website. Visit this at *www.fda.gov/ cder/cancer*. **There is a listing of cancer medicine trials on the World Wide Web at** *http://cancertrials.nci.nih.gov*. **The STAR (Study of Tamoxifen and Raloxifene) trial is underway. This is a National Cancer Institute study evaluating 19,000 women (enrollment started July 1, 1999, and the trial is now fully enrolled with women) who are at risk for breast cancer. They will be given either 20 mg per day of tamoxifen or 60 mg of raloxifene each day for 5 years. For more information, you can reach the National Cancer Institute at 1-800-422-6237. A substudy called Co-STAR will look at memory, mood, and sleep habits in those 65 or older. People who enroll receive a newsletter called** *Constellation*.

How This Drug Works: It is thought that by blocking the uptake of estradiol (estrogen), this drug removes or reduces a stimulus to breast cancer cells. It acts as a selective estrogen receptor modulator, or SERM. Newer thoughts include causing cells surrounding the cancer to release a substance called transforming growth factor-beta (TGF-beta), suppression of IGF-1, and inhibiting a protein kinase (protein kinase C) as well as calmodulin dependent cAMP phosphodiesterase.

▷ **Widely Used Guidelines That Involve This Medicine (representative sample):** Please look at the section at the very beginning of this profile called "Class." Next, turn to Table 22 and you will find guidelines listed by the class involved!

Available Dosage Forms and Strengths
Tablets — 10 mg, 20 mg
Tablets (Canada) — 15.2 mg, 30.4 mg

▷ **Usual Adult Dosage Ranges:** *Breast cancer:* 20–40 mg a day is used. If the 40 mg dose is undertaken, it is given as 20 mg twice a day. In order to get the medicine distributed (to steady state), a loading dose of 40 mg four times a day is used for one day, followed by 20 mg a day. Dosing is continued for 5 years. *Prevention of breast cancer:* At this time, both age and risk factors are used to determine the BENEFITS versus RISKS of giving the medicine. Health care professionals may obtain a *Gail Model Risk Assessment Tool by calling 1-800-544-2007. For reduction of breast cancer in high-risk women:*

20 mg daily for 5 years is given. The STAR trial is expected to provide further information. Some controversy exists regarding use of 10 mg every other day. Further study is needed.

Note: Actual dose and schedule must be determined for each patient individually.

Conditions Requiring Dosing Adjustments

Liver Function: Dose decreases are not defined in liver disease.

Kidney Function: Dose decreases are not thought to be needed in mild to moderate kidney disease. No studies are available in severe disease.

▷ **Dosing Instructions:** Best to take the tablet whole either on an empty stomach or with food. If you forget a dose: Take the missed dose as soon as you remember it, unless it's nearly time for your next dose—if that is the case, skip the missed dose and take the next dose right on schedule. DO NOT double up on doses. Talk with your doctor if you find yourself missing doses—there are effective beeper-based systems to help you remember your medicine.

Usual Duration of Use: Use on a regular schedule for 4 to 10 weeks usually determines effectiveness in controlling growth and spread of advanced breast cancer. In the presence of bone involvement, treatment for several months may be required to evaluate effectiveness. Ongoing use for prevention of breast cancer still requires careful examinations and long-term use. Ongoing use (months to years) requires physician supervision and periodic evaluation. Evaluation should continue even after the medicine is stopped as some undesirable effects may not appear until later.

Typical Treatment Goals and Measurements (Outcomes and Markers)

Breast cancer: Treatment of existing cancer seeks to attain a complete remission. The minimum goal is to shrink (regress) the size of the tumor and decrease the probability of spread. Checks of coagulation (such as clotting factor assay) can help define how activated the coagulation system has become. In breast cancer prophylaxis, the goal is to prevent breast cancer in females who carry significant risk factors for breast cancer.

▷ **This Drug Should Not Be Taken If**
- you had a serious allergic or adverse reaction to it before.
- you have active phlebitis or history of deep vein clot (thrombosis) or lung clot (pulmonary thrombosis).
- you have a significant deficiency of white blood cells or blood platelets.
- you have a ductal carcinoma in situ (DCIT—talk to your doctor) or require anticoagulant therapy and are at high risk for breast cancer.
- you are pregnant.

▷ **Inform Your Physician Before Taking This Drug If**
- you have a history of thrombophlebitis or pulmonary embolism.
- you become short of breath while taking this medicine.
- you take birth control pills.
- you have a history of abnormally high blood calcium levels.
- you have a history of any type of blood cell or bone marrow disorder.
- you have a history of breast cancer (benefit is thought to outweigh the risks, but prudent to inform your doctor).
- you have cataracts or other visual impairment.
- you have impaired liver function.
- you have high cholesterol.
- you plan to have surgery in the near future.

Possible Side Effects (natural, expected, and unavoidable drug actions)
Hot flashes—frequent.
Fluid retention, weight gain. Increased bone and/or tumor pain (flare)—tends to ease quickly.

▷ **Possible Adverse Effects** (unusual, unexpected, and infrequent reactions)
If any of the following develop, consult your physician promptly for guidance.

Mild Adverse Effects
Allergic reaction: skin rash.
Visual impairment—infrequent.
Increased calcium—infrequent.
Headache, dizziness, drowsiness, depression, fatigue, confusion—infrequent.
Nausea, vomiting—frequent.
Itching in genital area, loss of hair—infrequent.

Serious Adverse Effects
Initial "flare" of severe pain in tumor or involved bone—possible.
Development of thrombophlebitis, pulmonary embolism, heart attack, or stroke—increased risk.
Eye changes: corneal opacities, retinal injury—case reports.
Delusions—rare.
Increased uterine cancer risk (increased karyopyknotic index of vaginal epithelium)—possible, but many researchers now believe that the benefits far outweigh the risks.
Liver or other cancer (Brenner tumor)—questionable causation versus association.
Development of abnormally high blood calcium levels—possible.
Transient decreases in white blood cells and blood platelets—frequent.
Neutropenia or decrease in all blood cells (pancytopenia)—case reports.
Liver toxicity—rare.

▷ **Possible Effects on Sexual Function:** Premenopausal—altered timing and pattern of menstruation. Postmenopausal—vaginal bleeding, decreased libido (may be frequent). Breast tenderness and milk production in non-pregnant females (galactorrhea)—case report.
Abnormal and painful erections (priapism)—case reports.
This drug may be effective in treating the following conditions:
• male infertility due to abnormally low sperm counts.
• male breast enlargement and tenderness.
• chronic female breast pain (mastodynia).

Possible Effects on Laboratory Tests
Complete blood cell counts: decreased red cells, hemoglobin, white cells, and platelets.
Blood calcium level: increased.
Blood thyroid hormone levels: T3, T4, and free T4 increased.
Liver function tests: increased liver enzyme (AST/GOT), increased bilirubin (one case report).
Sperm count: increased or decreased.
Cholesterol and triglycerides: may be increased.
HDL: may be decreased.

CAUTION
1. If this drug is used prior to your menopause, it may induce ovulation and predispose you to pregnancy. Since this drug should not be used

during pregnancy, some method of contraception (other than oral contraceptives) is advised.

2. Do not take any form of estrogen while taking this drug; estrogens can inhibit tamoxifen's effectiveness.

3. Tamoxifen has been shown to cause an increased risk of uterine cancer. Women who have received or are receiving this drug should have regular gynecological examinations. Report menstrual irregularity, abnormal vaginal bleeding or vaginal discharge, and pelvic pain or pressure promptly to your doctor.

4. High-risk females in the BCPT were defined as a 5-year predicted risk greater than 1.67%. The model used (Gail Model) can be obtained by your health care professional from Zeneca by calling 1-800-345-4334 or by calling 1-800-544-2007. Even though this medicine is taken, all risk of breast cancer is NOT removed, and the usual detection and screening measures should be continued.

5. Case reports of undesirable lipid changes (increased triglycerides and cholesterol and decreased HDL) have been made. Periodic checks are prudent.

▷ **Advisability of Use During Pregnancy**
Pregnancy Category: D. See Pregnancy Risk Categories at the back of this book.
Animal Studies: No birth defects due to this drug reported.
Human Studies: Adequate studies of pregnant women are not available.
This drug can have estrogenic effects. It should not be used during pregnancy.

Advisability of Use If Breast-Feeding
Presence of this drug in breast milk: Unknown.
Avoid drug or refrain from nursing.

Habit-Forming Potential: None.

Effects of Overdose: Severe extension of the pharmacological effects.

Possible Effects of Long-Term Use: Development of abnormally high blood calcium levels.

Suggested Periodic Examinations While Taking This Drug (at physician's discretion)
Complete blood cell counts.
Measurements of blood calcium, cholesterol, and lipid levels.
Complete eye examinations if impaired vision occurs.
Liver function tests.
Women who have been given or are now receiving tamoxifen must have regular gynecological examinations.

▷ **While Taking This Drug, Observe the Following**
Foods: No restrictions.
Herbal Medicines or Minerals: Some patients use echinacea to attempt to boost their immune systems. Unfortunately, use of echinacea is not recommended in people with damaged immune systems. This herb may also actually weaken any immune system if it is used too often or for too long a time. Black cohosh estrogenic effects may have an undesirable effect on tamoxifen, and combination in not advisable. Ipriflavone blunted effectiveness of genestein (a closely related compound). Red clover extracts contain daidzein and genistein, both of which can blunt the benefits of tamoxifen on tumors. Do not take those extracts or red clover.
Beverages: No restrictions. May be taken with milk.

▷   *Alcohol:* No interactions expected.

Tobacco Smoking: No interactions expected. I advise everyone to quit smoking.

Marijuana Smoking: Animal studies show an increased suppression of the immune system; significance in humans is not known.

▷   *Other Drugs*

The following drugs may ***decrease*** the effects of tamoxifen:

- estrogens.
- oral contraceptives (those that contain estrogens).

Tamoxifen ***taken concurrently*** with

- clopidogrel (Plavix) may result in higher than expected tamoxifen levels; no reports of adverse effects from this reaction have been made, but caution is advised.
- cyclophosphamide (Cytoxan) may increase blood clot (thromboembolism) risk.
- cyclosporine (Sandimmune) may increase cyclosporine levels and cause toxicity.
- medicines that inhibit CYP2C9 (such as fluconazole, fluvastatin, and zafirlukast) may lead to increased tamoxifen levels—talk to your doctor about this.
- methotrexate (Mexate, Rheumatrex) may increase blood clot (thromboembolism) risk.
- mitomycin will cause increased risk of hemolytic uremic syndrome.
- pneumococcal and perhaps other vaccines will blunt the vaccine's immune response (benefit).
- ritonavir (Norvir) and perhaps other protease inhibitors (see Drug Classes) may lead to toxicity.
- warfarin (Coumadin) presents an increased risk of bleeding; increased frequency of INR (prothrombin time or protime) testing is needed.

▷   *Driving, Hazardous Activities:* This drug may cause dizziness or drowsiness. Restrict activities as necessary.

Aviation Note: The use of this drug ***may be a disqualification*** for piloting. Consult a designated Aviation Medical Examiner.

Exposure to Sun: No restrictions.

TAMSULOSIN (TAM su low sin)

Introduced: 1997   **Class:** Antiprostatism, alpha 1 (A) blocker   **Prescription:** USA: Yes   **Controlled Drug:** USA: No   **Available as Generic:** No

Brand Name: Flomax, Flomax SR

BENEFITS versus RISKS	
Possible Benefits	*Possible Risks*
MODEST IMPROVEMENT IN BENIGN PROSTATIC HYPERPLASIA	Headache
	Runny nose
ONCE-DAILY DOSING	Abnormal ejaculation
More selective for the genitourinary tract than other therapies	

▷ **Principal Uses**
> *As a Single Drug Product:* Uses currently included in FDA-approved labeling: Treats symptomatic benign prostatic hyperplasia (BPH).
> Other (unlabeled) generally accepted uses: (1) Appears to help swelling of the ureter (radiation induced urethritis) caused by radiation treatment of the prostate.

> **How This Drug Works:** Relaxes smooth muscle around the bladder neck and prostate (by binding to a very specific alpha 1A receptor), allowing opening of the urethra and increased urine flow.

▷ **Widely Used Guidelines That Involve This Medicine (representative sample):** Please look at the section at the very beginning of this profile called "Class." Next, turn to Table 22 and you will find guidelines listed by the class involved!

Available Dosage Forms and Strengths
> Capsules — 0.4 mg
> Sustained Release Capsules — 0.4 mg (Canada only)

▷ **Usual Adult Dosage Ranges:** Started with 0.4 mg once daily. If response is not acceptable after 2 to 4 weeks, the dose can be increased to 0.8 mg once a day.

> **Note: Actual dose and schedule must be determined for each patient individually.**

Conditions Requiring Dosing Adjustments
> *Liver Function:* No dose changes needed in moderate liver disease.
> *Kidney Function:* Dose changes not needed in those with creatinine clearance (see Glossary) as low as 10 mL/min. Not studied in more compromised kidney failure patients.

Dosing Instructions: Take this medicine half an hour after the same meal every day (helps maintain similar blood levels). It may make you drowsy. If you forget a dose: Take the missed dose as soon as you remember it, unless it is nearly time for your next dose—if that is the case, skip (omit) the missed dose and take the next scheduled dose right on schedule. DO NOT double doses. Do NOT break, chew, or crush the capsules. If you forget this medicine for several days, treatment should be resumed with the 0.4 mg dose and dose increased as previously required and scheduled.

Usual Duration of Use: Benefits may be seen very quickly with the first dose and with symptoms resolving within the first week of regular treatment. Use on a regular schedule for 14 weeks may be needed to see this drug's peak benefit.

Typical Treatment Goals and Measurements (Outcomes and Markers)
> *Benign Prostatic Hypertrophy (BPH):* Urologists use improvement in urinary flow as well as subjective measures such as relief of difficulty urinating and lowered feeling of urgency. There is a score set called the American Urological Association (AUA) symptom scores as well as the Boyarsky symptom scores. Digital rectal examination for prostate cancer should be done periodically.

Possible Advantages of This Drug: May give you symptomatic relief of benign prostatic hyperplasia (BPH) without surgery. Goes to work quickly (faster onset) than previously available medicines.

▷ **This Drug Should Not Be Taken If**
- you had an allergic reaction to it previously or if you are a woman or child.

▷ **Inform Your Physician Before Taking This Drug If**
- you have impaired liver function or liver disease.
- you have not had prostate cancer ruled out and this is a new prescription.
- you have kidney problems of any nature.
- your job requires balance and operation of hazardous machinery (this drug can cause dizziness and vertigo).

Possible Side Effects (natural, expected, and unavoidable drug actions)
Excessive lowering of blood pressure on standing (orthostatic hypotension).

▷ **Possible Adverse Effects** (unusual, unexpected, and infrequent reactions)
If any of the following develop, consult your physician promptly for guidance.

Mild Adverse Effects
Allergic reactions: skin rash, hives—rare.
Change in vision (amblyopia)—rare.
Runny nose—may be frequent.
Headache or dizziness—may be frequent.
Drowsiness—infrequent.
Back or joint pain (up to 8–11% in one trial).
Nausea or diarrhea—infrequent.
Slight decreases in red blood cell counts or hemoglobin—possible.
Increased liver function tests—rare (may normalize over time).

Serious Adverse Effects
Allergic reactions: hypersensitivity reactions—case reports.

Possible Effects on Sexual Function: Abnormal ejaculation (up to 18%) and rare cases of decreased libido have been reported. Rare priapism.

Possible Delayed Adverse Effects: Not reported.

Possible Effects on Laboratory Tests
Slight decreases in hemoglobin and red blood cells.
PSA: unchanged.
Some increased liver enzyme reports.

CAUTION
1. A digital rectal exam and other prostate cancer exams are prudent before this medicine is started. PSA will be falsely decreased by this medicine.

Precautions for Use
By Infants and Children: Safety and effectiveness for infants and children are not established.
By Those Over 60 Years of Age: No specific precautions other than changes related to decreased liver function.

▷ **Advisability of Use During Pregnancy**
Pregnancy Category: B. See Pregnancy Risk Categories at the back of this book.
Human Studies: Contraindicated in women.

Advisability of Use If Breast-Feeding
Unknown, but tamsulosin is NOT indicated for women.

Habit-Forming Potential: None.

Effects of Overdose: Extension effects of the pharmacological and adverse effects.

Possible Effects of Long-Term Use: Adverse effects of long-term use are similar to short-term use effects.

Suggested Periodic Examinations While Taking This Drug (at physician's discretion)

Patients should be checked (monitored) for signs and symptoms of orthostatic hypotension.

Patients should be monitored for improvement in symptoms of BPH.

Periodic digital rectal exams and PSA are needed.

While Taking This Drug, Observe the Following

Foods: If this medicine is taken on an empty stomach, the amount that can get into the body may be higher than if taken after a meal. While considered minor, current recommendations are to take it half an hour after the same meal daily.

Herbal Medicines or Minerals: Saw palmetto works by anti-androgenic and anti-inflammatory actions. The combination of this herb and tamsulosin has not been studied, but both drugs appear to work by different mechanisms. Talk to your doctor before combining.

Beverages: No restrictions.

▷ *Alcohol:* No restrictions.

Tobacco Smoking: No interactions expected. I advise everyone to quit smoking.

Marijuana Smoking: No interactions expected.

▷ *Other Drugs*

Tamsulosin **taken concurrently** with

- beta blockers (see Drug Classes) may increase extent of first dose orthostatic hypotension. Caution is advised.
- cimetidine (Tagamet) may increase tamsulosin blood levels and extent of first dose orthostatic hypotension as well as dizziness. Caution is advised.
- medicines that change liver enzymes in the cytochrome P450 class. The specific enzymes involved in removing tamsulosin have not been fully characterized, but combining medicines that change that liver enzyme system may have an effect on tamsulosin levels. Caution is advised.
- sildenafil (Viagra), vardenafil (Levitra), and tadalafil (Cialis) may excessively lower blood pressure and is NOT recommended.
- warfarin (Coumadin) may change the effects of tamsulosin or warfarin. More frequent checks of INR and careful patient check for unexpected adverse effects are prudent.

▷ *Driving, Hazardous Activities:* No restrictions.

Aviation Note: No restrictions.

Exposure to Sun: No restrictions.

Special Storage Instructions: Keep at room temperature. Avoid exposure to extreme humidity.

TEGASEROD (TAY gas err odd)

Introduced: 2003   **Class:** Diarrhea predominant irritable syndrome treatment, serotonin 4 (5HT 4 agonist), Antidiarrheal   **Prescription:** USA: Yes   **Controlled Drug:** USA: No   **Available as Generic:** No

Brand Name: Zelnorm

Author's Note: Information in this profile will be broadened as further data from use and comparative studies become available.

TERAZOSIN (ter AY zoh sin)

Introduced: 1987 **Class:** Antihypertensive **Prescription:**
USA: Yes **Controlled Drug:** USA: No **Available as Generic:** Yes
Brand Names: ✤Apo-Terazosin, Hytrin, Novo-Terazosin

BENEFITS versus RISKS

Possible Benefits	*Possible Risks*
EFFECTIVE TREATMENT OF MILD TO MODERATE HYPERTENSION	"First-dose" drop in blood pressure with fainting
LOWERED LOW-DENSITY LIPOPROTEINS AND TOTAL CHOLESTEROL	Fluid retention
LOWERED TRIGLYCERIDE LEVELS	
TREATS BENIGN PROSTATIC HYPERPLASIA	

**Author's Note: Data from the ALLHAT trial found that alpha blockers
such as this medicine are not drugs of first choice in high blood pressure. Information in this profile has been shortened for more widely
used medicines.**

TERBUTALINE (ter BYU ta leen)

Introduced: 1974 **Class:** Antiasthmatic, bronchodilator **Prescription:** USA: Yes **Controlled Drug:** USA: No; Canada: No
Available as Generic: Yes

Brand Names: Brethaire, Brethine, Bricanyl, ✤Bricanyl Spacer, ✤Med-
Broncodil

BENEFITS versus RISKS

Possible Benefits	*Possible Risks*
VERY EFFECTIVE RELIEF OF BRONCHOSPASM	Increased blood pressure
	Fine hand tremor
	Irregular heart rhythm (with excessive use)

▷ **Principal Uses**

As a Single Drug Product: Uses currently included in FDA-approved labeling:
Relieves acute bronchial asthma and reduces frequency and severity of
chronic, recurrent asthmatic attacks.

Other (unlabeled) generally accepted uses: (1) May have a role in helping
ease fetal distress in some patients; (2) used to help stop premature labor
and continue pregnancies to more than 36 weeks; (3) an alternative to
intravenous isoproterenol in therapy of status asthmaticus; (4) relieves
reversible bronchospasm associated with chronic bronchitis and emphysema.

How This Drug Works: Stimulates sympathetic nerve terminals dilating constricted bronchial tubes, improving the ability to breathe.

▷ **Widely Used Guidelines That Involve This Medicine (representative sample):** Please look at the section at the very beginning of this profile called "Class." Next, turn to Table 22 and you will find guidelines listed by the class involved!

Available Dosage Forms and Strengths

Aerosol (per actuation) — 0.2 mg

Aerosol (Canada) (per actuation) — 0.25 mg

Injection — 1 mg/mL

Tablets — 2.5 mg, 5 mg

▷ **Usual Adult and Children Over 12 Dosage Ranges:** *Aerosol:* 0.4 mg taken in two separate inhalations 1 minute apart; repeat every 4 to 6 hours as needed.

Tablets: 2.5 to 5 mg taken every 6 hours while the patient is awake. The total daily dose should not exceed 15 mg.

Use of the injectable IV form is no longer recommended for home intravenous use by the FDA. Some clinicians have undertaken under the skin (subcutaneous) use with a MiniMed 404-SP pump to give continuous under the skin (subcutaneous) doses of 50–100 micrograms per hour in conjunction with nursing and pharmaceutical care. This use generally goes on until the fetus is roughly 37 weeks old (e.g. for 6–8 weeks).

Note: Actual dose and schedule must be determined for each patient individually.

Conditions Requiring Dosing Adjustments

Liver Function: Extensively metabolized in the liver, but dosing guidelines in liver disease are not available.

Kidney Function: For patients with moderate to severe kidney failure, 50% of the usual dose can be taken at the usual time. In severe failure, the drug should not be used.

▷ **Dosing Instructions:** Tablets may be crushed and taken on an empty stomach or with food or milk. For aerosol, follow the written instructions carefully. Do not overuse. If you forget a dose: Use the inhaler as soon as you remember it, unless it's nearly time for your next dose—if that is the case, skip the missed dose and take the next dose right on schedule. Use the remaining doses for the day at evenly spaced dosing intervals, and then return to your usual schedule. Talk with your doctor if you find yourself missing doses. If you think your inhaler container (canister) is empty, get a bowl of cold water and place the canister in it—if the canister floats, there is no medicine left in it. If your doctor has prescribed this in order to keep you from delivering your infant too early, screening for glucose intolerance should be checked on at least one occasion after a week of treatment has been taken.

Usual Duration of Use: Individualized. Do not use beyond the time necessary to stop (terminate) episodes of asthma. Unlabeled use as a tocolytic in preterm labor often continues until 37 weeks of pregnancy.

Typical Treatment Goals and Measurements (Outcomes and Markers)

Asthma: Signs and symptoms of asthma such as difficulty breathing (dyspnea), cough, light-headedness, and wheezing should lessen. Forced expiratory volume at one second (FEV1) and/or peak expiratory flow rate (PEF) are checked by most pulmonologists as indicators of successful treatment. If the usual benefit is not realized after the time to peak effect (see above) was expected, call your doctor.

Possible Advantages of This Drug: Rapid onset of action. Long duration of action. Highly effective relief of asthma.

▷ **This Drug Should Not Be Taken If**
- you had an allergic reaction to any form of it previously.
- you currently have an irregular heart rhythm.
- you took a monoamine oxidase (MAO) type A inhibitor (see Drug Classes) in the last 14 days.

▷ **Inform Your Physician Before Taking This Drug If**
- you are overly sensitive to other drugs that stimulate the sympathetic nervous system.
- you are currently using epinephrine (Adrenalin, Primatene Mist, etc.) to relieve asthmatic breathing.
- you have a seizure disorder.
- you have liver or kidney failure.
- you have any type of heart or circulatory disorder, especially high blood pressure or coronary heart disease.
- you have diabetes or an overactive thyroid gland (hyperthyroidism).
- you are taking any form of digitalis or any stimulant drug.

Possible Side Effects (natural, expected, and unavoidable drug actions)
Aerosol—dryness or irritation of mouth or throat, altered taste. Tablet—nervousness, tremor, palpitation.

▷ **Possible Adverse Effects** (unusual, unexpected, and infrequent reactions)
If any of the following develop, consult your physician promptly for guidance.
Mild Adverse Effects
Allergic reaction: skin rashes.
Headache, dizziness, drowsiness, restlessness, insomnia—infrequent.
Rapid, pounding heartbeat; increased sweating; muscle cramps in arms and legs—infrequent to frequent.
Nausea, heartburn, vomiting—rare with oral form, frequent with IV.
Increased blood sugar—frequent (40% abnormal one-hour glucose).
Increased plasma insulin levels—possible.
Serious Adverse Effects
Rapid or irregular heart rhythm, intensification of angina, increased blood pressure—infrequent.
Chest pain with heartbeat changes (ST depression)—reported when oral and intravenous therapy is combined in preterm labor.
Lowered blood calcium or potassium (especially with intravenous use)—possible.
Liver toxicity—case reports.
Severe lowering of blood pressure (hypotension)—case reports.
Increased blood sugar—infrequent.
Ketoacidosis—case reports.
Fluid around the lungs (pulmonary edema)—case reports.

▷ **Possible Effects on Sexual Function:** None reported.

Natural Diseases or Disorders That May Be Activated by This Drug
Latent coronary artery disease, diabetes, or high blood pressure.

Possible Effects on Laboratory Tests
Blood total cholesterol and LDL cholesterol levels: no effect.

Blood HDL cholesterol level: increased.
Blood triglyceride levels: no effect.
Calcium may decrease.
Blood thyroid hormone levels: T3 increased; T4 decreased; free T4 no effect.
Glucose tolerance test: abnormal test.
Liver function tests: may be elevated.

CAUTION

1. Combination of this drug by aerosol with beclomethasone aerosol (Beclovent, Vanceril) may increase risk of fluorocarbon propellant (being phased out) toxicity. Best to use this aerosol 20 to 30 minutes before beclomethasone aerosol. This reduces toxicity risk and will help beclomethasone get into the lungs.
2. **Avoid excessive use of aerosol inhalation.** Excessive or prolonged inhalation use can reduce effectiveness and cause serious heart rhythm disturbances, including cardiac arrest.
3. Do not use this drug with epinephrine. These two drugs may be used alternately, allowing 4 hours between doses. Combined use with other medicines that have similar action also should be avoided (such as albuterol, pirbuterol, or salmeterol).
4. If you do not respond to your usually effective dose, ask your doctor for help. Do not increase the size or frequency of the dose without your physician's approval.

Precautions for Use

By Infants and Children: Manufacturer DOES NOT recommend use in those under 12 years of age.

By Those Over 60 Years of Age: Avoid excessive and continual use. If acute asthma is not relieved promptly, other drugs will be needed. Watch for nervousness, palpitations, irregular heart rhythm, and muscle tremors. Use with extreme caution if you have hardening of the arteries, heart disease, or high blood pressure.

▷ Advisability of Use During Pregnancy

Pregnancy Category: B. See Pregnancy Risk Categories at the back of this book.
Animal Studies: No significant birth defects reported in mouse and rat studies.
Human Studies: Adequate studies of pregnant women are not available.
Use only if clearly needed. Ask your physician for guidance.

Advisability of Use If Breast-Feeding

Presence of this drug in breast milk: Yes (a small amount of roughly 0.2% of the mom's dose).
Monitor nursing infant closely, and discontinue drug or nursing if adverse effects develop.

Habit-Forming Potential: None.

Effects of Overdose: Nervousness, palpitation, rapid heart rate, sweating, headache, tremor, vomiting, chest pain.

Possible Effects of Long-Term Use: Loss of effectiveness. See *CAUTION* for this drug.

Suggested Periodic Examinations While Taking This Drug (at physician's discretion)

Blood pressure measurements.
Evaluation of heart status.

▷ While Taking This Drug, Observe the Following

Foods: No restrictions.

Herbal Medicines or Minerals: Using St. John's wort, ma huang (no longer available for weight loss in the U.S.), bitter orange, country mallow, ephedrine-like compounds, mate, or kola while taking this medicine may result in unacceptable central nervous system stimulation. Fir or pine needle oil should NOT be used by asthmatics. Ephedra alone does carry a German Commission E monograph indication for asthma treatment. If you are allergic to plants in the Asteraceae family (aster, chrysanthemum, daisy, or ragweed), you may also be allergic to echinacea, chamomile, feverfew, and St. John's wort. Since part of the way ginkgo and ginseng work may be as MAO inhibitors, do not combine them with terbutaline.

Beverages: Avoid excessive use of caffeine-containing beverages: coffee, tea, mate, guarana, cola, and chocolate.

▷ *Alcohol:* No interactions expected.

Tobacco Smoking: No interactions expected. I advise everyone to quit smoking.

▷ *Other Drugs*

Terbutaline *taken concurrently* with
- monoamine oxidase (MAO) type A inhibitors may cause excessive increase in blood pressure and undesirable heart stimulation (see Drug Classes).
- succinylcholine (Anectine) may lead to increased neuromuscular blockade that may require neostigmine.
- theophylline (Theo-Dur, others) may cause decreased theophylline effectiveness.

The following drugs may *decrease* the effects of terbutaline:
- beta blockers (see Drug Classes)—may impair terbutaline's effectiveness.

▷ *Driving, Hazardous Activities:* Usually no restrictions. Use caution if excessive nervousness or dizziness occurs.

Aviation Note: The use of this drug *is a disqualification* for piloting. Consult a designated Aviation Medical Examiner.

Exposure to Sun: No restrictions.

Heavy Exercise or Exertion: Use caution—excessive exercise can induce asthma in some patients.

TERIPARATIDE (Ter ih PAIR a tyde)

Other Names: PTH, human PTH 1-34, hPTH 1-34, parathyroid hormone, PTH 1-34

Introduced: 2003   **Class:**   hormone, parathyroid   **Prescription:** USA: Yes   **Controlled Drug:**   USA: No; Canada: No   **Available as Generic:**   USA: No; Canada: No

Brand Name: Forteo

Author's Note: This medicine is the first prescription medicine used to treat osteoporosis that works by increasing bone formation (osteoblast action). Information in this profile will be broadened once more data and outcomes research are available.

TESTOSTERONE (Tes TOS tur own)

Other Names: Chlorotrianisene, conjugated estrogens, esterified estrogens, estradiol, estriol, estrone, estropipate, quinestrol

Introduced: 2000 (Gel)   **Class:**   Male sex hormone   **Prescription:**
USA: Yes   **Controlled Drug:**   USA: No; Canada: No   **Available as**
Generic: USA: No; Canada: No
Brand Names: AndroGel 1%, Andriol, Androderm, Testoderm

Author's Note: Information in this profile will be broadened once more data
and outcomes are available. A testosterone patch (see The Leading Edge,
next section) is being studied for increasing sex drive in women.

TETRACYCLINE ANTIBIOTIC FAMILY (te trah SI kleen)

Other Names: Doxycycline, tetracycline
Introduced: 1953, 1967   **Class:**   Antibiotic, tetracyclines   **Prescrip-**
tion: USA: Yes   **Controlled Drug:**   USA: No; Canada: No   **Available**
as Generic: Yes
Brand Names: Doxycycline: Adoxia, ✤Apo-Doxy, ✤Apo-Doxy-Tabs, Atridox
    (gum line delivery form), ✤Doryx, Doryx, Doxy Caps, Doxychel,
    ✤Doxycin, Doxy-Lemmon, Doxy 100, Doxy Tabs, Doxy 200, Monodox,
    ✤Novo-Doxylin, Periostat, Vibramycin, Vibra-Tabs, ✤Vibra-Tabs C-Pak,
    Tetracycline: Achromycin, Achromycin Ophthalmic, Achromycin V,
    ✤Acrocidin, Actisite, ✤Apo-Tetra, Aureomycin, Bristacycline, Contimycin,
    Cyclinex, Cyclopar, Lemtrex, ✤Medicycline, Mysteclin-F [CD], ✤Neo-
    Tetrine, ✤Nor-Tet, ✤Novo-Tetra, ✤Nu-Tetra, Panmycin, Retet, Robitet,
    SK-Tetracycline, Sumycin, Teline, Tetra-C, Tetracap, Tetra-Con, Tetracyn,
    Tetralan, Tetram, Tetrex-F, Tropicycline

BENEFITS versus RISKS

Possible Benefits	*Possible Risks*
EFFECTIVE TREATMENT OF INFECTIONS DUE TO SUSCEPTIBLE BACTERIA AND PROTOZOA	ALLERGIC REACTIONS, MILD TO SEVERE: ANAPHYLAXIS, DRUG-INDUCED HEPATITIS Drug-induced colitis Superinfections (bacterial or fungal) Blood cell disorders: hemolytic anemia, abnormally low white cell and platelet counts Kidney toxicity

---

▷ **Principal Uses**
    As a Single Drug Product: Uses currently included in FDA-approved labeling:
        (1) Treats a broad range of infections caused by susceptible bacteria and
        protozoa (short-term use); (2) treats severe, resistant pustular acne (long-
        term use) (tetracycline); (3) used in a sustained-release form (Actisite) to
        treat gum disease (periodontitis) in adults (tetracycline) and a doxycycline
        form (Periostat) and Atridox gel are used to treat gum disease (periodonti-
        tis); (4) doxycycline treats gonorrhea and syphilis in penicillin-allergic peo-
        ple; (5) helpful in acne; (6) helps prevent malaria in travelers; (7)
        tetracycline is the drug of choice for cholera; (8) doxycycline treats anthrax
        (including postexposure use), brucellosis, cholera, and plague.

Other (unlabeled) generally accepted uses: (1) Combination antibiotic treatment of duodenal ulcers caused by *Helicobacter pylori;* (2) used in vaginal and vulval cysts (Gartner's) and in vaginal hydrocele; (3) topical tetracycline is useful in chronic eye problems (blepharitis); (4) treats cancer (malignant) fluid (pericardial effusion) buildup around the heart; (5) has a role in acne rosacea in decreasing the number of papules or nodules; (7) doxycycline: (a) treats early (stage one) Lyme disease (one study found that 87% of people who took doxycycline within 72 hours of a tick bite DID NOT develop Lyme disease); (b) treats sexual assault victims; (c) treats prostatitis; (d) can help in some cases of PMS; (e) may treat some cases of male infertility of unexplained origin; (f) helps treat rheumatoid arthritis.

As a Combination Drug Product [CD]: Tetracycline is available combined with amphotericin B, an antifungal antibiotic that is provided to reduce the risk of developing an overgrowth of yeast organisms (superinfection) of the gastrointestinal tract.

How These Drugs Work: Prevent growth and multiplication of susceptible organisms by interfering with formation of essential proteins. Periostat seems to work by its anticolligenase and anti-inflammatory properties.

▷ **Widely Used Guidelines That Involve This Medicine (representative sample):** Please look at the section at the very beginning of this profile called "Class." Next, turn to Table 22 and you will find guidelines listed by the class involved!

Available Dosage Forms and Strengths

Doxycycline:

Capsules — 50 mg, 75 mg, 100 mg
Capsules, coated pellets — 100 mg
Capsule, delayed release — 100 mg
Gel — 10 mg
Injection (per vial) — 100 mg, 200 mg
Oral suspension — 25 mg/5 mL
Syrup — 50 mg/5 mL
Tablets — 50 mg, 100 mg

Tetracycline:

Capsules — 100 mg, 250 mg, 500 mg
Ointment — 3%
Ointment, ophthalmic — 10 mg/g
Periodontal fiber (per fiber) — 12.7 mg
Solution, topical — 2.2 mg/mL
Suspension, ophthalmic — 10 mg/mL
Suspension, oral — 125 mg/5 mL
Tablets — 250 mg, 500 mg

▷ **Usual Adult Dosage Ranges:**

Doxycycline: General infections from susceptible organisms: 100 mg every 12 hours the first day and then 100 mg once daily. Some severe infections may require ongoing therapy of 100 mg every 12 hours. *Anthrax:* 100 mg twice a day for 60 days (started in combination with one or two additional antibiotics intravenously and then switched to oral treatment when your doctor feels this is appropriate). Total daily dose should not exceed 300 mg.

Tetracycline: 250 to 500 mg every 6 hours, or 500 to 1,000 mg every 12 hours. The total daily dose should not exceed 4,000 mg (4 g).

Note: Actual dose and schedule must be determined for each patient individually.

Typical Treatment Goals and Measurements (Outcomes and Markers)

Infections: The most commonly used measures of serious infections are white blood cell counts and differentials (the kind of blood cells that occur most often in your blood), and temperature. Many clinicians look for positive changes in 24–48 hours. NEVER stop an antibiotic because you start to feel better. For many infections, a full 14 days is REQUIRED to kill the bacteria. Inhalational anthrax treatment continues for 60 days. The goals and time frame (see peak benefits above) should be discussed with you when the prescription is written.

Conditions Requiring Dosing Adjustments

Liver Function: Doxycycline: Patients with both liver and kidney compromise should have the dose decreased. Drug can cause liver problems, and a benefit-to-risk decision should be made for people with liver disease.

Tetracycline: Is a possible cause of hepatoxicity. A benefit-to-risk decision should be made for patients with compromised livers to use this drug. Daily maximum in liver disease is 1 g.

Kidney Function: Patients with mild to moderate kidney failure can take the usual dose every 8 to 12 hours. Patients with moderate to severe kidney failure take the usual dose every 12 to 24 hours. In severe kidney failure (creatinine clearance less than 10 mL/min), tetracycline should be avoided.

Malnutrition: Doxycycline: Lower than expected levels may occur in patients with malnutrition. If clinical progress is not as expected, the dose may need to be increased.

▷ **Dosing Instructions:** Immediate release forms may be crushed and the capsule opened and preferably taken on an empty stomach, 1 hour before or 2 hours after eating. However, to reduce stomach irritation, it may be taken with crackers that contain insignificant amounts of iron, calcium, magnesium, or zinc. Avoid all dairy products for 2 hours before and after taking this drug. (Unlike other tetracyclines, doxycycline absorption is not significantly changed by food or milk.) Sustained release or delayed release forms should NOT be crushed, chewed, or altered. Suspension forms should be shaken well before being taken and should be dosed using a calibrated dosing spoon or a dosing cup. Take at the same time each day, with a full glass of water. Take the full course prescribed. If you forget a dose: Take the missed dose as soon as you remember it, unless it's nearly time for your next dose—if that is the case, skip the missed dose and take the next dose right on schedule. DO NOT double up on doses. Taking your medicine exactly as prescribed will get the best results. Talk with your doctor if you find yourself missing doses.

Usual Duration of Use: The time required to control the acute infection and be free of fever and symptoms is 48 hours. This varies with the nature of the infection. Long-term use (months to years, as for treatment of acne) requires supervision and periodic evaluation. Treatment of stage one Lyme disease requires 3 to 4 weeks in adults even though one doxycycline dose may prevent a high percentage of Lyme infections.

Possible Advantages of These Drugs

Twice-a-day treatment for 7 days for chlamydia trachomatis. Provides coverage for many bioterror agents.

▷ **These Drugs Should Not Be Taken If**

- you are allergic to any tetracycline (see Drug Classes).
- you are pregnant or breast-feeding.
- you have severe liver disease.

▷ **Inform Your Physician Before Taking This Drug If**
- it is prescribed for a child under 8 years of age.
- you have a history of liver or kidney disease.
- you have systemic lupus erythematosus.
- you are taking any penicillin drug.
- you are taking any anticoagulant drug.
- you will have surgery with general anesthesia.

Possible Side Effects (natural, expected, and unavoidable drug actions)

Superinfections (see Glossary), often due to yeast organisms—these can occur in the mouth, intestinal tract, rectum, and/or vagina, resulting in rectal and vaginal itching. Tooth discoloration (when used in children less than 8 years old). Metallic taste in your mouth.

▷ **Possible Adverse Effects** (unusual, unexpected, and infrequent reactions)

If any of the following develop, consult your physician promptly for guidance.

Mild Adverse Effects

Allergic reactions: skin rash, hives, itching of hands and feet, swelling of face or extremities.

Loss of appetite, stomach irritation, taste disorders, nausea, vomiting, diarrhea—infrequent.

Warts—very rare and of questionable causality (tetracycline).

Irritation of mouth or tongue, black tongue, sore throat, abdominal cramping or pain—infrequent.

Serious Adverse Effects

Allergic reactions: anaphylactic reaction (see Glossary), asthma, fever, swollen joints and lymph glands.

Serious skin problems (Stevens-Johnson syndrome, Jarisch-Herxheimer reaction)—case reports.

Drug-induced hepatitis with jaundice—case reports.

Permanent discoloration and/or malformation of teeth if taken by children under 8, including unborn child and infant.

Drug-induced colitis, myasthenia gravis, or pancreatitis—case reports.

Worsening of existing systemic lupus erythematosus—case reports.

Rare blood cell disorders: hemolytic anemia (see Glossary); abnormally low white blood cell count, causing fever and infections; abnormally low blood platelet count—case reports.

Impairment of blood clotting—case reports.

Increased intracranial pressure (pseudotumor cerebri) or kidney problems—rare (tetracycline).

Drug-induced porphyria, esophageal ulcers, or low blood potassium—case reports (tetracycline).

▷ **Possible Effects on Sexual Function:** Decreased effectiveness of oral contraceptives taken concurrently (several case reports of pregnancy). Decreased male fertility—case reports (tetracycline).

▷ **Adverse Effects That May Mimic Natural Diseases or Disorders**

Drug-induced hepatitis may suggest viral hepatitis.

Natural Diseases or Disorders That May Be Activated by This Drug

Systemic lupus erythematosus.

Possible Effects on Laboratory Tests

Complete blood cell counts: decreased red cells, hemoglobin, white cells, and platelets; increased eosinophils (allergic reaction).

Blood lupus erythematosus (LE) cells: positive.

Blood amylase level: increased (toxic effect in pregnant women).

Liver function tests: increased enzymes (ALT/GPT, AST/GOT, alkaline phosphatase) or bilirubin.

Kidney function tests: increased blood creatinine and urea nitrogen (BUN) levels (kidney damage).

Urine sugar tests: false-positive results with Benedict's solution and Clinitest.

CAUTION

1. Antacids, dairy products, and preparations containing aluminum, bismuth, calcium, iron, magnesium, or zinc can prevent adequate absorption and reduce effectiveness significantly.
2. Troublesome and persistent diarrhea can occur. If diarrhea persists for more than 24 hours, call your doctor.
3. If general anesthesia is required while taking this drug, the choice of anesthetic agent must be selected carefully to prevent kidney damage.
4. Periostat form can still lead to vaginal or oral yeast (candida) infections.

Precautions for Use

By Infants and Children: If possible, tetracyclines should not be given to children under 8 years of age because of the risk of permanent discoloration and deformity of the teeth. Rarely, infants may develop increased intracranial pressure within the first 4 days of receiving this drug. Tetracyclines may inhibit normal bone growth and development.

By Those Over 60 Years of Age: Dose must be carefully individualized based on kidney function. Natural skin changes may predispose to severe and prolonged itching reactions in the genital and anal regions.

▷ **Advisability of Use During Pregnancy**

Pregnancy Category: D. See Pregnancy Risk Categories at the back of this book.

Animal Studies: Tetracycline causes limb defects in rats, rabbits, and chickens.

Human Studies: Information from studies of pregnant women indicates that this drug can cause impaired development and discoloration of teeth and other developmental defects.

It is advisable to avoid these drugs completely during entire pregnancy.

Advisability of Use If Breast-Feeding

Presence of these drugs in breast milk: Yes.

Avoid drug or refrain from nursing.

Habit-Forming Potential: None.

Effects of Overdose: Stomach burning, nausea, vomiting, diarrhea.

Possible Effects of Long-Term Use: Superinfections; impairment of bone marrow, liver or kidney function—rare.

Suggested Periodic Examinations While Taking This Drug (at physician's discretion)

Complete blood cell counts.

Liver and kidney function tests.

During extended use, sputum and stool examinations may detect early superinfection due to yeast organisms.

▷ **While Taking This Drug, Observe the Following**

Foods: Avoid cheeses, yogurt, ice cream, iron-fortified cereals and supplements, and meats for 2 hours before and after taking this drug.

Herbal Medicines or Minerals: Some patients use echinacea to attempt to boost their immune systems. Use of echinacea is not recommended in people with damaged immune systems. This herb may also actually weaken any immune system if it is used too often or for too long a time. No data exist for combination use with tetracyclines. Mistletoe has been used in similar fashion and there are also NO DATA for combining it with tetracyclines. Calcium, zinc, and iron can combine with these drugs and reduce absorption significantly. St. John's wort and this medicine can intensify reactions to the sun—extreme caution is advised.

Beverages: Avoid all forms of milk for 2 hours before and after taking.

▷ *Alcohol:* Reduces doxycycline blood levels. Alcohol should be avoided with doxycycline and perhaps another tetracycline substituted, particularly for those who have drinking problems. Alcohol is also best avoided if you have active liver disease.

Tobacco Smoking: No interactions expected. I advise everyone to quit smoking.

▷ *Other Drugs*

Tetracyclines may ***increase*** the effects of
- cyclosporine (Sandimmune, Neoral).
- digoxin (Lanoxin) and cause digitalis toxicity.
- lithium (Eskalith, Lithane, etc.) and increase the risk of lithium toxicity.
- oral anticoagulants such as warfarin (Coumadin) and make it necessary to reduce their dose; increased INR (prothrombin time or protime) testing is needed.

Tetracyclines may ***decrease*** the effects of
- birth control pills (oral contraceptives) and impair their effectiveness in preventing pregnancy.
- penicillins (see Drug Classes) and impair their effectiveness in treating infections.

Tetracyclines ***taken concurrently*** with
- furosemide (Lasix) increases blood urea nitrogen (BUN).
- isotretinoin (Accutane) may worsen tetracycline-caused increased intracranial pressure and cause additive toxicity.
- methoxyflurane anesthesia may impair kidney function.
- theophylline (Theo-Dur) may result in variable changes in drug levels; more frequent theophylline blood levels are needed if these medicines are to be combined.
- warfarin (Coumadin) poses an increased risk of bleeding; INR (prothrombin time or protime) testing should be checked more frequently and doses adjusted if needed.

The following drugs may ***decrease*** the effects of tetracyclines:
- antacids (aluminum or magnesium preparations, sodium bicarbonate, etc.)—may reduce drug absorption.
- bismuth subsalicylate (Pepto-Bismol, others).
- calcium supplements (various brands).
- carbamazepine (Tegretol).
- cholestyramine (Questran) and other cholesterol-lowering resins.
- colestipol (Colestid) and perhaps colesevelam (Welchol).
- iron, zinc, magnesium, and mineral preparations—may reduce drug absorption.
- phenobarbital.
- phenytoin (Dilantin) or fosphenytoin (Cerebyx).
- quinapril (Accupril).
- rifampin (Rifadin, others).
- sucralfate (Carafate).
- zinc salts.

▷   *Driving, Hazardous Activities:* Usually no restrictions. However, this drug may
      cause nausea or diarrhea. Restrict activities as necessary.
      Aviation Note: The use of these drugs *may be a disqualification* for piloting.
      Consult a designated Aviation Medical Examiner.
      Exposure to Sun: Use caution—some tetracyclines can cause photosensitivity
      (see Glossary).

THEOPHYLLINE (thee AHF ah lin)

Introduced: 1900   **Class:**   Antiasthmatic, bronchodilator, xanthines
Prescription: USA: Yes   **Controlled Drug:**   USA: No; Canada: No
Available as Generic: Yes

Brand Names: Accurbron, ✦Acet-Am, A.E.A., Aerolate, Aminodrox-Forte,
✦Apo-Oxtriphylline, ✦Aquaphyllim, ✦Asbron [CD], Asmalix, Azpan, Bro-
comar [CD], Bronchial Gelatin Capsule, Broncomar [CD], Bronkaid
Tablets [CD], Bronkodyl, Bronkolixir [CD], Bronkotabs, Bronkotabs [CD],
Constant-T, Duraphyl, Elixicon, Elixomin, Elixophyllin, For-Az-Ma [CD],
Isuprel Compound [CD], Labid, Lanophyllin, Lixolin, Lodrane, Lodrane
CR, Marax [CD], Marax DF [CD], Mudrane GG Elixir [CD], Phedral [CD],
Phyllocontin, Physpan, ✦PMS Theophylline, Primatene, ✦Pulmophylline,
Quadrinal [CD], Quibron [CD], Quibron Plus [CD], Quibron-T Dividose,
Quibron-300 [CD], Quibron-T/SR, Respbid, Slo-Bid, Slo-Bid Gyrocaps,
Slo-Phyllin, Slo-Phyllin GG [CD], Slo-Phyllin Gyrocaps, Somophyllin,
Somophyllin-12, Sustaire, Tedral [CD], Tedral SA [CD], T.E.H. [CD], T.E.P.,
Thalfed, Theobid Duracaps, ✦Theo-Bronc, Theochron, Theoclear, Theo-
clear L.A., Theocord, Theo-Dur, Theo-Dur Sprinkle, Theolair, Theolair-SR,
Theolate [CD], Theolixir, Theomar [CD], Theomax DF, Theon, Theophyl-
SR, Theospan-SR, Theo-SR, Theo-Time, Theo-24, Theovent, Theox,
Theozine, Therex [CD], Uni-Dur, ✦Uniphyl, Vitaphen [CD]

BENEFITS versus RISKS

Possible Benefits	*Possible Risks*
EFFECTIVE PREVENTION AND RELIEF OF ACUTE BRONCHIAL ASTHMA	NARROW TREATMENT RANGE FREQUENT STOMACH DISTRESS
MODERATELY EFFECTIVE CONTROL OF CHRONIC, RECURRENT BRONCHIAL ASTHMA	Gastrointestinal bleeding Central nervous system toxicity, seizures
Moderately effective symptomatic relief in chronic bronchitis and emphysema	Heart rhythm disturbances

---

▷ **Principal Uses**

   As a Single Drug Product: Uses currently included in FDA-approved labeling:
      (1) Used to relieve shortness of breath and wheezing of acute bronchial
      asthma and to prevent the recurrence of asthmatic episodes; (2) useful in
      relieving asthmalike symptoms associated with some types of chronic
      bronchitis, chronic obstructive pulmonary disease, and emphysema.

Other (unlabeled) generally accepted uses: (1) May have a role in combination therapy of cystic fibrosis; (2) can help decrease excessive production of red blood cells in kidney transplant patients; (3) may have a role in helping decrease the risk of sudden infant death syndrome (SIDS); (4) may have a supportive role with steroids and other agents in helping prevent rejection of transplanted kidneys; (5) can help ease essential tremor; (6) decreases risk of breathing cessation in neonatal apnea; (7) helps in treating SIDS children; (8) may have a role in treating sleep apnea; (9) one small study found it effective in stopping ACE inhibitor (see Drug Classes) cough.

As a Combination Drug Product [CD]: Available combined with several other drugs that manage bronchial asthma and related conditions. Ephedrine is added to enhance opening of the bronchi (bronchodilation), guaifenesin is added to thin mucus in the bronchial tubes (an expectorant effect), and mild sedatives such as phenobarbital are added to allay anxiety often seen in acute attacks of asthma.

How This Drug Works: By inhibiting the enzyme phosphodiesterase, this drug produces an increase in the tissue chemical cyclic AMP. This causes relaxation of the muscles in the bronchial tubes and blood vessels of the lung, resulting in relief of bronchospasm, expanded lung capacity, and improved lung circulation.

▷ **Widely Used Guidelines That Involve This Medicine (representative sample):** Please look at the section at the very beginning of this profile called "Class." Next, turn to Table 22 and you will find guidelines listed by the class involved!

Available Dosage Forms and Strengths
Capsules — 100 mg, 200 mg, 250 mg, 260 mg
Capsules, prolonged action — 50 mg, 60 mg, 65 mg, 75 mg, 100 mg, 125 mg, 130 mg, 200 mg, 250 mg, 260 mg, 300 mg
Elixir — 27 mg/5 mL, 50 mg/5 mL
Oral solution — 27 mg/5 mL, 53.3 mg/5 mL
Oral suspension — 100 mg/5 mL
Syrup — 27 mg/5 mL, 50 mg/5 mL
Tablets — 100 mg, 125 mg, 200 mg, 250 mg, 300 mg
Tablets, prolonged action — 50 mg, 60 mg, 65 mg, 75 mg, 100 mg, 125 mg, 130 mg, 200 mg, 225 mg, 250 mg, 260 mg, 300 mg, 350 mg, 400 mg, 450 mg, 500 mg, 600 mg

▷ **Recommended Dosage Ranges** (Actual dose and schedule must be determined for each patient individually.)

Infants and Children: Sudden asthma attack (an inhaled beta-2 agonist is the drug of choice to manage these acute symptoms, but for those not currently taking theophylline or having a dose in 12–24 hours) loading dose of the immediate release form dosed as 5 milligram per kilogram (mg/kg) of body mass. For acute attack (while currently taking theophylline) a theophylline lab level should be checked, and then one milligram per kilogram of body weight is given for each 2 microgram/milliliter increase in blood level that the clinician is seeking. Blood levels of theophylline should be checked after such dosing adjustments.

For ongoing use during acute attack, dose is based on age: After the loading dose is given, the ongoing dose is calculated based on age and body weight. For example, for those 1–9 years of age—4 mg per kg of body mass, every 6 hours. For those 9 to less than 16 years of age—3 mg per kg of body mass, every 6 hours when the Slo-Phyllin syrup or tablets are used.

For ongoing use to prevent asthma—dose is based on age: Once slow dosing increase is accomplished, daily doses are adjusted to reach blood levels of 10 to 15 mcg/mL.

16 to 60 Years of Age:

For acute attack of asthma (not currently taking theophylline): (an inhaled beta-2 agonist is the drug of choice): When the decision is made to add on theophylline (and no theophylline was given in the last 12–24 hours): Loading dose of 5 mg per kg of body mass. For acute attack while currently taking theophylline—a serum theophylline level should be checked, then one milligram per kilogram of body weight is given for each two microgram/milliliter increase in blood level that the clinician wants to achieve. Follow-up blood levels of theophylline should then be checked.

For maintenance during acute attack: For nonsmokers: 3 mg per kg of body mass, every 8 hours; for smokers: a loading dose as described above then 3 mg per kg of body mass, every 6 hours.

For chronic treatment to prevent recurrence of asthma: The goal is to obtain a usually therapeutic blood level of 10–20 mcg/mL. Dosing is started at 10 mg/kg/day, up to a maximum of 300 mg daily. If this dose is tolerated, a blood level should be checked in three days. Another increase as needed and tolerated by a step up to 13mg/kg per day up to a maximum of 450 mg/day (roughly 25%). Further incremental steps guided by patient tolerance and blood levels can be undertaken. The total daily calculated dose can be given every 12 hours using the Slo-bid or Theolair-SR forms. If patient response happens with a lower level, the patient response should be used as the guide. "Treat the patient, not the level."

For once daily dosing: The Slo-bid Gyrocap form may work in adult nonsmokers when they are given once a day. The strategy here is usually to establish a therapeutic blood level using the twice-daily approach, and then using that effective dose. The once-a-day dose is then twice the two-times-a-day dose. This current once-daily dose is started 12 hours after the last twice-a-day dose. Blood levels should be checked as the peak and trough levels may be higher or lower than with the twice-a-day approach. If problems consistent with toxicity happen, the patient should be returned to the twice-a-day dosing strategy.

Over 60 Years of Age: Theophylline is removed roughly 30% more slowly than in younger patients. Decreased doses and more frequent blood levels are prudent. For example: people in this population or those with cor pulmonale are given 2 mg/kg every eight hours, guided by blood levels.

Conditions Requiring Dosing Adjustments

Liver Function: The dose must be lowered and blood levels obtained frequently. Doses may need to be decreased by 50% in some cases.

Kidney Function: Lower doses and more frequent blood levels are indicated.

▷ **Dosing Instructions:** May be taken with or following food to reduce stomach irritation. The regular capsules may be opened, and the regular tablets may be crushed. The prolonged-action forms should be swallowed whole and not altered or chewed. Shake the oral suspension well before measuring each dose (using a dose cup or calibrated measuring spoon). Do not refrigerate liquid dose forms. Blood levels are critical for this medicine. If theophylline has been taken previously, a blood level is often checked and then clinicians use 1 mg/kg for each 2 mcg/mL increase in blood level that is wanted. If you forget a dose: Take the missed dose as soon as you remember it, unless it's nearly time for your next dose—if that is the case, skip the missed dose and take the next dose right on schedule. JUST THE RIGHT BLOOD LEVEL is very important for this medicine. DO NOT double up doses. Talk with your doctor and pharmacist if you find yourself forgetting this drug. Timers, phone call services, and beeper-based reminder services can be very helpful.

Usual Duration of Use: Use on a regular schedule for 48 to 72 hours usually determines effectiveness in controlling the breathing impairment associated with bronchial asthma and chronic lung disease. Long-term use requires supervision and periodic physician evaluation.

Typical Treatment Goals and Measurements (Outcomes and Markers)
Asthma: Signs and symptoms of asthma such as difficulty breathing (dyspnea), cough, light-headedness, and wheezing should lessen. Exercise ability should increase. Forced expiratory volume at one second (FEV1) and/or peak expiratory flow rate (PEF) are checked by most lung doctors (pulmonologists) as indicators of successful treatment. Blood levels are used to guide dosing (10–20 mcg/mL). If the usual benefit is not realized, or if symptoms improve and then worsen, call your doctor.

▷ **This Drug Should Not Be Taken If**
- you have had an allergic reaction to it or to aminophylline, dyphylline, or oxtriphylline.
- you have active peptic ulcer disease.
- you have an uncontrolled seizure disorder.
- you had a blood level drawn and it is in the "toxic" range.

▷ **Inform Your Physician Before Taking This Drug If**
- you have had an unfavorable reaction to any related medicine (xanthine; see Drug Classes).
- you have a seizure disorder of any kind.
- you have a history of peptic ulcer disease.
- you have a history of underactive thyroid (hypothyroidism).
- you have impaired liver (may lower blood proteins and lead to toxicity with "normal" levels) or impaired kidney function.
- you take any of the drugs listed in the Other Drugs section below.
- you have hypertension, heart disease, or any type of heart rhythm disorder.

Possible Side Effects (natural, expected, and unavoidable drug actions)
Nervousness, insomnia, rapid heart rate, increased urine volume (caffeine-like effects).

▷ **Possible Adverse Effects** (unusual, unexpected, and infrequent reactions)
If any of the following develop, consult your physician promptly for guidance.
Mild Adverse Effects
Allergic reactions: skin rash, hives.
Headache, dizziness, irritability, tremor, fatigue, weakness—infrequent.
Loss of appetite, nausea, vomiting (may be an early warning of toxicity), abdominal pain, diarrhea, excessive thirst—infrequent.
Stuttering—case report.
Flushing of face—case reports.
Serious Adverse Effects
Allergic reaction: severe skin rash (Stevens-Johnson syndrome)—case reports.
Idiosyncratic reactions: marked anxiety, confusion, behavioral disturbances.
Central nervous system toxicity: muscle twitching, seizures—dose-related.
Fever—possible (if in children and of sudden onset and lasting more than 24 hours—call your doctor as a 50% decrease in dose may be needed).
Heart rhythm abnormalities, rapid breathing, low blood pressure—variable and dose-related.

Gastrointestinal bleeding—rare.

Defects in clotting (coagulation)—case reports.

Drug-induced abnormal urine production (SIADH) or porphyria—case reports.

Worsening of ulcers—possible.

Liver toxicity—case reports.

▷ **Possible Effects on Sexual Function:** None reported.

Natural Diseases or Disorders That May Be Activated by This Drug

Latent peptic ulcer disease.

Possible Effects on Laboratory Tests

Blood uric acid level: increased.

Fecal occult blood test: positive (large doses may cause stomach bleeding).

Triglycerides: may be increased with prolonged use.

CAUTION

1. This drug should not be taken at the same time as other antiasthmatic drugs unless your doctor prescribes the combination. Serious overdose could result.
2. If you develop severe weakness or confusion, irregular heartbeats, shakes (tremors), or muscle twitching while taking this medicine—CALL YOUR DOCTOR immediately.
3. Influenza vaccines may delay the elimination of this drug and cause accumulation to toxic levels.

Precautions for Use

By Infants and Children: Do not exceed recommended doses. Watch for toxicity: irritability, agitation, tremors, lethargy, fever, vomiting, rapid heart rate and breathing, seizures. Blood level tests are needed during long-term use.

By Those Over 60 Years of Age: Small starting doses are indicated. You may be at increased risk for stomach irritation, nausea, vomiting, or diarrhea. When used concurrently with coffee (caffeine) or nasal decongestants, this drug may cause excessive stimulation and a hyperactivity syndrome.

▷ **Advisability of Use During Pregnancy**

Pregnancy Category: C. See Pregnancy Risk Categories at the back of this book.

Animal Studies: Significant birth defects due to this drug reported in mice.

Human Studies: Adequate studies of pregnant women are not available. No increase in birth defects reported in 394 exposures to this drug.

Avoid this drug during the first 3 months. Use it otherwise only if clearly needed. Ask your physician for guidance.

Advisability of Use If Breast-Feeding

Presence of this drug in breast milk: Yes, and at roughly the same concentration of the mother's.

Talk to your doctor about this benefit-to-risk decision. The peak concentration for the infant, and therefore the expected peak effect, would happen 1–3 hours after nursing. Refraining from the medicine or refraining from nursing may be needed depending on the infant's ability to tolerate theophylline.

Habit-Forming Potential: None.

Effects of Overdose: Nausea, vomiting, restlessness, irritability, confusion, delirium, seizures, high fever, weak pulse, coma.

Possible Effects of Long-Term Use: Gastrointestinal irritation.

Suggested Periodic Examinations While Taking This Drug (at physician's discretion)

Periodic testing of blood theophylline levels (see Therapeutic Drug Monitoring, Chapter 2). Time to sample blood for theophylline level: 2 hours after regular (standard) dose forms; 5 hours after sustained-release dose forms. Recommended therapeutic range: 10 to 20 mcg/mL.

▷ **While Taking This Drug, Observe the Following**

Foods: No restrictions.

Herbal Medicines or Minerals: Avoid using St. John's wort, ma huang, ephedrine-like compounds, kola, mate, and guarana (principle active ingredient of guarana and mate is caffeine—and use should be avoided). The other listed products, if taken while taking theophylline, may result in increased sensation of jitteriness or nervousness (central nervous system stimulation). There is one case report of decreased removal (clearance) of theophylline from the body if it is combined with St. John's wort. Caution and more frequent testing of blood levels are prudent. Fir or pine needle oil should NOT be used by asthmatics. Ephedra alone does carry a German Commission E monograph indication for asthma treatment. If you are allergic to plants in the Asteraceae family (aster, chrysanthemum, daisy, or ragweed), you may also be allergic to echinacea, chamomile, feverfew, and St. John's wort. Ipriflavone can increase theophylline levels, requiring theophylline dosage adjustments. Talk to your doctor BEFORE adding any herbal medicine to theophylline.

Beverages: Avoid excessive use of caffeine-containing beverages: coffee, tea, cola, guarana, mate, or chocolate; this combination could cause nervousness and insomnia.

▷ *Alcohol:* Large doses may decrease removal by up to 30%. May have additive effect on stomach irritation.

Tobacco Smoking: May hasten the elimination of this drug and reduce its effectiveness. I advise everyone to quit smoking.

Marijuana Smoking: May hasten the elimination of this drug and reduce its effectiveness. Higher doses may be necessary to maintain a therapeutic blood level.

▷ *Other Drugs*

Theophylline may *decrease* the effects of
- adenosine (Adenocard).
- benzodiazepines (See Drug Classes).
- lithium (Lithane, Lithobid, etc.).
- zafirlukast (Accolate).

Theophylline *taken concurrently* with
- halothane (anesthesia) may cause heart rhythm abnormalities.
- phenytoin (Dilantin) may cause decreased effects of both drugs. Monitor blood levels and adjust doses as appropriate.
- tacrolimus (Prograf) may cause increased levels of tacrolimus—more frequent tacrolimus blood levels are prudent.

The following drugs may *increase* the effects of theophylline:
- allopurinol (Lopurin, Zyloprim).
- amiodarone (Cordarone).
- birth control pills (oral contraceptives—estrogens).
- capsaicin (Zostrix, others).
- cimetidine (Tagamet).
- clarithromycin (Biaxin) or azithromycin (Biaxin).

- corticosteroids (see Drug Classes).
- diltiazem (Cardizem).
- disulfiram (Antabuse).
- doxycycline and other tetracyclines.
- ephedrine (various).
- erythromycin (E-Mycin, Erythrocin, etc.).
- famotidine (Pepcid).
- flu vaccine (influenza vaccine).
- fluoroquinolone antibiotics such as ciprofloxacin (Cipro), enoxacin (Penetrex—greatest increase of roughly 50%), grepafloxacin (Raxar), norfloxacin (Noroxin), ofloxacin (Floxin), perfloxacin (Perflacine-France), and trovafloxacin (Trovan) because of their elimination by or effect on the P450 1A2 liver enzyme.
- fluvoxamine (Luvox).
- furosemide (Lasix).
- imipenem/cilastatin (Primaxin).
- interferon alfa-2A or 2B.
- ipriflavone (various).
- isoniazid (INH).
- methotrexate (Mexate).
- mexiletine (Mexitil).
- nicotine (Nicorette, Pro-Step, others).
- pentoxifylline (Trental).
- propafenone (Rythmol).
- ranitidine (Zantac).
- riluzole (Rilutek).
- sertraline (Zoloft).
- tacrine (Cognex).
- thiabendazole.
- ticlopidine (Ticlid).
- troleandomycin (TAO).
- verapamil (Calan, Verelan).
- viloxazine.
- zafirlukast (Accolate).
- zileuton (Zyflo)—may require 50% dose decreases.

The following drugs may *decrease* the effects of theophylline:
- barbiturates (phenobarbital, etc.).
- beta blockers (see Drug Classes).
- carbamazepine (Tegretol).
- isoproterenol.
- fosphenytoin (Cerebyx) or phenytoin (Dilantin).
- lansoprazole (Prevacid).
- primidone (Mysoline).
- rifampin (Rifadin, Rimactane, etc.).
- ritonavir (Norvir) and perhaps other protease inhibitors (see Drug Classes).
- sulfinpyrazone (Anturane).
- terbutaline (Brethine, others).

▷ *Driving, Hazardous Activities:* This drug may cause dizziness. Restrict activities as necessary.

Aviation Note: The use of this drug *may be a disqualification* for piloting. Consult a designated Aviation Medical Examiner.

Exposure to Sun: No restrictions.

Occurrence of Unrelated Illness: Sudden viral respiratory infections or even fever may slow drug removal. Watch for signs of toxicity, as dosing must be changed if this occurs. More frequent blood levels are needed. Seizure disorders may be worsened by this medicine. Use with extreme caution by seizure patients. Theophylline used with extreme caution in active peptic ulcer disease or heart arrhythmias (cardiac, not including slow or brad- yarrhythmias).

Discontinuation: Avoid prolonged or unnecessary use of this drug. When your asthma resolves, withdraw this drug gradually over several days.

THIAZIDE DIURETICS FAMILY

Bendroflumethiazide   (ben droh FLOO meh THI a zide)   **Chlorothiazide** (kloroh THI azide)   **Chlorthalidone**   (KLOR thal i dohn)   **Hydro- chlorothiazide**   (hi droh klor oh THI a zide)   **Hydroflumethiazide**   (hi droh flu meh THI a zide) **Methyclothiazide** (METH i klo THI a zide)   **Meto- lazone** (me TOHL a zohn)   **Trichlormethiazide**   (tri klor me THI a zide)

Introduced   1960, 1957, 1960, 1959, 1961, 1959, 1974, 1962, respectively **Class**   Antihypertensive, diuretic, thiazides   **Prescription**   USA: Yes **Controlled Drug:**   USA: No; Canada: No   **Available as Generic**   USA: Yes, hydrochlorothiazide and combination with triamterene and with bisoprolol also; Canada: Yes

Brand Names: *Bendroflumethiazide*: Naturetin, *Chlorothiazide*: Aldochlor [CD], Diachlor, Diupres [CD], Diurigen, Diuril, SK-Chlorothiazide, ♣Supres [CD], *Chlorthalidone*: ♣Apo-Chlorthalidone, Combipres [CD], Demi-Regroton [CD], Hygroton, ♣Hygroton-Resperpine [CD], Hylidone, ♣Novothalidone, Regroton [CD], ♣Tenoretic[CD], Thalitone, ♣Uridon, *Hydrochlorothiazide*: Atacand HCT [CD], Aldactazide [CD], Aldoril D30/D50 [CD], Aldoril-15/25 [CD], ♣Apo-Amilzide, ♣Apo-Hydro, ♣Apo- Methazide [CD], ♣Apo-Triazide [CD], Apresazide [CD], Apresoline- Esidrix [CD], Avalide [CD], Capozide [CD], ♣Co-Betaloc [CD], Diaqua, ♣Diuchlor H, Dyazide [CD], Esidrex, Ezide, H-H-R, H.H.R., HydroDiuril, Hydromal, Hydro-Par, Hydropres [CD], Hydroserpine [CD], Hydroserpine Plus [CD], Hydro-T, Hydro-Z-50, Hyzaar [CD], Inderide [CD], Inderide LA [CD], ♣Ismelin-Esidrex [CD], Lopressor HCT [CD], Maxzide [CD], Maxzide-25 [CD], M Dopazide [CD], Microzide, Mictrin, ♣Moduret [CD], Moduretic [CD], ♣Natrimax, ♣Neo-Codema, Normozide [CD], ♣Novo- Doparil [CD], ♣Novo-Hydrazide, ♣Novo-Spirozine [CD], ♣Novo- Triamzide [CD], Oretic, Oreticyl [CD], ♣PMS Dopazide [CD], Prinzide [CD], Ser-Ap-Es [CD], Serpasil-Esidrex [CD], SK-Hydrochlorothiazide, Thiuretic, Timolide [CD], Trandate HCT [CD], Unipres [CD], Uniretic [CD] ♣Urozide, Vaseretic [CD], ♣Viskazide [CD], Zestoretic [CD], Ziac [CD], Zide, *Hydroflumethiazide*: Diucardin, Saluron, *Methyclothiazide*: Aquatensen, ♣Duretic, Enduron, *Metolazone*: Diulo, Microx, Mykrox, Zaroxolyn, *Trichlormethiazide*: Diurese, Marazide II, Metahydrin, Naqua, Naquival [CD]

BENEFITS versus RISKS	
Possible Benefits	*Possible Risks*
EFFECTIVE, WELL-TOLERATED DIURETICS	Loss of body potassium and magnesium (especially with higher doses)
POSSIBLY EFFECTIVE IN MILD HYPERTENSION	
ENHANCES EFFECTIVENESS OF OTHER ANTIHYPERTENSIVES	Cardiac arrhythmias caused by decreased electrolytes (studied in chlorthalidone and hydrochlorothiazide)
Beneficial in treatment of diabetes insipidus	
Helps build stronger bones and avoid fractures	Increased blood sugar, uric acid, or calcium
ALLHAT DATA SHOWED THAT CHLORTHALIDONE WAS BETTER THAN AMLODIPINE AT PREVENTING HEART FAILURE AND ALSO HELPED PREVENT MAJOR HEART ATTACK. CHLORTHALIDONE ALSO HELPED MORE THAN LISINOPRIL IN PREVENTING STROKE, HEART FAILURE, AND NEED FOR MEASURES TO OPEN HEART ARTERIES	Rare blood cell disorders
	Rare liver toxicity (chlorothiazide or hydrochlorothiazide)

▷ **Principal Uses**

As a Single Drug Product: Uses currently included in FDA-approved labeling: (1) Increases the volume of urine (diuresis) to correct fluid retention (edema) seen in congestive heart failure, corticosteroid or estrogen use, and certain types of liver and kidney disease; (2) starting therapy for high blood pressure (hypertension—noncombination forms).

Author's Note: One large study showed that hydrochlorothiazide achieves benefits (outcomes) in decreasing left ventricular size equal to more expensive agents, such as ACE inhibitors. A review of 10 studies found that diuretics versus beta blockers should be the first-line medicines for treating high blood pressure in the elderly. The current JNC VII also recommends diuretics as first-line medicines (compelling reasons may modify this).

Other (unlabeled) generally accepted uses: (1) Prevention of kidney stones that contain calcium; (2) may help decrease the frequency of hip fractures in the elderly; (3) methyclothiazide has been used to help maintain blood calcium levels in Paget's disease; (4) may have a role in helping prevent osteoporosis (by correcting abnormally high elimination of calcium in the urine or hypercalciuria); (5) used in diabetes insipidus (nephrogenic) in decreasing the urine volume.

As Combination Drug Products [CD]: Used to treat blood pressure that has not responded to single-drug therapy by combining beta blockers, ACE inhibitors, or angiotensin II receptor blockers with this diuretic.

How These Drugs Work: By increasing removal of salt and water in the urine, these drugs reduce fluid volume and body sodium. They also relax walls of smaller arteries. The combined effect of these two actions (reduced blood volume in expanded space) lowers blood pressure. May also have a role in increasing a prostaglandin that the kidney makes.

▷ **Widely Used Guidelines That Involve This Medicine (representative sample):** Please look at the section at the very beginning of this profile called "Class." Next, turn to Table 22 and you will find guidelines listed by the class involved!

Available Dosage Forms and Strengths

Bendroflumethiazide:

Tablets — 5 mg, 10 mg

Chlorothiazide:

Injection — 500 mg/20 mL
Oral suspension — 250 mg/5 mL
Tablets — 250 mg, 500 mg

Chlorthalidone:

Tablets — 15 mg, 25 mg, 50 mg, 100 mg

Chlorthalidone combinations:

Tablets — 25 mg chlorthalidone, 50 mg
atenolol (Tenoretic)

Hydrochlorothiazide:

Solution — 50 mg/5 mL
Solution, intensol — 100 mg/mL
Tablets — 12.5 mg, 25 mg, 50 mg, 100 mg

Hydrochlorothiazide combinations:

Bisoprolol and hydrochlorothiazide — 2.5 mg/6.25 mg, 5 mg/6.25 mg, 10
mg/6.25 mg
Candesartan and hydrochlorothiazide — 16 mg/12.5 mg, 32 mg/12.5 mg
Losartan and hydrochlorothiazide — 50 mg/12.5 mg, 100 mg/12.5 mg

Methyclothiazide:

Tablets — 2.5 mg, 5 mg

Metolazone:

Tablets — 0.5 mg, 2.5 mg, 5 mg, 10 mg

Trichlormethiazide:

Tablets — 2 mg, 4 mg

▷ **Usual Adult Dosage Ranges:** *Bendroflumethiazide:* As antihypertensive—12.5 to 5 mg daily, in a single dose.

Chlorothiazide: As antihypertensive—500 to 1,000 mg per day to start, and 500 to 2,000 mg daily as a maintenance dose. As a diuretic—500 to 2,000 mg per day, using the smallest effective dose. Daily maximum is 2,000 mg.

Chlorthalidone: As antihypertensive—15 mg as a starting dose, then increased as needed and tolerated in 15 mg steps to 30 mg daily, and then up to 45 mg daily if needed. Some other forms are only available in 25 mg increments and are started as a half of one tablet to one tablet. As a diuretic—30 to 60 mg daily and then the smallest effective dose is used (maintenance dose). Some clinicians use 60 mg every other day. Some patients have required 120 mg daily.

Hydrochlorothiazide: As antihypertensive—12.5 to 100 mg daily initially; 12.5 to 200 mg daily for maintenance. As diuretic—variable; 12.5 to 200 mg daily. Many patients require 100–200 mg; the smallest effective dose should be determined (see CAUTION below). The total daily dose should not exceed 200 mg. Microzide is a once-daily formulation (12.5 mg) of this medicine. Combination forms are started using the lowest dose combination form and then are increased as needed and tolerated.

Author's Note: Many patients with mild to moderate high blood pressure get acceptable blood-pressure-lowering results from 12.5 mg of hydrochlorothiazide or 15 mg of chlorthalidone. If results are obtained with this dose, it can minimize loss of potassium and magnesium as well!

Methyclothiazide: As antihypertensive or diuretic—2.5 to 5 mg daily. Maximum daily diuretic dose is 10 mg. Pediatric dose—0.05 to 0.2 mg per kg of body mass daily.

Trichlormethiazide: As antihypertensive or diuretic—therapy may be started with 1 to 4 mg twice daily. Usual maintenance dose is 1 to 4 mg once daily.

Note: Actual dose and schedule must be determined for each patient individually.

Conditions Requiring Dosing Adjustments

Liver Function: Electrolyte balance is critical in liver failure. These drugs may precipitate encephalopathy. Hydrochlorothiazide and chlorothiazide are also a rare cause of cholestatic jaundice and should be used with caution in liver failure.

Kidney Function: These drugs can be used with caution by patients with mild kidney failure and are not effective for patients with moderate failure. They should not be used in severe kidney failure; they can be a rare cause of kidney damage.

▷ **Dosing Instructions:** The tablets may be crushed and taken with or following meals to reduce stomach irritation. For liquid forms, dosing should be accomplished using a calibrated dosing spoon or dose cup. Suspensions should be well shaken BEFORE EACH dose. All forms are best taken in the morning to avoid nighttime urination. If you forget a dose: Take the missed dose as soon as you remember it, unless it's nearly time for your next dose—if that is the case, skip the missed dose and take the next dose right on schedule. DO NOT double up on doses. Talk with your doctor if you find yourself missing doses because the best results come from keeping your blood pressure under tight control.

Usual Duration of Use: Regular use for up to 4 weeks determines full benefits in lowering high blood pressure. Long-term use requires follow-up with your doctor. If goals for blood pressure are not met, dose increases, combination treatment, or changing medicines is appropriate. Take control of blood pressure for life.

Typical Treatment Goals and Measurements (Outcomes and Markers)

Blood Pressure: Guidelines (JNC VII) define normal blood pressure (BP) as **less than** 120/80 and **pre-hypertension** as 120/80 to 139/89. This new range is intended to help doctors encourage lifestyle changes (or, in the case of people with a risk factor for high blood pressure, start treatment) much earlier—so that damage to blood vessels, heart, kidneys, sexual potency, or eyes might be minimized or avoided altogether. Stage 1 hypertension is 140/90 to 159/99, and stage 2 hypertension equal to or greater than 160/100 mm Hg. These guidelines also recommend that clinicians work with their patients to agree on the goals and a plan of treatment. The first-ever guidelines for blood pressure (hypertension) in African Americans recommends that MOST black patients be started on TWO antihypertensive medicines with the goal of lowering blood pressure to 130/80 for those with high risk for heart and blood vessel disease or with diabetes. The American Diabetes Association also recommends 130/80 as the target for diabetics and less than 125/75 for those who spill more than one gram of protein into their urine. Most clinicians try to achieve a BP that confers the best balance of lower cardiovascular risk and avoids the problem of too low a blood pressure. Blood pressure duration is generally increased with beneficial restriction of sodium. If goals are not met, it is not unusual to intensify doses or add on medicines.

Possible Advantages of These Drugs

Hydrochlorothiazide was studied in more than 1,100 Veterans Administration patients with mild to moderate high blood pressure. It was found to have met blood pressure reduction goals while offering decreased left ventricular mass. These outcomes or results were accomplished using low-dose therapy, avoiding many of the undesirable changes in blood chemistry that can be seen with higher doses. This was also accomplished at a fraction of the direct cost of ACE inhibitors or calcium channel blockers. Results from ALLHAT (NHLBI study) also show equal results (efficacy)in blood pressure lowering by chlorthalidone versus two nondiuretics—an ACE inhibitor (lisinopril) and calcium channel blocker (amlodipine). Consideration must be given to the expense of laboratory monitoring required when using these medicines. Diuretics (based on individual clinical considerations) are drugs of first choice for African Americans with high blood pressure versus prior preference given to calcium channel blockers. May strengthen bones.

▷ **These Drugs Should Not Be Taken If**
- you had an allergic reaction to any form of them previously or are allergic to sulfonamides (chlorthalidone).
- your kidneys are not making urine.

▷ **Inform Your Physician Before Taking These Drugs If**
- you are allergic to any form of sulfa drug.
- you are pregnant or planning pregnancy.
- you have a history of kidney or liver disease.
- you have a history of pancreatitis or lupus erythematosus.
- you have developed swelling (angioedema) of the tongue, face, or throat (medicine should be stopped).
- you have asthma or allergies to other medicines.
- you have had testing of electrolytes ordered by another physician, which your doctor has not seen.
- you develop muscle cramps, weakness, or abnormal heartbeats while taking one of these medicines.
- you have diabetes, gout, or lupus erythematosus.
- you are allergic to the dye tartrazine, as some of these medicines contain it.
- you take any form of cortisone, digitalis, oral antidiabetic drug, or insulin.
- you will have surgery with general anesthesia.

Possible Side Effects (natural, expected, and unavoidable drug actions)

Light-headedness on arising from sitting or lying position (see Orthostatic Hypotension in Glossary). Increased blood sugar or uric acid level; decreased blood potassium, zinc, or magnesium level. Decreased blood magnesium, combined with loss of potassium, may lead to increased risk of sudden cardiac death (high doses for extended periods).

▷ **Possible Adverse Effects** (unusual, unexpected, and infrequent reactions)

If any of the following develop, consult your physician promptly for guidance.

Mild Adverse Effects

Allergic reactions: skin rashes, hives, drug fever (see Glossary).

Muscle aches—case report.

Headache, dizziness, blurred or yellow vision—infrequent.

Reduced appetite, indigestion, nausea, vomiting, diarrhea—infrequent.

Serious Adverse Effects

Allergic reactions: hepatitis with jaundice (see Glossary), anaphylactic reaction (see Glossary), severe skin reactions.

Inflammation of the pancreas—case reports.

Bone marrow depression (see Glossary): fever, sore throat, abnormal bleeding/bruising—case reports.

Data from studies of hydrochlorothiazide and chlorthalidone suggest that potassium and magnesium loss associated with higher-dose therapy increases the risk of sudden cardiac death.

Acute gout in some patients (because these medicines decrease uric acid removal).

Loss of blood glucose control—possible.

Short-term (less than 1 year) increase in serum lipids (returns to pretreatment levels in about 1 year).

▷ **Possible Effects on Sexual Function:** Decreased libido (hydrochlorothiazide, chlorthalidone); impotence (bendroflumethiazide, chlorothiazide, hydrochlorothiazide, chlorthalidone)—case reports.

▷ **Adverse Effects That May Mimic Natural Diseases or Disorders**

Liver reaction may suggest viral hepatitis.

Natural Diseases or Disorders That May Be Activated by These Drugs

Diabetes, gout, systemic lupus erythematosus. Those with asthma or drug allergies are more likely to have allergic reactions.

Possible Effects on Laboratory Tests

Complete blood counts: decreased red cells, hemoglobin, white cells, and platelets.

Blood amylase level: increased (possible pancreatitis).

Blood calcium or uric acid level: increased.

Blood sodium and chloride levels: decreased.

Blood cholesterol and triglyceride levels: increased, short term.

Blood glucose level: increased.

Glucose tolerance test (GTT): decreased.

Blood lithium level: increased.

Blood potassium and magnesium level: decreased.

Blood urea nitrogen (BUN) level: increased with long-term use.

Liver function tests (hydrochlorothiazide and chlorothiazide): increased liver enzymes (ALT/GPT, AST/GOT, and alkaline phosphatase), increased bilirubin.

CAUTION

1. One study found a strong association between higher doses of hydrochlorothiazide and chlorthalidone and combination drugs containing these diuretics and electrolyte loss and sudden cardiac death. This appeared to be a result of magnesium and potassium loss and may be circumvented by close following of those minerals (electrolytes). Electrolytes should be closely followed.

2. Take these exactly as prescribed. Excessive loss of sodium and potassium can lead to loss of appetite, nausea, fatigue, weakness, confusion, and tingling in the extremities.

3. If you take digitalis (digitoxin, digoxin), adequate potassium is critical. Periodic testing and high-potassium foods may be needed to prevent potassium deficiency—a potential cause of digitalis toxicity (see Table 13, High-Potassium Foods, Section Six).

Precautions for Use

By Infants and Children: Overdose could cause serious dehydration. Significant potassium loss can occur within the first 2 weeks of drug use.

By Those Over 60 Years of Age: Starting doses may be as low as 12.5 mg or 15 mg for chlorthalidone. Increased risk of impaired thinking, orthostatic hypotension, potassium loss, and blood sugar increase. Overdose or extended use can cause excessive loss of body water, thickening (increased viscosity) of blood, and increased tendency for the blood to clot—predisposing to stroke, heart attack, or thrombophlebitis (vein inflammation with blood clot).

▷ Advisability of Use During Pregnancy

Pregnancy Category: Metolazone: B by manufacturer, D by other researchers. Thalitone is B by the manufacturer, but D by one researcher. All other thiazides in this class are D. See Pregnancy Risk Categories at the back of this book. Some combination forms are C during the first trimester and D during the second and third trimesters.

Animal Studies: No birth defects found in rat studies.

Human Studies: Reports are conflicting and inconclusive.

Use of thiazides can cause maternal complications that may cause adverse fetal effects, including death. They should not be used in pregnancy unless a very serious complication occurs for which these drugs work. Ask your doctor for guidance.

Advisability of Use If Breast-Feeding

Presence of these drugs in breast milk: Yes.

Avoid drugs or refrain from nursing.

Habit-Forming Potential: None.

Effects of Overdose: Dry mouth, thirst, lethargy, weakness, muscle cramping, nausea, vomiting, drowsiness progressing to stupor or coma.

Possible Effects of Long-Term Use: Impaired balance of water, salt, magnesium, and potassium in blood and body tissues. Impaired tolerance of glucose. Pathological changes in parathyroid glands with increased blood calcium levels and decreased blood phosphate levels.

Suggested Periodic Examinations While Taking These Drugs (at physician's discretion)

Complete blood cell counts.

Measurements of blood levels of sodium, potassium, chloride, magnesium, sugar, and uric acid.

Kidney and liver function tests.

Repeat bone mineral density test (2 years after starting therapy) if this drug is used to decrease calcium loss.

▷ While Taking These Drugs, Observe the Following

Foods: Ask your doctor if you need to eat foods rich in potassium. See Table 13, High-Potassium Foods, Section Six, if needed. Follow your physician's advice regarding the use of salt.

Herbal Medicines or Minerals: Ginseng, bitter orange, country mallow, hawthorn, saw palmetto, ma huang (no longer on the U.S. market for weight loss), mate, guarana, and licorice may cause increased blood pressure. Licorice can also cause potassium loss and is especially NOT to be combined with a thiazide. Indian snakeroot has a German Commission E monograph indication for hypertension, but has not been studied with thiazides. Eleuthero root and ephedra should be avoided by people living with hypertension. Calcium and garlic may lower blood pressure. Use caution and work with your doctor to make sure blood pressure is not lowered too much. Calcium may also accumulate to a greater degree than expected since thiazides decrease removal of calcium in the urine. Because St. John's wort and some of these medicines may increase sun sensitivity, the combination is NOT advised. Talk to your doctor BEFORE combining any herbal medicine with these medicines. Diuretics are well known for depleting magnesium, zinc, and potassium. These minerals should be routinely checked and supplemented if the medicines have lowered blood mineral levels.

Beverages: No restrictions. This drug may be taken with milk.

▷ *Alcohol:* Use with caution—alcohol may exaggerate the blood-pressure-lowering effects of these drugs and cause orthostatic hypotension.

Tobacco Smoking: No interactions expected. I advise everyone to quit smoking.

▷ *Other Drugs*

These drugs may ***increase*** the effects of
- other antihypertensive drugs; dose adjustments may be necessary to prevent excessive lowering of blood pressure (may also be used to combination therapy benefit).
- fluconazole (Diflucan) (HCTZ report).
- lithium (Lithobid, others) and cause lithium toxicity.

These drugs may ***decrease*** the effects of
- oral anticoagulants such as warfarin (Coumadin); increased frequency of INR (prothrombin time) testing is needed.
- oral antidiabetic drugs (sulfonylureas—see Drug Classes and others); dose adjustments may be needed for better blood sugar control.

These drugs ***taken concurrently*** with
- allopurinol (Zyloprim) may decrease kidney function.
- amphotericin B (Abelcet, Fungizone) may result in additive potassium loss; increased frequency of laboratory testing is needed.
- calcium may result in the milk-alkali syndrome with increased calcium, alkalosis, and kidney failure.
- carbamazepine (Tegretol) may result in low sodium levels and symptomatic hyponatremia.
- cortisone or other corticosteroid medicines may result in excessive potassium loss with resultant heart rhythm changes and lethargy.
- cyclophosphamide (Cytoxan) may increase immunosuppression.
- digitalis preparations (digitoxin, digoxin) require careful monitoring and dose changes to prevent low potassium levels and bad heart rhythm.
- dofetilide (Tikosyn) and hydrochlorothiazide—do not combine.
- methotrexate (Mexate) may increase immunosuppression.
- nonsteroidal anti-inflammatory drugs (see Drug Classes), such as sulindac (Clinoril) and naproxen (Naprosyn, Aleve, Anaprox, others), may result in decreased thiazide effectiveness.
- probenecid (various) may result in increased thiazide blood levels. Checks of thiazide response are prudent.

The following drugs may ***decrease*** the effects of these thiazides:
- cholestyramine (Cuemid, Questran)—may interfere with their absorption.
- colestipol (Colestid)—may interfere with their absorption.

Take cholestyramine and colestipol 1 hour before any oral diuretic.

▷ *Driving, Hazardous Activities:* Use caution until the possible occurrence of orthostatic hypotension, dizziness, or impaired vision has been determined.

Aviation Note: The use of these drugs *may be a disqualification* for piloting. Consult a designated Aviation Medical Examiner.

Exposure to Sun: These drugs can cause photosensitivity (see Glossary). Use caution until sensitivity has been determined.

Exposure to Heat: **Caution**—excessive perspiring could cause additional loss of salt and water from the body.

Heavy Exercise or Exertion: Avoid exertion that produces light-headedness, excessive fatigue, or muscle cramping. Isometric exercises can raise blood pressure significantly. Ask your doctor for help regarding participation in this form of exercise.

Occurrence of Unrelated Illness: Vomiting or diarrhea can produce a serious imbalance of important body chemistry. Ask your doctor for help.

Discontinuation: These drugs should not be stopped abruptly following long-term use; sudden discontinuation can cause serious thiazide-withdrawal fluid retention (edema). The dose should be reduced gradually. It may be advisable to discontinue this drug 5 to 7 days before major surgery. Ask your physician, surgeon, and/or anesthesiologist for guidance.

THIAZOLIDINEDIONE FAMILY (THIGH ah zoh li dean die ohn)

Rosiglitazone   (ROSS ih glit a zoan)   **Pioglitazone**   (PEE oh glit a zoan)

Introduced: 1999,   1999   **Class:**   Antidiabetic,   thiazolidinedione
Prescription: USA: Yes   **Controlled Drug:**   USA: No; Canada: No
Available as Generic: No

Brand Name: *Rosiglitazone:* Avandamet [CD], Avandia, *Pioglitazone:* Actos

Author's Note: The FDA required modifying the warnings, precautions, and adverse reactions section of the labels for both Actos and Avandia. Health care professionals were alerted to the fact that either medicine can lead to fluid retention when used alone or when combined with insulin. Cases of congestive heart failure (CHF) have been reported, and were more likely in people who had diabetes for a longer amount of time, had preexisting medical conditions (such as ischemic heart disease, CHF, and vascular disease), took higher doses of the medicine, and were older. What this means is that people taking these medicines should be watched for signs and symptoms of heart failure (see cautions below).

BENEFITS versus RISKS

Possible Benefits	*Possible Risks*
COMBINATION USE OF ROSIGLITAZONE OR PIOGLITAZONE WITH METFORMIN MAY SLOW DIABETES PROGRESSION AS WELL AS HELP AVOID LONG-TERM COMPLICATIONS OF DIABETES ITSELF	FLUID RETENTION (CHF—see CURRENT CAUTION)
	Low blood sugar (possible)
	Worsening of existing heart failure
	Case reports of both medicines and heart failure (because of fluid retention)
DECREASED INSULIN RESISTANCE	
EFFECTIVE CONTROL OF BLOOD SUGAR (GLUCOSE)	
POSSIBLE AVOIDANCE OF LONG-TERM EFFECTS (BLOOD VESSEL, NERVE, KIDNEY, HIGH BLOOD PRESSURE, AND HEART ADVERSE EFFECTS) FROM DIABETES	
FAVORABLE SIDE EFFECT PROFILES VERSUS TROGLITAZONE	
ROSIGLITAZONE AVOIDS CYP3A4 ELIMINATION OF PIOGLITAZONE (uses CYP2C8 and has fewer potential drug-drug interactions)	
ROSIGLITAZONE MAY HAVE A BENEFICIAL EFFECT ON PLATELETS	
May have a role in some kinds of infertility where insulin resistance may be part of the problem (such as polycystic ovary syndrome or PCOS)	

▷ **Principal Uses**

As a Single Drug Product: Uses currently included in FDA-approved labeling: (1) Helps control Type 2 diabetes mellitus (adult, maturity-onset); (2) helps people who have not responded to diet alone or to a maximum dose of metformin (Glucophage); (3) either medicine can be used in combination with metformin, a sulfonylurea, or insulin; (4) rosiglitazone available combined with metformin in a single pill.

Other (unlabeled) generally accepted uses: (1) May help improve resistance to insulin and may help some patients with syndromes such as Werner syndrome or PCOS where insulin resistance is part of the problem; (2) rosiglitazone may be effective if used with a sulfonylurea.

How These Drugs Work: Work to make insulin more effective (decrease cellular resistance as a peroxisome proliferator activated receptor gamma activator—PPAR gamma). This increases the number of GLUT-4 transporters. Probably also work to decrease local and systemic lipid availability. Data presented at the American Diabetes Association 63rd scientific sessions appear to show that rosiglitazone has an effect in decreasing repeat blockage of wire mesh tubes (stents) that have been implanted in patients with coronary artery blockages (see Choi in Sources). This implies that rosiglitazone has an anti-inflammatory effect (some later data show an antiplatelet effect).

▷ **Widely Used Guidelines That Involve This Medicine (representative sample):** Please look at the section at the very beginning of this profile called "Class." Next, turn to Table 22 and you will find guidelines listed by the class involved!

Available Dosage Forms and Strengths
Rosiglitazone:
   Tablets — 1 mg (Canada), 2 mg, 4 mg, 8 mg
Pioglitazone:
   Tablets — 15 mg, 30 mg, and 45 mg

▷ **Usual Adult Dosage Ranges**
Rosiglitazone: Used alone (monotherapy): Initially 4 mg once daily or separated into two 2 mg given twice daily. The dose may be increased, if needed and tolerated, after 12 weeks to 4 mg twice daily or 8 mg once daily.
Combined with metformin: Same as monotherapy.
Combined with insulin: 4 mg daily which is also the maximum dose. If excessive lowering of the sugar (glucose) happens (less than 100 mg/deciliter), insulin dosing is decreased by 10–25% AND subsequently further adjusted to blood sugar response.
Pioglitazone: Used alone in Type 2 diabetes, the starting dose is 15 or 30 mg once a day. If the response is not at target, the dose may be slowly increased to 45 mg once a day.
Combined with insulin: The starting dose is 15 or 30 mg once a day. Once pioglitazone is started, if low blood sugar (hypoglycemia) happens or if plasma sugar (glucose) is 100 mg/deciliter or less, the dose of insulin should be lowered by 10 to 25%. Close patient follow-up for signs and symptoms of heart failure is needed. If this medicine is combined with metformin, the prior metformin dose can be continued as hypoglycemia is unlikely.
Combined with a sulfonylurea: 15 or 30 mg once daily is used. The sulfonylurea dose will have to be decreased if hypoglycemia occurs.
Note: Actual dose and schedule must be determined for each patient individually.

Conditions Requiring Dosing Adjustments
Liver Function:
   Rosiglitazone: Should NOT be started if there is active liver disease or if ALT is more than 2.5 times the upper normal limit. In mild to moderate liver disease, rosiglitazone blood levels and the time rosiglitazone stays in the body increase. Decreases in dose or increases in dosing interval are required.
   Pioglitazone: Should NOT be used in people with increased liver enzymes (transaminases such as an alanine aminotransferase more than 2.5 times the upper normal) or in patients with clinical signs/symptoms/evidence of active liver disease.
Kidney Function:
   Rosiglitazone or pioglitazone: Dosing changes are probably not needed in kidney compromise.

▷ **Dosing Instructions:** May be taken with or without food. Skipping meals while taking these medicines is NOT advised, as the medicine will still continue to increase insulin sensitivity even if the sugar (glucose) from a meal is not there—making hypoglycemia more likely. The tablets may be crushed to make it easier to take. If you are taking these medicines with the maximum dose of metformin, lower ongoing doses of rosiglitazone or pioglitazone may be effective for you. If you are taking these medicines with a sulfony-lurea and low blood sugar occurs, the sulfonylurea dose will have to be decreased. If you develop signs and symptoms of heart failure (swelling of the ankles, shortness of breath, etc.), call your doctor. If you forget a dose: Take the missed dose as soon as you remember it, unless it's nearly time for your next dose—if that is the case, skip the missed dose and take the next dose right on schedule. DO NOT double doses. Talk with your doctor if you find yourself missing doses. Taking these medicines the right way and keeping blood sugar in tight control gets the best long-term results.

Usual Duration of Use: Use on a regular schedule for 12 weeks usually deter-mines peak effectiveness in controlling diabetes for rosiglitazone. Benefits for both medicines as checked by hemoglobin A1C (glycosylated hemoglo-bin) or charts of sugar patterns in your glucose meter. Insulin resistance may require longer therapy. Failure to respond after the 12-week period requires a dose increase for rosiglitazone and failure to respond after an acceptable period for pioglitazone also requires a dose increase. Effective use can only be determined by periodic measurement of the blood sugar. See your doctor on a regular basis.

Typical Treatment Goals and Measurements (Outcomes and Markers)

Blood sugar: The general goal for blood sugar is to return it to the usual "nor-mal" range (generally 80–120 mg/dL), while avoiding risks of excessively low blood sugar. One study (the United Kingdom Prospective Diabetes Study or UKPDS) used a fasting plasma sugar (glucose) of less than 108 mg/dL. The Diabetes Control and Complications Trial (DCCT) attempted to achieve near normal glycosylated hemoglobin and found reduced unde-sirable small blood vessel (microvascular) changes. Using glycosylated hemoglobin as a marker or resolution of insulin resistance will require a longer time period to response than blood sugar.

Fructosamine and glycosylated hemoglobin: Fructosamine levels (a measure of the past 2 to 3 weeks of blood sugar control) should be less than or equal to 310 micromoles per liter. Glycosylated hemoglobin or hemoglobin A1C (a measure of the past 2–3 months of blood sugar control) should be less than or equal to 7.0%. Some clinicians now advocate 6.5% or lower as a target in order to help avoid diabetes complications. Work with your doctor to get the best individualized results and make certain you know the signs and symptoms of hypoglycemia and what to do about them if hypoglycemia occurs.

Possible Advantages of These Drugs

Offer a novel mechanism of action. Appear to avoid the liver damage poten-tial of troglitazone. Rosiglitazone does not use the CYP3A4 enzyme (a more widely used enzyme) for removal from the body (uses CYP2C8) and therefore has fewer potential drug-drug interactions than pioglitazone (which uses both). Pioglitazone may have a more favorable effect on good and bad cholesterol. Rosiglitazone has current data that show it helps avoid repeat clogging (restenosis) of stents placed in patients with blockages in their coronary arteries (may have an antiplatelet effect as well).

▷ **These Drugs Should Not Be Taken If**
- you have had an allergic reaction to them previously.
- you have active liver disease or if ALT (ask your doctor about this blood test) is more than 2.5 times the upper normal limit.
- you have Type 1 diabetes (monotherapy) or are in ketoacidosis.

▷ **Inform Your Physician Before Taking This Drug If**
- you are over 60 years old.
- your diabetes has been unstable or brittle in the past.
- you are pregnant or have been unable to ovulate (both drugs may cause ovulation to restart in premenopausal women with insulin resistance who previously did not ovulate). Adequate contraception will be needed.
- you do not know how to recognize or treat hypoglycemia (see Glossary).
- you have an infection and a fever.
- you have a deficiency of red blood cells (anemia)—ask your doctor.
- you have liver or kidney damage.
- you have NYHA class III or IV heart failure.
- you have or develop an accumulation of fluid in your body (edema).
- you are nursing your child.
- you develop an unusually quick increase in weight or swelling of the legs or shortness of breath (possible signs and symptoms of heart failure). **Call your doctor immediately if this occurs.**

Possible Side Effects (natural, expected, and unavoidable drug actions)
   If drug dose is excessive or food intake is delayed or inadequate, abnormally low blood sugar (hypoglycemia) may occur. Fluid accumulation—increasing risk of heart failure.

▷ **Possible Adverse Effects** (unusual, unexpected, and infrequent reactions)
   If any of the following develop, consult your physician promptly for guidance.
   Mild Adverse Effects
   Allergic reactions: not reported—rare.
   Headache—infrequent.
   Hypoglycemia—possible.
   Weight gain—possible.
   Muscle aches—infrequent (pioglitazone).
   Fluid retention (edema)—infrequent.
   Increased liver enzymes—very rare (happened within the first two weeks of treatment).
   Diarrhea—rare.
   Serious Adverse Effects
   Allergic reactions: not reported.
   Idiosyncratic reactions: not reported.
   Congestive heart failure or worsening of existing heart failure—possible due to increased retention of body fluid. Either drug alone or in combination of Actos (pioglitazone) with insulin can cause this. If you have an unusually quick weight gain, swelling of the legs or ankles, or unexplained shortness of breath (possible signs or symptoms of heart failure)—**Call your doctor immediately.**
   Retinopathy aggravation—case report (pioglitazone).
   Hypoglycemia—possible.
   Anemia—possible—usually mild.
   Liver toxicity—very rare.

▷ **Possible Effects on Sexual Function:** If insulin resistance has been a cause of infertility, these drugs may enable you to become fertile.

▷ **Adverse Effects That May Mimic Natural Diseases or Disorders**
   Fluid accumulation may mimic edema from congestive heart failure.

Natural Diseases or Disorders That May Be Activated by This Drug
   Increased fluid in the body (plasma volume expansion) may worsen congestive heart failure.

Possible Effects on Laboratory Tests

Complete blood cell count: decreased red cells, hemoglobin, and hematocrit— mild.

Blood glucose, fructosamine, or glycosylated hemoglobin level: decreased.

Liver function tests (ALT): possibly increased.

LDL: increased by up to 19% for rosiglitazone at the 8 mg dose (inconsistent change for pioglitazone).

Total cholesterol: increased.

HDL: increased (beneficial effect) by up to 14% for rosiglitazone and 19% for pioglitazone.

CAUTION

1. These drugs must be regarded as only one part of the total program for the management of your diabetes. It is not a substitute for a properly prescribed diet, insulin, and regular exercise.
2. A similar medicine caused serious liver reactions. While these medicines HAVE NOT caused such reactions, liver enzyme testing is required.
3. These drugs may cause you to ovulate if insulin resistance has been the cause of a failure to ovulate.
4. If you develop shortness of breath, unusually quick weight gain, or swelling of the ankles or any other signs or symptoms of heart failure— **call your doctor immediately.**
5. The American Diabetes Association (ADA) defines diabetes as two fasting blood sugars in a row more than 125 mg/dL. This more conservative approach reflects current information saying that complications start at lower blood sugar levels than previously thought. The concept of prediabetes (formerly impaired glucose tolerance) is described in the Glossary. British data advocated that statin type medicines could cut the risk of heart attack and stroke by a third (even in people with normal cholesterol)—yet these medicines are underused in diabetics. Talk to your doctor about this.

Precautions for Use

By Infants and Children: Safety and efficacy have not been established in this age group.

By Those Over 65 Years of Age: Any medicine with the potential to lower blood sugar should be used with caution in this age group and monitored closely to prevent hypoglycemic reactions. Repeated episodes of hypoglycemia in the elderly can cause brain damage. Clinical trials did not reveal differences in safety or effectiveness in those over 65 for either medicine. Because older people are more likely to have heart problems, patients should be aware of signs and symptoms (such as shortness of breath and quick weight gain) as possible drug-induced accumulation of fluid and possible heart failure.

▷ Advisability of Use During Pregnancy

Pregnancy Category: C (both medicines). See Pregnancy Risk Categories at the back of this book.

Animal Studies: Rosiglitazone in treated rats and rabbits (during mid-late gestation) showed growth retardation and was associated with fetal death. Pioglitazone in treated rats and rabbits showed delayed parturition and embryotoxicity at high doses.

Human Studies: Adequate studies of pregnant women are not available for either medicine.

Because uncontrolled blood sugar levels during pregnancy are associated with a higher incidence of birth defects, many experts recommend that insulin (instead of an oral agent) be used as necessary to control diabetes during the entire pregnancy.

Advisability of Use If Breast-Feeding
Presence of this drug in breast milk: Yes for rosiglitazone, unknown for pioglitazone.
Avoid drug or refrain from nursing.

Habit-Forming Potential: None.

Effects of Overdose: Limited experience is available for both medicines. Single doses of rosiglitazone of 20 mg by mouth were well tolerated. One pioglitazone patient took 180 mg for 7 days without any reported ill effects. If an overdose occurs of either drug, supportive treatment consistent with the patient's signs and symptoms should be provided.

Possible Effects of Long-Term Use: Normalization of fructosamine, hemoglobin A1C, decreased LDL, increased HDL. Pioglitazone may have a more favorable effect on good and bad cholesterol.

Suggested Periodic Examinations While Taking These Drugs (at physician's discretion)
Complete blood cell counts.
Liver function (serum transaminases) must be tested at the beginning of treatment, every 2 months for the first year, and then periodically thereafter. If signs or symptoms of liver problems (light stools, yellow eyes or skin, etc.) begin, serum transaminases should be measured.
Routine testing of blood sugar levels at intervals recommended by your physician is prudent. Finger stick testing accurately reflects the blood sugar and helps ensure better control (tighter control) of blood glucose. One novel device uses a laser to "stick" the finger (see www.cellrobotics.com). The laser is painless and appears to avoid toughening the skin like a lancet. One blood sugar machine can also test glycated protein (fructosamine). If you are ill, increased frequency of finger stick blood glucose testing may be indicated. A handheld machine called A1cNow enables pharmacists and physicians to check hemoglobin A1C in the office or pharmacy in 8 minutes! Additionally, a device called a Glucowatch Biographer uses a pad and a watchlike device to painlessly check blood sugar (see www.cygnus.com). Periodic evaluation of heart and circulatory system (diabetes is a large risk factor for heart and blood vessel disease).
Ankle Brachial Index (see Glossary).
Fructosamine (now available as a finger stick self-test).
Glycosylated hemoglobin.
HDL and LDL and fractions.
Checks for decline in heart status, edema, or congestive heart failure. Drugs should be discontinued if decline in heart (cardiac) status happens.

▷ **While Taking These Drugs, Observe the Following**
Foods: Follow the diabetic diet prescribed by your physician. Rice bran has been checked in a small (57 subjects) study of Type 1 and Type 2 diabetics. The benefit was a 30% lowering of sugar. This might be a new complementary care option.
Herbal Medicines or Minerals: Using chromium may change the way your body is able to use sugar. Some health food stores advocate vanadium as mimicking the actions of insulin, but possible toxicity and need for rigorous studies presently preclude recommending it. Caution: St. John's wort may change blood sugar. DHEA may change sensitivity to insulin or insulin resistance. Aloe, fenugreek, bitter melon, eucalyptus, hawthorn, ginger, garlic, ginseng, guar gum, glucomannan, licorice, nettle, and yohimbe may

change blood sugar. Since this may require adjustment of hypoglycemic medicine dosing, talk to your doctor BEFORE combining any of these herbal medicines with this medicine. Echinacea pupurea (injectable) and blonde psyllium seed or husk should NOT be taken by people living with diabetes. Psyllium increases risk of excessively low blood sugar. Surprisingly, boiled stems of the Optuntia streptacantha prickly pear cactus appears to be able to lower blood sugar. Ongoing effects and effects on A1C are not known. Red sage is used for blood sugar effects, but is unproven.

Beverages: As directed in the diabetic diet. May be taken with milk.

▷ *Alcohol:* Single doses did not increase risk of sudden lowering of blood sugar (hypoglycemia). Use with caution. Repeated or large doses of alcohol can lower blood sugar, and chronic high doses can impact liver function.

Tobacco Smoking: No interaction expected. I advise everyone to quit smoking.

▷ *Other Drugs*

The following drugs may ***decrease*** the effects of rosiglitazone:
- beta blocker (see drug classes).
- cholestyramine (Questran).
- corticosteroids (see Drug Classes).
- thiazide diuretics (see Drug Classes).

These medicines ***taken concurrently*** with
- birth control pills (oral contraceptives) lead to loss of control with one medicine in this same class. Pills containing ethinyl estradiol or norethindrone may not work with pioglitazone.
- medicines metabolized by CYP2C8 or decreasing this enzyme may increase blood levels of rosiglitazone.
- medicines that increase levels of CYP2C8 may decrease the effects of rosiglitazone.
- medicines metabolized by CYP3A4 or inhibiting this enzyme (such as many macrolide antibiotics, azole antifungals, protease inhibitors, and zafirlukast or zileuton) may increase blood levels of pioglitazone.
- medicines that increase levels of CYP3A4 (such as carbamazepine, fosphenytoin, phenytoin, rifampin, or dexamethasone) may decrease the effects of pioglitazone.
- protease inhibitors (PIs—see Drug Classes) may result in loss of glucose control because PIs as a class can cause glucose intolerance.
- sulfonylureas (see Drug Classes) can work to effectively lower blood sugar, but may also lower blood sugar too much. Combination use requires blood sugar checks and adjustments of sulfonylurea dosing if the blood sugar goes too low. This is also true of other medicines that lower blood sugar.

▷ *Driving, Hazardous Activities:* Regulate your dose schedule, eating schedule, and physical activities very carefully to prevent hypoglycemia. Be able to recognize the early symptoms of hypoglycemia so that you can avoid hazardous activities and take corrective measures.

Aviation Note: Diabetes ***is a disqualification*** for piloting. Consult a designated Aviation Medical Examiner.

Exposure to Sun: Not defined.

Occurrence of Unrelated Illness: Acute infections, illnesses causing vomiting or diarrhea, serious injuries, and surgical procedures can interfere with diabetic control and may require insulin. If any of these conditions occur, call your doctor promptly.

Discontinuation: Talk with your doctor before changing the dosing schedule of this medicine or considering stopping these medicines.

THIORIDAZINE (thi oh RID a zeen)

Introduced: 1959   **Class:** Antipsychotic; tranquilizer, major; phenothiazines   **Prescription:** USA: Yes   **Controlled Drug:** USA: No; Canada: No   **Available as Generic:** USA: Yes; Canada: Yes

Brand Names: ✤Apo-Thioridazine, Mellaril, Mellaril-S, Millazine, ✤Novo-Ridazine, ✤PMS-Thioridazine, SK-Thioridazine

---

BENEFITS versus RISKS

Possible Benefits	*Possible Risks*
EFFECTIVE CONTROL OF ACUTE MENTAL DISORDERS	TARDIVE DYSKINESIA (SERIOUS TOXIC BRAIN EFFECT) with long-term use
Relief of anxiety, agitation, and tension	NEUROLEPTIC MALIGNANT SYNDROME
Behavior problems that are resistant to other medicines	MAY PROLONG HEARTBEAT INTERVALS AND LEAD TO FATAL HEART RHYTHM PROBLEMS
	Liver damage with jaundice (infrequent)
	Blood cell disorder: abnormally low white blood cell count

▷ **Principal Uses**

As a Single Drug Product: Uses currently included in FDA-approved labeling: (1) Helps manage symptoms of psychotic disorders, moderate to marked depression with significant anxiety and nervous tension, and agitation, anxiety, depression, and exaggerated fears in the elderly; (2) used in severe behavioral problems in children characterized by hyperexcitability, short attention span, and rapid swings in mood (temper tantrums); (3) eases agitation in Alzheimer's disease.

Other (unlabeled) generally accepted uses: (1) May have a role in treating alcohol withdrawal in patients who cannot tolerate benzodiazepines; (2) can be used to treat unexplained infertility; (3) may help control premature ejaculation and nocturnal emissions in men; (4) can help borderline personality disorder; (5) of use in some chronic pain syndromes; (6) may be of use in hypersexuality.

Author's Note: Information in this profile has been shortened to make room for more widely used medicines.

THIOTHIXENE (thi oh THIX een)

Introduced: 1967   **Class:** Tranquilizer, major; thioxanthenes   **Prescription:** USA: Yes   **Controlled Drug:** USA: No; Canada: No   **Available as Generic:** USA: Yes; Canada: No

Brand Name: Navane

Author's Note: Information in this profile has been shortened to make room for more widely used medicines.

TICLOPIDINE (ti KLOH pi deen)

Introduced: 1985   **Class:**   Antiplatelet

Author's Note: Because of more widespread use of clopidogrel, this profile has been truncated.

TIMOLOL (TI moh lohl)

Introduced: 1972   **Class:**   Anti-anginal, antiglaucoma, antihypertensive, beta blocker   **Prescription:**   USA: Yes   **Controlled Drug:**   USA: No; Canada: No   **Available as Generic:**   USA: Yes; Canada: No

Brand Names: ✦Apo-Timolol, ✦Apo-Timop, Betimol, Blocadren, Cosopt [CD], ✦Dom-Timolol, ✦Novo-Timolol, ✦Timolide [CD], Timoptic, Timoptic Ocudose, Timoptic-XE, ✦Xalacom

Author's Note: Benefit-to-Risk profile considerations are generally much more relaxed for eye (ophthalmic) forms as adverse systemic effects are much less likely.

```
BENEFITS versus RISKS

        Possible Benefits                    Possible Risks
EFFECTIVE, WELL-TOLERATED          CONGESTIVE HEART FAILURE IN
  ANTI-ANGINAL DRUG                  ADVANCED HEART DISEASE
EFFECTIVE ANTIGLAUCOMA             Worsening of angina in coronary
  DRUG                               heart disease (if drug is abruptly
ANTIHYPERTENSIVE DRUG in mild       withdrawn)
  to moderate hypertension         Masking of low blood sugar
EFFECTIVE PREVENTION OF             (hypoglycemia) in drug-treated
  MIGRAINE HEADACHES                diabetes
EFFECTIVE ADJUNCTIVE              Provocation of asthma in asthmatics
  PREVENTION (SECONDARY
  PREVENTION) OF RECURRENT
  HEART ATTACK
Used in glaucoma combined with
  dorzolamide or latanoprost
```

▷ **Principal Uses**

As a Single Drug Product: Uses currently included in FDA-approved labeling: (1) Treats classical effort-induced angina, certain types of heart rhythm disturbance, and high blood pressure; (2) lowers increased internal eye pressure in chronic open-angle glaucoma; (3) beneficial when taken within 24 hours and thereafter in decreasing the size of the heart damage, decreasing arrhythmias, and preventing repeat heart attacks (myocardial infarction); (4) reduces frequency and severity of migraines.

Other (unlabeled) generally accepted uses: (1) Has been used by people who are afraid to fly on airplanes (air travel phobia); (2) may help decrease incidence of abnormal heart rhythms in the atria of the heart (atrial fibrillation and flutter); (3) helps prevent abnormally increased intraocular pressure after cataract surgery; (4) used in patients with detached (not torn) retinas.

As a Combination Drug Product [CD]: Available combined with hydrochlorothiazide to treat high blood pressure. Combination product includes two drugs with different mechanisms of action. This provides better effectiveness and convenience for long-term use. Available (Cosopt) with dorzolamide as an eye drop, adding the benefit of a carbonic anhydrase inhibitor—decreases formation of the fluid (aqueous humor of the eye) by slowing bicarbonate formation as well as beta blockade from timolol. The beta blockade from timolol is also added to latanoprost (increases uveoscleral outflow) in the Xalacom form.

How This Drug Works: Blocks certain actions of the sympathetic nervous system:
- reducing heart rate and contraction force, lowering blood ejection pressure and reducing oxygen needs of the heart, increasing blood flow to the heart (myocardial perfusion).
- reducing degree of blood vessel wall contraction, lowering blood pressure.
- prolonging conduction time of nerve impulses through the heart, of benefit in managing certain heart rhythm disorders.
- slowing formation of fluid (aqueous humor) in the anterior eye chamber, improving its drainage from the eye, lowering the internal eye pressure.

▷ **Widely Used Guidelines That Involve This Medicine (representative sample):** Please look at the section at the very beginning of this profile called "Class." Next, turn to Table 22 and you will find guidelines listed by the class involved!

Available Dosage Forms and Strengths
> Eye solutions — 0.25%, 0.5%
> Eye solution combo — timolol 0.5% and 2% dorzolamide (Cosopt)
> Eye solution combo — timolol 5 mg/mL and 50 mcg/mL latanoprost (Xalacom)
> Timoptic-XE — 2.5 mg/mL and 5 mg/mL
> Tablets — 5 mg, 10 mg, 20 mg

▷ **Usual Adult Dosage Ranges:** *Anti-anginal and antihypertensive:* Initially 10 mg two times daily; increase dose gradually every 7 days as needed and tolerated. Usual maintenance dose is 10 to 20 mg once a day or divided into two equal doses and taken twice daily. The total daily dose should not exceed 60 mg. Used alone or in combination with a water pill (diuretic).
Migraine headache prevention: Initially 10 mg two times daily; increase dose as needed to 10 mg in the morning and 20 mg at night.
Preventing repeat heart attack: 10 mg twice daily.
Anti-glaucoma: One drop in affected eye twice daily.
> **Author's Note: Timoptic-XE form is a clear gel and is used as one drop, once daily.**
> **Note: Actual dose and schedule must be determined for each patient individually.**

Combination: Cosopt: One drop twice a day

Combination: Xalacom: One drop a day.

Conditions Requiring Dosing Adjustments
Liver Function: Prudent to decrease systemic (nonophthalmic) doses in people with liver diseases.
Kidney Function: Patients with kidney compromise should be followed closely and the dose decreased if the medication appears to be accumulating.

▷ **Dosing Instructions:** Systemic forms: Preferably taken 1 hour before eating to maximize absorption. Immediate release tablets may be crushed. Do not stop this drug abruptly. Eyedrops or gel must be used on an ongoing basis.

Wash your hands before using the eye drops and do not touch the dropper end. If you forget a dose: Take the missed dose as soon as you remember it, unless it's 4 hours or less until your next dose—if that is the case, skip the missed dose and take the next dose right on schedule. DO NOT double up on doses. Talk with your doctor and pharmacist if you find yourself missing doses—there are beeper-based systems, phone call reminders, and other products to help you remember your medicines.

Usual Duration of Use: Use on a regular schedule for 10 to 14 days usually determines effectiveness in preventing angina, controlling heart rhythm disorders, and lowering blood pressure. Peak benefit may require continual use for 6 to 8 weeks. The long-term use of pill forms will be determined by the course of your symptoms and response to an overall treatment program (weight reduction, salt restriction, smoking cessation, etc.). Ophthalmic forms start to work in 15 to 20 minutes, but require ongoing doses to keep eye pressure low. Follow-up with your doctor is mandatory.

Typical Treatment Goals and Measurements (Outcomes and Markers)

Blood Pressure: Guidelines (JNC VII) define normal blood pressure (BP) as **less than** 120/80 and **pre-hypertension** as 120/80 to 139/89. This new range is intended to help doctors encourage lifestyle changes (or, in the case of people with a risk factor for high blood pressure, start treatment) much earlier—so that damage to blood vessels, heart, kidneys, sexual potency, or eyes might be minimized or avoided altogether. Stage 1 hypertension is 140/90 to 159/99, and stage 2 hypertension equal to or greater than 160/100 mm Hg. These guidelines also recommend that clinicians work with their patients to agree on the goals and a plan of treatment. The first-ever guidelines for blood pressure (hypertension) in African Americans recommends that MOST black patients be started on TWO antihypertensive medicines with the goal of lowering blood pressure to 130/80 for those with high risk for heart and blood vessel disease or with diabetes. The American Diabetes Association also recommends 130/80 as the target for diabetics and less than 125/75 for those who spill more than one gram of protein into their urine. Most clinicians try to achieve a BP that confers the best balance of lower cardiovascular risk and avoids the problem of too low a blood pressure. Blood pressure duration is generally increased with beneficial restriction of sodium. If goals are not met, it is not unusual to intensify doses or add on medicines.

Glaucoma: Ophthalmologists measure intraocular pressure (IOP) and then check IOP lowering once this medicine is started. The chamber angle can be checked prior to treatment.

Possible Advantages of This Drug: XE form for eye (ophthalmic) use actually forms a clear gel from the initial application of a solution. Once-daily dosing is expected to help people remember to take their medicine (adherence benefit).

▷ **This Drug Should Not Be Taken If**
- you have bronchial asthma or severe obstructive lung disease.
- you have had an allergic reaction to it previously.
- you have Prinzmetal's variant angina (coronary artery spasm).
- you have congestive heart failure.
- you have an abnormally slow heart rate or a serious form of heart block.
- you took a monoamine oxidase (MAO) type A (see Drug Classes) in the last 14 days.

▷ **Inform Your Physician Before Taking This Drug If**
- you had an adverse reaction to a beta blocker (see Drug Classes).
- you have a history of serious heart disease or impaired circulation.
- you have a history of hay fever (allergic rhinitis), asthma, chronic bronchitis, or emphysema.
- you have a history of overactive thyroid function (hyperthyroidism).
- you have a history of low blood sugar (hypoglycemia).
- you have impaired liver or kidney function.
- you have Raynaud's phenomenon.
- you have diabetes or myasthenia gravis.
- you currently take digitalis, quinidine or reserpine, or any calcium-channel-blocker drug (see Drug Classes).
- you plan to have surgery under general anesthesia in the near future.

Author's Note: Above contraindications and precautions apply for the systemic form. For ophthalmic:

▷ **This Drug Should Not Be Taken If**
- you are allergic to timolol, latanoprost, dorzolamide, or any substance in the eye drop.
- you have asthma or chronic obstructive pulmonary disease (COPD).
- you have severe slow heartbeat (bradycardia), overt heart failure, second- or third-degree AV block, or are in cardiogenic shock.

▷ **Inform Your Physician Before Taking This Drug If**
- you have congestive heart failure.
- you have a history of ongoing bronchitis or emphysema.
- you have diabetes or hypothyroidism.
- you have risk factors for macular edema (lens capsule tear, aphakia, or pseudoaphakia).
- you have contact lenses (remove them before instilling and do not put them back in for 15–20 minutes), an inflammatory eye condition, or an eye infection.
- you have a history of sulfonamide allergy (if taking dorzolamide combination eyedrop).

Possible Side Effects (natural, expected, and unavoidable drug actions)
Lethargy and fatigability, cold extremities, slow heart rate, light-headedness in upright position (see Orthostatic Hypotension in Glossary).

▷ **Possible Adverse Effects** (unusual, unexpected, and infrequent reactions)
If any of the following develop, consult your physician promptly for guidance.
Mild Adverse Effects
Allergic reactions: skin rash, itching.
Loss of hair involving the scalp, eyebrows, and/or eyelashes. This effect can occur with use of the oral tablets or the eyedrops (used to treat glaucoma). Regrowth occurs with discontinuation of this drug.
Headache, dizziness, visual disturbances, vivid dreams—infrequent.
Indigestion, nausea, vomiting, diarrhea—infrequent.
Numbness and tingling in extremities, joint pain—case reports.
Serious Adverse Effects
Allergic reactions: laryngospasm, severe dermatitis.
Idiosyncratic reactions: acute behavioral disturbances—depression, hallucinations.
Chest pain, shortness of breath, precipitation of congestive heart failure—case reports.

Induction of bronchial asthma (in asthmatic individuals)—possible.

May mask warning signs of impending low blood sugar (hypoglycemia) in drug-treated diabetes.

Drug-induced myasthenia gravis—case reports.

Periodic cramping of the leg (intermittent claudication)—possible.

Stopping of breathing (respiratory arrest)—case report.

Author's Note: Some of the eyedrop combination or timolol forms or eye gel form can get into your body. While the listed possible reactions are mainly for the forms taken by mouth (oral), they may possibly (although much less likely) happen with the eye forms.

▷ **Possible Effects on Sexual Function:** Decreased libido, impaired erection, impotence—case reports.

Note: All of these effects can occur with the use of timolol eyedrops at recommended dose, albeit less often.

▷ **Adverse Effects That May Mimic Natural Diseases or Disorders**
Reduced blood flow to extremities may resemble Raynaud's phenomenon (see Glossary).

Natural Diseases or Disorders That May Be Activated by This Drug
Prinzmetal's variant angina, Raynaud's phenomenon, intermittent claudication, myasthenia gravis (questionable).

Possible Effects on Laboratory Tests
None reported.

CAUTION

1. ***Do not stop this drug suddenly*** without the knowledge and guidance of your doctor. Carry a note stating that you take this drug.
2. Ask your doctor or pharmacist before using nasal decongestants usually present in over-the-counter cold preparations and nose drops (less likely to be any problem with the eye forms of this medicine). With systemic use of timolol, these can cause sudden increases in blood pressure when taken concurrently with beta-blocker drugs.
3. Report development of tendency to emotional depression.

Precautions for Use
By Infants and Children: Safety and effectiveness for those under 12 years of age are not established. However, if this drug is used, watch for low blood sugar (hypoglycemia) during periods of reduced food intake.
By Those Over 60 Years of Age: High blood pressure should be reduced without creating risks associated with excessively low blood pressure. Small starting doses and frequent blood pressure checks are needed. Sudden, rapid, and excessive lowering of blood pressure can predispose to stroke or heart attack. Watch for dizziness, unsteadiness, falling, confusion, hallucinations, depression, or urinary frequency.

▷ **Advisability of Use During Pregnancy**
Pregnancy Category: C. See Pregnancy Risk Categories at the back of this book.
Animal Studies: No significant increase in birth defects due to this drug.
Human Studies: Adequate studies of pregnant women are not available.
Avoid use during the first 3 months if possible. Use only if clearly needed. Ask your physician for guidance.

Advisability of Use If Breast-Feeding
Presence of this drug in breast milk: Yes.
Monitor nursing infant closely, and discontinue drug or nursing if adverse effects develop.

Habit-Forming Potential: None.

Effects of Overdose: Weakness, slow pulse, low blood pressure, fainting, cold and sweaty skin, congestive heart failure, possible coma, and convulsions.

Possible Effects of Long-Term Use: Reduced heart reserve and eventual heart failure in susceptible people with advanced heart disease. Contraindicated in overt heart failure.

Suggested Periodic Examinations While Taking This Drug (at physician's discretion)
Complete blood cell counts (because of adverse effects of other drugs of this class).
Measurements of blood pressure.
Evaluation of heart function.
Lowering of eye (intraocular) pressure with ophthalmic forms.

▷ **While Taking This Drug, Observe the Following**
Foods: No restrictions. Avoid excessive salt intake.
Herbal Medicines or Minerals: Ginseng, guarana, bitter orange, country mallow, hawthorn, saw palmetto, ma huang (no longer on the U.S. market for weight loss), goldenseal, yohimbe, and licorice may also cause increased blood pressure. Excessive caffeine from coffee, mate, or guarana may also increase blood pressure. Dong quai and St. John's wort may inhibit liver removal of this medicine. Combination is NOT advisable. Calcium and garlic may help lower blood pressure. Use caution and work with your doctor to make sure blood pressure is not lowered too much. Indian snakeroot has a German Commission E monograph indication for hypertension—talk to your doctor. Eleuthero root and ephedra should be avoided by people living with hypertension. Scopolia root has glaucoma as a possible side effect. DO NOT COMBINE. Henbane and belladonna should also be avoided. Talk to your doctor BEFORE combining any herbals with this drug.
Beverages: No restrictions. May be taken with milk.
▷ *Alcohol:* Use with caution. Alcohol may exaggerate this drug's ability to lower blood pressure and may increase its mild sedative effect.
Tobacco Smoking: Nicotine may reduce this drug's effectiveness. I advise everyone to quit smoking.
▷ *Other Drugs*
Timolol may ***increase*** the effects of
• amiodarone (Cordarone) and cause cardiac arrest and bradycardia.
• other antihypertensive drugs and cause excessive lowering of blood pressure; dose adjustments may be necessary (for example, alpha-1 blockers or dihydropyridine calcium channel blockers). Calcium channel blockers (such as diltiazem or verapamil) may also change heart electrical conduction (AV Conduction).
• ergot derivatives, increasing risk of decreased blood flow to arms and legs (peripheral ischemia).
• lidocaine (Xylocaine, etc.).
• reserpine (Ser-Ap-Es, etc.) and cause sedation, depression, slowing of the heart rate, and lowering of blood pressure.
• verapamil (Calan, Isoptin) and cause excessive depression of heart function; monitor this combination closely.
Timolol may ***decrease*** the effects of
• theophyllines (Aminophyllin, Theo-Dur, etc.) and reduce their antiasthmatic effectiveness.

Timolol *taken concurrently* with
- clonidine (Catapres) requires close monitoring for rebound high blood pressure if clonidine is withdrawn while timolol is still being taken.
- epinephrine (Adrenalin, etc.) may cause marked rise in blood pressure and slowing of the heart rate.
- insulin may hide the symptoms of hypoglycemia (see Glossary).
- methyldopa may have paradoxical increases in blood pressure.
- oral hypoglycemic agents (see Oral Antidiabetic Drugs in Drug Classes) such as acetohexamide (Dymelor) and glipizide (Glucotrol) may result in prolonged low blood sugar.
- quinidine (Quinaglute, others) may lead to excessive slowing of the heart.
- venlafaxine (Effexor) may result in increased risk of timolol toxicity.

Timolol/latanoprost form *taken concurrently* with
- pilocarpine will blunt latanoprost results.
- thimerosal will lead to precipitation of the eye drop. Separate doses by 5–10 minutes.

The following drugs may *increase the effects* of timolol:
- chlorpromazine (Thorazine, etc.).
- cimetidine (Tagamet).
- fluoxetine (Prozac).
- fluvoxamine (Luvox).
- methimazole (Tapazole).
- propylthiouracil (Propacil).
- ritonavir (Norvir) and perhaps other protease inhibitors (see Drug Classes).
- zileuton (Zyflo).

The following drugs may *decrease the effects* of timolol:
- antacids (when taken at the same time).
- barbiturates (phenobarbital, etc.).
- indomethacin (Indocin) and possibly other aspirin substitutes, or NSAIDs—may impair timolol's antihypertensive effect.
- rifabutin (Mycobutin).
- rifampin (Rifadin, Rimactane).

▷ *Driving, Hazardous Activities:* Use caution until the full extent of dizziness, lethargy, and blood pressure change has been determined.

Aviation Note: The use of this drug *may be a disqualification* for piloting. Consult a designated Aviation Medical Examiner.

Exposure to Sun: No restrictions.

Exposure to Heat: Caution is advised. Hot environments can exaggerate the effects of this drug.

Exposure to Cold: Caution is advised. Cold environments can worsen circulatory deficiency in the extremities that may occur with this drug. The elderly should be careful to prevent hypothermia (see Glossary).

Heavy Exercise or Exertion: It is advisable to avoid exertion that produces light-headedness, excessive fatigue, or muscle cramping. The use of this drug may intensify the hypertensive response to isometric exercise.

Occurrence of Unrelated Illness: Fever can lower blood pressure and require adjustment of dose. Nausea or vomiting may interrupt the dosing schedule. Ask your doctor for help.

Discontinuation: It is advisable to avoid sudden discontinuation of this drug in all situations; this is especially true in the presence of coronary artery disease. If possible, gradual reduction of dose over a period of 2 to 3 weeks is recommended. Ask your physician for specific guidance.

TOLBUTAMIDE (tohl BYU ta mide)

Introduced: 1956   **Class:** Antidiabetic, sulfonylureas   **Prescription:** USA: Yes   **Controlled Drug:** USA: No; Canada: No   **Available as Generic:** Yes

Brand Names: ✤Apo-Tolbutamide, ✤Mobenol, ✤Novo-butamide, Oramide, Orinase, Orinase Diagnostic, SK-Tolbutamide

Warning: The brand names Orinase, Ornade, and Ornex sound similar; this can lead to serious medication errors. Orinase is tolbutamide, used to treat diabetes. Ornade is chlorpheniramine and phenylpropanolamine, used to treat nasal and sinus congestion. Ornex is acetaminophen and phenylpropanolamine, used to treat head colds and sinus pain. Make sure you get the correct drug.

Author's Note: The information in this profile has been shortened to make room for more widely used medicines.

TOLCAPONE (TOHL ka poan)

Introduced: 1998   **Class:** COMT inhibitor, anti-Parkinsonism   **Prescription:** USA: Yes   **Controlled Drug:** USA: No   **Available as Generic:** No

Brand Names: Tasmar

Author's Note: The information in this profile will be broadened in subsequent editions once concerns about possible liver toxicity are resolved.

TOLMETIN (TOHL met in)

Please see the acetic acid (nonsteroidal anti-inflammatory drug) family profile.

TOLTERODINE (tol TER oh dyne)

Introduced: 1998   **Class:** Muscarinic receptor antagonist, overactive bladder treatment   **Prescription:** USA: Yes   **Controlled Drug:** USA: No   **Available as Generic:** No

Brand Names: Detrol, Detrol LA, ✤Detrol SR, ✤Unidet

```
┌─────────────────────────────────────────────────────────────────┐
│                      BENEFITS versus RISKS                        │
│        Possible Benefits                    Possible Risks        │
│  EFFECTIVE TREATMENT OF            CONSTIPATION                    │
│    OVERACTIVE BLADDER              Dry mouth or throat             │
│  CONTROLS URGE TO URINATE          Blurred vision                 │
│  LOWERS FREQUENCY OF                                               │
│    URINATION                                                      │
│  DECREASES UNEXPECTED                                              │
│    URGENT DESIRE TO URINATE                                        │
│    (URGE INCONTINENCE)                                             │
│  ONCE DAILY FORM OFFERS                                            │
│    INCREASED CONTROL AND                                           │
│    ADHERENCE                                                       │
└─────────────────────────────────────────────────────────────────┘
```

▷ **Principal Uses**

As a Single Drug Product: Uses currently included in FDA-approved labeling: (1) Treats symptoms of overactive bladders; (2) used to decrease excessive urination (urinary frequency); (3) eases unexpected urgent desire to urinate followed by inability to control the bladder (urinary urgency, urge incontinence).

Other (unlabeled) generally accepted uses: None at present.

How This Drug Works: Acts as an anticholinergic agent (competitive muscarinic receptor antagonist) with some selective action on the bladder. This effect increases volume of residual urine and decreases maximum detrusor pressure. This makes it more difficult to urinate, easing overactive bladder symptoms and helping urge incontinence.

▷ **Widely Used Guidelines That Involve This Medicine (representative sample):** Please look at the section at the very beginning of this profile called "Class." Next, turn to Table 22 and you will find guidelines listed by the class involved!

Available Dosage Forms and Strengths

Capsules, extended release (LA, SR) — 2 mg, 4 mg

Tablets — 1 mg, 2 mg

▷ **Usual Adult Dosage Ranges:** Started with 2 mg twice a day. The dose may be lowered to 1 mg twice a day if the higher dose is not tolerated. People taking drugs inhibiting liver enzymes CYP3A4 and CYP2D6 should also be given 1 mg twice daily as other medicines can cause tolterodine to accumulate. *Detrol LA* form is dosed at 4 mg once daily. As with the immediate-release form, the dose is decreased (to 2 mg once daily) for those taking drugs inhibiting CYP 3A4 or 2D6 or in people with lowered kidney or liver function.

Note: Actual dose and schedule must be determined for each patient individually.

Conditions Requiring Dosing Adjustments

Liver Function: Dose should be decreased to 1 mg twice a day of the immediate-release form or 2 mg once daily of Detrol LA in liver disease. (As this drug undergoes cytochrome P-450 2D6 and CYP3A4 metabolism.)

Kidney Function: Used with caution. The drug was not studied in kidney disease, but dose should be decreased to 1 mg of the immediate-release form twice daily or to 2 mg once daily of Detrol LA.

▷ **Dosing Instructions:** The immediate release tablet may be crushed and taken without regard to food (food does increase bioavailability—53% on average—but this is not thought to be clinically significant). The LA or SR form or any other extended release forms should not be crushed, altered, or chewed. If you forget a dose: Take the missed dose as soon as you remember it, unless it's nearly time for your next dose—if that is the case, skip the missed dose and take the next dose right on schedule. DO NOT double up on doses. Talk with your doctor if you find yourself missing doses.

Usual Duration of Use: Initial response to this medicine happens in about an hour. The clinical trials leading to FDA approval showed some benefits of use on a regular schedule in one trial at 4 weeks and peak and consistent benefits at 12 weeks. It is important to follow up with your doctor regarding side effects (dose may need to be decreased) and therapeutic benefits.

Typical Treatment Goals and Measurements (Outcomes and Markers)

Bladder Activity: Most urologists use patient reports of lowered desire or frequency of urination as a hallmark of successful therapy. A general sense of decreased need to urinate immediately (urgency) is also useful. Some physicians will use a bladder diary to help define, in absolute terms, the beneficial effects of this medicine. More invasive cystometry can also be used.

Possible Advantages of This Drug

May be more selective for the bladder than other medicines. If bladder selectivity stands up, this medicine may be a drug of choice based on more favorable cardiovascular profile—especially in people with heart disease or in elderly patients.

▷ **This Drug Should Not Be Taken If**
- you are allergic to tolterodine.
- you retain urine abnormally (retention of urine).
- you have a problem with retaining food or fluid in the stomach (gastric retention).
- you have narrow-angle glaucoma that is not controlled.

▷ **Inform Your Physician Before Taking This Drug If**
- you have liver or kidney disease.
- you have a history of ulcerative colitis.
- you have narrow-angle glaucoma controlled by medicines.
- your job requires visual acuity.
- you have heart or blood vessel disease (edema and slight increased heart rate possible, but generally a more favorable profile than other medicines for this condition).
- you have had a bowel obstruction or ulcerative colitis.
- you are breast-feeding your child.
- you are prone to constipation.
- you will have surgery under general anesthesia soon.

Possible Side Effects (natural, expected, and unavoidable drug actions)

Dry mouth, nasal congestion, indigestion (dyspepsia), constipation—may be frequent.

▷ **Possible Adverse Effects** (unusual, unexpected, and infrequent reactions)

If any of the following develop, consult your physician promptly for guidance.

Mild Adverse Effects

Allergic reaction: skin rash.

Dizziness or headache—infrequent.

Blurred vision and increased light sensitivity—rare to infrequent.

Decreased salivation—infrequent.

Fast heart rate (tachycardia)—reported.
Dryness of hands or feet—infrequent.
Edema—reported.
Serious Adverse Effects
Allergic reactions: anaphylactoid reactions.
Passing out (syncope)—case reports in clinical trials.
Liver toxicity—case report (possibly a hypersensitivity reaction).
Hallucinations—case reports.
Cerebrovascular disorder—case reports, possibly related to the drug in clinical trials.
Urinary retention—case reports.

▷ **Possible Effects on Sexual Function:** None defined.

Natural Diseases or Disorders That May Be Activated by This Drug
Tendency to constipation may be worsened.
Narrow-angle glaucoma may be worsened.

Possible Effects on Laboratory Tests: Liver function tests may be increased.

CAUTION
1. Some people (about 7% of the population) are poor metabolizers of this drug. This means that the medicine may accumulate and more of an effect from a "normal dose" will be seen in those people. Once this pattern is identified, doses will need to be decreased to avoid getting too much of the medicine from a "normal" dose.
2. Talk to your doctor or dentist about sugarless candy or other measures to take if dry mouth becomes a problem.
3. If you are prone to constipation, it may be prudent to start a medicine to address possible constipation if this medicine is started.

Precautions for Use
By Infants and Children: Safety and effectiveness not established in pediatrics.
By Those Over 60 Years of Age: No dosage change is recommended by the manufacturer. Mean blood concentrations of the drug and its metabolite were increased by 20–50%, but no overall safety differences were seen between older and younger patients who were studied.

▷ **Advisability of Use During Pregnancy**
Pregnancy Category: C. See Pregnancy Risk Categories at the back of this book.
Animal Studies: No birth defects found in mice studies.
Human Studies: Adequate studies of pregnant women are not available.
Use this drug only if clearly needed. Ask your doctor for help.

Advisability of Use If Breast-Feeding
Presence of this drug in breast milk: Yes in mice, unknown in humans.
Stop the medicine or discontinue nursing.

Habit-Forming Potential: None.

Effects of Overdose: Severe central anticholinergic effects.

Possible Effects of Long-Term Use: None reported.

Suggested Periodic Examinations While Taking This Drug (at physician's discretion)
Follow-up on decreased urination versus adverse effects.
Baseline liver function test and follow up with any change in stool color, abdominal pain, yellowing of the skin, or dark urine would be prudent.

▷ **While Taking This Drug, Observe the Following**
Foods: Grapefruit is not advisable.

Herbal Medicines or Minerals: Since St. John's wort and tolterodine may increase sun sensitivity, the combination is NOT advised. Caffeine-containing beverages as well as kola, mate, guarana, ephedra, and ma huang may increase blood pressure, eventually leading to possible increased fluid removal and increased need to urinate. Caution is advised.

Beverages: Grapefruit juice is not advisable. May be taken with water or milk. See caffeine note above (coffee and some teas). Some teas also contain substances that act as mild diuretics.

▷ *Alcohol:* Alcohol can increase loss of water from the body. This can work against the action of this medicine.

Tobacco Smoking: Nicotine may work counter to this medicine. Avoid all forms of tobacco.

▷ *Other Drugs*

Tolterodine **taken concurrently** with

• other medicines that inhibit CYP3A4 or CYP2D6 (such as macrolide antibiotics [erythromycin and clarithromycin], itraconazole, ketoconazole, voriconazole [Vfend], and others) may lead to excessive blood levels and toxicity risk.

• fluoxetine (Prozac) may lead to tolterodine toxicity.

• warfarin (Coumadin) may lead to increased bleeding risk. More frequent laboratory tests (INRs) are prudent with dosing adjusted as needed.

▷ *Driving, Hazardous Activities:* This drug may cause blurred vision and dizziness. Restrict activities as necessary.

Aviation Note: The use of this drug **may be a disqualification** for piloting. Consult a designated Aviation Medical Examiner.

Exposure to Sun: May increase sensitivity of your eyes to the sun.

Heavy Exercise or Exertion: Excessive exertion is cooled by sweating. This medicine may lead to drying of skin and decreased perspiration.

Discontinuation: Ask your doctor for help.

TOPIRAMATE (TOH peer ah mate)

Introduced: 1999 **Class:** Anticonvulsant, mood stabilizer **Prescription:** USA: Yes **Controlled Drug:** USA: No; Canada: No **Available as Generic:** USA: No

Brand Names: Topamax, Topamax Sprinkle

BENEFITS versus RISKS	
Possible Benefits	*Possible Risks*
EFFECTIVE MANAGEMENT OF SEIZURES THAT RESIST THERAPY	CHANGES IN THINKING
	Weight loss
INCREASE IN SEIZURE-FREE DAYS	
MANAGEMENT OF PARTIAL SEIZURES	
MANAGEMENT OF SEIZURES ASSOCIATED WITH LENNOX-GASTAUT SYNDROME	
Weight loss	

▷ **Principal Uses**

As a Single Drug Product: Uses currently included in FDA-approved labeling: (1) Adjunctive combination therapy of generalized (tonic-clonic, partial onset) seizures in adults and children (2–16); (2) adjunctive combination treatment of Lennox-Gastaut syndrome in patients 2 years old and older.

Other (unlabeled) generally accepted uses: (1) May have a role in treating binge eating; (2) could have a role in bipolar disorder; (3) some case-based use in Tourette's syndrome; (4) because weight gain happens with selective serotonin reuptake inhibitors (SSRIs), this medicine may have beneficial effects in fighting weight gain in adults (may be an undesirable effect in children).

How This Drug Works: The exact mechanism of action is not exactly known. It appears to block the action of nerve cells (neurons) by blocking sodium channels—this keeps the nerve cells from firing excessively. Topiramate works to help a compound that inhibits nerves (an inhibitory neurotransmitter called gamma-aminobutyric acid or GABA). It also has the effect of increasing GABA concentrations. Lastly, this medicine works against a chemical called kainate and a corresponding activator called glutamate. Weight loss specifics are not identified.

▷ **Widely Used Guidelines That Involve This Medicine (representative sample):** Please look at the section at the very beginning of this profile called "Class." Next, turn to Table 22 and you will find guidelines listed by the class involved!

Available Dosage Forms and Strengths

Capsules — 15 mg, 25 mg

Coated tablets — 25 mg, 100 mg, 200 mg

▷ **Recommended Dosage Ranges** (Actual dose and schedule must be determined for each patient individually.)

Infants and Children: Lennox-Gastaut, partial onset, or tonic-clonic (generalized) seizures (2–16 years old): Dosing is accomplished on a weight basis and is started with 1–3 mg/kg each night or 25 mg, whichever is less. This dosing is continued for 7 days and effectiveness checked. Subsequently, doses can be increased as needed and tolerated by steps of 1–3 mg/kg/24 hours. If dosing is increased, the total daily dose is equally divided into two doses, given in the morning and at night. If additional increases are needed the same 1–3mg/kg/24 hour step is taken, but at intervals of 7–14 days. Ongoing (maintenance) doses are generally in the range of 5–9 mg/kg per day. The total dose is separated into two equal doses. The Topamax Sprinkle capsule form offers the advantage of being opened and sprinkled on food (roughly a teaspoon) and taken right away.

17 years old or older: For Lennox-Gastaut, partial onset, or tonic-clonic (generalized) seizures: Dosing is started with 50 mg in the evening. Similar to the pediatric dosing, increases are typically made in steps, and in this case, increased as needed and tolerated to 50 mg in the morning and 50 mg in the evening, then 50 mg in the morning and 100 mg in the evening, and so on. In patients receiving medicines known to interact, dosing should be guided by blood levels and patient tolerance and adjusted as needed. Doses more than 800 mg twice a day have NOT been used.

Over 65 Years of Age: Same dosing as 16 to 65, but because kidney function tends to decline as we age, it is prudent to more slowly increase (titrate) this medicine, check blood levels, and carefully follow patients in this population.

Conditions Requiring Dosing Adjustments

Liver Function: This medicine is changed in the liver, but specific guidelines for dosing are not currently available. Prudent to start slowly (low dose), obtain blood levels, and assess current recommendations if a decision is made to start this medicine in patients with compromised liver function.

Kidney Function: Most of this medicine (once changed or glucuronidated) is removed by the kidneys. Used with caution and with more frequent blood levels (in severe kidney failure).

Author's Note: Information in this profile will be broadened in subsequent editions if clinical studies and results warrant this. This medicine is generally removed more quickly in children than in adults. A given dose in children could lead to a lower level than that seen in adults.

TRAMADOL (TRAM ah doll)

Introduced: 1996   **Class:** Analgesic   **Prescription:** USA: Yes
Controlled Drug: USA: Yes; Canada: No   **Available as Generic:** USA: Yes; Canada: No
Brand Names: Ultram, Ultracet [CD]

BENEFITS versus RISKS	
Possible Benefits	*Possible Risks*
EFFECTIVE TREATMENT OF PAIN	DROWSINESS
MINIMAL SIDE EFFECTS VERSUS	May decrease the seizure threshold
MORPHINE-LIKE AGENTS	Constipation
(OPIOIDS)	

▷ **Principal Uses**

As a Single Drug Product: Uses currently included in FDA-approved labeling: Used to provide symptomatic relief in all types of pain.

Other (unlabeled) generally accepted uses: (1) May have a role in pain where depression is also a therapeutic problem; (2) might have a role as an adjunct to anesthesia; (3) eases fibromyalgia pain.

As a Combination Drug Product [CD]: Available combined with acetaminophen (325 mg) for sudden (acute) pain.

How This Drug Works: Increases the availability of serotonin and norepinephrine in certain brain centers and also works at opioid (see Glossary) centers, thereby relieving pain.

▷ **Widely Used Guidelines That Involve This Medicine (representative sample):** Please look at the section at the very beginning of this profile called "Class." Next, turn to Table 22 and you will find guidelines listed by the class involved!

Available Dosage Forms and Strengths
Tablets — 50 mg
Tablets combined form — 37.5 mg tramadol, 325 mg acetaminophen

▷ **Usual Adult Dosage Ranges:** 50 to 100 mg every 4 to 6 hours. Many patients respond to 150 to 300 mg daily. The total daily dose should not exceed 400 mg. German data found clinicians using 0.7 mg per kg per dose and 5.6 mg per kg of body mass per day as a maximum for those over 18 years of age.

Ultracet form: Used for short-term (5 days or less) management of sudden (acute) pain. Two tablets are given every 4–6 hours up to a daily maximum of 8 tablets.

Note: Actual dose and schedule must be determined for each patient individually.

Conditions Requiring Dosing Adjustments

Liver Function: Patients with cirrhosis should be closely watched for adverse effects and may take only 50 mg every 12 hours of the tramadol form. The Ultracet form HAS NOT BEEN STUDIED and should not be used in that population at present.

Kidney Function: For patients with creatinine clearances less than 30 mL/min, usual dose is taken every 12 hours, and the daily maximum is 200 mg for the tramadol form. The Ultracet form has not been studied in this population, but previous tramadol dosing suggests use of no more than 2 Ultracet tablets every 12 hours.

▷ **Dosing Instructions:** May be taken without regard to meals. The tablet may be crushed. If excessive drowsiness or dizziness occurs, call your doctor. If you forget a dose: Take the missed dose as soon as you remember it, unless it's nearly time for your next dose—if that is the case, skip the missed dose and take the next dose right on schedule. DO NOT double doses. Talk with your doctor if you find yourself missing doses.

Usual Duration of Use: Peak effect usually happens in half an hour. Use on a regular schedule depends on the condition treated. Many chronic pain syndromes are treated with combinations of medicines. Long-term use requires supervision by your doctor. Ultracet form is only approved for use up to five days.

Typical Treatment Goals and Measurements (Outcomes and Markers)

Pain: Most clinicians treating pain use a device called an algometer to check your pain. This looks like a small ruler, but lets the clinician better understand your pain. The goals of treatment then relate to where the level of pain started (for example, a rating of 7 on a 0 to 10 scale) and what the cause of the pain was. I use the PQRSTBG (see Glossary) method. Pain medicines may also be used together (in combination) in order to get the best result or outcome. If your pain control is not acceptable to YOU (remember, in hospitals and outpatient settings, etc., pain control is a patient right and the fifth vital sign), call your doctor. It is not unusual to have an immediate-release rescue dose available and then some percentage of previous day use added back to an extended-release form. Pain can be dynamic, and adjustments are often required.

Possible Advantages of This Drug

Avoids narcotic (opioid) side effects.

▷ **This Drug Should Not Be Taken If**

• you have had an allergic reaction to it previously.
• you are allergic to codeine or similar compounds.
• you have a history of seizures or take medicines that may make seizures more likely.
• you are intoxicated by morphinelike drugs or alcohol.
• you are taking, or have taken within the last 14 days, a monoamine oxidase (MAO) inhibitor.

▷ **Inform Your Physician Before Taking This Drug If**

• you have a history of alcoholism, epilepsy, narcotic addiction, or thyroid gland problems.

- you are prone to constipation.
- you have impaired liver or kidney function.
- you are pregnant or breast-feeding your infant.
- you plan to have surgery under general anesthesia in the near future.

Possible Side Effects (natural, expected, and unavoidable drug actions)
Drowsiness, light-headedness on standing (orthostatic hypotension)—rare.
Blurred vision, dry mouth, constipation—infrequent to frequent.

▷ **Possible Adverse Effects** (unusual, unexpected, and infrequent reactions)
If any of the following develop, consult your physician promptly for guidance.

Mild Adverse Effects
Allergic reaction: skin rash.
Rapid heart rate, palpitations—case reports.
Nausea, vomiting, diarrhea—infrequent to frequent.
Sweating—frequent.
Urinary retention—possible.

Serious Adverse Effects
Allergic reaction: anaphylaxis—case reports.
Behavioral effects: confusion, hallucinations—case reports.
Abnormal ECG, myocardial ischemia, or palpitations—reported.
Seizures—increased risk, especially in those with seizure disorders or in those who take medicines that can make seizures more likely (should not be used).
Serotonin syndrome—case reports.
Movement problem (ataxia)—one case report with a 100 mg dose.
Lowered blood pressure—possible and dose-related.

▷ **Possible Effects on Sexual Function:** Decreased male or female libido—possible.

Possible Effects on Laboratory Tests
Liver enzymes: increased.

CAUTION
1. If you experience a significant degree of mouth dryness while using this drug, consult your dentist regarding the risk of gum erosion or tooth decay. Ask for guidance in ways to keep the mouth comfortably moist.
2. If you have breathing problems (such as chronic obstructive pulmonary disease [COPD]), you may be at greater risk for respiratory depression.
3. DO NOT take this medicine if you are allergic to codeine (more likely to have a serious reaction).

Precautions for Use
By Infants and Children: Safety and effectiveness for use by those under 18 years of age have not been established.
By Those Over 60 Years of Age: Lower starting doses and adjustment to calculated creatinine clearance are prudent. During the first 2 weeks of treatment, observe for confusion or disorientation. Be aware of possible unsteadiness and incoordination that may predispose to falling. This drug may enhance prostatism (see Glossary).

▷ **Advisability of Use During Pregnancy**
Pregnancy Category: C. See Pregnancy Risk Categories at the back of this book.
Animal Studies: Fetal deaths and birth defects reported at doses 3 to 15 times the human dose.
Human Studies: Adequate studies of pregnant women are not available.
Avoid this drug completely during the first 3 months. Ask your physician for guidance.

Advisability of Use If Breast-Feeding
Presence of this drug in breast milk: Yes.
Avoid drug or refrain from nursing.

Habit-Forming Potential: May cause psychological or physical dependence.

Effects of Overdose: Marked drowsiness, weakness, confusion, tremors, stupor, coma, possible seizures.

Possible Effects of Long-Term Use: May increase likelihood of dependence.

Suggested Periodic Examinations While Taking This Drug (at physician's discretion)
Heart rate and blood pressure.
Bowel and bladder status.
Evaluation for tremor or hallucination.
Liver function tests.

▷ **While Taking This Drug, Observe the Following**
Foods: No restrictions.
Herbal Medicines or Minerals: Kava kava and valerian (questions are unresolved for liver toxicity as well) may worsen drowsiness. Since ginseng may act as an MAO inhibitor, DO NOT combine. St. John's wort can change (inducing or increasing) P450 enzymes, blunting the effects of this medicine. Talk to your doctor BEFORE you combine any herbal medicines with tramadol.
Beverages: No restrictions. May be taken with milk.
▷ *Alcohol:* Avoid completely. This drug can markedly increase the intoxicating effects of alcohol and accentuate its depressant action on brain functions.
Tobacco Smoking: No interactions expected. I advise everyone to quit smoking.
▷ *Other Drugs*
Tramadol may ***increase*** the effects of
- antihypertensive drugs and cause excessive lowering of blood pressure; dose adjustments may be necessary.
- drugs with sedative effects and cause excessive sedation (see Antihistamines, Opioids, Antianxiety Drugs, etc., in Drug Classes).
- tricyclic or SSRI antidepressants (see Drug Classes), leading to seizures or leading to serotonin syndrome.
- warfarin (Coumadin), requiring dose adjustment; more frequent INR (protime) tests are prudent.
Tramadol ***taken concurrently*** with
- some antipsychotic medicines (see Drug Classes, such as molindone-Moban) may result in excessive risk of seizures.
- carbamazepine (Tegretol) may lower tramadol benefits.
- clonidine will lessen tramadol's therapeutic effect.
- clozapine (Clozaril) may increase seizure risk.
- cyclobenzaprine (Flexeril) increases seizure risk.
- digoxin (Lanoxin) may lead to digoxin toxicity. Extremely careful patient follow-up and more frequent checks of digoxin levels are needed.
- fluoxetine (Prozac) may result in an increased seizure risk.
- fluvoxamine (Luvox) may result in an increased seizure risk.
- medicines that increase CYP2D6 will decrease benefits of tramadol, while those that decrease or inhibit CYP2D6 will increase effects of tramadol and may also increase chances of adverse effects.
- monoamine oxidase (MAO) inhibitors (see Drug Classes) may result in serious side effects (seizures, cardiovascular collapse)—DO NOT COMBINE.

- other drugs that cause central nervous system depression (see Benzodiazepines, Opioids, and Tranquilizers in Drug Classes) may have additive effects.
- other drugs that increase seizure risks may have additive effects.
- some phenothiazines (see Drug Classes) may result in excessively lowered blood pressure or increased seizure risk.
- quinidine (Quinaglute, others) may change tramadol levels.
- ritonavir (Norvir) and perhaps other protease inhibitors (see Drug Classes) may lead to toxicity.
- sertraline (Zoloft) increases seizure risk.
- venlafaxine (Effexor) increases seizure risk.

▷ *Driving, Hazardous Activities:* This drug may cause dizziness or drowsiness. Restrict activities as necessary.

Aviation Note: The use of this drug *is a disqualification* for piloting. Consult a designated Aviation Medical Examiner.

Exposure to Sun: No restrictions.

Discontinuation: It is advisable to discontinue this drug gradually. Ask your physician for guidance in dose reduction over an appropriate period of time.

TRAVOPROST (TRAV oh prost)

Introduced: 2001   **Class:**   Prostaglandin   analogue,   antiglaucoma
Prescription: USA: Yes   **Controlled Drug:**   USA: No; Canada: No
Available as Generic: No
Brand Name: Travatan

BENEFITS versus RISKS	
Possible Benefits	*Possible Risks*
EFFECTIVE REDUCTION OF INTERNAL EYE PRESSURE FOR CONTROL OF ACUTE AND CHRONIC GLAUCOMA CONTROL OF OCULAR HYPERTENSION ONCE DAILY DOSING HELPS ADHERENCE	Mild side effects with systemic absorption possible with eye use Pigmentation of the iris (appears to be less than latanoprost)

▷ **Principal Uses**

As a Single Drug Product: Uses currently included in FDA-approved labeling: (1) Used to manage glaucoma in patients who are intolerant of or who are not adequately controlled by other intraocular pressure–lowering medicines; (2) lowers increased pressure in the eye (intraocular pressure). Other (unlabeled) generally accepted uses: None as yet.

How This Drug Works: This medicine is changed to (hydrolyzed) to trovoprost free acid (the active form), which subsequently lowers pressure in the eye by increasing outflow from the uveoscleral area without changing aqueous flow.

▷ **Widely Used Guidelines That Involve This Medicine (representative sample):** Please look at the section at the very beginning of this profile called

"Class." Next, turn to Table 22 and you will find guidelines listed by the class involved!

Available Dosage Forms and Strengths
Eyedrop solutions — 0.004% or 40 mcg per mL.

▷ **Usual Adult Dosage Ranges:** For open-angle glaucoma or ocular hypertension: One drop (0.004%) in the eye each evening (once every 24 hours).

Note: Actual dose and dosing schedule must be determined for each patient individually.

Conditions Requiring Dosing Adjustments
Liver Function: The drug is changed to the active form by substances (esterases) in the eye and then in the liver to inactive substances that are removed by the kidneys. Dose changes in liver disease are not defined.

Kidney Function: Changed drug (metabolites) removed by the kidney, but dosing changes in kidney failure are not defined.

▷ **Dosing Instructions:** Remove contact lenses and do not replace them for at least 15 minutes after putting this medicine into your eye. To avoid excessive absorption into the body, press finger against inner corner of the eye (to close off the tear duct) during and for 1 minute after dropping the medicine in. Be careful not to touch the dropper to the eye. If you forget a dose: Take the missed dose as soon as you remember it, unless it's nearly time for your next dose—if that is the case, skip the missed dose and take the next dose right on schedule. DO NOT double doses. Talk with your doctor and pharmacist if you find yourself missing doses.

Usual Duration of Use: Use on a regular schedule for a day usually sees an effect in lowering the pressure in the eye. A week may be required for the full benefits of the medicine to be realized. Long-term use (months to years) requires physician supervision and may require combination therapy if pressure rises again.

Typical Treatment Goals and Measurements (Outcomes and Markers)
Glaucoma: Ophthalmologists measure intraocular pressure (IOP), and then check IOP lowering once this medicine is started. The chamber angle can be checked prior to treatment. A drop in intraocular pressure is common during ongoing use.

▷ **This Drug Should Not Be Taken If**
- you have had an eye infection with herpes simplex (case report authors suggest avoiding latanoprost, and since travoprost is similar, it is prudent to follow the same action).
- you have had an allergic reaction to it previously or to the benzalkonium chloride that is in it.

▷ **Inform Your Physician Before Taking This Drug If**
- you wear contact lenses.
- you have had an eye infection in the last three months.
- you have some of the risk factors for fluid accumulation in the macula (macular edema). Talk to your doctor about this.
- you are pregnant or plan pregnancy.
- you have sudden (acute) angle closure of the eye.

Possible Side Effects (natural, expected, and unavoidable drug actions)
Burning of the eyes or irritation—frequent (usually mild).
Pigmentation of the eye (iridial) has been reported in up to 5% of people who use this medicine. May happen with greater frequency in people with

mixed-color eyes (blue-brown, green-brown, and yellow-brown). This is apparently caused by increased melanin and may be permanent.

Redness of the eye (ocular hyperemia)—up to 50% of patients. Often this is mild, but has led to patients having to stop the medicine roughly 3% of the time.

▷ **Possible Adverse Effects** (unusual, unexpected, and infrequent reactions)

If any of the following develop, consult your physician promptly for guidance.

Mild Adverse Effects

Allergic reactions: itching of the eyes, eyelid itching and/or swelling, or rash. Change in visual acuity—infrequent.

Serious Adverse Effects

Angina pectoris and/or slow heart rate—infrequent (up to 5%).

▷ **Possible Effects on Sexual Function:** None reported.

Natural Diseases or Disorders That May Be Activated by This Drug

Not defined.

Possible Effects on Laboratory Tests

None reported.

Precautions for Use

By Those Over 60 Years of Age: No age-specific changes presently needed.

▷ **Advisability of Use During Pregnancy**

Pregnancy Category: C. See Pregnancy Risk Categories at the end of book.

Human Studies: Adequate studies of pregnant women are not available. Discuss use with your doctor BEFORE using this drug.

Advisability of Use If Breast-Feeding

Presence of this drug in breast milk: Yes, in rats; unknown in humans. Watch infant closely and stop drug or nursing if adverse effects develop.

Habit-Forming Potential: None.

Effects of Overdose: Not defined.

Possible Effects of Long-Term Use: Pigmentation of the iris.

Suggested Periodic Examinations While Taking This Drug (at physician's discretion)

Measurement of internal eye pressure on a regular basis.

Check for early signs of pigmentation.

▷ **While Taking This Drug, Observe the Following**

Foods: No restrictions.

Herbal Medicines or Minerals: Scopolia root has glaucoma as a possible side effect. DO NOT COMBINE. Henbane, ephedra, and belladonna should also be avoided.

Beverages: No restrictions.

▷ *Alcohol:* No restrictions except prudence in alcohol use.

Tobacco Smoking: No interactions expected. I advise everyone to quit smoking.

Marijuana Smoking: Sustained additional decrease in internal eye pressure.

▷ *Other Drugs*

Travoprost *taken concurrently* with

- other eyedrops should be separated by at least 5 minutes.
- thimerosal (various) may cause a precipitation. DO NOT combine eyedrops containing thimerosal with latanoprost. Separate doses by 5 minutes or more.

▷ *Driving, Hazardous Activities:* This drug may cause blurry vision for a time. Restrict activities as necessary.

Aviation Note: The use of this drug **may be a disqualification** for piloting. Consult a designated Aviation Medical Examiner.

Exposure to Sun: This medicine may make your eyes sensitive to the sun. Wear sunglasses. See the table in the back of this book about other medicines that may cause such sensitivity—effects may be additive if these medicines are combined.

Discontinuation: Do not stop regular use of this drug without consulting your physician.

TRAZODONE (TRAZ oh dohn)

Introduced: 1967 **Class:** Antidepressants **Prescription:** USA: Yes **Controlled Drug:** USA: No; Canada: No **Available as Generic:** USA: Yes; Canada: Yes

Brand Names: Desyrel, ✤Alti-Trazodone, ✤Apo-Trazodone, ✤Desyrel Dividose, ✤Novo-Trazodone, ✤PMS-Trazodone, Trialodine

Author's Note: Information in this profile has been shortened to make room for more widely used medicines.

TRIAMCINOLONE (tri am SIN oh lohn)

Introduced: 1985 **Class:** Antiasthmatic, cortisone-like drugs **Prescription:** USA: Yes **Controlled Drug:** USA: No; Canada: No **Available as Generic:** Yes

Brand Names: Amcort, Aristocort, Aristocort R, Aristoform D, ✤Aristospan, Articulose LA, ✤Aureocort, Azmacort, Cenocort, Cenocort Forte, Flutex, ✤Kenacomb, Kenacort, Kenaject, Kenalog, Kenalog H, Kenalog IN, Kenalone, Mycogen II, Mycolog [CD], Mycomar, Mytrex [CD], Mytriacet II [CD], Nasacort, Nasacort AQ, SK-Triamcinolone, TAC-D, TAC-40, Triacet, ✤Triaderm Mild, ✤Triaderm Regular, Triam-A, Triam-Forte, Triamolone 40, Triderm, Tri-Kort, Trilog, Tristoject, ✤Viaderm-K.C.

Author's Note: This profile will focus on inhalation, oral, topical, and nasal forms as injections that are not self-administered. Talk with your doctor about any questions on those forms.

BENEFITS versus RISKS

Possible Benefits	*Possible Risks*
EFFECTIVE CONTROL OF SEVERE, CHRONIC BRONCHIAL ASTHMA	Yeast infections of mouth and throat
EFFECTIVE SUPPRESSION OF A VARIETY OF INFLAMMATORY DISORDERS	Suppression of normal cortisone production
POSSIBLE REDUCTION IN SYSTEMIC STEROID USE	Euphoria and psychotic episodes
	Cushing's syndrome ("moon face," obesity, and "buffalo hump")
EFFECTIVE TREATMENT OF SEASONAL OR PERENNIAL ALLERGIC RHINITIS IN ADULTS AND CHILDREN	Muscle wasting (with long-term use)
	Osteoporosis (with long-term use)
	Increased infection susceptibility
	Aseptic bone necrosis (osteonecrosis) is an area of controversy, unclear onset, patient risk factors, and correlation versus causation (see Controversies in Medicine, below)

▷ **Principal Uses**

As a Single Drug Product: Uses currently included in FDA-approved labeling: (1) Inhaler form is used to treat chronic bronchial asthma in people who require cortisone-like drugs for asthma control—this is better than cortisone taken by mouth (swallowed) or injection because it works more locally on the respiratory tract, not requiring systemic distribution; this helps prevent some serious adverse effects that usually result from the long-term use of cortisone taken for systemic effects; (2) tablet form can be used in a variety of inflammatory disorders; (3) tablet form is used to ease drug reactions; (4) used as part of combination treatment of acute lymphocytic leukemia in children; (5) used in autoimmune hemolytic anemia; (6) nasal inhaler form helps adults and children with symptoms of seasonal or perennial allergic rhinitis; (7) combined with antibiotics in some countries for use as a wound dressing; (8) injection form can be given into a large muscle or into an afflicted joint itself.

Other (unlabeled) generally accepted uses: (1) May have a role in postherpetic nerve pain (neuralgia); (2) corticosteroids may be of use with *Pneumocystis carinii* pneumonia in extreme cases where conventional therapy has not worked; (3) may help Guillain-Barré syndrome; (4) can help myasthenia gravis; (5) short-term therapy of psoriasis; (6) injection form relieves pseudogout.

As a Combination Drug Product [CD]: Available combined with antibiotics in some countries as a wound dressing.

How This Drug Works: By increasing the amount of cyclic AMP in appropriate tissues, this drug may thereby increase the concentration of epinephrine, which is an effective bronchodilator and antiasthmatic. Additional benefit is due to the drug's ability to reduce local allergic reaction and inflammation in the lining tissues of the respiratory tract.

▷ **Widely Used Guidelines That Involve This Medicine (representative sample):**
Please look at the section at the very beginning of this profile called "Class." Next, turn to Table 22 and you will find guidelines listed by the class involved!

Available Dosage Forms and Strengths

Inhalation aerosol (per metered spray) — 0.1 mg

Nasal inhaler — 55 mcg per actuation

Injection — 25 mg per mL
Nasal spray — 55 mcg or 100 mcg per metered
dose (100 mcg is Canada only)
Tablets — 1 mg, 2 mg, 4 mg, 8 mg
Topical cream — 0.025%, 0.1%, 0.25%
Topical ointment — 0.1%, 0.5%
Topical ointment — 0.25%, 0.5%

▷ **Recommended Dosage Ranges** (Actual dose and schedule must be determined for each patient individually.)

Infants and Children:

Up to 6 years of age: Dose not established.

6 to 12 years of age: Inhalation: 0.1 to 0.2 mg (one or two metered sprays) three or four times a day. Adjust dose as needed and tolerated. Limit total daily dose to 1.2 mg (12 metered sprays).

12 to 60 Years of Age:

Inhalation: Initially 0.2 mg (two metered sprays) three or four times a day. For severe asthma—1.2 to 1.6 mg (12 to 16 metered sprays) per day, in divided doses. Adjust dose as needed and tolerated. It is usually used as two inhalations three to four times a day. Results are better when used in this fashion versus on an as-needed basis. Limit total daily dose to 1.6 mg (16 metered sprays).

Intranasal: In treating perennial or seasonal allergic rhinitis, the recommended dose in children more than 12 years old and also in adults: two sprays in each nostril daily (220 mcg per day). If acceptable relief has not been accomplished in 4–7 days, the dose can be increased to 440 mcg a day (four sprays in each nostril daily). If relief still is not adequate, after 21 days, an alternate treatment should be considered. If relief is accomplished (signs and symptoms under control), the dose is lowered to one spray in each nostril once a day (110 mcg for the Nasacort form). For the Nasacort AQ form, dosing is started at 220 mcg a day (given as two sprays in each nostril). Once symptoms are under control, dosing is decreased to 110 mcg a day as an ongoing dose (one spray in each nostril).

Tablets: 4 to 48 mg daily for inflammatory conditions, depending on the nature and severity of the condition.

Topical cream: 0.025% is usually applied to the affected area two to four times a day.

Over 60 Years of Age: Same as 12 to 60 years of age.

Conditions Requiring Dosing Adjustments

Liver Function: This drug is metabolized in the liver. Dosing changes in liver compromise are not defined.

Kidney Function: Dosing adjustments do not appear warranted for patients with compromised kidneys.

▷ **Dosing Instructions:** Inhalation form: May be used as needed without regard to eating. Shake the container well before using. Carefully follow the printed patient instructions provided with the unit. Rinse the mouth and throat (gargle) with water thoroughly after each inhalation; do not swallow the rinse water. The Nasacort AQ form is water-based for treatment of allergic rhinitis and does not contain chlorofluorocarbon propellants.

Oral tablets: May cause stomach upset and can be taken with meals or snacks.

If you forget a dose: Take, use, or apply the missed dose as soon as you remember it, unless it's nearly time for your next dose—if that is the case, skip the missed dose and take the next dose right on schedule. DO NOT double up on doses. Talk with your doctor if you find yourself missing doses.

Usual Duration of Use: Use on a regular schedule for 1 to 2 weeks usually determines effectiveness in controlling severe, chronic asthma. Symptom relief in allergic or perennial rhinitis often happens in a few days. Long-term use varies with the problem being treated, systemic or local therapy, patient reaction, disease flare, and tapering; all are salient factors.

Typical Treatment Goals and Measurements (Outcomes and Markers)

Asthma: Frequency and severity of asthma attacks should ease. Some clinicians also use decreased frequency of rescue inhaler use as a further clinical indicator. It is critical that this medicine is used regularly to get the best results. Lung (pulmonary function) testing (FEV1 and others) and improvement in those tests also helps define results in asthma. Lastly, clinical signs and symptoms such as wheezing, tightness in the chest, and exercise tolerance should all move in favorable directions.

An additional goal of therapy is to use the lowest effective dose. Some people keep their improvements when doses are lowered, while others relapse. Those with a less than twofold improvement in airway response and people who stay in the moderate to severe asthma range despite appropriate dosing may be more likely to relapse if dosing decrease attempts are made. If the usual benefit of ongoing use is not realized, call your doctor.

Inflammation: The general goal is to relieve the swelling and the inflammatory response. Topical use in skin conditions gives a local effect to benefit discomfort, itching, and swelling.

Allergic rhinitis: Symptoms such as itchy, runny nose, sore throat, and postnasal drip should all ease once this medicine begins to work. Because there may be some seasonality to the pollen or molds that can cause rhinitis, talk to your doctor about exactly how he or she wants you to use this medicine.

▷ **This Drug Should Not Be Taken If**
- you have had an allergic reaction to it previously.
- you are having severe acute asthma or status asthmaticus that requires immediate relief and you have been prescribed the inhaler form of this medicine alone.
- you have a form of nonallergic bronchitis with asthmatic features.
- you have a systemic fungal infection.
- the dental paste form has been prescribed and you have a bacterial, viral, or fungal mouth infection.

▷ **Inform Your Physician Before Taking This Drug If**
- you are now taking, or have recently taken, any cortisone-related drug (including ACTH by injection) for any reason (see Drug Classes).
- you have a history of tuberculosis of the lungs.
- you have chronic bronchitis or bronchiectasis.
- you have diabetes, glaucoma, myasthenia gravis, or peptic ulcer disease.
- you have unexplained joint pain (such as in the knee, hip, or shoulder) while taking or after taking this medicine systemically. This could be an early sign of osteonecrosis. Call your doctor right away.
- you have had unexpected surgery (may delay wound healing).
- you have osteoporosis.
- you have an underactive thyroid (hypothyroidism).
- you think you may have an active infection of any kind, especially a respiratory infection, as this medicine can blunt your immune system.

- you are taking any of the following drugs: warfarin, oral antidiabetic drugs, insulin, or digoxin.

Possible Side Effects (natural, expected, and unavoidable drug actions)
Yeast infections (thrush) of the mouth and throat. Irritation of mouth, tongue, or throat. May cause euphoria, manic-depressive illness, or paranoid states with long-term oral use. Can cause a syndrome (Cushing's) characterized by "moon face," obesity, and poorly controlled high blood pressure.

▷ **Possible Adverse Effects** (unusual, unexpected, and infrequent reactions)
If any of the following develop, consult your physician promptly for guidance.
Mild Adverse Effects
Allergic reaction: skin rash.
Easy bruising (ecchymosis)—infrequent.
Swelling of face, hoarseness, voice change, cough—possible to infrequent.
Serious Adverse Effects
Allergic reactions—rare.
Bronchospasm, asthmatic wheezing—rare.
Can be a cause of high blood pressure with long-term use.
Edema or swelling, especially with kidney or heart vessel disease—infrequent.
Decrease of circulating T lymphocytes—possible.
Drug-induced seizures, ulcer development, pancreatitis, or osteoporosis—possible to infrequent.
Increased intracranial pressure (pseudotumor cerebri)—rare.
Necrosis of bone (osteonecrosis, avascular necrosis, or aseptic necrosis)—Questions remain as to correlation versus causation, but may be more likely with high initial corticosteroid doses, long-term treatment, and cumulative doses of 4.32 grams. May also happen with short-term, modest doses. Individual patient risk factors and/or diseases or conditions appear to be important. Call your doctor if unexplained joint pain happens.
Osteoporosis—possible with long-term use.
Electrolyte disturbances (decreased blood potassium)—infrequent.
Excessive thyroid activity (hyperthyroidism).
Cataract formation or muscle wasting has occurred with long-term use.
Decreased growth in children, especially with high-dose and long-term therapy—possible.
Elevated blood sugar—possible.
Toxic megacolon—rare.
Toxic psychosis has occurred with other steroids.
Author's Note: The inhalation, nasal, and topical cream forms avoid many of the systemic side effects of oral systemic use.

▷ **Adverse Effects That May Mimic Natural Diseases or Disorders:**
Pattern of symptoms resembling Cushing's syndrome. Osteoporosis may resemble bone loss after menopause.

▷ **Possible Effects on Sexual Function:** None reported.

Natural Diseases or Disorders That May Be Activated by This Drug
Latent amebiasis, congestive heart failure, diabetes, glaucoma, hypertension, myasthenia gravis, peptic ulcer.
Cortisone-related drugs (used by inhalation) that produce systemic effects can impair immunity and lead to reactivation of "healed" or quiescent tuberculosis of the lungs. Individuals with a history of tuberculosis should be observed closely during use of cortisone-like drugs by inhalation. Other

dormant or existing infections (such as threadworm—Strongyloides) may become more active.

Possible Effects on Laboratory Tests

Blood calcium levels: decreased.

Blood total cholesterol levels: increased.

Blood glucose or sodium levels: increased.

Glucose tolerance test: decreased.

Blood potassium levels: decreased.

Fecal occult blood: may be positive with tablet and systemic use (secondary to GI irritation).

CAUTION

1. This drug is NOT for the immediate relief of acute asthma.
2. If you were using any cortisone-related drugs for asthma *before* switching to this inhaler, you may need to restart the former cortisone-related drug if you are injured, get an infection, or require surgery. Tell your doctor about prior use of cortisone-related drugs.
3. If you experience a return of severe asthma while using this drug, call your doctor immediately. Additional treatment with cortisone-related drugs by mouth or injection may be required.
4. Carry a card noting (if applicable) that you have used cortisone-related drugs within the past year. During periods of stress, resumption of cortisone treatment may be required.
5. Approximately 5 to 10 minutes should separate the inhalation of bronchodilators such as albuterol, epinephrine, pirbuterol, etc. (which should be used first), and the inhalation of this drug. This sequence will permit greater penetration of triamcinolone into the bronchial tubes. This will also reduce the possibility of adverse effects from the propellants used in the two inhalers.
6. A variety of patient risk factors appear to be important in possible development of osteonecrosis. Talk to your doctor about the current list. If you develop knee, hip, joint, or back pain while taking this medicine—especially if therapy is long term—call your doctor.

Controversies in Medicine: Medicines in this class have had conflicting reports regarding correlation with or causation of aseptic bone necrosis (osteonecrosis-ON). There appear to be patient risk factors, possible delayed onset with occurrence even after the medicine is stopped, and some diseases or conditions where corticosteroids are often used and ON is more frequent than in the general population. It is unclear if this is because of the disease or condition or the use of corticosteroids. Previous data regarding cumulative dosing (4.32 grams) appear controversial, with more recent case reports of 6 days of treatment with some doses being associated with ON. Some existing and emerging patient risk factors, including alcohol use versus abuse, initial high doses, HIV positive patients who weight trained, systemic lupus erythematosus, some clotting disorders, and high homocysteine levels, amongst others, appear to increase risk. Early research regarding use of alendronate (Fosamax) to treat ON appears to show that it is important for patients to quickly return to their doctors if unexplained joint pain (such as in the hip or knee) happens. Some centers note that ON has been poorly studied, and while the weight of data in growing, it is yet too early to say more than ON is correlated with corticosteroid use.

Precautions for Use

By Infants and Children: Safety and effectiveness for use of the oral inhaler by those under 6 years of age have not been established. To ensure adequate penetration of the drug and obtain maximal benefit, the use of a spacer device is recommended for inhalation therapy in children.

By Those Over 60 Years of Age: Individuals with chronic bronchitis or bronchiectasis should be observed closely for the development of lung infections. Systemic use may be associated with greater risk of adverse effects from ongoing dosing. Avoid this if possible.

▷ **Advisability of Use During Pregnancy**

Pregnancy Category: C. See Pregnancy Risk Categories at the back of this book.

Animal Studies: Rat and rabbit studies reveal significant toxic effects on the embryo and fetus and multiple birth defects due to this drug.

Human Studies: Adequate studies of pregnant women are not available.

Limit use to very serious illness for which no satisfactory treatment alternatives are available.

Advisability of Use If Breast-Feeding

Presence of this drug in breast milk: expected to be safe.

Ask your doctor for guidance.

Habit-Forming Potential: With recommended dose, a state of functional dependence (see Glossary) is not likely to develop.

Effects of Overdose: Indications of cortisone excess (due to systemic absorption)—fluid retention, flushing of the face, stomach irritation, nervousness.

Possible Effects of Long-Term Use: Significant suppression of normal cortisone production with systemic use.

Suggested Periodic Examinations While Taking This Drug (at physician's discretion)

Inspection of mouth and throat for evidence of yeast infection.

Assessment of the status of adrenal gland function (cortisone production).

X-ray of the lungs of people with a prior tuberculosis history.

Check of growth rate in children.

Bone mineral density tests to assess osteoporosis. Check of bone status relative to osteonecrosis if unexplained joint pain occurs. (MRI may be prudent).

▷ **While Taking This Drug, Observe the Following**

Foods: No specific restrictions beyond those advised by your physician.

Herbal Medicines or Minerals: Increased calcium and vitamin D are prudent. During long-term use, take a vitamin D and vitamin C supplement. During wound repair, take a zinc supplement. Potassium loss may need to be replaced. Ask your doctor if glucosamine makes sense for you if you are taking the oral form. Hawthorn, garlic, ginger, ma huang, ginseng, guar gum, fenugreek, glucomannan, and nettle may change blood sugar. Since this medicine can also change blood sugar, caution is advised.

Fir or pine needle oil should NOT be used by asthmatics. Ephedra alone does carry a German Commission E monograph indication for asthma treatment, but both ephedra and ephedra containing products (such as ma huang) can decrease corticosteroid benefits. If you are allergic to plants in the Asteraceae family (aster, chrysanthemum, daisy, or ragweed), you may also be allergic to echinacea, chamomile, feverfew, and St. John's wort. Echinacea and ginseng can increase the function of the immune system, blunting benefits of this medicine. Licorice may inhibit liver removal of this medicine, leading to excessive steroid effects. Talk to your doctor BEFORE combining any herbal medicine with triamcinolone.

Beverages: No specific restrictions.

▷ *Alcohol:* Use caution if you are prone to peptic ulcers. Talk to your doctor to get his or her approval of drinking beer, wine, or other liquor while taking this medicine. Controversy exists as to any alcohol use versus abuse as a risk factor for osteonecrosis.

Tobacco Smoking: No interactions expected. I advise everyone to quit smoking.

▷ *Other Drugs*

The following drugs may ***increase*** the effects of triamcinolone:
- inhalant bronchodilators—albuterol, bitolterol, epinephrine, pirbuterol, etc.
- oral bronchodilators—aminophylline, ephedrine, terbutaline, theophylline, etc.

The following drugs may ***decrease*** the effects of triamcinolone:
- carbamazepine (Tegretol)—increases triamcinolone metabolism and may result in decreased effectiveness.
- phenobarbital (various).
- phenytoin (Dilantin) or fosphenytoin (Cerebyx)—increases triamcinolone metabolism and may result in decreased effectiveness.
- primidone (Mysoline)—increases steroid metabolism and may result in decreased triamcinolone metabolism.
- rifampin (Rifadin).

Triamcinolone ***taken concurrently*** with
- amphotericin B (Abelcet) may lead to additive potassium loss.
- aspirin may result in increased removal of aspirin from the body and may also lead to increased stomach irritation or ulceration. This effect may be immediate or delayed. Patients should be checked for loss of aspirin benefits and stomach upset of GI bleeding.
- cyclosporine (Sandimmune) may result in changes in the blood levels of both medicines.
- human growth hormone (HGH) may blunt HGH benefits.
- insulin (various forms) may lead to loss of glucose control.
- neuromuscular blocking agents (such as pancuronium—Pavulon, or vercuronium—Norcuron) may prolong muscle weakness.
- oral hypoglycemic agents (see Oral Antidiabetic Drugs in Drug Classes) may result in loss of glucose control.
- thiazide diuretics (see Drug Classes) can result in loss of glucose control.
- vaccines (flu, rabies, rotavirus, others) may result in a less than optimal vaccine response.
- warfarin (Coumadin) can result in variation in the degree of anticoagulation; increased INR (prothrombin time or protime) testing is indicated.

▷ *Driving, Hazardous Activities:* No restrictions.

Aviation Note: The use of this drug and the disorder for which this drug is prescribed ***may be disqualifications*** for piloting. Consult a designated Aviation Medical Examiner.

Exposure to Sun: No restrictions.

Occurrence of Unrelated Illness: Acute infections, serious injuries, and surgical procedures can create an urgent need for the administration of additional supportive cortisone-related drugs given by mouth and/or injection. Notify your physician immediately in the event of new illness or injury of any kind.

Special Storage Instructions: Store at room temperature. Avoid exposure to temperatures above 120°F (49°C). Do not store or use this inhaler near heat or open flame.

Discontinuation: **Do not stop this drug abruptly after chronic use.** Ask your doctor for help about gradual, individualized withdrawal. Some clinicians change from daily to every other day therapy for 4 weeks BEFORE starting to lower the dose in a stepwise fashion. Many patients tolerate dose reductions of 2.5 mg of prednisone (other steroids are calculated on the basis of prednisone equivalents) with those decreases made every 3–7 days. If a disease flare occurs (worsening of symptoms), the dose should be increased to the last dose before the disease flare and should be tapered more slowly down to 5–10 mg or lower. Some clinicians use 8 A.M. predose plasma cortisol to guide tapering. If this lab test is less than 10 mcg/deciliter, tapering is continued until the daily prednisone equivalent is 2–5 mg. In general, if long-term treatment or high doses were used, prednisone equivalents should be tapered over 9–12 months. For up to 2 years after stopping this drug, you may require it again if you have an injury, surgery, or an illness.

TRIAMTERENE (tri AM ter een)

Introduced: 1964   **Class:** Diuretic   **Prescription:** USA: Yes
Controlled Drug: USA: No; Canada: No   **Available as Generic:** Yes
Brand Names: ✤Apo-Triazide [CD], Dyazide [CD], Dyrenium, Maxzide [CD], Maxzide-25 [CD], ✤Novo-Triamzide [CD], ✤Nu-Triazide, ✤Riva-Zide

---

BENEFITS versus RISKS

Possible Benefits	*Possible Risks*
EFFECTIVE PREVENTION OF POTASSIUM LOSS WHEN USED ADJUNCTIVELY WITH OTHER DIURETICS	ABNORMALLY HIGH BLOOD POTASSIUM LEVEL WITH EXCESSIVE USE
EFFECTIVE DIURETIC IN REFRACTORY CASES OF FLUID RETENTION WHEN USED ADJUNCTIVELY WITH OTHER DIURETICS	Possible blood cell disorders: megaloblastic anemia, abnormally low white blood cell and platelet counts
	Possible kidney stone formation

Principal Uses

As a Single Drug Product: Uses currently included in FDA-approved labeling: (1) Used in combination with other drugs to treat high blood pressure (primarily used in situations where it is advisable to prevent loss of potassium from the body); (2) used as combination therapy of congestive heart failure or liver and kidney disorders accompanied by excessive fluid retention (edema). Other (unlabeled) generally accepted uses: None.

As a Combination Drug Product [CD]: Available in combination with hydrochlorothiazide, a different kind of diuretic that promotes potassium loss from the body. Triamterene is used to counteract the potassium-losing (wasting) effect of the thiazide diuretic.

How This Drug Works: By inhibiting the enzyme system that starts the sodium-potassium exchange process, this drug prevents reabsorption of sodium and excretion of potassium by the kidney. This leads to excretion of sodium (and water with it) and potassium retention.

▷ **Widely Used Guidelines That Involve This Medicine (representative sample):** Please look at the section at the very beginning of this profile called

"Class." Next, turn to Table 22 and you will find guidelines listed by the class involved!

Available Dosage Forms and Strengths
Capsules — 50 mg, 100 mg
Capsules — triamterene 37.5 mg and hydrochlorothiazide 25 mg.

▷ **Usual Adult Dosage Ranges:** Initially 50 to 100 mg twice daily. The dose is then adjusted according to individual response. The usual ongoing dose is 100 to 200 mg daily, divided into two doses. The total daily dose should not exceed 300 mg.
Dyazide combination—one or two capsules daily for high blood pressure.
Note: Actual dose and schedule must be determined for each patient individually.

Conditions Requiring Dosing Adjustments
Liver Function: Dose should be reduced and used with extreme caution in liver disease.
Kidney Function: Patients with mild to moderate kidney failure may take the usual dose every 12 hours. In severe or progressive kidney failure, this medication should not be used.

▷ **Dosing Instructions:** May be taken with or following meals to promote absorption of the drug and reduce stomach irritation. The capsule may be opened. If you forget a dose: Take the missed dose as soon as you remember it, unless it's nearly time for your next dose—if that is the case, skip the missed dose and take the next dose right on schedule. DO NOT double doses. Talk with your doctor if you find yourself missing doses as the best control of blood pressure comes from taking your medicine exactly as prescribed.

Usual Duration of Use: Use on a regular schedule for 3 to 5 days usually determines effectiveness in clearing edema and for 2 to 3 weeks usually determines its effect on hypertension. Long-term use (months to years) requires physician supervision and periodic evaluation. Take control of your blood pressure by taking this medicine!

Typical Treatment Goals and Measurements (Outcomes and Markers)
Blood Pressure: Guidelines (JNC VII) define normal blood pressure (BP) as **less than** 120/80 and **pre-hypertension** as 120/80 to 139/89. This new range is intended to help doctors encourage lifestyle changes (or, in the case of people with a risk factor for high blood pressure, start treatment) much earlier—so that damage to blood vessels, your heart, kidneys, sexual potency, or eyes might be minimized or avoided altogether. Stage 1 hypertension is 140/90 to 159/99, and stage 2 hypertension equal to or greater than 160/100 mm Hg. These guidelines also recommend that clinicians work with their patients to agree on the goals and a plan of treatment. The first-ever guidelines for blood pressure (hypertension) in African Americans recommends that MOST black patients be started on TWO antihypertensive medicines with the goal of lowering blood pressure to 130/80 for those with high risk for heart and blood vessel disease or with diabetes. The American Diabetes Association also recommends 130/80 as the target for diabetics and less than 125/75 for those who spill more than one gram of protein into their urine. Most clinicians try to achieve a BP that confers the best balance of lower cardiovascular risk and avoids the problem of too low a blood pressure. Blood pressure duration is generally increased with beneficial restriction of sodium. If goals are not met, it is not unusual to intensify doses or add on medicines.

▷ **This Drug Should Not Be Taken If**
  • you have had an allergic reaction to it previously or you have a sulfa drug allergy.
  • you have severely impaired liver or kidney function.
  • your kidney disease is progressive or you have a creatinine clearance greater than 2.5 mg/dL (ask your doctor).
  • your blood potassium level is significantly elevated (ask your doctor).

▷ **Inform Your Physician Before Taking This Drug If**
  • you have a history of liver or kidney disease.
  • you have diabetes or gout.
  • you are taking any of the following: antihypertensives, a digitalis preparation, another diuretic, lithium, or a potassium preparation.
  • you have a history of glucose-6-phosphate dehydrogenase (G6PD) deficiency (ask your doctor).
  • you have a history of blood cell disorders.
  • you will have surgery with general anesthesia.

Possible Side Effects (natural, expected, and unavoidable drug actions)
  With excessive use: abnormally high blood potassium levels, abnormally low blood sodium levels, dehydration. Blue coloration of the urine (of no significance).

▷ **Possible Adverse Effects** (unusual, unexpected, and infrequent reactions)
  If any of the following develop, consult your physician promptly for guidance.
  Mild Adverse Effects
  Allergic reactions: skin rash, itching.
  Headache, dizziness, unsteadiness, weakness, drowsiness, lethargy—infrequent.
  Dry mouth, nausea, vomiting, diarrhea—infrequent.
  Serious Adverse Effects
  Allergic reaction: anaphylactic reaction (see Glossary).
  Symptomatic potassium excess: confusion, numbness, tingling in lips and extremities, fatigue, weakness, shortness of breath, slow heart rate, low blood pressure—possible.
  Blood cell disorders: megaloblastic anemia, abnormally low white blood cell count, or abnormally low blood platelet count—case reports.
  Hemolytic anemia—in those with deficiency of G6PD in red cells.
  Abnormal urine production (SIADH)—case reports.
  Formation of kidney stones and kidney toxicity—rare.
  Liver toxicity—rare.

▷ **Possible Effects on Sexual Function:** None reported.

Possible Effects on Laboratory Tests
  Complete blood cell counts: decreased red cells, hemoglobin, white cells, and platelets; increased eosinophils (allergic reaction).
  Blood glucose level: increased in diabetics.
  Blood lithium, potassium, or uric acid level: increased.
  Liver function tests: Increased—rare.
  Kidney function tests: increased blood creatinine and urea nitrogen (BUN) levels (kidney damage).

CAUTION
  1. Do not take potassium supplements or increase your intake of potassium-rich foods while taking this drug.

2. Patients who take quinidine (Quinaglute, others) may have falsely increased laboratory test results if fluorescent measurement techniques are used.
3. Do not stop this drug abruptly unless abnormally high blood levels of potassium develop.
4. Avoid liberal use of salt substitutes with potassium in them (potential causes of potassium excess).

Precautions for Use

By Infants and Children: This drug is not recommended for use in children.

By Those Over 60 Years of Age: Natural decline in kidney function may predispose to potassium retention. Watch for potassium excess: slow heart rate, irregular heart rhythms, low blood pressure, confusion, drowsiness. Excessive use of diuretics can cause harmful loss of body water (dehydration), increased viscosity of the blood, and an increased tendency of the blood to clot, predisposing to stroke, heart attack, or thrombophlebitis.

▷ **Advisability of Use During Pregnancy**

Pregnancy Category: B by one manufacturer, D by one researcher. See Pregnancy Risk Categories at the back of this book.

Animal Studies: No birth defects due to this drug were reported.

Human Studies: Adequate studies of pregnant women are not available.

This drug should not be used during pregnancy unless a very serious complication of pregnancy occurs for which this drug is significantly beneficial.

Advisability of Use If Breast-Feeding

Presence of this drug in breast milk: Yes.

Avoid drug or refrain from nursing.

Habit-Forming Potential: None.

Effects of Overdose: Thirst, drowsiness, fatigue, nausea, vomiting, confusion, irregular heart rhythm, low blood pressure.

Possible Effects of Long-Term Use: Potassium accumulation to abnormally high blood levels.

Suggested Periodic Examinations While Taking This Drug (at physician's discretion)

Complete blood cell counts.

Measurements of blood sodium, potassium, and chloride levels.

Kidney function tests.

▷ **While Taking This Drug, Observe the Following**

Foods: Diets high in high-potassium foods (see Table 13, Section Six) may cause problems. Avoid excessive restriction of salt.

Herbal Medicines or Minerals: Ginseng, bitter orange, country mallow, hawthorn, saw palmetto, ma huang (no longer available for weight loss in the U.S.), goldenseal, and yohimbe may increase blood pressure. Caffeine excess from guarana and mate may blunt medicine benefits. Calcium and garlic may help lower blood pressure. Use caution and work with your doctor to make sure blood pressure is not lowered too much. Indian snakeroot has a German Commission E monograph indication for hypertension—talk to your doctor. Eleuthero root and ephedra should be avoided by people living with hypertension. Licorice can increase risk of excessive lowering of potassium (hypokalemia) if combined with a diuretic such as triamterene. **CAUTION:** St. John's wort may also lead to unexpected sensitivity to the sun (photosensitivity).

Beverages: Excessive caffeine may blunt benefits. May be taken with milk.

▷ *Alcohol:* Use with caution. Alcohol may enhance drowsiness and the blood-pressure-lowering effect of this drug.

Tobacco Smoking: No interactions expected. I advise everyone to quit smoking.

▷ *Other Drugs*

Triamterene may *increase* the effects of
- amantadine (Symmetrel).
- digoxin (Lanoxin).
- metformin (Glucophage).
- methotrexate (Mexate), leading to bone marrow toxicity.
- valsartan (Diovan), leading to potassium toxicity.

Triamterene *taken concurrently with*
- captopril (Capoten) or other ACE inhibitors may cause excessively high blood potassium levels.
- cyclosporine (Sandimmune) SHOULD NOT BE COMBINED.
- dofetilide (Tikosyn) may lead to excessive dofetilide levels. Careful patient monitoring and more frequent dofetilide levels are indicated if these medicines are combined as they both are removed from the body by the same mechanism.
- folic acid may reduce folic acid benefits.
- histamine (H2) blockers (see Drug Classes) may decrease triamterene absorption and its therapeutic effects.
- indomethacin (Indocin) may increase the risk of kidney damage.
- lithium may cause accumulation of lithium to toxic levels.
- NSAIDs (see Drug Classes) may blunt the blood-pressure-lowering effect of triamterene.
- potassium preparations may cause excessively high blood pressure.
- spironolactone (various) may lead to excessively high potassium. Combination use is NOT advisable.
- tacrolimus (Prograf) may lead to excessively high blood potassium levels. Combination should be avoided.

▷ *Driving, Hazardous Activities:* This drug may cause dizziness and drowsiness. Restrict activities as necessary.

Aviation Note: The use of this drug *may be a disqualification* for piloting. Consult a designated Aviation Medical Examiner.

Exposure to Sun: Use caution—this drug may cause photosensitivity (see Glossary).

Discontinuation: With high-dose or prolonged use, it is best to slowly withdraw this drug. Stopping it suddenly may cause rebound potassium removal and potassium deficiency. Ask your doctor for help.

TRICHLORMETHIAZIDE (tri KLOR meth i a zide)

Please see the thiazide diuretics family profile.

TRIFLUOPERAZINE (tri flu oh PER a zeen)

Introduced: 1958 **Class:** Tranquilizer, major; phenothiazines **Prescription:** USA: Yes **Controlled Drug:** USA: No; Canada: No **Available as Generic:** USA: Yes; Canada: No

Brand Names: ✤Apo-Trifluoperazine, ✤Novo-Flurazine, ✤Solazine, Stelabid [CD], Stelazine, Suprazine, ✤Terfluzine

Author's Note: Information in this profile has been truncated to make room for more widely used medicines.

TRIMETHOPRIM (tri METH oh prim)

Introduced: 1966 **Class:** Anti-infective **Prescription:** USA: Yes **Controlled Drug:** USA: No; Canada: No **Available as Generic:** USA: Yes; Canada: No

Brand Names: Alti-Trimethoprim, ✤Apo-Sulfatrim [CD], ✤Apo-Sulfatrim DS [CD], Bactrim [CD], Bactrim DS [CD], Bethaprim [CD], Comoxol [CD], ✤Coptin [CD], Cotrim [CD], ✤Novo-Trimel [CD], ✤Novo-Trimel DS [CD], ✤Nu-Cotrimox, Polytrim, Proloprim, ✤Protrin [CD], ✤Protrin DF [CD], ✤Roubac [CD], Septra [CD], Septra DS [CD], SMZ-TMP [CD], Sulfatrim D/S, Trimpex, Uroplus DS [CD], Uroplus SS [CD]

BENEFITS versus RISKS	
Possible Benefits	*Possible Risks*
EFFECTIVE TREATMENT OF INFECTIONS DUE TO SUSCEPTIBLE MICROORGANISMS	Blood cell disorders: megaloblastic anemia, methemoglobinemia, abnormally low white cells or platelets
Effective adjunctive prevention and treatment of *Pneumocystis carinii* pneumonia (AIDS related)	May increase homocysteine with ongoing use

---

▷ **Principal Uses**

As a Single Drug Product: Uses currently included in FDA-approved labeling: (1) Treats or prevents certain infections of the urinary tract not complicated by the presence of kidney stones or obstructions to the normal flow of urine; (2) treats eye infections caused by sensitive organisms; (3) cotrimoxazole, Septra, and Bactrim forms approved to treat and prevent PCP pneumonia.

Other (unlabeled) generally accepted uses: (1) Used in combination with dapsone to treat *Pneumocystis carinii* pneumonia in AIDS patients; (2) may have a role in combination therapy of resistant acne; (3) prevention (prophylaxis) of urinary tract infections.

As a Combination Drug Product [CD]: Available combined with sulfamethoxazole (cotrimoxazole is used in some countries to identify this combination). Treats certain urinary tract infections, middle ear infections, chronic bronchitis, acute enteritis, and certain types of pneumonia. It is now used as primary prevention and treatment of *Pneumocystis carinii* pneumonia associated with AIDS.

How This Drug Works: Prevents growth and multiplication of susceptible organisms by inactivating enzyme systems needed for formation of essential nuclear elements and cell proteins.

▷ **Widely Used Guidelines That Involve This Medicine (representative sample):** Please look at the section at the very beginning of this profile called "Class." Next, turn to Table 22 and you will find guidelines listed by the class involved!

Available Dosage Forms and Strengths
Ophthalmic — 1 mg/mL
Oral suspension, combination (per 5 mL) — 40 mg trimethoprim/200 mg sulfamethoxazole
Tablets — 100 mg, 200 mg
Tablets, combination — 80 mg trimethoprim/400 mg sulfamethoxazole, 160 mg trimethoprim/800 mg sulfamethoxazole

▷ **Usual Adult Dosage Ranges:** *Orally for infections:* 100 mg every 12 hours for 10 days. For certain pneumonias, the same dose is taken every 6 hours. The total daily dose should not exceed 640 mg.

Ophthalmic: One drop in the affected eye every 3 hours (up to six doses a day) for 7 to 10 days.

Note: Actual dose and schedule must be determined for each patient individually.

Conditions Requiring Dosing Adjustments
Liver Function: Used with caution by patients with both liver and kidney disease.
Kidney Function: Patients with mild kidney compromise can take the usual dose every 12 hours. Patients with stable moderate to more compromised kidney failure (creatinine clearances of 15 to 50 mL/min) can take the usual dose every 18 hours. Should NOT be used in severe or worsening kidney failure.

▷ **Dosing Instructions:** The tablet may be crushed and may be taken with or following food if necessary to reduce stomach irritation. The suspension form should be shaken well and dosed using a calibrated medicine spoon or dosing cup. If you forget a dose: Take the missed dose as soon as you remember it, unless it's nearly time for your next dose—if that is the case, skip the missed dose and take the next dose right on schedule. DO NOT double up on doses. Talk with your doctor if you find yourself missing doses as compliance ensures the best treatment results or best possible prevention of infection.

Usual Duration of Use: Use on a regular schedule for 7 to 14 days usually determines effectiveness in controlling responsive infections. Duration will depend on the nature of the infection. Prevention of (prophylaxis) of PCP in HIV-positive patients with the combination form will be ongoing.

Typical Treatment Goals and Measurements (Outcomes and Markers)
Infections: The most commonly used measures of serious infections are white blood cell counts and differentials (the kind of blood cells that occur most often in your blood), and temperature. Many clinicians look for positive changes in 24–48 hours. NEVER stop an antibiotic because you start to feel better. For treating infections, the full course is REQUIRED to kill the bacteria. Prophylaxis (for example of PCP) often requires ongoing use. The goals and timeframe (see peak benefits above) should be discussed with you when the prescription is written.

Currently a Drug of Choice
When combined with sulfamethoxazole, for preventing pneumonia (due to *Pneumocystis carinii*) in patients with AIDS.

▷ **This Drug Should Not Be Taken If**
- you have had an allergic reaction to it previously.
- you have an anemia due to folic acid deficiency (megaloblastic anemia).

▷ **Inform Your Physician Before Taking This Drug If**
  • you have a history of folic acid deficiency.
  • you have impaired liver or kidney function.
  • you are pregnant or breast-feeding.
  • you have a history of cardiovascular disease. This medicine may increase homocysteine levels.

Possible Side Effects (natural, expected, and unavoidable drug actions)
  None with short-term use.

▷ **Possible Adverse Effects** (unusual, unexpected, and infrequent reactions)
  If any of the following develop, consult your physician promptly for guidance.
  Mild Adverse Effects
  Allergic reactions: skin rash, itching, drug fever (see Glossary).
  Headache, abnormal taste, sore mouth or tongue, nausea, vomiting, cramping, diarrhea—infrequent.
  Serious Adverse Effects
  Allergic reactions: severe dermatitis with peeling of skin (toxic epidermal necrolysis).
  Blood cell disorders: megaloblastic anemia, methemoglobinemia, abnormally low white blood cell and platelet counts—rare.
  Worsening of hyperkalemia (increased blood potassium)—possible.
  Kidney or liver toxicity—rare.
  Aseptic meningitis (of questionable causal relationship)—case reports.

▷ **Possible Effects on Sexual Function:** None reported.

Possible Effects on Laboratory Tests
  Complete blood cell counts: decreased red cells, hemoglobin, white cells, and platelets.
  INR (prothrombin time): increased (when taken concurrently with warfarin).

CAUTION
  1. Resistance may develop. If you do not show significant improvement within 2 days, call your physician.
  2. Comply with your physician's request for periodic blood counts during long-term therapy.
  3. This medicine may increase homocysteine levels. Talk to your doctor about checking levels if you will be taking this medicine on an ongoing basis. Taking a multivitamin appears prudent (B vitamins have a role in helping decrease homocysteine).

Precautions for Use
  By Infants and Children: Safety and effectiveness for those under 2 months of age are not established.
  By Those Over 60 Years of Age: The natural decline in liver and kidney function may require smaller doses. If you develop itching reactions in the genital or anal areas, report this promptly.

▷ **Advisability of Use During Pregnancy**
  Pregnancy Category: C. See Pregnancy Risk Categories at the back of this book.
  Animal Studies: Birth defects due to this drug reported in rat and rabbit studies.
  Human Studies: Adequate studies of pregnant women are not available.
  Avoid use of drug during the first 3 months and during the final 2 weeks of pregnancy. Use this drug otherwise only if clearly needed. Ask your physician for guidance.

Advisability of Use If Breast-Feeding
Presence of this drug in breast milk: Yes, but in small amounts.
Talk to your doctor about the best course of action.

Habit-Forming Potential: None.

Effects of Overdose: Headache, dizziness, confusion, depression, nausea, vomiting, bone marrow depression, possible liver toxicity with jaundice.

Possible Effects of Long-Term Use: Impaired production of red and white blood cells and blood platelets.

Suggested Periodic Examinations While Taking This Drug (at physician's discretion)
Complete blood cell counts.

▷ **While Taking This Drug, Observe the Following**
Foods: Since this medicine may increase homocysteine levels, a multivitamin appears prudent.

Herbal Medicines or Minerals: Some patients use echinacea to attempt to boost their immune systems. Unfortunately, echinacea is not recommended in people with damaged immune systems. This herb may also actually weaken any immune system if it is used too often or for too long a time. DO NOT take mistletoe herb, oak bark, or F.C. of marshmallow root and licorice extracts. Pure cranberry juice may help keep harmful bacteria from attaching to the bladder wall and may be useful in combination with antibiotics in helping to prevent urinary tract infections. TALK to your doctor BEFORE adding any herbal medicine.

Beverages: No restrictions. May be taken with milk.

▷ *Alcohol:* No interactions expected.

Tobacco Smoking: No interactions expected, but I advise everyone to quit smoking.

▷ *Other Drugs*
Trimethoprim may ***increase*** the effects of
- abacavir/lamivudine/zidovudine (Trizivir) combined with this medicine will have the lamivudine and zidovudine components increased.
- ACE inhibitors (see Drug Classes), resulting in dangerously increased potassium levels.
- amantadine (Symmetrel) and also result in increased levels of trimethoprim, resulting in toxicity.
- cyclosporine (Sandimmune) and result in increased kidney toxicity.
- dapsone and result in dapsone or trimethoprim toxicity.
- digoxin (Lanoxin), leading to toxicity.
- dofetilide (Tikosyn) may lead to heart toxicity. Avoid this combination.
- lamivudine (Epivir) and adjustments in lamivudine doses may be required.
- leukovorin (Leukovorin calcium for injection) will blunt treatment (increase treatment failure) for leukovorin.
- metformin (Glucophage) and other cationic drugs.
- methotrexate (Mexate), leading to toxicity.
- phenytoin (Dilantin) or fosphenytoin (Cerebyx) can cause phenytoin or fosphenytoin toxicity.
- procainamide (Procan SR) and result in procainamide toxicity.
- tolbutamide (Orinase), leading to increased risk of hypoglycemia.
- zidovudine (AZT), leading to increased toxicity risk.

Cotrimoxazole form may ***increase*** the effects of
- medicines such as class I, IA, or III antiarrhythmics (dofetilide [Tikosyn], clarithromycin, cotrimoxazole, ondansetron, ziprazidone, zolmitriptan,

and others) may lead to prolongation of the QTc interval and undesirable effects. Combination is not recommended.

The following drugs may *decrease* the effects of trimethoprim:

- cholestyramine (Questran) and perhaps other cholesterol-lowering medicines (see Drug Classes) of the same class—these will bind trimethoprim and blunt its beneficial effects by inhibiting absorption.
- rifampin (Rifadin, Rimactane).
- ritonavir (Norvir).

▷ *Driving, Hazardous Activities:* No restrictions.

Aviation Note: The use of this drug is *probably not a disqualification* for piloting. Consult a designated Aviation Medical Examiner.

Exposure to Sun: No restrictions.

VALPROIC ACID (val PROH ik A sid)

Introduced: 1967 **Class:** Anticonvulsant, mood stabilizer **Prescription:** USA: Yes **Controlled Drug:** USA: No; Canada: No **Available as Generic:** USA: Yes; Canada: Yes

Brand Names: ✦Alti-Valproic, ✦Apo-Divalproex, ✦Apo-Valproic, Atemperator, Depa, Depakene, Depakote (divalproex sodium), Depakote ER, Depakote Sprinkle, Deproic, ✦Dom-Divalproex ✦Epival, Myproic, ✦Novo-Divalproex, ✦Novo-valproic, ✦Nu-Valproic, Rhoproic, Valproic

---

BENEFITS versus RISKS

Possible Benefits	*Possible Risks*
EFFECTIVE CONTROL OF MULTIPLE SEIZURE TYPES: ABSENCE SEIZURES, TONIC-CLONIC SEIZURES, MYOCLONIC SEIZURES, PSYCHOMOTOR SEIZURES, WHEN USED ADJUNCTIVELY WITH OTHER ANTISEIZURE DRUGS	LIVER TOXICITY, INFREQUENT BUT MAY BE SEVERE
	Reduction of blood platelets and impaired platelet function with risk of bleeding
HELPS CONTROL REFRACTORY MIGRAINES	Possible pancreatitis or liver toxicity
USED AS A MOOD STABLIZER IN SOME PSYCHIATRIC PATIENTS (EASING MANIA)	

▷ **Principal Uses**

As a Single Drug Product: Uses currently included in FDA-approved labeling: (1) Used to manage the following types of epilepsy: simple and complex absence seizures (petit mal), tonic-clonic seizures (grand mal), myoclonic seizures, and complex partial seizures (psychomotor, temporal lobe epilepsy)—sometimes used adjunctively with other anticonvulsants as needed; (2) used for people who do not respond to medicine once they have a migraine or have more than two migraines a month; (3) valproic acid and divalproex sodium (Depakote) are approved for use in treating mania; (4) eases mania in AIDS; (5) helps kleptomania.

Author's Note: The American Psychiatric Association updated their 1994 treatment guidelines for bipolar disorder (see American Psychiatric

Association in Sources). Valproate (Depakote form) approved for mania secondary to bipolar problems. This drug or lithium is recommended as first choices for most people.

Other (unlabeled) generally accepted uses: (1) Can help relieve the symptoms of trigeminal neuralgia; (2) can have a role in intractable hiccups; (3) some use in patients with epilepsy and hepatic porphyria.

How This Drug Works: It is thought that by increasing the availability of the nerve impulse transmitter gamma-aminobutyric acid (GABA), this drug suppresses the spread of abnormal electrical discharges that cause seizures. May also act by lowering undesirable nerve excitation caused by aspartate or by a direct action on nerve (neuronal) membranes.

▷ **Widely Used Guidelines That Involve This Medicine (representative sample):** Please look at the section at the very beginning of this profile called "Class." Next, turn to Table 22 and you will find guidelines listed by the class involved!

Available Dosage Forms and Strengths

Capsules — 250 mg

Capsules, sprinkle — 125 mg

Solution — 200 mg/ mL

Syrup — 250 mg/5 mL

Tablets, enteric coated — 125 mg, 250 mg, 500 mg

Tablets, extended release — 250 mg, 500 mg (Depakote ER form)

▷ **Usual Adult Dosage Ranges:** Starting dose is 10–15 mg per kg of body mass per day. The dose is increased cautiously by 5 to 10 mg per kg of body mass daily, every 7 days as needed and tolerated. The usual daily dose is from 1,000 mg to 1,600 mg in divided doses. The total daily dose should not exceed 60 mg per kg of body mass. Blood levels are used to guide ongoing dosing. *For migraines:* Starting dose is 250 mg, which is then slowly increased, as needed and tolerated, to 500 to 1000 mg daily in divided doses. For the extended release tablet: 500 mg once a day to start for 7 days, then increased to 1,000 mg a day as needed and tolerated. *For mania:* Depakote is dosed as 750 mg daily in divided doses. In adults, a loading dose of 20 mg per kg of body weight per day has been used in acute mania to achieve blood levels of 80 mg/liter. Dosing is adjusted to find the lowest effective dose.

Note: Actual dose and schedule must be determined for each patient individually.

Typical Treatment Goals and Measurements (Outcomes and Markers)

Seizures: The general goal for this medicine is effective seizure control. Neurologists tend to define effectiveness on a case-by-case basis depending on the seizure type and patient factors. If seizure control is not effective, it's not unusual to use combination treatment. For this medicine, a balance must be struck between too little medicine and too much medicine. Blood levels are used to make sure that the amount of medicine is in just the right range.

For mania: Return of more appropriate affect and ability in activities of daily living (ADLs).

Conditions Requiring Dosing Adjustments

Liver Function: This medicine SHOULD NOT be taken by patients with significant liver compromise or liver disease.

Kidney Function: No dosing changes thought to be needed in kidney disease, but it is prudent to get more frequent blood levels (free levels) and adjust dosing as needed.

▷ **Dosing Instructions:** Preferably taken 1 hour before meals, although it may be taken with or following food if necessary to prevent stomach irritation.

The regular capsule should not be opened, and the tablet should not be crushed in order to avoid irritation that this medicine can cause to the mouth and throat. The sprinkle capsule may be opened and the contents sprinkled on soft food, then best taken right away. Some remainders of the sprinkle form may be seen in your stool. Do not give the syrup in carbonated beverages. Dilute in water or milk. The solution and syrup have different concentrations. Make sure you have the correct product. Any liquid form should be dosed using a calibrated measuring spoon or dose cup. The extended release tablet should not be altered. If you forget a dose: Take the missed dose as soon as you remember it, unless it's nearly time for your next dose—if that is the case, skip the missed dose and take the next dose right on schedule. DO NOT double up on doses. Talk with your doctor if you find yourself missing doses. The best seizure control comes from keeping this medicine in just the right range. This most often results from taking just the right dose at just the right time.

Usual Duration of Use: Use on a regular schedule for 2 weeks usually determines effectiveness in reducing the frequency and severity of seizures. Long-term use (months to years) requires physician supervision and periodic evaluation. Use in seizure cases will be ongoing, as will use in migraine prevention.

▷ **This Drug Should Not Be Taken If**
  • you have had an allergic reaction to it previously.
  • you have active liver disease.
  • you are pregnant.
  • you have an active bleeding disorder.

▷ **Inform Your Physician Before Taking This Drug If**
  • you have a history of liver disease, impaired liver function, or pancreatitis.
  • you have a history of any type of bleeding disorder.
  • you are pregnant or planning pregnancy or are breast-feeding your infant.
  • you have myasthenia gravis or pancreatitis.
  • you are taking anticoagulants, other anticonvulsants, or antidepressants—either the tricyclic type or monoamine oxidase (MAO) type A inhibitors (see Drug Classes).
  • you develop yellow skin or eyes, loss of seizure control, unusual weakness or dizziness, or unusual bleeding or bruising while taking this medicine.
  • you will have surgery or dental extraction.

Possible Side Effects (natural, expected, and unavoidable drug actions)
  Drowsiness and lethargy, excessive lowering of blood pressure on standing (postural hypotension).

▷ **Possible Adverse Effects** (unusual, unexpected, and infrequent reactions)
  If any of the following develop, consult your physician promptly for guidance.
  Mild Adverse Effects
  Allergic reaction: skin rash—rare.
  Headache, dizziness, confusion, unsteadiness, tremor—dose-related.
  Slurred speech—infrequent.
  Nausea, indigestion, stomach cramps, diarrhea—infrequent.
  Weight gain—case reports.
  Bedwetting at night—case reports.
  Lowering of zinc, carnitine, and selenium—possible.
  Temporary loss of scalp hair—case reports.
  Serious Adverse Effects
  Idiosyncratic reactions: bizarre behavior, psychosis, hallucinations.
  Drug-induced hepatitis with jaundice (see Glossary).

Children less than 2 years old have considerably increased risk of fatal liver toxicity (hepatotoxicity).

Leukemia-like cells in the circulation (acute promyelocytic leukemia (APML)—case report.

Blood ammonia level or blood glucose—increased.

Drug-induced pancreatitis, porphyria, lowered thyroid gland function (hypothyroidism)—case reports.

Selenium, zinc, and carnitine levels—decreased.

Reduced formation of blood platelets, impaired platelet function, and anemia (including pure red cell aplasia)—case reports.

Clotting (coagulation) defects—case reports (one case of lung bleeding).

Worsening of demylinating disease—case report.

Increased pressure in the head (pseudotumor cerebri)—case reports.

Movement problems (ataxia, extrapyramidal symptoms, others)—reported.

Can cause a Reye's-like syndrome.

▷ **Possible Effects on Sexual Function:** Altered timing and pattern of menstruation. Female breast enlargement with milk production (galactorrhea). Polycystic ovary syndrome (PCOS)—case reports. Decreased libido—case reports. Decreased effectiveness of oral contraceptives taken concurrently—CAUTION.

▷ **Adverse Effects That May Mimic Natural Diseases or Disorders**

Liver reactions may suggest viral hepatitis.

Possible Effects on Laboratory Tests

Complete blood cell counts: decreased white cells and platelets.

Sodium levels: may be decreased.

Homocysteine: may be increased.

Bleeding time or INR (prothrombin time): increased.

Blood amylase level: increased (possible pancreatitis).

Liver function tests: increased enzymes (ALT/GPT, AST/GOT, alkaline phosphatase) or bilirubin.

CAUTION

1. The capsules and tablets should be swallowed whole to avoid irritation of the mouth and throat.
2. Carnitine, selenium, and zinc supplementation may be needed. Talk to your doctor.
3. This drug can impair normal blood-clotting mechanisms. In the event of injury, dental extraction, or need for surgery, inform your physician or dentist that you are taking this drug.
4. Because this drug can impair the normal function of blood platelets, it is best to avoid aspirin (which has the same effect).
5. Because this drug can lead to pancreatitis, patients are best told about signs of pancreatitis and to call their doctor if they happen.
6. Over-the-counter drug products that contain antihistamines (allergy and cold remedies, sleep aids) can enhance sedation.
7. This medicine may increase homocysteine—it is prudent to get a blood test for this.

Precautions for Use

By Infants and Children: The concurrent use of aspirin with this drug can cause abnormal bleeding or bruising. Children with mental retardation, organic brain disease, or severe seizure disorders may be at increased risk for severe liver toxicity while taking this drug. Observe closely for the development of fever that could indicate the onset of a drug-induced Reye's syndrome (see

Glossary). Avoid concurrent use of clonazepam (Klonopin); the combined use could result in continuous petit mal episodes.

By Those Over 60 Years of Age: Start treatment with small doses and increase dose cautiously. Observe closely for excessive sedation, confusion, or unsteadiness that could predispose to falling and injury.

▷ **Advisability of Use During Pregnancy**

Pregnancy Category: D. See Pregnancy Risk Categories at the back of this book.

Animal Studies: Palate and skeletal birth defects reported in mouse, rat, and rabbit studies.

Human Studies: Adequate studies of pregnant women are not available. There have been several reports of birth defects attributed to the use of this drug during early pregnancy.

Talk to your doctor about the advantages and disadvantages of using this drug. If it is used, it is advisable to keep the dose as low as possible.

Advisability of Use If Breast-Feeding

Presence of this drug in breast milk: Yes, at roughly 1–10% of the mother's serum level.

Talk to your doctor about this benefit-to-risk decision.

Habit-Forming Potential: None.

Effects of Overdose: Increased drowsiness, weakness, unsteadiness, confusion, stupor progressing to coma.

Possible Effects of Long-Term Use: Coagulation changes, bone marrow depression.

Suggested Periodic Examinations While Taking This Drug (at physician's discretion)

Complete blood cell counts and baseline liver function tests should be done before treatment is started. During treatment, blood counts should be repeated every month and liver function tests repeated frequently (your doctor will define this)—particularly during the first 6 months of therapy. Amylase or patient sign and symptom instruction for possible pancreatitis is prudent.

Because homocysteine may be increased (a risk factor for heart disease), periodic check of homocysteine is prudent.

▷ **While Taking This Drug, Observe the Following**

Foods: No restrictions.

Herbal Medicines or Minerals: Using kola, guarana, mate, or ma huang (no longer on the U.S. market for weight loss) may result in unacceptable central nervous system stimulation. Valerian and kava kava may interact to increase drowsiness and also have current concerns about possible liver effects (as well as eucalyptus) and therefore are not presently recommended. St. John's wort may also cause increased sun sensitivity—caution is advised. Replacement of zinc and selenium is prudent. Carnitine replacement (intravenous) is needed in valproic acid–caused (induced) liver toxicity and overdose. Carnitine replacement may also be needed in infants and young children taking multiple seizure medicines as well as epileptic patients on a ketogenic diet who have low carnitine (hypocarnitinemia). Evening primrose oil and a contaminant in some ginkgo preparations can lead to increased seizure risk and are not advisable. Talk to your doctor and pharmacist BEFORE adding any herbals.

Beverages: Do not administer the syrup in carbonated beverages; this could liberate the valproic acid and irritate the mouth and throat. This drug may be taken with milk.

▷ *Alcohol:* Alcohol can increase the sedative effect of this drug. Also, this drug can increase the depressant effects of alcohol on brain function. Avoid alcohol.

Tobacco Smoking: No interactions expected. I advise everyone to quit smoking.

▷ *Other Drugs*

Valproic acid may ***increase*** the effects of

- anticoagulants (warfarin-Coumadin, etc.) and increase the risk of bleeding; increased frequency of INR (prothrombin time or protime) testing is needed.
- antidepressants (both monoamine oxidase [MAO] type A inhibitors and tricyclics) and cause toxicity.
- benzodiazepines (such as alprazolam).
- nimodipine (Nimotop) and cause nimodipine toxicity.
- phenobarbital and cause barbiturate intoxication.
- phenytoin (Dilantin) or fosphenytoin (Cerebyx), and cause phenytoin or fosphenytoin toxicity.
- zidovudine (AZT) and may lead to zidovudine toxicity.

Valproic acid ***taken concurrently*** with

- acyclovir (Zovirax) may lower valproic acid levels.
- antacids (Maalox) will decrease absorption and lower therapeutic benefits of valproic acid.
- antiplatelet drugs—aspirin, dipyridamole (Persantine), sulfinpyrazone (Anturane)—may enhance the inhibition of platelet function and increase the risk of bleeding.
- aspirin can lead to valproic acid toxicity.
- carbamazepine (Tegretol) may have a variable effect on blood levels; more frequent blood level testing is advised.
- cholestyramine (various) may blunt valproic acid benefits.
- clonazepam (Klonopin) may result in repeated episodes of absence seizures (absence status).
- cyclosporine (Sandimmune) may increase risk of liver toxicity.
- erythromycin (Ery-Tab, others) may increase the level of valproic acid and result in toxicity; the newer macrolides (azithromycin or clarithromycin) may also cause problems.
- felbamate (Felbatol) can lead to increased valproic acid levels.
- fluoxetine (Luvox) can lead to increased valproic acid levels. Blood levels and dosing adjusted to levels are prudent.
- isoniazid (INH) can cause valproic acid or isoniazid toxicity.
- rifampin (Rifater) may lead to valproic acid toxicity.
- ritonavir (Norvir) can lead to loss of valproic acid benefits.

▷ *Driving, Hazardous Activities:* This drug may cause drowsiness, dizziness, or confusion. Restrict activities as necessary.

Aviation Note: The use of this drug ***is a disqualification*** for piloting. Consult a designated Aviation Medical Examiner.

Exposure to Sun: Caution: This drug has caused photosensitivity.

Discontinuation: Do not stop this drug suddenly. Abrupt withdrawal can cause repetitive seizures that are difficult to control.

VANCOMYCIN (van koh MI sin)

Introduced: 1974   **Class:** Anti-infective, glycopeptideantibiotic   **Pre-scription:** USA: Yes   **Controlled Drug:** USA: No; Canada: No   **Available as Generic:** USA: Yes; Canada: Yes

Brand Names: ✤PMS-Vancomycin, Vancocin, Vancoled, Vancor

Author's Note: Vancomycin is used to treat a variety of serious infections. It is given intravenously to treat some infections and orally to treat others. In the past, the information provided in this profile was limited to the use of vancomycin taken by mouth. Since resistant organisms have necessitated increased use of this medicine by vein (intravenously), this profile has been expanded to help patients understand vancomycin's broadened role in infectious disease.

BENEFITS versus RISKS

Possible Benefits	*Possible Risks*
TREATS SERIOUS INFECTIONS CAUSED BY RESISTANT GRAM-POSITIVE ORGANISMS SUCH AS STAPH AND STREP	KIDNEY TOXICITY (WITH COMBINED AMINOGLYCOSIDE USE)
TREATS ANTIBIOTIC-ASSOCIATED PSEUDOMEMBRANOUS COLITIS (ORAL FORM)	Ringing in ears (tinnitus) Loss of hearing

---

▷ **Principal Uses**

As a *Single Drug Product:* Uses currently included in FDA-approved labeling: (1) Oral form is used in antibiotic-associated pseudomembranous colitis caused by *Clostridium difficile;* (2) the oral form is also used in enterocolitis caused by staphylococcal organisms; (3) the intravenous form is used to treat a variety of serious infections, such those in heart valves, bones (osteomyelitis), endocarditis, and meningitis, including those caused by methicillin-resistant *Staphylococcus aureus* (MRSA) and other susceptible bacteria.

Other (unlabeled) generally accepted uses: (1) May have a role preventing central venous catheter infections (combined with heparin flush) in immunosuppressed pediatric patients; (2) recommended by the CDC as one of the additional antibiotics to be part of combination therapy for inhalational, oropharyngeal, or gastrointestinal anthrax cases in the case of intentional bioterrorist release.

How This Drug Works: By inhibiting the formation of bacterial cell walls and the production of RNA, this drug destroys susceptible strains of infecting bacteria.

▷ **Widely Used Guidelines That Involve This Medicine (representative sample):** Please look at the section at the very beginning of this profile called "Class." Next, turn to Table 22 and you will find guidelines listed by the class involved!

Available Dosage Forms and Strengths

Capsules — 125 mg, 250 mg

Intravenous — 500 mg/15 mL, 1 g/15 mL

Oral solution — 250 mg/5 mL teaspoonful and 500 mg/5 mL

▷ **Recommended Dosage Ranges** (Actual dose and schedule must be determined for each patient individually.)

Infants and Children: 10 mg per kg of body mass every 6 hours, for 5 to 10 days. The total daily dose should not exceed 2,000 mg (2 g). Repeat course as necessary.

12 to 60 Years of Age: Intravenous: Many clinicians use a 15-mg-per-kg-of-body-mass loading dose and then calculate ongoing doses based on individual patient height, weight, kidney function, and suspected bacteria (bacterial pathogen). Calculations are made in order to attain a peak blood level of 30–40 mcg/mL and a lowest blood level (trough) of 5–10 mcg/mL.

Oral dosing for pseudomembranous colitis caused by *Clostridium difficile:* 125 mg by mouth every 6 hours for 10 days.

Over 60 Years of Age: Intravenous dosing: The loading dose is the same as for younger patients. Ongoing doses may be much smaller and may need to be taken much less often than in younger patients (such as once a day or once every 2 days) because of the age-related declines in kidney function.

Oral dosing: Same as 12 to 60 years of age (vancomycin in pseudomembranous colitis is not absorbed).

Conditions Requiring Dosing Adjustments

Liver Function: The liver is not involved in the elimination of vancomycin.

Kidney Function: Oral vancomycin is minimally absorbed. Intravenous vancomycin MUST be given/taken in decreased doses or increased intervals in kidney compromise. This drug is also a potential cause of kidney failure and should only be taken if other alternatives are not available. Daily measures of kidney function and more frequent blood levels are indicated if this medicine is used by patients with compromised kidneys.

▷ **Dosing Instructions:** Oral form may be taken with or following food to reduce stomach irritation. Because of this drug's unpleasant taste, it is preferable to swallow the capsule whole without alteration. Use a measuring device to ensure accuracy of dose when taking the oral solution. Observe the expiration date. If you forget a dose: For oral dosing: Take the missed dose as soon as you remember it, unless it's nearly time for your next dose—if that is the case, skip the missed dose and take the next dose right on schedule. Take any remaining doses for the day at evenly spaced intervals, then return to your usual dosing schedule. For intravenous home therapy: If you miss a dose, call the home IV service or your doctor for instructions. Talk with your doctor if you find yourself missing doses because the best results come from taking this medicine right on time and keeping the blood levels or intestinal levels high enough to kill the infecting organism.

Usual Duration of Use

Oral use: Use on a regular schedule for 48 to 72 hours usually determines effectiveness in controlling infection in the colon. If response is prompt, treatment may be limited to 10 days. If symptoms warrant, oral treatment for *Clostridium difficile* diarrhea may have to be continued for 14 to 21 days. See your doctor on a regular basis.

Intravenous use: The length of treatment depends on the severity and site of the infection (for example, bone infections such as osteomyelitis may take 6 weeks to cure, and anthrax cases 60 days).

Typical Treatment Goals and Measurements (Outcomes and Markers)

Infections: The most commonly used measures of serious infections are white blood cell counts and differentials (the kind of blood cells that occur most often in your blood), and temperature. Many clinicians look for positive changes in 24–48 hours. NEVER stop an antibiotic because you start to feel better. For many infections, a full 14 days is REQUIRED to kill the bacteria. The goals and timeframe (see peak benefits above) should be discussed with you when the prescription is written.

Currently a "Drug of Choice"

For treating metronidazole-treatment failures in antibiotic-associated pseudomembranous colitis caused by *Clostridium difficile* and in cases of methicillin-resistant *Staphylococcus aureus* (MRSA).

▷ ## This Drug Should Not Be Taken If

- you have had an allergic reaction to it previously.

▷ ## Inform Your Physician Before Taking This Drug If

- you have a history of Crohn's disease or ulcerative colitis.
- you have impaired kidney function.
- you are pregnant.
- you have any degree of hearing loss.
- you are taking cholestyramine (Questran) or colestipol (Colestid) and are prescribed the oral form.

Possible Side Effects (natural, expected, and unavoidable drug actions)

Bitter, unpleasant taste for the oral form. Kidney damage with long-term, high-dose use of the intravenous form. Red-man syndrome (lowering of blood pressure, sudden rash of neck, chest, face, and extremities) and even cardiac arrest have occurred with too rapid vancomycin infusions. Doses should be given over 1 hour.

▷ ## Possible Adverse Effects (unusual, unexpected, and infrequent reactions)

If any of the following develop, consult your physician promptly for guidance.

Mild Adverse Effects

Allergic reaction: skin rash (with large doses or prolonged use).

Nausea, vomiting—infrequent with oral form and rare with intravenous form.

Chills—infrequent.

Serious Adverse Effects

Allergic reactions: anaphylaxis.

Serious skin rashes (exfoliative dermatitis or Stevens-Johnson syndrome).

Ringing or buzzing in ears, sensation of ear fullness, loss of hearing—toxicity sign.

Lowering of white blood cells—reversible and seen with the intravenous form.

Lowering of white blood cells (granulocytes) and platelets—case reports and reversible with granulocyte colony stimulating factor (GCSF).

Cardiac arrest—rare.

Hearing loss—may be reversible and more likely with high-dose or long-term use.

Kidney toxicity—may be dose-dependent and more likely with higher doses and long-term use.

Pseudomembranous colitis—possible with the IV form.

Thrombophlebitis—infrequent with the intravenous form.

▷ ## Possible Effects on Sexual Function: None reported.

Natural Diseases or Disorders That May Be Activated by This Drug

Latent hearing loss, kidney failure.

Possible Effects on Laboratory Tests

Serum creatinine: increased (a sign of kidney toxicity).

CAUTION
1. Report promptly the development of fullness, ringing, or buzzing in either ear. This may indicate the onset of nerve damage that could lead to hearing loss.
2. Do not take any medication to stop your diarrhea without calling your doctor. The bacterial toxin that causes colitis is eliminated by diarrhea; stopping the elimination could intensify and prolong your illness.
3. Blood levels MUST be used to guide intravenous dosing. Keep all appointments for laboratory work.

Precautions for Use
By Infants and Children: Some cases may require doses up to 50 mg per kg of body mass daily.
By Those Over 60 Years of Age: You may be more susceptible to drug-induced hearing loss. Use the minimum course of treatment required to cure your colitis or other infection.

▷ **Advisability of Use During Pregnancy**
Pregnancy Category: C. See Pregnancy Risk Categories at the back of this book.
Animal Studies: Rat and rabbit studies reveal no drug-induced birth defects.
Human Studies: Adequate studies of pregnant women are not available.
Use this drug only if clearly needed. Ask your doctor for help.

Advisability of Use If Breast-Feeding
Presence of this drug in breast milk: Yes.
Avoid drug or refrain from nursing.

Habit-Forming Potential: None.

Effects of Overdose: Possible nausea, vomiting, ringing in ears.

Possible Effects of Long-Term Use: Hearing loss.

Suggested Periodic Examinations While Taking This Drug (at physician's discretion)
Hearing tests.
Measures of kidney function and blood vancomycin levels with intravenous use.

▷ **While Taking This Drug, Observe the Following**
Foods: No restrictions.
Herbal Medicines or Minerals: Some patients use echinacea to attempt to boost their immune systems. Unfortunately, use of echinacea is not recommended in people with damaged immune systems. This herb may also actually weaken any immune system if it is used too often or for too long a time.
Beverages: No restrictions. May be taken with milk.
▷ *Alcohol:* No interactions expected. Use sparingly; alcohol may aggravate colitis.
Tobacco Smoking: No interactions expected. I advise everyone to quit smoking.
▷ *Other Drugs*
The following drugs may *decrease* the effects of vancomycin:
• cholestyramine (Questran).
• colestipol (Colestid).
Vancomycin *taken concurrently* with
• aminoglycoside antibiotics (see Drug Classes), such as gentamicin or tobramycin, may cause additive toxicity risk to the ears and kidneys.
• cyclosporine (Sandimmune) may result in increased toxicity risk.
• metformin (Glucophage) or other cationic drugs poses an increased risk of lactic acidosis.

- other medicines that cause kidney toxicity may pose an additive toxicity risk.
- rapacuronium (Raplon) can lead to extended neuromuscular blockade requiring neostigmine use.
- succinylcholine (Anectine) can lead to extended neuromuscular blockade requiring neostigmine use.
- warfarin (Coumadin) may cause increased bleeding risk; increased INR (prothrombin time or protime) testing is needed.

▷ *Driving, Hazardous Activities:* Usually no restrictions.

Aviation Note: The use of this drug is **probably not a disqualification** for piloting. Consult a designated Aviation Medical Examiner.

Exposure to Sun: No restrictions.

Special Storage Instructions: Refrigerate the oral solution. A home IV service will explain storage of the intravenous form.

Observe the Following Expiration Times: Provided on your prescription label by your pharmacist.

Discontinuation: To be determined by your physician.

VARICELLA VIRUS VACCINE (VAIR a sell ah)

Introduced: 1995   **Class:** Vaccine   **Prescription:** USA: Yes
Controlled Drug: USA: No; Canada: No   **Available as Generic:** USA: No; Canada: No
Brand Name: Varivax

BENEFITS versus RISKS	
Possible Benefits	*Possible Risks*
PREVENTION OF VARICELLA (CHICKEN POX)	Rash Soreness at the injection site Anaphylactic reaction

▷ **Principal Uses**

As a Single Drug Product: Uses currently included in FDA-approved labeling: Prevention of chicken pox and shingles.

Other (unlabeled) generally accepted uses: (1) Prevention of herpes zoster (in people more than 55 years old) who have previously had chicken pox.

How This Drug Works: By stimulating the immune system, the vaccine prepares the body to fight any exposure to the wild-type virus.

▷ **Widely Used Guidelines That Involve This Medicine (representative sample):** Please look at the section at the very beginning of this profile called "Class." Next, turn to Table 22 and you will find guidelines listed by the class involved!

Available Dosage Forms and Strengths

Vaccine: Single-dose vials with a final dose of 1350 plaque-forming units (PFU) per 0.5 mL.

How to Store

This product must be kept frozen prior to use.

▷ **Recommended Dosage Ranges** (Actual dose and schedule must be determined for each patient individually.)

Infants and Children (One Year to 12 Years Old): Children 1 year to 12 years old are
given 0.5 mL injected under the skin. Those 13 or older should be given a first
shot of 0.5 mL, followed by a second shot 4 to 8 weeks after the first one. In
people who fail to develop immunity (usually happens in about 30 days),
revaccination to take place 3 months after the first attempt should be tried.

Otherwise Healthy Adults: Same as the children's dose for 13 and older, providing the patient has not had chicken pox.

Over 55 Years of Age: Not studied.

**Author's Note: The Centers for Disease Control (CDC) Immunization
Practices Committee has recommended that all children 12 to 18
months old should be given varicella vaccine if they have not previously contracted chicken pox. The vaccine is also recommended by
the committee for children 19 months to 13 years old. Finally, adults
or adolescents who have not had chicken pox and are at risk for exposure may also be given the vaccine. Current recommendations for vaccines in general can be found at** *www.cdc.gov/nip/recs/child-schedule.htm.*
**Teens and adults not protected are 10–20 times more likely than chil-
dren to have complications of chicken pox. Those who are immunosuppressed (including HIV or AIDS) should NOT be given the vaccine.**

Conditions Requiring Dosing Adjustments

Liver Function: Not a consideration.

Kidney Function: Not a consideration.

▷ **Dosing Instructions:** This vaccine is to be injected under the skin. It may be
given with measles, mumps, and rubella vaccine. If you forget to get vaccinated: Talk with your pediatrician about vaccine schedules. It's always better to PREVENT a disease or condition than to have to treat it.

Usual Duration of Benefit: Exposure to chicken pox 5 years after vaccination
may result in 20% of patients developing mild disease. More experience is
needed before the question of repeat vaccination (booster) is answered. At
present a booster dose is NOT recommended. Immunity may last 10 years.

Typical Treatment Goals and Measurements (Outcomes and Markers)

Immune response/protection from varicella (chicken pox): The general goal is to
challenge the immune system of the person receiving the vaccination
enough to elicit an immune response that will protect the person from the
virus itself. For example, earlier generations "expected" to get many childhood diseases. Subsequently, measles, mumps, and varicella vaccines were
created, and possible death (mortality) and problems (morbidity) may be
avoided by getting the shots. The varicella vaccine is important as it probably protects adults from shingles later in life. Clinical markers include
gpELISA of greater than 0.3 and avoidance of varicella infection despite
subsequent exposure. Check of cell-mediated immunity (CMI) by delayed
hypersensitivity or a specific white blood cell (lymphocyte transformation)
may give a more accurate picture of immune status.

Possible Advantages of This Drug

Prevention of chicken pox when in childhood and avoidance of shingles later
in life as an adult. Nerve pain from shingles (postherpetic neuralgia) is
severe.

Currently a "Drug of Choice"

For prevention of chicken pox. Some company-based information can be
obtained by calling 1-800-Merck-RX or 1-800-637-2579.

▷ **This Drug Should Not Be Taken If**
- you have a history of anaphylactic reaction to neomycin, or to the first shot in the two-shot series.
- you have a history of blood diseases or leukemia or have HIV/AIDS.
- you are taking medicines that suppress the immune system.
- you have tuberculosis that has not been treated.
- you are allergic to eggs, gelatin, or any other vaccine component.
- you are pregnant (avoid pregnancy for 3 months after vaccine).
- you have an active infection.

▷ **Inform Your Physician Before Taking This Drug If**
- you are planning pregnancy in the near future.
- you have a condition that may require steroids.
- you have had blood or plasma transfusions (vaccination should be delayed for 5 months).
- you take salicylates (aspirin, others) on a regular basis. This should NOT be done for 6 weeks following vaccination, as it is a risk for Reye's syndrome.
- you live with someone who has a depressed immune system (such as an AIDS patient). Because this vaccine is a live-virus vaccine, you may be infectious to them.

Possible Side Effects (natural, expected, and unavoidable drug actions)
Pain at the injection site, fever—infrequent to frequent.

▷ **Possible Adverse Effects** (unusual, unexpected, and infrequent reactions)
If any of the following develop, consult your physician promptly for guidance.
Mild Adverse Effects
Allergic reaction: skin rash.
Varicella-like rash—infrequent.
Headache, irritability, fatigue, and loss of appetite—rare to infrequent.
Increased sensitivity to light (photophobia)—case reports.
Chills, stiff neck, and joint pain (arthralgia)—infrequent.
Nausea, vomiting—rare.
Serious Adverse Effects
Allergic reactions: anaphylactic reaction, serious skin rashes (Stevens-Johnson syndrome or TENS)—case reports.
Idiosyncratic reactions: none reported.
Febrile seizures—case reports.
Thrombocytopenic purpura—case reports.
Herpes zoster—possible.
Pneumonitis—case report and of questionable causation.
May be possible for a recently vaccinated person to transmit varicella to a susceptible contact—one case report.

▷ **Possible Effects on Sexual Function:** None reported.

Possible Delayed Adverse Effects: None reported.

▷ **Adverse Effects That May Mimic Natural Diseases or Disorders**
Rash may resemble chicken pox.

Natural Diseases or Disorders That May Be Activated by This Drug
Herpes zoster not activated but has occurred rarely after some patients received the shot or a booster.

Possible Effects on Laboratory Tests
None reported.

CAUTION
> **Do not** give aspirin or other salicylates (INCLUDING HERBALS SUCH AS WHITE WILLOW BARK) to patients who have recently received the vaccine. The risk of Reye's syndrome is associated with such aspirin use.

Precautions for Use
> *By Infants and Children:* Safety and effectiveness for use by those under 12 months of age have not been established.
> *By Those Over 60 Years of Age:* Not studied.

▷ **Advisability of Use During Pregnancy**
> *Pregnancy Category:* C. See Pregnancy Risk Categories at the back of this book.
> *Animal Studies:* Have not been conducted with this vaccine.
> *Human Studies:* Information from adequate studies of pregnant women is not available.
> The manufacturer says that the vaccine should not be given to pregnant women, and pregnancy should be avoided for 3 months following vaccination.

Advisability of Use If Breast-Feeding
> Presence of this drug in breast milk: Expected.
> Vaccine viewed as appropriate by American Academy of Pediatrics if the risk of exposure of the mother is high. Avoid drug or refrain from nursing.

Habit-Forming Potential: None.

Effects of Overdose: Not defined.

Possible Effects of Long-Term Use: Not intended for long-term use.

Suggested Periodic Examinations While Taking This Drug (at physician's discretion)
> Immunity check.

▷ **While Taking This Drug, Observe the Following**
> *Foods:* No restrictions.
> *Herbal Medicines or Minerals:* Some patients use echinacea to attempt to boost their immune systems. Unfortunately, use of echinacea is not recommended in people with damaged immune systems. This herb may also actually weaken any immune system if it is used too often or for too long a time. Mistletoe has also not been studied and cannot be recommended. White willow bark contains aspirin-like chemicals. DO NOT take this for 6 weeks after getting the vaccine.
> *Beverages:* No restrictions.
▷ *Alcohol:* No interactions expected.
> *Tobacco Smoking:* No interactions expected. I advise everyone to quit smoking.
▷ *Other Drugs*
> Varicella vaccine *taken concurrently* with
> - acyclovir (Zovirax) may result in a blunted immune benefit from the vaccine.
> - adalimumab (Humira) may result in a blunted immune benefit from the vaccine.
> - aspirin or any salicylates (various) may result in Reye's syndrome—DO NOT take aspirin for 6 weeks after vaccination.
> - chemotherapy (various) may lead to infection risk by the vaccine.
> - corticosteroids (see Drug Classes) may result in extreme reactions.
> - etanercept (Enbrel) may blunt immune response to varicella vaccine.
> - hepatitis B immune globulin may blunt immune response to varicella vaccine.

- immune globulins (such as varicella-zoster immune globulin, rabies, or tetanus immune globulin) may blunt beneficial response to the vaccine.
- immunosuppressant medicines (such as cyclosporine [Sandimmune], sirolimus [Rapamune], or tacrolimus [Prograf]) may result in blunted beneficial vaccine response as well as unexpected reactions, sometimes extreme reactions.
- infliximab (Remicade) may increase risk of varicella infection from varicella vaccine itself.
- leflunomide (Arava) may blunt immune response to varicella vaccine. Rapid elimination procedure for leflunomide may be needed.
- mesalamine (Asacol) may result in risk of Reye's syndrome—DO NOT take salicylates for 6 weeks after vaccination.
- olsalazine (Dipentum) may result in risk of Reye's syndrome—DO NOT take salicylates for 6 weeks after vaccination.

▷ *Driving, Hazardous Activities:* This drug may cause soreness at the injection site. Restrict activities as necessary.

Aviation Note: The use of this drug *is probably not a disqualification* for piloting. Consult a designated Aviation Medical Examiner.

Exposure to Sun: No restrictions.

Occurrence of Unrelated Illness: This vaccination should not be given in the presence of any other active infection.

Special Storage Instructions: This vaccine must be stored frozen.

Author's Note: A Vaccine Adverse Event Reporting System (VAERS) can be reached with a free call to 1-800-822-7967.

VENLAFAXINE (ven la FAX een)

Introduced: 1993   **Class:** Antidepressant   **Prescription:** USA: Yes   **Controlled Drug:**   USA: No; Canada: No   **Available as Generic:** USA: No

Brand Names: Effexor, Effexor XR

```
┌─────────────────────────────────────────────────────────────────┐
│                     BENEFITS versus RISKS                         │
│        Possible Benefits                    Possible Risks        │
│  EFFECTIVE TREATMENT OF           INCREASED BLOOD PRESSURE        │
│    DEPRESSION                     Seizures                        │
│  BETTER SIDE-EFFECT PROFILE       Constipation                   │
│    THAN TRICYCLIC ANTI-           Increased heart rate            │
│    DEPRESSANTS                    Increased serum lipids          │
│  RAPID ONSET OF EFFECT                                            │
│  EXCELLENT REMISSION RATE IN                                      │
│    MAJOR DEPRESSION                                               │
│  HELPS PREVENT RELAPSE AND                                        │
│    RECURRENCE OF DEPRESSION                                       │
│  EFFECTIVE TREATMENT OF                                           │
│    ANXIETY                                                        │
│  TREATS GENERALIZED ANXIETY                                       │
│    DISORDER                                                       │
│  TREATMENT OF SOCIAL ANXIETY                                      │
│    DISORDER                                                       │
│  Second-line treatment of children                               │
│    who have both depression and                                  │
│    ADHD (XR form)                                                │
│  May decrease hot flashes in cancer                              │
│    survivors and after menopause                                │
└─────────────────────────────────────────────────────────────────┘
```

▷ **Principal Uses**

As a Single Drug Product: Uses currently included in FDA-approved labeling: (1) Treatment of depression; (2) treatment of generalized anxiety disorder; (3) treatment of social anxiety disorder (also called social phobia); (4) prevention of relapse and recurrence of depression.

Other (unlabeled) generally accepted uses: (1) May be useful in obsessive-compulsive disorder; (2) may treat chronic fatigue syndrome; (3) may have a role in easing hot flashes in cancer survivors and after menopause; (4) second-line treatment in children who have both depression and ADHD; (5) can be helpful in premenstrual dysphoric disorder (PMDD); (6) case-based use in neuropathic pain and nerve pain from chemotherapy with a more favorable side-effect profile than tricyclic antidepressants.

How This Drug Works: This bicyclic (second-generation) antidepressant inhibits the return (reuptake) of nerve transmitters (serotonin, norepinephrine, and dopamine) and helps return normal mood and thinking. This medicine is actually a mixture of two forms called isomers. The positive isomer works mostly as a serotonin uptake inhibitor.

▷ **Widely Used Guidelines That Involve This Medicine (representative sample):** Please look at the section at the very beginning of this profile called "Class." Next, turn to Table 22 and you will find guidelines listed by the class involved!

Available Dosage Forms and Strengths

Tablets — 25 mg, 37.5 mg, 50 mg, 75 mg, 100 mg

Tablets, extended release — 37.5 mg, 75 mg, 100 mg, 150 mg (100 mg in Canada)

Tablets, sustained release — 100 and 150 mg (Canada only)

▷ **Recommended Dosage Ranges** (Actual dose and schedule must be determined for each patient individually.)

Infants and Children: Safety and efficacy for those under 18 years of age are not established.

18 to 60 Years of Age: For depression and generalized anxiety disorder: Start with 75 mg per day, as 25 mg doses three times daily taken with food. If needed and tolerated, the dose may be increased at 4-day intervals in steps up to a maximum of 225 mg per day. Some hospitalized patients have been given a maximum of 375 mg per day. The XR form is started at 37.5 milligrams per day. Dose increases of 75 mg/day can be made at intervals of at least 4 days. Daily maximum is 225 mg per day. In general, conversion from immediate release to venlafaxine XR can be done using the total immediate release daily dose and converting that to the nearest equal dose of the XR form.

For reducing hot flashes in cancer survivors: 12.5 mg twice daily.

Over 60 Years of Age: Low starting doses and slow increases are indicated. Natural declines in kidney function may lead to drug accumulation at higher doses. May worsen constipation.

Conditions Requiring Dosing Adjustments

Liver Function: Total daily dose must be reduced by 50% for patients with moderate liver compromise. Further dose decreases and individualized dosing is needed in liver cirrhosis.

Kidney Function: Patients with compromised kidneys (creatinine clearance of 10 to 70 mL/min) should take 75% of the usual daily dose.

▷ **Dosing Instructions:** Best to take this medicine with food. The XR form should NOT be crushed or chewed. If you forget a dose: Take the missed dose as soon as you remember it, unless it's nearly time for your next dose—if that is the case, skip the missed dose and take the next dose right on schedule. DO NOT double up on doses. Because this medicine must reach an equilibrium (or steady state) in the brain, it is very important to take it exactly as prescribed to get the best results in helping depression. Talk with your doctor if you find yourself missing doses.

Usual Duration of Use: Regular use for 2 weeks usually determines benefits in treating depression, but up to 6 weeks may be needed to see the peak benefits. Decreasing hot flashes in cancer survivors may take several weeks. Long-term use requires follow-up by your doctor.

Typical Treatment Goals and Measurements (Outcomes and Markers)

Depression: The general goal: to at least help lessen the degree and severity of depression, letting patients return to their daily lives. Specific measures of depression involve testing or inventories (such as the Hamilton Depression) and can be valuable in helping check benefits from this medicine. In using this medicine for short-term treatment of social anxiety disorder (SAD), the Liebowitz Social Anxiety Scale (LSAS) is often used.

Possible Advantages of This Drug

Effective treatment of depression with fewer side effects than other currently available agents. Starts to have a therapeutic effect more rapidly than other available agents. One study of 1,108 patients with major depression found a 45% remission rate. Works on both serotonin and norepinephrine nerve transmitters (neurotransmitters) unlike other antidepressants that may only impact serotonin.

▷ **This Drug Should Not Be Taken If**
- you had an allergic reaction to any form of it previously.
- you are taking a monoamine oxidase (MAO) inhibitor (see Drug Classes).

▷ **Inform Your Physician Before Taking This Drug If**
  • you have a history of high blood pressure.
  • you've recently had a heart attack.
  • you have a history of abnormally increased lipids (hyperlipidemia).
  • you are planning pregnancy.
  • you have a history of seizures.
  • you have a history of suicide attempts or think about suicide.
  • you have trouble sleeping.
  • you have a history of hypomania or mania.
  • you are unsure how much to take or how often to take this medicine.

Possible Side Effects (natural, expected, and unavoidable drug actions)
  Constipation and headache. Sleepiness, weight loss, dry mouth. Small
  increases in cholesterol (2–3 mg/dL). A withdrawal syndrome is possible if
  this medicine is stopped abruptly. Best to slowly decrease (taper) the dose
  over 2–4 weeks or longer.

▷ **Possible Adverse Effects** (unusual, unexpected, and infrequent reactions)
  **If any of the following develop, consult your physician promptly for
  guidance.**
  Mild Adverse Effects
  Allergic reactions: Possible.
  Palpitations or fast heart rate—rare.
  Nausea and vomiting—infrequent.
  Weight decrease—infrequent.
  Dizziness (may disappear without treatment), fatigue, and headache—
  infrequent to frequent.
  Anxiety, somnolence, or insomnia (may stop on its own).
  Blurred vision—possible.
  Spontaneous and easy bruising (ecchymosis)—case report.
  Sweating—possible (benztropine eased one case).
  Serious Adverse Effects
  Allergic reactions: Possible.
  Idiosyncratic reactions: one case report of lowered white blood cells (agran-
  ulocytosis).
  Liver toxicity—case reports.
  SIADH and very low sodium—case reports.
  Increased blood pressure—case reports.
  Serotonin syndrome—case reports.
  Neuroleptic malignant syndrome—case report.
  Rhabdomyolisis—case report.
  Mania—case reports.
  Seizures—very rare during premarketing studies.

▷ **Possible Effects on Sexual Function:** Delayed orgasm, abnormal ejaculation,
  priapism, impotence, and erectile failure—all rare.

Possible Delayed Adverse Effects: None reported.

▷ **Adverse Effects That May Mimic Natural Diseases or Disorders**
  None reported.

Natural Diseases or Disorders That May Be Activated by This Drug
  None reported.

Possible Effects on Laboratory Tests
  Serum cholesterol: increased slightly.

CAUTION

1. This drug should not be taken with MAO inhibitors (see Glossary). If you have recently stopped an MAO inhibitor, 14 days should pass before venlafaxine is started.

2. Because the half life of this medicine is relatively short, if this medicine needs to be stopped, best to slowly decrease (taper) it over 2–4 weeks or longer.

3. Pediatric and adult patients treated with this medicine should be closely watched for worsening depression or suicidal thinking. The FDA has required makers of antidepressants such as this one to alert health care professionals to the fact that children and adults with major depression may develop worsening depression or suicidal thoughts and behavior whether they take medicine for depression or do not take it. Patients should be carefully followed for such clinical worsening (particularly when treatment is started or doses are increased or decreased).

▷ **Advisability of Use During Pregnancy**

Pregnancy Category: C. See Pregnancy Risk Categories at the back of this book.

Animal Studies: There was an increase in stillborn rats at 10 times the usual human dose.

Human Studies: Adequate studies of pregnant women are not available.

Ask your doctor for guidance.

Advisability of Use If Breast-Feeding

Presence of this drug in breast milk: Yes.

Monitor nursing infant closely, and discontinue drug or nursing if adverse effects develop.

Habit-Forming Potential: None.

Effects of Overdose: Nausea, vomiting, constipation, seizure potential.

Possible Effects of Long-Term Use: None noted.

Suggested Periodic Examinations While Taking This Drug (at physician's discretion)

Blood pressure checks, periodic lipid panels, resolution of depression.

▷ **While Taking This Drug, Observe the Following**

Foods: No restrictions.

Herbal Medicines or Minerals: Since venlafaxine and St. John's wort may act to increase serotonin, the combination is not advised (St. John's wort may also cause fast heart rate). Since part of the way ginseng and ginkgo work may be as MAO inhibitors, do not combine ginseng or ginkgo with venlafaxine. Ma huang, yohimbe, Indian snakeroot, and kava kava are also best avoided while taking this medicine. Talk to your doctor BEFORE combining any herbals with this medicine.

Nutritional Support: No special support indicated.

Beverages: Since venlafaxine is metabolized in the liver and grapefruit juice has been shown to inhibit the removal (metabolism) of some other medications, caution is advised. Water is the best liquid to take this medicine with.

▷ *Alcohol:* May increase somnolence if combined.

Tobacco Smoking: No interactions expected. I advise everyone to quit smoking.

Marijuana Smoking: Additive effect on somnolence, one case of mania following combination with fluoxetine. DO NOT COMBINE.

▷   *Other Drugs*
    Venlafaxine ***taken concurrently*** with
- beta blockers (see Drug Classes) may result in larger than expected pharmacological effects from the beta blockers; because these agents are metabolized in the liver and venlafaxine may block this metabolism, caution is advised.
- calcium channel blockers (see Drug Classes) may result in toxicity; because these agents are metabolized in the liver and venlafaxine may block this metabolism, caution is advised.
- cimetidine (Tagamet) may lead to venlafaxine toxicity.
- dextromethorphan (the DM in many cough and cold preparations) may result in dextromethorphan or venlafaxine toxicity. Caution is advised.
- dofetilide (Tikosyn) may result in dofetilide toxicity.
- MAO inhibitors (see Drug Classes) may lead to undesirable side effects—DO NOT COMBINE.
- medicines such as class I, IA, or III antiarrhythmics (dofetilide [Tikosyn], clarithromycin, cotrimoxazole, ondansetron, ziprazidone, and others) may lead to added prolongation of the QTc interval and undesirable effects. Combination is not recommended.
- quinidine (Quinaglute, others) may result in venlafaxine toxicity.
- ritonavir (Norvir) may lead to venlafaxine toxicity.
- drugs with sedative properties will increase those effects.
- paroxetine (Paxil—a SSRI) or SNRIs can lead to a serotonin syndrome if a sufficient time does not pass between stopping a first medicine and starting an alternative therapy. The time required (washout) may vary patient to patient, but the generally accepted time is 2 weeks.
- sibutramine (Meridia) increases toxicity risk (serotonin syndrome)—DO NOT COMBINE.
- sumatriptan (Imitrex), naratriptan (Amerge), rizatriptan (Maxalt) or zolmitriptan (Zomig), almotriptan (Axert), or other "triptans" may lead to incoordination and weakness—DO NOT COMBINE.
- tramadol (Ultram) may increase the risk of seizures.
- tricyclic antidepressants (see Drug Classes) may result in toxicity; because these agents are metabolized in the liver and venlafaxine may block this metabolism, caution is advised.
- warfarin (Coumadin) may result in bleeding; more frequent INR (prothrombin time or protime) testing is needed. Ongoing warfarin doses should be adjusted to laboratory results.
- zolpidem (Ambien) may increase risk of hallucinations—DO NOT COMBINE.

▷   *Driving, Hazardous Activities:* This drug may cause somnolence. Restrict activities as necessary.
    Aviation Note: The use of this drug ***is a disqualification*** for piloting. Consult a designated Aviation Medical Examiner.
    Exposure to Sun: No restrictions.
    Exposure to Heat: No restrictions.
    Discontinuation: If this medicine is to be stopped, the dose should be slowly lowered over 2–4 weeks or longer on your doctor's advice. Tapering over this time helps your body best adjust to not having this medicine, minimizing risk of undesirable discontinuation symptoms.

VERAPAMIL (ver AP a mil)

Introduced: 1967   **Class:** Anti-anginal, antiarrhythmic, antihypertensive, calcium channel blocker   **Prescription:** USA: Yes   **Controlled Drug:** USA: No; Canada: No   **Available as Generic:** USA: Yes (verapamil SR); Canada: Yes

BrandNames: ✤Alti-Verapamil, ✤Apo-Verap, Calan, Calan SR, ✤Chronovera, Covera-HS, ✤Dom-Verapamil SR, ✤Gen-Verapamil, Isoptin, Isoptin SR, ✤Med-Verapamil, ✤Novo-Veramil, ✤Nu-Verap, ✤PMS-Verapamil, Tarka [CD], Verelan, Verelan PM

Controversies in Medicine: Medicines in this class have had many conflicting reports. The FDA has held hearings on the calcium channel blocker (CCB) class. Amlodipine got the first FDA approval to treat high blood pressure or angina in people with congestive heart failure. Early research at New York University found that a calcium channel blocker called nifedipine is a cause of reversible male infertility. CCBs are currently second-line agents for high blood pressure according to the JNC VII (see Glossary).

BENEFITS versus RISKS

Possible Benefits	*Possible Risks*
EFFECTIVE PREVENTION OF BOTH MAJOR TYPES OF ANGINA	Congestive heart failure
	Low blood pressure (infrequent)
EFFECTIVE CONTROL OF HEART RATE IN CHRONIC ATRIAL FIBRILLATION AND FLUTTER	Heart rhythm disturbance
	Fluid retention
	Constipation
EFFECTIVE PREVENTION OF PAROXYSMAL ATRIAL TACHYCARDIA (PAT)	Liver damage without jaundice
	Swelling of male breast tissue
EFFECTIVE TREATMENT OF HYPERTENSION	

▷ **Principal Uses**

As a Single Drug Product: Uses currently included in FDA-approved labeling: Used to treat (1) angina pectoris due to coronary artery spasm (Prinzmetal's variant angina) that occurs spontaneously and is not associated with exertion; (2) classical angina of effort (due to atherosclerotic disease of the coronary arteries) in individuals who have not responded to or cannot tolerate the nitrates and beta-blocker drugs customarily used to treat this disorder; (3) abnormally rapid heart rate due to chronic atrial fibrillation or flutter; (4) recurrent paroxysmal atrial or supraventricular tachycardia; (5) primary hypertension.

Other (unlabeled) generally accepted uses: (1) May help decrease abnormal scar (keloid) formation; (2) prevents abnormal heart rhythms that occur after surgery; (3) relieves symptoms of and may help reverse hypertrophic cardiomyopathy; (4) may help decrease the severity or occurrence of cluster headaches; (5) helps control symptoms of panic attacks; (6) can be of use in postischemic-acute-kidney failure; (7) may stop the progression of abnormal buildup on the inside of blood vessels (atherosclerosis); (8) may help decrease severity and occurrence of nocturnal leg cramps; (9) can help stuttering; (10) may have a role in treating Tourette's syndrome.

As a Combination Drug Product [CD]: This drug is available in combination (Tarka brand) with an ACE inhibitor (trandolapril). The combination offers benefits of two different mechanisms of action in the same medicine in treating high blood pressure.

How This Drug Works: By blocking passage of calcium through certain cell walls (which is necessary for the function of nerve and muscle tissue), this drug slows the spread of electrical activity through the heart and inhibits the contraction of coronary arteries and peripheral arterioles. As a result of these combined effects, this drug prevents spontaneous coronary artery spasm (Prinzmetal's type of angina).

- reduces heart rate and contraction force during exertion, thus lowering the oxygen requirement of the heart muscle; this reduces the occurrence of effort-induced angina (classical angina pectoris).
- reduces degree of contraction of peripheral arterial walls, resulting in relaxation and lowering of blood pressure. This further reduces the workload of the heart during exertion and contributes to the prevention of angina.
- slows the rate of electrical impulses through the heart and thereby prevents excessively rapid heart action (tachycardia).

▷ **Widely Used Guidelines That Involve This Medicine (representative sample):** Please look at the section at the very beginning of this profile called "Class." Next, turn to Table 22 and you will find guidelines listed by the class involved!

Available Dosage Forms and Strengths

Caplets, sustained-release — 120 mg, 180 mg, 240 mg
Capsules, sustained-release — 120 mg, 180 mg, 240 mg, 360 mg
Injection — 5 mg/2 mL
Tablets — 40 mg, 80 mg, 120 mg
Tablets, combination (Tarka) — 1 mg trandolapril/240 mg verapamil,
2 mg trandolapril/180 mg verapamil,
2 mg trandolapril/240 mg verapamil,
4 mg trandolapril/240 mg verapamil
(also available in extended release in the same doses)
Tablets, extended-release — 180 mg, 240 mg, 360 mg
Tablets, sustained-release — 120 mg, 180 mg, 240 mg
Tablets, timed-release (Verelan PM) — 100 mg, 200 mg, 300 mg

▷ **Usual Adult Dosage Ranges:** Hypertension: Initially 80 mg three times daily. The dose may be increased gradually at 1- to 7-day intervals as needed and tolerated. The usual maintenance dose is from 240 to 360 mg daily in three or four divided doses. The prolonged-action (sustained-release) dose forms permit once-a-day dosing. The total daily dose should not exceed 360 mg.

Once-a-day treatment may be initiated with one prolonged-action capsule of 120 mg or one tablet of 180 mg (particularly the elderly or patients of small stature).

The Covera HS form is given as one 180 mg extended-release tablet at bedtime. If adequate response is not obtained, the dose may be increased to 240 mg at bedtime. Dose may be subsequently increased as needed and tolerated to a maximum of 480 mg. The lowest effect or trough effect would be best evaluated just before bedtime.

The Verelan PM form is designed to be taken at bedtime. Dosing generally starts at 100 mg at bedtime as a conservative strategy.

Tarka form: Talk to your doctor.

Note: Actual dose and schedule must be determined for each patient individually.

Conditions Requiring Dosing Adjustments

Liver Function: Blood levels should be obtained to guide dosing. In liver disease, dose should be decreased to 20–50% of usual doses at the usual times. This drug is also a rare cause of liver damage. Electrocardiogram changes may provide an early indication of increasing blood levels.

Kidney Function: In severe kidney compromise, the dose should be decreased by 50–75%.

Heart (Myocardial) Dysfunction: Intravenous doses (0.0001 mg/kg/minute) are started and adjusted (titrated) against heart rate. Also adjusted if you are taking digoxin or a beta blocker.

▷ **Dosing Instructions:** Preferably taken with meals and with food at bedtime. The regular tablet may be crushed for administration. Most prolonged-action dose forms (capsules and tablets) should be swallowed whole and not altered. Both Calan and Isoptin SR forms can be cut in half without changing the release rate of the medicine. Neither form should be crushed or cut into fourths. Verelan capsules may be taken without regard to food intake. The Verelan PM form IS NOT a sleeping pill. The PM is meant to stand for bedtime dosing. If you forget a dose: Take the missed dose as soon as you remember it, unless it's nearly time for your next dose—if that is the case, skip the missed dose and take the next dose right on schedule. DO NOT double up on doses. Talk with your doctor if you find yourself missing doses.

Usual Duration of Use: Use on a regular schedule for 2 to 4 weeks usually determines effectiveness in reducing the frequency and severity of angina. Reduction of elevated blood pressure may be apparent within the first 1 to 2 weeks. For long-term use (months to years), the smallest effective dose should be used. Periodic physician evaluation is needed to keep blood pressure in the target range.

Typical Treatment Goals and Measurements (Outcomes and Markers)

Blood Pressure: Guidelines (JNC VII) define normal blood pressure (BP) as **less than** 120/80 and **pre-hypertension** as 120/80 to 139/89. This new range is intended to help doctors encourage lifestyle changes (or, in the case of people with a risk factor for high blood pressure, start treatment) much earlier—so that damage to blood vessels, heart, kidneys, sexual potency, or eyes might be minimized or avoided altogether. Stage 1 hypertension is 140/90 to 159/99, and stage 2 hypertension equal to or greater than 160/100 mm Hg. These guidelines also recommend that clinicians work with their patients to agree on the goals and a plan of treatment. The first-ever guidelines for blood pressure (hypertension) in African Americans recommends that MOST black patients be started on TWO antihypertensive medicines with the goal of lowering blood pressure to 130/80 for those with high risk for heart and blood vessel disease or with diabetes. The American Diabetes Association also recommends 130/80 as the target for diabetics and less than 125/75 for those who spill more than one gram of protein into their urine. Most clinicians try to achieve a BP that confers the best balance of lower cardiovascular risk and avoids the problem of too low a blood pressure. Blood pressure duration is generally increased with beneficial restriction of sodium. If goals are not met, it is not unusual to intensify doses or add on medicines.

Abnormal Heartbeats: The general goal is to return the heart to a normal rhythm or at least to markedly reduce the occurrence of abnormal heartbeats. In life-threatening arrhythmias, the goal is to abort the abnormal beats and return the pattern to normal. Success at ongoing suppression may involve ambulatory checks of heart rate and rhythm for a day (such as in Holter monitoring). This kind of testing involves placement of adhesive-backed temporary electrodes on the skin in several positions around the heart. A small heart rate and rhythm (EKG or ECG) recording device is carried around via a shoulder strap and records what the heart is doing over 24 hours. Once the recording is made, a scanning machine reviews the record, tallies abnormal heartbeats or rhythms, and gives a close and extended look at how the heart is reacting or benefiting from the medicines that the patient is taking. Repeat measurements can be made if doses are changed to check the success at keeping the heart in normal sinus rhythm!

Possible Advantages of This Drug

No adverse effects on blood levels of glucose, potassium, or uric acid. Does not increase blood cholesterol or triglyceride levels. Does not impair capacity for exercise. The 360 mg strength of Verelan allows once-daily dosing for those patients who require more than 240 mg daily. The company has noted that there is no increase in side effects when comparing the 240 mg capsules to the newer 360 mg ones.

The Verelan PM and the Covera HS forms are specifically made to reach their peak levels in the body in the morning—the thinking here is that since heart attacks most often happen in the morning, they may actually be related to early morning increases in heart rate and blood pressure. These medicines seek to avoid low medicine blood levels at a time when it appears they are needed most.

Currently a "Drug of Choice"

In people who have contraindications for beta blockers and in whom a blood vessel spasm (vasospastic) underlying cause (mechanism) is suspected.

▷ This Drug Should Not Be Taken If

- you have had an allergic reaction to it previously.
- you have active liver disease.
- you have a "sick sinus" syndrome (and do not have an artificial pacemaker).
- you have a fast heart rate (ventricular tachycardia) arising in the ventricles.
- you have atrial fibrillation or flutter.
- you have been told that you have a second- or third-degree heart block or congestive heart failure.
- you have low blood pressure (systolic pressure below 90).

▷ Inform Your Physician Before Taking This Drug If

- you have had an unfavorable response to any calcium channel blocker.
- you are currently taking any other drugs, especially digitalis or a beta-blocker drug (see Drug Classes).
- you have had a recent stroke or heart attack.
- you have a history of congestive heart failure, angina, or heart rhythm disorders.
- you have aortic stenosis (ask your specialist).
- the left side of your heart is very weak (ejection fraction less than 30% or pulmonary wedge pressure more than 20 mm Hg—ask your doctor).
- you have poor circulation to your extremities or gangrene.
- you develop a skin reaction while taking this medicine. Some reactions have gone on to more serious problems (such as erythema multiforme).

- you have impaired liver or kidney function.
- you have a history of drug-induced liver damage.

Possible Side Effects (natural, expected, and unavoidable drug actions)

Low blood pressure, fluid retention—rare. Change in how well platelets work (antiplatelet effect)—may be significant if combined with aspirin. Constipation (up to 42%).

▷ **Possible Adverse Effects** (unusual, unexpected, and infrequent reactions)

If any of the following develop, consult your physician promptly for guidance.

Mild Adverse Effects

Allergic reactions: skin rash, hives, itching, aching joints.

Flushing—infrequent.

Headache—frequent.

Dizziness, fatigue—infrequent.

Nausea, indigestion, constipation—rare to infrequent.

Abnormal growth of the gums—infrequent to frequent.

Sensation of numbness or coldness in the extremities—case reports.

Hair color change—case report.

Cough—rare.

Serious Adverse Effects

Allergic reaction: skin rash (Stevens-Johnson syndrome)—possible.

Serious disturbances of heart rate and/or rhythm, congestive heart failure—rare.

Drug-induced liver damage without jaundice—case reports

Antiplatelet effect and extended time to form blood clots—possible.

Lung problems (pulmonary edema).

Excessive lowering of blood pressure—case reports.

Unmasking of parkinsonism or movement disorders—rare.

Low blood sugar—possible.

▷ **Possible Effects on Sexual Function:** Altered timing and pattern of menstruation.

Male breast enlargement and tenderness (gynecomastia)—case reports.

Impotence—frequent.

Possible Effects on Laboratory Tests

Blood total cholesterol and HDL cholesterol levels: no effect in some; decreased in others.

Blood LDL cholesterol or triglyceride level: no effect.

Glucose tolerance test (GTT): decreased.

Liver function tests: increased enzymes (ALT/GPT, AST/GOT), increased bilirubin (case reports).

CAUTION

1. Be sure to inform all doctors and other health care professionals who provide medical care for you that you take this drug. Carry a card in your wallet or purse that says you are taking this drug.

2. You may use nitroglycerin and other nitrate drugs as needed to relieve acute episodes of angina pain. If angina attacks become more frequent or intense, call your doctor promptly.

3. If this drug is used concurrently with a beta-blocker drug, you may develop excessively low blood pressure (may be required in some resistant blood pressure patients).

4. This drug may cause swelling of the feet and ankles. This may not be indicative of either heart or kidney dysfunction.

Precautions for Use

By Infants and Children: Safety and effectiveness for those under 12 years of age are not established.

By Those Over 60 Years of Age: You may be more susceptible to weakness, dizziness, fainting, and falling. Take necessary precautions to prevent injury. Report promptly any changes in your pattern of thirst and urination.

▷ **Advisability of Use During Pregnancy**

Pregnancy Category: C. See Pregnancy Risk Categories at the back of this book.

Animal Studies: Toxic effects on the embryo and retarded growth of the fetus (but no birth defects) reported in rat studies.

Human Studies: Adequate studies of pregnant women are not available.

Avoid this drug during the first 3 months. Use during the final 6 months only if clearly needed. Ask your doctor for help.

Advisability of Use If Breast-Feeding

Presence of this drug in breast milk: Yes.

Discuss the benefits and risks of nursing your infant. Most clinicians find breast milk drug levels to be insignificant. Monitor infant for adverse effects.

Habit-Forming Potential: None. A withdrawal syndrome is possible (increased frequency and severity of angina). If the medicine must be stopped, it should be slowly decreased—NOT stopped abruptly.

Effects of Overdose: Flushed and warm skin, sweating, light-headedness, irritability, rapid heart rate, low blood pressure, loss of consciousness.

Possible Effects of Long-Term Use: None reported.

Suggested Periodic Examinations While Taking This Drug (at physician's discretion)

Evaluations of heart function, including electrocardiograms.

Liver and kidney function tests, with long-term use.

▷ **While Taking This Drug, Observe the Following**

Foods: DO NOT take this medicine with grapefruit or grapefruit juice. Avoid excessive salt intake.

Herbal Medicines or Minerals: Ginseng, guarana, mate, bitter orange, country mallow, hawthorn, saw palmetto, ma huang, goldenseal, yohimbe, and licorice may also cause increased blood pressure. Excessive caffeine and added caffeine from guarana can worsen blood pressure, will also stay in your body longer than expected, and are not recommended. Garlic and calcium may work to lower blood pressure, but calcium may reverse the benefits off verapamil. Some dosing changes may be needed. St. John's wort may work to lower calcium channel blocker levels (because it increases P-glycoprotein in the gut). This combination may also increase sun sensitivity. Eleuthero root and ephedra (no longer on the U.S. market for weight loss) should be avoided by people living with hypertension. Indian snakeroot has a German Commission E monograph indication for hypertension. Discuss any plans for herbal medicines or minerals with your doctor BEFORE adding them.

Beverages: Caffeine levels will be increased if caffeine-containing beverages are consumed while you are on verapamil. DO NOT take this medicine with grapefruit or grapefruit juice. May be taken with milk.

▷ *Alcohol:* Use with caution until combined effects have been determined. Alcohol may exaggerate the drop in blood pressure and change the elimination of alcohol (experienced by some patients). This may lead to an exaggerated effect of alcohol.

Tobacco Smoking: Nicotine can reduce the effectiveness of this drug. Avoid all forms of tobacco.

Marijuana Smoking: Possible reduced effectiveness of this drug; mild to moderate increase in angina; possible changes in electrocardiogram, confusing interpretation.

▷ *Other Drugs*

Verapamil may *increase* the effects of
- buspirone (Buspar).
- carbamazepine (Tegretol) and cause carbamazepine toxicity.
- digitoxin and digoxin (Lanoxin) and cause digitalis toxicity.
- lovastatin (Mevacor), simvastatin (Zocor), and other HMG CoA reductase inhibitors that use cytochrome P 450 3A4 for removal.
- neuromuscular blocking agents (such as pancuronium—Pavulon, or vecuronium—Norcuron) and may prolong muscle weakness.
- sirolimus (Rapamune).
- tacrolimus (Prograf).
- tretinoin (Vesanoid).
- tricyclic antidepressants (see Drug Classes).
- vincristine (Oncovin).

Verapamil *taken concurrently* with
- amiodarone (Cordarone) may result in cardiac arrest.
- aspirin (various) may result in excessive verapamil levels and excessive lowering of blood pressure.
- beta blockers (see Drug Classes) may affect heart rate and rhythm adversely. Careful monitoring by your physician is necessary if these drugs are taken concurrently.
- calcium supplements (various) may blunt the therapeutic benefits of verapamil—separate calcium and verapamil dosing by 2 hours.
- cilostazol (Pletal) may result in cilostazol toxicity. Lower cilostazol doses are prudent.
- colesevelam (Welchol) will decrease the therapeutic blood level of verapamil.
- cyclosporine (Sandimmune) may result in cyclosporine toxicity and renal compromise.
- dantrolene will cause elevated blood potassium and depression of the heart.
- dofetilide (Tikosyn) may result in dofetilide toxicity. Checks of dofetilide levels and dosing adjustments to levels are prudent.
- disopyramide (Norpace) can cause congestive heart failure.
- flecainide (Tambocor) may have additive heart effects (excessively low heart rate or cardiogenic shock).
- lithium (Lithobid, others) may result in lithium toxicity and mania.
- medicines such as class I, IA, or III antiarrhythmics—amiodarone (Cordarone), dofetilide (Tikosyn), clarithromycin, cotrimoxazole, ondansetron, ziprazidone and others—may lead to prolongation of the QTc interval and undesirable effects. Combination is not recommended (see amiodarone note above regarding extreme caution if these two medicines are combined or if transition is made from quinidine to amiodarone).
- midazolam (Versed) may result in midazolam toxicity. Lower doses (by 50%) and careful patient monitoring are critical.
- NSAIDs (see Drug Classes) may blunt the therapeutic effect of verapamil on blood pressure.
- oral hypoglycemic agents (see Oral Antidiabetic Drugs in Drug Classes) may lead to excessively low blood sugar.

- phenytoin (Dilantin) may result in decreased effectiveness of verapamil.
- prazosin (Minipres, others) may increase risk of orthostatic hypotension.
- quinidine (Quinaglute, others) can result in quinidine toxicity.
- rifampin (Rifadin, others) will decrease the therapeutic benefits of verapamil.
- sulfinpyrazone increases the removal of verapamil and lessens its therapeutic effects.
- terazosin (Hytrin) can lead to excessive decreases in blood pressure.
- theophylline (Theo-Dur, others) can lead to theophylline toxicity.
- warfarin (Coumadin) or other oral anticoagulants may increase risk of stomach or intestinal (GI) hemorrhage. More frequent INR tests are indicated.

The following drugs may *increase* the effects of verapamil:
- cimetidine (Tagamet) and other histamine (H2) blocking drugs (see Drug Classes).
- clarithromycin (Biaxin).
- quinupristin/dalfopristin (Synercid).
- ritonavir (Norvir), amprenavir (Agenerase), atazanavir (Reyataz), and perhaps other protease inhibitors (see Drug Classes).
- tricyclic antidepressants (see Drug Classes).

▷ *Driving, Hazardous Activities:* Usually no restrictions. This drug may cause dizziness. Restrict activities as necessary.

Aviation Note: Coronary artery disease *is a disqualification* for piloting. Consult a designated Aviation Medical Examiner.

Exposure to Sun: Use caution until sensitivity has been determined. This drug may cause photosensitivity (see Glossary).

Exposure to Heat: Caution is advised. Hot environments can exaggerate the blood pressure–lowering effects of this drug. Observe for light-headedness or weakness.

Heavy Exercise or Exertion: This drug may improve your ability to be more active without resulting angina pain. Use caution and avoid excessive exercise that could impair heart function in the absence of warning pain.

Discontinuation: **Do not stop this drug abruptly.** Consult your physician regarding gradual withdrawal to prevent the development of rebound angina.

WARFARIN (WAR far in)

Introduced: 1941   **Class:**   Anticoagulant, coumarins   **Prescription:** USA: Yes   **Controlled Drug:**   USA: No; Canada: No   **Available as Generic:**   USA: Yes; Canada: Yes

Brand Names: ♣Apo-Warfarin, Athrombin-K, Carfin, Coumadin, ♣Gen-Warfarin ♣Lin-Warfarin, PanWarfarin, Sofarin, ♣Taro-warfarin, Warnerin

---

BENEFITS versus RISKS

Possible Benefits	*Possible Risks*
EFFECTIVE PREVENTION OF BOTH ARTERIAL AND VENOUS THROMBOSIS (THEREFORE STROKE PREVENTION)	NARROW TREATMENT RANGE Dose-related bleeding Skin and soft tissue hemorrhage with tissue death
EFFECTIVE PREVENTION OF EMBOLIZATION IN THROMBOEMBOLIC DISORDERS	
HELPS PREVENT RECURRENCE OF HEART ATTACK	
HELPS PREVENT STROKES IN PATIENTS WITH ATRIAL FIBRILLATION	
TREATS ACUTE CORONARY SYNDROME	
HELPS PREVENT BLOOD CLOTS AFTER MITRAL VALVE REPLACEMENT	
May have a role in helping to prevent cancer	

▷ **Principal Uses**

As a Single Drug Product: Uses currently included in FDA-approved labeling: Used in (1) acute thrombosis (clot) or thrombophlebitis of the deep veins; (2) acute pulmonary embolism, resulting from blood clots that originate anywhere in the body; (3) atrial fibrillation, to prevent clotting of blood inside the heart that could result in embolization of small clots to any part of the body (leading to heart attack or stroke); (4) after a sudden (acute) myocardial infarction (heart attack), to prevent undesirable clotting and embolization and a repeat (recurrence) of heart attack; (5) mitral valve replacement; (6) helping prevent blood clots in the lungs (pulmonary embolism) that may start after hip replacement surgery.

Other (unlabeled) generally accepted uses: (1) Helps prevent embolization from the heart in people with artificial heart valves or coronary angioplasty; (2) may help patients with low blood platelets caused by heparin; (3) one case report of benefits in treatment-resistant migraines; (4) a study of 854 patients (after suffering a first blood clot) who were then treated with warfarin appeared to have a lower risk of newly diagnosed cancer, and this possible chemoprotective effect must be further evaluated; (5) prevention of stroke (INR=1.6–2.6) in patients who have already had one.

How This Drug Works: The coumarin anticoagulants interfere with the production of four essential blood-clotting factors by blocking the action of vitamin K. This leads to a deficiency of these clotting factors in circulating blood and inhibits blood-clotting mechanisms. Mechanism in possibly decreasing cancer risk is not known.

▷ **Widely Used Guidelines That Involve This Medicine (representative sample):** Please look at the section at the very beginning of this profile called "Class." Next, turn to Table 22 and you will find guidelines listed by the class involved!

Available Dosage Forms and Strengths
> Injection — 5 mg
> Tablets — 1 mg, 2 mg, 2.5 mg, 3 mg, 4 mg, 5 mg, 6 mg, 7.5 mg, 10 mg
> Tablets (Canada) — 25 mg

▷ **Usual Adult Dosage Ranges:** Initially a starting (induction) dose of 2 to 5 mg daily is used. A large loading dose is inappropriate and may be hazardous—hence an induction dose is used in the aforementioned range and then the ongoing dose is decided based on INR (prothrombin time or protime) results and the condition being treated. Defined ranges exist for treating or preventing problems with various diagnoses. The usual ongoing maintenance dose range is 2 to 10 mg daily, adjusted to maintain the prothrombin time (protime) to 1.2 to 2 times the control value, which corresponds to an International Normalized Ratio (INR) of 2.0 to 3.0 for most indications (1.5 to 5.0 is a possible INR range).

Note: Actual dose and schedule must be determined for each patient individually.

Author's Note: Many patients have their anticoagulation managed in a special service called an anticoagulation clinic. The manufacturer of the Warfarin brand offers a database called Coumacare, which is used to closely follow patients.

Conditions Requiring Dosing Adjustments
Liver Function: Blood testing (prothrombin times) should be obtained to guide dosing. This drug is only used when extremely careful followup is possible and a cautious benefit-to-risk decision is made.
Kidney Function: This drug should be used with caution in renal compromise, as warfarin may cause microscopic kidney stones
Congestive Heart Failure (CHF): This drug should be used with caution in CHF because the liver may become overloaded (congested) and the response to anticoagulation may be exaggerated.

▷ **Dosing Instructions:** The tablet may be crushed and is preferably taken when the stomach is empty and at the same time each day to ensure uniform results. If you forget a dose: Take the missed dose as soon as you remember it. If you don't remember until the next day, skip the missed dose and take the next dose right on schedule. Let your doctor know you missed a dose. Be honest if you find yourself missing doses; there are timers and beeper-based systems that can be very helpful.

Usual Duration of Use: Use on a regular schedule for 3 to 5 days usually determines effectiveness in providing significant anticoagulation. An additional 10 to 14 days is required to determine the optimal maintenance dose for each person. INR ranges vary according to the condition warranting use of warfarin in the first place. The appropriate duration of therapy is controversial and should be discussed with your doctor according to the condition being treated. Ongoing use (months to years) requires physician supervision. Patient self-testing (INR) monitors are now available and can empower people taking warfarin.

Typical Treatment Goals and Measurements (Outcomes and Markers)
Anticoagulation: The goal of anticoagulation is to prevent further extension of an existing clot or to prevent a clot in patients who are at risk for getting a blood clot. Additionally, a balance must be struck between thinning the blood enough to avoid an undesirable blood clot and thinning it so much

that bleeding occurs. The INR (a ratio involving a prothrombin time test and standardization to make results "the same" lab to lab) is used to check to what degree the blood has been made less likely to clot by warfarin.

While you are taking this medicine you will have blood drawn on a regular basis to make sure that your blood is in the right range. Many patients refer to anticoagulation as being "thin" enough and to warfarin as a blood thinner. The key, however, is to make the blood less likely to form abnormal clots, yet have it retain enough of an ability to clot to keep you from bleeding. For example, the Antithrombotic Therapy in Acute Coronary Syndrome (ACTACS) study reported that when INR is adjusted to a range of between 2 and 3, the frequency of bleeding complications was about the same (not statistically different) for aspirin alone (162.5 mg) or aspirin plus warfarin in people with chest pain (ischemic pain) due to unstable angina or non-Q-wave heart attack (myocardial infarction).

▷ **This Drug Should Not Be Taken If**
- you have had an allergic reaction to it previously.
- you have an active peptic ulcer or active ulcerative colitis.
- you are pregnant, and are experiencing eclampsia or a threatened abortion.
- you have had recent anesthesia (lumbar block) to the spine.
- you've had a spinal tap (lumbar puncture).
- you have arterial aneurysm.
- you have malignant hypertension.
- you have low blood platelets.
- you have infective pericarditis or endocarditis.
- you have liver disease.
- you have esophageal varices (ask your doctor).
- you have had a recent stroke.

▷ **Inform Your Physician Before Taking This Drug If**
- you are now taking any other drugs, either prescription drugs or over-the-counter drug products.
- you are planning pregnancy.
- you have a history of a bleeding disorder.
- you have congestive heart failure.
- you have high blood pressure.
- you have abnormally heavy or prolonged menstrual bleeding.
- you have a thyroid problem (low or excessive thyroid activity may have an altered response to this medicine).
- you have diabetes.
- you are using an indwelling catheter.
- you have impaired liver or kidney function.
- you will have surgery or dental extraction.

Possible Side Effects (natural, expected, and unavoidable drug actions)
Minor episodes of bleeding may occur even though dose and INR or prothrombin times are well within the recommended range.

▷ **Possible Adverse Effects** (unusual, unexpected, and infrequent reactions)
If any of the following develop, consult your physician promptly for guidance.
Mild Adverse Effects
Allergic reactions: skin rash, hives.
Loss of scalp hair (alopecia)—case reports.
Loss of appetite, nausea, vomiting, cramping, diarrhea—case reports.

Serious Adverse Effects

Allergic reactions: drug fever (see Glossary).

Idiosyncratic reactions: bleeding into skin and soft tissues, causing gangrene of breast, toes, and localized areas of necrosis anywhere—rare.

Hereditary warfarin resistance—rare.

Abnormal bleeding from nose, gastrointestinal tract (one case of esophageal ulcer), lungs, urinary tract, uterus, or other sites—possible and dose-related.

Pericardial tamponade—case reports.

Hemolytic anemia—rare.

Adrenal gland problems (adrenal insufficiency)—case reports.

Sudden nerve damage (femoral neuropathy)—case reports.

Kidney problems (tubulointerstitial nephritis)—case reports.

Liver toxicity (viral hepatitis-like syndrome)—case report.

▷ **Possible Effects on Sexual Function:** Extended erections (priapism).

▷ **Adverse Effects That May Mimic Natural Diseases or Disorders**

Drug-induced fever may suggest infection.

Natural Diseases or Disorders That May Be Activated by This Drug

Bleeding from "silent" peptic ulcer, intestinal or bladder polyp or tumor.

Possible Effects on Laboratory Tests

Complete blood cell counts: decreased red cells, hemoglobin, and white cells.

Eosinophils: increased in one case report.

Bleeding time: increased.

INR (prothrombin time): increased (desirable when in therapeutic range).

Blood uric acid level: increased (in men).

Liver function tests: increased liver enzymes (ALT/GPT, AST/GOT, and alkaline phosphatase).

CAUTION

1. Always carry a personal identification card that includes a statement that *you are taking an anticoagulant drug. A medicine alert bracelet is also prudent.*

2. While taking this drug, always consult your physician **before** starting any new drug, changing the dose schedule of any drug, or stopping any drug.

3. Data from the Agency for Health Care Policy and Research have shown that expanded use of warfarin could cut in half the 80,000 strokes that occur every year in patients who have atrial fibrillation.

4. **If** you start taking the brand, it is prudent to keep taking the brand. Conversely, if you have your anticoagulation adjusted using the generic form, it is prudent to continue the generic. Changing from one form to the other may result in differences in degree of anticoagulation.

5. **If** you choose to use acetaminophen while taking this medicine, talk to your doctor about adjusting the warfarin and INR testing.

6. Hereditary or acquired warfarin resistance is possible.

7. Some herbal medicines can lead to additive bleeding problems. Avoid garlic, ginkgo, ginseng, and echinacea (amongst others—see below) prior to any surgery and while you are taking this medicine.

8. Checks of INR are MANDATORY while you are taking this medicine. Home monitors can be extremely helpful by increasing access to INR tests. They are available from CoaguCheck (1-800-852-8766—Roche) and ProTime (1-800-631-5945—International Technodyne). Read more in Table 18.

Precautions for Use

By Those Over 60 Years of Age: Small starting doses are mandatory. Watch regularly for excessive drug effects: prolonged bleeding from shaving cuts, bleeding gums, bloody urine, rectal bleeding, excessive bruising. Some study data reveal that the beneficial effects of this medicine are not as widely known as needed and it is underprescribed for those over 60.

▷ **Advisability of Use During Pregnancy**

Pregnancy Category: X. See Pregnancy Risk Categories at the back of this book.

Animal Studies: Fetal hemorrhage and death due to this drug have been reported in mice.

Human Studies: Information from studies of pregnant women indicates fetal defects and fetal hemorrhage due to this drug. The manufacturers state that this drug is contraindicated during entire pregnancy.

Advisability of Use If Breast-Feeding

Presence of this drug in breast milk: Yes, but in inactive forms.

Breast-feeding appears to be safe. Checking the infant for warfarin effects is prudent in those infants at risk for such effects (vitamin K deficient).

Habit-Forming Potential: None.

Effects of Overdose: Episodes of bleeding, from minor surface bleeding (nose, gums, small lacerations) to major internal bleeding (vomiting blood, bloody urine or stool).

Possible Effects of Long-Term Use: Blue toe syndrome.

Suggested Periodic Examinations While Taking This Drug (at physician's discretion)

Regular determinations of INR (prothrombin time or protime) are essential to safe dose and proper control.

Urine analysis for blood.

Stool guaic test for hidden (occult) blood.

▷ **While Taking This Drug, Observe the Following**

Foods: A larger intake than usual of foods rich in vitamin K may reduce the effectiveness of this drug and make larger doses necessary. Foods rich in vitamin K include asparagus, bacon, beef liver, cabbage, fish, cauliflower, and green leafy vegetables. Vitamin C in high doses has some conflicting reports of warfarin resistance. Vitamin E (high dose) may increase risk of bleeding. Mango fruit was reported to cause up to a 38% increase in INR in one report. Papaya also increased INR. Talk to your doctor before eating these fruits.

Herbal Medicines or Minerals: Because many herbal products are extracts from plants with a variety of active compounds in addition to those listed on the label—and since many compounds can have activity as anticoagulants—herbal medicines in general SHOULD NOT be combined with warfarin.

Specifically, angelica root, anise, borage seed oil, devil's claw, papain, ginseng, ginger, ginkgo, horse chestnut, ipriflavone, alfalfa, red clover, clove oil, evening primrose oil, feverfew, passionflower herb, salvia root (danshen), skull cap, willow bark, cinchona bark, white willow bark, turmeric, and garlic may also change clotting, so combining those herbals with these medicines cannot be recommended. Dong quai appears to have a true pharmacodynamic interaction with warfarin (potentiation), and since it is as yet uncharacterized, these medicines should not be combined. Boldo-Fenugreek caused more than a 50% increase in INR in one case report (patient also had the same problem when the medicines were introduced a second time). Co-enzyme Q10 (ubiquinone) and green tea may decrease warfarin benefits. Herbal medicine such as eucalyptus, kava, or valerian with known impact on liver function (so critical to anticoagulation) are best NOT combined. TALK TO YOUR DOCTOR BEFORE taking any herbal medicine with warfarin—but, again, any combination is not advisable.

Beverages: No restrictions. May be taken with milk.

▷ *Alcohol:* Limit alcohol to one drink daily. Note: Heavy users of alcohol with liver damage may be very sensitive to anticoagulants and require smaller than usual doses.

Tobacco Smoking: Heavy smokers may require relatively larger doses of this drug. I advise everyone to quit smoking.

▷ *Other Drugs*

Warfarin may ***increase*** the effects of
- oral hypoglycemic agents (see Oral Antidiabetic Drugs in Drug Classes).
- phenytoin (Dilantin) or fosphenytoin (Cerebyx).

Warfarin may ***decrease*** the effects of
- cyclosporine (Sandimmune, others).
- phenytoin (Dilantin) or fosphenytoin (Cerebyx).

The following drugs may ***increase*** the effects of warfarin:
- abciximab (Reopro).
- acarbose (Precose).
- acetaminophen (Tylenol, others—especially if more than 2,275 mg per week is taken).
- allopurinol (Zyloprim).
- alteplase (Activase) and is contraindicated if the prothrombin time is more than 15 seconds.
- amiodarone (Cordarone).
- amprenavir (Agenerase), atazanavir (Reyataz), ritonavir (Norvir), and saquinavir (Invirase).
- androgens (see Drug Classes).
- aprepitant (Emend).
- argatroban (Acova).
- aspirin and some other NSAIDs (see Drug Classes).
- azithromycin (Zithromax).
- bismuth subsalicylate (Pepto-Bismol).
- some calcium channel blockers (various) have been associated with an increased risk of stomach and intestine (gastrointestinal) hemorrhage. This risk may be exacerbated by warfarin use.
- capsaicin (Zostrix, others).
- carbamazepine (Tegretol).
- cephalosporins (see Drug Classes).
- chloral hydrate (Noctec).
- chloramphenicol (Chloromycetin).
- cimetidine (Tagamet).
- ciprofloxacin and other quinolone antibiotics (see Drug Classes).
- cisapride (Propulsid).
- clarithromycin (Biaxin).
- clofibrate (Atromid-S).
- clopidogrel (Plavix).
- cloxacillin (various).
- cotrimoxazole (Bactrim).
- COX-II inhibitors (celecoxib, rofecoxib, and valdecoxib).

- dextrothyroxine.
- dirithromycin and other macrolide antibiotics (see Drug Classes).
- disopyramide (Norpace).
- disulfiram (Antabuse).
- enoxaparin (Lovenox) and other low molecular weight heparins (see Drug Classes).
- eptifibatide (Integrelin).
- erythromycin (various).
- felbamate (Felbatol).
- fluconazole (Diflucan).
- fluoxetine (Prozac).
- fluvastatin (Lescol), lovastatin (Advicor, Mevacor), rosuvastatin (Crestor), and simvastatin (Zocor).
- fluvoxamine (Luvox).
- fosphenytoin (Cerebyx) or phenytoin (Dilantin).
- gemfibrozil (Lopid).
- glucagon.
- heparin (various).
- HMG CoA-reductase inhibitors (see Drug Profiles).
- imatinib (Gleevec).
- influenza vaccine (various).
- isoniazid (INH).
- itraconazole (Sporanox), ketoconazole (Nizoral), and voriconazole (Vfend).
- mesna (Mesnex).
- methyltestosterone (any 17-alkylated androgen).
- metronidazole (Flagyl).
- miconazole (Monistat).
- minocycline.
- nonsteroidal anti-inflammatory drugs (see Drug Classes).
- omeprazole (Prilosec).
- oral anticoagulants—low molecular weight heparins, etc. (see Drug Classes).
- orlistat (Xenical).
- paroxetine (Paxil).
- propafenone (Rythmol).
- propranolol (Inderal).
- propoxyphene (various).
- quetiapine (Seroquel).
- quinidine (Quinaglute).
- raloxifene (Evista)—more frequent INR checks are prudent.
- ranitidine (Zantac).
- salicylates (aspirin, etc.).
- sertraline (Zoloft).
- streptokinase.
- sulfinpyrazone (Anturane).
- sulfonamides (see Drug Classes).
- tamoxifen (Nolvadex).
- tamsulosin (Flomax).
- terbinafine (Lamisil).
- testosterone (various).
- tetracyclines (see Drug Classes).
- thyroid hormones (various).
- thrombolytic drugs (such as alteplase).

- tramadol (Ultram).
- traztuzumab (Herceptin).
- tricyclic antidepressants (see Drug Classes).
- vancomycin (Vancoled).
- vitamin E (higher doses).
- zafirlukast (Accolate).
- zileuton (Zyflo).
- zotepine (Nipolept).

The following drugs may **_decrease_** the effects of warfarin:
- antithyroid agents (various) by decreasing prior high rates of clotting factor metabolism.
- azathioprine (Imuran).
- barbiturates (see Drug Classes).
- birth control pills (oral contraceptives).
- carbamazepine (Tegretol).
- chlordiazepoxide (Librium).
- cholestyramine (Questran).
- estrogens (various).
- ethchlorvynol (Placidyl).
- glutethimide (Doriden).
- griseofulvin (Gris-PEG).
- phenobarbital (various).
- phytonadione (vitamin K).
- primidone (Mysoline).
- rifampin (Rifadin).
- spironolactone.
- sucralfate (Carafate).
- telmisartan (Micardis)—slight decrease.
- thiazide diuretics (see Drug Classes).
- vitamin K.

▷ _Driving, Hazardous Activities:_ No restrictions.
Aviation Note: The use of this drug **_is a disqualification_** for piloting. Consult a designated Aviation Medical Examiner.
Exposure to Sun: No restrictions.
Discontinuation: Do not stop this drug abruptly unless abnormal bleeding occurs. Ask your physician for guidance regarding gradual reduction in dose over a period of 3 to 4 weeks.

ZALCITABINE (zal SIT a been)

Other Names: Dideoxycytidine, DDC

Introduced: 1987   **Class:**   Antiviral,   anti-AIDS   **Prescription:**
USA: Yes   **Controlled   Drug:**   USA: No; Canada: No   **Available   as**
Generic: USA: No

Brand Name: Hivid

Author's Note: Information in this profile has been shortened to make room for more widely used medicines.

ZALEPLON (ZAH la plon)

Introduced: 1999 **Class:** Hypnotic, nonbenzodiazepine **Prescription:** USA: Yes **Controlled Drug:** USA: C-IV*; Canada: Prescription **Available as Generic:** USA: No
Brand Names: Sonata, ✽Starnoc

BENEFITS versus RISKS

Possible Benefits	*Possible Risks*
GIVES SHORT-TERM RELIEF OF INSOMNIA WITH MINIMAL SLEEP DISRUPTION (REM)	Habit-forming potential with prolonged use
REDUCES SLEEP LATENCY	
MAY BE TAKEN AT BEDTIME OR LATER (AS LONG AS 4 HOURS OF TIME IN BED ARE LEFT)	
SHORT HALF-LIFE (AVOIDS HANGOVER EFFECT)	

▷ **Principal Uses**

As a Single Drug Product: Uses currently included in FDA-approved labeling: Treatment of insomnia in adults for up to 35 days (newer and longer period of approved use).

Other (unlabeled) generally accepted uses: None at present.

How This Drug Works: This drug attaches (binds) to a specific receptor (GABA-BZ subunit modulation) and reduces the time it takes to fall asleep.

▷ **Widely Used Guidelines That Involve This Medicine (representative sample):** Please look at the section at the very beginning of this profile called "Class." Next, turn to Table 22 and you will find guidelines listed by the class involved!

Available Dosage Forms and Strengths

Tablets — 5 mg, 10 mg

▷ **Recommended Dosage Ranges** (Actual dose and schedule must be determined for each patient individually.)

Infants and Children: Safety and efficacy for those under 18 years of age are not established.

18 to 60 Years of Age: 10 mg is taken immediately before bedtime. If patients are of small stature (low weight), it is prudent to use 5 mg as a starting dose. Patients should be reevaluated after taking this drug for 7–10 days. Maximum length of use was 28 days in clinical studies. Current approval is for 35 days. Patients of low body weight should be given 5 mg as a starting dose. Dose may be increased slowly to a maximum of 20 mg as needed and tolerated.

Over 60 Years of Age: Therapy should be started with 5 mg taken at bedtime. The dose may be cautiously increased to 10 mg at bedtime.

Conditions Requiring Dosing Adjustments

Liver Function: The dose should be reduced by 50% in mild to moderate liver compromise (5 mg).

---

*See Schedules of Controlled Drugs at the back of this book.

Kidney Function: No changes thought to be needed in mild compromise. This medicine HAS NOT been studied in severe kidney insufficiency.

▷ **Dosing Instructions:** The tablet may be crushed. Best taken on an empty stomach (taking it with a high-fat meal delays absorption). Do not stop this drug abruptly if taken more than 7 days. If you forget a dose: Take the missed dose as soon as you remember it, as long as you will be in bed for another 4 hours.

Usual Duration of Use: Use on a regular schedule for 2 nights usually determines effectiveness in treating insomnia. Your physician should assess the benefit of this drug after 7 to 10 days. Current recommended maximum length of use is 35 days.

Typical Treatment Goals and Measurements (Outcomes and Markers)

Insomnia: The general goal is to decrease the amount of time it takes between the time you go to bed and the time you fall asleep (shortened sleep latency). Additionally, the number of times that you wake up is expected to decrease, enabling a full night of sleep. How alert you feel in the morning is also a consideration. Many other hypnotics with longer half-lives also have significant effects the next morning ("hangover" effects). Two scales often used are the Stanford Sleepiness Scale (SSS) and the Saint Mary Hospital Sleep Questionnaire (SMHSQ).

Possible Advantages of This Drug

Low occurrence of adverse effects. Short half-life. No difference between a dummy pill (placebo) and this medicine was seen when patients were checked for next-day sleepiness. Now approved for up to 35 days of insomnia treatment.

▷ **This Drug Should Not Be Taken If**

- you had an allergic reaction to it previously or to tartrazine (yellow number 5).
- you have severe liver compromise.

▷ **Inform Your Physician Before Taking This Drug If**

- you have abnormal liver or kidney function.
- you are pregnant or planning pregnancy or are breast-feeding your infant.
- you have a history of alcoholism or drug abuse.
- you have a serious lung problem (respiratory impairment).
- you have a history of serious depression or mental disorder.
- you are elderly or are debilitated.
- you are unsure how much to take or how often to take this medicine.

Possible Side Effects (natural, expected, and unavoidable drug actions)

Sleepiness.

▷ **Possible Adverse Effects** (unusual, unexpected, and infrequent reactions)

If any of the following develop, consult your physician promptly for guidance.

Mild Adverse Effects

Allergic reactions: Itching and rash.

Drowsiness and dizziness—possible and dose related.

Psychomotor impairment—possible and dose related.

Fever—rare.

Blurred vision—dose related—rare.

Rebound insomnia—possible, dose dependent, and appears to resolve by the second night.

Lowered white blood cell counts—rare and transitory and of questionable causation.

Nausea, anorexia, or indigestion—infrequent.

Muscle aches (myalgia)—infrequent.

Increased liver enzymes—rare and transient and of questionable causality.

Serious Adverse Effects

Allergic reactions: not defined.

Peripheral edema or chest pain—reported.

Abnormal thoughts or hallucinations—very rare.

▷ **Possible Effects on Sexual Function:** Dysmenorrhea—very rare.

Possible Effects on Laboratory Tests

Liver function tests: possibly increased SGOT, SGPT, and CPK.

CAUTION

1. This drug works quickly. It is best to take it just before bedtime.
2. Do not drink alcohol while taking this drug.
3. Withdrawal (see Glossary) may occur, even if this drug was only taken for a week or two. Ask your doctor for advice before stopping zaleplon.
4. You may experience trouble going to sleep for 1 or 2 nights after stopping this drug (rebound insomnia). This effect usually doesn't last long (short term).
5. Sleep disturbances may be a symptom of underlying psychological problems. Tell your doctor if unusual behaviors or odd thoughts occur.
6. Drugs that depress the central nervous system may produce additive effects with this drug. Ask your doctor or pharmacist before combining other prescription or nonprescription drugs with zaleplon.

Precautions for Use

By Infants and Children: Safety and effectiveness for those under 18 years of age are not established.

By Those Over 60 Years of Age: The starting dose should be decreased to 5 mg. Since this drug works quickly, it is best taken immediately before going to bed. You may be at increased risk for falls if the drug remains in your system in the morning. Watch for lethargy, unsteadiness, nightmares, and paradoxical agitation and anger.

▷ **Advisability of Use During Pregnancy**

Pregnancy Category: C. See Pregnancy Risk Categories at the back of this book.

Animal Studies: In rats, there was increased stillbirth and postnatal death as well as slower growth and development in offspring of females treated with 7 mg per kg per day during the later part of pregnancy and throughout lactation.

Human Studies: Adequate studies of pregnant women are not available.

Use during pregnancy is not recommended.

Advisability of Use If Breast-Feeding

Presence of this drug in breast milk: Yes, in small amounts.

Avoid drug or refrain from nursing.

Habit-Forming Potential: This drug may cause dependence (see Glossary).

Effects of Overdose: One case of 100 mg taken in combination with a benzodiazepine reported that the patient recovered without ill effects. Supportive and symptomatic care is recommended.

Possible Effects of Long-Term Use: Psychological and/or physical dependence.

Suggested Periodic Examinations While Taking This Drug (at physician's discretion)

Liver function tests.

▷ **While Taking This Drug, Observe the Following**
    Foods: This drug is best taken on an empty stomach because food delays absorption.

    Herbal Medicines or Minerals: Kava kava and valerian (no longer recommended because of liver toxicity questions) may exacerbate central nervous system depression (avoid this combination). Kola nut, Siberian ginseng, mate, guarana, ephedra, and ma huang may blunt the benefits of this medicine. While St. John's wort is indicated for anxiety, it is also thought to increase (induce) cytochrome P450 enzymes and could tend to blunt zaleplon effectiveness.

    Beverages: Avoid caffeine-containing beverages: coffee, tea, cola, chocolate.

▷   *Alcohol:* This drug should not be combined with alcohol.

    Tobacco Smoking: Nicotine is a stimulant and should be avoided. I advise everyone to quit smoking.

    Marijuana Smoking: May cause additive drowsiness.

▷   *Other Drugs*

        Zaleplon ***taken concurrently*** with

- cimetidine (Tagamet, others) may increase zaleplon effects (inhibits aldehyde oxidase and CYP3A4—both methods that the body uses to eliminate this drug). A starting dose of 5 mg and careful patient follow-up are needed if these medicines are combined.
- medicines that inhibit both aldehyde oxidase (primary removal mechanism) and CYP3A4 will inhibit removal of zaleplon and may lead to zaleplon toxicity.
- medicines that induce both aldehyde oxidase (primary removal mechanism) and CYP3A4 will blunt benefits of zaleplon by decreasing blood levels.
- rifampin (Rifater, others) may decrease zaleplon benefits.
- ritonavir (Norvir) and perhaps other protease inhibitors (see Drug Classes) may lead to toxicity.

        Zaleplon may ***increase*** the effects of

- chlorpromazine (Thorazine).
- narcotics or other CNS-depressant drugs (see Drug Classes for Opioids, Phenothiazines, Antihistamines, and Benzodiazepines).

▷   *Driving, Hazardous Activities:* This drug may cause drowsiness and impair coordination. Restrict activities as necessary.

    Aviation Note: The use of this drug ***is a disqualification*** for piloting. Consult a designated Aviation Medical Examiner.

    Discontinuation: This drug should not be stopped abruptly, even after a week of use. Ask your doctor for help regarding an appropriate withdrawal schedule.

ZIDOVUDINE (zi DOH vyoo deen)

Other Names: AZT, azidothymidine, compound S, ZDV

Introduced: 1987 **Class:** Antiviral, anti-HIV **Prescription:** USA: Yes **Controlled Drug:** USA: No; Canada: No **Available as Generic:** USA: No; Canada: Yes

Brand Names: ✤Apo-Zidovudine, Combivir [CD], ✤Novo-AZT, Retrovir, Trizivir [CD]

BENEFITS versus RISKS

Possible Benefits	*Possible Risks*
DELAYED PROGRESSION OF DISEASE IN HIV-INFECTED PATIENTS WHEN COMBINATION TREATMENT IS USED	SERIOUS BONE MARROW DEPRESSION
	Brain toxicity
	Lip, mouth, and tongue sores
REDUCED INCIDENCE OF INFECTIONS (OPPORTUNISTIC) WITH COMBINATION THERAPY	
COMBIVIR AND TRIZIVIR FORMS ENCOURAGE COMPLIANCE BY COMBINING TWO OR THREE MEDICINES IN ONE PILL	
REDUCED POSSIBILITY OF TRANSMISSION OF HIV FROM MOTHER TO FETUS (ZIDOVUDINE)	

▷ **Principal Uses**

As a Single Drug Product: Uses currently included in FDA-approved labeling: (1) Used to treat selected patients who have acquired immunodeficiency syndrome (AIDS)—this drug is not a cure for HIV; (2) approved to help prevent transmission of HIV from mother to infant; (3) approved for combination therapy with other agents; (4) approved for children 3 months or older who have laboratory values that indicate HIV infection or HIV immunosuppression; (5) approved for use in HIV-positive patients who are as yet asymptomatic.

Author's Note: Adherence—taking medicines for HIV exactly on time and in the right amount—is ABSOLUTELY critical to getting the best possible results or outcomes. The antiretroviral therapy guidelines from NIAID take into account how easily the medicine treating HIV can fit into a patient's life (twice-daily dosing is a distinct advantage). Structured therapy interruptions (STI) or structured interruptions of therapy (SIT) are controversial. Combination therapy has become a standard of care.

Other (unlabeled) generally accepted uses: (1) Used to treat Kaposi's sarcoma; (2) helps remove hairy leukoplakia in the mouth; (3) may prevent HIV in health care workers exposed to the AIDS virus (combined with other HIV medicines); (4) appears to increase AIDS-related low platelet counts; (5) may have a role treating adult T-cell leukemia or lymphoma with interferon alpha.

As a Combination Drug Product [CD]: This drug is available in combination (Combivir—lamivudine and zidovudine; Trizivir—abacavir, lamivudine, and zidovudine). The combinations offer two different and three different medicines in the same pills.

How This Drug Works: By interfering with essential enzyme systems, this drug is thought to prevent the growth and reproduction of HIV particles within tissue cells, thus limiting the severity and extent of HIV infection.

▷ **Widely Used Guidelines That Involve This Medicine (representative sample):**
Please look at the section at the very beginning of this profile called "Class." Next, turn to Table 22 and you will find guidelines listed by the class involved!

Available Dosage Forms and Strengths
Capsules — 100 mg
Injection — 10 mg/mL
Syrup — 50 mg/5 mL
Tablet (Combivir) — lamivudine 150 mg
— zidovudine 300 mg
Tablet (Trizivir) — abacavir 300 mg
— lamivudine 150 mg
— zidovudine 300 mg

▷ **Usual Adult Dosage Ranges:** *HIV infection:* The product information insert for zidovudine recommends 600 mg daily, divided into equal doses in combination with other antiretroviral agents. Further, 500 mg as 100 mg every 4 hours while awake or 600 mg daily divided into equal doses is suggested. Combivir form—one tablet twice daily. Trizivir form—one tablet twice daily in people weighing more than 40 kg.

Prevention of maternal-fetal transmission in pregnancy: Once the mother has passed 14 weeks of pregnancy—100 mg by mouth five times per day until the start of labor. During labor, AZT is given intravenously (2 mg per kg of body mass), followed by 1 mg per kg of body mass per hour. This dose is continued until the umbilical cord is clamped. The infant then receives 1.5 mg per kg of body mass every 6 hours. The CDC recommends combination therapy for pregnant women.

Note: Actual dose and administration schedule must be determined for each patient individually.

Conditions Requiring Dosing Adjustments
Liver Function: Dose decreased by 50% or the dosing interval doubled in significant liver disease. Drug can be a rare cause of liver damage, and patients should be followed closely.

Kidney Function: Specific guidelines for dose adjustments in patients with compromised kidneys are not available. This drug should be used with caution in kidney compromise.

Granulocytopenia: If counts of this type of white blood cell are less than 750/mL cubed or if there is a decrease in number of this kind of cell of more than 50% of what a patient starts with, this medicine may need to be stopped until the bone marrow recovers.

Anemia: If the hemoglobin drops more than 25% from the starting point or is less than 7.5 g per deciliter, zidovudine may have to be stopped. Occurrence increases with higher doses and/or lower CD4 counts. Erythropoietin may help reduce the need for blood transfusions.

▷ **Dosing Instructions:** Preferably taken on an empty stomach, but may be taken with or following food. Take exactly as prescribed. Zidovudine capsule may be opened and the contents mixed with food just prior to taking it. Best to take the capsule with at least 120 mL of water, and patients should then NOT lie down for an hour. If you forget a dose: Take the missed dose as soon as you remember it, unless it's nearly time for your next dose—if that is the case, skip the missed dose and take the next dose right on schedule. DO NOT double up on doses. Talk with your doctor and pharmacist if you find yourself missing doses. IT IS ABSOLUTELY CRITICAL to take HIV medicines exactly as prescribed. There are beeper-based and phone-based systems that can be a great help in complicated medication schedules.

Usual Duration of Use: Use on a regular schedule for 10 to 12 weeks usually determines effectiveness in improving the course of symptomatic AIDS infection. Long-term use requires periodic physician evaluation of response (viral load and CD4) and dose adjustment. It is not uncommon for antiretrovirals to be changed during HIV treatment based on genotypic, phenotypic, or viral burden checks.

Typical Treatment Goals and Measurements (Outcomes and Markers)

HIV: Goals for HIV treatment presently are maximum suppression of viral replication, maximum lowering of the amount of virus in your body (viral load or burden), and maximum patient survival. The loftier goal of eradication of HIV from the body does not appear possible given the medicines presently available. Long-term survival is achievable for many patients. Markers of successful therapy include undetectable viral load, increased CD4 cells, absence of indicator or opportunistic infections (OIs), and, in the case of the HIV-positive patient, failure of the infection to progress to AIDS.

Possible Advantages of This Drug

Combination form gives a three-drug combination while preserving the protease inhibitor class.

▷ **This Drug (These Drugs) Should Not Be Taken If**
  • you have had a serious allergic reaction to it previously.
  • you have a serious degree of uncorrected bone marrow depression.

▷ **Inform Your Physician Before Taking This Drug (These Drugs) If**
  • you have a history of either folic acid or vitamin B_{12} deficiency.
  • you have impaired liver or kidney function.
  • you take other drugs that can have a bad effect on the bone marrow (are myelosuppressive).

Possible Side Effects (natural, expected, and unavoidable drug actions)

None reported.

▷ **Possible Adverse Effects** (unusual, unexpected, and infrequent reactions)
If any of the following develop, consult your physician promptly for guidance.

Mild Adverse Effects

Allergic reactions: skin rash, hives, itching.

Headache, weakness, drowsiness, dizziness, nervousness, insomnia—infrequent.

Nausea, diarrhea, vomiting, altered taste, lip sores, swollen mouth or tongue—infrequent (incidence higher with combination forms).

Paresthesias, muscle aches, fever, sweating—infrequent.

Serious Adverse Effects

Allergic reactions: one case report of toxic epidermolysis for zidovudine. **A severe and life-threatening hypersensitivity reaction (3–5%) has been reported with abacavir (Trizivir form only).**

Confusion, loss of speech, twitching, tremors, seizures (representing brain toxicity)—infrequent.

Eye problems (macular edema)—case reports.

Muscle toxicity (myopathy)—infrequent.

Mania or seizures—rare.

Muscle toxicity of the heart (cardiomyopathy)—case reports.

Bone marrow depression (see Glossary): fatigue, weakness, fever, sore throat, abnormal bleeding or bruising.

Anemia occurs most commonly after 4 to 6 weeks of treatment; abnormally low white blood cell counts occur after 6 to 8 weeks of treatment—infrequent.

Esophageal ulcers (patients should take this medicine with at least 120 mL of water and not lie down for an hour)—possible.

Liver toxicity—infrequent.

Increased blood sugar (Trizivir form)—may be frequent.

Increased triglycerides (Trizivir form)—frequent (up to 25% in some populations).

▷ **Possible Effects on Sexual Function:** None reported.

Possible Delayed Adverse Effects: Significant anemia and deficient white blood cell counts may develop after this drug has been discontinued. Myopathy, increased triglycerides, blood sugar increases.

▷ **Adverse Effects That May Mimic Natural Diseases or Disorders**
Seizures may suggest the possibility of epilepsy.

Possible Effects on Laboratory Tests
Complete blood cell counts: decreased red cells, hemoglobin, white cells, and platelets

Triglycerides (Trizivir form)—frequent increases

Blood glucose (sugar) (Trizivir form)—may be increased frequently.

CAUTION
1. These drugs are not a cure for AIDS, nor do they protect completely against other infections or complications. Follow your doctor's instructions. Take all medications exactly as prescribed.
2. These drugs do not reduce the risk of transmitting AIDS to others through sexual contact or contamination of the blood. The use of an effective condom is mandatory. Needles for drug administration should not be shared.
3. Triglyceride and blood sugar increases should be followed with combination forms.
4. Follow-up viral burden and CD4 tests are critical. Medicines that have failed MUST be changed (salvage therapy).

Precautions for Use
By Infants and Children: Zidovudine syrup is used in HIV-infected pediatric patients who are greater than 3 months old. The usual dose is 180 mg per square meter.

By Those Over 60 Years of Age: Impaired kidney function will require dose reduction.

▷ **Advisability of Use During Pregnancy**
Pregnancy Category: C. See Pregnancy Risk Categories at the back of this book.

Animal Studies: Rat studies reveal no birth defects.

Human Studies: Adequate studies of pregnant women are not available.
Consult your physician for specific guidance. This medicine has been shown to dramatically reduce the transference of HIV from mother to infant. If the decision is made to use this medicine in pregnancy, cases should be reported to 1-800-258-4263.

Advisability of Use If Breast-Feeding
Presence of this drug in breast milk: Unknown.
Breast-feeding may pass the HIV to the infant. DO NOT BREAST-FEED.

Habit-Forming Potential: None.

Effects of Overdose: Nausea, vomiting, diarrhea, bone marrow depression.

Possible Effects of Long-Term Use: Serious anemia and loss of white blood cells. Muscle toxicity (myopathy).

Suggested Periodic Examinations While Taking This Drug (at physician's discretion)

Complete blood cell counts before starting treatment and weekly thereafter until tolerance is established.

Checks of phenotypic or genotypic analysis of the viral population encompassing the infection.

Continual monitoring for bone marrow depression is necessary during entire course of treatment.

Periodic CD4 counts or measurements of viral load are indicators that treatment is failing and demand change of antiretroviral therapy.

▷ **While Taking This Drug, Observe the Following**

Foods: No restrictions.

Herbal Medicines or Minerals: Some patients use echinacea to attempt to boost their immune systems. Unfortunately, use of echinacea is not recommended in people with damaged immune systems. This herb may also actually weaken any immune system if it is used too often or for too long a time. Use of mistletoe is also not recommended.

Beverages: No restrictions. May be taken with milk.

▷ *Alcohol:* No interactions expected with zidovudine or Combivir, but the Trizivir form contains abacavir. Abacavir blood levels are significantly increased when combined with alcohol, and this combination should be avoided.

Tobacco Smoking: No interactions expected. I advise everyone to quit smoking.

▷ *Other Drugs*

The following drugs may ***increase*** the effects of zidovudine and enhance its toxicity:

- acetaminophen (Tylenol, others), although reports have NOT been consistent.
- acyclovir (Zovirax).
- amphotericin B (Fungizone).
- aspirin.
- benzodiazepines (see Drug Classes).
- cidefovir (Vistide), which is given with probenecid, may lead to increased zidovudine levels because of the probenecid.
- cimetidine (Tagamet).
- cotrimoxazole (various).
- fluconazole (Diflucan).
- ganciclovir (Cytovene).
- indomethacin (Indocin).
- interferon alpha, beta-1-A and natural.
- methadone (Dolophine).
- morphine (various).
- probenecid (Benemid).
- sulfonamides (see Drug Classes).

Zidovudine ***taken concurrently*** with

- dapsone may suppress bone marrow and increase risk of blood (hematologic) toxicity; more frequent complete blood counts are warranted.
- didanosine may result in increased risk of myelosuppression.
- doxorubicin (various) and other chemotherapy increases risk of bone marrow depression.
- filgrastim (Neupogen) may help maintain the white blood cell count.
- flucytosine (Ancobon) may suppress bone marrow and increase risk of blood (hematologic) toxicity; more frequent complete blood counts are warranted.

- fosphenytoin (Cerebyx) or phenytoin (Dilantin) may change blood levels of all drugs. Phenytoin levels and more, frequent complete blood counts are warranted.
- ganciclovir (Cytovene) may suppress bone marrow and increase risk of blood (hematologic) toxicity; more frequent complete blood counts are warranted.
- nimodipine (Nimotop) can increase toxicity to nerves.
- other nucleoside analogs for HIV may lower the ability of other HIV treatment requiring phosphorylation to become active.
- pyrazinamide (Rifater, others) may lower concentrations of pyrazinamide and increase risk of progression of tuberculosis. Pyrazinamide levels and dosing adjustments are prudent.
- rifabutin (Mycobutin) and rifampin (Rifadin) can lead to decreased zidovudine blood levels. Zidovudine levels may need to be increased if these medicines are combined.
- ritonavir (Norvir) may lower zidovudine levels.
- stavudine (D4T) may lessen effectiveness, as both agents are cell cycle specific.
- trimexate may cause additive hematological toxicity.
- valproic acid (Depakene) increases zidovudine blood levels. Lower doses of zidovudine and change from fixed dosage forms may be needed if valproic acid is required.

▷ *Driving, Hazardous Activities:* This drug may cause dizziness or fainting. Restrict activities as necessary.

Aviation Note: The use of this drug *is a disqualification* for piloting. Consult a designated Aviation Medical Examiner.

Exposure to Sun: No restrictions.

Discontinuation: Do not stop this drug without your physician's knowledge and guidance.

ZIPRASIDONE (ZIH praise ih dohn)

Introduced: 2001 **Class:** Atypical antipsychotic agent, neuroleptic
Prescription: USA: Yes **Controlled Drug:** USA: No; Canada: No
Available as Generic: USA: No; Canada: No
Brand Name: Geodon

BENEFITS versus RISKS	
Possible Benefits	*Possible Risks*
TREATMENT OF SCHIZOPHRENIA	PROLONGATION OF THE QT
LESS WEIGHT GAIN THAN OTHER	INTERVAL OF THE HEART
AVAILABLE NEUROLEPTIC	ABNORMAL HEART RHYTHMS
MEDICINES	Blood sugar changes (glucose
EFFECTIVE TREATMENT OF	dysregulation)
CERTAIN MENTAL DISORDERS	Abnormal lowering of blood pressure
LOW OCCURRENCE OF	on standing (postural hypotension)
MOVEMENT DISORDERS	Involuntary movement disorder
(EXTRAPYRAMIDAL)	Neuroleptic malignant syndrome
	(possible)

▷ **Principal Uses**

As a *Single Drug Product:* Uses currently included in FDA-approved labeling: (1) Manages adult schizophrenia; (2) helps sudden (acute) episodes of schizoaffective disorder in adults.

Other (unlabeled) generally accepted uses: (1) May have a role in easing sudden (acute) bipolar mania (see Keck, P.E. in Sources).

How This Drug Works: Goes to work at serotonin (also known as 5HT-2A) and dopamine D2 (D2 agonist) sites. This medicine also is active at 5HT-1A-type sites "Ziprasidone," which might account for greater protection against movement (extrapyramidal), disorders, all of which help restore more normal thinking and mood.

▷ **Widely Used Guidelines That Involve This Medicine (representative sample):** Please look at the section at the very beginning of this profile called "Class." Next, turn to Table 22 and you will find guidelines listed by the class involved!

Available Dosage Forms and Strengths

Capsules — 20 mg, 40 mg, 60 mg, 80 mg

▷ **Recommended Dosage Ranges** (Actual dose and schedule must be determined for each patient individually.)

Infants and Children: Safety and efficacy for those less than 18 years of age are not established.

18 to 60 Years of Age: Starting dose is 20 mg, taken twice a day with food. Dose can be increased as needed and tolerated after as little as 2 days, but preferably after several weeks (gives more time to see improvement from a given dose) in steps up to a dose of 80 mg twice a day. The lowest effective dose should be used. Doses greater than 80 mg twice per day are not recommended.

Over 60 Years of Age: No specific dosing changes thought to be needed. Additionally, no changes thought to be needed in mild to moderate kidney problems (CrCl of 60 down to 10 mL/min), which encompasse the "usual" age-related decline in kidney function. Because older patients may be more susceptible to sudden decreases in blood pressure (orthostatic hypotension), careful attention must be paid to blood pressure and development of adverse effects in this population.

Conditions Requiring Dosing Adjustments

Liver Function: No dose change needed for mint to moderate (Child-Pugh A or B) liver compromise.

Kidney Function: No changes thought to be needed for those with creatinine clearance from 10 mL/minute to 60 mL/min.

▷ **Dosing Instructions:** The capsule should not be broken, chewed, or crushed, and is best taken with food or milk in order to ease stomach irritation. Also best taken at the same time in order to help keep the level of medicine in your body about the same. If you forget a dose: Take the medicine right away, unless it's almost time for your next dose. If it is nearly time for your next dose, skip the missed dose, take the next scheduled dose right on time, and then continue your usual dosing schedule from there on. DO NOT double up on doses. Talk with your doctor if you find yourself missing doses.

Usual Duration of Use: Use on a regular schedule for at least 14 days is required to reach steady-state levels and help define how well a given dose will work. Given severity of symptoms and symptom control, some clinicians increase doses in as little as 48 hours. Peak benefits may take 4 weeks to be seen. Ongoing use requires physician supervision and checks of ongoing results.

Typical Treatment Goals and Measurements (Outcomes and Markers)

Schizophrenia: The general goal: to ease the severity of symptoms in order to let the patient resume his or her usual activities. There should be lessened intrusion of abnormal thinking into more normal life. As in depression, scales such as the Brief Psychiatric Rating Scale (BPRS) and the Scale for Assessment of Negative Symptoms (SANS) can help assess the benefits of this medicine.

Possible Advantages of This Drug

Information from the ZEUS research (Ziprasidone Extended Use in Schizophrenia) found that the use of ziprasidone decreased the number of people who had repeat problems (relapsed) who previously had ongoing, stable schizophrenia.

▷ This Drug Should Not Be Taken If

- you have had an allergic reaction to it previously.
- you have had a heart attack (MI) recently, have a history of abnormal heartbeats (arrhythmia), have a history of long QT syndrome present at birth (congenital), are taking a QT interval prolonging medicine (see Glossary), or have heart failure that is not compensated (talk to your doctor).

▷ Inform Your Physician Before Taking This Drug If

- you have had neuroleptic malignant syndrome.
- your liver is compromised.
- you have constitutionally low blood pressure, take medicine to treat high blood pressure, or have cardiovascular or cerebrovascular disease.
- you have a history of prediabetes or diabetes.
- you are pregnant.
- you have a history of breast cancer.
- you have low blood magnesium or potassium.
- you plan to have surgery under general or spinal anesthesia in the near future.

Possible Side Effects (natural, expected, and unavoidable drug actions)

Prolonging of the QT interval (dose related), decreased blood pressure on standing (postural hypotension)—possible.

▷ Possible Adverse Effects (unusual, unexpected, and infrequent reactions)

If any of the following develop, consult your physician promptly for guidance.

Mild Adverse Effects

Allergic reactions: skin rash, itching—rare.

Weight gain—rare.

Headache, drowsiness, or dizziness—rare to infrequent.

Movement urgency, feeling like you have to keep moving (akathesia)—may be frequent.

Runny nose—possible.

Constipation, nausea, or vomiting—infrequent to frequent.

Sugar changes (increased-hyperglycemia/diabetes)—possible with all atypical antipsychotics (risk not available).

Drug-induced increased liver enzymes—rare.

Serious Adverse Effects

Allergic reactions: Not defined.

Movement disorders—possible (less than other medicines).

New-onset diabetes mellitus and/or blood sugar problems (increased sugar or hyperglycemia, glucose dysregulation)—possible with all antipsychotics and possible ketoacidosis—frequency not available.

Neuroleptic malignant syndrome—case reports.

▷ **Possible Effects on Sexual Function:** Case reports of extended and painful erections (priapism), amenorrhea, and vaginitis.

▷ **Adverse Effects That May Mimic Natural Diseases or Disorders**

Nervous system reactions may suggest true Parkinson's disease. Liver reactions may suggest viral hepatitis. Blood sugar changes resemble diabetes.

Possible Effects on Laboratory Tests

Prolactin levels: Increased.

Blood sugar: Increased.

Liver function tests: Mildly increased liver enzymes (ALT/GPT, AST/GOT, and alkaline phosphatase).

CAUTION

1. Other medicines (nonprescription or prescription) that can cause drowsiness or central nervous system effects may react unfavorably with this medicine. Talk with your doctor or pharmacist before combining any medicines.

2. Since this medicine can cause orthostatic hypotension, some high blood pressure (antihypertensive) medicines may have a greater than expected effect if taken with ziprazidone.

3. Given reports of glucose changes, caution should be used with people already having a problem regulating blood sugar and more careful monitoring undertaken.

Precautions for Use

By Infants and Children: Safety and effectiveness for those under 18 years of age are not established.

By Those Over 60 Years of Age: No clinically significant differences have been identified.

▷ **Advisability of Use During Pregnancy**

Pregnancy Category: C. See Pregnancy Risk Categories at the back of this book.

Human Studies: Adequate studies of pregnant women are not available.

Use of this drug is a benefit-to-risk decision. Ask your doctor for guidance.

Advisability of Use If Breast-Feeding

Presence of this drug in breast milk: Unknown in humans.

Avoid drug or refrain from nursing.

Habit-Forming Potential: Not defined.

Effects of Overdose: Treatment of what the patient develops (symptomatic management).

Possible Effects of Long-Term Use: Not defined.

Suggested Periodic Examinations While Taking This Drug (at physician's discretion)

Liver function tests.

Careful inspection of the tongue for early evidence of fine, involuntary, wavelike movements that could be the beginning of tardive dyskinesia.

Sitting and standing blood pressure checks may be advisable when therapy is started, to assess orthostatic hypotension.

Blood sugar and A1C—particularly when starting treatment, then periodically.

▷ **While Taking This Drug, Observe the Following**

Foods: Avoid eating grapefruit while taking this medicine. Follow prescribed diet. See grapefruit warning below.

Herbal Medicines or Minerals: Current data from a small study of 40 patients (See Emsley, R. in Sources) found that add-on therapy with one of the components of fish oil (eicosapenteanoic acid or EPA) helped schizophrenic patients (Positive and Negative Syndrome Scale scores) and was well-tolerated. More study is needed.

Using kola, guarana, mate, bitter orange, country mallow, or ma huang may result in unacceptable central nervous system stimulation. St. John's wort may impact one of the liver enzymes that helps remove this medicine, leading to reduced benefits. Do not combine. Since part of the way ginkgo and ginseng work may be as MAO inhibitors, do not combine them with ziprasidone. Belladonna may lead to excessive anticholinergic actions. Betel nut may make movement disorders more likely. DHEA use may blunt medicine benefits. Given more recent concerns regarding blood sugar and this medicine: Using chromium may change the way your body is able to use sugar. Some health food stores advocate vanadium as mimicking the actions of insulin, but possible toxicity and need for rigorous studies presently preclude recommending it. DHEA may change sensitivity to insulin or insulin resistance. Aloe, bitter melon, eucalyptus, fenugreek, ginger, garlic, ginseng, glucomannan, guar gum, hawthorn, licorice, nettle, and yohimbe may change blood sugar. Surprisingly, boiled stems of the *Opuntia streptacantha* prickly pear cactus appear to be able to lower blood sugar. Ongoing effects and effects on A1C are not known. Red sage is used for blood sugar effects, but is unproven. Psyllium increases risk of excessively low blood sugar. Echinacea purpurea (injectable) and blonde psyllium seed or husk should NOT be taken by people living with diabetes. Talk to your doctor before adding ANY herbals.

Beverages: Grapefruit juice may decrease metabolism of ziprasidone and lead to toxicity. May be taken with milk or water.

▷ *Alcohol:* Not defined.

Marijuana Smoking: Expected to cause an increase in drowsiness; accentuation of orthostatic hypotension; increased risk of precipitating latent psychoses, confusing the interpretation of mental status and drug responses.

▷ *Other Drugs*

Ziprasidone *taken concurrently* with
- activated charcoal will decrease absorption of ziprasidone. (May be of use in overdoses.)
- amprenavir (Agenerase) may increase either medicine.
- any medicine that has central nervous system activity may result in additive effects.
- benzodiazepines (see Drug Classes) may magnify the orthostatic hypotension problem caused by ziprasidone.
- carbamazepine (Tegretol) causes up to a 35% decrease in blood level of ziprasidone in the body; dosing increases in ziprasidone appear prudent.
- fluoroquinolone antibiotics (see Glossary) may lead to abnormal heart rhythm.
- medicines that *decrease* or inhibit cytochrome P450 3A4 may lead to ziprasidone toxicity.
- medicines that *increase* cytochrome P450 3A4 will blunt ziprasidone benefits.
- medicines that *change* or modify the QT interval such as dofetilide

(Tikosyn) and other medicines such as class I, IA, or III antiarrhythmics; chloral hydrate (Noctec, others); chlorpromazine; clarithromycin; cotrimoxazole; ondansetron; ziprazidone; zolmitriptan; and others may lead to prolongation of the QTc interval and undesirable effects (see QT interval in Glossary). Combination is not recommended.

The following drugs may **decrease** the effects of ziprasidone:
- Medicines that increase (induce) cytochrome P450 3A4 may blunt ziprasidone benefits.

▷ *Driving, Hazardous Activities:* This drug may cause drowsiness or dizziness. Restrict activities as necessary.

Aviation Note: The use of this drug **may be a disqualification** for piloting. Consult a designated Aviation Medical Examiner.

Exposure to Sun: No problems reported.

Exposure to Heat: This medicine can cause problems in regulating body temperature (core temperature homeostasis). If you work or are frequently in a hot environment, be careful to replace enough fluids to avoid dehydration.

Heavy Exercise or Exertion: Since this medicine may cause problems in temperature regulation, caution is advised.

Discontinuation: Do not stop this medicine without first talking to your doctor.

ZOLPIDEM (ZOL pi dem)

Introduced: 1993   **Class:** Hypnotic, imidazopyridine   **Prescription:** USA: Yes   **Controlled Drug:**   USA: C-IV*; Canada: Prescription   **Available as Generic:**   USA: No
Brand Name: Ambien

BENEFITS versus RISKS

Possible Benefits	*Possible Risks*
GIVES SHORT-TERM RELIEF OF INSOMNIA WITH MINIMAL SLEEP DISRUPTION (REM)	Habit-forming potential with prolonged use

---

▷ **Principal Uses**

As a Single Drug Product: Uses currently included in FDA-approved labeling: Short-term treatment of insomnia in adults.

Other (unlabeled) generally accepted uses: (1) Long-term (more than 1 year) treatment of insomnia has been accomplished successfully in limited trials; (2) use in treating insomnia resulting from some antidepressants (SSRIs—see Drug Classes) has been investigated.

How This Drug Works: This drug attaches (binds) to a specific receptor (omega-1) and reduces the time it takes to fall asleep (latency) and increases total sleep time while producing a pattern and benefit of sleep that is similar to normal sleep patterns. Lowers the cyclic alternating pattern (CAP) rate.

*See Schedules of Controlled Drugs at the back of this book.

▷ **Widely Used Guidelines That Involve This Medicine (representative sample):** Please look at the section at the very beginning of this profile called "Class." Next, turn to Table 22 and you will find guidelines listed by the class involved!

Available Dosage Forms and Strengths
Tablets — 5 mg, 10 mg

▷ **Recommended Dosage Ranges** (Actual dose and schedule must be determined for each patient individually.)
Infants and Children: Safety and efficacy for those under 18 years of age are not established.
18 to 60 Years of Age: 10 mg is taken immediately before bedtime. Patients should be reevaluated after taking this drug for 7–10 days, and again if this medicine is needed for more than 14–21 days.
Over 60 Years of Age: Therapy should be started with 5 mg taken at bedtime. The dose may be cautiously increased to 10 mg at bedtime. In general, any given dose will lead to about 50% higher peak concentrations. Confusion and falls are more likely in this population.

Conditions Requiring Dosing Adjustments
Liver Function: The dose should be reduced by half (50%) in liver compromise.
Kidney Function: No changes thought to be needed.

▷ **Dosing Instructions:** The tablet may be crushed. Best taken on an empty stomach. Do not stop this drug abruptly if taken more than 7 days. If you forget a dose: Because this medicine is taken when you can't sleep, a specific schedule is usually not required. Some patients take this medicine just before going to sleep, while others take it only if they can't sleep. DO NOT double up on doses.

Usual Duration of Use: Use on a regular schedule for 2 nights usually determines effectiveness in treating insomnia. Your physician should assess the benefit of this drug after a week to 10 days. Use needed for more than 14–21 days should again be reevaluated.

Typical Treatment Goals and Measurements (Outcomes and Markers)
Insomnia: The general goal is to decrease the amount of time it takes between the time you go to bed and the time you fall asleep (sleep latency). Additionally, the number of times that you wake up is expected to decrease, enabling a full night of sleep. How alert you feel in the morning is also a consideration, as many other hypnotics with longer half-lives also have significant effects the next morning ("hangover" effects). Two scales often used are the Stanford Sleepiness Scale (SSS) and the Saint Mary Hospital Sleep Questionnaire (SMHSQ).

Possible Advantages of This Drug
Low occurrence of adverse effects. May produce less of an undesirable effect on normal sleep patterns (sleep architecture).
Author's Note: The National Institute of Mental Health has an information page on anxiety. It can be found on the World Wide Web (*www.nimh.nih.gov/anxiety*).

Currently a "Drug of Choice"
For short-term management of insomnia in adults.

▷ **This Drug Should Not Be Taken If**
• you had an allergic reaction to it previously.

▷ **Inform Your Physician Before Taking This Drug If**
- you have abnormal liver or kidney function.
- you are pregnant or planning pregnancy.
- you have a history of alcoholism or drug abuse.
- you have a serious lung problem (respiratory impairment).
- you have a history of serious depression or mental disorder.
- you are unsure how much to take or how often to take this medicine.

Possible Side Effects (natural, expected, and unavoidable drug actions)
Drowsiness. Rebound insomnia may happen the first night after this medicine is stopped.

▷ **Possible Adverse Effects** (unusual, unexpected, and infrequent reactions)
If any of the following develop, consult your physician promptly for guidance.
Mild Adverse Effects
Allergic reaction: skin rash.
Drowsiness and dizziness—rare.
Central nervous system reactions (confusion, nightmares), sleep walking (somnambulism)—case reports.
Nausea and diarrhea—infrequent.
Elevation of liver function tests—rare.
Muscle tremors—infrequent.
Blurred vision, double vision—infrequent.
Serious Adverse Effects
Allergic reactions: not defined.
Abnormal thoughts or hallucinations—case reports.
One well-designed study found that use in elderly patients (mean age was 82) nearly doubled the number of hip fractures in that patient population—fall precautions are prudent.
Paradoxical aggression, agitation, or suicidal thoughts—rare.

▷ **Possible Effects on Sexual Function:** None reported.

Possible Effects on Laboratory Tests
Liver function tests: increased SGOT, SGPT, and CPK.

CAUTION
1. This drug works quickly. It is best to take it just before bedtime.
2. Do **not** drink alcohol while taking this drug.
3. This medicine does not work to resolve anxiety. Your doctor should talk to you about NOT using it excessively if anxiety is a root cause of your sleep problem.
4. Withdrawal (see Glossary) may occur, even if this drug was only taken for a week or two. Ask your doctor for advice before stopping zolpidem.
5. You may experience trouble going to sleep for 1 or 2 nights after stopping this drug (rebound insomnia). This effect is usually short term.
6. Sleep disturbances may be a symptom of underlying psychological problems. Tell your doctor if unusual behaviors or odd thoughts occur.
7. Drugs that depress the central nervous system may produce additive effects with this drug. Ask your doctor or pharmacist before combining other prescription or nonprescription drugs with zolpidem.

Precautions for Use
By Infants and Children: Safety and effectiveness for those under 18 years of age are not established.

By Those Over 60 Years of Age: The starting dose should be decreased to 5 mg. Since this drug works quickly, it is best taken immediately before going to bed. You may be at increased risk for falls if the drug remains in your system in the morning. Watch for lethargy, unsteadiness, nightmares, and paradoxical agitation and anger.

▷ **Advisability of Use During Pregnancy**

Pregnancy Category: B. See Pregnancy Risk Categories at the back of this book.

Animal Studies: In rats, abnormal skull bone formation was reported. In rabbits, abnormal bone formation was found.

Human Studies: Adequate studies of pregnant women are not available.
Use during pregnancy is not advisable. Ask your doctor for guidance.

Advisability of Use If Breast-Feeding

Presence of this drug in breast milk: Yes.
Avoid drug or refrain from nursing.

Habit-Forming Potential: This drug may cause dependence (see Glossary).

Effects of Overdose: Marked change from lethargy to coma. Cardiovascular and respiratory compromise was also reported. The drug flumazenil may help reverse symptoms.

Possible Effects of Long-Term Use: Psychological and/or physical dependence.

Suggested Periodic Examinations While Taking This Drug (at physician's discretion)

Liver function tests. Checks of sleep hygiene.

▷ **While Taking This Drug, Observe the Following**

Foods: This drug should not be taken with food (food slows the time to beneficial effects).

Herbal Medicines or Minerals: Kava kava and valerian (no longer widely recommended because of liver toxicity concerns) may exacerbate central nervous system depression (avoid this combination). Kola nut, Siberian ginseng, mate, guarana, ephedra, and ma huang may blunt the benefits of this medicine. While St. John's wort is indicated for anxiety, it is also thought to increase (induce) cytochrome P450 enzymes and could tend to blunt zolpidem effectiveness.

Beverages: Avoid caffeine-containing beverages: coffee, tea, cola, chocolate.

▷ *Alcohol:* This drug should not be combined with alcohol.

Tobacco Smoking: Nicotine is a stimulant and should be avoided. I advise everyone to quit smoking.

Marijuana Smoking: May cause additive drowsiness.

▷ *Other Drugs*

Zolpidem ***taken concurrently*** with
- azole antifungals (itraconazole, ketoconazole, fluconazole, voriconazole [Vfend], and others) may lead to zolpidem toxicity.
- bupropion (Wellbutrin) may increase risk of hallucinations.
- desipramine (Norpramin) may increase risk of hallucinations.
- fluoxetine (Prozac, SARAFEM) may increase risk of hallucinations.
- rifampin (Rifater, others) may decrease zolpidem benefits.
- ritonavir (Norvir) and perhaps other protease inhibitors (see Drug Classes) may lead to zolpidem toxicity.
- sertraline (Zoloft or venlafaxine [Effexor]) may increase risk of hallucinations.

Zolpidem may *increase* the effects of
- chlorpromazine (Thorazine).
- narcotics or other CNS-depressant drugs (see Drug Classes for Opioids, Phenothiazines, Antihistamines, and Benzodiazepines).

▷ *Driving, Hazardous Activities:* This drug may cause drowsiness and impair coordination. Restrict activities as necessary.

Aviation Note: The use of this drug *is a disqualification* for piloting. Consult a designated Aviation Medical Examiner.

Discontinuation: This drug should not be stopped abruptly, even after a week of use. Ask your doctor for help regarding an appropriate withdrawal schedule.

Author's Note: This marks the end of the medicine profiles in this edition. Your Guide continues with MANY helpful tables (including one new table on Guidelines, which can help you more fully understand how national experts suggest medicines should be used, and three broadened tables to help you and your family) as well as a glossary of medical terms. YOU should be the center of health care. Become a smart patient by knowing your medicines, what they are supposed to do, and how long any medicine should take to help!

THE LEADING EDGE

This section, like my website (*www.medicineinfo.com*), is designed to help you become more fully aware of medicines that show promise, are moving along toward approval, and may just become the next best thing! Some are novel applications of approved medicines or are unapproved medicines that are FDA-approvable are also presented. The Leading Edge will help explain new information about concepts in how medicines are packaged for better delivery into the body.

A few interesting medicines or therapeutic products still in early clinical trials are included as "stars on the horizon." It is impossible to predict which medicines or delivery systems will achieve final FDA approval or will be used in specific medicines, but many successful ones will be covered in subsequent editions of this book.

Please be aware that many medicines or delivery systems that could be covered in a given year may be omitted simply because of space limitations. The author will select those that in his opinion offer the most potential benefit to his readers in helping them become powerful patients.

ATHEROSCLEROSIS VACCINE (ATH er oh skler oh sis)

Novel Approach
We've all heard that high levels of "bad" cholesterol are harmful. There are numerous profiles in this book outlining medicines (HMG-CoA reductase inhibitors) that block formation of or otherwise work to lower harmful cholesterol.

A vaccine is being tested against CETP (cholesterol ester transfer protein—now in phase two clinical trials) by a company named Avant. The company was granted patent 6,410,022 on June 25, 2002. The hope of the vaccine is that it may improve the ratio of good (HDL) to bad (LDL) cholesterol.

EXENATIDE (EX ann ih tyde)

Novel Approach
Data presented at the June 15, 2003, American Diabetes Association meeting may realize its promise. Exenatide (a GLP-1 analog called synthetic exendin-4) may help diabetics reach their A1C goal in a novel way and is moving along toward approval. Visit *www.medicineinfo.com* for updates.

EZETIMIBE/SIMVASTATIN (IH zet ah maybe/SIM vah sta tin)

Novel Approach
Combining two medicines in one pill makes it easier to remember them (increases adherence). This novel combination to be called Vytorin does this, and works on both the cholesterol in your diet AND on the cholesterol that your liver makes! Given the new lower cholesterol goals (less than 70 mg/dL) for very high risk patients and trouble many patients have reaching the <100 mg/dL goal, Vytorin may be a key new treatment.

HDAC (HISTONE DEACETYLASE) INHIBITORS

Star on the Horizon
Researching one problem (in this case, cancer) can often lead to a fundamental understanding of another. It's well known that the heart is a muscle. Like any muscle, it can grow or hypertrophy. Unfortunately, unlike the muscle in your arms, the wall of the chest limits how much the muscle can grow. If the heart muscle (left ventricle) gets too big, it can fail. HDAC inhibitors may work to help prevent this prevalent problem. Further research is needed to define their role and drug candidates, but the future appears promising.

HDL (HIGH-DENSITY LIPOPROTEIN) THERAPY

Star on the Horizon
A small company studying ApoA-I Milano/phospholipid complex, or AIM (Esperion Therapeutics), was bought out by Pfizer. The research on reverse cholesterol transport is continuing. This novel approach requires an injection, yet gave some remarkable results in the last round of research. Additional details are available at the company website at *www.pfizer.com*. I'll also update you on *www.medicineinfo.com* as well as progress continues.

HUMAN GENOME (JEE nohm)

Star on the Horizon
The promise of the genome is still unrealized—yet developing medicines that actually correct the underlying CAUSE of a disease or condition is still very, very real. Interestingly, some 20 diseases cause more than 80% of deaths around the world, and about 200–300 genes are responsible for these diseases. One prevalent example might be found in the fact that about every 3 weeks we in essence get a new heart from the same genes; if it would be possible to eliminate a "bad" gene from a gene pair, it might be possible to reverse some heart disease!

INSULIN, ORAL (IN sue lyn)

Medication Delivery
Data continue to evolve on this new insulin delivery system that promises to replace an insulin shot with a sprayer that is actually sprayed into the mouth. The company has reached an agreement for development of Oralin in Australia, India, and China. Generex Biotechnology (*www.generex.com*) may have Oralin available outside the United States on an aggressive timeframe. Blood sugar control without a shot may soon be here!

PKC INHIBITORS

Star on the Horizon
People living with diabetes are prone to developing painful nerve damage known as neuropathy (specifically, diabetic peripheral neuropathy). A family of compounds known as PKC inhibitors and an investigational compound from Lilly known as LY 333531 appear to show great promise. LY 333351 is currently being studied (Phase Three) for neuropathy and for a diabetic eye problem. For more information, visit *www.lilly.com*. There is a clinical trials support number (1-877-285-4559).

RIMONABANT (RIH mon ah bant)

Novel Approach
This medicine works on a novel receptor (endocannabinoid). Amazingly, it appears to accomplish two highly desirable effects. For people who smoke, it works to ease cravings for tobacco products. For those of us with a weight problem, it eases food cravings. Could there be one pill that eases two very prevalent problems? Time will tell, but early data look very very good. Considering that obesity is a major risk factor for cardiovascular disease and smoking is a major risk factor for stroke AND cardiovascular disease, rimonabant (brand is expected to be Accomplia) could be a major inroad to helping prevent heart attacks and strokes. The medicine is being researched by Sanofi Pharmaceuticals (*www.sanofi.com*).

RUBOXISTAURIN MESYLATE (Ruh BOX ih star ihn)

Star on the Horizon

PKC Beta inactivators continue to be of interest. Ruboxistaurin (LY333531) continues to be researched in delaying vision loss in diabetic patients with moderate to severe diabetic retinopathy (nonproliferative). This is important because almost half of diabetics develop some degree of retinopathy. These undesirable changes in the small blood vessels of the retina can lead to macular edema and visual impairment or even blindness. Present timing for submission to the FDA is 2005. Visit *www.medicineinfo.com* for updates!

TESTOSTERONE (Tess TOSS tuhr own)

Star on the Horizon

Some of us have heard of testosterone and think of it as a male sex characteristic hormone. This hormone is indeed part of the reason for secondary gender characteristics such as a man's beard. Did you know it has a role in WOMEN— particularly in sexuality? Procter & Gamble is investigating a patch form of testosterone in order to increase sex drive and sexual satisfaction in women. Work has progressed far enough that a 24-week study of 533 women was reported at the 2004 Endocrine Society of America meeting. The study showed that this patch (called Intrinsa) gave a 49% boost in sexual desire and a 51% frequency of what the participants called satisfying sexual activity. If progress continues as expected, the medicine may be available in 2005.

XIMELAGATRAN (ZI mel ag a tran)

Novel Approach

We've all had a cut that healed and have been thankful for that clot and scab. Unfortunately, if you get a clot on the inside of one of your blood vessels it can lead to a heart attack or stroke. For people who are likely to form an undesirable clot, a medicine to fight that (called an anticoagulant) is often used. Unfortunately, existing pill forms of anticoagulants must be closely checked with laboratory tests. They also have numerous drug interactions. The "new kid" on the scene is shaping up to be ximelagatran (Exanta). While it is still experimental, it is moving through the steps toward approval. Visit *www.medicineinfo.com* for more information.

DRUG CLASSES

Throughout the drug profiles, I often refer you to various drug classes. Use this section to protect yourself and your family. Medicines in the same class often share important characteristics in their chemistry, how they work in the body, and even the problems or side effects that they may cause. Any drug (or all drugs) in a given class can be expected to behave in a similar way. This knowledge helps you prevent interactions or unanticipated or hazardous adverse effects.

Each drug class is named, followed by an alphabetic listing of the generic names of the medicines in the class. Following each generic name (and enclosed in parentheses) is the widely recognized brand name(s) of that particular drug. A complete listing is not possible. If your medicine is not present, call your doctor or pharmacist to get the generic name of the drug that concerns you. The generic name listings are sufficiently complete to serve the scope of this book.

ACE (Angiotensin-Converting Enzyme) Inhibitors

benazepril (Lotensin)
captopril (Capoten)
cilazapril (investigational)
enalapril (Vasotec)
enalapril/felodipine (Lexxel)
fosinopril (Monopril)
lisinopril (Prinivil, Zestril)
lisinopril/hctz (Prinzide, Zestoretic)
moexipril (Univasc)
moexipril/hydrochlorothiazide
  (Uniretic)
perindopril (Aceon)
quinapril (Accupril)
ramipril (Altace)
spirapril (Renormax)
trandolapril (Mavik)
trandolapril/verapamil (Tarka)

Adrenocortical Steroids (Cortisone-like Drugs)

amcinonide (Cyclocort)
beclomethasone (Beclovent, Vanceril)
betamethasone (Celestone)
budesonide (Pulmicort)
cortisone (Cortone)
dexamethasone (Decadron)
fludrocortisone (Florinef)
flunisolide (AeroBid, Nasarel)
fluorometholone (FML)
fluticasone (Flonase)
halcinonide (Halog)

halobetasol (Ultravate)
hydrocortisone (Cortef)
medrysone (HMS Ophthalmic
    Suspension)
methylprednisolone (Medrol)
mometasone (Elocon)
paramethasone (Haldrone)
prednisolone (Delta-Cortef)
prednisone (Deltasone)
rimexalone (Vexol)
triamcinolone (Aristocort, Azmacort)

Alpha-Glucosidase Inhibitors

acarbose (Precose)

miglitol (Glyset)

Amebicides (Anti-Infectives)

chloroquine (Aralen)
emetine
iodoquinol (Yodoxin)

metronidazole (Flagyl)
paromomycin (Humatin)

Aminoglycosides (Anti-Infectives)

amikacin (Amikin)
gentamicin (Garamycin)
kanamycin (Kantrex)

neomycin (Mycifradin, Neobiotic)
paromomycin (Humatin)
tobramycin (Tobicin)

Amphetamine-like Drugs

amphetamine
amphetamine/dextroamphetamine
    (Adderall)
benzphetamine (Didrex)
dextroamphetamine (Dexedrine)
diethylpropion (Tenuate, Tepanil)
methamphetamine (Desoxyn)

methylphenidate (Ritalin)
phendimetrazine (Adipost, Anorex,
    Plegine)
phenmetrazine (Preludin)
phentermine (Adipex-P, Fastin)
phentermine resin complex (Ionamin)
phenylpropanolamine (Dexatrim)

Analgesics (Pain relievers)

acetaminophen (Datril, Tylenol)
acetaminophen/propoxyphene
    (Darvocet-N 100)
aspirin
capsaicin (Zostrix)
COX II inhibitors (rofecoxib-Vioxx,
    celecoxib-Celebrex,
    etoricoxib,valdecoxib-Bextra)
Fentanyl (Duragesic)
Gabapentin (Neurontin)

lidocaine/prilocaine cream (Emla)
morphine (Kadian, MS-Contin, Avinza)
oxycodone (Oxycontin)
propoxyphene (Darvon)
tramadol (Ultram)
zinconotide (investigational)
See also Nonsteroidal Anti-
    Inflammatory Drugs (NSAIDs) and
    Opioid Drugs

Androgens (Male Sex Hormones)

fluoxymesterone (Halotestin)
methyltestosterone (Android,
  Metandren, Oreton)

testosterone (Androderm, Andriol,
  AndroGel, Depotest, Testoderm,
  Testone)

Anemia Treatments (Blood Modifiers, Hematinics)

erythropoetin alpha (Procrit)
pegfilgrastim (Neulasta)

filgrastim (Neupogen)

Angiotensin-II-Receptor Antagonists (also known as ARBS)

candesartan (Atacand)
candesartan/HCTZ (Atacand HCT)
eprosartan (Teveten)
irbesartan (Avapro)
irbesartan/HCTZ (Avalide)

losartan (Cozaar)
losartan/HCTZ (Hyzaar)
telmisartan (Micardis)
valsartan (Diovan)
valsartan/HCTZ (Diovan HCT)

Anorexiants (Appetite Suppressants)

mazindol (Mazanor, Sanorex)
sibutramine (Meridia)

See also Amphetamine-like Drugs

Anti-Acne Drugs

adapalene (Differin)
azelaic acid (Azelex)
benzoyl peroxide (Epi-Clear, others)
erythromycin (Eryderm)
isotretinoin (Accutane)

sodium sulfacetamide 10% lotion
  (Klaron)
tetracycline (Achromycin V)
tretinoin (Retin-A)

Anti-AIDS/HIV Drugs (Anti-Retrovirals)

abacavir (Ziagen)
abacavir/lamivudine/zidovudine (Trizivir)
amprenavir (Agenerase or VX-1478)
atazanavir (Reyataz)
delavirdine (Rescriptor)
didanosine (DDI, Videx)
efavirenz (Sustiva)
emtricitabine (FTC)
hydroxyurea (Droxia)
indinavir (Crixivan)
integrase (Zintevir)

lamivudine (3TC, Epivir)
lopinavir/ritonvair (Kaletra)
nelfinavir (Viracept)
nevirapine (Viramune)
ritonavir (Norvir)
saquinavir (Invirase)
stavudine (D4T, Zerit)
T-20 (enfuvirtide-Fuzeon)
zalcitabine (dideoxycytidine, DDC,Hivid)
zidovudine (AZT, Retrovir)
tenofovir (Viread)

Antialcoholism Drugs

disulfiram (Antabuse)

naltrexone (Trexan, ReVia)

Anti-Alzheimer's Drugs

donepezil (Aricept)
galantamine (Reminyl)
ginkgo biloba (herbal product)
memantine (Namenda)

metrifonate (Bilarcil)
rivastigmine (Exelon)
tacrine (Cognex)
vitamin E (various brands)

Anti-Anginal Drugs

bepridil (Vascor)
diltiazem (Cardizem)
nicardipine (Cardene)
nifedipine (Adalat, Procardia)

nitrates (see class below)
verapamil (Calan, Isoptin)
See also Beta Blockers

Antianxiety Drugs

buspirone (Buspar)
chlormezanone (Trancopal)
hydroxyzine (Atarax, Vistaril)
lorazepam (Ativan)

meprobamate (Equanil, Miltown)
paroxetine (Paxil)—generalized and
adult social anxiety disorder
See also Benzodiazepines

Antiarrhythmic Drugs (Heart-Rhythm Regulators)

Class or Group One

disopyramide (Norpace)
flecainide (Tambocor)
mexiletine (Mexitil)
procainamide (Procan SR, Pronestyl)

quinidine (Quinaglute, Quinidex,
    Quinora)
propafenone (Rythmol)
tocainide (Tonocard)

Class or Group Two

acebutolol (Sectral)
propranolol (Inderal)

sotalol (Betapace)

Class or Group Three

amiodarone (Cordarone)
dofetilide (Tikosyn)

ibutilide (Corvert)
sotalol (Betapace)

Class or Group Four

diltiazem (Cardizem)

verapamil (Calan, Isoptin)

Miscellaneous

adenosine (Adenocard)

digoxin (Lanoxin)

Antiarthritics

Adalimumab (Humira)
aspirin
azathioprine (Imuran; rheumatoid only)
chloroquine (Aralen; rheumatoid only)
COX-II inhibitor family
etanercept (Enbrel)
infliximab (Remicade)

leflunomide (Arava)
penicillamine (Cuprimine)
See also Nonsteroidal Anti-Inflammatory
    Drugs (NSAIDs) and Adrenocortico-
    steroids
anakinra (Kineret)

Antiasthmatic Drugs

Anti-IgE

Omalizumab (Xolair)

Anti-Inflammatory Agents, Corticosteroids

beclomethasone (Beclovent, Vanceril)
flunisolide (AeroBid)
fluticasone (Flovent)

fluticasone/salmeterol (Advair Diskus)
triamcinolone (Azmacort)

Anti-Leukotrienes

montelukast (Singulair)
zafirlukast (Accolate)

zileuton (Zyflo)

Bronchodilators

albuterol (Proventil, Ventolin)
aminophylline (Phyllocontin)
bitolterol (Tornalate)
dyphylline (Lufyllin)
ephedrine (Efed II)
epinephrine (Adrenalin, Bronkaid Mist, Primatene Mist)
formoterol (Foradil)
ipratropium
isoetharine (Bronkosol, Dey-Lute)

isoproterenol (Isuprel)
metaproterenol (Alupent, Metaprel)
oxtriphylline (Choledyl)
pirbuterol (Maxair)
salmeterol (Serevent) (see combination form above)
terbutaline (Brethaire, Brethine, Bricanyl)
theophylline (Bronkodyl, Elixophyllin, Slo-Phyllin, others)

Combination Agents

fluticasone/salmeterol (Advair Diskus)

Mast-Cell-Stabilizing Agents

cromolyn sodium (Gastrocrom, Intal)

nedocromil (Tilade)

Preventive Agents

cromolyn (Intal)

nedocromil (Tilade)

Xanthines

theophylline (Slo-bid, Theo-Dur)

Anti-Attention-Deficit-Hyperactivity-Disorder Drugs

amphetamine and dextroamphetamine (Adderall)
atomoxetine (Strattera)
bupropion (Wellbutrin)
clonidine (Catapres)

desipramine (Norpramin)
dexmethylphenidate (Focalin)
methylphenidate (Concerta, Metadate, Methylin, Ritalin)
pemoline (Cylert)

Anti-Benign-Prostatic-Hyperplasia Drugs

doxazosin (Cardura)
finasteride (Proscar)
prazosin (Minipres)

saw palmetto (various)—herbal product
tamsulosin (Flomax)
terazosin (Hytrin)

Antibiotics

See specific antibiotic class
  (Cephalosporins, Ketolides, Macrolides,
  Penicillins, Tetracyclines, etc.)

Anticancer Drugs (Antineoplastics or Chemotherapy)

anastrozole (Arimidex)
capecitabine (Zeloda)
chlorambucil (Leukeran)
cyclophosphamide (Cytoxan)
flutamide (Eulexin)
hydroxyurea (Hydrea)

liposomally encapsulated doxorubicin
  (Evacet) (investigational)
mercaptopurine (Purinethol)
methotrexate (Rheumatrex)
tamoxifen (Nolvadex)

Signal Transduction Inhibitor Chemotherapy

imatinib STI571 (Gleevec)

Anti-Canker-Sore Drugs

amlexanox (Apthasol)

Anticholesterol Drugs

See Cholesterol-Reducing Drugs
See HMG-CoA Reductase Inhibitors

See "The Leading Edge" section of this
  book

Anticholinergic Drugs (Atropine-like Drugs)

atropine
belladonna
hyoscyamine
scopolamine
See also the specific drug class:

Antidepressant Drugs, Tricyclic
Antihistamines, some
Anti-Parkinsonism Drugs, some
Antispasmodics, Synthetic, some
Muscle Relaxants, some

Anticoagulant Drugs

anisindione (Miradon)
dicumarol
fondaparinux (Arixtra)
low-molecular-weight heparins
  (ardeparin-Normiflo,
  dalteparin-Fragmin,
  enoxaparin-Lovenox,

tinzaparin-Innohep)
warfarin (Coumadin and generic)
Ximelagatran (Exanta)

Anticonvulsant Drugs (Antiepileptic Drugs)

acetazolamide (Diamox)
carbamazepine (Tegretol)
clonazepam (Klonopin)
clorazepate (Tranxene)
diazepam (Valium)
ethosuximide (Zarontin)
ethotoin (Peganone)
felbamate (Felbatol)
gabapentin (Neurontin)
lamotrigine (Lamictal)
levetiracetam (Keppra)
mephenytoin (Mesantoin)
methsuximide (Celontin)
oxcarbamazepine (Trileptal)
paramethadione (Paradione)
phenacemide (Phenurone)
phenobarbital (Luminal)
phensuximide (Milontin)
phenytoin (Dilantin)
primidone (Mysoline)
topiramate (Topamax)
trimethadione (Tridione)
valproic acid (Depakene)
zonisamide (Zonegran)

Anti-Cystic-Fibrosis Agents (Recombinant DNase)

dornase alfa (Pulmozyme)

Antidepressant Drugs

Bicyclic Antidepressants

fluoxetine (Prozac, Prozac Weekly)

venlafaxine (Effexor)

Tetracyclic Antidepressants

maprotiline (Ludiomil)

mirtazapine (Remeron)

Tricyclic Antidepressants

amitriptyline (Elavil, Endep)
amoxapine (Asendin)
clomipramine (Anafranil)
desipramine (Norpramin, Pertofrane)
doxepin (Adapin, Sinequan)
imipramine (Tofranil)
nortriptyline (Aventyl, Pamelor)
protriptyline (Vivactil)
trimipramine (Surmontil)

Other Antidepressants

bupropion (Wellbutrin, Wellbutrin SR)
fluoxetine/olanzapine (Symbyax—used in
  depression in bipolar disorder)
fluvoxamine (Luvox)
hypericum (St. John's wort)
nefazodone (Serzone)
paroxetine (Paxil)
sertraline (Zoloft)
trazodone (Desyrel)
See also Monoamine Oxidase (MAO)
  Inhibitors

Antidiabetic Drugs

Oral

See Alpha-Glucosidase Inhibitors,
  Biguanides, D-phenylalanine derivatives,
Meglitinides, Sulfonylureas and
Thiazolindinediones

Injectable

Insulin (various)

Mouth (Oral) Spray

insulin (Oralin—investigational)

Antidiarrheal Drugs

loperamide

tegaserod (diarrhea predominant irritable bowel syndrome)

Antiemetic Drugs (Anti-Motion-Sickness, Anti-Nausea Drugs)

aprepitant (Emend)
chlorpromazine (Thorazine)
cyclizine (Marezine)
dimenhydrinate (Dramamine)
diphenhydramine (Benadryl)
ginger (various)
granisetron (Kytril)
hydroxyzine (Atarax, Vistaril)

meclizine (Antivert, Bonine)
ondansetron (Zofran)
palonosetron (Aloxi)
prochlorperazine (Compazine)
promethazine (Phenergan)
scopolamine (Transderm Scop)
trimethobenzamide (Tigan)

Substance-P-Blocking Antiemetics

Aprepitant (Emend)

Antiepileptic Drugs

See Anticonvulsant Drugs

Antifungal Drugs (Anti-Infectives)

amphotericin B (Fungizone)
butenafine (Mentax)
caspofungin (Cancidas)
fluconazole (Diflucan)
flucytosine (Ancobon)
griseofulvin (Fulvicin, Grifulvin, Grisactin)
itraconazole (Sporanox)

ketoconazole (Nizoral)
lipid-associated amphotericin
  B(Abelcet)
miconazole (Monistat)
nystatin (Mycostatin)
terbinafine (Lamisil)
tioconazole (Vagistat-1)

Antiglaucoma Drugs

acetazolamide (Diamox)
betaxolol (Betoptic)
bimatoprost (Lumigan)
brimonidine (Alphagan)
brinzolamide (Azopt)
dipivefrin (Propine)
dorzolamide (Trusopt)
dorzolamide and timolol (Cosopt)
epinephrine (Glaucon)

latanoprost (Xalatan)
levobetaxolol (Betaxon)
levobunolol (Betagan)
metipranolol (Optipranolol)
pilocarpine (Pilocar)
timolol (Betimol, Timoptic,
Timoptic-XE)
travaprost (Travatan)

Antigout Drugs

allopurinol (Zyloprim)
colchicine
diclofenac (Cataflam, Voltaren)
fenoprofen (Nalfon)
ibuprofen (Advil, Motrin, Nuprin, Rufin)
indomethacin (Indocin)
ketoprofen (Orudis)

mefenamic acid (Ponstel)
naproxen (Anaprox, Naprosyn)
oxaprozin (Daypro)
piroxicam (Feldene)
probenecid (Benemid)
sulfinpyrazone (Anturane)
sulindac (Clinoril)

Antihistamines

astemizole (Hismanal) (nowremoved from
    the market)
azatadine (Optimine)
azelastine (Astelin)
brompheniramine (Dimetane, others)
carbinoxamine (Clistin, Rondec)
cetirizine (Zyrtec)
chlorpheniramine (Chlor-Trimeton,
    Teldrin)
clemastine (Tavist)
cyclizine (Marezine)
cyproheptadine (Periactin)
desloratadine (Clarinex)

dimenhydrinate (Dramamine)
diphenhydramine (Benadryl)
doxylamine (Unisom)
hydroxyzine (Atarax)
loratadine (Claritin, Claritin Extra)
meclizine (Antivert, Bonine)
orphenadrine (Norflex)
pheniramine (component of Triaminic)
promethazine (Phenergan, others)
pyrilamine (component of Triaminic)
tripelennamine (Pyribenzamine, PBZ)
triprolidine (component of Actifed and
    Sudahist)

Nonsedating or Minimally Sedating

astemizole (Hismanal) (now removed from
    the market)
cetirizine (Zyrtec)

desloratadine (Clarinex)
fexofenadine (Allegra)
loratadine (Claritin)

Antihypertensive Drugs

amlodipine/benazepril (Lotrel)
bisoprolol/hydrochlorothiazide (Ziac)
carvedilol (Coreg)
clonidine (Catapres)
doxazosin (Cardura)
enalapril/felodipine (Lexxel)
eplerenone (Inspra)
guanabenz (Wytensin)
guanadrel (Hylorel)
guanethidine (Ismelin)
guanfacine (Tenex)
hydralazine (Apresoline)

hydrochlorothiazide/benazepril
    (Lotensin)
methyldopa (Aldomet)
minoxidil (Loniten)
prazosin (Minipres)
ramipril/felodipine (Altace plus Felodipine
reserpine (Serpasil)
terazosin (Hytrin)
See also ACE Inhibitors, Angiotensin-
    II-Receptor Antagonists, Beta
    Blockers, Calcium Blockers, and
    Diuretics

Anti-Impotence Drugs

alprostadil injection (Caverject)
apomorphine (Uprima)
sildenafil (Viagra)

tadalafil (Cialis)
vardenafil (Levitra)

Anti-Infective Drugs

See the specific anti-infective drug
   classes:
Amebicides
Aminoglycosides
Antifungal Drugs
Antileprosy Drugs
Antimalarial Drugs
Antituberculosis Drugs

Antiviral Drugs
Cephalosporins
Fluoroquinolones
Macrolide Antibiotics
Oxazolidinones
Penicillins
Sulfonamides
Tetracyclines

Anti-Infective Drugs, Miscellaneous

atovaquone (Mepron)
chloramphenicol (Chloromycetin)
clindamycin (Cleocin)
colistin (Coly-Mycin S)
daptomycin (Cedecin)
furazolidone (Furoxone)
lincomycin (Lincocin)
linezolid (Zyvox)

nalidixic acid (NegGram)
nitrofurantoin (Furadantin,
   Macrodantin)
novobiocin (Albamycin)
pentamidine (Pentam-300)
trimethoprim (Proloprim, Trimpex)
vancomycin (Vancocin)

Anti-Infective Drugs, Topical

mupirocin (Bactroban)

Antileprosy Drugs (Anti-Infectives)

clofazimine (Lamprene)

dapsone

Antimalarial Drugs (Anti-Infectives)

chloroquine (Aralen)
doxycycline (Vibramycin)
hydroxychloroquine (Plaquenil)
mefloquine (Lariam)
primaquine

pyrimethamine (Daraprim)
quinacrine (Atabrine)
quinine
sulfadoxine (Fansidar)

Antimigraine Drugs

almotriptan (Axert)
acetylsalicylic acid (aspirin-Excedrin
   Migraine)
atenolol (Tenormin)
eletriptan (Replax)
ergotamine (Ergostat)
frovatriptan (Miguard)
methysergide (Sansert)
metoprolol (Lopressor)
nadolol (Corgard)

naratriptan (Amerge)
nifedipine (Procardia)
propranolol (Inderal)
rizatriptan benzoate (Maxalt, Maxalt MLT)
sumatriptan (Imitrex)
timolol (Blocadren)
valproic acid (Divalproex)
verapamil (Calan, Isoptin)
zolmatriptan (Zomig, Zomig nasal spray)

Anti-Motion-Sickness/Antinausea Drugs

See Antiemetic Drugs

Anti-Myasthenics

neostigmine

Antimycobacterial Agents

rifabutin (Mycobutin)

Anti-Osteoporotics

alendronate (Fosamax)
antiestrogens (SERM)
calcitonin (Miacalcin)
calcium (various brands)
estrogen (various brands)
pravastatin (Pravachol—one study
    reported improvement—not an
    FDA-approved use)

raloxifene (Evista)
risedronate (Actonel)
synthetic conjugated estrogens
teriparatide (Forteo)
tiludronate (Skelid)
zoledronic acid (Zoledronate—
    investigational)

Anti-Parkinsonism Drugs

amantadine (Symmetrel)
benztropine (Cogentin)
bromocriptine (Parlodel)
diphenhydramine (Benadryl)
levodopa (Dopar, Larodopa)
levodopa/bensarazide (Prolopa)
levodopa/carbidopa (Sinemet, Sinemet CR)
pergolide (Permax)
prampexole (Myrapex)

ropinirole (Requip)
selegiline (Eldepryl)
tolcapone (Tasmar)
trihexyphenidyl (Artane)
vitamin E (various)
Catechol O-Methyl Tranferase (COMT)
    Drugs
tolcapone (Tasmar)

Antiplatelet Drugs (Platelet Aggregation Inhibitors)

aspirin
aspirin/dipyridamole (Aggrenox)
clopidogrel (Plavix)
dipyridamole (Persantine)

sulfinpyrazone (Anturane)
ticlopidine (Ticlid)
tirofiban (Aggrastat)

Antipsoriatic Drugs

acitretin (Soriatane)
alefacept (Amavive)
efalizumab (Raptiva)
etanercept (Enbrel)

etretinate
infliximab (Remicade)
methotrexate

Antipsychotic Drugs (Neuroleptics, Major Tranquilizers)
Note: Some are atypical antipsychotics

aripiprazole (Abilify)
chlorprothixene (Taractan)
clozapine (Clozaril)
haloperidol (Haldol)
loxapine (Loxitane)
molindone (Moban)
olanzapine (Zyprexa)

pimozide (Orap)
quetiapine (Seroquel)
risperidone (Risperdal)
thiothixene (Navane)
ziprasidone (Geodon)
See also Phenothiazines and
    Thienobenzodiazepines

Antipyretic Drugs (Fever-Reducing Drugs)

acetaminophen
aspirin
See also COX II inhibitors

See also Nonsteroidal Anti-Inflammatory
    Drugs (NSAIDs)

Anti-Sickle-Cell Anemia Drugs

hydroxyurea (Droxia, Hydrea)

Antispasmodics, Synthetic

anisotropine (Valpin)
clidinium (Quarzan)
glycopyrrolate (Robinul)
hexocyclium (Tral)
isopropamide (Darbid)

mepenzolate (Cantil)
methantheline (Banthine)
methscopolamine (Pamine)
propantheline (Pro-Banthine)
tridihexethyl (Pathilon)

Antituberculosis Drugs

aminosalicylate sodium (Sodium P.A.S.)
capreomycin (Capastat)
cycloserine (Seromycin)
ethambutol (Myambutol)
ethionamide (Trecator-SC)
isoniazid (Laniazid, Nydrazid)

pyrazinamide
rifabutin (Mycobutin)
rifampin (Rifadin, Rimactane, Rifater)
rifapentine (Priftin)
streptomycin

Antitussive Drugs (Cough Suppressants)

benzonatate (Tessalon)
codeine (various brands)
dextromethorphan (Hold DM, Suppress)
diphenhydramine (Benylin)

hydrocodone (Hycodan)
hydromorphone (Dilaudid)
promethazine (Phenergan)

Antiulcer Drugs

Antacids

various brands

Antibiotics

amoxicillin
clarithromycin
metronidazole

tetracycline
See Histamine (H2) Blockers
See Proton Pump Inhibitors

Miscellaneous Antiulcer Drugs

amoxicillin/clarithromycin/
lansoprazole (Prevpac)
bismuth subsalicylate (Pepto-Bismol,
  others)

misoprostol (Cytotec)
ranitidine bismuth citrate (Tritec)
sucralfate (Carafate)

Antiviral Drugs (Anti-Infectives)

Abacavir (Ziagen)
Abacavir, lamivudine, zidovudine
  (Trizivir)
acyclovir (Zovirax)
amantadine (Symmetrel)
amprenavir (Agenerase)
atazanavir (Reyataz)
cidofovir (Vistide)
didanosine (Videx)
docosanol (Abreva)
efavirenz (Sustiva)
emtricitabine (FTC)
enfuvirtide (Fuzeon)
famciclovir (Famvir)
foscarnet (Foscavir)
ganciclovir (Cytovene)
indinavir (Crixivan)
lamivudine (Epivir, Epivir HBV)

tenofovir (Viread)
lopinavir/ritonavir (Kaletra)
nelfinavir (Viracept)
nevirapine (Viramune)
oseltamivir (Tamiflu)
penciclovir (Denavir)
peginterferon alpha-2a (Pegasys)
ribavirin (Copegus, Virazole)
rimantadine (Flumadine)
ritonavir (Norvir)
saquinavir (Invirase)
stavudine (Zerit)
valacyclovir (Valtrex)
vidarabine (Vira A)
zalcitabine (Hivid)
zanamivir (Relenza)
zidovudine (Retrovir)

Appetite Suppressants

See Anorexiants

Aromatase inhibitors

anastrozole (Arimidex)

Atropine-like Drugs

See Anticholinergic Drugs

Barbiturates

amobarbital (Amytal)
aprobarbital (Alurate)
butabarbital (Butisol)
mephobarbital (Mebaral)
metharbital (Gemonil)

pentobarbital (Nembutal)
phenobarbital (Luminal, Solfoton)
secobarbital (Seconal)
talbutal (Lotusate)

Benzodiazepines

alprazolam (Xanax)
bromazepam (Lectopam)
chlordiazepoxide (Libritabs, Librium)
clonazepam (Klonopin)
clorazepate (Tranxene)
diazepam (Valium, Vazepam)
estazolam (Prosom)
flurazepam (Dalmane)
halazepam (Paxipam)

ketazolam (Loftran)
lorazepam (Ativan)
midazolam (Versed)
nitrazepam (Mogadon)
oxazepam (Serax)
prazepam (Centrax)
quazepam (Doral)
temazepam (Restoril)
triazolam (Halcion)

Beta Blockers (Beta-Adrenergic-Blocking Drugs)

acebutolol (Sectral)
atenolol (Tenormin)
betaxolol (Kerlone)
bisoprolol (Zebeta)
bisoprolol/hydrochlorothiazide (Ziac)
carteolol (Cartrol)
carvedilol (Coreg)

labetalol (Normodyne, Trandate)
metoprolol (Lopressor)
nadolol (Corgard)
penbutolol (Levatol)
pindolol (Visken)
propranolol (Inderal)
timolol (Blocadren)

Biguanides (Oral Antidiabetic Drugs)

metformin (Glucophage)

Bisphosphonates

alendronate (Fosamax)
risedronate (Actonel)

tiludronate (Skelid)
zoledronate (Zometra)

Blood Flow Agents

cilostazol (Pletal)
ginkgo biloba (various)

pentoxifylline (Trental)

Bowel Anti-Inflammatory Drugs (Inflammatory Bowel Disease Suppressants)

azathioprine (Imuran)
infliximab (Avakine)
mesalamine (Rowasa, Asacol)

metronidazole (Flagyl)
olsalazine (Dipentum)
sulfasalazine (Azulfidine)

Bronchodilators

See Antiasthmatic Drugs

Calcium Blockers (Calcium-Channel-Blocking Drugs)

amlodipine (Norvasc)

bepridil (Vascor)

diltiazem (Cardizem, Tiazac)

felodipine (Plendil)

isradipine (DynaCirc)

mibefradil (Posicor) (removed by the
company)

nicardipine (Cardene, Cardene SR)

nifedipine (Adalat CC, Procardia XL)

nimodipine (Nimotop)

nisoldipine (Sular)

verapamil (Calan, Isoptin, Verelan)

Cardiac Hormones (Anti–Congestive Heart Failure)

Nesiritide (Natrecor)

Cephalosporins (Anti-Infectives)

cefaclor (Ceclor)

cefadroxil (Duricef, Ultracef)

cefamandole (Mandol)

cefatrizine (Cefaperos)

cefazolin (Ancef, Kefzol, Zolicef)

cefdinir (Omnicef)

cefepime (Maxipime)

cefixime (Suprax)

cefmetazole (Zefazone)

cefonicid (Monocid)

cefoperazone (Cefobid)

ceforanide (Precef)

cefotaxime (Claforan)

cefotetan (Cefotan)

cefoxitin (Mefoxin)

cefpodoxime (Vantin)

cefprozil (Cefzil)

ceftazidime (Fortaz, Tazidime, Tazicef)

ceftibuten (Cedax)

ceftizoxime (Cefizox)

ceftriaxone (Rocephin)

cefuroxime (Ceftin, Kefurox, Zinacef)

cephalexin (Keflex, Keftab)

cephalothin (Keflin)

cephapirin (Cefadyl)

cephradine (Anspor, Velosef)

loracarbef (Cefobid)

moxalactam (Moxam)

Cholesterol-Reducing Drugs

APO-A Milano (investigational)

atorvastatin (Lipitor)

cholestyramine (Questran, Prevalite)

clofibrate (Atromid-S)

colesevelam (Welchol)

colestipol (Colestid)

dextrithyroxiune (Choloxin)

ezetimibe (Zetia)

ezetimibe/simvastatin (Vytorin)

fenofibrate (Tricor)

fluvastatin (Lescol)

gemfibrozil (Lopid)

lovastatin (Mevacor)

niacin/lovastatin (Advicor)

niacin (Nicobid, Slo-Niacin, others)

pravastatin (Pravachol)

rosuvastatin (Crestor)

simvastatin (Zocor)

Cortisone-like Drugs

See Adrenocortical Steroids

Cough Suppressants

See Antitussive Drugs

COX II Inhibitors

celecoxib (Celebrex)
etoricoxib (investigational; Arcoxia)

rofecoxib (Vioxx)
valdecoxib (Bextra)

Decongestants

ephedrine (Efedron, Ephedrol)
naphazoline (Naphcon, Vasocon)
oxymetazoline (Afrin, Duration, others)
phenylephrine (Neo-Synephrine, others)

phenylpropanolamine (Propadrine, Propagest, others)
pseudoephedrine (Afrinol, Sudafed, others)
tetrahydrozoline (Tyzine, Visine, others)
xylometazoline (Otrivin)

Digitalis Preparations

deslanoside (Cedilanid-D)
digitoxin (Crystodigin)

digoxin (Lanoxicaps, Lanoxin)

Direct Thrombin Inhibitors

argatroban (Argatroban)

ximelagatran (Exanta)

Disease-Modifying Antirheumatic Drugs (DMARDs)

adalimumab (Humira)
etanercept (Enbrel)

leflunomide (Arava)
methotrexate (Rheumatrex)

Diuretics

acetazolamide (Diamox)
amiloride (Midamor)
bumetanide (Bumex)
chlorthalidone (Hygroton)
ethacrynic acid (Edecrin)
furosemide (Lasix)

indapamide (Lozol)
metolazone (Diulo, Zaroxolyn)
spironolactone (Aldactone)
triamterene (Dyrenium)
See also Thiazide Diuretics

Dopamine System Stabilizers

aripiprazole (Abilify)

D-phenylalanine derivative oral hypoglycemics

nateglinide (Starlix)

Endocannabinoid

rimonabant (Accomplia—investigational)

Ergot Derivatives

bromocriptine (Parlodel)
ergotamine (Bellergal)

methysergide (Sansert)
pergolide (Permax)

Estrogens (Female Sex Hormones)

chlorotrianisene (Tace)
diethylstilbestrol (DES, Stilphostrol)
estradiol (Estrace, Estraderm, others)
estrogens, conjugated (Premarin, Prempro)
estrogens, esterified (Estratab, Menest)
estrone (Theelin, others)
estropipate (Ogen)

ethinyl estradiol (Estinyl)
quinestrol (Estrovis)
plant-derived synthetic conjugated estrogens, A (Cenestin)
plant-derived synthetic conjugated estrogens, B (Enjuvia)

Female Sex Hormones

See Estrogens and Progestins

Female Sexual Enhancers

Testosterone patch (Intrinsa)

Fever-Reducing Drugs

See Antipyretic Drugs

5-Alpha-Reductase Inhibitors

finasteride (Proscar)

saw palmetto (various)

Fluoroquinolones (Anti-Infectives)

balofloxacin (pending)
ciprofloxacin (Cipro)
fleroxacin (Quinodis [Germany])
gatiloxacin (Tequin)
grepafloxacin (Raxar)
levofloxacin (Levaquin)

lomefloxacin (Maxaquin)
moxifloxacin (Avelox)
norfloxacin (Noroxin)
ofloxacin (Floxin)
sparfloxacin (Zagam)
trovafloxacin (Trovan)

Fusion Inhibitors (Anti-HIV, Anti-Infectives)

enfuvirtide (Fuzeon)

Gastrointestinal Drugs

Miscellaneous

cisapride (Propulsid)
infliximab (Avakine)

metoclopramide (Reglan)

Ulcer Preventatives

misoprostol (Cytotec)

Hair Growth Stimulants
finasteride (Proscar, Propecia)   minoxidil (Rogaine)

Heart Rhythm Regulators
See Antiarrhythmic Drugs

Hematopoietic Agents
filgrastim (Neupogen)   pegfilgrastim (Neulasta)

HMG-CoA reductase inhibitors
atorvastatin (Lipitor)   pravastatin (Pravachol)
fluvastatin (Lescol)   rosuvastatin (Crestor)
lovastatin (Mevacor)   simvastatin (Zocor)

Hormones

Miscellaneous
nafarelin (Synarel)   See also Estrogens and Progestins for
See also Androgens for male sex hormones   female sex hormones

H2 Blockers (Histamine [H2] Blocking Drugs)
cimetidine (Tagamet, Tagamet HB 200)   nizatidine (Axid, Axid AR)
famotidine (Pepcid, Pepcid AC, Pepcid-   ranitidine (Zantac, Zantac 75)
   Complete)

Hypnotic Drugs (Sedatives/Sleep Inducers)
acetylcarbromal (Paxarel)   paraldehyde (Paral)
chloral hydrate (Aquachloral, Noctec)   propiomazine (Largon)
estazolam (Prosom)   quazepam (Doral)
ethchlorvynol (Placidyl)   temazepam (Restoril)
ethinamate (Valmid)   triazolam (Halcion)
flurazepam (Dalmane)   zaleplon (Sonata)
glutethimide (Doriden)   zolpidem (Ambien)
methyprylon (Noludar)   See also Barbiturates

Immunosuppressants
azathioprine (Imuran)   hydroxychloroquine (Plaquenil)
chlorambucil (Leukeran)   leflunomide (Arava)
cyclophosphamide (Cytoxan)   serolimus (Rapamune)
cyclosporine (Sandimmune)   tacrolimus (Prograf)

Interleukin One Receptor Antagonists
Anakinra (Kineret)

Ketolide Antibiotics (Anti-Infectives)

Telithromycin (Ketek; investigational)

Low-Affinity NMDA Receptor Antagonists

Memantine (Namenda)

Macrolide Antibiotics (Anti-Infectives)

azithromycin (Zithromax)
clarithromycin (Biaxin)
dirithromycin (Dynabac)

erythromycin (E-Mycin, Ilosone,
Erythrocin, E.E.S.)
troleandomycin (TAO)

Male Sex Hormones

See Androgens

Mast-Cell-Stabilizing Agents

See Antiasthmatic Drugs

Meglitinides

Netaglinide (Starlix)

repaglinide (Prandin)

Mixed Amphetamines

Amphetamine/dextroamphetamine
  (Adderall)

Monoamine Oxidase (MAO) Inhibitor Drugs (Type A: Antidepressants)

isocarboxazid (Marplan)
phenelzine (Nardil)

tranylcypromine (Parnate)

Mood Stabilizers

Lithium (lithobid, others)
Oxcarbazepine (Trileptal)

Valproic acid (Depakote, others)

Muscarinic Receptor Antagonists (Anti-Incontinence)

tolteradine (Detrol)

Muscle Relaxants (Skeletal Muscle Relaxants)

baclofen (Lioresal)
carisoprodol (Rela, Soma, others)
chlorphenesin carbamate (Maolate)
chlorzoxazone (Paraflex, Parafon Forte)
cyclobenzaprine (Flexeril)
dantrolene (Dantrium)

diazepam (Valium)
meprobamate (Equanil, Miltown, others)
metaxalone (Skelaxin)
methocarbamol (Robaxin, others)
orphenadrine (Norflex, others)

Neuramidase Inhibitors

oseltamivir (Tamiflu)

zanamivir (Relenza)

Nitrates

amyl nitrate (amyl nitrate generic,
Vaporole, others)
erythrityl tetranitrate (Cardilate)
isosorbide dinitrate (Isordil,
Sorbitrate, others)

isosorbide mononitrate (Ismo, Imdur)
nitroglycerin (Nitrostat, Nitrolingual,
Nitrogard, Nitrong, others)
pentaerythritol tetranitrate (Duotrate,
Peritrate)

Nonnucleoside Reverse Transcriptase Inhibitors

delavirdine (Rescriptor)
efavirenz (Sustiva)

nevirapine (Viramune)

Nonnucleotide Reverse Transcriptase Inhibitors

tenofovir (Viread)

Nonsteroidal Anti-Inflammatory Drugs (NSAIDs)

Aspirin substitutes

Acetic Acids

bromfenac sodium (Duract)
diclofenac potassium (Cataflam)
diclofenac sodium (Voltaren)
etodolac (Lodine)
indomethacin (Indochron E-R, Indocin,
Indocin SR)

ketorolac (Toradol)
meloxicam (Mobic)
nabumetone (Relafen)
sulindac (Clinoril)
tolmetin (Tolectin, Tolectin DS)

Fenamates

meclofenamate (Meclomen)

mefenamic acid (Ponstel)

Oxicams

piroxicam (Feldene)

Propionic Acids

diflunisal (Dolobid)
fenoprofen (Nalfon)
flurbiprofen (Ansaid)
ibuprofen
ketoprofen (Orudis, Oruvail)
naproxen (Naprosyn)

naproxen sodium (Aleve, Anaprox,
    Anaprox DS)
oxaprozin (Daypro)
oxyphenbutazone (Oxalid)
suprofen (Profenal)

Opioid Antagonists

naltrexone (ReVia)

Opioid Drugs (Narcotics)

alfentanil (Alfenta)
codeine
fentanyl (Actiq, Sublimaze, Duragesic)
hydrocodone (Hycodan)
hydromorphone (Dilaudid)
levorphanol (Levo-Dromoran)
meperidine (Demerol)

methadone (Dolophine)
morphine (Astramorph, Duramorph, MS
    Contin, Roxanol, Avinza)
oxycodone (OxyContin, Roxicodone)
oxymorphone (Numorphan)
propoxyphene (Darvon)
sufentanil (Sufenta)

Pain Syndrome Modifiers (also Adjuvants)

carbamazepine (Tegretol)
gabapentin (Neurontin)
phenytoin (Dilantin)

samarium-EDTMP (Quadramet)
strontium-89 (Metastron)

Penicillins (Anti-Infectives)

amoxicillin (Amoxil, Larotid, Polymox,
    Trimox, others)
amoxicillin/clavulanate (Augmentin)
ampicillin (Omnipen, Polycillin, Principen,
    Totacillin)
ampicillin/sulbactam (Unasyn)
bacampicillin (Spectrobid)
carbenicillin (Geocillin, Geopen, Pyopen)
cloxacillin (Cloxapen, Tegopen)
dicloxacillin (Dynapen, Pathocil, Veracillin)

methicillin (Staphcillin)
mezlocillin (Mezlin)
nafcillin (Nafcil, Unipen)
oxacillin (Prostaphlin)
penicillin G (Pentids, others)
penicillin V (Pen Vee K, V-Cillin K,
    Veetids, others)
piperacillin (Pipracil)
ticarcillin (Ticar)
ticarcillin/clavulanate (Timentin)

Phenothiazines (Antipsychotic Drugs)

acetophenazine (Tindal)
chlorpromazine (Thorazine)
fluphenazine (Permitil, Prolixin)
mesoridazine (Serentil)
perphenazine (Trilafon)
prochlorperazine (Compazine)

promazine (Sparine)
thioridazine (Mellaril)
trifluoperazine (Stelazine)
triflupromazine (Vesprin)
ziprasidone (Geodon)

Potassium Replacement Products

K-Dur

Potassium chloride (various)

Progestins (Female Sex Hormones)

ethynodiol

hydroxyprogesterone (Duralutin, Gesterol L.A., others)

medroxyprogesterone (Amen, Curretab, Prempro, Premphase, Provera)

megestrol (Megace)

norethindrone (Micronor, Norlutate, Norlutin)

norgestrel (Ovrette)

progesterone (Gesterol 50, Progestaject)

Protease Inhibitors

amprenavir (Agenerase)

atazanavir, (Reyataz)

indinavir (Crixivan)

lopinavir/ritonvair (Kaletra)

nelfinavir (Viracept)

ritonavir (Norvir)

saquinavir (Fortovase, Invirase)

Proton Pump Inhibitors (H/K ATPase Inhibitors)

esomeprazole (Nexium)

lansoprazole (Prevacid, Prevpac)

omeprazole (Prilosec)

pantoprazole (Protonix)

rabeprazole (Aciphex)

Radiopharmaceuticals

samarium-EDTMP (Quadramet)

strontium-89 (Metastron)

Renin-angiotensin Aldosterone System Modulator (Anti-Hypertensive)

eplerenone (Inspra)

Salicylates

aspirin

choline salicylate (Arthropan)

magnesium salicylate (Doan's, Magan, Mobidin)

salsalate (Amigesic, Disalcid, Salsitab)

sodium salicylate

sodium thiosalicylate (Rexolate, Tusal)

Sedatives/Sleep Inducers

See Hypnotic Drugs

Selective Estrogen Receptor Modulators (SERMs)

raloxifene (Evista)

tamoxifen (Nolvadex)

Selective Serotonin Reuptake Inhibitors (SSRIs)

citalopram (Celexa)
escitalopram (Lexapro)
fluoxetine (Prozac)
fluvoxamine (Luvox)
nefazodone (Serzone)

paroxetine (Paxil)
sertraline (Zoloft)
trazodone (Desyrel)
venlafaxine (Effexor)

Smoking Cessation Adjuncts

bupropion (Zyban)
nicotine (Nicorette, various patch brands
  such as Nicotrol)

rimonabant (Accomplia—investigational)
varenicline (investigational)

Sulfonamides (Anti-Infectives)

multiple sulfonamides (Triple Sulfa No. 2)
sulfacytine (Renoquid)
sulfadiazine
sulfamethizole (Thiosulfil)
sulfamethoxazole (Gantanol)

sulfasalazine (Azulfidine)
sulfisoxazole (Gantrisin)
COX II Inhibitor
celecoxib (Celebrex)

Sulfonylureas (Oral Antidiabetic Drugs)

acetohexamide (Dymelor)
chlorpropamide (Diabinese)
glimepiride (Amaryl)
glipizide (Glucotrol)

glyburide (DiaBeta, Micronase)
tolazamide (Ronase, Tolamide, Tolinase)
tolbutamide (Orinase)

Tetracyclines (Anti-Infectives)

demeclocycline (Declomycin)
doxycycline (Doryx, Doxychel,
  Vibramycin)
methacycline (Rondomycin)

minocycline (Minocin)
oxytetracycline (Terramycin)
tetracycline (Achromycin V, Panmycin,
  Sumycin)

Thiazide Diuretics

bendroflumethiazide (Naturetin)
benzthiazide (Aquatag, Exna, Marazide)
chlorothiazide (Diuril)
cyclothiazide (Anhydron)
hydrochlorothiazide (Esidrix, HydroDiuril,
  Oretic)

hydroflumethiazide (Diucardin, Saluron)
methyclothiazide (Enduron, Aquatensen)
polythiazide (Renese)
trichlormethiazide (Metahydrin, Naqua)

Thiazolidinediones

pioglitazone (Actos)
rosiglitazone (Avandia)

troglitazone (Rezulin—
  no longer available in the United States)

Thienobenzodiazepines

olanzapine (Zyprexa)

Thyroid Hormones

levothyroxine (Synthroid)

liothyronine (Cytomel)

Tranquilizers, Major

See Antipsychotic Drugs

Tranquilizers, Minor

See Antianxiety Drugs

Vaccines (Immune Modulators)

influenza vaccine (Fluogen, Flu-Shield, Fluzone, FluMist)
lyme disease vaccine (LYMErix)

pneumococcal vaccine (Prevnar)
varicella virus vaccine (Varivax)

Vasodilators (Peripheral Vasodilators)

cyclandelate (Cyclospasmol)
ethaverine (Ethaquin, Isovex)
isoxsuprine (Vasodilan)

nylidrin (Arlidin)
papaverine (Cerespan, Pavabid)

Weight Loss Agents (Miscellaneous)

orlistat (Xenical)

rimonabant (Accomplia)

Xanthines (Bronchodilators)

aminophylline (Phyllocontin, Truphylline)
dyphylline (Dilor, Lufyllin)

oxtriphylline (Choledyl)
theophylline (Bronkodyl, Slo-Phyllin, Theolair, others)

A GLOSSARY
OF
MEDICINE-RELATED TERMS

A Glossary of Medicine-Related Terms

absolute risk This is generally used in conjunction with diseases. The absolute risk of a disease over a given time period is the actual number of people (usually in two groups that are compared) who will get a disease.

ace (usually seen as ACE) A term used by clinicians to refer to the class of medicines for high blood pressure called angiotensin-converting enzyme inhibitors (such as ramipril or Altace).

acute coronary syndrome (ACS) A term from cardiology used to describe sudden problems that happen to the heart. ACS encompasses heart attack (acute myocardial infarction or AMI), Unstable Angina (UA—the leading reason people are admitted to a coronary care unit in the U.S.), and Non ST-Segment Elevation MI (NSTEMI).

addiction This is generally recognized as intense drug dependence, with uncontrollable drug-seeking behavior, *tolerance* for pleasure-giving effects, and *withdrawal* if the drug is withheld. This is *physical dependence* where the drug is incorporated into the fundamental biochemistry of the brain. Some clinicians characterize this as a loss of control (centrality) of drug use with continued drug use by those addicted even though it proves to be harmful. (See the terms dependence and tolerance for accounts of physical and psychological dependence.)

adherence (Prior term: compliance. European term: concordance.) How appropriately a patient takes their medicine according to the way it was prescribed. For example: If a medicine is to be taken three times a day and the patient actually takes it three times a day, they are perfectly adherent to their medicine (100% adherent).

adverse effect or reaction An abnormal, unexpected, infrequent, and often unpredictable injurious response to a medicine. This does not include a pharmacological action, even though some may be undesirable and unintended. (See side effect.) Adverse reactions are those due to drug *allergy*, individual *idiosyncrasy*, and *toxic* effects of drugs on tissues (see allergy [drug], idiosyncrasy and toxicity).

allergy (drug) An abnormal medicine response that happens after antibodies* are made to the drug itself. People with history of hay fever, asthma, hives, or eczema are more likely to develop medicine allergies. Allergies can develop slowly, or they can appear suddenly and require lifesaving medical attention.

*Antibodies are proteins that combine with foreign substances. Protective antibodies destroy bacteria and neutralize toxins. Injurious antibodies react with foreign substances, such as drugs, to cause release of histamine, a chemical causing allergic reactions.

alternative delivery system (ADS) A term describing a variety of health care forms other than the established fee-for-service model, such as HMOs, PPOs, and others.

analgesic A medicine used to relieve pain. There are three types:
- simple nonnarcotics, which block production of chemicals that cause or worsen pain (prostaglandins, etc.)—examples are acetaminophen, aspirin, nonsteroidal anti-inflammatory drugs (Motrin, Advil, etc.), and the new COX II inhibitors
- narcotic analgesics or opioids, which relieve pain by blunting pain perception in the brain—examples are morphine, codeine, and hydrocodone (natural derivatives of opium) and meperidine or pentazocine (synthetic drug products)
- local anesthetics, which relieve pain by making sensory nerve endings insensitive to pain—such as phenazopyridine (Pyridium)

anaphylactic (anaphylactoid) reaction Signs and symptoms that indicate an extreme hypersensitivity to a medicine. Anaphylactic reactions often involve several body systems. Mild symptoms include itching, hives, congestion, nausea, cramping, or diarrhea. Sometimes these precede severe problems, such as choking, shortness of breath, and loss of consciousness (usually referred to as anaphylactic shock). Anaphylactic reactions can happen after a very small dose; they may develop suddenly and can be rapidly fatal. They are true medical emergencies. Any adverse effect appearing within 20 minutes after taking a drug should be considered an early sign of anaphylactic reaction. Get medical attention immediately! (See allergy [drug] and hypersensitivity.)

ankle brachial index (ABI) A way of checking for blood vessel disease known as peripheral vascular disease. The ABI is normal if it is more than 1. Most clinicians find an ABI of less than 0.9 to be very suggestive of peripheral vascular disease (PVD). Some 30% of people with PVD have cramping when they walk which is called intermittant claudication.

antihypertensive A medicine used to lower high blood pressure. *Hypertension* describes blood pressure above a normal range. It is not nervous or emotional tension. Currently, the National Heart, Lung, and Blood Institute or NHLBI describes three stages of hypertension. Optimal is 120/80 for those without diabetes and 130/80 for those living with diabetes. Stage one hypertension begins at 149/89. There are also categories a, b, and c within those numerical ranges, which seek to stratify risk factors onto blood pressure ranges. Medicines to treat hypertension fall into several major groups:
- drugs that increase urine production (the diuretics)
- drugs that relax blood vessel walls
- drugs that reduce sympathetic nervous system activity

Some clinicians classify antihypertensives based on their site or mechanism of action—for example, ACE inhibitors that inhibit angiotensin converting enzyme, or ARBs—antihypertensives that act as angiotensin two (AT1 subtype) receptor blockers. Please note—although high blood pressure often does not have any symptoms, you MUST treat it for life. Take your medicine EXACTLY as prescribed.

antipyretic A medicine that lowers body temperature. It reduces fever by working on the hypothalamus of the brain. This leads to dilation of blood vessels (capillary beds) in the skin and brings heated blood to the skin surface for cooling. Sweat glands are also stimulated to cool the body through evaporation. An antipyretic may also be a pain reliever (analgesic, such as acetaminophen) or analgesic and anti-inflammatory (aspirin).

aplastic anemia Also known as pancytopenia, where production of the three types of blood cells is seriously impaired. Aplastic anemia can occur from unknown causes, but about half of reported cases are caused by drugs or chemicals. A delay of 1 to 6 months may occur between the use of a drug and anemia. Symptoms include lower red blood cells (anemia), resulting in fatigue and pallor; deficiency of white blood cells (leukopenia), predisposing to infections; and low blood platelets (thrombocytopenia), which can cause spontaneous bruising or bleeding. Treatment is difficult. Even with the best of care, half the cases may be fatal. Aplastic anemia is rare, but anyone taking a drug that can cause it should have periodic complete blood cell counts. For a listing of causative drugs, see Table 5, Section Six.

ARB A common term used to refer to the class of medicines known as angiotensin receptor blockers.

aspirin resistance A new term used to describe the occurance of a second heart attack in some patients DESPITE the appropriate and ongoing use of aspirin. A study by Eikelboom et al. in circulation (see Sources) postulated that roughly one in five people are able to make a compound called thromboxane A2 even though they are taking aspirin as directed. The researchers suggested that people who have had a heart attack get a test of urinary 11-dehydro thromboxane B2 to find out if they make excessive thromboxane A2 and may be candidates for increased aspirin dosing. More research is needed to determine the required dose as well as who to test and when.

Bad Med Syndrome (BMS) The decreased quality of life, decrease in expected beneficial medicine results, loss of time from work, unnecessary stays in the hospital, or additional treatment resulting from medicines themselves or from the improper use of medicines. Improper use includes drug interactions resulting from inappropriate medicine combinations, too low a dose (subtherapeutic dosing), too high a dose (overdose), as well as taking the medicine "every once in a while" when it was prescribed for ongoing use.

   No one intends to cause Bad Med Syndrome (BMS), yet patients, pharmacists, physicians, other health care providers, and many organizations all contribute to it. I believe it will take a team effort to solve it.

bioavailability How fast and how much active medicine is absorbed into the blood. Two types of measurements—blood levels after it was taken and how long the drug stays in the blood—show how much drug is available to work and for how long. The two major factors that govern bioavailability are (1) the chemical and physical characteristics of the dose, and (2) how well the digestive system of the person taking it works. A medicine that falls apart quickly in a normal stomach or small intestine produces blood levels quite promptly. Such a drug product has good bioavailability. Drugs such as metoclopramide or cisapride that slow the gastrointestinal system may act to actually increase the amount of drug that gets into the body.

bioequivalence The ability of a drug product to cause its intended therapeutic effect is related to bioavailability. When a medicine is made by several manufacturers, it is critical to pick the one that has the bioavailability needed to work. While the drug in medicines from different firms may be the same chemical, don't assume that they are equally available.

   Bioavailability depends mostly on physical characteristics of how a medicine is made. These determine how well a drug falls apart and releases its active drug component(s). Drug products that have the same drug but are combined with different inert additives, coated with different substances, or enclosed in different capsules may or may not have the same bioavailability. Those that do are termed bioequivalent and can be relied upon to give the same result.

   If you consider having your prescription filled with a generic, ask your physician and pharmacist for help. This requires professional judgment in each case. In some cases, reasonable differences in bioavailability are acceptable. For serious illnesses, or when blood levels must be kept in a narrow range, it is essential to use the drug product that has been shown to have reliable bioavailability. This has been a major area of controversy for blood thinners (anticoagulants) and medicines used to control seizures.

blood platelets The smallest of the blood cells made by bone marrow. Platelets are normally present in very large numbers. They are the basis of normal blood clotting and prevent excessive bruising or bleeding if you are injured. Platelets preserve smaller blood vessel walls. If there is damage, platelets seal small holes in vessel walls. Some drugs and chemicals may lower the platelet count. Many slow formation; other medicines hasten destruction. If the platelet count gets too low, blood begins to leak through the walls of smaller vessels. This shows as scattered bruises in the skin of the thighs or legs and is called purpura. Bleeding happens anywhere, internally as well as into the tissues immediately beneath the skin. For a listing of causative drugs, see Table 5, Section Six.

body mass index (BMI) A calculation used to measure the relative degree of a patient's obesity. This measurement is used in deciding the appropriateness of using sibutramine (Meridia). BMI is calculated using weight in kilograms divided by height in meters squared. If the BMI is greater than 30 kg per square meter or is 27 kg per square meter with other risk factors such as diabetes, sibutramine is approved for use in weight loss considering those additional factors.

bone marrow depression A decrease in the ability of bone marrow to make blood cells. This can be an adverse reaction to medicines or chemicals. Bone marrow makes most of the body's blood cells: red blood cells (erythrocytes), white blood cells (leukocytes), and platelets (thrombocytes). Each type of cell has one or more functions, critical to life and health.

Drugs that depress bone marrow may impair all types of blood cells right away or only one type selectively. Blood tests can show drug effects on bone marrow. If fewer red blood cells are made, anemia results, causing weakness, cold intolerance, and shortness of breath. Low white blood cells lowers resistance to infection (fever, sore throat, or pneumonia). If platelets fall to very low levels, the blood loses its ability to clot quickly. Bruising or prolonged bleeding may happen. Any of these symptoms require immediate studies of blood and bone marrow. For a listing of causative drugs, see Table 5, Section Six.

brand name The registered trade name given to a medicine by its manufacturer. Each company creates a trade name to distinguish its brand of the generic drug from its competitors'. A brand name designates a proprietary drug— one that is protected by patent or copyright. Generally, brand names are shorter, easier to pronounce, and more readily remembered than their generic counterparts.

capitation A system where a set amount of money is used to cover the cost of health care for a given person. For instance, a health plan or hospital is paid monthly on a negotiated per-person rate, and the plan or hospital provides all health services for the people in the plan.

cause-and-effect relationship An association between a medicine and a biological event—most commonly a side effect or an adverse effect. Important factors are when the drug was given, the use of multiple drugs and their possible interactions, the effects of the disease being treated, the physiological and psychological patient factors, and the influences of unrecognized disorders or malfunctions.

The majority of adverse drug reactions occur sporadically, unpredictably, and infrequently in the general population. A *definite* cause-and-effect relationship between medicine and reaction is shown when (1) the adverse effect immediately follows dosing of the drug, (2) the adverse effect disappears after the drug is stopped (dechallenge) and reappears when the medicine is used again (rechallenge), or (3) the adverse effects are clearly the expected and predictable toxic consequences of drug overdose.

There is also a large gray area of "probable," "possible," and "coincidental" associations. Clarification of cause-and-effect relationships requires observation over a long period of time, followed by sophisticated statistical analysis. Some news stories are based on suggestive but incomplete data. Though early warning is in the public interest, these stories should make clear whether the presumed relationship is based on definitive criteria or is inferred. It is critical to avoid losing valuable medicines because of poorly designed studies that find their way to the news.

The most competent techniques for evaluating cause-and-effect relationships of adverse drug reactions have been devised by the Division of Tissue Reactions to Drugs, a research unit of the Armed Forces Institute of Pathology:

No association	5.0%
Coincidental	14.5%
Possible	33.0%
Probable	30.0%
Causative	17.5%

It is significant that expert evaluation of 2,800 drug-related cases concluded that only 47.5% could be substantiated as causative or probably causative.

contraindication A condition or disease that precludes the use of a medicine. Some contraindications are absolute, meaning that the drug should NEVER be used in a particular situation. Other contraindications are relative, meaning that using the drug requires expert consideration of all factors.

coordinated performance measurement for the management of adult diabetes A term used to describe a great new consensus reached by the American Medical Association (AMA), the Joint Commission on Accreditation of Healthcare Organizations (JCAHO), and The National Committee on Quality Assurance (NCQA). This body of information was released in April 2001 and seeks to look at how typical measures, markers, or preventive measures used in diabetes (such as lipid management, hemoglobin A1C, and flu shots) should be approached to get the best frequency of testing and avoidance of disease progression or incidental or at risk infections.

covered lives A term used by health maintenance organizations to indicate how many people have enrolled in their plan. From the HMO's point of view, a minimum number of covered lives is needed to support a certain number of family practice physicians, specialists, and so on. Understanding their logic helps explain why some HMOs have one specialist while others have several.

COX-II Inhibitor A medicine that inhibits the action of cyclooxygenase or COX type two. While type one COX can have some protective functions in the body, COX-II is an enzyme that works to make compounds that lead to swelling (inflammation). If COX-II is blocked, inflammation is prevented or relieved.

creatinine clearance A measure of how well the kidneys are eliminating waste, toxins, and impurities from the body. A low creatinine clearance (such as 20 mL per minute or mL/min) means poorer kidney function; a high creatinine clearance (such as 120 mL/min) means better kidney function. People who have low creatinine clearances often receive lower initial doses and smaller increases of medicines that are removed by the kidneys.

critical or clinical pathway An assortment of coordinated measures taken by a health care organization to effectively group care of specific diseases or conditions. All diagnostic tests, treatments, discharge plans, and other factors are carefully studied, and practice is aimed at giving the best patient results in the most cost-effective manner.

dependence A term identifying *psychological dependence* (or *habituation*) and *physical dependence* (or *addiction*). In addition, functional dependence—the need to use a drug continuously in order to sustain a particular body function—is included.

Psychological dependence is a form of neurotic behavior—an "emotional" dependence. This characterizes itself as an obsession to satisfy a particular desire. Psychological dependence is also seen in many more socially acceptable patterns such as entertainment, sports, and collecting. Unfortunately, we often see an increasing reliance on medicines to cope with everyday problems: pills for frustration, nervous stomach, tension headache, and insomnia. This compulsive abuse shows little or no tendency to increase the dose (see tolerance) and minor or nonexistent physical symptoms if the medicine is taken away (withdrawn). Some clinicians include psychological dependence in their definition of addiction.

Physical dependence, which is true addiction, includes two elements: tolerance and withdrawal. Addicting drugs provide relief from anguish and pain, but can also cause a physiological tolerance requiring increased doses or repeated use to remain effective. These two features foster its becoming a functioning component in brain biochemistry. (Thus some authorities prefer the term chemical dependence.) Sudden removal of the medicine causes a major upheaval in body chemistry, provoking a withdrawal syndrome— intense mental and physical pain—that is the hallmark of addiction. True addiction is rare, and fear of addiction, even with potent narcotics, should never stand in the way of effective pain control.

Functional dependence differs from both psychological and physical dependence. It occurs when a drug relieves a distressing condition and provides a sense of well-being. Drugs that cause functional dependence are often used for symptom relief. The most familiar example of functional dependence is the "laxative habit." Some types of constipation are made worse by the wrong laxative, and natural bowel function fades as the colon becomes more and more dependent on the laxative drug.

disease management An approach to prevention and treatment of a specific condition that checks how often it happens in a population, organizes resources, and allocates money to reach the best balance of dollars spent and results achieved.

disulfiramlike (Antabuse-like) reaction Symptoms resulting from the interaction of alcohol and a medicine causing the "Antabuse effect." Symptoms include intense facial flushing, severe throbbing headache, shortness of breath, chest pains, nausea, repeated vomiting, sweating, and weakness. If a large enough amount of alcohol is present, the reaction may progress to blurred vision, vertigo, marked drop in blood pressure, and loss of consciousness. Severe reactions may lead to convulsions and death. The reaction can last from 30 minutes to several hours, depending upon the amount of alcohol in the body. As the symptoms subside, the person is exhausted and often sleeps for several hours.

diuretic A medicine that increases urine volume. Diuretics work in several ways to accomplish this. Diuretics are used to (1) remove excess water from the body (as in congestive heart failure and some types of liver and kidney disease) and (2) treat hypertension by promoting excretion of sodium from the body.

divided doses The total daily dose of a medicine is split into smaller individual doses over the course of a day.

DMARD A Disease-Modifying Antirheumatic Drug. These medicines represent a true breakthrough in rheumatoid arthritis (RA) because they actually attack the cause of RA. For example, leflunomide (Arava) works to shut down T-cells destroying tissue, and etanercept (Enbrel) works to bind tumor necrosis factor (TNF) so that it can't harm joints.

dosage forms and strengths This information category in the individual Drug Profiles (Section Two) uses several abbreviations to designate measurements of weight and volume:

mcg = microgram =1,000,000th of a gram (weight)
mg = milligram = 1,000th of a gram (weight)
mL = milliliter =1,000th of a liter (volume)
gm = gram = 1,000 milligrams (weight)
There are approximately 65 mg in 1 grain.
There are approximately 5 mL in 1 teaspoon.
There are approximately 15 mL in 1 tablespoon.
There are approximately 30 mL in 1 ounce.
One milliliter of water weighs 1 g.
There are approximately 454 g in 1 pound.

drug, drug product Terms used interchangeably to describe a medicine (in any form) used in medical practice. The term *drug* refers to the single chemical that provokes a specific response when put in a biological system—the "active" ingredient. A *drug product* is the dosage form—tablet, capsule, elixir, etc.—that has the active drug mixed with inactive ingredients to provide convenient dosing. Drug products that have one active ingredient are called single-entity drugs. Drug products with two or more active ingredients are called combination drugs ([CD] in the brand names in the Drug Profiles, Section Two).

drug class A group of drugs that are similar in chemistry, method of action, and use. Because of their common characteristics, many drugs in a class will cause the same side effects and have similar potential for related adverse reactions and interactions. Variations among members within a drug class can occur. This can let choices be made if certain benefits are desired or particular side effects are to be minimized. Examples: antihistamines and phenothiazines (see Drug Classes, Section Four).

drug family A group of medicines that are similar in chemistry, method of action, and purpose. In *The Essential Guide,* drug families are identified by entries such as the Minimally Sedating Antihistamine Family. This allows you to easily compare the drugs meeting the criteria for listing in the book.

drug fever Increased body temperature caused by a medicine. Drugs can cause fever by allergic reactions, tissue damage, acceleration of tissue metabolism, constriction of skin blood vessels, and direct action on the brain. The most common form of drug fever is allergic. It may be the only allergic symptom, or it may include skin rash, hives, joint swelling and pain, enlarged lymph glands, hemolytic anemia, or hepatitis. The fever usually appears about 7 to 10 days after starting the drug and varies from low-grade to alarmingly high levels. It may be sustained or intermittent, but it usually lasts for as long as the medicine is taken. Although many drugs can cause fever, the following are more commonly responsible:

allopurinol	novobiocin
antihistamines	para-aminosalicylic acid
atropine-like drugs	penicillin
barbiturates	pentazocine
coumarin anticoagulants	phenytoin
hydralazine	procainamide
iodides	propylthiouracil
isoniazid	quinidine
methyldopa	rifampin
nadolol	sulfonamides

drug recall Removal of a medicine by the FDA. There are three classes of recalls (see *www.fda.gov*). Used when use of or exposure to a product will do the following:
Class I will cause serious adverse health consequenses or death.

Class II may cause medically reversible or temporary adverse health consequences, or is used where probability of serious health consequences are remote.

Class III is unlikely to cause adverse health effects.

EBCT Electron Beam Computed Tomography (also known as ultra-fast CAT scan) is an X-ray based technique with great utility in helping diagnose heart disease. The result of an EBCT scan is a "virtual tour" of the coronary arteries and a calcium score. Low calcium scores are associated with decreased risk of heart attacks, while high scores are cause for concern.

evidence-based medicine An important concept in therapeutics that impacts which medicines are used and how they are used. This involves combining recent best research (evidence) with knowledge of how disease happens (pathophysiology), patient preferences, and clinical expertise in order to come up with the best individualized medicine for any given patient. Fortunately, development and use of evidence-based medicine skills are now being integrated into U.S. medical schools.

extension effect An unwanted but predictable medicine response that is a result of mild to moderate overdose. It is an exaggeration of the drug's pharmacological action; it can be thought of as a mild form of dose-related toxicity (see overdosage and toxicity).

Example: The continued "hangover" of mental sluggishness that persists in the morning is a common extension effect of a long-acting sleep-inducing medicine (a hypnotic such as Dalmane) taken the night before.

FDA-approvable A stage in the Food and Drug Administration's review and approval process. A medicine is considered FDA-approvable once the panel that reviewed the supporting data submitted to the FDA finds that data acceptable. In general, at this point only final details need to be resolved before the medicine becomes FDA-approved and is made available for general use.

FDA-review status A description of chemical types and review status has been developed by the FDA. Chemical types are divided into:

1. New molecular entity
2. New ester, new salt form, or other covalent derivative
3. New formulation
4. New combination
5. New manufacturer
6. New indication
7. Drug already marketed, but without an approved NDA

The review process is divided into:

Fast track: Critical review for a new treatment for a life-threatening condition (such as a new HIV/AIDS drug).

Priority review: Significant improvement compared to marketed products in the treatment, diagnosis, or prevention of a disease.

Standard review: The medicine appears to have therapeutic qualities similar to those of one or more already marketed drugs.

fructosamine A new term in diabetes, which is also known as glycated protein. Fructosamine is used in conjunction with glycosylated hemoglobin (hemoglobin A1C) to check to see how well blood sugar has been controlled. Unlike A1C, fructosamine gives a picture of glucose control for prior weeks versus months. There is a home glucose meter that tests fructosamine.

generic name The official, common, or public name used to describe an active medicine. Generic names are coined by committees of drug experts and are approved by governmental agencies for national and international use. Many drug products are marketed only under a generic name. The drugs most commonly prescribed as generics are listed below, ranked in descending order of new or refill prescriptions issued.

amoxicillin
hydrocodone/acetaminophen
furosemide
albuterol aerosol
trimethoprim/Sulfa

cephalexin
acetaminophen/codeine
propoxyphene-N/acetaminophen
triamterene/HCTZ
ibuprofen

genetic diversity This is actually a descriptive term used to identify ways in which a given person's genetic makeup differs from the expected sequences of the human genome. Snippets of nuclear material are analyzed, and once variant sequences are identified, in time we may be able to remove them and restore people to health.

genetic therapy Perhaps the most promising area of therapy in medicine today. Healthy genetic material is isolated and inserted into appropriate but diseased cells. For example, normal lung genes are given to a person with cystic fibrosis. Still very experimental, it may someday allow people suffering with genetically based diseases or conditions to receive therapy that changes the affected genes and actually *cures* those conditions. The latest approaches are working on causing the heart to grow new blood vessels and actually reversing congestive heart failure by the AC-6 gene. One of the true breakthroughs in medicine for this edition was the complete identification of the human genome by a private U.S. company. There are some 3 billion base pairs, and an estimated 40,000 genes in the human genome. Some 20 diseases cause more than 80% of deaths around the world. About 200–300 genes are responsible for these diseases. Considering that about every 3 weeks we in essence get a new heart from the same set of genes, if controlling the genes becomes a reality—-we can possibly knock out heart disease!

habituation A form of drug dependence based upon strong psychological gratification. Ongoing use of mood-altering drugs or those relieving minor discomforts results from a compulsive need to feel pleasure and satisfaction or to escape emotional distress. If these drugs are abruptly stopped, a withdrawal does not result. Thus habituation is a *psychological dependence*. (See dependence for more on psychological and physical dependence.)

hemolytic anemia Lower red blood cells and hemoglobin caused by premature destruction (hemolysis) of red blood cells. One way that this happens is from a genetic lowering of glucose-6-phosphate dehydrogenase (G6PD), a needed enzyme. If patients with this condition are given antimalarial medicines or sulfa drugs, red cells will be destroyed. One type of drug-induced hemolytic anemia is a form of allergy. Many widely used medicines (such as quinidine and levodopa) can cause hemolytic destruction of red cells as an allergic reaction. Hemolytic anemia can occur abruptly or silently. The acute form lasts about 7 days and shows as fever, pallor, weakness, dark-colored urine, and varying degrees of jaundice. If drug-induced hemolytic anemia is mild, there may be no symptoms (see idiosyncrasy and allergy [drug]). For drugs that may cause this, see Table 5, Section Six.

hepatitis-like reaction Some medicines may cause liver damage similar to viral hepatitis. Symptoms of drug-induced hepatitis and viral hepatitis are often so similar that only laboratory tests can tell the difference. Hepatitis from drugs may be allergy, or it may be a toxic adverse effect. Serious liver reactions usually lead to jaundice (see jaundice). For drugs that can cause this, see Table 8, Section Six.

HMO Abbreviation for Health Maintenance Organization—a health care system that provides a broad spectrum of medical therapies and services by a collective group of people in a common organization.

hospitalist A relatively new term used to denote a physician who specializes in working in a hospital as opposed to a doctor who primarily has an office-based practice. The intent here is to create a group of doctors who are very familiar with critical paths, streamlining, and other hospital methods to make length of stay as appropriate as possible.

hypersensitivity Overresponsiveness to medicines. Used in this sense, it means that the response is appropriate but the degree of response is exaggerated. More widely used today to identify allergy. To have *hypersensitivity* to a drug is to be allergic to it (see allergy [drug]). Some people develop cross-hypersensitivity. This means that allergy to one drug will also lead to a reaction to other closely related medicines.

> *Example:* A *hypersensitive* patient had seasonal hay fever and asthma since childhood. His *allergy* to penicillin developed after his third treatment. The *hypersensitivity* was a diffuse, measles-like rash. When he was later given a cephalosporin antibiotic (chemically related to penicillins), he developed the same rash.

hypnotic A medicine used to cause sleep. Classes include antihistamines, barbiturates, benzodiazepines, and several unrelated compounds. In the past 15 years, benzodiazepines have largely replaced barbiturates. In general, they are safer and have lower dependence potential. Tolerance to the hypnotic effect can happen after several weeks of continual use, so hypnotics should be used for short periods of time.

hypoglycemia Sugar (glucose) in blood below the normal range. Since the brain only runs on sugar, the brain can be seriously impaired by too low a sugar level. Early warnings include headache, mild drunkenness feeling, hunger, and an inability to think clearly. If blood sugar falls further, nervousness and confusion develop. Weakness, numbness, trembling, sweating, and rapid heartbeat follow. If blood sugar drops further, impaired speech and unconsciousness, with or without convulsions, will follow. Treatment for any low blood sugar (hypoglycemia) is important. If you take a medicine that can cause hypoglycemia, it is prudent to know the symptoms and what to do if hypoglycemia occurs.

hypothermia When internal body temperature falls below 98.6°F or 37°C. By definition, hypothermia is a body temperature of less than 95 degrees F or 35 degrees C. The elderly and debilitated are more prone to hypothermia. Most cases are initiated by room temperatures below 65 degrees F or 18.3 degrees C. This can develop suddenly, can mimic a stroke, and has a mortality rate of 50%. Some drugs, such as phenothiazines, barbiturates, and benzodiazepines, may make hypothermia more likely.

idiosyncrasy An abnormal medicine response that happens in people with a defect in body chemistry (often hereditary) that produces an effect totally unrelated to the drug's normal action. This is not a form of allergy. Some defects responsible for idiosyncratic drug reactions are well understood; others are not.

> *Example:* Some 100 million people (including 10% of African Americans) have a low glucose-6-phosphate dehydrogenase (G6PD) in red blood cells. The cells then disintegrate when exposed to sulfonamides (Gantrisin, Kynex), nitrofurantoin (Furadantin, Macrodantin), probenecid (Benemid), quinine, and quinidine. This can lead to a serious anemia.

immunosuppressive A medicine that suppresses the immune system. Immuno-suppression may be an intended drug effect, such as cyclosporine preventing the rejection of a transplanted kidney. In other cases, it is an unwanted side effect, as in the long-term use of cortisone-like drugs (to control asthma) suppressing the immune system. Chronic disorders thought to be autoimmune—such as rheumatoid arthritis, ulcerative colitis, and systemic lupus erythematosus—may be eased by immunosuppressive medicines.

INR This is a term used in blood thinning or anticoagulation. It stands for International Normalized Ratio. The intent of the INR is to remove the problem of testing variation in reagents from laboratory to laboratory in coagulation results. The INR helps make a coagulation test (protime number and then calculated ratio) mean the same thing for a patient being tested in New York or Omaha. The sequence happens like this: Blood is drawn from the patient, and a prothrombin time or protime test is done. The protime number is then put into a calculation that standardizes the result. The end of the math is an INR, a ratio that tells a clinician to what degree the ability of the blood to clot (coagulate) has been changed by warfarin or a clotting factor problem.

interaction A change in a medicine that results when a second drug (altering the action of the first) is given to the same person. Some interactions can enhance the effect of either drug, giving a response similar to overdose. Other interactions may reduce drug effectiveness and cause inadequate response. A third interaction can produce an unrelated toxic response with no increase or decrease in the interacting drugs. Many interactions can be anticipated, and appropriate adjustments in dose can be made to prevent or minimize fluctuations in drug response.

jaundice A yellowing in the color of skin (and the white portion of the eyes) that occurs when bile accumulates in blood because of impaired liver function. Jaundice can happen from a wide variety of diseases or may be an adverse reaction to a medicine. Jaundice due to a drug is always a serious adverse effect. If you take a medicine that can cause jaundice, watch closely for any change in urine or feces color. Dark discoloration of urine or pale (lack of color) stools may be early indication of developing jaundice. If this happens, call your doctor promptly. Lab tests can clarify the nature of the jaundice. Table 8, Section Six, lists causative medicines.

JNC VI A national committee of experts that meets to try to establish a framework of medicines used to treat high blood pressure. The committee reviews the currently available medicines and attempts to organize possible treatments into a logical approach for lowering high blood pressure and prolonging lives.

JNC VII The current (as of 2003) guidelines from a national committee of experts at the National Insitutes of Health (NIH) that summarized current best studies into guidelines to help clinicians work to control blood pressure. The current guidelines (published in the *Journal of The American Medical Association* [*JAMA*], 2003) developed key changes such as a category called prehypertention, which starts at 120/80 and tries to tell us that even with what used to be considered "normal" blood pressure, damage can be done to blood vessels. Pre-hypertension seeks to foster a talk between clinicians and patients at an earlier point and to start lifestyle changes (such as exercise and diet) to get blood pressure under control earlier. Find the guidelines at *www.nhlbi.nih.gov/guidelines/hypertension/index.htm.*

low-dose medications A group of medicines that have been found to be effective in some patients in doses that are lower than the doses recommended by the manufacturer. This area of therapeutics is controversial and results from the gap between valid and valuable research publication and the time it takes for a manufacturer to send needed data to the FDA and for the FDA to review and approve changes to the labeling of the medicine. Some of the controversy also revolves around varying opinion as to required outcomes from treatment from medicines.

low molecular weight heparins A group of blood-thinning (anticoagulant) medicines used to prevent abnormal blood clots (venous thromboembolisms or VTEs). New recommendations from the Sixth American College of Chest Physicians may lead to increased use of these medicines versus unfractionated heparins to prevent these clots (VTEs) in high risk patients.

lupus erythematosus (LE) A serious disease, seen in two forms: one limited to skin (discoid LE) and the other involving several body systems (systemic LE). Both forms occur mostly in young women. About 5% of cases of discoid form convert to the systemic form. Systemic LE is an immune disorder that can be chronic, with progressive inflammation destroying connective tissue of the skin, blood vessels, joints, brain, heart muscle, lungs, and kidneys. Altered proteins in the blood lead to antibody formation that attacks the person's own organs or tissues. Low white blood cells and platelets often occur. The course of systemic LE is usually quite protracted and unpredictable. There is no cure, but acceptable management may be achieved in some cases by judicious use of cortisone-like drugs.

Several medicines can start a form of systemic LE quite similar to that which occurs spontaneously. Symptoms may appear as early as 2 weeks or as late as years after starting the drug. Initial symptoms are usually low-grade fever, skin rashes of various kinds, aching muscles, and multiple joint pains. Chest pains (pleurisy) are fairly common. Enlargement of the lymph glands occurs less frequently. Symptoms usually subside if the drug is stopped, but laboratory evidence of the reaction may persist for many months.

medication map (MM) A new concept in medicines pioneered by Dr. Rybacki. One of the flaws in current drug information is that it is provided for individual medicines when patients actually often take medicines during the same day and in combination as well. Patients are not given a schedule that organizes their medicines into a framework that works well with their usual day. The medication map seeks to organize any and all of the medicines a patient takes into a clear schedule using the best possible times, combinations, and results or outcomes data. A medication map helps avoid drug-drug, drug-food, and drug-activity interactions, and gives the patient the best possible quality of life.

national cholesterol education program (NCEP) A program of the National Institutes of Health that works to standardize the approach to cholesterol laboratory values, treatments, and patient care using evidence-based medicine principles. The guidelines ATP III (Adult treatment panel, version three) were released in 2001 and could help save thousands of lives when successfully implemented.

neuroleptic malignant syndrome (NMS) A rare, serious, sometimes fatal idiosyncratic reaction to neuroleptic (antipsychotic) medicines. Symptoms include hyperthermia (temperatures of 102 to 104°F), marked muscle rigidity, and coma. Rapid heart rate and breathing, profuse sweating, tremors, and seizures can also occur. Two-thirds of cases happen in men, one-third in women. Mortality rate is 15 to 20%.

The following drugs may cause this reaction:

amantadine (Symmetrel)	levoda + carbidopa (Sinemet)
amitripyline + perphenazine (Triavil)	lithium (Lithobid)
	loxapine (Loxitane)
amoxapine (Asendin)	metoclopramide (Reglan, Octamide)
bromocriptine (Parlodel)	molindone (Moban)
carbamazepine (Tegretol)	oral contraceptives (combination)
chlorpromazine (Thorazine)	paroxetine (Paxil)
chlorprothixine (Taractan)	perphenazine (Etrafon, Trilafon)
clomipramine (Anafranil)	pimozide (Orap)
clozapine (Clozaril)	prochlorperzine (Compazine)
cyclobenzaprine	risperidone (Risperdal)
doxepin (Asendin)	sertraline (Zoloft)
fluoxetine (Prozac)	thioridazine (Mellaril)
fluphenazine (Permitil, Prolixin)	thiothixene (Navane)
fluvoxamine (Luvox)	trifluoperazine (Stelazine)
haloperidol (Haldol)	trimeprazine (Temaril)
imipramine (Tofranil, etc.)	zotepine (Nipolept)

orthostatic hypotension A type of low blood pressure related to body position or posture (also called postural hypotension). People who get orthostatic hypotension may have normal blood pressure lying down, but on sitting upright or standing will feel light-headed, dizzy, and as if they are going to faint. These symptoms come from inadequate blood flow (oxygen supply) to the brain.

Many medicines may cause orthostatic hypotension. Tell your doctor if you have this effect so that changes can be made. If this situation isn't corrected, severe falls or injury may result. It is prudent to avoid sudden standing, prolonged standing, vigorous exercise, and exposure to hot environments. Alcoholic beverages should be used cautiously until combined effects with the drug in use have been determined.

outcomes research A concept in health care evaluation that considers the benefits (gauged by a variety of measures) of using a particular medicine versus another. This may lead to the least expensive drug actually not being the drug of choice, because the outcomes from therapy don't stand up over time or may result in significant treatment failure.

outcomes survey short-form 36 (SF-36) A check of quality of life that is often used to find out the impact of rheumatoid arthritis (RA) on patients. Improvements in SF-36 can help clinicians decide how beneficial a medicine is for a particular patient.

overdose The meaning of this term is not limited to doses exceeding the normal range recommended by a manufacturer. The "best" dose of many medicines varies greatly from person to person. An average dose for most people can be an overdose for some and an underdose for others. Factors such as age, body size, nutritional status, and liver and kidney function have significant impact on dosing.

Drugs with narrow safety margins often give signs of overdose if removal of the daily dose is delayed. Massive overdose—as in accidental ingestion of drugs by children or with suicides—is referred to as poisoning.

over-the-counter (OTC) drugs Medicines that can be bought without prescriptions. Many people do not look upon OTC medicines as drugs. It is important to remember that OTC medicines can have a variety of actions. OTC drugs may react with one another and can also react with prescription medicines. Serious problems can arise when (1) the patient fails to tell the doctor about OTC drug(s) he or she is taking ("because they really aren't drugs") and (2) the doctor fails to specify that his or her question about which medicines are being taken includes all OTC drugs and herbal meds as well. During any treatment, patients need to talk with their doctor or pharmacist about any OTC drug that he or she wishes to take. The major classes of OTC drugs for internal use include:

allergy medicines (antihistamines)	menstrual aids
antacids	motion sickness remedies
antiworm medicines	pain relievers
aspirin and aspirin combinations	salt substitutes
aspirin substitutes	sedatives and tranquilizers
asthma aids	sleeping pills
cold medicines (decongestants)	smoking cessation products
cough medicines	stimulants (caffeine)
diarrhea remedies	sugar substitutes (saccharin)
digestion aids	tonics
diuretics	vaginal yeast infection medicines
heartburn medicines	vitamins
iron laxatives	weight-reduction aids
laxatives	

paradoxical reaction A medicine response that does not follow the known pharmacology of a drug. These effects are due to individual sensitivity and can occur at any age. They are seen more commonly in children and the elderly.

Example: An 80-year-old man was sent to a nursing home after his wife died. He had trouble adjusting to his new environment and was agitated and irritable. He was given diazepam (Valium) to relax him, starting with small doses. On the second day he became confused. The dose of diazepam was increased. On the third day he began to wander, talked incessantly, and was angry when attempts were made to help him. Suspecting a paradoxical reaction, his health care provider stopped the diazepam. All behavioral disturbances subsided in 3 days.

Parkinson-like disorders (Parkinsonism) A group of symptoms resembling Parkinson's disease. The typical features of Parkinsonism include a fixed, emotionless facial expression (mask-like in appearance); trembling hands, arms, or legs; and stiffness of extremities that produces rigid posture and gait. Parkinsonism is a fairly common adverse effect that occurs in about 15% of patients who take large doses of phenothiazines or use them over an extended period. If found early, the Parkinson-like features will lessen or disappear with lower doses or different medicines. In some cases, Parkinson-like changes may become permanent.

peripheral neuritis (peripheral neuropathy) A group of symptoms that results from injury to nerve tissue in the extremities. A variety of drugs or chemicals can cause this. The sensation of numbness and tingling usually starts in the toes and fingers and is accompanied by altered sensation to touch. Vague discomfort from aching sensations to burning pain is also seen. Severe forms of peripheral neuritis may include loss of muscular strength and coordination. Isoniazid can cause this condition.

If vitamin B_6 (pyridoxine) is not given with isoniazid, peripheral neuritis may occur. Vitamin B_6 can be both preventive and curative in this form of drug-induced peripheral neuritis.

Since peripheral neuritis can also be a late complication of many viral infections, care must be taken to avoid assigning a cause-and-effect relationship to a medicine that is not responsible for the nerve injury (see cause-and-effect relationship). See Table 10, Section Six, for further discussion of drug-induced nerve damage.

Peyronie's disease A permanent deformity of the penis caused by dense fibrous (scar-like) tissue within in the penile vessels that become engorged with blood during an erection. During sexual arousal, inelastic fibrous tissue causes painful downward bowing of the penis that hampers or precludes intercourse. This condition has been caused by phenytoin (Dilantin, etc.) and with most members of the beta-blocker drugs (see Drug Classes, Section Four). For a listing of causative medicines, see Table 11, Section Six.

pharmacoeconomics The discipline within pharmacology that studies the issues of costs versus benefits, utilizing a variety of measures: material and personnel costs, treatment outcomes, quality of patient life, etc. Study results are used in deciding where and how health care resources should be utilized.

pharmacogenomics The use of knowledge of the human genome, actions of genes, and the way that certain genes are active or inactive in a disease to design medicines. This new area also takes into account the concept of individualizing an approach to patients based on THEIR specific genes. The first medicine to result from pharmacogenomics is imatinib or Gleevec (see drug profile). This medicine is a signal transduction inhibitor that works to turn off a gene that is active in leukemia and a rare kind of stomach tumor.

pharmacology The medical science relating to development and use of drugs as well as their composition and action in animals and humans. Used in its broadest sense, pharmacology embraces related sciences of medicinal chemistry, experimental therapeutics, and toxicology.

photosensitivity A drug-induced skin change resulting in a rash or exaggerated sunburn on exposure to the sun or ultraviolet lamps. The reaction is confined to uncovered areas of skin, giving a clue to the nature of its cause. For a list of causative medicines, see Table 2, Section Six.

porphyria Hereditary disorders where excessive amounts of respiratory pigments known as porphyrins are made. (One porphyrin is part of hemoglobin in red blood cells.) Two forms of porphyria—acute intermittent porphyria and cutaneous porphyria—can be activated by medicines. Acute intermittent porphyria involves nervous system damage. An attack can include fever, rapid heart rate, vomiting, pain in the abdomen and legs, hallucinations, seizures, paralysis, and coma. Some examples of causative drugs include barbiturates, sulfa drugs, chlordiazepoxide (Librium), chlorpropamide (Diabinese), methyldopa (Aldomet), and phenytoin (Dilantin).

Cutaneous porphyria involves skin and liver damage. Symptoms include red and blistered skin, followed by crusting, scarring, and excessive hair growth. Repeated liver damage can lead to cirrhosis. This form of porphyria can be caused by chloroquine, estrogen, oral contraceptives, and excessive iron.

PQRSTBG A mnemonic used to help clinicians who manage pain remember critical factors. **P**alliative tells what makes pain better. **Q**uality refers to the nature of the pain. **R**adiation tells them if the pain moves from one part of the body to another. **S**everity tells the relative intensity of the pain. **T**emporal refers to how the pain changes over the course of the day. **B**owel is there to remind clinicians that narcotic pain relievers can also cause constipation. **G**oals refer to clinician expectations, and critically to what the patient and family want as a benefit from the therapy that is chosen.

pre-diabetes A situation that is commonly found before people develop true diabetes. This pre-diabetic condition is characterized by blood sugar (glucose) levels that are higher than normal, but not elevated enough to make the diagnosis of diabetes. The most critical aspect of this state is that some degree of damage to the heart and blood vessels (circulatory system) probably happens in pre-diabetes. The American Diabetes Association (*www.diabetes.org*) has a risk test and great information on warning signs.

priapism Prolonged, painful erection of the penis usually on sexual arousal. It is caused by obstruction to drainage of blood through the veins at the root of the penis. Erection may last for 30 minutes to a few hours and then subside, or it may persist for up to 30 hours and require surgical drainage. More than half of priapism from drugs results in permanent impotence. Sickle-cell anemia may predispose to priapism, and those with this disorder should avoid all medicines that may cause priapism.

Drugs reported to induce priapism include:

anabolic steroids (male hormone–like drugs: Anadrol, Anavar, Android, Halotestin, Metandren, Oreton, Testred, Winstrol)

chlorpromazine (Thorazine)

cocaine

guanethidine (Ismelin)

heparin

levodopa (Sinemet)

molindone (Moban)

prazosin (Minipres)

prochlorperzine (Compazine)

trazodone (Desyrel)

trifluoperazine (Stelazine)

warfarin (Coumadin)

prostatism The difficulties that happen with an enlarged prostate. As the prostate enlarges, it constricts the urethra (outflow passage) and impedes urination. This causes a lower size and force of the urinary stream, hesitancy, interruption, and incomplete bladder emptying. Atropine and medicines with atropine-like effects can impair the bladder's ability to compensate for the prostate gland, intensifying all of the above symptoms.

pseudoaddiction The development of drug-seeking behavior (see addiction), but only for pain control. Pseudoaddiction is a characteristic of less than optimal pain control and tends to resolve with adequate pain control.

QT interval medicines This new term is used to describe drugs that can have an effect on part of the heartbeat (QT interval) and pose a complicated benefit-to-risk decision in people with heart rhythm problems or who are at increased risk for heart rhythm problems (such as the elderly, people with existing heart disease, women, those with low magnesium or potassium, and others). These medicines have led to such concern that the FDA will now require all new medicines to be tested for QT interval prolongation. Representative medicines include: arsenic trioxide; chlorpromazine; class I, IA, or III antiarrhythmics; clarithromycin; clindamycin; cotrimoxazole; dofetilide; dolasetron; droperidol; erythromycin; fluconaxzole; fluoxetine; foscarnet; gatifloxacin, moxifloxacin or sparfloxacin; halofantrine; haloperidol; isradipine; ketoconazole; levomethadyl (Orlaam); mesoridazine; octreotide (Santostatin); ondansetron; pentamidine; phenothiazines in general; pimozide; quinidine; risperidone; sotolol; sulfamethoxazole; tacrolimus; thioridazine; tricyclic antidepressants; trimethoprim; venlafaxine; ziprazodone; zotepine; and others.

Raynaud's phenomenon Intermittent episodes of reduced blood flow to fingers or toes, with resulting paleness, discomfort, numbness, and tingling. Stress or exposure to cold can cause attack. It can occur as part of a systemic disorder (lupus erythematosus, scleroderma), or it can occur without apparent cause (Raynaud's disease). Beta-adrenergic blockers and products that contain ergotamine can lead to Raynaud-like symptoms in predisposed people.

relative risk A comparison made between two groups of people in specific populations to see if a specific disease or risk factor for a disease is associated with an increase, no change, or a decrease in the disease rate in the specific populations.

reverse cholesterol transport The moving of cholesterol from the body to the liver. A particularly important example is when cholesterol is absorbed from dietary sources, formed into compounds that can be deposited onto blood vessels—leading to atherosclerosis. The RCT pathway takes these atherogenic substances off the blood vessels or from the circulation and moves them to the liver, where they are made into needed chemicals or cell walls.

Reye (Reye's) syndrome A sudden, often fatal, childhood illness where the brain swells and the liver degenerates. It usually develops during a viral infection (flu), measles, or chicken pox. Cases have been seen with lupus (SLE). Symptoms include fever, headache, delirium, loss of consciousness, and seizures. It is one of the 10 major causes of death in children ages 1 to 10 years. Those younger than 18 may be affected. The syndrome may be due to combined effects of viral infection and chemical toxins in a genetically predisposed child. Medicines that have been used prior to symptoms include salicylates (aspirin) and drugs to control nausea and vomiting. This is why salicylates (aspirin and aspirin-like medicines) should be avoided in children with flu-like infections, chicken pox, or measles. Some clinicians question use of any NSAID. Remember to look for salicylates in combination cold or flu products and inflammatory bowel drugs. Valproic acid (a seizure medicine) can cause a Reye-like syndrome. Acetaminophen appears to be the medicine of choice in those less than 18 with fever from a sudden viral illness.

secondary effect A complication of medicine use that does not occur as part of the drug's primary pharmacological activity. Secondary effects are unwanted consequences and are adverse effects.

   Example: Cramping of leg muscles can be a secondary effect of diuretic (urine-producing) drug treatment for high blood pressure. Excessive loss of potassium renders the muscle vulnerable to painful spasm during exercise.

SIADH A Syndrome of Inappropriate Antidiuretic Hormone excretion. This may be caused by medicines and is repeatedly cited where appropriate in the text. Since antidiuretic hormone (ADH) works to control the amount of water that the body retains, excessive ADH causes the body to retain water. This can be very serious, as the excessive water dilutes minerals such as sodium, which is critical for life.

side effect A normal, expected, and predictable response to a drug. Side effects are part of a medicine's pharmacological activity and are unavoidable. Most side effects are undesirable. The majority cause minor annoyance and inconvenience; a few can be hazardous.

STEMI ST Segment Elevation Myocardial Infarction. A type of heart attack where the severity of damage leads to changes in the electrical pattern of the heart.

superinfection (suprainfection) A second infection superimposed on an initial infection. The superinfection is caused by organisms not killed by the drug(s) used to treat the original (primary) infection. This kind of infection usually happens during or following use of a broad-spectrum antibiotic. The disturbance of the normal balance of bacteria permits overgrowth of organisms usually found in numbers too small to cause disease. The superinfection may also require treatment, using those medicines that are effective against the offending organism.

> *Example:* A woman is given an antibiotic for a sinus infection. This medicine changes the bacteria usually present in her vagina, allowing yeast to grow. The yeast infection must then be treated with a second medicine.

tardive dyskinesia A drug-induced nervous system disorder with involuntary and bizarre movements of eyelids, jaws, lips, tongue, neck, and fingers. It can happen after use of potent medicines for mental illness. It may occur in any age group but is more common in the middle-aged and especially in chronically ill older women. Once it starts, it may be irreversible. To date, there is no way of identifying who may develop this reaction. The abnormal movement (dyskinesia) is not associated with decline in mental function.

tolerance A situation where the body adapts to a medicine and reacts to it less vigorously over time. Tolerance can be beneficial or harmful in treatment.

> *Example:* Beneficial tolerance happens when someone with hay fever finds that drowsiness from their antihistamine gradually disappears after 4 or 5 days of continuous use. Harmful tolerance occurs when the patient with "shingles" (herpes zoster) finds that the usual dose of pain medicine no longer works to relieve pain.

toxicity Capacity of a drug to impair body functions or damage tissues. Most drug toxicity is related to total dose: the larger the dose, the greater the toxic effects. Some medicines are toxic in normal doses. Toxic effects due to overdose are often a harmful extension of normal pharmacological actions and may be predictable and preventable.

treat to goal An important yet widely underused concept. One of the features in this edition of the *Guide* is the concept of treatment goals, measurements, and outcomes. Treating to goal means that when a particular medicine is considered, results and timeframes to achieve those goals are set and communicated to the patient. If goals are NOT achieved, medication doses can often be increased (if not at maximum), new medicines can be added, or different non-pharmacological approaches may be tried in order to reach the goal. A good example is treatment of high cholesterol (hyperlipidemia). It is not enough to find elevated cholesterol, start a medicine (such as an HMG-CoA reductase inhibitor or statin), and forget about it. The treatment goal of the medicine (such as getting the LDL to less than 130 mg/dL or HDL to more than 40 mg/dL) should be explained, the medicine started, and then cholesterol rechecked in a reasonable interval (such as 3 months). If the goal is achieved, and the treatment well tolerated, the medicine should be continued. If the goal is not reached and a medicine such as Pravachol (Pravastatin) is being used, it is reasonable (depending on the starting dose) to increase the dose and then recheck the cholesterol in 3 months. The process then continues until the National Cholesterol Education Program (NCEP) target or the target chosen by your doctor is reached.

trough-to-peak ratio (T/P) A concept used to check dosing of medicines for high blood pressure. The T/P ratio is calculated by dividing the blood pressure level immediately before the next drug dose (trough) by the largest blood pressure drop during the time between doses. A result greater than 50% means that the effect of the medicine over the entire time between doses is ideal.

tyramine A chemical present in many common foods and beverages that raises blood pressure. Normally, enzymes in the body neutralize tyramine (monoamine oxidase [MAO] type A). If the action of MAO type A is blocked, substances such as tyramine can cause alarming and dangerous increases in blood pressure.

Several medicines can block monoamine oxidase type A. They are called monoamine oxidase (MAO) type A inhibitors (see Drug Classes, Section Four). If you take one of these drugs and your diet includes foods or beverages high in tyramine, sudden increases in blood pressure may happen. Talk with your doctor or pharmacist about an appropriate diet and before combining any other medicine with an MAO inhibitor.

The following foods and beverages have been reported to contain varying amounts of tyramine. Unless their tyramine content is known to be insignificant, they should be avoided altogether while taking an MAO type A inhibitor drug.

FOODS	BEVERAGES
aged cheeses of all kinds	beer (unpasteurized)
avocado	Chianti wine
banana skins	sherry wine
bean curd	vermouth
bologna	
"Bovril" extract	
broad bean pods	
chicken liver (unless fresh and used at once)	
chocolate	
figs, canned	
fish, canned	
fish, dried and salted	
herring, pickled	
liver, if not very fresh	
"Marmite" extract	
meat extracts	
meat tenderizers	
pepperoni	
raisins	
raspberries	
salami	
shrimp paste	
sour cream	
soy sauce	
yeast extracts	

Note: *Any* high-protein food that is aged or has undergone breakdown by putrefaction probably contains tyramine and could produce a hypertensive crisis in anyone taking MAO type A inhibitor drugs.

VIPPS seal A term used in reference to pharmacies on the Internet. This seal is presently a hallmark of a valid pharmacy on the Internet from which to get prescriptions filled. The term stands for Verified Internet Pharmacy Practice Site. You will usually see this seal pictured prominently on a site that has achieved this credential!

viral load or viral burden A term used in reference to AIDS patients to describe the amount of HIV virus present in the body at any given time. The amount of virus relates to how well drug therapy is working, and can be a reason to change medicines if the load increases.

WHO pain ladder A therapeutic scheme using increasing strengths and combinations of pain medicines (analgesics) that includes NSAIDs, opiates, and adjuvant drugs to control pain as specified by the World Health Organization (WHO). It is not an absolute treatment scheme, but it should be used to organize the approach to effective pain prevention.

wnl (usually seen as WNL) A term often used to refer to laboratory results, which means within normal limits.

WOMAC A widely used approach to measure the health status of osteoarthritis patients. This scale is the Western Ontario and McMaster University index, or WOMAC. What it does is work to check (assess) the therapeutic scheme using increasing strengths and combinations of pain medicines (analgesics) that include NSAIDs, opiates, and adjuvant drugs to control pain as specified by the World Health Organization (WHO). It is not an absolute assessment scheme but, when used correctly, organizes patient information into a rational approach to checking how compromised the patient is before the medicine is added and then allows an objective follow-up check on how well the medicine is working.

Young mania rating scale (Y-MRS) A tool used by psychiatric clinicians to assess the severity of mania. Often used in bipolar disorder as a clinical outcomes measurement.

TABLES OF MEDICINE INFORMATION

TABLE 1

Medicines That May Adversely Affect the Fetus and Newborn Infant

In 1961, a decision was made to use thalidomide to try to make pregnancy less stressful, and pregnant women more relaxed. Despite these laudable intentions, this became the thalidomide DISASTER of 1961. What was not known then was that thalidomide (and many other drugs) caused birth defects or even fetal death if used during pregnancy (possible teratogens or embryocidal medicines). This does NOT mean that the medicines are "bad" medicines. For example, extremely effective medicines such as the "statins" (HMG-CoA reductase inhibitors) for lowering cholesterol should NEVER be taken during pregnancy (Category X) yet they save many, many lives when people have high cholesterol. Interestingly, thalidomide itself has seen a resurrection because it fights an important body chemical called Tumor Necrosis Factor (or TNF). It still should NEVER be used in pregnancy, but now has a valuable role treating erythema nodosum leprosum (ENL).

Our understanding of how drugs can affect the fetus or newborn infant continues to grow, and the list of the drugs that can cause significant harm to the unborn and newborn child has gotten larger and larger. In many cases, it is not possible to clearly separate adverse effects due to the mother's disease or disorder from those that may be caused by medicines. Based on current knowledge, it is strongly recommended that only those drugs that confer clear and essential benefits should be used during pregnancy. The FDA started an interdisciplinary task force in 1997 to revise the current pregnancy drug labeling system, but at the time of this writing has not released a new system (please see the existing FDA system and a note regarding possible changes at the end of this book). Some medicines have pregnancy registries sponsored by the company that makes the product. Where possible, I have included the 800 numbers for pregnancy registries, as I consider them to be a good idea if the decision is made to use a medicine in pregnancy. Talk to your doctor for more information.

Drugs that *probably* cause adverse effects when taken during the *first* trimester

aminopterin	finasteride	misoprostol
anticonvulsants*	fluorouracil	opioid analgesics*
antithyroid drugs	HMG-CoA reductase	progestins*
cytarabine	inhibitors*	quinine
danazol	iodides	streptomycin
diethylstilbestrol	isotretinoin	testosterone
ethanol (large amounts and	kanamycin	thalidomide
for long periods)	mercaptopurine	warfarin
etretinate	methotrexate	

Drugs that *possibly* cause adverse effects when taken during the *first* trimester

angiotensin-converting	lithium	piperazine
enzyme inhibitors*	mebendazole	rifampin
busulfan	monoamine oxidase	tetracyclines*
chlorambucil	(MAO) inhibitors*	
estrogens*	oral contraceptives	

*See Drug Class, Section Four.

Drugs that *probably* cause adverse effects when taken during the *second* and *third* trimesters

amiodarone
androgens*
angiotensin-converting
   enzyme inhibitors*
antithyroid drugs
aspirin
benzodiazepines*
chloramphenicol
estrogens*
ethanol (large amounts and
   for long periods)

finasteride
HMG-CoA reductase
   inhibitors*
iodides
kanamycin
lithium
nonsteroidal anti-
   inflammatory drugs*
opioid analgesics*
phenothiazines*
progestins*

rifampin
streptomycin
sulfonamides*
sulfonylureas*
tetracyclines*
thalidomide
thiazide diuretics*
tricyclic antidepressants*
warfarin

Drugs that *possibly* cause adverse effects when taken during the *second* and *third* trimesters

acetazolamide
clemastine
diphenhydramine

ethacrynic acid
fluoroquinolones*
haloperidol

hydroxyzine
promethazine

TABLE 2

Medicines That May Increase Sensitivity to the Sun (Photosensitivity)

Some drugs can sensitize skin to ultraviolet light. This can cause the skin to react with a rash or exaggerated burn on exposure to sun or ultraviolet lamps. If you are taking any of the following drugs, ask your doctor for help about sun exposure and sun blocks. Phototoxicity may be the next level of this reaction, possibly with repeat exposure.

acetazolamide
acetohexamide
alprazolam
amantadine
amiloride
aminobenzoic acid
amiodarone
amitriptyline
amoxapine
barbiturates
bendroflumethiazide
benzocaine
benzophenones
benzoyl peroxide
benzthiazide
captopril
carbamazepine
chlordiazepoxide
chloroquine
chlorothiazide
chlorpromazine

chlorpropamide
chlortetracycline
chlorthalidone
ciprofloxacin
clindamycin
clofazimine
clofibrate
clomipramine
cyproheptadine
dacarbazine
dapsone
demeclocycline
desipramine
desoximetasone
diethylstilbestrol
diflunisal
diltiazem
diphenhydramine
disopyramide
doxepin
doxycycline

enoxacin
estrogen
etretinate
flucytosine
fluorescein
fluorouracil
fluphenazine
flutamide
furosemide
glipizide
glyburide
gold preparations
griseofulvin
haloperidol
hexachlorophene
hydrochlorothiazide
hydroflumethiazide
ibuprofen
imipramine
indomethacin
isotretinoin

*See Drug Class, Section Four.

Drugs That May Increase Sensitivity to the Sun (cont.)

ketoprofen	oxyphenbutazone	tetracycline
lincomycin	oxytetracycline	thiabendazole
lomefloxacin	para-aminobenzoic acid	thioridazine
maprotiline	perphenazine	thiothixene
mesoridazine	phenelzine	tolazamide
methacycline	phenobarbital	tolbutamide
methotrexate	phenylbutazone	tranylcypromine
methyclothiazide	phenytoin	trazodone
methyldopa	piroxicam	tretinoin
metolazone	polythiazide	triamterene
minocycline	prochlorperazine	trichlormethiazide
minoxidil	promazine	trifluoperazine
nabumetone	promethazine	triflupromazine
nalidixic acid	protriptyline	trimeprazine
naproxen	pyrazinamide	trimethoprim
nifedipine	quinidine	trimipramine
norfloxacin	quinine	triprolidine
nortriptyline	St. John's wort	vinblastine
ofloxacin	sulfonamides	
oral contraceptives	sulindac	

TABLE 3

Medicines That May Adversely Affect Behavior

Medicines can alter mood and emotional stability. They can also cause unpredictable patterns of thinking or behavior. These responses are relatively infrequent, but the nature and degree of mental disturbance can be alarming as well as dangerous for both patient and family.

Such paradoxical responses are often of an idiosyncratic nature, and someone with a history of a serious mental or emotional disorder is more likely to experience bizarre reactions. In some cases, it may be hard to separate the disorder being treated from an effect of one (or more) medicines the patient may be taking. If in doubt, it is best to talk with your doctor.

Medicines reported to impair *concentration* and/or *memory*

acyclovir	barbiturates*	MAO inhibitors*
anticonvulsants	benzodiazepines*	phenytoin
antihistamines*	isoniazid	primidone
anti-parkinsonism drugs*	monoamine oxidase	scopolamine

Medicines reported to cause *confusion, delirium*, or *disorientation*

acetazolamide	antidepressants*	bromides
acyclovir	antihistamines*	carbamazepine
amantadine	antipsychotics	chloroquine
aminophylline	atropine-like drugs*	cimetidine
amphetamines	barbiturates*	clonidine
amphotericin B	benzodiazepines*	cortisone-like drugs*
anticholinergics	beta adrenergic blockers (some)	

*See Drug Class, Section Four.

Medicines reported to cause *confusion, delirium,* or *disorientation* (cont.)

cycloserine
dantrolene
digitalis
digitoxin
digoxin
disulfiram
diuretics
ethchlorvynol
ethinamate
fenfluramine
fluoroquinolone
   antibiotics*
glutethimide
histamine (H2) receptor
   antagonists

interferons
isoniazid
lamotrigine
levodopa
lidocaine
liposomal amphotericin B
lisinopril
melatonin
meprobamate
mesalamine
methyldopa
metoclopramide
narcotic pain relievers
   (analgesics)
NSAIDs*

para-aminosalicylic acid
phenelzine
phenothiazines*
phenytoin
piperazine
primidone
propranolol
quinidine
reserpine
scopolamine
tacrine
theophylline
tricyclic antidepressants
zolpidem

Medicines reported to cause *paranoid thinking*

acyclovir
amphetamine-like medicines
anticholinergic drugs
benzodiazepines
bromides
cocaine

cortisone-like drugs*
cycloserine
dextromethorphan (when
   abused in high doses)
diphenhydramine
disopyramide

disulfiram
isoniazid
levodopa
propafenone
propranolol
tricyclic antidepressants

Medicines reported to cause *schizophrenic-like behavior*

amphetamines*
anabolic steroids
cimetidine (case reports and
   in elderly or debilitated)

ciprofloxacin (case reports
   and idiosyncratic)
ephedrine
fenfluramine

phenmetrazine
phenylpropanolamine

Medicines reported to cause *manic-like behavior*

antidepressants*
clarithromycin (case
   reports)
cortisone-like drugs*

levodopa
metoclopramide (case
   reports)
monoamine oxidase (MAO)
   inhibitors*

selective serotonin
reuptake inhibitors (SSRIs)
   (when drug is stopped)

Some medicines have mood-altering *side effects*, although they are prescribed for altogether unrelated conditions. Emotional and behavioral secondary effects will be quite unpredictable and vary enormously from person to person. However, the following experiences have been seen with sufficient frequency to establish recognizable patterns.

Medicines reported to cause *nervousness* (anxiety and irritability)

amantadine
amphetamine-like drugs*
   (appetite suppressants)
anabolic steroids
antihistamines*

aripiprazole (Abilify)
caffeine
chlorphenesin
cimetidine (case reports in
   elderly)

cocaine
cortisone-like drugs*
ephedrine
epinephrine
isoproterenol

*See Drug Class, Section Four.

Medicines reported to cause *nervousness* (cont.)

levodopa
liothyronine (in excessive
    dosage)
methylphenidate
methysergide

monoamine oxidase (MAO)
    inhibitors*
nylidrin
oral contraceptives
selective serotonin reuptake
    inhibitors (SSRIs)

theophylline
thyroid (in excessive
    dosage)
thyroxine (in excessive
    dosage)

Medicines reported to cause *emotional depression*

amantadine
amphetamines* (on
    withdrawal)
baclofen
benzodiazepines*
beta adrenergic blockers
    (some)
calcium channel blockers
    (case reports)
carbamazepine
chloramphenicol
cimetidine
clonidine
clotrimazole
cortisone-like drugs*
cycloserine
digitalis
digitoxin
digoxin
diphenoxylate
estrogens

ethionamide
fenfluramine (on
    withdrawal)
fluoroquinolone
    antibiotics
fluphenazine
guanethidine
haloperidol
HMG-CoA reductase
    inhibitors
    (case reports)
hydrocortisone
indomethacin
isoniazid
isotretinoin
levodopa
methsuximide
methyldopa
methysergide
metoclopramide (case
    reports)

metoprolol
oral contraceptives
peginterferon alfa-2A
phenylbutazone
procainamide
progesterones
propranolol
raloxifene
reserpine
ribavirin (in combination
    with peginterferon
    alfa-2A)
sulfonamides*
thiazide diuretics (may
    start after weeks to
    months)
tretinoin
vinblastine (possibly dose
    related)
vitamin D (in excessive
    dosage)

Medicines reported to cause *euphoria*

amantadine
aminophylline
amphetamines
antihistamines* (some)
antispasmodics, synthetic*
aspirin
barbiturates*
benzphetamine
cephalosporins (increased
    risk with kidney disease)
chloral hydrate
clorazepate

codeine
cortisone-like drugs*
diethylpropion
diphenoxylate
dronabinol
ethosuximide
flurazepam
ginseng (sign of abuse)
haloperidol
levodopa
meprobamate
methysergide

monoamine oxidase (MAO)
    inhibitors*
morphine
opioids
pargyline
pentazocine
phenmetrazine
propoxyphene
scopolamine
tybamate

Medicines reported to cause *excitement*

acetazolamide
amantadine
amphetamine-like drugs*
antidepressants*

antihistamines*
atropine-like drugs*
barbiturates* (paradoxical
    response)

benzodiazepines*
    (paradoxical
    response)
cortisone-like drugs

*See Drug Class, Section Four.

Medicines reported to cause *excitement* (cont.)

cycloserine
diethylpropion
digitalis
ephedrine
epinephrine
ethinamate (paradoxical
 response)
ethionamide

glutethimide (paradoxical
 response)
isoniazid
isoproterenol
levodopa
meperidine and MAO
 inhibitor drugs*
methyldopa and MAO
 inhibitor drugs*

methylphenidate
methyprylon (paradoxical
 response)
nalidixic acid
orphenadrine
quinine
scopolamine

TABLE 4

Medicines That May Adversely Affect Vision

A significant percentage of all adverse drug effects involve visual changes or eye damage. Some effects, such as blurring of vision or double vision, may occur shortly after starting a drug. More subtle and serious effects, such as cataract development or damage to the retina or optic nerve, may not happen until a drug has been in use for a long time. Some changes are irreversible. If you are taking a drug that can affect the eye, promptly report any eye discomfort or change in vision.

Medicines reported to cause *blurring of vision*

acetazolamide
antiarthritic/anti-
 inflammatory drugs
antidepressants*
antihistamines*
atropine-like drugs*
chlorthalidone

ciprofloxacin
cortisone-like drugs*
diethylstilbestrol
etretinate
fenfluramine
norfloxacin
oral contraceptives

phenytoin
sildenafil
sulfonamides*
tetracyclines*
thiazide diuretics*

Medicines reported to cause *double vision*

Allopurinol
antidepressants*
antidiabetic drugs*
antihistamines*
aspirin
atacurium
barbiturates*
benzodiazepines*
bromides
bupivicaine
carbamazepine
carisoprodol
chlordiazepoxide
chloroquine
chlorprothixene
ciprofloxacin
clomiphene

colchicine
colistin
cortisone-like drugs*
dicloxacillin
digitalis
digitoxin
digoxin
ethanol
ethionamide
ethosuximide
etretinate
fenoprofen
guanethidine
hydroxychloroquine
ibuprofen
indomethacin
isoniazid

levodopa
mephenesin
methocarbamol
methsuximide
morphine
nalidixic acid
nicotine
nitrofurantoin
norfloxacin
oral contraceptives
organophosphates
orphenadrine
oxyphenbutazone
pentazocine
phenelzine
phenothiazines*
phensuximide

*See Drug Class, Section Four.

Medicines reported to cause *double vision* (cont.)

phentermine
phenylbutazone
phenytoin

primidone
propranolol
quinidine

sedatives/sleep inducers*
thiothixene
tranquilizers*

Medicines reported to cause *farsightedness*

ergot
penicillamine

sulfonamides* (possibly)
tolbutamide (possibly)

Medicines reported to cause *nearsightedness*

acetazolamide
aspirin
carbachol
chlorthalidone
codeine
cortisone-like drugs*

ethosuximide
methsuximide
morphine
oral contraceptives
penicillamine
phenothiazines*

phensuximide
spironolactone
sulfonamides*
tetracyclines*
thiazide diuretics*

Medicines reported to *alter color vision*

acetaminophen
amodiaquine
amyl nitrite
aspirin
atropine
barbiturates*
belladonna
chloramphenicol
chloroquine
chlorpromazine
chlortetracycline
ciprofloxacin
cortisone-like drugs*
digitalis
digitoxin
digoxin
disulfiram
epinephrine
ergotamine
erythromycin
ethchlorvynol

ethionamide
etretinate
griseofulvin
fluphenazine
furosemide
hydroxychloroquine
ibuprofen
indomethacin
isocarboxazid
isoniazid
mefenamic acid
mesoridazine
methysergide
nalidixic acid
norfloxacin
oral contraceptives
oxyphenbutazone
paramethadione
pargyline
penicillamine
pentylenetetrazol

perphenazine
phenacetin
phenylbutazone
primidone
prochlorperazine
promazine
promethazine
quinacrine
quinidine
quinine
reserpine
sildenafil
sodium salicylate
streptomycin
sulfonamides*
thioridazine
tranylcypromine
trifluoperazine
triflupromazine
trimeprazine
trimethadione

Medicines reported to cause *sensitivity to light* (photophobia)

amiodarone
antidiabetic drugs*
atropine-like drugs*
bromides
chloroquine
chlorpropamide
cimetidine
ciprofloxacin
clomiphene

digitoxin
doxepin
ethambutol
furosemide
ethionamide
ethosuximide
etretinate
gold salts
hydroxychloroquine

lithium
mephenytoin
methsuximide
monoamine oxidase
(MAO) inhibitors*
nalidixic acid
tricyclic antidepressants
norfloxacin
oral contraceptives

*See Drug Class, Section Four.

Medicines reported to cause *sensitivity to light* (photophobia) (cont.)

paramethadione	quinidine	tetracyclines*
phenothiazines*	quinine	tolbutamide
rabies vaccine	sildenafil	trimethadione

Medicines reported to cause *halos around lights*

amyl nitrite	digoxin	paramethadione
chloroquine	hydrochloroquine	phenothiazines*
cortisone-like drugs*	nitroglycerin	quinacrine
digitalis	norfloxacin	trimethadione
digitoxin	oral contraceptives	

Medicines reported to cause *visual hallucinations*

amantadine	digitalis	pargyline
amphetamine-like drugs*	digoxin	pentazocine
amyl nitrite	disulfiram	phenothiazines*
antihistamines*	ephedrine	phenylbutazone
aspirin	furosemide	phenytoin
atropine-like drugs*	gabapentin	primidone
barbiturates*	griseofulvin	propranolol
benzodiazepines*	haloperidol	quinine
bromides	hydroxychloroquine	sedatives/sleep inducers*
carbamazepine	indomethacin	sulfonamides*
cephalexin	isosorbide	tetracyclines*
cephaloglycin	levodopa	tricyclic antidepressants*
chloroquine	nialamide	tripelennamine
cycloserine	oxyphenbutazone	

Medicines reported to impair the use of *contact lenses*

brompheniramine	dexbrompheniramine	furosemide
carbinoxamine	dexchlorpheniramine	oral contraceptives
chlorpheniramine	dimethindene	terfenadine
cyclizine	latanoprost	travaprost
cyproheptadine	diphenhydramine	tripelennamine

Medicines reported to cause *cataracts* or *lens deposits*

allopurinol	methotrimeprazine	thioridazine
busulfan	perphenazine	thiothixene
chlorpromazine	phenmetrazine	trifluoperazine
chlorprothixene	pilocarpine	triflupromazine
cortisone-like drugs*	prochlorperazine	trimeprazine
fluphenazine	promazine	
mesoridazine	promethazine	

TABLE 5

Medicines That May Cause Blood Cell Dysfunction or Damage

All blood cells come from and mature in the bone marrow: red blood cells (erythrocytes), white blood cells (leukocytes), and blood platelets (thrombocytes).

*See Drug Class, Section Four.

There are three kinds of white blood cells: granulocytes, monocytes (macrophages), and lymphocytes. Drugs that affect formation or development of blood cells can (1) act on any stage of cell production, (2) impair one cell type or line, and/or (3) influence all cell lines. Some medicines can damage mature cells in the bloodstream; some result in lower hemoglobin.

Medicines that cause inevitable (dose-dependent) *aplastic anemia* (see Glossary)

actinomycin D	cytarabine	mercaptopurine
azathioprine	doxorubicin	methotrexate
busulfan	epirubicin	mitomycin
carboplatin	etoposide	mitoxantrone
carmustine	fluorouracil	plicamycin
chlorambucil	hydroxyurea	procarbazine
cisplatin	lomustine	thioguanine
cyclophosphamide	melphalan	thiotepa

Medicines that may cause idiosyncratic (dose-independent) *aplastic anemia*

amodiaquine	mepacrine	pyrimethamine
benoxaprofen	oxyphenbutazone	sulfonamides*
carbimazole	penicillamine	sulindac
chloramphenicol	phenylbutazone	thiouracils
chlorpromazine	phenytoin	trimethoprim/
gold	piroxicam	sulfamethoxazole
indomethacin	prothiaden	

Medicines that may *impair red blood cell production* (only)

azathioprine	isoniazid	sulfasalazine
carbamazepine	methyldopa	sulfathiazol
chloramphenicol	penicillin	sulfonamides*
chlorpropamide	pentachlorophenol	sulfonylureas*
dapsone	phenobarbital	thiamphenicol
fenoprofen	phenylbutazone	tolbutamide
gold	phenytoin	trimethoprim/
halothane	pyrimethamine	sulfamethoxazole

Medicines that may significantly *reduce granulocyte cell counts* (various mechanisms)

acetaminophen	chloroquine	gentamicin
acetazolamide	chlorothiazide	gold
allopurinol	chlorpromazine	hydralazine
amitriptyline	chlorpropamide	hydrochlorothiazide
amodiaquine	chlorthalidone	imipramine
benzodiazepines*	cimetidine	indomethacin
captopril	clindamycin	isoniazid
carbamazepine	dapsone	levamisole
carbimazole	desipramine	meprobamate
cephalosporins*	disopyramide	methimazole
chloramphenicol	ethacrynic acid	methyldopa

*See Drug Class, Section Four.

Medicines that may significantly *reduce granulocyte cell counts* (cont.)

oxyphenbutazone
penicillamine
penicillins*
pentazocine
phenacetin
phenothiazines*
phenylbutazone
phenytoin
procainamide

propranolol
propylthiouracil
pyrimethamine
quinidine
quinine
ranitidine
rifampin
sodium aminosalicylate
streptomycin

sulfadoxine
sulfadoxine/pyrimethamine
sulfonamides*
tetracyclines*
tocainide
tolbutamide
trimetophrim
    sulfanethoxazole
vancomycin

Medicines that cause lower hemoglobin

Alpha-interferon–2A

Medicines that may significantly *reduce blood platelet counts*

acetazolamide
actinomycin
allopurinol
alpha-interferon
amiodarone
ampicillin
aspirin
aztreonam
carbamazepine
carbenicillin
cephalosporins*
chenodeoxycholic acid
chloroquine
chlorothiazide
chlorpheniramine
chlorpropamide
chlorthalidone
cimetidine
clonazepam
cotrimoxazole
cyclophosphamide
danazol
desferrioxamine
diazepam
diazoxide

diclofenac
digoxin
diltiazem
enalapril
fluconazole
furosemide
gentamicin
glyburide
gold
heparin
hydrochlorothiazide
imipramine
isoniazid
isotretinoin
levamisole
lisinopril
meprobamate
methyldopa
mianserin
minoxidil
mitomycin
morphine
nitrofurantoin
oxprenolol
oxyphenbutazone

penicillamine
penicillin
phenylbutazone
phenytoin
piroxicam
primidone
procainamide
procarbazine
quinidine
quinine
ranitidine
rifampin
sodium aminosalicylate
sulfasalazine
sulfonamides*
thioguanine
tobramycin
tocainide
trimethoprim
trimetrexate
valproate (valproic acid)
vancomycin
vincristine

Medicines that cause *hemolytic anemia* due to glucose-6-phosphate dehydrogenase (G6PD) deficiency of red blood cells

acetanilid
dapsone
methylene blue
nalidixic acid
naphthalene
niridazole

nitrofurantoin
pamaquine
phenazopyridine
phenylhydrazine
primaquine
sulfacetamide

sulfamethoxazole
sulfanilamide
sulfapyridine
thiazolsulfone
toluidine blue

*See Drug Class, Section Four.

Medicines that may cause *hemolytic anemia* by other mechanisms

antimony	para-aminosalicylic acid	ribavirin
chlorpropamide	penicillamine	rifampin
cisplatin	phenazopyridine	sulfasalazine
mephenesin	quinidine	
methotrexate	quinine	

Medicines that may cause *megaloblastic anemia*

acyclovir	metformin	primidone
alcohol	methotrexate	pyrimethamine
aminopterin	neomycin	sulfasalazine
azathioprine	nitrofurantoin	tetracycline
colchicine	nitrous oxide	thioguanine
cycloserine	oral contraceptives	triamterene
cytarabine	para-aminosalicylic acid	trimethoprim
floxuridine	pentamidine	vinblastine
fluorouracil	phenformin	vitamin A
hydroxyurea	phenobarbital	vitamin C (large doses)
mercaptopurine	phenytoin	zidovudine

Medicines that may cause *sideroblastic anemia*

alcohol	isoniazid	pyrazinamide
chloramphenicol	penicillamine	
cycloserine	phenacetin	

TABLE 6

Medicines That May Cause Heart Dysfunction or Damage

Drugs may damage either heart structure or function. Heart problems themselves often decide the nature of adverse drug effects. Some are direct pharmacological actions of a drug on heart tissues, and others are caused indirectly by altering chemical balances that diminish how well the heart works (as with potassium or magnesium loss from diuretics).

Medicines that may cause or contribute to *abnormal heart rhythms* (arrhythmias)

aminophylline	bronchodilators*	diuretics*
amiodarone	carbamazepine	dofetilide
amitriptyline	chlorpromazine	doxepin
antiarrhythmic drugs*	cimetidine	droperidol
aripiprazole	cisapride (use is now	encainide
arsenic trioxide	limited)	erythromycin (intravenous)
astemizole (no longer on	clarithromycin	fentolterol
the U.S. market)	digitoxin	felbamate
bepridil	digoxin	flecainide
beta adrenergic blockers*	diltiazem	fluoxetine
beta-adrenergic	disopyramide	fluvoxamine

*See Drug Class, Section Four.

Medicines that may cause or contribute to *abnormal heart rhythms* (cont.)

foscarnet
fosphenytoin
gatifloxacin
grepafloxacin (no longer on
   the U.S. market)
halofantrene
haloperidol
ibutilide
indapamide
isoproterenol
isradipine
ketanserin
levofloxacin
levomethadyl
lidocaine
maprotiline
methyldopa
mesoridazine
mexiletine
milrinone
moexipril/hctz
moxifloxacin
naratriptan
nicardipine
octreotide
pentamidine
phenothiazines*
pimozide

prenylamine
procainamide
quetiapine
quinidine
QTc blockers: arsenic
   trioxide; chlorpromazine;
   class I, IA, or III
   antiarrhythmics; clarithromycin; clindamycin;
   cotrimoxazole; dofetilide;
   dolasetron; droperidol;
   erythromycin;
   fluconaxzole; fluoxetine;
   foscarnet; gatifloxacin,
   moxifloxacin or
   sparfloxacin; halo-
   fantrine; haloperidol;
   isradipine; ketoconazole;
   levomethadyl (Orlaam);
   mesoridazine; octreotide
   (Santostatin);
   ondansetron; pentami-
   dine; phenothiazines in
   general; pimozide;
   quinidine; risperidone;
   sotolol; sulfamethoxa-
   zole; tacrolimus;
   thioridazine; tricyclic

antidepressants;
   trimethoprim; venla
   faxine; ziprazodone;
   zotepine; and others
ranitidine
risperidone
salmeterol
sertraline
sotalol
sparfloxacin
sumatriptan
tacrolimus
tamoxifen
terbutaline
terfenadine (no longer
   on the U.S. market)
theophylline
thiazide diuretics*
thioridazine
tizanidine
trazodone
tricyclic antidepressants
   (such as Elavil,
   Sinequan, Tofranil)*
venlafaxine
verapamil
ziprasidone
zolmitriptan

Medicines that may *depress heart function* (reduce pumping efficiency)

beta adrenergic blockers*
beta blockers still used
   post-MI
cocaine
daunorubicin

diltiazem
disopyramide
doxorubicin
epinephrine
flecainide

fluorouracil
isoproterenol
nifedipine
verapamil

Medicines that may *reduce coronary artery blood flow* (reduce oxygen supply to heart muscle)

amphetamines*
beta adrenergic blockers*
   (abrupt withdrawal)
cocaine

ergotamine
fluorouracil
nifedipine
oral contraceptives

ritodrine
vasopressin
vinblastine
vincristine

Medicines that may *impair healing of heart muscle* following heart attack (myocardial infarction)

adrenocortical steroids*
nonsteroidal
   anti-inflammatory drugs (NSAIDs)*

*See Drug Class, Section Four.

Medicines that may cause *heart valve damage*

dexfenfluramine (Redux)
ergotamine
fen-phen
  (fenfluramine-
  phenteramine)

pergolide (permax)
methysergide
minocycline (blue-black
  pigmentation)

Medicines that may cause *pericardial disease*

actinomycin D
anthracyclines
bleomycin
cisplatin
cyclophosphamide

cytarabine
fluorouracil
hydralazine
methysergide
minoxidil

phenylbutazone
practolol
procainamide
sulfasalazine

TABLE 7

Medicines That May Cause Lung Dysfunction or Damage

Lung damage from medicines may be difficult to distinguish from natural diseases or disorders that involve lung function or structure. Type A reactions are those due to known pharmacological drug actions; Type B are unexpected and unpredictable allergic or idiosyncratic reactions.

Medicines that may adversely affect *blood vessels of the lung*

Drugs that may cause thromboembolism

chlorpromazine
estrogens*

oral contraceptives
  (high-estrogen type)

Drugs that may cause pulmonary hypertension

amphetamines*
dexfenfluramine (Redux)
fenfluramine
oral contraceptives

sibutramine (Meridia)
  (carries a warning on
  the label, but effect has
  NOT been reported)

tryptophan

Drugs that may cause vasculitis (blood vessel damage) with or without hemorrhage

aminoglutethimide
amphotericin
cocaine

febarbamate
nitrofurantoin
penicillamine

phenytoin

Drugs that may cause adult respiratory distress syndrome (ARDS)

bleomycin
codeine
cyclophosphamide
dextropropoxyphene

heroin
hydrochlorothiazide
methadone
mitomycin

naloxone
ritodrine
terbutaline
vinblastine

*See Drug Class, Section Four.

Medicines that may adversely affect the *bronchial tubes*

Drugs that may cause bronchoconstriction (asthma)

acetaminophen
aspirin
beta adrenergic blockers*
carbachol
cephalosporins*
chloramphenicol
deanol
demeclocycline
erythromycin

griseofulvin
maprotiline
methacholine
methoxypsoralen
metoclopramide
morphine
neomycin
neostigmine
nitrofurantoin

nonsteroidal anti-
    inflammatory drugs*
penicillins*
pilocarpine
propafenone
pyridostigmine
streptomycin
tartrazine (coloring agent)

Drugs that may cause bronchiolitis (with permanent obstruction of small bronchioles)

penicillamine   sulfasalazine

Medicines that may *damage lung tissues*

Drugs that may cause acute allergic-type pneumonitis

ampicillin
bleomycin
cephalexin
chlorpropamide
gold
imipramine
mephenesin
mercaptopurine
metformin

methotrexate
metronidazole
mitomycin
nalidixic acid
nitrofurantoin
nomifensine
nonsteroidal anti-
    inflammatory drugs*
para-aminosalicylic acid

penicillamine
penicillin
phenylbutazone
phenytoin
procarbazine
sulfonamides*
tetracycline
vinblastine

Medicines that may cause *chronic pneumonitis and/or fibrosis* (scarring)

amiodarone
azathioprine
BCNU
bleomycin
bromocriptine
busulfan
carmustine
CCNU
chlorambucil

cyclophosphamide
ergotamine
gold
hexamethonium
lomustine
mecamylamine
melphalan
mercaptopurine
methysergide

nitrofurantoin
peginterferon alfa-2A
pentolinium
practolol
ribavirin
sulfasalazine
tocainide
tolfenamic acid

Medicines that may *damage the pleura*

bromocriptine   methysergide   practolol

*See Drug Class, Section Four.

TABLE 8

Medicines That May Cause Liver Dysfunction or Damage

The liver often changes drugs into forms easily removed from the body. Medicines can hurt liver structure or function. Reactions range from mild and transient changes in liver function tests to complete liver failure and death. Many medicines may affect the liver in more than one way. Careful liver monitoring is required.

Medicines that may cause *acute dose-dependent liver damage* (resembling acute viral hepatitis)

acetaminophen (overdose)	salicylates (such as	6-mercaptopurine
amiodarone	aspirin—doses over 2 g	
niacin	daily)	

Medicines that may cause *acute dose-independent liver* damage (resembling acute viral hepatitis)

acebutolol	indomethacin	phenytoin
allopurinol	isoniazid	piroxicam
atenolol	ketoconazole	probenecid
carbamazepine	labetalol	pyrazinamide
cimetidine	maprotiline	quinidine
cocaine	metoprolol	quinine
dantrolene	mianserin	ranitidine
diclofenac	naproxen	rifampin
diltiazem	nifedipine	sulfonamides*
disulfiram	para-aminosalicylic acid	sulindac
enflurane	penicillins*	tricyclic antidepressants*
ethambutol	phenelzine	trovafloxacin
ethionamide	phenindione	valproic acid
halothane	phenobarbital	verapamil
ibuprofen	phenylbutazone	

Medicines that may cause *acute fatty infiltration of the liver*

adrenocortical steroids*	phenothiazines*	tetracyclines*
antithyroid drugs	phenytoin	valproic acid
isoniazid	salicylates*	
methotrexate	sulfonamides*	

Medicines that may cause *cholestatic jaundice*

acetaminophen	chlordiazepoxide	diazepam
actinomycin D	chlorpromazine	diclofenac
amitriptyline	chlorpropamide	disopyramide
amoxicillin/clavulanate	cimetidine	enalapril
azathioprine	cloxacillin	erythromycin (estolate)
captopril (case reports)	cyclophosphamide	estradiol
carbamazepine	cyclosporine	flecainide
carbimazole	danazol	flurazepam
cephalosporins*	desipramine	flutamide

*See Drug Class, Section Four.

Medicines that may cause *cholestatic jaundice* (cont.)

glyburide
gold
griseofulvin
haloperidol
imipramine
indomethacin
ketoconazole
mercaptopurine
methyltestosterone
nafcillin
niacin
nifedipine
nitrofurantoin

nonsteroidal anti-
    inflammatory drugs*
norethandrolone
oral contraceptives
oxacillin
penicillamine
phenothiazines*
phenytoin
piroxicam
propoxyphene
propylthiouracil
rifampin
sulfonamides*

sulindac
tamoxifen
thiabendazole
tolazamide
tolbutamide
tricyclic antidepressants*
trimethoprim/sulfamethox-
    azole
troleandomycin
verapamil
zidovudine

Medicines that may cause *liver granulomas* (chronic inflammatory nodules)

allopurinol
aspirin
carbamazepine
chlorpromazine
chlorpropamide
diltiazem
disopyramide

gold
hydralazine
isoniazid
methyldopa
nitrofurantoin
penicillin
phenylbutazone

phenytoin
procainamide
quinidine
ranitidine
sulfonamides*
tolbutamide

Medicines that may cause *chronic liver disease*

Drugs that may cause active chronic hepatitis

acetaminophen (chronic
    use, large doses)
dantrolene

isoniazid
methyldopa
nitrofurantoin

salicylates (aspirin)
trazodone

Drugs that may cause liver cirrhosis or fibrosis (scarring)

methotrexate
methyldopa

nicotinic acid

vitamin A

Drugs that may cause chronic cholestasis (resembling primary biliary cirrhosis)

chlorpromazine/valproic
    acid (combination)
chlorpropamide/
    erythromycin
    (combination)

imipramine
phenothiazines*
phenytoin

thiabendazole
tolbutamide

Medicines that may cause *liver tumors* (benign and malignant)

anabolic steroids
androgens (C17-substituted
    kinds)

danazol
oral contraceptives
testosterone

thorotrast

*See Drug Class, Section Four.

Medicines that may cause *damage to liver blood vessels*

adriamycin
anabolic steroids
azathioprine
carmustine
cyclophosphamide/
  cyclo-sporine
  (combination)

dacarbazine
herbal teas
  (some)
mercaptopurine
methotrexate
mitomycin
oral contraceptives

thioguanine
vincristine
vitamin A
  (excessive doses)

Medicines that can cause *idiosyncratic liver damage*

acarbose
acebutolol (case reports)
amoxicillin/clavulanate
carbamazepine
chlorpromazine

dacarbazine
kava kava
leflunomide
procainamide
propylthiouracil

sulfonamides
troglitazone
trovafloxacin
valproic acid

TABLE 9

Medicines That May Cause Kidney Dysfunction or Damage

The kidneys perform two major drug functions: (1) alteration of the drug to help remove it, and (2) elimination of the drug from the body in the urine. As with effects on the liver, many drugs can harm the kidneys in several ways. Careful monitoring is prudent when taking any of the drugs listed below.

Medicines that may primarily *impair kidney function* (without damage)

amphotericin
angiotensin-converting-
  enzyme inhibitors* (with
  renal artery stenosis;
  with congestive heart
  failure)
beta adrenergic blockers*
ceftazidime
colchicine

demeclocycline
diuretics/NSAIDs* (avoid
  this combination)
glyburide
isofosfamide
lithium/tricyclic anti
  depressants* (avoid this
  combination)
methoxyflurane

nifedipine
nitroprusside
nonsteroidal
  anti-inflammatory
  drugs (NSAIDs)*
rifampin
vinblastine

Medicines that may cause *acute kidney failure* (due to kidney damage)

Drugs that may damage the kidney filtration unit (the nephron)

acetaminophen (excessive
  dosage)
allopurinol
aminoglycoside
antibiotics*
amphotericin
bismuth thiosulfate
carbamazepine

cisplatin
cyclosporine
enalapril
ergometrine
hydralazine
methy-CCNU
metronidazole
mitomycin

oral contraceptives
penicillamine
phenytoin
quinidine
rifampin
streptokinase
sulfonamides*
thiazide diuretics*

*See Drug Class, Section Four.

Medicines that may cause *acute interstitial nephritis*

allopurinol
amoxicillin
ampicillin
aspirin
azathioprine
aztreonam
captopril
carbamazepine
carbenicillin
cefaclor
cefoxitin
cephalexin
cephalothin
cephapirin
cephradine
cimetidine
ciprofloxacin
clofibrate
cloxacillin
diazepam

diclofenac
diflunisal
fenoprofen
foscarnet
furosemide
gentamicin
glafenine
ibuprofen
indomethacin
ketoprofen
mefenamate
methicillin
methyldopa
mezlocillin
minocycline
nafcillin
naproxen
oxacillin
penicillamine
penicillin

phenindione
phenobarbital
phenylbutazone
phenytoin
piroxicam
pirprofen
pyrazinamide
rifampin
sodium valproate
sulfamethoxazole
sulfinpyrazone
sulfonamides*
sulindac
thiazide diuretics*
tolmetin
trimethoprim
vancomycin
warfarin

Medicines that may cause *muscle destruction* and associated *acute kidney failure*

adrenocortical steroids*
alcohol
amphetamines*
amphotericin
aristolochic acid (prompted
  removal of several herbal
  products from the mar-
  ket by the FDA)

carbenoxolone
chlorthalidone
clofibrate
cocaine
cytarabine
fenofibrate
haloperidol
halothane

heroin
lovastatin
opioid analgesics*
pentamidine
phenothiazines*
streptokinase
suxamethonium

Medicines that may cause kidney damage resembling *glomerulonephritis or nephrosis*

captopril
fenoprofen
gold
ketoprofen

lithium
mesalamine
penicillamine
phenytoin

practolol
probenecid
quinidine

Medicines that may cause *chronic interstitial nephritis and papillary necrosis* (analgesic kidney damage)

acetaminophen
aspirin

phenacetin
(All with long-term use)

*See Drug Class, Section Four.

Medicines that may cause or contribute to *urinary tract crystal or stone formation*

acetazolamide
acyclovir
cytotoxic drugs
dihydroxyadenine
magnesium trisilicate
mercaptopurine
methotrexate

methoxyflurane
phenylbutazone
probenecid
salicylates*
sulfonamides*
thiazide diuretics*
triamterene

uricosuric drugs
vitamin A
vitamin C
vitamin D
warfarin
zoxazolamine

TABLE 10

Medicines That May Cause Nerve Dysfunction or Damage

Medicines may affect any part of the nervous system from the brain to peripheral nerves. The extent of benefits or problems varies widely from person to person.

Medicines that may cause *significant headache*

albuterol
amyl nitrate
bepridil
bromocriptine
caffeine
cilostazol
clonidine
cocaine
delavirdine
ergotamine (prolonged use)
etretinate
felodipine
fluticasone
fluvoxamine
HMG-CoA reductase
   inhibitors

hydralazine
ibuprofen
indomethacin
labetalol
liposomal amphotericin B
lithium
lomefloxacin
mesalamine
naproxen
nifedipine
nisoldipine
nitrofurantoin
nitroglycerin
oral contraceptives
perhexiline
peginterferon alfa-2A

propranolol
ranitidine
sertraline
sibutramine
sildenafil
stavudine
sulindac
terbutaline
tetracyclines*
theophylline
tolmetin
trimethoprim/
   sulfamethoxazole
valacyclovir

Medicines that may cause *seizures (convulsions)*

acyclovir
alprostadil
amantadine
amitriptyline
ampicillin
antihistamines (some first-
   generation forms in high
   dose)
baclofen
bromocriptine
bupropion
carbamazepine
   (exacerbation of absence)

carbenicillin
cephalosporins*
chloroquine
cimetidine
ciprofloxacin and other fluoroquinolone antibiotics
cisapride
clozapine
cocaine
cycloserine
dantrolene
dextromethorphan (high
   doses and when abused)

disopyramide
disulfuram
enoxacin
ephedra (ma Huang now
   removed from the market)
ethosuximide
ether
gabapentin
halothane
imipenem-cilastatin
   (Primaxin) and other
   carbapenem antibiotics
indomethacin

*See Drug Class, Section Four.

Medicines that may cause *seizures (convulsions)* (cont.)

isoniazid
levodopa
lidocaine
lindane
lithium
mefenamic acid
meperidine (Demerol)
metronidazole (high doses)
morphine (high-dose
    intravenous)

nalidixic acid
ofloxacin
oxacillin
paclitaxel
penicillins* (synthetic)
phenobarbital
phenothiazines*
pseudoephedrine
pyrimethamine
tacrine

terbutaline
theophylline
ticarcillin
tramadol
tricyclic antidepressants*
venlafaxine
vincristine

Medicines that may cause *stroke*

amitriptyline
anabolic steroids
cocaine

estrogens
nicotine
oral contraceptives

phenylpropanolamine
sumatriptan
trazodone

Medicines that may cause features of *parkinsonism*

amitriptyline
amodiaquine
atypical antipsychotics (see
    Drug Classes)
chloroquine
chlorprothixene
clozapine
desipramine

diazoxide
diltiazem
diphenhydramine
droperidol
fluoxetine
haloperidol
imipramine
levodopa

lithium
methyldopa
metoclopramide
phenothiazines*
reserpine
thiothixene
trifluperidol
valproic acid

Medicines that may cause *acute dystonias* (acute involuntary movement syndromes—AIMS)

carbamazepine
chlorzoxazone
fluoxetine

haloperidol
metoclopramide
phenothiazines*

phenytoin
propranolol
tricyclic antidepressants*

Medicines that may cause *tardive dyskinesia* (see Glossary)

Atypical antipsychotics
haloperidol

phenothiazines*

thiothixene

Medicines that may cause *neuroleptic malignant syndrome* (NMS)

See this term in the Glossary for a list of causative drugs.

Medicines that may cause *peripheral neuropathy* (see Glossary)

amiodarone
amitriptyline
amphetamines*
amphotericin
anticoagulants*
carbutamide
chlorambucil
chloramphenicol
chloroquine

chlorpropamide
cimetidine
cisplatin
clioquinol
clofibrate
colchicine
colistin
cytarabine
dapsone

didanosine
disopyramide
disulfiram
emetine
ergotamine
ethambutol
ethanol
glutethimide
gold

*See Drug Class, Section Four.

Medicines that may cause *peripheral neuropathy* (cont.)

hydralazine
imipramine
indomethacin
isoniazid
lamotrigine
losartan
methaqualone
methimazole
methysergide
metronidazole
nalidixic acid
nelfinavir

nitrofurantoin
nitrofurazone
paclitaxel
penicillamine
penicillin
perhexiline
phenelzine
phenylbutazone
phenytoin
podophyllin
procarbazine
propranolol

propylthiouracil
ritonavir
stavudine
streptomycin
sulfonamides*
sulfoxone
thalidomide
tolbutamide
vinblastine
vincristine

Drugs that may cause a *myasthenia gravis syndrome*

aminoglycoside
   antibiotics*
amitriptyline
azithromycin (exacerbation
   of existing MG)
beta adrenergic blockers*
codeine

erythromycin (exacerbation
   of existing MG)
lithium
morphine
norfloxacin (exacerbation
   of existing MG)
penicillamine

phenytoin
polymixin B
procainamide
tetracycline
trihexyphenidyl

TABLE 11

Medicines That May Adversely Affect Sexuality

Many commonly used drugs can cause obvious or subtle changes on one or more aspects of sexual expression. Patients may be unaware that sexual changes can be related to medicines and are often reluctant to talk about them. Sexual dysfunction may also be a result of the disorder being treated or an undetected problem. Diabetes, kidney failure, hypertension, depression, and alcoholism may reduce libido and cause failure of erection. Many drugs used to treat these conditions may worsen subclinical sexual dysfunction. This requires the closest cooperation between therapist and patient in order to correctly assess possible cause-and-effect relationships and change therapy appropriately.

Possible Drug Effects on Male Sexuality

1. Increased libido
   androgens (replacement therapy in deficiency states)
   baclofen (Lioresal)
   bupropion (Wellbutrin)
   chlordiazepoxide (Librium) (antianxiety effect)
   diazepam (Valium) (antianxiety effect)
   haloperidol (Haldol)
   levodopa (Larodopa, Sinemet) (may be an indirect effect due to improved
      sense of well-being)
   sildenafil (Viagra) (may be an effect of confidence from the drug)

*See Drug Class, Section Four.

2. Decreased libido
   amphetamines
   antihistamines
   barbiturates
   chlordiazepoxide (Librium) (sedative effect)
   chlorpromazine (Thorazine), 10% to 20% of users
   cimetidine (Tagamet)
   clofibrate (Atromid-S)
   clonidine (Catapres), 10% to 20% of users
   danazol (Danocrine)
   diazepam (Valium) (sedative effect)
   disulfiram (Antabuse)
   estrogens (therapy for prostatic cancer)
   fenfluramine (Pondimin)
   finasteride (Propecia, Proscar)
   heroin
   licorice
   medroxyprogesterone (Provera)
   methyldopa (Aldomet), 10% to 15% of users
   metoclopramide (Reglan), 80% of users
   perhexiline (Pexid)
   prazosin (Minipres), 15% of users
   propranolol (Inderal), rarely
   reserpine (Serpasil, Ser-Ap-Es)
   spironolactone (Aldactone)
   tricyclic antidepressants

3. Impaired erection (impotence)
   amitriptyline
   amphetamines
   angiotensin-converting enzyme (ACE) inhibitors
   anticholinergics
   antihistamines
   baclofen (Lioresal)
   barbiturates (when abused)
   beta blockers*
   captopril
   chlordiazepoxide (Librium) (in high dosage)
   chlorpromazine (Thorazine)
   cimetidine (Tagamet)
   citalopram (Celexa)
   clofibrate (Atromid-S)
   clonidine (Catapres)
   cocaine
   diazepam (Valium) (in high dosage)
   digitalis and its glycosides
   disopyramide (Norpace)
   disulfiram (Antabuse), uncertain
   estrogens (therapy for prostatic cancer)
   ethacrynic acid (Edecrin)

*See Drug Class, Section Four.

ethionamide (Trecator-SC)
fenfluramine (Pondimin)
Finasteride (Proscar)
furosemide (Lasix)
gabapentin (Neurontin)
guanethidine (Ismelin)
haloperidol (Haldol)
heroin
hydrochlorothiazide (ESPECIALLY if combined with a beta blocker)
hydroxyprogesterone (therapy for prostatic cancer)
indomethacin
itraconazole
licorice
lisinopril
lithium (Lithonate)
losartan (Cozaar)
marijuana
mesoridazine (Serentil)
methantheline (Banthine)
methyldopa (Aldomet)
metoclopramide (Reglan)
mirtazapine (Remeron)
monoamine oxidase (MAO) type A inhibitors*
perhexiline (Pexid)
pravastatin
prazosin (Minipres), infrequently
reserpine (Serpasil, Ser-Ap-Es)
simvastatin
spironolactone (Aldactone)
telmisartan (Micardis)
thiazide diuretics
thioridazine (Mellaril)
tricyclic antidepressants
venlafaxine (Effexor)

4. Impaired ejaculation
   anticholinergics
   barbiturates (when abused)
   chlorpromazine (Thorazine)
   clonidine (Catapres)
   cocaine
   estrogens (therapy for prostatic cancer)
   guanethidine (Ismelin)
   heroin
   mesoridazine (Serentil)
   methyldopa (Aldomet)
   monoamine oxidase (MAO) type A inhibitors*
   phenoxybenzamine (Dibenzyline)
   phentolamine (Regitine)
   reserpine (Serpasil, Ser-Ap-Es)

*See Drug Class, Section Four.

thiazide diuretics*
thioridazine (Mellaril)
tricyclic antidepressants*

5. Decreased testosterone
adrenocorticotropic hormone (ACTH)
barbiturates
digoxin (Lanoxin)
haloperidol (Haldol)—increased testosterone with low dosage, decreased testosterone with high dosage
lithium (Lithonate)
marijuana
medroxyprogesterone (Provera)
monoamine oxidase (MAO) type A inhibitors*
spironolactone (Aldactone)

6. Impaired spermatogenesis (reduced fertility)
adrenocorticosteroids (prednisone, etc.)
androgens (moderate to high dosage, extended use)
antimalarials
aspirin (abusive, chronic use)
chlorambucil (Leukeran)
cimetidine (Tagamet)
colchicine
cotrimoxazole (Bactrim, Septra)
cyclophosphamide (Cytoxan)
estrogens (therapy for prostatic cancer)
marijuana
medroxyprogesterone (Provera)
methotrexate
metoclopramide (Reglan)
monoamine oxidase (MAO) type A inhibitors
niridazole (Ambilhar)
nitrofurantoin (Furadantin)
spironolactone (Aldactone)
sulfasalazine (Azulfidine)
testosterone (moderate to high dosage, extended use)
vitamin C (doses of 1 g or more)

7. Testicular disorders
Swelling
—tricyclic antidepressants
Inflammation
—oxyphenbutazone (Tandearil)
Atrophy
—androgens (moderate to high dosage, extended use)
—chlorpromazine (Thorazine)
—cyclophosphamide (Cytoxan) (in prepubescent boys)
—spironolactone (Aldactone)

*See Drug Class, Section Four.

8. Penile disorders
    Priapism (see Glossary)
    —alfentanil
    —anabolic steroids (male hormone-like drugs)
    —chlorpromazine (Thorazine)
    —clozapine (Clozaril)
    —cocaine
    —fluphenazine (Prolixin)
    —guanethidine (Ismelin)
    —haloperidol (Haldol)
    —heparin
    —hydralazine (Apresoline)
    —levodopa (Sinemet)
    —mesoridazine (Serentil)
    —molindone (Moban)
    —phenelzine (Nardil)
    —phenytoin (Dilantin)
    —prazosin (Minipres)
    —prochlorperazine (Compazine)
    —risperidone (Risperdal)
    —tamoxifen (Nolvadex)
    —thioridazine (Mellaril)
    —trazodone (Desyrel)
    —trifluoperazine (Stelazine)
    —warfarin (Coumadin)
    Peyronie's disease (see Glossary)
    —beta blockers*
    —phenytoin (Dilantin, etc.)

9. Gynecomastia (excessive development of the male breast)
    anabolic steroids
    androgens (partial conversion to estrogen)
    busulfan (Myleran)
    captopril
    carmustine (BiCNU)
    chlormadinone
    chlorpromazine (Thorazine)
    chlortetracycline (Aureomycin)
    cimetidine (Tagamet)
    clonidine (Catapres), infrequently
    diazepam
    diethylstilbestrol (DES)
    digitalis and its glycosides
    diltiazem
    enalapril
    estrogens (therapy for prostatic cancer)
    ethionamide (Trecator-SC)
    finasteride (Propecia, Proscar)
    fluphenazine
    griseofulvin (Fulvicin, etc.)
    haloperidol (Haldol)

*See Drug Class, Section Four.

    heroin
    human chorionic gonadotropin
    indinavir (Crixivan)
    isoniazid (INH, Nydrazid)
    marijuana
    mestranol
    methyldopa (Aldomet)
    metoclopramide (Reglan)
    nifedipine
    omeprazole (Prilosec)
    penicillamine
    phenelzine (Nardil)
    phenothiazines
    reserpine (Serpasil, Ser-Ap-Es)
    spironolactone (Aldactone)
    thioridazine (Mellaril)
    tricyclic antidepressants (TCAs)
    verapamil
    vincristine (Oncovin)

10. Feminization (loss of libido, impotence, gynecomastia, testicular atrophy)
    conjugated estrogens (Premarin, etc.)

11. Precocious puberty
    anabolic steroids
    androgens
    isoniazid (INH)

Possible Drug Effects on Female Sexuality

1. Increased libido
    androgens
    chlordiazepoxide (Librium) (antianxiety effect)
    diazepam (Valium) (antianxiety effect)
    mazindol (Sanorex)
    oral contraceptives (freedom from fear of pregnancy)

2. Decreased libido
    See list of drug effects on male sexuality. Some of these may have potential
      for reducing libido in the female. The literature is sparse on this subject.

3. Impaired arousal and orgasm
    anticholinergics
    clonidine (Catapres)
    methyldopa (Aldomet)
    monoamine oxidase (MAO) inhibitors*
    tricyclic antidepressants*

4. Breast enlargement
    penicillamine
    tricyclic antidepressants*

*See Drug Class, Section Four.

5. Galactorrhea (spontaneous flow of milk)
   amphetamine
   chlorpromazine (Thorazine)
   cimetidine (Tagamet)
   haloperidol (Haldol)
   heroin
   methyldopa (Aldomet)
   metoclopramide (Reglan)
   oral contraceptives
   phenothiazines
   reserpine (Serpasil, Ser-Ap-Es)
   sulpiride (Equilid)
   tricyclic antidepressants*

6. Ovarian failure (reduced fertility)
   anesthetic gases (operating room staff)
   cyclophosphamide (Cytoxan)
   cytostatic drugs
   danazol (Danocrine)
   medroxyprogesterone (Provera)

7. Altered menstruation (menstrual disorders)
   adrenocorticosteroids (prednisone, etc.)
   androgens
   barbiturates (when abused)
   chlorambucil (Leukeran)
   chlorpromazine (Thorazine)
   cyclophosphamide (Cytoxan)
   danazol (Danocrine)
   estrogens
   ethionamide (Trecator-SC)
   haloperidol (Haldol)
   heroin
   isoniazid (INH, Nydrazid)
   marijuana
   medroxyprogesterone (Provera)
   metoclopramide (Reglan)
   oral contraceptives
   phenothiazines
   progestins
   radioisotopes
   rifampin (Rifadin, Rifamate, Rimactane)
   spironolactone (Aldactone)
   testosterone
   thioridazine (Mellaril)
   vitamin A (in excessive dosage)

8. Virilization (acne, hirsutism, lowering of voice, enlargement of clitoris)
   anabolic drugs
   androgens

*See Drug Class, Section Four.

haloperidol (Haldol)
oral contraceptives (lowering of voice)

9. Precocious puberty
estrogens (in hair lotions)
isoniazid (INH, Nydrazid)

TABLE 12

Medicines That May Interact With Alcohol

Alcohol may interact with a wide variety of drugs. The most important problem happens when the depressant action on the brain of sedatives, sleep-inducing drugs, tranquilizers, and narcotic medicines is intensified by alcohol. Alcohol may also reduce drug benefits or lead to toxic effects. Some drugs may increase the intoxicating effects of alcohol, further impairing mental alertness, judgment, coordination, and reaction time.

The intensity and significance can vary greatly from one person to another and from one occasion to another. This is because many factors influence what happens when drugs and alcohol interact. Factors include variations in sensitivity to drugs, the chemistry and quantity of the drug, the type and amount of alcohol consumed, and the sequence in which drugs and alcohol are taken. If you need to use any of the drugs in the following table, ask your doctor for help about alcohol use.

Medicines with which it is advisable to avoid alcohol completely

Drug name or class	Possible interaction with alcohol
amphetamine	excessive rise in blood pressure with alcoholic beverages containing tyramine**
antidepressants	excessive sedation, increased intoxication
barbiturates*	excessive sedation
bromides	confusion, delirium, increased intoxication
calcium carbimide	disulfiram-like reaction**
carbamazepine	excessive sedation
chlorprothixene	excessive sedation
chlorzoxazone	excessive sedation
disulfiram	disulfiram-reaction**
ergotamine	reduced effectiveness of ergotamine
fenfluramine	excessive stimulation of nervous system with some beers and wines
furazolidone	disulfiram-like reaction**
haloperidol	excessive sedation
MAO inhibitors*	excessive rise in blood pressure with alcoholic beverages containing tyramine**
meperidine	excessive sedation
meprobamate	excessive sedation

*See Drug Class, Section Four.
**See Glossary.

Medicines with which it is advisable to avoid alcohol completely (cont.)

Drug name or class	Possible interaction with alcohol
methotrexate	increased liver toxicity and excessive sedation
metronidazole	disulfiram-like reaction**
narcotic drugs	excessive sedation
oxyphenbutazone	increased stomach irritation and/or bleeding
pentazocine	excessive sedation
pethidine	excessive sedation
phenothiazines*	excessive sedation
phenylbutazone	increased stomach irritation and/or bleeding
procarbazine	disulfiram-like reaction**
propoxyphene	excessive sedation
reserpine	excessive sedation, orthostatic hypotension**
sleep-inducing drugs (hypnotics) —carbromal —chloral hydrate —ethchlorvynol —ethinamate —flurazepam —glutethimide —methaqualone —methyprylon —temazepam —triazolam	excessive sedation
thiothixene	excessive sedation
tricyclic antidepressants*	excessive sedation, increased intoxication
trimethobenzamide	excessive sedation

Medicines with which alcohol should be used only in small amounts (use cautiously until combined effects have been determined)

Drug name or class	Possible interaction with alcohol
acetaminophen (Tylenol, etc.)	increased liver toxicity
antiarthritic/anti-inflammatory drugs	increased stomach irritation and/or bleeding
anticoagulants (coumarins)*	increased anticoagulant effect
antidiabetic drugs (sulfonylureas)*	increased antidiabetic effect, excessive hypoglycemia**
antihistamines*	excessive sedation
antihypertensives*	excessive orthostatic hypotension**
aspirin (large doses or continuous use)	increased stomach irritation and/or bleeding
benzodiazepines*	excessive sedation

(continued)

*See Drug Class, Section Four.
**See Glossary.

Medicines with which alcohol should be used only in small amounts (cont.)

Drug name or class	Possible interaction with alcohol
carisoprodol	increased alcoholic intoxication
diethylpropion	excessive nervous system stimulation with alcoholic beverages containing tyramine**
dihydroergotoxine	excessive lowering of blood pressure
diphenoxylate	excessive sedation
dipyridamole	excessive lowering of blood pressure
diuretics*	excessive orthostatic hypotension**
ethionamide	confusion, delirium, psychotic behavior
fenoprofen	increased stomach irritation and/or bleeding
griseofulvin	flushing and rapid heart action
ibuprofen	increased stomach irritation and/or bleeding
indomethacin	increased stomach irritation and/or bleeding
insulin	excessive hypoglycemia**
iron	excessive absorption of iron
isoniazid	decreased effectiveness of isoniazid, increased incidence of hepatitis
lithium	increased confusion and delirium (avoid all alcohol if any indication of lithium overdosage)
methocarbamol	excessive sedation
methotrimeprazine	excessive sedation
methylphenidate	excessive nervous system stimulation with alcoholic beverages containing tyramine**
metoprolol	excessive orthostatic hypotension**
nalidixic acid	increased alcoholic intoxication
naproxen	increased stomach irritation and/or bleeding
nicotinic acid	possible orthostatic hypotension**
nitrates* (vasodilators)	possible orthostatic hypotension**
nylidrin	increased stomach irritation
orphenadrine	excessive sedation
phenelzine	increased alcoholic intoxication
phenoxybenzamine	possible orthostatic hypotension**
phentermine	excessive nervous system stimulation with alcoholic beverages containing tyramine**
phenytoin	decreased effect of phenytoin
pilocarpine	prolongation of alcohol effect
prazosin	excessive lowering of blood pressure
primidone	excessive sedation
propranolol	excessive orthostatic hypotension**
sulfonamides*	increased alcoholic intoxication

*See Drug Class, Section Four.
**See Glossary.

Medicines with which alcohol should be used only in small amounts (cont.)

Drug name or class	Possible interaction with alcohol
sulindac	increased stomach irritation and/or bleeding
tolmetin	increased stomach irritation and/or bleeding
tranquilizers (mild)	excessive sedation
—chlordiazepoxide	
—clorazepate	
—diazepam	
—hydroxyzine	
—meprobamate	
—oxazepam	
—phenaglycodol	
—tybamate	
tranylcypromine	increased alcoholic intoxication

Medicines capable of producing a disulfiramlike reaction when used concurrently with alcohol**

antidiabetic drugs (sulfonylureas)*
calcium carbimide
chloral hydrate
chloramphenicol
disulfiram
furazolidone
metronidazole
nifuroxime
nitrofurantoin
procarbazine
quinacrine
sulfonamides*
tinidazole
tolazoline

*See Drug Class, Section Four.
**See Glossary.

TABLE 13

High-Potassium Foods

Drugs that cause loss of potassium are often used to treat conditions that also require a reduced intake of sodium. The high-potassium foods listed below have been selected for compatibility with a sodium-restricted diet (500 to 1,000 mg of sodium daily). Water pills (diuretics) may also cause loss of magnesium. Make sure magnesium is tested if you take a diuretic and discuss the results with your doctor.

Beverages

orange juice	skim milk	tomato juice
prune juice	tea	whole milk

Breads and Cereals

brown rice	muffins	waffles
cornbread	oatmeal	
griddle cakes	shredded wheat	

Fruits

apricot	fig	orange
avocado	honeydew melon	papaya
banana	mango	prune

Meats

beef	haddock	rockfish
chicken	halibut	salmon
codfish	liver	turkey
flounder	pork	veal

Vegetables

baked beans	parsnips	tomato
lima beans	radishes	white potato
mushrooms	squash	
navy beans	sweet potato	

TABLE 14

Your Personal Drug Profile

I have spoken to countless patients who were sure that they knew how much of their medicines to take, and when to take them, only to learn that they were not only taking the wrong dose, but had also been taking a second medicine too many or too few times a day. Knowing as much as possible about your body and your medicines can save your life. Please take the time to fill out this profile with the latest information. **Medicine never does you any good if you forget to take it. Take control of that chronic disease or condition by finding the goals and taking the medicine.** Also, make time to copy the Medication Map and have your doctor or pharmacist fill it in and discuss it with you. Make sure you work with your doctor to fit your medicines into your life.

Name: _____

Age: _____

Weight in kilograms (pounds divided by 2.2): _____

Height in inches: _____

Prescription drug allergies: _____

_____

Nonprescription drug allergies: _____

_____

Food allergies: _____

_____

My kidneys* are: normal _____

mildly _____   moderately _____   severely _____   compromised.

My liver* is: normal _____

mildly _____   moderately _____   severely _____   compromised.

Conditions or diseases that I have or have had: _____

_____

Prescription and nonprescription medications I take regularly: _____

_____

*Make certain your dose is decreased if the drug is eliminated by an organ (such as the liver or kidneys) with which you have a problem. To determine which organs are involved, refer to the drug profile and, in particular, the Conditions Requiring Adjustments section for each medication you are taking.

Prescription and nonprescription medications I take periodically: _____

_____

I find it very difficult _____ to remember to take medicines.

I find it very easy _____ to remember to take medicines.

I become constipated rarely _____ occasionally _____ never _____.

Urination is usually easy _____ rather difficult _____ difficult _____.

The phone number of the nearest Poison Control Center is _____.

I sleep well _____ OK _____ poorly _____ little _____ on most nights.

I have _____ have never _____ had blood problems in the past.

I am considering becoming _____ might be _____ am _____ pregnant.

I want the medications that offer the best balance of price and outcomes for my specific medical history and present conditions.

TABLE 15

The Medication Map

Getting four new prescriptions often means that you will get four brief patient package inserts or papers stapled to the pharmacy bag when you pick up your prescriptions. Rarely does anyone take the time to understand YOUR INDIVID-UAL day and select medicines based on how your day REALLY works or help you fit the medicines into the way that you actually live. I believe that this is a critical cause of drug interactions, irrational drug combinations, and taking the medicine incorrectly. It also dooms to failure what otherwise might be brilliant use of medicines.

This reality contributes to the more than 100 billion dollars spent EACH YEAR and leads to the more than 100,000 deaths caused by the medicine itself. I can't begin to count the number of times I've found that medicines prescribed three times a day were actually only taken twice a day or less. The cure can easily become the disease.

Use the map below to talk with your doctor or pharmacist to schedule your prescription, nonprescription, or herbal medicines as you really plan or are able to take them. Make sure the timing and combinations are OK! Important questions to ask include:

Have all of these medicines been checked for drug interactions?

Do I really need to take all of these medicines at this time?

Are there newer medicines that might have fewer possible side effects or that might treat the conditions or diseases being treated more effectively (get better results or outcomes)?

Are there medicines that only need to be taken twice or once daily that could be substituted for one or more of those I take now?

Can food react with any of the medicines I take?

Midnight	Medicine and dose planned:	
1 A.M.	Medicine and dose planned:	
2 A.M.	Medicine and dose planned:	
3 A.M.	Medicine and dose planned:	
4 A.M.	Medicine and dose planned:	
5 A.M.	Medicine and dose planned:	
6 A.M.	Medicine and dose planned:	
7 A.M.	Medicine and dose planned:	*Morning Meal Time:*
8 A.M.	Medicine and dose planned:	
9 A.M.	Medicine and dose planned:	
10 A.M.	Medicine and dose planned:	
11 A.M.	Medicine and dose planned:	
12 noon	Medicine and dose planned:	*Lunch or Brunch Time:*
1 P.M.	Medicine and dose planned:	
2 P.M.	Medicine and dose planned:	
3 P.M.	Medicine and dose planned:	
4 P.M.	Medicine and dose planned:	
5 P.M.	Medicine and dose planned:	
6 P.M.	Medicine and dose planned:	*Evening Meal Time:*
7 P.M.	Medicine and dose planned:	
8 P.M.	Medicine and dose planned:	
9 P.M.	Medicine and dose planned:	*Snack Time (if any):*
10 P.M.	Medicine and dose planned:	
11 P.M.	Medicine and dose planned:	

TABLE 16

Medicines Removed from the Market

Once again, either the FDA or the companies that make medicines have seen fit to remove some medicines from the market. I've included prior removals for continuity. While removals could be seen as disconcerting, it also shows that the Phase Four (reporting after a drug is FDA-approved) system sometimes works. This also means that, more than ever, you need to be a partner in your health care! Talk to your doctor right away if you suspect you are having a reaction to one of your medicines. It is literally impossible for the FDA to check EVERY medicine against one that is pending approval for possible drug interactions or side effects. Encourage your doctor to report serious new adverse effects to the company that makes the drug or to the FDA (FDA MedWatch can be reached at 1-800-332-1088). The listings will give the general category to which the medicine belongs, the generic name and at least one brand name, and the reason for removal. While the Web address and location give a rough idea of the date of removal, beginning with the 2002 edition, removals will have the FDA MedWatch removal report date with each new listing.

Antibiotics

grepafloxacin (Raxar)   Reason removed: Risks of adverse effects (abnormal
                               heart rhythms or arrhythmias) outweighed the
                               benefits.
sparfloxacin (Zagam)   Reason removed: Drug interactions, safety profile.

Antidepressant Drugs (Depression Treatments)

nefazodone (Serzone) Reason removed: Declining sales. This medicine was previously removed from the market in several other countries because of liver toxicity. The company voluntarily removed the medicine.

Antidiabetic Drugs (Diabetes Treatments)

troglitazone (Rezulin) Reason removed: Negative publicity regarding liver damage and death precluded effective use of the product. The FDA requested and the company voluntarily removed the medicine.

Antipsoriatic Drugs (Psoriasis Treatments)

etretinate (Tegison) Reason removed: Newer medicines available.

Cholesterol-Reducing Drugs

probucol (Lorelco) Reason removed: More effective medicines available.
cerivastatin (Baycol) Reason removed: Reports of sometimes fatal muscle damage (rhabdomyolysis). FDA MedWatch report date 8/9/01: *www.fda.gov/ medwatch/safety/2001safety01.html#bayco2.*

Gastrointestinal Medicines (GERD, Heartburn)

cisapride (Propulsid) Reason removed: Serious cardiovascular side effects and drug interactions with multiple drugs. More information can be found at *www.fda.gov/medwatch/safety/2000/safety00.htm#propul.*

Herbal Medicines (Various indications and there have been a variety of herbs and herbal products)

Aristolochic Acid (Akebia Trifoliata Caulis-Mu Tong and Asarum Sieboldii Herba cum Radix-Xi Xin) Reason removed: Aristolochic acid has been found to be a potent carcinogen and has been associated with several kidney failure cases. More information can be found at *www.fda.gov/medwatch/safety/2001/ safety01.htm#aristo.*

Ephedra (ma huang remains as part of traditional Chinese medicine (TCM) Reason removed: The benefit-to-risk profile for weight loss was evaluated in the context of the Rand and other reports. Visit *www.fda.gov* and enter Ephedra in the search box.

High Blood Pressure Medicines (Antihypertensives)

mibefradil (Posicor) Reason removed: Serious drug interactions with multiple drugs. More information is at *www.fda.gov/bbs/topice/answers/ans00876.html.*

Immunosuppressant

cyclosporine (Gegraf form only) Reason removed: Found NOT to be bioequivalent to Neoral when mixed with apple juice. More information is at *www.fda.gov.*

Irritable Bowel Syndrome Treatment

alosetron (Lotronex) Reason removed: Voluntarily withdrawn because of serious bowel impactions, ischemic colitis cases, and deaths. More information is available from the FDA at *www.fda.gov*. Subsequently, patient groups started a petition drive to have this medicine **reconsidered** for use in the United States. On June 7, 2002, the FDA announced approval of a supplemental New Drug Application (sNDA) that permitted the marketing of alosetron (Lotronex) with restrictions. Restrictions include a prescribing program for prescribers, restriction to treatment of women with severe diarrhea predominant Irritable Bowel Syndrome (IBS) and who have failed to respond to conventional IBS therapy, patient education, and event reporting as well as assessment of the risk management program and other measures. For more information, go to *www.fda.gov/bbs/topics/NEWS/2002/NEW00814.html*.

Minimally Sedating Antihistamines

astemizole (Hismanal)	Reason removed: Voluntarily withdrawn because of serious drug interactions with multiple drugs. More information is available at *http://www.fda.gov/bbs/topics/answers/ans00961.html*.
terfenadine (Seldane)	Reason removed: Voluntarily withdrawn because of serious drug interactions with multiple drugs. Find more info at: *www.fda.gov/bbs/topics/answers/ans00843.html*.

Vaccines

Rotavirus vaccine (RotaShield)	Reason removed: Withdrawn because it can cause the bowel to collapse or telescope onto itself (intussusception). Find out more at *www.fda.gov*.

Weight Loss Agents (Anorexiants)

dexfenfluramine (Redux)	Reason removed: Possible heart valve damage.
fenfluramine (Pondimin)	Reason removed: Possible heart valve damage. Questions and answers about this can be found at *www.fda.gov/cder/news/fenphenqa2.htm*.

TABLE 17

Helpful, Balanced, and Objective Web Sites

There has been an explosion of information available on the Internet. Unfortunately, like information found elsewhere, all of it is NOT reliable. From my own activities in research, and from my experience with MY Web site, I'm please to augment this new table that tells you about Web sites that I've found to offer balanced, objective, and scientifically rigorous information. I've also added three sites that have been highly rated in a survey by the Rowin Group. Happy surfing, and ALWAYS TALK TO YOUR HEALTH CARE PROVIDER BEFORE YOU CHANGE ANY THERAPY.

To find information on AFFORDING YOUR MEDICINES (many companies have programs based on income for help getting the medicine)

For your doctor or prescriber (sponsored by a Robert Wood Johnson grant): *www.rxassist.org*.

For YOU to fill out a form and find out more about getting your medicine at a reduced price or free: *www.helpingpatients.org.*

For YOU to find out more about companies offering medicines at reduced prices based on income: *www.needymeds.com.*

For YOU to find out more about the new Medicare Prescription Drug Program: *www.medicare.gov.*

To find information on Taking your Medicines (adherence, compliance, or concordance)

www.4woman.gov
www.acog.org
www.nwhn.org
www.fda.gov/womens/tttc.html
www.health.gov/healthypeople
www.medicineinfo.com
www.medscape.com
www.aarp.org
www.talkaboutrx.org
www.americanheart.org/CAP/

To find information on Addiction

www.asam.org
www.samhsa.gov
www.paimed.org

To find information on AIDS

www.amfar.org
www.cdc.org
www.Hopkins-aids.edu

To find information on Anxiety

www.nimh.nih.gov/anxiety

To find information on Arthritis

www.arthritis.org
www.niams.nih.gov
www.rheumatology.org
www.hopkins-arthritis.som.jhmi.edu
www.arthritis.ca/home.html

To find information on Attention Deficit/Hyperactivity Disorder Guidelines

www.pediatrics.org

To find information on Bacteria that have become resistant to treatment

www.fda.gov/oc/opacom/hottopics/anti_resist.html

To find information on Cancer

www.cancer.org
www.clinicaltrials.gov
www.fda.gov/cder/cancer
www.cancertrails.nci.nih.gov
www.fda.gov/bs/topics/NEWS/2001/NEW00766.html
www.cancer.med.upenn.edu

To find information on Colon Cancer

www.cancer.gov/cancerinfo/pdg/treatment/colon/HealthProfessional

To find information on Counterfeit Medicines

www.fda.gov/medwatch/safety/2001/sero_faked.html
www.amgen.com/news/news01/release01510.html
www.gene.com/gene/products/nutropin_aq/product_update.html

To find information on How to Stop Smoking (Cessation)

www.lungusa.org

To find information on Cholesterol-Reducing Drugs

www.americanheart.org
www.americanheart.org/getwiththeguidelines.html
www.acc.org
www.nhlbi.nih.gov

To find information on cold sores (Herpes simplex)

www.coldsource.com

To find highly rated Consumer-Oriented Web sites (breast cancer treatment, heartburn/ulcer treatment, and high cholesterol treatment)

www.nolvadex.com
www.prevacid.com
www.zocor.com

To find the FDA

www.fda.gov

To find information on Health Care Policy and Research

www.ahcpr.gov

To find information on the Heart and Heart Health

www.acc.org
www.americanheart.org
www.clevelandclinic.org
www.mendedhearts.org
www.sln.fi.edu/biosci/heart.html
www.med.yale.edu/library/heartbk/

To find information for Patients and Families After a Heart Attack

www.mendedhearts.org
www.americanheart.org

To find information on Herpes (Genital)

www.denavir.com
www.famvir.com
Herpeshelp: *www.zovirax.com*
www.idsa.org
www.valtrex.com

To find information on Hospital Accreditation

www.jcaho.org

To find High Blood Pressure Medicines (Antihypertensives)

www.americanheart.org
www.cdc.gov
www.acc.org
www.nhlbi.nih.gov
www.nhlbi.nih.gov/hbp
www.nhlbi.nih.gov/guidelines/hypertensoin/index.htm
www.ash-us.org

To find out about Herbal Supplements and Disease/Structure Function Claims and Prudent Steps Regarding Herbals

http://vm.cfsan.fda.gov/;sllrd/fr000106.html
www.talkaboutrx.org

To find information on Guidelines (national)

www.guidelines.gov

To find information on Immunizations (shots)

www.cdc.gov/nip/recs/child-schedule.htm

To find information on Macular Degeneration

www.macular.org
www.maculardegeneration.org
www.maculardisease.org

To find information on Medicines for our Canadian neighbors

www.hc-sc.gc.ca
www.gov.on.ca
www.canadianpainsociety.ca
www.heartandstroke.ca

To find information on Menopause

www.acog.org
www.americanheart.org
www.asrm.org
www.menopause.org
www.4woman.gov

To find out about Nutrition

www.americanheart.org
www.eatright.org

To find out about Osteoporosis

www.nof.org
www.asbmr.org
www.iscd.org
www.strongerbones.org

To find information about Pain and Pain Guidelines

www.ahcpr.gov
www.ampainsoc.org
www.jcaho.org/standard/pm_hap.html

www.painandhealth.org
www.pain.com
www.painmed.org

To find information on Pediatrics

www.aap.org
www.tchin.org

To find information on Pharmacies on the Internet (see VIPPS Seal in the glossary—tells you that a site on the Internet is a valid pharmacy)

www.pharmacyandyou.org

To find information on Pre-diabetes and Diabetes

www.diabetes.org

To find information on Pregnancy and Medicine Effects

www.fda.gov/womens/registries/default.htm

To find information on Reproductive Health/Contraception

www.acog.org
www.amwa.org
www.nwhn.org
www.plannedparenthood.org
www.americanheart.org (as contraception impacts cardiovascular system)

To find information on Research Involving Medicines

www.clinicaltrials.gov

To find information on Rheumatoid Arthritis

The American College of Rheumatology: *www.acr.org*
The Arthritis Foundation: *www.arthritis.org*

To find information on timing for shots (Immunizations)

www.cdc.gov/nip/recs/child-schedule.htm

To find information on Strokes

www.apacure.com
www.strokes.org
www.strokeassociation.org

To find information on Transplantation

www.otf.org

To find information on Health Around the World

www.cdc.gov
www.who.org

To find information on Weight Control

www.americanheart.org/heart_and_stroke_A_Z_guide/obesity.html
www.eatright.org
www.naaso.org

TABLE 18

Smart Patients and Home Test Kits

"You'll need to go to the hospital laboratory and get that checked." I remember telling many patients about blood tests, blood levels, and a variety of other reasons that they would need to have blood taken when I was telling them about their new prescriptions. Fortunately, there has been an explosion of new technology to give the power of checking results from medicines to YOU! This is a wonderful development. Not only does it help save some money in the long run—but it also puts you in the driver's seat. I'll take a hard look at some common diseases or conditions where lab tests are needed in the next edition and will bring you awareness of devices or strategies (some Web or smart card enabled or enhanced) to help make sure you are getting the benefits while avoiding the risks of your medicines. The focus for this edition will be on taking your medicines (adherence)!

To find information on taking your medicines (adherence, compliance, or concordance)

www.4woman.gov
www.acog.org
www.health.gov/healthypeople
www.medicineinfo.com
www.medscape.com
www.aarp.org
www.talkaboutrx.org
www.americanheart.org/CAP/

Very clearly, the group at e-pill has taken a lead role in a range of devices from beeper-based systems to a beeping pill bottle cap that tells you it is time to take control of that disease or condition by taking your medicine! Find out more by visiting *www.epill.com.* **Call them at 1-800-549-0095.**

TABLE 19

Running a Risk: Recognizing and Regaining Control of Heart Disease Risk Factors

The National Cholesterol Education Adult Treatment Panel number three (NCEP ATP III) is without a doubt a blueprint of rational steps to take to control your risk of heart disease. There have been many many reviews of these steps as well as of the risk factors themselves. I'll update this table once the more practical approaches have been sorted out.

For now, there are a number of sites that can help you calculate the 10-year risk of death (based on a large study typically referred to as Framingham). I had the opportunity to meet Joseph Scheese from Scientific Software Tools, Inc., at the recent American Diabetes Association meeting. What Joe showed me was not only the most impressive risk tool I have seen, but it also provided input on important new technologies such as electron beam computed tomography (EBCT—see *www.healthwisecenter.com*) and a host of new risk factors that are also important. Because I think that some of the risk factors will change, I will take the most conservative step of

1) referring you to your doctor to have this very important discussion about heart disease risk factors and preventing heart disease. Clearly, your doctor who has your individual patient history, laboratory results, and results from existing medicines is in the best position to give you the most valuable estimation of risk. There are also a host of emerging risk factors that are important to talk to your doctor about (such as small LDL particles and at least seven different kinds of LDL, HDL subspecies of at least five different kinds, homocysteine, CRP, and apolipoproteins)!

2) referring you to the National Heart, Lung and Blood Institute (NHLBI) at *www.nhlbi.nih.gov*, where the new guidelines were created. The actual guidelines can be seen at *www.nhlbi.nih.gov/guidelines/cholesterol/atp3_rpt.htm*. From the NCEP ATP III report: critical factors to learn more about include: LDL cholesterol, total cholesterol, and HDL cholesterol. Additionally, diabetes, clinical heart disease, peripheral artery disease, carotid artery disease, aneurysm of the abdominal aorta, and people with more than a 20% 10-year risk of MI or CHD death confer high risk for coronary heart disease. Other than LDL, low HDL, family history of premature heart disease, cigarette smoking, blood pressure greater than or equal to 140/90, and even taking medicines for high blood pressure count as added risks, although medicines help control the pressure. Importantly, risk factors that can be changed: the modifiable include inactivity, hypertension, cigarette smoking, being overweight, and having an artery-clogging (atherogenic) diet.

    The factors in the 10-year risk tables that are used to determine heart attack (MI) or CHD death risk as a percentage (based on the data gathered from the Framingham study) are a starting point to help you become a powerful patient in controlling risk: total cholesterol, smoking (please try to quit), HDL, blood pressure, and age (risk increases as we get older).

3) promising you that if there is any way possible to integrate the Scientific Software Tool into my *www.medicineinfo.com* site, I will work with Joe and his colleagues to bring you this important feature!

4) pointing out to you that one of the most important risk factors to emerge in heart disease is called C Reactive Protein (CRP)! A study published in the November 14, 2002, *New England Journal of Medicine* (see Ridker, P.M. in the Sources section) found that bad cholesterol (low density lipoprotein, or LDL) and CRP were very useful in finding people at risk for heart and blood vessel (cardiovascular) problems. More importantly, a researcher named Paul Ridker determined that CRP and LDL determine and define risk for DIFFERENT groups. The way that I think of this is that people with low LDL and CRP are at low risk. People with high levels of LDL and CRP are at high risk. The critical point is that those with low LDL and high CRP are at higher risk for heart and blood vessel problems than people with high LDL and low CRP. This research was of such importance that a new set of guidelines (albeit conservative ones) was released by the American Heart Association for who should be tested for CRP levels. Many of you know that I have a terrible family history for diabetes and heart disease. When I discussed this with my doctor and a CRP was checked, it came back very elevated. Fortunately, a high CRP can be treated effectively. Stains, also known as HMG-CoA reductase inhibitors (see Drug Classes), work very well in this area. Most clinicians would also add on low-dose aspirin as well in order to further decrease risk.

5) encouraging you to go to *www.nhlbi.nih.gov*. Click on Health Assessment Tools. Click on Body Mass Index (BMI) Calculator, and check your body mass index (you'll need height and weight). If you are not in the desired range, talk with your doctor about making a plan over the next year to work on this!

6) encouraging you to go to *www.nhlbi.nih.gov*. Click on Health Assessment Tools. Click on 10-Year Heart Attack Risk Calculator to check your 10-year risk of heart disease (you'll need to know age, gender, smoking history, your total cholesterol, HDL cholesterol, and systolic blood pressure [the first number in a blood pressure—for example, in a 120/80, the 120 is the systolic pressure]). Talk to your doctor about the results and make a clear plan with measurable goals on how you will address the results and lower risk in the future.

TABLE 20

Living Longer (Longevity) with Therapeutic Lifestyle Changes

The NCEP ATP 3 report increased awareness of therapeutic lifestyle changes and how these changes can help YOU control your risk of heart disease! The new high blood pressure guidelines, JNC VII, can be seen at *www.nhlbi.nih.gov/guidelines/hypertension/index.htm*. Once again, LIFESTYLE changes pop up.

Once again, I want to encourage you to be a powerful patient and have a discussion with your doctor about therapeutic lifestyle changes that apply to YOU. Interestingly, the latest guidelines from the National Institutes of Health recommend that doctors *work with patients* to agree on blood pressure goals and to develop a plan for treatment (see Chobanian, A.V. in Sources).

1) You can find the full ATP III guidelines at *www.nhlbi.nih.gov/guidelines/cholesterol/atp3_rpt.htm*. When you make that next appointment with your doctor, make it clear that you want to spend time talking about the ATP III guidelines and therapeutic lifestyle changes! Because of the need to individualize lifestyle changes to YOU and your specific situation, I think this discussion is best undertaken with your doctor.

2) To find the specific general lifestyle changes, please visit the full ATP III guidelines and look specifically at Section FIVE, Parts One through Six. Once again, this is a blueprint for general changes that can (with the help of your doctor, lipid clinic nurse, and specially trained pharmacists) be adjusted specifically to you to get THE BEST POSSIBLE RESULTS. Be a smart patient and use therapeutic lifestyle changes in combination with medicines to be healthier!

3) The current high blood pressure guidelines (JNC VII—see Chobanian, A.V. in Sources) advocate the use of the DASH diet (Dietary Approaches to Stop Hypertension), aerobic exercise, moderate alcohol intake, and lower sodium in order to help control blood pressure. While I know it isn't easy, losing some weight (YOU DON'T HAVE TO DO IT ALL AT ONCE) helps lower risk of diabetes, can help keep prehypertension in an even lower range, and can lower those blood pressure numbers by 5–20 mm of Hg for each 10 kg. The National Heart, Lung, and Blood Institute (NHLBI), from a committee of the NHLBI and National Institutes of Health-NIH, which is called the Coordinating Committee of the NHLBI National High Blood Pressure Education Program (NHBPEP), has consumer-friendly information and resources at *www.nhlbi.nih.gov/hbp*.

For now, even doing more in the sense of exercising, even if you don't lose weight, may make the kind of cholesterol that your body makes change to a more desirable form!

TABLE 21

How to Get Help with the Cost of Medicines (Programs and Web Sites)

"How am I going to afford these medicines?" So many patients have asked me this over the years. I've decided to focus on the issue and identify some strategies, programs, and Web sites that can help! The Medicare Prescription Drug benefit is easing into place. My understanding is that the full program will take shape by 2006. In the meantime, here are some added sources of help.

Strategies:

The immediate problem is affording the medicines actually starts with your doctor.

1) In the office
   a. Ask the price question early. A great study by Blue Cross and Shield (*www.bcbsm.com*) in Michigan found that savings from patients who asked for generics could be more than 50%. Ask your doctor!
   b. Some states offer coverage. Roughly 30 have some kind of benefit at the time of this writing. Visit the National Conference of State Legislatures (*www.ncsl.org/programs/health/drugaid.htm*).
   c. Dual-price substitution. Once the medicine is chosen and the prescription almost written, it's important to ask about the expense. Did you know that sometimes, there are actually different prices for the same medicine? It's true—and it's called dual-price substitution. There are some new office-based programs that your doctor may have that can pick between various brand names to find the best price!
2) Local area on aging (1-800-677-1116) can help with community-based services. Visit the eldercare Web site at *www.eldercare.gov.*
3) Hospital-based programs (social services): While you are still in the hospital, ask your doctor to find out about available social services. So many times, social services can arrive right at the bedside, help with paperwork, and make sense of your situation.
4) The VA. Did you forget that you have a family member who is a vet? It's easy to lose track of the prescription medicine benefit that may be available to YOU. Call the VA at 1-877-222-8387. You can also visit the VA on the web at *www.va.gov.*
5) Controversial strategies: There are so many controversial aspects about going to or ordering medicines (even with a valid prescription) from another country. At the time of this writing, the situation is so fluid that I will only mention that the FDA has a statement on this at *www.fda.gov.*
   a. Canada or Mexico: A service called *www.pharmacychecker.com* appears to give objective information on medicines from these other sources. Membership is $19.95 for a year and $15.00 for a 90-day trial.
6) General information on special programs from the pharmaceutical companies could be a phone call away. Try 1-800-762-4636 or go to the Web at *www.pharma.org.* the new site that I've become aware of is *www.helping-patients.org*

Programs: There are a huge variety of company programs. Some of the companies are:

Abbott Laboratories (see Together Rx Card)

Bristol Myers Squibb Patient Assistance Foundation, Inc.
C/O McKesson P.O. Box 52112
Phoenix, Arizona 85072-2112
Phone: 1-800-736-0003
Fax: 1-800-736-1611
On the Web at: *www.bms.com*

GlaxoSmithKline
On the Web at: *www.togetherrx.com*

Lilly Answers Card
Phone: 1-877-795-4559
On the Web at: *www.lillyanswers.com*

Kos Pharmaceutical:
To contact the company, call: 1-305-577-3464
On the Web at: *www.kospharm.com*

Merck Patient Assistance Program:
To enroll, call: 1-800-727-5400
On the Web at: *www.merck.com/pap/pap/consumer/request_application.jsp*

Monarch Pharmaceutical:
Phone: 1-800-776-3637
Via King Pharmaceutical
On the Web at: *wwwkingpharm.com*

Novartis:
www.togetherrx.com

Pfizer for Living Share Card
To enroll, call: 1-800-717-6005
Fax: 1-800-736-1611
On the Web at: *www.pfizersharecard.com*

Schering Plough SP-Cares Patient Assistance Program:
To enroll, call: 1-800-656-9485
On the Web at: *www.sgp.com/scheringplough/corp/spcares.jsp*

Multiple Company Programs:

Together Rx Card: **Founding members include Abbott Laboratories, Astra Zeneca, Aventis, Bristol-Myers Squibb, GlaxoSmithKline, Janssen Pharmaceutica, Novartis, and Ortho-McNeil Pharmaceutical:**
Medicines covered by this program for the individual companies are shown on the Web at *www.togetherrx.com/allience.html* and are also listed on their individual company Web sites (www dot the name of the company dot com).

Balanced and Objective Web Sites:

www.rxassist.org: This site was started by a group from Brown University that was funded by a Robert Wood Johnson Foundation grant. It was originally intended for doctors, but has a listing of consumer friendly sources that are very helpful.
www.needymeds.com: This site was started by a physician and a nurse who wanted to provide a resource for patients.

www.medicare.gov: Because we finally have a Medicare prescription drug benefit, it certainly makes great sense to visit their site and check up on their progress. At the time of this writing, the program is a collection of medication assistance cards with some additional help available based on income. Visit my site at *www.medicineinfo.com* for more helpful information.

TABLE 22

Important National Guideline: Roadmaps to Success

Guidelines are a snapshot of expert opinion. They are a collective approach—one road that can lead patients to recovery. Medicines relate to guidelines in many senses, but it is crucial to know that study after study shows that despite proven benefits, many patients are NOT getting all of the medicines that they need. Simply put, the guidelines are not being followed. This means that you may not be getting the best chance at preventing a heart attack, stroke, or worsening disease. In order to help you fight this problem, I've created a new section in every profile. For this edition, this table will cover some of the most prevalent medicine families and guidelines that mention them. I expect that this table will grow in coming editions and will help you understand more of the options, evidence base that supports the medicines, and other factors that will help you partner with your doctor to make the best choices!

How to use this new feature: Find your medicine in the book:

1. Go to the beginning of the drug profile and find the section called "Class." For example, aspirin belongs to the pain reliever (analgesic) class and also belongs to the antiplatelet class,
2. Write the class names down. Next go to the Principal Uses section. Write down the principal uses.
3. Next, return to this table and find the class name or the principal use. Underneath the class name or in the principal use disease or condition will be representative guidelines that relate to your medicine! Just a short trip to the Internet will let you read much more on the background of both the guideline and your medicine. For example, the guidelines that relate to aspirin will take you to some pain management guidelines from the American Pain Society. Because aspirin is also used to help prevent heart attacks (by making platelets less likely to form undesirable clots), looking at the antiplatelet class will give you a URL for guidelines on preventing a first or second heart attack!
4. Since this first version of the table is not as broad as it eventually will be: If your condition is not covered in the Essential Eleven, go to *www.guidelines.gov* and enter the disease or condition you are interested in. Another great approach is to go to the national organization that covers the disease or condition (for example, if you are interested in osteoporosis, visit the National Osteoporosis Foundation on the Web at *www.nof.org* and enter "guidelines" in the search engine). For other conditions, follow the same approach, visit the national site for the disease or condition, enter the search term "guidelines" in the search section of the Web site. Some national sites actually have a pull-down or click-on section called guidelines!

An Essential Eleven: Guidelines for common conditions

ADHD
Anxiety
Asthma
Bronchitis, infectious disease, HIV/AIDS
Cancer
Cardiology:
    Antiplatelet medicines
    Heart attacks: primary and secondary
    Hypertension
    Cholesterol
Depression
Diabetes:
    Obesity
Osteoarthritis
Pain
Strokes

To find guidelines on Attention Deficit Hyperactivity Disorder

www.clinicaltrials.gov A source for current research on ADHD. Enter the search term ADHD.
www.guidelines.gov An objective national guideline clearinghouse site. Enter the search term ADHD.

National organizations that are involved:

American Academy of Pediatrics: *www.aap.org*

National Headquarters:	Washington, D.C. Office:
141 Northwest Point Boulevard	Department of Federal Affairs
Elk Grove Village, IL 60007-1098	601 13th Street, NW
USA	Suite 400 North
Phone: 847-434-4000	Washington, DC 20005 USA
Fax: 847-434-8000	Phone: 202-347-8600
Email: (Customer Service: csc@aap.org)	Fax: 202-393-6137
(Practice Guidelines: guidelines@aap.org)	

The National Institute of Mental Health: *www.nimh.nih.gov* (*www.nimh.nih.gov/healthinformation/adhdmenu.cfm*)
Office of Communications
6001 Executive Boulevard, Room 8184, MSC 9663
Bethesda, MD 20892-9663
Phone: 301-443-4513/1-866-615-6464 (toll free)/301-443-8431 (TTY)
Fax: 301-443-4279
Email: *nimhinfo@nih.gov*

Representative current guideline:

Clinical Practice Guideline:
Treatment of the School-Aged Child With Attention-Deficit/Hyperactivity Disorder
Subcommittee on Attention-Deficit/Hyperactivity Disorder and Committee on Quality Improvement
(*Pediatrics* Vol. 108 No 4 October 2001, 1033–1044)

To find guidelines on Anxiety

www.clinicaltrials.gov A source for current research on these medicines; enter "anxiety."
www.guidelines.gov A guideline clearinghouse site; enter "anxiety."

National organizations that are involved:
The National institute of Mental Health: *www.nimh.nih.gov*
Office of Communications
6001 Executive Boulevard, Room 8184, MSC 9663
Bethesda, MD 20892-9663
Phone: 301-443-4513/1-866-615-6464 (toll free)/301-443-8431 (TTY)
Fax: 301-443-4279
Email: nimhinfo@nih.gov

The American Academy of Family Physicians: *www.aafp.org*
11400 Tomahawk Creek Parkway
Leawood, KS 66211-2672
Mailing Address:
P.O. Box 11210
Shawnee Mission, KS 66207-1210
Phone: 800-274-2237/913-906-6000
Email: fp@aafp.org

Representative current guidelines or information:

Anxiety Disorders Five major types: *www.nimh.nih.gov/healthinformation/anxietymenu.cfm*
Major depression, panic disorder, and generalized anxiety disorder in adults in primary care.
Institute for Clinical Systems Improvement-Private Nonprofit Organization. 1996 (revised 2002 May)

To find guidelines on Asthma and Asthma Medicines

www.clinicaltrials.gov A source for current research. Enter the search term asthma.
www.guidelines.gov A guideline clearing house site. Enter the search term asthma.

National organizations that are involved:

U.S. Department of Health and Human Services: *www.cdc.gov/hchs/products/pubs/pubd/hestats/asthma/asthma.htm*
1600 Clifton Road
Atlanta, GA 30333
Phone: 404-639-3311
Public Inquiries: 404-639-3534/800-311-3435

The Agency for Healthcare Research and Quality: *www.ahrq.gov*
540 Gaither Road
Rockville, MD 20850
Phone: 301-427-1364
Email: info@ahrq.gov

Representative current guideline:

National Asthma Education and Prevention Program
Expert panel report: guidelines for the diagnosis and management of asthma
update on selected topics—2002
(*Journal of Allergy Clin Immunol* 2002;110(5suppl):S142–S219.)

To find guidelines on Bronchitis, Infectious disease, and HIV/AIDS

www.clinicaltrials.gov A source for current research on these infections/information categories.
www.guidelines.gov A guideline clearinghouse site. Enter the search term you are interested in.

National organizations that are involved:

The Infectious Disease Society of America (a resource for all of the above infections): *www.idsociety.org*
66 Canal Center Plaza
Suite 600
Alexandria, VA 22314
Phone: 703-299-0200
Fax: 703-299-0204
Email: info@idsociety.org

Representative current guideline:

The University of Chicago: *www.journals.uchicago.edu/IDSA/guidelines*
The Department of Health and Human Services and their AIDSinfo site: *www.aidsinfo.nih.gov/guidelines/default_db2.asp?id=50*

Representative current guideline:

Guidelines for the Use of Antiretroviral Agents in HIV-infected Adults and Adolescents—March 23, 2004
Accessed from *www.aidsinfo.nih.gov* on June 29, 2004.

To find guidelines on Cancer (organized by the location or site of the cancer)

www.clinicaltrials.gov A source for current research on cancer by site (such as breast cancer).
www.guidelines.gov A guideline clearinghouse site. Once again, enter the location or site of the cancer you are interested in.

National organizations that are involved:

The National Comprehensive Cancer Network: *www.nccn.org*
Business & Professional Inquiries
500 Old York Road, Suite 250
Jenkintown, PA 19046
Phone: 215-690-0300
Fax: 215-690-0280

Treatment Guidelines for Patients
888-909-NCCN
888-909-6226

The American Cancer Society: *www.cancer.org*
Phone: 800-ACS-2345 (contact your local chapter)

Representative current guideline(s):

NCCN Breast Cancer Treatment Guidelines for Patients
Supportive Care
NCCN Cancer Pain Treatment Guidelinees Patients

To find guidelines on various aspects of Heart Disease (Cardiology):

Antiplatelet medicines:
www.clinicaltrials.gov A source for current research on these medicines
www.guidelines.gov A guideline clearinghouse site

National organizations that are involved:

The American College of Chest Physicians: *www.chestnet.org*
3300 Dundee Road
Northbrook, IL 60062-2348
847-498-1400/800-343-2227

The American College of Cardiology: *www.acc.org*
Heart House
911 Old Georgetown Road
Bethesda, MD 20814-1699
Phone: 800-253-4636 ext. 694/301-897-5400
Fax: 301-897-9745
Email: (Customer service) resource@acc.org

The American Heart Association: *www.americanheart.org*
National Center
7272 Greenville Avenue
Dallas, TX 75231
Phone: 800-AHA-USA-1/800-242-8721
AHA Professional Membership: 800-787-8984 (outside the United States: 301-223-2307)

Representative current guideline:

Search the specific condition on the national site above:

For example:

Antithrombotic Therapy (will lead to)

Antithrombotic Therapy in Peripheral Arterial Occlusive Disease
(*Chest.* 2001;119:283S-299S)

Heart attacks:
 Preventing a first heart attack (primary prevention)
www.clinicaltrials.gov A source for current research on these medicines
www.guidelines.gov A guideline clearing house site

National organizations that are involved:
The American College of Chest Physicians: *www.chestnet.org*
3300 Dundee Road

Northbrook, IL 60062-2348
847-498-1400/800-343-2227
The American College of Cardiology: *www.acc.org*
Heart House
911 Old Georgetown Road
Bethesda, Maryland 20814-1699
Phone: 800-253-4636 ext. 694/301-897-5400
Fax: 301-897-9745
Email: (Customer service) resource@acc.org

The American Heart Association: *www.americanheart.org*
National Center
7272 Greenville Avenue
Dallas, TX 75231
Phone: 800-AHA-USA-1/800-242-8721
AHA Professional Membership: 800-787-8984 (outside the United States: 301-223-2307)

Representative current guideline:

Search the specific aspect you are looking for. For example:

Primary prevention of heart disease in women
STEMI (a kind of heart attack)

Preventing a second heart attack (secondary prevention)

www.clinicaltrials.gov A source for current research on these medicines
www.guidelines.gov A guideline clearinghouse site

National organizations that are involved:

The American College of Chest Physicians: *www.chestnet.org*
3300 Dundee Road
Northbrook, IL 60062-2348
847-498-1400/800-343-2227

The American College of Cardiology: *www.acc.org*
Heart House
911 Old Georgetown Road
Bethesda, MD 20814-1699
Phone: 800-253-4636 ext. 694/301-897-5400
Fax: 301-897-9745
Email (customer service): resource@acc.org

The American Heart Association: *www.americanheart.org*
National Center
7272 Greenville Avenue
Dallas, TX 75231
Phone: 800-AHA-USA-1/800-242-8721
AHA Professional Membership: 800-787-8984 (outside the United States: 301-223-2307)

Representative current guideline:

Go to *www.americanheart.org* and enter the search term "secondary prevention."

Controlling high blood pressure (Hypertension)

www.clinicaltrials.gov A source for current research on these medicines
www.guidelines.gov A guideline clearing house site

National organizations that are involved:

The National Heart, Lung and Blood Institute (NHLBI): *www.nhlbi.nih.gov*
NHLBI Health Information Center
P.O. Box 30105
Bethesda, MD 20824-0105
Phone:301-592-8573/240-629-3255 (TTY)
Fax: 301-592-8563
Email: nhlbiinfo@nhlbi.nih.gov

The American College of Cardiology: *www.acc.org*
Heart House
911 Old Georgetown Road
Bethesda, MD 20814-1699
Phone: 800-253-4636 ext. 694/301-897-5400
Fax: 301-897-9745
Email (customer service): resource@acc.org

The American Heart Association: *www.americanheart.org*
National Center
7272 Greenville Avenue
Dallas, TX 75231
Phone: 800-AHA-USA-1/800-242-8721
AHA Professional Membership: 800-787-8984 (outside the United States: 301-223-2307)

Representative current guideline:

JNC VII

Controlling abnormal kinds and amounts of Cholesterol

www.clinicaltrials.gov A source for current research on these medicines
www.guidelines.gov A guideline clearinghouse site

National organizations that are involved:

The National Heart, Lung and Blood Institute (NHLBI): *www.nhlbi.nih.gov*
NHLBI Health Information Center
P.O. Box 30105
Bethesda, MD 20824-0105
Phone:301-592-8573/240-629-3255 (TTY)
Fax: 301-592-8563
Email: nhlbiinfo@nhlbi.nih.gov

The American College of Cardiology: *www.acc.org*
Heart House
911 Old Georgetown Road
Bethesda, MD 20814-1699
Phone: 800-253-4636 ext. 694/301-897-5400
Fax: 301-897-9745
Email (customer service): resource@acc.org

The American Heart Association: *www.americanheart.org*
National Center
7272 Greenville Avenue
Dallas, TX 75231
Phone: 800-AHA-USA-1/800-242-8721
AHA Professional Membership: 800-787-8984 (outside the United States: 301-223-2307)

Representative current guideline:
NCEP ATP3
The National Cholesterol Education Program Adult treatment Panel Three

To find guidelines on Depression Medicines

www.clinicaltrials.gov A source for current research on these medicines
www.guidelines.gov A guideline clearinghouse site

National organizations that are involved:

The National Institute of Mental Health and the National Institute of Health:
www.nimh.nih.gov
Office of Communications
6001 Executive Boulevard, Room 8184, MSC 9663
Bethesda, MD 20892-9663
Phone: 301-443-4513/866-615-6464/301-443-8431 (TTY)
Fax: 301-443-4279
Email: nimhinfo@nih.gov

Representative current guideline:

Visit their web site and enter the search term "depression."

To find guidelines on Diabetes Medicines

www.clinicaltrials.gov A source for current research on these medicines
www.guidelines.gov A guideline clearing house site

National organizations that are involved:

The American Diabetes Association: *www.diabetes.org*
ATTN: National Call Center
1701 North Beauregard Street
Alexandria, Virginia 22311
Phone: 800-DIABETES (1-800-342-2383)
Email: AskADA@diabetes.org

The American College of Cardiology (risk factor for heart disease): *www.acc.org*
Heart House
911 Old Georgetown Road
Bethesda, MD 20814-1699
Phone: 800-253-4636 ext. 694/301-897-5400
Fax: 301-897-9745
Email (customer service): resource@acc.org

The American Heart Association (risk factor for heart disease):
www.americanheart.org
National Center
7272 Greenville Avenue
Dallas, TX 75231

Phone: 800-AHA-USA-1/800-242-8721
AHA Professional Membership: 800-787-8984 (outside the United States: 301-223-2307)

Representative current guideline:

The recent update was published in the January 2004 issue of *Diabetes Care*.

To find guidelines on Obesity and being overweight (a risk factor for diabetes)

www.clinicaltrials.gov A source for current research on these medicines
www.guidelines.gov A guideline clearinghouse site

National organizations that are involved:

The National Heart Lung and Blood Institute: *www.nhlbi.nih.gov/guidelines/obesity/ob_home.htm*

NHLBI Health Information Center
P.O. Box 30105
Bethesda, MD 20824-0105
Phone:301-592-8573/240-629-3255 (TTY)
Fax: 301-592-8563
Email: nhlbiinfo@nhlbi.nih.gov

The American Diabetes Association: *www.diabetes.org*
ATTN: National Call Center
1701 North Beauregard Street
Alexandria, Virginia 22311
Phone: 800-DIABETES (1-800-342-2383)
Email: AskADA@diabetes.org

The American Heart Association (various diets for heart patients):
www.americanheart.org
National Center
7272 Greenville Avenue
Dallas, TX 75231
Phone: 800-AHA-USA-1/800-242-8721
AHA Professional Membership: 800-787-8984 (outside the United States: 301-223-2307)

www.nhlbisupport.com/bmi. Body mass index calculator from NHLBI

Representative current guideline:

Visit *www.nhlbi.nih.gov/guidelines/obesity/ob_home.htm*.

To find guidelines on Osteoarthritis (the wear-and-tear kind of arthritis)

www.clinicaltrials.gov The site to search for current studies of osteoarthritis
www.guidelines.gov The site to search for this kind of arthritis

National organizations that are involved:

The American College of Rheumatology: *www.rheumatology.org*
1800 Century Place, Suite 250
Atlanta, GA 30345-4300
Phone: 404-633-3777
Fax: 404-633-1870

The Arthritis Foundation: *www.arthritis.org*
P.O. Box 7669
Atlanta, GA 30357-0669
Phone: 800-283-7800

The Americana Academy of Orthopaedic Surgeons: *www.aaos.org*
6300 North River Road
Rosemont, IL 60018-4262
Phone: 847-823-7186/800-346-AAOS
Fax: 847-823-8125 (Fax on demand 800-999-2939)
Email: Public Inquiries—pemr@aaos.org; Customer Service—custserv@aaos.org

Representative current guideline:

Visit *www.rheumatology.org* and enter the search term "osteoarthritis."

To find guidelines on Pain Management

www.clinicaltrials.gov
www.guidelines.gov

National organizations that are involved:

The American Pain Society: *www.ampnsoc.org*
4700 W. Lake Avenue, Glenview, IL 60025-1485
Phone: 847-375-4715
Fax: 847-375-6315
Email: info@ampainsoc.org

Representative current guideline:

Principles of Analgesic Use in the Treatment of Acute Pain and Cancer Pain
(A National Chapter of the International Association for the Study of Pain.)

To find guidelines on Strokes

www.clinicaltrials.gov The site for clinical studies
www.guidelines.gov The site for guideline searches

National organizations that are involved:

The American College of Chest Physicians: *www.chestnet.org*
3300 Dundee Road
Northbrook, IL 60062-2348
847-498-1400/800-343-2227

The National Stroke Association: *www.stroke.org*
9707 E. Easter Lane
Englewood, CO 80112
Phone: 1–800–STROKES (1–800–787–6537)
AHA Professional Membership: 800-787-8984 (outside the United States: 301-223-2307)

Representative current guideline:

Visit *www.stroke.org* and enter the search term "guidelines."

Sources

The following sources were consulted in the compilation and revision of this book:

Abramowicz, M., ed. *The Choice of Antibacterial Drugs: The Medical Letter on Drugs and Therapeutics.* 1999. New Rochelle, NY: The Medical Letter.

Abramowicz, M., ed. *Drug Interactions: The Medical Letter on Drugs and Therapeutics.* Vol. 41 (issue 1056), July 2, 1999. New Rochelle, NY: The Medical Letter.

Abramowicz, M., ed. *Drugs of Choice: The Medical Letter on Drugs and Therapeutics.* 1997. New Rochelle, NY: The Medical Letter.

Abramowicz, M., ed. *Drugs of Choice: The Medical Letter on Drugs and Therapeutics.* 1999. New Rochelle, NY: The Medical Letter.

Abramowicz, M., ed. *Drugs of Choice: The Medical Letter on Drugs and Therapeutics.* 2001. New Rochelle, NY: The Medical Letter.

Abramowicz, M., ed. *Rofecoxib for Osteoarthritis Pain: The Medical Letter on Drugs and Therapeutics.* Vol. 41 (issue 1056), July 2, 1999. New Rochelle, NY: The Medical Letter.

Abramowicz, M., ed. *Some Drugs That Cause Psychiatric Symptoms: The Medical Letter on Drugs and Therapeutics.* 1998. New Rochelle, NY: The Medical Letter.

Ackerman B.H. and Kasbekar N. Disturbances of Taste and Smell Induced by Drugs. *Pharmacotherapy* 17(3):482–496. 1997.

ACR Cinical Guidelines Committee, ed† C. Guidelines for RA Management. *Arthritis & Rheumatism.* 39; 5:713–722, May 1996.

Adami H.O. and Trichopoulos D. Obesity and Mortality from Cancer. *New England Journal of Medicine.* 2003; 348(17):1623–4.

Adrogue H.J. and Madias N.E. Hyponatremia. *New England Journal of Medicine* 342(21):1581–1589. 2000.

Adult Treatment Panel 3 (ATP III). Third Report of the National Cholesterol Education Program (NCEP) Expert Panel on Detection, Evaluation, and Treatment of High Blood Cholesterol in Adults. June, 2001. The National Institutes of Health.

Advances in Osteoporosis. 1996, 1997.

Agarwala S., et al. Alendronate in the treatment of avascular necrosis of the hip. Rheumatology. 2002; 41:346–357.

AIDS Clinical Care. 1997, 1998, 1999, 2000. Boston: Massachusetts Medical Society.

Albert, C.H., et al. Blood levels of long-chain n-3fatty acids and the risk of sudden death. *New England Journal of Medicine.* 346(15):1113–1118. 2002.

Alikhan R., et al. Risk Factors for Venous Thromboembolism in Hospitalized Patients With Acute Medical Illness: Analysis of the MEDENOX Study. *Arch Intern Med.* 2004; 164:963–968.

Altshuler, L.L., et al. Does thyroid supplementation accelerate tricyclic antidepressant response? A review and meta-analysis of the literature. *American Journal of Psychiatry.* 2001; 158:1617–1622.

Altshuler, L.L., et al. Impact of Antidepressant Discontinuation After Acute Bipolar Depression Remission on Rates of Depressive Relapse at 1-Year Follow-Up. *Am J Psychiatry 2003; 160:1252–1262.*

Amended report from NAMS Advisory Panel on Postmenopausal Hormone Therapy. *Menopause* 2003; 10:6–12.

American Academy of Pediatrics Subcommittee on Attention-Deficit/Hyperactivity Disorder and Committee on Quality Improvement. Clinical Practice Guideline: treatment of the school-aged child with attention-deficit/hyperactivity disorder. *Pediatrics. 2004; 108: 1033–1044.*

American Botanical Society. *The Complete German Commission E Monographs Therapeutic Guide to Herbal Medicines.* 1st ed. 1998. Austin, Texas: American Botanical Council and Integrative Medicine Communications.

American College of Cardiology. ACC/AHA Guideline Update for the Management of Patients with Unstable Angina and NonST-Segment Elevation Myocardial Infarction (NSTEMI). CD-Rom released March, 2002.

American Heart Association. *2001 Heart and Stroke Statistical Update.* Dallas, Texas: American Heart Association, 2000.

American Heart Association. *2002–2003 Heart and Stroke Statistical Update.* Dallas, Texas: American Heart Association, 2001, 2002.

American Heart Association. *Get With the Guidelines.* On www.americanheart.org. Dallas, Texas: American Heart Association, 2001.

American Journal of Clinical Nutrition. Harper, A. E., ed. Physiologically Active Food Components: Their Role in Optimizing Health and Aging. June 2000. Weston, MA.

American Journal of Hospice and Palliative Care. Enk, R., ed. 1998. Weston, MA.

American Medical Association (AMA), Joint Commission on Accreditation of Healthcare Organizations (JCAHO) and the National Committee for Quality Assurance (NCQA). *Coordinated Performance Measurement for the Management of Adult Diabetes.* April 2001, pages 1–42. 2001.

American Pain Society Arthritis Pain Management Panel. *Guidelines for the Management of Pain in Osteoarthritis, Rheumatoid Arthritis, and Juvenile Chronic Arthritis.* American Pain Society, Glenview IL, 2002.

American Pain Society Quality of Care Committee. *Quality Improvement Guidelines for the Treatment of Acute Pain and Cancer Pain.* Journal of the American Medical Association, December 20, 1995, pp. 1874–1880.

American Pharmaceutical Association Special Report: A Review of the Sixth Report of the Joint National Committee on Prevention, Detection, Evaluation, and Treatment of High Blood Pressure. 1998. Washington, DC: American Pharmaceutical Association.

American Psychiatric Association. *American Psychiatric Association Practice Guidelines for the Treatment of Psychiatric Disorders: Compendium 2002.* American Psychiatric Publishing, Inc. Washington, D.C.

Andersen, K., et al. Aspirin non-responsiveness as measured by PFA-100 in patients with coronary artery disease. Thromb Res 2003; 108:37–42.

Anderson, A.S., et al. Current Management of Chronic Heart Failure. *Postgraduate Medicine.* 109(3):35–61. March, 2001.

Andrade, A. and Flexner, C. Genes, Ethnicity, and Efavirenz Response: Clinical Pharmacology Update from the 11th CROI, Hopkins HIV Report, May 2004, 6(3):1–12.

Andre, M., et al. Phase III randomized study comparing 5 or 10 microg per kg per day of filgrastim for mobilization of peripheral blood progenitor cells with chemotherapy, followed by intensification and autologous transplantation in patients with nonmyeloid malignancies. *Transfusion.* 2003 Jan. 43(1):50–7.

Annals of Pharmacotherapy. 1996–1998. Cincinnati, OH: Harvey Whitney Books.

Antman, E.M., and Anbe, D.T.; Armstrong, P.W.; Bates, E.R.; Green, L.A.; Hand, M.; Hochman, J.S.; Krumholz, H.M.; Kushner, F.G.; Lamas, G.A.; Mullany, C.J.; Ornato, J.P.; Pearle, D.L.; Sloan, M.S.; Smith, S.C., Jr. *ACC/AHA Guidelines for the Management of Patients with ST-elevation Myocardial Infarction.* Executive summary: A report of the ACC/AHA Task Force on Practice Guidelines (Committee to Revise the 1999 Guidelines on the Management of Patients with Acute Myocardial Infarction). *Circulation* 2004; 110. *www.acc.org* (accessed July 11, 2004).

Antonicelli, R. et al. Smooth blood pressure control obtained with extended-release felodipine in elderly patients with hypertension: evaluation by 24-hour ambulatory blood pressure monitoring. *Drugs Aging.* 2002; 19(7):541–51.

Aparasu, R.R. and Flinginger, S. E. Inappropriate Medication Prescribing for the Elderly by Office-Based Physicians. *Annals of Pharmacotherapy.* 31:823–836. July/August, 1997.

Arango, C., et al. Olanzapine Effects on Auditory Sensory Gating in Schizophrenia. *Am J Psychiatry.* 2003; 160:2066–2068.

ARRIVE Registry: Advanced Resuscitation of Refractory VT/VF I.V. Amiodarone Evaluation. Accessed from www.Cordarone.com/news/arrive.asp. April, 2003.

Asztalos, B.F., et al. High-density lipoprotein subpopulations in pathologic conditions. *American Journal of Cardiology* 2003 April 3; 91(7A):12E–17E.

Ascott-Evans, B.H., et al. Alendronate prevents loss of bone density associated with discontinuation of hormone replacement therapy. *Archives Internal Medicine 2003.* 163:789–794.

Avorn, J., et al. Persistence of use of lipid-lowering medications: a cross-national study. *JAMA.* 18:1458–62. May 13, 1998.

Bacon, et al. Training and supporting pharmacists to supply progestogen-only emergency contraception. *Journal of Family Planning and Reproductive Health Care* 2003 April, 29(2):17–22

Baigent, C., et al. Selective Cyclooxygenase 2 Inhibitors, Aspirin, and Cardiovascular Disease. *Arthritis & Rheumatism* 48; 1:12–20. January 2003.

Baker, D.E. Pegylated interferon plus ribavirin for the treatment of chronic hepatitis C. *Review in Gastroenterology Discord* Spring 2003; 3(2):93–109.

Balkrishnan, R., et al. Predictors of medication adherence and associated health care costs in an older population with type 2 diabetes mellitus: a longitudinal cohort study. *Clin Ther.* 2003 Nov; 25(11):2958–71.

Ballantyne, C.M., et al. Effect of Ezetimibe Coadministered With Atorvastatin in 628 Patients With Primary Hypercholesterolemia. A Prospective, Randomized, Double-Blind Trial. *Circulation.* April 28, 2003 (epub ahead of print).

Banzer J.A., et al. Results of cardiac rehabilitation in patients with diabetes mellitus. *Am J Cardiol.* 2004 Jan 1; 93(1):81–84.

Barbieri, R.L., et al. Insulin stimulates androgen accumulation in incubations of ovarian stroma obtained from women with hyperandrogenism. *Journal of Clinical Endocrinology and Metabolism* 1986; 62:904–10.

Baron, J.A., et al. Calcium Supplements for the Prevention of Colorectal Adenomas. *New England Journal of Medicine.* 340:101–107. January 14, 1999.

Baron, J.A., et al. A Randomized Trial of Aspirin to Prevent Colorectal Adenomas. *New England Journal of Medicine 2003.* 348:891–899.

Barrett-Connor, E., et al. Raloxifene and cardiovascular events in osteoporotic postmenopausal women: Four-year results from the MORE (Multiple Outcomes of Raloxifene Evaluation) randomized trial. *JAMA Feb. 20, 2002; 287:847–857.*

Barrett-Connor, E., et al. Women and Heart Disease: The Role of Diabetes and Hyperglycemia. *Arch Intern Med* 2004; 164:934–942.

Bartlett, J. *The Johns Hopkins Hospital 1996 Guide to Medical Care of Patients with HIV Infection.* Baltimore: Williams and Wilkins.

Bartlett, J. *Medical Management of HIV Infection: 1998 Edition.* Baltimore: Port City Press.

Bartlett, J., et al. *The Hopkins HIV Report.* Volume 13, Number 3 (Updated Guidelines for Managing HIV in Pregnancy From the USPHS Task Force and Update from the 8th CROI: Adverse Effects of HAART and Structured Treatment Interruption, Number 4. The Johns Hopkins University AIDS Service, Division of Infectious Diseases. 2001.

Bartlett, J.G. and Gallant, J.E. 2000–2001 *Medical Management of HIV Infection.* Baltimore: Port City Press.

Bartlett, J.G. and Gallant, J.E. 2003 *Medical Management of HIV Infection.* Johns Hopkins University, Baltimore.

Bates, D., et al. Effect of Computerized Physician Order Entry and a Team Intervention on Prevention of Serious Medication Errors. *Journal of the American Medical Association.* 280(15):1311–1316. October 21, 1998.

Bays, H., et al. *The ADVOCATE Study.* The 51st Scientific Session of the American College of Cardiology National Meeting. Atlanta, GA, March 2002.

Beard, S.L. HMG-CoA Reductase Inhibitors: Assessing Differences in Drug Interactions and Safety Profiles. *Journal of the American Pharmaceutical Association Sept/Oct 2000.* 40(5):637–644. 2000.

Beckman, S.E., et al., Consumer Use of St. John's Wort: A Survey on Effectiveness, Safety and Tolerability. *Pharmacotherapy 2000.* 20(5):568–574. 2000.

Beebe, L.H. Health Promotion in Persons with Schizophrenia: Atypical Medications. *J Am Psychiatr Nurses Assoc 2003. 9,115–122.*

Belch, J.J., et al. Critical issues in peripheral arterial disease detection and management: a call to action. *Archives of Internal Medicine* 2003:163(8)884–892.

Bell, N.H., et al. Alendronate Increases Bone Mass and Reduces Bone Markers in Post-menopausal African-American Women. *Journal of Clinical Endocrinology and Metabolism* June 2002, 87(6):2792–2797.

Berchou, R.C. and Scheife, R.T. Contemporary Issues in the Pharmacotherapy of Parkinson's Disease. *Pharmacotherapy the Journal of Human Pharmacology and Drug Therapy.* Vol. 20, No. 1 Part 2, January, 2000.

Berger, K., et al. Light-to-Moderate Alcohol Consumption and the Risk of Stroke Among U.S. Male Physicians. *New England Journal of Medicine.* 341(21):1557. November 18, 1999.

Berkow, R., ed. *The Merck Manual.* 15th ed. 1996. Rahway, NJ: Merck, Sharp, and Dohme Research Laboratories.

Berthold-Gouni, I. and Berthold, H.K. Policosanol: Clinical pharmacology and therapeutic significance of a new lipid-lowering agent. *American Heart Journal.* 2002; 143:356–365.

Bittner, V. Treatment of dyslipidemia in pre- and postmenopausal women with and without known atherosclerotic cardiovascular disease. *Current Cardiology Report 2001 Sept; 3(5):401–407.*

Black, C. and Jick, H. Etiology and Frequency Rhabdomyolysis. *Pharmacotherapy* 2002; 22(12):1524–1526.

Black, D., et al. The Effects of Parathyroid Hormone and Alendronate Alone or in Combination in Postmenopausal Osteoporosis. *The New England Journal of Medicine.* 349:13. Sept 2003.

Black, S., et al. Efficacy, safety and immunogenicity of heptavalent pneumococcal conjugate vaccine in children. *Pediatric Infections Disease Journal* 2000; 19(3):187–195.

Blair, S.N., et al. Incremental Reduction of Serum Total Cholesterol and Low-Density Lipoprotein Cholesterol With the Addition of Plant Stanol Ester-Containing Spread to Statin Therapy. *Journal of the American College of Cardiology.* 86(1):46–52. 2000.

Bloch, Y., et al. Hyperglycemia from olanzapine treatment in adolescents. *Journal of Child and Adolescent Psychopharmacology.* 2003 Spring; 13(1):97–102.

Bone, H.G. Ten Years' Experience with Alendronate for Osteoporosis in Postmenopausal Women. *New England Journal of Medicine 2004 March; 12(350):1189–1199.*

Bonnick, S. L. *The Osteoporosis Handbook.* 1994. Dallas: Taylor Publishing.

Boothby, L.A. and Doering, P.L. FDA Labeling System for Drugs in Pregnancy. *The Annals of Pharmacotherapy.* Vol. 35, No. 11, November 2001.

Borenstein, D. *Back in Control: A Conventional and Complimentary Prescription for Eliminating Back Pain.* M. Evans, New York. 2001.

Bosch, J., et al. Use of ramipril in preventing stroke: double blind randomised trial. *British Medical Journal.* 2002; 324:699–703.

Boton, R., et al. Prevalence, pathogenesis and treatment of renal dysfunction associated with chronic lithium therapy. *American Journal of Kidney Diseases* 1987; 10(5):329–45.

Boullata, J.I. and Nace, A.M. Safety Issues with Herbal Medicine. *Pharmacotherapy: The Journal of Human Pharmacology and Drug Therapy.* 20(3):257–269. 2000.

Bowden, C.L. A Placebo-Controlled 18-Month Trial of Lamotrigine and Lithium Maintenance Treatment in Recently Manic or Hypomanic Patients with Bipolar I Disorder. *Archives of General Psychiatry* April 2003; 60:392–400.

Bowes, J. Concomitant Administration of Drugs Known to Decrease the Systemic Availability of Gatifloxacin. *Pharmacotherapy* 2002; 22(6):800–801

Braunstein, J.B. Tight control: The risk-versus-benefit game. *Diabetes Forecast.* April 1, 2002. Accessed from the American Diabetes Association web site at *www.diabetes.org.*

Braunwald, E., et al. ACC/AHA Guidelines for the Management of Patients with Unstable Angina and Non-ST-Segment Elevation Myocardial Infarction. *Journal of the American College of Cardiology vol. 36, 2000: 970–1062.*

Braunwald, E. Application of current guidelines to the management of unstable angina and non-ST-elevation myocardial infarction. *Circulation.* 2003 Oct 21;108(16 suppl 1): III28–37.

Braunwald, E., et al. ACC/AHA Guidelines for the Management of Patients with Unstable Angina and Non-ST-Segment Elevation Myocardial Infarction. CD-Rom distributed at March, 2002 ACC meeting.

Bressan, R.A., et al. Is Regionally Selective D2/D3 Dopamine Occupancy Sufficient for Atypical Antipsychotic Effect? An In Vivo Quantitative [123 I] Epidepride SPET Study of Amisulpride-Treated Patients. *Am J Psychiatry* 2003; 160:1413–1420.

Briggs, G.G., Bodendorfer, T.W., Freeman, R.K., and S.J. Yaffee. *Drugs in Pregnancy and Lactation.* 1983. Baltimore: Williams and Wilkins.

Brodaty, H., et al. A Randomized Placebo-Controlled Trial of Risperidone for the Treatment of Aggression, Agitation and Psychosis of Dementia. *Journal of Clinical Psychiatry* 2003; 64:134–143.

Brooke, M.H. *A Clinician's View of Neuromuscular Diseases.* 2nd ed. 1986. Baltimore: Williams and Wilkins.

Bull, S.A., et al. Discontinuing or Switching Selective Serotonin-Reuptake Inhibitors. *The Annals of Pharmacotherapy* 2002; 36:578–584.

Burke, L. E. and Ockene, I. S. *Compliance in Healthcare and Research.* The American Heart Association. Futura Publishing Company, Armonk, NY 2000.

Business Wire: June 28, 2001. Roche and Trimeris Correct Previous Announcement on Complete Enrollment in T-20 Phase III Clinical Trial. Nutley, NJ and Durham, NC.

Buttgereit, F., et al. Standardised nomenclature for glucocorticoid dosages and glucocorticoid treatment regimens: current questions and tentative answers in rheumatology. *Annals of Rheumatological Diseases* 2002; 61:718–722.

Cabana, M.D., et al. Why Don't Physicians Follow Clinical Practice Guidelines? A Framework for Improvement. *Journal of the American Medical Association,* 282:1458–1465.

Calabrese, L.H. Molecular differences in anticytokine therapies. *Clinical and Experimental Rheumatology.* 2003 Mar–Apr; 21(2):241–8.

Califf, R.M., et al. Underuse of aspirin in a referral population with documented coronary artery disease. *American Journal of Cardiology* 2002; 89:653–661.

Calle, E.E., et al. Overweight, Obesity and Mortality from Cancer in a Prospectively Studied Cohort of US Adults. *New England Journal of Medicine* 2003; 348(17):1625–1638.

Canadian Pharmaceutical Association, St. Paul's Hospital British Columbia Center of Excellence for HIV-AIDS. 1997, 1998. Vancouver, BC: Canadian Pharmaceutical Association.

Cannon, C.P., Braunwald, E., McCabe, C.H., et al. Intensive versus Moderate Lipid Lowering with Statins after Acute Coronary Syndromes. *New Engl J Med* 2004 April; 350(15): 1495–1504.

Cape, R. *Aging: Its Complex Management.* 1978. Hagerstown, MD: Harper and Row.

CAPRIE Steering Committee. A randomised, blinded trial of clopidogrel versus aspirin in patients at risk of ischaemic events (CAPRIE). Lancet 1996; 348:1329–1339.

Caring for the Dying. 1996. American Board of Internal Medicine.

Carmona, R., et al. Pharmacological Treatment of Social Anxiety Disorder. *Essent Psychopharmacol* 5:3, 2003, 141–155.

Carnahan, R.M., et al. Ziprasidone, a New Atypical Antipsychotic Drug. *Pharmacotherapy* 2001; 21(6):717–730. 2001.

Caron, M.F., and White, M. Evaluation of the Antihyperlipidemic Properties of Dietary Supplements. *Pharmacotherapy* 2001; 21(4):481–487. 2001.

Centorrino, F., et al. Pilot Comparison of Extended- Release and Srandard Perpartions of Divalproex Sodium in Patients With Bipolar and Schizoaffective Disorders. *Am J Psychiatry 2003; 160:1348–1350.*

Cha, J.K., et al. Changes in platelet p-selectin and in plasma C-reactive protein in acute atherosclerotic ischemic stroke treated with a loading dose of clopidogrel. *Journal of Thrombosis and Thrombolysis* 2002 Oct; 14(2):145–50.

Chan, A.W., Chew, D.P., et al. Relation of inflammation and benefit of statins after percutaneous coronary interventions. *Circulation* 2003. (Accessed at *circulation* on line November 2003).

Chan, F.K.L., et al. Celecoxib Versus Diclofenac and Omeprazole in Reducing the Risk of Recurrent Ulcer Bleeding in Patients with Arthritis. *New England Journal of Medicine* 2002; 347(26):2104–2110.

Chavez, M.L. Natural Medicines An Evidence-Based Approach. *The Rx Consultant.* 11(1): 1–8. 2001.

Cheng, J.W.M., et al. Patient-Reported Adherence to Guidelines of the Sixth Joint National Committee on Prevention, Detection, Evaluation and Treatment of High Blood Pressure. *Pharmacotherapy* 2001; 21(7):828–841. 2001.

Cheshire, W.P. Defining the Role for Gabapentin in the Treatment of Trigeminal Neuralgia: A Retrospective Study. *The Journal of Pain* 2002; 3(2):137–142. 2002.

Chin, R.L., et al. Etanercept (Enbrel®) therapy for chronic inflammatory demyelinating polyneuropathy. *J Neurol Sci.* 2003 June 15; 210(1–2):19–21.

Chlebowski, R.T., et al. Influence of Estrogen Plus Progestin on Breast Cancer and Mammographyin Healthy Postmenopausal Women. *Journal of the American Medical Association* 2003; 289:3243–3253.

Chobanian, A.V., et al. The Seventh Report of the Joint National Committee on Prevention, Detection, Evaluation and Treatment of High Blood Pressure. *Journal of the American Medical Association* 2003; 289: (DOI 10.1001/jama.289.19.2560), Early Release Article posted May 14, 2003.

Choi, S.L., et al. The American Diabetes Association 63rd Scientific Sessions. Chicago, 2003.

Chow, C.C., et al. Oral Alendronate Increases Bone Mineral Density in Postmenopausal Women with Primary Hyperparathyroidism. *Journal of Clinical Endocrinology and Metabolism,* Feb 2003, 88(2):581–587.

Cice, G., et al. Sustained-release diltiazem reduces myocardial ischemic episodes in end-stage renal disease: a double-blind, randomized, crossover, placebo-controlled trial. *Journal of the American Society of Nephrology.* 2003 Apr; 14(4):1006–11.

Classen, D.C., et al. Adverse Drug Events in Hospitalized Patients. *Journal of the American Medical Association.* 277:301–306. 1997.

Clin-Alert. 1996–1997. Medford, NJ: Clin-Alert.

Clinisphere. Facts and Comparisons 2.0. 1999. St. Louis: Facts and Comparisons.

Cohen, J.D. PREDICT study results of a simulated study with OTC Pravachol. *Paper presentation: American Society for Clinical Pharmacology and Therapeutics.* Atlanta, GA. March 24, 2002.

Cohen, M.M., et al. Emergency contraception: models to increase accessibility. *Journal of Obstetrics and Gynecology of Canada.* 2003 Jun: 25(6):499–504.

Compendium of Pharmaceuticals and Specialties. 26th ed. 1991. Ottawa: Canadian Pharmaceutical Association.

Conroy, W.E., et al. Lipid Screening in Adults. Working to prevent coronary artery disease. *Postgraduate Medicine.* 107(4):229–235. April, 2000.

Considerations for Antiretroviral Therapy in Women, HIV/AIDS Treatment Information Service. National Library of Medicine. February 4, 2002. Accessed from *www.hivatis.org* June 23, 2002.

Cooper, S.M. Improving Outcomes in Osteoarthritis. *Postgraduate Medicine.* 105(6):29–38. 1999.

Coull, B.M., et al. Anticoagulants and Antiplatelet Agents in Acute Ischemic Stroke. *Stroke* 2002;33:1934.

Cranor, C.W., Barry, B.A., Christensen, D.B. The Asheville Project: Long-Term Clinical and Ecomomic Outcomes of a Community Pharamcy Diabetes Care Program. *J Am Pharm Assoc.* 2003; 43:173–84.

Cranor, C.W., Christensen, D.B. The Asheville Project: Short-Term Outcomes of a Community Pharmacy Diabetes Care Program. *J Am Pharm Assoc.* 2003; 43:149–59.

Cranor, C.W. The Asheville Project: Long-Term Outcomes of a Community Pharmacy Diabetes Care Program. *Journal of the American Pharmaceutical Association, March/April* 2003, Vol. 43, No. 2.

Cromwell, W.C. and Ziakja, P.E. Development of tachyphylaxis among patients taking HMG CoA reductase inhibitors. *American Journal of Cardiology 2000; 86:1123–1127.*

Crouse, J.R., et al. A Randomized Trial Comparing the Effect of Casein With That of Soy Protein Containing Varying Amounts of Isoflavones on Plasma Concentrations of Lipids and Lipoproteins. *Archives of Internal Medicine* 159: 2070–2076. September 27, 1999.

Cumming, R.G., et al. Use of Inhaled Corticosteroids and the Risk of Cataracts. *New England Journal of Medicine.* 337(1):8–14. 1997.

Cunnane, G., et al. Infections and biological therapy in rheumatoid arthritis. *Best Practice Residency of Clinical Rheumatology.* 2003 April; 17(2):345–63.

Cunningham, C.K., et al. Development of resistance mutations in women on standard antiretroviral therapy who received intrapartum nevirapine to prevent perinatal HIV-1 transmission: a substudy of Pediatric AIDS Clinical Trials Group Protocol 316. *Journal of Infectious Diseases* 2002 (in press at the time of this writing).

Cupp, M.J. Herbal Remedies: Adverse Effects and Drug Interactions. *American Family Physician.* 59(5):1239–1244. 1999.

Dahlof, B., et. al. Cardiovascular morbidity and mortality in patients with diabetes in the Losartan Intervention For Endpoint reduction in hypertention study (LIFE): a randomized trial against atenolol. *The Lancet.* 359(9311): March 23, 2002. Accessed from *www.lancet.com* March 24, 2002.

Daniels, J.B., ed. *Infectious Disease in Clinical Practice.* 1997. Baltimore: Williams and Wilkins.

Davis, E.A. and Pathak, D.S. Psychometric Evaluation of Four HIV Disease-Specific Quality-of-Life Instruments. *Annals of Pharmacotherapy.* 159:546–552. May, 2001.

Davis, S.M., et al. Statistical Approaches to Effectiveness Measurement and Outcome-Driven Re-Randomizations in the Clinical Antipsychotic Trials of Intervention Effectiveness (CATIE) Studies. *Schizophrenia Bulletin* 29(1):73–80, 2003.

DeBattista, C. and Solvason, H.B. When the First SSRI Fails:A Review of Switching Strategies in Patients Resistant to an Initial SSRI. *Esssent Psychopharmacol* 5:3, 2003, 217–224.

De Deyn, P.P., et al. A randomized trial of risperidone, placebo, and haloperidol for behavioral symptons of dementia. *Neurology* 1999; 53:946–955.

De Koning, J.S., et al. Deprivation and systematic stroke prevention in general practice: an audit among general practitioners in the Rotterdam region, The Netherlands. *Eur J Public Health.* 2003 Dec; 13(4):340–6.

Depression in Primary Care. Volume 1: Detection and Diagnosis. 1993. Washington, DC: U.S. Department of Health and Human Services.

DeRosier, J., et al. Using Health Care Failure Mode and Effect Analysis. The Joint Commission of Accreditation of Healthcare Organizations, Chicago, IL, 2002.

Diabetes Control and Complications Trial (DCCT). The effect of intensive treatment of diabetes on the development and progression of long-term complications in insulin-dependent diabetes mellitus. *New England Journal of Medicine 1993; 329:977–986.*

Diabetes Control and Complication Trial. Retinopathy and Nephropathy in Patients with Type 1 Diabetes Four Years After a Trial of Intensive Therapy. *The New England Journal of Medicine.* 342(6):381–389. February 10, 2000.

Digoxin Investigation group (DIG) as accessed June, 2003. *Journal of the American Medical Association 2003.* 289:871–878.

DiGregorio, J.G., et al. *Handbook of Pain Management.* 1991. Westchester, NY: Medical Surveillance.

Digwood-Lettieri, S., et al. Levofloxacin-Induced Toxic Epidermal Necrolysis in an Elderly Patient. *Pharmacotherapy* 2002; 22(6):789–793.

Dodds Ashley, E.S., et al. Patient Detection of a Drug Dispensing Error by Use of Physician-Provided Drug Samples. *Pharmacotherapy* 2002; 22(12):1642–1643.

Dorian, P., et al. Amiodarone as Compared with Lidocaine for Shock-Resistant Ventricular Fibrillation. *New England Journal of Medicine.* 346(12):884–890. 2002.

Douglas, J.G., et al. Management of High Blood Pressure in African Americans. *Arch Intern Med* 2003; 163(5):525–541.

Douketis, J.D., et al. Low-Molecular-Weight Heparin as Bridging Anticoagulation During Interruption of Warfarin: Assessment of a Standardized Periprocedural Anticoagulation Regimen. *Arch Intern Med.* 2004; 164:1319–1326.

Drazen J.M. Inappropriate Advertising of Dietary Supplements. *New England Journal of Medicine* 2003; 348(9):777–8.

Drug Information Journal. 1996–1998.

Drug Interactions Newsletter. 1997. Spokane, WA: Applied Therapeutics.

DrugLink. 1998. St. Louis: J. B. Lippincott, Facts and Comparisons.

Drug Newsletter. 1998. St. Louis: J. B. Lippincott, Facts and Comparisons.

Drugs and Therapy Perspectives. 1996–1997.

Drug Therapy: Physicians Prescribing Update. 1992. Lawrenceville, NJ: Excerpta Medica.

Dukes, M.N.G., ed. *Meyler's Side Effects of Drugs.* 11th ed. 1988. Amsterdam: Excerpta Medica.

Eastell, R., et al. Treatment of Postmenopausal Osteoporosis. *New England Journal of Medicine.* 338(11):736–746. 1998.

Eikelboom, J.W., Hankey, G.J. Aspirin resistance: a new independent predictor of vascular events? *Journal of the American College of Cardiology.* 2003. Mar 19; 41(6):966–968.

Eikelboom, J.W., Hirsh, J., et al. Aspirin-resistant thromboxane biosynthesis and the risk of myocardial infarction, stroke or cardiovascular death in patients at high risk for cardiovascular events. *Circulation* 2002 (accessed at www.circulationaha.org).

Elhilali, M.M., Nickel, J.C. Benign prostatic hyperplasia: from A-Z. *Canadian Journal of Urology.* 2003 Apr; 10(2):1799–802.

Epstein, F. H., et al. Acute-Phase Proteins and Other Systemic Responses to Inflammation. *New England Journal of Medicine.* 340(6):448–454. February 11, 1999.

Erkinjuntti, T., et al. Efficacy of galantamine in probable vascular dementia and Alzheimer's disease combined with cerebrovascular disease: a randomised trial. *The Lancet 2002.* April 13. 359:1283–1290.

Ernst, E. The Risk-Benefit Profile of Commonly Used Herbal Therapies: Ginkgo, St. John's Wort, Ginseng, Echinacea, Saw Palmetto and Kava. *Annals of Internal Medicine 2002.* 136: 42–53.

Erramouspe, J. and Heyneman, A. Treatment and Prevention of Otitis Media. *The Annals of Pharmacotherapy.* 34:1452. 2001.

Eskola, J., et al. Efficacy of a pneumococcal conjugate vaccine against acute otitis media. *New England Journal of Medicine* 2001; 344(6):403–409.

Essock, S.M., et al. Randomized Controlled Trials in Evidence-Based Mental Health Care: Getting the Right Answer to the Right Question. *Schizophrenia Bulletin* 20(1):115–123, 2003.

Farrell, B., and B. Farrell, eds. *Pain in the Elderly.* 1996. International Association for the Study of Pain Press.

Fathi, R., et al. A randomized trial of aggressive lipid reduction for improvement of myocardial ischemia, symptom status, and vascular function in patients with coronary artery disease not amenable to intervention. *American Journal of Medicine* 2003 Apr 15; 114(6):445–53.

Favus, M., ed. *Primer on the Metabolic Bone Diseases and Disorders of Mineral Metabolism.* 3rd ed. 1996. Philadelphia, New York: Lippincott-Raven.

FDA Arthritis Advisory Committee Hearing. February 7, 2001; Gaithersburg, MD.

FDA Drug Bulletin. 1996–1997. Rockville, MD: Department of Health and Human Services, Food and Drug Administration.

FDA News. July 16, 2003. FDA Announces Intiative to Heighten Battle Against Counterfeit Drugs. Rockville, MD: Department of Health and Human Services, Food and Drug Administration (http://www.fda.gov/bbs/to[pics/NEWS/2003/NEW00926.html).

FDA News Digest. July 16, 2001. Guidance on Levothyroxine Sodium Products. Rockville, MD: Department of Health and Human Services, Food and Drug Administration.

FDA Summary. April, 2002. ACTOS [pioglitazone HCl]; AVANDIA [rosiglitazone maleate].

FDA Talk Paper T02–18. April 11, 2002. FDA Approves New Indication and Label Changes for the Arthritis Drug, Vioxx. Food and Drug Administration, Rockville, MD.

FDA Talk Paper T03–39. May 27, 2003. WHIMS Study on Estrogen/Progestin. Food and Drug Administration, Rockville, MD.

Ferguson, T.B., et al. Preoperative B-blocker use and mortality and morbidity following CABG surgery in North America. *Journal of the American Medical Association.* 287(17): 2221–2227. May 1, 2002.

Finkelstein, J.S., et al. Effects of Parathyroid Hormone, Alendronate, or Both on Bone Density in Osteoporotic Men. *Presentation Number: 1007*.ASBMR: 24TH Annual Meeting 2003.

Fischer, M.A., and Avorn, J. Economic consequences of underuse of generic drugs: evidence from Medicaid and implications for prescription drug benefit plans. *Health Serv Res*. Aug 2003. 38(4): 1051–63.

Fitzgerald, G.A., and Patrono, C. The Coxibs, Selective Inhibitors of Cyclooxygenase-2. *The New England Journal of Medicine*. August 9, 2000. Vol 345(6). Content.*nejm.org/cgi/content/short/345/6/433*.

Fleischhacker, W.W., et al. Treatment of Schizophrenia With Long-Acting Injectable Risperidone: A 12-month Open-Label Trial of the First Long- Acting Second-Generation Antipsychotic. *J Clin Psychiatry* 64:10, October 2003,1250–1257.

Fonseca, V., et al. Addition of nateglinide to rosiglitazone monotherapy suppresses mealtime hyperglycemia and improves overall glycemic control. *Diabetes Care*. 2003 Jun; 26(6):1685–90.

Frackiewicz, Edyta J. Endometriosis: An Overview of the Disease and Its Treatment. *Journal of the American Pharmaceutical Association*. Vol. 40, No. 5, September/October 2000.

Frackiewicz, E. J., and Cutler, N. Women's Health Care During the Perimenopause. *Journal of the American Pharmaceutical Association*. Vol. 40, No. 6. November/December 2000.

Francis, G.S., ed. *The Cleveland Clinic Heart Advisor*. 3(4):3. 2000.

Fraunfelder, F. T. Drug-Induced Ocular Side Effects and Drug Interactions. 3rd ed. 1989. Philadelphia: Lea and Febiger.

Freedman, R. Schizophrenia. *N Engl Med* 2003; 349:1738–49.

Frick, A., et al. Omeprazole reduces clozapine plasma concentrations—a case report. *Pharmacopsychiatry*. 2003 May; 36(3):121–3.

Gandhi, T.K., et al, Adverse Drug Events in Ambulatory Care. *New England Journal of Medicine* 2003; 348:1556–64.

Ganju, V. Implementation of Evidence-Based Practices in State Mental Systems: Implications for Research and Effectiveness Studies. *Schizophrenia Bulletin* 29(1):125–131, 2003.

Ganz, D.A., et al. Adherence to guidelines for oral anticoagulation after venous thrombosis and pulmonary embolism. *J Gen Intern Med*. 2000 Nov; 15(11):776–81.

Gardiner, S.J., et al. Transfer of Olanzapine into Breast Milk, Calculation of Infant Drug Dose, and Effect on Breast-Fed Infants. *Am J Psychiatry* 2003; 160:1428–1431.

Garg, R.K., and Sorrentino M.D., Beta blockers for CHF. *Postgraduate Medicine*. 109(3): 49–57. 2001.

Garrett, G.D., Martin, A.L. The Asheville Project:Participants' Perceptions of Factors Contributing to the Success of a Patient Self-Management Diabetes Program. *J Am Pharm Assoc. 2003; 43:185–90*.

Geber, J., et al. Optimizing Drug Therapy in Patients with Cardiovascular Disease: The Impact of Pharmacist-Managed Pharmacotherapy Clinics in a Primary Care Setting. *Pharmacotherapy* 2002; 22(6):738–747.

Geddes, J. Generating Evidence to Inform Policy and Practice: The Example of the Second Generation "Atypical" Antipsychotics. *Schizophrenia Bulletin* 29(1):105–114, 2003.

Generali, M.S., ed., et al. *Clini-Alert Reporting on Adverse Clinical Events*. 38(7):1–8. 2000.

Gerberding, J.L. Occupational Exposure to HIV in Health Care Settings. *New England Journal of Medicine* 2003; 348(9):826–33.

Ghandi, S.K., et al. The Pathogenesis of Acute Pulmonary Edema Associated with Hypertension. *New England Journal of Medicine* 344(1):17–22. January 4, 2001.

Gilbert, D.L., et al. Tic reduction with pergolide in a randomized controlled trial in children. *Neurology 2003*. Feb 25; 60(4):606–611.

Ginsberg, H.N. Treatment for patients with the metabolic syndrome. *American Journal of Cardiology* 2003 Apr 3; 91(7A):29E-39E. Review.

Glasser, S.P., et al. Bedtime dosing of diltiazem. *52nd* Scientific Session of the American College of Cardiology 2003 March 30, 2003. Chicago.

Glassman, A.H., et al. Sertraline treatment of major depression in patients with acute MI or unstable angina. *JAMA 2002*. 288 (6):701–709.

Gleason, P.P., et al. Medical Outcomes and Antimicrobial Costs With the Use of the American Thoracic Society Guidelines for Outpatients With Community Acquired Pneumonia. *Journal of the American Medical Association*. 278 (1):32–39. 1997.

Gloth, M.J. Treatment of Pain in Older Patients. *Patient Care.* March 30, 1999: 62–68.

Goldman, S.A., et al. Minimizing the Risks of Drug Interactions. *Patient Care.* March 30, 1999: 26–68.

Goodman, L.S., and A. Gilman, eds. *The Pharmacological Basis of Therapeutics.* 9th ed. 1996. New York: Macmillan.

Goodwin, F.K. and Ghaemi, S.N. The Course of Bipolar Disorder and the Nature of Agitated Depression. *Am J Psychiatry* 160:12, Dec. 2003: 2077–2079.

Gorman, J.D., et al. Treatment of ankylosing spondylitis by inhibition of tumor necrosis factor alpha. *New England Journal of Medicine* 2002. 346:1249–1256.

Gorski, E.D. and Willis, K.C. Report of Three Case Studies with Olanzapine for Chronic Pain. *Journal of Pain.* 2003; 4(3):166–8.

Goulding, M.R. Inappropriate Medication Prescribing for Elderly Ambulatory Care Pateints. *Archives of Internal Medicine 2004.* 164(3):305–312.

Gourang, P.P. and Kasiar, J.B. Syndrome of Inappropriate Antidiuretic Hormone-Induced Hyponatremia Associated with Amiodarone. *Pharmacotherapy* 2002; 22(5):649–651.

Graham, A.S. Cytochrome P450 Drug Interactions. *The Rx Consultant.* 8(2):1–8. 1999.

Graham, I.M., et al. Plasma Homocysteine as a Risk Factor for Vascular Disease. *Journal of the American Medical Association.* 277(22):1775–1781. 1997.

Grau, A.J., et al. Platelet function under aspirin, clopidogrel, and both after ischemic stroke: a case-crossover study. *Stroke* 2003 Apr; 34(4):849–54.

Graumlich, J.F., MD. Preventing gastrointestinal complications of NSAIDS. *Postgraduate Medicine* 109(5):117–128. May 2001.

Gray, S.L., et al. Medication Adherence in Elderly Patients Receiving Home Health Services Following Hospital Discharge. *The Annals of Pharmacotherapy.* 35(5):539–545. May 2001.

Greenland, P. Beating High Blood Pressure with Low-Sodium DASH. *New England Journal of Medicine.* 344(1):53–55. January 4, 2001.

Greenspan, S.L., et al. Alendronate Improves Bone Mineral Density in Elderly Women with Osteoporosis Residing in Long-Term Care Facilities. *Annals of Internal Medicine.* 2002; 136:742–746.

Greenspan, S.L., et al. Significant Differential Effects of Alendrontate, Estrogen or Combination Therapy on the Rate of Bone Loss after Discontinuation of Treatment of Postmenopausal Osteoporosis. *Annals of Internal Medicine.* 2002; 137:875–883.

Greenspan, S.L., et al. Alendronate plus estrogen and Bone Mineral Density in Elderly Women. *JAMA.* 2003; 136:742–746.

Griffiths, M.C., ed. *USAN* 1989. Rockville, MD: United States Pharmacopeial Convention.

Griffiths, M.C., ed. *The USP Dictionary of Drug Names.* 1988. Rockville, MD: United States Pharmacopeial Convention.

Grim, S.A., et al. Late-Onset Drug Fever Associated with Minocycline: Case Report and Review of the Literature. *Pharmacotherapy.* 2003; 23(12):1531–1537.

Grundy, S.M., and Cleeman, J.L.; Merz, N.B.; Brewer, Jr; Clark, L.T.; Hunninghake, D.B.; Pasternak, R.C.; Smith, S.C.; Stone, N.J., for the Coordinating Committee of the National Cholesterol Education Program. Endorsed by the National Heart, Lung, and Blood Institute, American College of Cardiology Foundation, and American Heart Association. *Implications of Recent Clinical Trials for the National Cholesterol Education Program Adult Treatment Panel III Guidelines.* Circulation. 2004; 110:227–239.

Guay, D.R.P. Cefdinir: An expanded Spectrum Oral Cephalosporin. *The Annals of Pharmacotherapy 2000.* 34:1469–1477. 2000.

Guidelines for the Use of Antiretroviral Agents in HIV Infected Adults and Adolescents. February 4, 2002. Accessed from *www.hivatis.org* June 24, 2002.

Gum, P.A., et al. A prospective, double-blinded determination of the natural history of aspirin resistance among stable patients with cardiovascular disease. *Journal of the American College of Cardiology* 2003; 41:961–5.

Hagg, S., et al. Long-term combination treatment with clozapine and filgrastim in patients with clozapine-induced agranulocytosis. *International Clinical Psychopharmacology.* 2003 May; 18(3):173–4.

Hambrecht, M.D., et al. Effect of Exercise on Coronary Endothelial Function in Patients With Coronary Artery Disease. *New England Journal of Medicine.* 342(7):454–460. 2000.

Hamelin, B.A., et al. Influence of the menstrual cycle on the timing of acute coronary events in premenopausal women. *Am J Med* 2003; 114:599–602.

Handbook of Clinical Drug Data. 1993. Hamilton, IL: Drug Intelligence Publications.

Handbook of Nonprescription Drugs. 11th ed. 1996. Washington, DC: American Pharmaceutical Association.

Hanlon, J.T., et al. Inappropriate Drug Use Among Community-Dwelling Elderly. *Pharmacotherapy 2000.* 20(5):575–582. 2000.

Hansten, P.D. *Drug Interactions.* 6th ed. 1992. Philadelphia: Lea and Febiger.

Hansten, P.D. and Horn, J.R. *The Top 100 Drug Interactions. A Guide to Patient Management.* 2001. Edmonds: H&H Publications.

Hart, S. Influence of B-Blockers on Mortality in Chronic Heart Failure. *The Annals of Pharmacotherapy.* 34:1440–1451. 2001.

Hasketh, P. L., ed. *The Journal of Oncology.* 1998. Cedar Knolls, NJ: National Medical Information Network.

Hawkins, David. Clinical trials with factor Xa inhibition in the prevention of postoperative venous thromboemolism. *American Journal of Health Systems Pharmacists.* 60:7. Nov 2003.

Hayden, F., et al. Inhaled Zanamivir for the Prevention of Influenza in Families. *New England Journal of Medicine.* 343(18):1282–1289. 2000.

Hays, J., et al. Effects of Estrogen plus Progestin on Health-Related Quality of Life. *New England Journal of Medicine* 2003, 348; 19:1839–54.

Hecht, H.S., et al. Electron Beam Tomography and National Cholesterol Education Program Guidelines in Asymptomatic Women. *Journal of the American College of Cardiology.* 37(6):1506–1511. 2001.

Heck, A.M., et al. Orlistat, a New Lipase Inhibitor for the Management of Obesity. *Pharmacotherapy the Journal of Human Pharmacology and Drug Therapy.* 20(3):270–279. 2000.

Heeschen, C., et al. Withdrawal of statins increases event rates in patients with acute coronary syndromes. *Circulation 2002; 10.1161/01. CIR.0000012530.68333C8.*

Heinonen, O.P., Slone, D., and S. Shapiro. *Birth Defects and Drugs in Pregnancy.* 1977. Littleton, MA: PSG Publishing.

Herrerias, C.T., et al. The Child with ADHD. Using the AAP Clinical Practice Guideline. *American Family Physician.* 63(9):1803–1812. 2001.

Hilleman, D.E. and Bauman, J.L. Role of Antiarrhythmic Therapy in Patients at Risk for Sudden Cardiac Death: An Evidence-Based Review. *Pharmacotherapy 2001.* 21(5): 556–574. 2001.

Hlatky, M.A., et al. Quality-of-life and depressive symptoms inpostmenopausal women after receiving hormone therapy: results from the Heart and estrogen/progesting Replacement Study (HERS) trial. *JAMA 2002* Feb 6; 287:591–7.

Hoff, P.M., et al. Comparison of oral capecitabine versis intravenous fluorouracil plus leucovorin as the first-line treatment of 605 patients with metastatic colorectal cancer: results of a randomized phase III study. *Journal of Clinical Oncology* 19(8):2282–92, 2001.

Hollister, L.E. *Clinical Pharmacology of Psychotherapeutic Drugs.* 2nd ed. 1983. New York: Churchill Livingstone.

Horsfield, S.A., et al. Fluoxentine's effects of cognitive performance in patients with traumatic brain injury. *International Journal of Psychiatry in Medicine.* 2002; 32(4):337–44.

The Hospice Journal. 1998. New York: The Haworth Press.

Horlan, C., et al. Frequency of Inappropriate Metformin Prescriptions. *Journal of the American Medical Association 2002* May 15, vol. 287(19): 2504 (Research Letter).

Houston Miller, N., et al. The Multilevel Compliance Challenge: Recommendations for a Call to Action. *Circulation* 95: 1085–1090. The American Heart Association 1997.

Hu, F., et al. Fish and Omega-3 Fatty Acid Intake and Risk of Coronary Heart Disease in Women. *JAMA* 2002; 287:1815–1821. April 10, 2002.

Hui, C.H., et al. Successful peripheral blood stem cell mobilisation with filgrastim in patients with chronic myeloid leukaemia achieving complete cytogenetic response with imatinib, without increasing disease burden as measured by quantitative real-time PCR. *Leukemia.* 2003 May; 17(5):821–8.

Hunninghake, D.B. Postdischarge lipid management of coronary artery disease patients according to the new National Cholesterol Education Program Guidelines. *American Journal of Cardiology 2001 Oct 18;* 18; 88(8A):37K-41K.

Hunt, L.W. How to manage difficult asthma cases. *Postgraduate Medicine* May 2001; 109(5): 61–68.

Hussar, D.A. New Drugs of 2000. *Journal of the American Pharmaceutical Association.*41(2): 229–280. The American Pharmaceutical Association. March/April 2001.

Hutubessy, R., et al. Generalized cost-effectiveness analysis for national-level priority setting in the health sector. *Cost Eff Resour Alloc.* 2003 Dec 19(epub ahead of print).

Hypericum Depression Trial Study Group. Effect of Hypericum perforatum (St. John's wort) in Major Depressive Disorder A Randomized Controlled Trial. *JAMA* 2002; 287: 1807–1853. April 10, 2002.

Im, J. Asthma. *The Rx Consultant.* XI(3):1–8. 2002.

Influenza and Pneumococcal Vaccination Levels Among Adults Aged Greater Than or Equal to 65. *Morbidity and Mortality Weekly Report.* 47:797–802. October 2, 1998.

International Drug Therapy Newsletter. 1997. Baltimore: Ayd Medical Communications.

Irwin, R.S. and Madison, J.M. Systemic Corticosteroids for Acute Exacerbations of Chronic Obstructive Pulmonary Disease. *New England Journal of Medicine.* 2003; 348(26): 2679–2681.

Isensee, B., et al. Smoking Increases the Risk of Panic. *Arch Gen Psychiatry. 2003;* 60:692–700.

Ismail, S. and Tariot, P. Long-Term Benefits of Early Pharmacologic Treatment in Alzheimer's Disease. *Essent Psychopharmacol.* 5:2. 2003.

Jaeger, J., et al. The Multidimensional Scale of Independent Functioning: A New Instrument for Measuring Functional Disability in Psychiatric Populations. *Schizophrenia Bulletin* 29(1):153–167, 2003.

Jakkula, M., et al. A Randomized Trial of Chinese Herbal Medicines for the Treatment of Symptomatic Hepatitis C. *Arch Intern Med.* 2004;164:1341–1346.

Janne, P.A. and Mayer, R.J. Chemoprevention of Colorectal Cancer. *New England Journal of Medicine.* 2000; 342(26):1960–1968.

Jefferson, J.W. Potassium supplementation in lithium patients: a timely intervention or premature speculation? *Journal of Clinical Psychiatry* 1992 Oct; 53(10):370–2.

Jefferson, J.W. and Greist, J.H. *Primer of Lithium Therapy.* 1977. Baltimore: Williams and Wilkins.

Jellin, J.M., et al. *The Pharmacist's Letter.* 17(1):1–6. 2001.

Johnson, M.D., et al. Clinically Significant Drug Interactions: What You Need to Know Before Writing Prescriptions. *Postgraduate Medicine.* 105(2):193–222. 1999.

Jones, P. Results of the STELLAR (Statin Therapies for Elevated Lipid Levels compared Across doses to Rosuvatstatin) trial. AAC (American College of Cardiology) national meeting April 2003.

Jonsson, B., et al. Health economics in the Hypertension Optimal Treatment (HOT) study: costs and cost-effectiveness of intensive blood pressure lowering and low-dose aspirin in patients with hypertension. *Journal of Internal Medicine.* 2003 Apr; 253(4):472–80.

Jorenby, D.E., Ph.D., et al. A Controlled Trial of Sustained-Release Bupropion, a Nicotine Patch, or Both for Smoking Cessation. *New England Journal of Medicine.* 340(9): 685–691. 1999.

Journal of Acquired Immune Deficiency Syndromes. 1999. Hagerstown, MD: Lippincott-Raven.

Journal of the American Medical Association. 1997–1999.

Journal of Bone and Mineral Research. 1996–2000. Malden, MA: Blackwell Science, Inc.

Journal of the National Cancer Institute. 1999. Cary, NC: Oxford University Press.

Journal Watch. 1996–2000. Waltham, MA: The Massachusetts Medical Society.

Journal Watch: Women's Health. 1996–2000. Waltham, MA: The Massachusetts Medical Society.

Kagan, R., et al. Preliminary results of the EFFECT (Efficacy of Fosamax versus Evista Comparison Trial). ACOG (American College of Obstetrics and Gynecology) national meeting April 22, 2003.

Kane, J.M., et al. Long-Acting Injectable Risperidone: Efficacy and Safety of the First Long-Acting Atypical Antipsychotic. *Am J Psychiatry* 2003; 160:1125–1132.

Kane, M.P., et al. Cholesteral and Glycemic Effects of Niaspan in Patients with Type 2 Diabetes. *Pharmacotherapy* 2001; 21(12):1473–1478.

Kaplan, N.M. *Management of Hypertension*. 6th ed. 1995. Durant, OK: Essential Medical Information Systems.

Kashyap, M.L., et al. Long-term Safety and Efficacy of a Once-Daily Niacin/Lovastatin Formulation for Patients With Dyslipidemia. *The American journal of Cardiology*. 89: 672–678. March 15, 2002.

Kawano, K.H., et al. Administration of nifedipine CR immeidately after awakening prevents a morning surge in hypertensive patients. Case report of three cases. *Blood Press Suppl 2003*. May; 1:44–48.

Keck, P.E., et al. A Placebo-Controlled, Double-Blind Study of the Efficacy and Safety of Aripiprazole in Patients With Acute Bipolar Mania. *American Journal of Psychiatry* 2003; 160(9):1651–1658.

Keck, P.E., et al. Ziprasidone in the Treatment of Acute Bipolar Mania: A Three-Week, Placebo-Controlled, Double-Blind, Randomized Trial. *American Journal of Psychiatry* 2003; 160:741–748

Keefe, Richard S.E., et al. Neurocognitive Assessment in the Clinical Antipsychotic Trials of Intervention Effectiveness (CATIE) Project Schizophrenia Trial: Development, Methodology, and Rationale. *Schizophrenia Bulletin* 29(1):45–55, 2003.

Kelly, William N. Can the Frequency and Risks of Fatal Adverse Drug Events Be Determined? *Pharmacotherapy*. 21(5). May 2001.

Kim, S.S. Role of fluoxetine in anorexia nervosa. *Annals of Pharmacotherapy*. 2003 Jun; 37(6):890–902.

Kindsvater, S., et al. Effects of coadministration of aspirin or clopidogrel on exercise testing in patients with heart failure receiving angiotensin-converting enzyme inhibitors. *American Journal of Cardiology*. 2003 Jun 1; 91(11):1350–2.

Klippel, J. H., ed. Systemic Lupus Erythematosus Demographics, Prognosis and Outcome. *Journal of Rheumatology Suppl* 48:67–71. 1997.

Knight, E.L., et al. Predictors of uncontrolled hypertension in ambulatory patients. *Hypertension 2001 Oct;* 38(4):809–814. 2001.

Knowler, W.C., et al. Reduction in the Incidence of Type 2 Diabetes With Lifestyle Intervention or Metformin. *New England Journal of Medicine*. 346(6):393–403. 2002.

Koda-Kimbal (Lloyd Yee Young). *Applied Therapeutics: The Clinical Use of Drugs*. 6th ed. 1995. Vancouver, WA: Applied Therapeutics.

Koller, E., et al. Clozapine-associated Diabetes. *The American Journal of Medicine*. December 2001. 111.

Koller, E.A., and Doraiswamy, P.M. Olanzapine-Associated Diabetes Mellitus. *Pharmacotherapy* 2002; 22(7):841–852.

Koller, E.A., et al. Risperidone-Associated Diabetes Mellitus: A Pharmacovigilance Study. *Pharmacotherapy*. 2003; 23(6):735–744.

Koller, W.C., ed. *Handbook of Parkinson's Disease*. 1987. New York: Marcel Dekker.

Kolodny, R.C., Masters, W.H., and V.E. Johnson. *Textbook of Sexual Medicine*. 1979. Boston: Little, Brown.

Koo, M.M., Krass, I., and Aslani, P. Factors Influencing Consumer Use of Written Drug Information. *Ann Pharmacother* 2003; 37:259–267.

Kovacs, J.A., and Masur, H. Prophylaxis Against Opportunistic Infections in Patients with Human Immunodeficiency Virus Infection. *NEJM*. 342(19):1416–1429. May 11, 2000.

Kwon, H.J., et al. Case reports of heart failure after therapy with a tumor necrosis factor antagonist. *Annals of Internal Medicine*. 2003 May 20; 138(10):807–11.

Lakrye, E.M., et al. The benefits of finasteride for hirsute women with polycystic ovary syndrome or idiopathic hirsutism. *Gynecology and Endocrinology*. 2003 Feb; 17(1):57–63.

Lambing, C.L. Osteoporosis prevention, detection, and treatment. A mandate for primary care physicians. *Postgraduate Medicine*. 107(7):37–56. June, 2000.

Larouche, S.J., et al. Lovastatin 10 mg efficacy in nonprescription studies. *Paper presentation: American Society for Clinical Pharmacology and Therapeutics*. Orlando, FL. March 7, 2001.

Lau, W.C., et al. Atorvastatin Reduces the Ability of Clopidogrel to Inhibit Platelet Aggregation: A New Drug-Drug Interaction. *Circulation*, Jan 2003; 107:32–37.

Laurie, S. and Khan, D. Inhaled corticosteroids as first-line therapy for asthma. *Postgraduate Medicine* May 2001; 109(5):44–56.

Lauten, W.B., et al. Usefulness of quinapril and irbesartan to improve the anti-inflammatory response of atorvastatin and aspirin in patients with coronary heart disease. *American Journal of Cardiology*. 2003 May 1;91(9):1116–9.

Lawrence, R.A. *Breast-Feeding*. 1980. St. Louis: Mosby.

Leaf, A., et al. Clinical prevention of sudden cardiac death by n-3polyunsaturated fatty acids and mechanism of prevention of arrhythmias by n-3 fish oils. *Circulation 2003.* as accessed from *http//circ.ahjajournals.org* [10.1161/01. CIR.0000069566.78305.33].

Lebowitz, B.D., et al. Approaches to Multisite Clinical Trials: The National Institute of Mental Health Perspective. *Schizophrenia Bulletin* 29, (1):7–13, 2003.

Lee, C.R., et al. Surrogate End Points in Heart Failure. *The Annals of Pharmacotherapy 2002.* 479–488.

Lee, T.H. A Broader Concept of Medical Errors. *New England Journal of Medicine*. 2002; 347(24):1965–6.

Leon, A.C., et al., Prospective Study of Fluoxetine Treatment of Suicidal Behavior in Affectively Ill Subjects. *American Journal of Psychiatry*. 156:195–201. 1999.

Lepore, L., et al. Drug-induced systemic lupus erythematosus associated with etanercept therapy in a child with juvenile idiopathic arthritis. *Clinical and Experimental Rheumatology*. 2003 Mar-Apr; 21(2):276–7.

Levien, T.L., et al. Nateglinide Therapy for Type 2 Diabetes Mellitus. *The Annals of Pharmacotherapy;* 35:1426–34. 2001.

Li, C.I., et al. Relationship Between Long Durations and Different Regimens of Hormone therapy and Risk of Breast Cancer. *JAMA* 2003; 289:3254–3263.

Lieberman, M.L. *The Sexual Pharmacy*. 1988. New York: New American Library.

Lindsay, R., et al. Effect of lower doses of conjugated equine estrogens with and without medroxyprogesterone acetate on bone in early postmenopausal women. *Journal of the American Medical Association* 2002; 287:2668–76.

Lipsy, R.J. The National Cholesterol Education Program Adult Treatment Panel III Guidelines. *JMCP, Vol. 9 No. 1 January/February 2003.*

Long, J.W. *Clinical Management of Prescription Drugs*. 1984. Philadelphia: Harper and Row.

Long, J.W. *The Essential Guide to Chronic Illness*. 1997. New York: HarperCollins.

Lonn, E.M. Effects of Ramipril and Vitamin E on Atherosclerosis. The Study to Evaluate Carotid Ultrasound Changes in Patients Treeated With Ramipril and Vitamin E (SECURE). *Circulation. 2001; 103:919–925.*

Love, N., et al. Symposium: A New Era in Breast Cancer. *Postgraduate Medicine*. 105(6): 43–103. 1999.

Lowy, F.D. Staphylococcus Aureus Infections. *New England Journal of Medicine*. 339 (8): 520–532. August 20, 1998.

Lucas, G.M., Chaisson, R.E. and Moore, R.D. Comparison of initial combination antiretroviral therapy with a single protease inhibitor, ritonavir and saquinavir, or efaviranz. *AIDS*. 15(13): pp 1679–1686. September, 2001.

Lucas, R.A., et al. Rhabdomyolysis Associated with Cerivastatin: Six Cases within Three Months at One Hospital. *Pharmacotherapy* 2002; 22(6):771–774.

Lyketsos, C.G., et al. Treating Depression in Alzheimer Disease. *Arch Gen Psychiatry* 2003; 60: 737–746.

Lynch, H.T. and Chapelle, A. Hereditary Colorectal Cancer. *New England Journal of Medicine* 2003. 348:919–932.

MacDonald, T.M., Wei, L. Effect of ibuprofen on cardioprotective effect of aspirin. *Lancet 2003;* 361:573–574.

Maddin, S., ed. *Current Dermatologic Therapy*. 1982. Philadelphia: W. B. Saunders.

Mahtabjafari, M., Masih, M., and Emerson, A.E. The value of pharmacist involvement in point-of-care service, walk-in lipid screening program. *Pharmacotherapy*. 21(11):1403–1406. 2001.

Maj, M., et al. Agitated Depression in Bipolar I Disorder: Prevalence, Phenomenology, and Outcome. *Am J Psychiatry* 2003; 160:2134–2140.

Maksymowych, W.P., et al. Canadian Rheumatology Association Consensus on the Use of Anti-Tumor Necrosis Factor-a Directed Therapies in the Treatment of Spondyloarthritis. *J Rheumatol.* 2003 Jun; 30(6):1356–1363.

Mancia, G., et al. An Ambulatory Blood Pressure Monitoring Study of the Comparative Antihypertensive Efficacy of Two Angiotensin II Receptor Antagonists. *Blood Pressure Monitoring.* May/June 2002, 7:135–142. 2002.

Marchioli, R., et al. Early Protection against sudden death by n-3 polyunsaturated fatty acids after myocardial infarction. Time-course analysis of the gruppo Italiano per lo Studio della Sopravvivenza nell-iInfarcto Miocardico (GISSI)-Prevenzione. *Circulation [10.1161/01. CIR.0000014682.14181. F2].2002.*Accessed at *www.circ.ahajournals.org/.*

Marcus, A.O. Lipid Disorders in Patients with Type 2 Diabetes Meeting the Challenges of Early, Aggressive Treatment. *Postgraduate Medicine.* 110(1):111–123. 2001.

Marder, S.R., et al. Maintenance Treatment of Schizophrenia With Risperidone or Haloperidol: 2-Year Outcomes. *Am J Psychiatry* 2003; 160:1405–1412.

Mario, F.D., et al. Rabeprazole in a one-week eradication therapy of Helicobacter pylori: Comparison of different dosages. *Journal of Gastroenterology and Hepatology.* 2003 Jul; 18(7):783–786.

Marso, S.P., Griffin, B.P., and Topol, E.J. *Manual of Cardiovascular Medicine.* 2000. Philadelphia: Lippincott Williams & Wilkins.

Martin, W.R. and Fuller, R.E. Suspected Chromium Picolinate-Induced Rhabdomyolysis. *Pharmacotherapy.* 18(4):860–862. 1998.

Mathis, A.S., et al. Risk Stratification in Non-ST Segment Elevation Acute Coronary Syndromes with Special Focus on Recent Guidelines. *Pharmacotherapy.* 21(8):954–987. 2001.

Mayeuz, R., and Sano, M. Treatment of Alzheimer's Disease. *New England Journal of Medicine.* 341(22):1670–1679. November 25, 1999.

Mayo Clinic Proceedings. 1996–2000.

McCabe, S. Advances in the Pharmacologist Treatment of Bipolar Affective Disorders. *Perspectives in Psychiatric Care* Vol. 39, No. 3, July-September, 2003.

McConnell, J.D., Roehrborn, C.G., and Bautista, O.M., et al. The long-term effect of doxazosin, finasteride and combination therapy on the clnical progression of benign prostatic hyperplasia. *New Engl J Med* 2003; 349(25)2387–2398.

McEvoy, G. K., ed. *American Hospital Formulary Service: Drug Information 1997.* Bethesda, MD: American Society of Hospital Pharmacists.

McKenney, J. ATP 3 Review. *Journal of American Pharmaceutical Association 2001.* 41(4):596–606.

McMinn, J.R. Jr., et al. Complete recovery from refractory immune thrombocytopenic purpura in three patients treated with etanercept. *American Journal of Hematology.* 2003 Jun; 73(2):135–40.

McNulty, S.J., et al. A randomized trial of sibutramine in the management of obese type 2 diabetic patients treated with metformin. *Diabetes Care.* 2003; 26:125–31.

Mease, P.J. Etanercept, a TNF antagonist for treatment for psoriatic arthritis and psoriasis. *Skin Therapy Lett.* 2003 Jan; 8(1):1–4.

Medical Letter on Drugs and Therapeutics. 1998, 1999, 2001, 2002. New Rochelle, NY: The Medical Letter.

Mehta, S.R., M.D., et al. The Clopidogrel in Unstable Angina to Prevent Recurrent Ischemic Events (CURE) trial programme; rationale, design and baseline characteristics including a meta-analysis of the effects of thienopyridines in vascular disease CURE study investigators. *European Heart Journal* 2000; 21:2022–2041.

Melmon, K.L., and Morrelli, H. F. *Clinical Pharmacology.* 2nd ed. 1978. New York: Macmillan.

Michaels, A.D., et al. Effects of intravenous nesiritide on human coronary vasomotor regulation and myocardial oxygen uptake. *Circulation* 2003; 107(21):2697–2701.

Michelson, D., et al. Atomoxetine in the treatment of children and adolescents with attention deficit/hyperactivity disorder: a randomized, placebo-controlled, dose-response study. *Pediatrics.2001*;108e83 (Accessed from *www.pediatrics.org* April, 2002).

Michelson, M. D., et al. Bone Mineral Density in Women with Depression. *New England Journal of Medicine.* 335(16): 1176–1181. 1996.

Micromedex: Drugex. 1999, 2000, 2001, 2002. Englewood, CO: Computerized Clinical Information System.

Milgrom, H., et al. Treatment of Allergic Asthma with Monoclonal Anti-IgE Antibody. *New England Journal of Medicine.* 341(26): 1964–1972. December 23, 1999.

Miller, C. D., et al. Hypoglycemia in patients with type 2 diabetes mellitus. *Archives of Internal Medicine.* 161: 1653–1659. July, 9, 2001.

Mintzer, J.E. and Kersharw, P. The efficacy of galantamine in the treatment of Alzheimer's disease: comparison of patients previously treated with acetylcholinesterase inhibitors to patients with no prior exposure.

Modi, P., et al. *The Evolving Role of Oral Insulin Spray (RapidMist) in the Treatment of Diabetes.* 5th International Congress of Immunology. Madrid, India February 2001.

Modi, P., et al. *The Role of Oral Insulin Combined with Metformin in the Treatment of Diabetes.* American Association National Meeting. Philadelphia, PA, June 2001.

Mohler, S. R. *Medication and Flying: A Pilot's Guide.* 1982. Boston: Boston Publishing.

Mojtabai, R., et al. Atypical Antripsychotics in First Admission Schizophrenia: Medications Continuation and Outcomes. *Schizophrenia Bulletin.* 2003; 29(3):519–530.

Mongthuong, T.T., et al. Role of Coenzyme Q10 in Chronic Heart Failure, Angina, and Hypertension. *Pharmacotherapy* 2001; 21(7):797–806.

Montserrat, V. L., et al. Cost-Effectiveness Results from the US Carvedilol Heart Failure Trials Program. *The Annals of Pharmacotherapy;* 35:846–851. 2001.

Morbidity and Mortality Weekly Report (MMWR): Prevention and Control of Influenza. Vol. 48, No. RR-4 April 30, 1999. Washington, DC: U.S. Department of Health and Human Services.

Morbidity and Mortality Weekly Report (MMWR): Report of the NIH Panel to Define Principles of Therapy of HIV Infection and Guidelines for the Use of Antiretroviral Agents in HIV-Infected Adults and Adolescents. April 24, 1998. Washington, DC: U.S. Department of Health and Human Services, CDC Atlanta, Georgia.

Morgan, T., Anderson, A. The effects of nonsteroidal anti-inflammatory drugs on blood pressure in patients treated with different antihypertensive drugs. *J Clin Hypertens (Greenwich).* 2003 Jan-Feb; 5(1):53–7.

Morgan, T.O., Anderson, A. Different drug classes have variable effects on blood pressure depending on the time of day. *Am J Hypertens.* 2003 Jan; 16(1):46–50.

Mosca, L., et al. ACC/AHA Guideline Update for the Management of Patients With Unstable Angina and Non-ST-Segment Elevation Myocardial Infarction-2002:Summary Article. *Circulation.* 2002; 106:1893.

Mosca, L., et al. Design and Methods of the Raloxifene Use for The Heart (RUTH) Study. *The American Journal of Cardiology 2001.* 88:392–395.

Mosca, L., et al. Guide to Preventive Cardiology for Women. *Circulation.* 1999; 99: 2480–2484. 1999.

Mosher, M. *Clinical Management of Hypertension.* Fourth Edition. 1999. Caddo, OK: Professional Communications, Inc.

Mossad, S. B. Prophylactic and Symptomatic Treatment of Influenza Current and Developing Options. *Postgraduate Medicine* 109. 97–105. January 2001.

Mukherjee, D., Nissen, S.E. and Topol, E.J. Risk of Cardiovascular Events Associated With Selective COX-2 Inhibitors. *Journal of the American Medical Association.* 286(8); August 22/29, 2001. accessed from *www.jama.ama-assn.org/issues/v286n8/rfull/jsc10193.html.*

Mukherjee, D., et al. NSAIDS, but not COX IIs inhibit aspirin benefits. *New England Journal of Medicine.* 109. 97–105. December 20, 2001.

Munzenberger, P.J., and Vinuya R.Z. Impact of an Asthma Program on the Quality of Life of Children in an Urban Setting. *Pharmacotherapy* 2002; 22(8):1055–1062.

Murphy, J. E. *Clinical Pharmacokinetics.* 1993. Bethesda, MD: American Society of Hospital Pharmacists.

Nallamothu, M., Fendrick, M. Rubenfire, et al. Lowering Elevated Homocysteine Levels Could Result in Substantial Clinical Benefits at a Reasonable Cost. *Archives of Internal Medicine* 160. 3406–3412. December 11, 2000.

National Center for Complementary and Alternative Medicine. NCCAM Consumer Advisory on Ephedra. accessed 4/6/03 at *www.nccam.nih.gov/health/alerts/ephedra/consumeradvisory.htm.*

National Center for Health Statistics, CDC. *Leading Causes of Death.* 2001. *www.cdc.gov/nchs/fastats/icod.htm.*

National Institutes of Health's (NIH, NHLBI) Guidelines for Diagnosis and Management of Asthma. 1997.

Nemeroff, C.B., Improving Antidepressant Adherence, *J Clin Psychiatry.* 2003 Dec; 64 (suppl 18):25–30.

Nephropathy, urinary tract cancer from herbal products containing aristolochic acid. FDA. *www.cfsan.fd.gov/;sldms/ds-bot3.* html. *Pharmacy Today.* Page 5, June 2001.

Nerhood, R.C. Making a Decision about ERT/HRT. *Postgraduate Medicine.* 109(3):167–178. 2001.

Ness, J., Aronow, W.S. Prevalence of coexistence of coronary artery disease, ischemic stroke, and peripheral arterial disease in older persons, mean age 80 years, in an academic hospital-based geriatrics practice. *J Am Geriatr Soc.* 1999; 47:1255–1256.

New England Journal of Medicine. 1997–2003.

Nichol, K.L., et al. Influenza vaccination and reduction in hospitalizations for cardiac disease and stroke among the elderly. *NEJM* 2003; 348(14):1322–1332.

Nielsen, J.W., MD, et al. Optimal Antidepressant Dosing. Practical framework for selection, titration, and duration of therapy. *Postgraduate Medicine.* 108(5):111–115. Oct. 2000.

Nierenberg, Andrew A. Predictors of response to antidepressants, General principles and clinical implications. *Psychiatric Clinics of North America. 2003;* 345–352.

O'Donnell, M. and Hirsch, J. Establishing an Ooptimal Therapeutic Range for Coumarins: Filling in the Gaps. *Archives of Internal Medicine.* March 2004. 164:6.

O'Laughlin, J., et al. The Role of Community Pharmacists in Health Education and Disease Prevention: A Survey of Their Interests and Needs in Relation to Cardiovascular Disease. *Preventive Medicine.* 28:324–331. 1999.

Olfsom, M, et al. Relationship Between Antidepressant Medication Treatment and Suicide in Adolescents. *Arch Gen Psychiatry.* 2003; 60:978–982.

Olin, B.R., ed. *Facts and Comparisons.* 1997, 1998, 2000. St. Louis: J. B. Lippincott, Facts and Comparisons.

Olin, B.R., ed. 1992. *Patient Drug Facts.* St. Louis: J. B. Lippincott, Facts and Comparisons.

Owens, R. C. Risk Assessment for Antimicrobial Agent-Induced QTc Interval Prolongation and Torsades de Pointes. *Pharmacotherapy 2001; 21(3):301–319.*

Packard, K.A., et al. Comparison of Gemfribrozil and Fenofibrate in Patients with Dyslipidemic Coronary Heart Disease. *Pharmacotherapy* 2002; 22(12):1527–1532.

Pain Forum: Official Journal of the American Pain Society. 1997, 1998, 2000. Secaucus, NJ: Churchill Livingstone.

Palacioz, K. P., et al. Drug-Induced Long QT Interval. *Detail-Document 170401 Therapeutic Resource Center. Pharmacist's Letter/Prescriber's Letter 2001.*

Paradiso-Hardy, F.L., Gordon, W.L., Jackevicius, C.A., et al. The importance of in-hospital statin therapy for patients with acute coronary syndromes. *Pharmacotherapy* 2003 Apr; 23(4):506–13.

Paris, D., Townsend, K.P., Humphrey, J., et al. Statins inhibit Abeta-neurotoxicity in vitro and Abeta-induced vasoconstriction and inflammation in rat aortae. *Atherosclerosis* 2002 Apr:161(2):293–299.

Park, P.J., et al. The performance of a risk score in predicting undiagnosed hyperglycemia. *Diabetes Care* 2002 June: 25(6):84–988.

Park, S.J., et al. A Paclitaxel-Eluting Stent for the Prevention of coronary Restenosis. *New England Journal of Medicine.* 2003; 348(16):1537–45.

Patel, T.N., et al. Use of Aspirin and Ibuprofen Compared With Aspirin and the Risk of Myocardial Infarction. *Arch Intern Med.* 2004; 164:852–856.

Pearson, T.A., et al. Markers of Inflammation and Cardiovascular Disease. *Circulation* 2003; 107(3):499

Pearson, V.E. Galantamine: A New Alzheimer Drug with a Past Life. *The Annals of Pharmacotherapy;* 35:1406–13. 2001.

Penzak, et al. Depression in patients with HIV infection. *American Journal of Health System Pharm.* 57:376–389. Feb 15, 2000.

Perazella, M.A. COX-2 Inhibitors and the Kidney. Hospital Practice, March 15, 2001.

Pham, J.V., and Puzantian T. Ecstacy: Dangers and Controversies. *Pharmacotherapy* 2001; 21(12):1561–1565.

Physicians' Desk Reference. Electronic Library 2000.1, version 5.1 AT. Montvale, NJ: Medical Economics.

Physician's GenRX. 1996. Version 96.1a. St. Louis, MO: Mosby.

Physician's Therapeutics and Drug Alert. 1998–2001.

Pickar, D. Pharmacogenomics of psychiatric drug treatment. *Psychiatric Clin N Am* 26(2003):303–321.

Pitt, B., et al. Eplerenone, a Selective Aldosterone Blocker, in Patients with Left Ventricular Dysfunction after Myocardial Infarction. *N Engl J Med* 2003:348(14):1309–1321.

Pletcher, M.J., et al. Using the Coronary Artery Calcium Score to Predict Coronary Heart Disease Events: A Systematic Review and Meta-analysis. *Arch Intern Med.* 2004; 164:1285–1292.

Poole-Wilson, P.A., et al. Comparison of carvedilol and metoprolol on clinical outcomes in patients with chronic heart failure in the Carvedilol or Metoprolol European Trail (COMET): randomized controlled trial. Lancet 2003 Jul 5; 362 (9377):7–13.

Portnoy, J.M. Immunotherapy for inhalant allergies. *Postgraduate Medicine* May 2001; 109(5):89–106.

Posey, M.L. Proving That Pharmaceutical Care Makes a Difference in Community Pharmacy. *Journal of the American Pharmaceutical Association, March/April 2003, Vol. 43, No. 2*

Postgraduate Medicine: The Journal of Applied Medicine for the Primary Care Physician. 1998–2000.

Potkin, S.G., et al. Aripirazole, an Antipsychotic With a Novel Mechanism of Action, and Risperidone vs Placebo in Patients With Schizphrenia and Schizoaffective Disorder. *Arch Gen Psychiatry.* 2003; 60:681–690.

Practice Guideline for the Treatment of Patients With Alzheimer's Disease and Other Dementias of Late Life. 1997. Washington, DC: American Psychiatric Association.

Pratt, D.S., and Kaplan, M.M. Evaluation of Abnormal Liver-Enzyme Results in Asymptomatic Patients. *New England Journal of Medicine.* 342(17):1266–1271. April 27, 2000.

Principles of Analgesic Use in the Treatment of Acute Pain and Cancer Pain. 3rd ed. 1996. Glenview, IL: American Pain Society.

Principles of Analgesic Use in the Treatment of Acute Pain and Cancer Pain. 4th ed. 1999. Glenview, IL: American Pain Society.

Qtcdrugs.org. International Registry for Drug-Induced Arrhythmias "drugs to avoid in patients with congenital Long QT syndrome." June 2001.

Quality Improvement Guidelines for the Treatment of Acute Pain and Cancer Pain. 1995. Glenview, IL: American Pain Society Quality of Care Committee.

Quilliam, B.J., et al. Quantifying the Effect of Applying the NCEP ATP III Criteria in a Managed Care Population Treated With Statin Therapy. *J Manag Care Pharm.* 2004; 10(3):244–250.

Quintiliani, R., et al. Optimizing Antiinfective Transition Therapy In Community-Acquired Pneumonia. *Pharmacotherapy.* 21(7) Part two: 1–108S. July 2001.

Quitkin, F.M., et al. When Should a Trial of Fluoxetine for Major Depression Be Declared Failed? *Am J Psychiatry* 2003; 160:734–740.

Raj, P.P. *Practical Management of Pain.* 1986. Chicago: Year Book Medical Publishers.

Rakel, R.E., ed. *Conn's Current Therapy* 1992. Philadelphia: W. B. Saunders.

Rational Drug Therapy and Pharmacology for Physicians. 1990. Bethesda, MD: American Society for Pharmacology and Experimental Therapeutics.

Ratnapalan, S., et al. Digoxin-carvedilol interactions in children. *J Pediatr 2003.* 142(5):572–574.

Ratthore, S.S., Krumholz, H.M. Digoxin therapy for heart failure: safe for women? *Italian Heart Journal 2003.* 4(3):148–151.

Reisberg, B., et al. Memantine in Moderate-to-Severe Alzheimer's Disease. *New Engl J Med* April 2003; 348(14):1333–1341.

Reiss, R.A., et al. Point-of-Care Laboratory Monitoring of Patients Receiving Different Anticoagulant Therapies. *Pharmacotherapy* 2002; 22(6):677–685.

Relkin, N.R., et al. A large, community-based, open label trial of donepezil in the treatment of Alzheimer's disease. *Dement Geriatr Cogn Disord* 2003; 16(1):15–24.

Rejnmark, L., et al. Dose-effect relations of and loop- and thiazide-diuretics on calcium homeostasis: a randomized, double-blinded Latin-square multiple cross-over study in postmenopausal osteopenic woman. *European Journal of Clinical Investigation* 2003 Jan; 33(1):41–50.

Rendell, M.S. and Kirchain, W.R. Pharmacotherapy of Type 2 Diabetes Mellitus. *The Annals of Pharmacotherapy 2000;* 34:878–895.

Reynolds, J.E.F., ed. *Martindale: The Extra Pharmacopoeia.* 29th ed. 1997. London: The Pharmaceutical Press.

Rhee, S.M., et al. *Use of Complementary and Alternative Medicines by Ambularory Patients.* Arch Intern Med. 2004; 164:1004–1009.

Ridker, P.M., et al. Comparison of C-reactive protein and low-density lipoprotein cholesterol levels in the prediction of first cardiovascular events. *New England Journal of Medicine 2002.* 347:1557–1565.

Robless, P.A., et al. Increased platelet aggregation and activation in peripheral arterial diseaase. *European Journal of Vascular and Endovascular Surgery* 2003 Jan; 25(1):16–22.

Rodrigo, B.A., et al. Is Regionally Selective D2/D3 Dopamine Occupancy Sufficient for Atyipcal Effect?An In Vivo Quantitive [123I]Epidepride SPET Study of Amisulpride-Treated Patients. *Am J Psychiatry* 2003; 160:1413–1420.

Rogers, C.S., and McCue, J.D., eds. *Managing Chronic Disease.* 1987. Oradell, NJ: Medical Economics Books.

Rojas-Fernandez, C.H., et al. Implications of Amyloid Precursor Protein and Subsequent Beta-Amyloid Production to the Pharmacotherapy of Alzheimer's Disease. *Pharmacotherapy* 2002; 22(12):1547–1563.

Romanelli F., et al. Human Immunodeficiency Virus Drug Resistance Testing: State of the Art in Genotypic and Phenotypic Testing of Antiretrovirals. *Pharmacotherapy 2000;* 20(2):151–157.

Romano, M.J., et al. Life-Threatening Isradipine Poisoning in a Child. *Pharmacotherapy* 202; 22(6):766–770.

Rosenberg, J. and Federiuk, C. Optimal digoxin range for men is 0.5 to 0.8 ng/mL. *Journal of Family Practice* 2003; 52(5):360–361.

Rosenheck, R., et al. Changing Environments and Alternative Perspectives in Evaluating the Cost-Effectiveness of New Antipsychotic Drugs. *Schizophrenia Bulletin* 29(1):81–93, 2003.

Ross, S.D. Discontinuation of Antihypertensive Drugs Due to Adverse Events: A Systemic Review and Meta-Analysis. *Pharmacotherapy 2001;* 21(8):940–953.

Russo, R.L. and D'Aprille, M. Role of Antimicrobial Therapy in Acute Exacerbations of Chronic Obstructive Pulmonary Disease. *The Annals of Pharmacotherapy.* 35, 576–580. May 2001.

Roth, M.T., et al. Asthma Exacerbation After Administration of Nicotine Nasal Spray for Smoking Cessation. *Pharmacotherapy* 2002; 22(6):779–782.

Rothbard, A.B., et al. Trends in the Rate and Type of Antipsychotic Medications Prescribed to Persons With Schizophrenia. *Schizophrenia Bulletin* 2003; 29(3):531–540.

Rybacki, J.J. Letter to the editor. *Journal of the American Medical Association.* 277(17):1351. 1997.

Rybacki, J.J. "What was the CURE trial?" Good News and New Medicines. 3(2): page 3 on www.medicineinfo.com. April 2001.

Rybacki, J.J. Improving Cardiovascular Health in Postmenopausal Women by Addressing Medication Adherence Issues. *The Journal of The American Pharmaceutical Association.* 42:63–73. January/February, 2002.

Saag, K.G. Resolved: Low-dose glucocorticoids are neither safe nor effective for the long-term treatment of rheumatoid arthritis. *Arthritis Care & Research.* 45: pp 468–471. October 2001.

Sacks, F.M., et al. Effects on Blood Pressure of Reduced Dietary Sodium and the Dietary Approaches to Stop Hypertension (DASH) Diet. *New England Journal of Medicine.* 344(1):3–10. January 4, 2001.

Safar, M.E. and Smulyan, H. Hypertension in women. *Am J Hypertens.* 2004 Jan; 17(1):82–87.

Sandler, R.S., et al. A Randomized Trial of Aspirin to Prevent Colorectal Adenomas in Patients with Previous Colorectal Cancer. *New England Journal of Medicine 2003.* 348:883–890.

Sanford, J., et al. *The Sanford Guide to HIV/AIDS Therapy.* 5th ed. 1996. Antimicrobial Therapy, Inc. Vienna, VA: Lippincott-Raven.

Sarner, L. et al. Acute Onset lactic acidosis and pancreatitis in the third trimester of pregnancy in HIV-1 positive women taking antiretroviral medication. *Sex Transm Inf* 2002; 78(1):58–59.

Sauer, G.C. *Manual of Skin Diseases.* 5th ed. 1985. Philadelphia: J. B. Lippincott.

Scan Newsletter. 1996–1998. Norwich, NY: Society for Clinical Densitometry.

Schaefer, D.C., and Cheskin, L.J. Constipation in the Elderly. *Am Fam Physician.* 1998 Sept. 15.

Schapowal, A. Randomized controlled trial of butterbur and cetirizine for treating seasonal allergic rhinitis. *British Medical Journal.* 2002; 324:144. www.bmj.org.

Schardein, J.L. *Drugs as Teratogens.* 1976. Cleveland: CRC Press.

Scheife, R.T., et al. Low Molecular Weight Heparins for Venous Thromboembolism: Making an Evidence-based Treatment Choice. *Pharmacotherapy.* 21(6), Part 2. June 2001.

Scheife, R.T., et al. New Strides in Asthma. *Pharmacotherapy.* 21(3), Part 2. March 2001.

Schneeweiss, S., et al. Outcomes of reference pricing for angiotensin-converting-enzyme inhibitors. *New England Journal of Medicine 2002.* 346:822–829.

Schneider, Lon, S., et al. Clinical Antipsychotic Trials of Intervantion Effectiveness (CATIE): Alzheimer's Disease Trial. *Schizophrenia Bulletin, 29(1):57–72, 2003.*

Schubert, I., et al., Development of indicators for assessing the qulity of prescribing of lipid-lowering drugs: data from the pharmacotherapeutic quality circles in Hesse, Germany. *International Journal of Clinical and Pharmacological Therapy 2001 Nov;* 39(11):492–498.

Schwartz, G.G., et al. Effects of Atorvastatin on Early Recurrent Ishcemic Events in Acute Coronary Syndromes the MIRACL Study: A randomized Controlled Trial. *Journal of the American Medical Association.* 285(13). April 4, 2001. Accessed from *www.jama.ama-assn.org.*

Scientific American Medicine. 1999. CD-ROM. New York: Enigma Information Systems.

Second Scientific Forum on Quality of Care and Outcomes Research in Cardiovascular Disease and Stroke. April 2000. The American Heart Association Councils on Clinical Cardiology, Cardiovascular Nursing, Cardiovascular Disease in the Young, Cardio-Thoracic and Vascular Surgery, Epidemiology and Prevention, High Blood Pressure Research and the American College of Cardiology. Abstracts. Washington, DC.

Semla, T. P., et al. *Geriatric Dosage Handbook.* 1993. Cleveland: Lexi-comp.

Shalansky, S.J. and Levy, A.R. Effect of Number of Mediations on Cardiovascular Therapy Adherence. Ann Pharmacother 2002; 36:1532–1539.

Shavelle, D. M., et al. Exercise Testing and Electron Beam Computed Tomography in the Evaluation of Coronary Artery Disease. *Journal of the American College of Cardiology.* 36(1). 2000.

Shekelle, P.G., et al. Efficacy of ACE inhibitors and beta blockers in the management of left ventricular systolic dysfunction according to race, gender and diabetic status. A meta-analysis of major clinical trials. *Journal of the American College of Cardiology* 2003; 41:1529–1538.

Shepard, J.E. Effects of Estrogen on Cognition, Mood, and Degenerative Brain Diseases. *Journal of the American Pharmaceutical Association* 41(2):221–228. March/April 2001.

Shepard, T.H. *Catalog of Teratogenic Agents.* 6th ed. 1989. Baltimore: Johns Hopkins University Press.

Sherman, J., et al. Adherence to Oral Montelukast and Inhaled Fluticasone in Children with Persistent Asthma. *Pharmacotherapy.*21(12):1464–1467. December 2001.

Sickle Cell Disease: Screening, Diagnosis, Management and Counseling in Newborns and Infants. 1993. Washington, DC: U.S. Department of Health and Human Services.

Siddiqui, A., et al. Lack of Physician Concordance With Guidelines on the Perioperative Use of B-Blockers. *Archives of Internal Medicine.* March 2004. 164:6.

Silver, H., et al. Add-on Fluvoxamine Improves Primary Negative Symptoms: Evidence for Specificity From Response Analysis of Individual Symptoms. *Schizophrenia Bulletin,* 2003, 29(3):541–546.

Silverstein, F.E., et al. Gastrointestinal toxicity with celecoxib vs nonsteroidal anti-inflammatory drugs for osteoarthritis and rheumatoid arthritis. The CLASS study: a randomized controlled trial. *JAMA 2000.* 284(10):1247–1255.

Simpson, S.H., et al. Economic Impact of Community Pharmacist Intervention in Cholesterol Risk Management: An Evaluation of the Study of Cardiovascular Risk Intervention by Pharmacists. *Pharmacotherapy.* 21(5):627–635. Mar 1, 2001.

Skaehill, P.A. Tacrolimus in Dermatologic Disorders. *The Annals of Pharmacotherapy.* 35: 582–588. May 2001.

Slatkin, N.E., et al. Donepezil in the treatment of opioid-induced sedation: report of six cases. J Pain Symptom Management 2001; 21(5):425–438.

Sleeper, R., et al. Psychotropic Drugs and Falls: New Evidence Pertaining to Serotonin Reuptake Inhibitors. *Pharmacotherapy 2000.* 20(3):308–317. 2000.

Smith, L. H., and Thier, S. O. *Pathophysiology: The Biological Principles of Disease.* 2nd ed. 1985. Philadelphia: W. B. Saunders.

Snyder, L., et al. Leukotriene Modifier Use and Asthma Severity: How is a New Medication Being Used by Adults With Asthma? *Archives of Internal Medicine.* March 2004. 164:6.

Solvason, H.B., et al. Predictors of response in anxiety disorders. *Psychiatric Clinics of North America.* 2003; 26:411–433.

Song, J.C., et al. Pharmacologic, Pharmacokinetic and Therapeutic Differences Among Angiotensin II Receptor Antagonists. *Pharmacotherapy: The Journal of Human Pharmacology and Drug Therapy.* 20(2):130–39. 2000.

Sorensen, S. J., and S. R. Abel. Comparison of the Ocular Beta-Blockers. *Annals of Pharmacotherapy.* 30:43–54. 1997.

Sotiriou, C.G. and Cheng, J. Beneficial Effects of Statins in Coronary Artery Disease—Beyond Lowering Cholesterol. *The Annals of Pharmacotherapy.* 34:1432–1439. 2000.

Spanheimer, R.G. Reducing Cardiovascular Risk in Diabetes: Which Factors to Modify First? *Postgraduate Medicine.* 109(4):26–36. 2001.

Spath, P. L., ed. *Clinical Paths, Tools for Outcomes Management.* 1994. Chicago: The American Hospital Association.

Speight, T. M., and N.H.G. Holford, eds. *Avery's Drug Treatment.* 4th ed. 1997. Auckland, NZ: Adis International.

Spencer, et al. Declining Length of Hospital Stay for Acute Myocardial Infarction and Post-discharge Outcomes. *Archives of Internal Medicine.* 164. April 2004.

Spinler, S.A. New Recommendations from the 1999 American College of Cardiology/American Heart Association Acute Myocardial Infarction Guidelines. *The Annals of Pharmacotherapy.* 35:589–588. May 2001.

Spruill, W.J., et al. Determining institution-specific costs of thromboembolic events with an algorithm and spreadsheet. *Am J Health-Syst Pharm.* 2003; 60:1741–9.

Statins in rheumatoid arthritis: Reduction in CV risk, but also in RA disease activity. June 2004.

Steimer, W., et al. Digoxin Assays: frequent, substantial, and potentially dangerous interference by spironolactone, canrenone and other steroids. *Clinical Chemistry* 2002; 48(3): 507–516.

Stein, E.A. The power of statins: aggressive lipid lowering. *Clin Cardiol.* 2003 Apr; 26(4 Suppl 3):III25–31.

Steinberger, J., Daniels, S.R. Obesity, Insulin Resistance, Diabetes, and Cardiovascular Risk in Children. *Circulation.* 2003; 107:1448.

Steinhubl, S.R., et al. Early and Sustained Dual Oral Antiplatelet Therapy Following Percutaneous Coronary Intervention: A Randomized Controlled Trial. *Journal of the American Medical Association* 2002; 288:2411–2420.

Stempel, et al. Inhaled Corticosteroids and Growth: How Big a Dose of Caution. *Contemporary Pediatrics.* 338(11):736–746. March, 2002.

Sterling, T.R. *The Hopkins HIV Report.* Volume 14, Number 2 When to start HAART: Still a Controversy. The Johns Hopkins University AIDS Service, Division of Infectious Diseases. March, 2002.

Stoupakis, G. and Klapholz, M. Natriuretic peptides: biochemistry, physiology, and therapeutic role in heart failure. *Heart Disease* 2003; May-June; 5(3):215–223.

Straka, R. J., et al. Assessment of hypercholesterolemia control in a managed care organization. *Pharmacotherapy.* 21(7):818–827. 2001.

Straus, S.E. Herbal Medicines—What's In the Bottle? *New England Journal of Medicine* 2002; 347(25):1997–8.

Stroup, S.T., et al. The National Institute of Mental Health Clinical Antipsychotic Trials of Intervention Effectiveness(CATIE) Project:Schizophrenia Trial Design and Protocol Debelopment. *Schizophrenia Bulletin, 29(1):15–31, 2003.*

Struckman, D.R. and Rivey, M.P. Combined Therapy with an Angiotensin II Receptor Blocker and an Angiotensin-Converting Enzyme Inhibitor in Heart Failure. *The Annals of Pharmacotherapy.* 35:242–248. 2001.

Sumpton, J.E. and Moulin, D.E. Treatment of Neuropathic Pain with Venlafaxine. *The Annals of Pharmacotherapy.* 35(5):557–559. May 2001.

Swartz, M.S., et al. Assessing Clinical and Functional Outcomes in the Clincal Antipsychotic Trials of Intervention Effectiveness (CATIE) Schizophrenia Trial. *Schizophrenia Bulletin, 29(1):33–43, 2003.*

Swash, M., and Schwartz, M. S. *Neuromuscular Diseases.* 2nd ed. 1988. Berlin: Springer-Verlag.

Swenson, C.N., and Fundak, G. Observational cohort study of switching warfarin sodium products in a managed care organization. *Am Jrn Health Syst. Pharm.* 57:452–455. Mar 1, 2000.

Szefler, S., et al. (The Childhood Asthma Research Group) Long-term Effects of Budesonide or Nedocromil in Children with Asthma. *New England Journal of Medicine.* 343(15): 1054–1069.

Tacconelli, S., et al. The Biochemical Selectivity of Novel COX-2 Inhibitors in Whole Blood Assays of COX-isozyme Activity. *Current Medical Research and Opinions* 2002;18(8): 503–511.

Tariot, P.N., et al. Memantine Treatment in Patients With Moderate to Severe Altxheimer Disease Already Recieveing Donepezil. *JAMA, 2004; 291:317–324.*

Tarle, M., et al. Early diagnosis of prostate cancer in finasteride treated BPH patients. *Anticancer Res.* 2003 Jan-Feb; 23(1B):693–6.

Tatro, D. S., ed. *Drug Interaction Facts.* 1997. St. Louis: J. B. Lippincott, Facts and Comparisons.

Taylor, A.J., et al. Lipid-Lowering Efficacy, Safety, and Costs of a Large-Scale Therapeutic Statin Formulary Conversion Program. *Pharmacotherapy* 2001; 21(9):1130–1139.

Tecce, M.A., et al. Heart disease in older women. Gender differences affect diagnosis and treatment. *Geriatrics.* 2003 Dec; 58(12):33–9.

Temple, M.E., and Nahata, M.C. Treatment of Pediatric Hypertension. *Pharmacotherapy.* 20(2):140–150. 2000.

Terry, M.B., Gammon, M.D., Zhang, F.F., et al. Association of Frequency and Duration of Aspirin Use and Hormone Receptor Status With Breast Cancer risk. *JAMA* 2004; 291(20):2433–2440.

Teter, C.J., et al. A Comprehensive Review of MDMA and GHB: Two Common Club Drugs. *Pharmacotherapy* 2001; 21(12):1486–1513.

Teter, C.J., et al. Ilicit Methylphenidate Use in an Undergraduate Student Sample: Prevalence and Risk Factors. *Pharmacotherapy* 2003; 23(5):609–617.

Thompson, I.M., et al. The Influence of Finasteride on the Development of Prostate Cancer. *NEJM.* 2003 July 17. as accessed in early release form: *http://content.nejm.org/content/abstract/NEJM0a030660v1.*

Thordsen, D. J., and Welty, T. E., eds. *Clinical Abstracts: Current Therapeutic Findings.* 1998. Cincinnati, OH: Harvey Whitney Books.

Tohen, M., et al. Olanzapine Versus Divalproex Sodium for the Treatment of Acute Mania and Maintenance of Remission: A 47- Week Study. *Am J Psychiatry; 160:1263–1271.*

Trachtman, H., et al. Clinical trial of extended-release felodipine in pediatric essential hypertension. *Pediatr Nephrol.* 2003 Jun; 18(6):548–53.

Tran, M.T., et al. Role of Coenzyme Q10 in Chronic Heart Failure, Angina, and Hypertension. *Pharmacotherapy 2001;* 21(7)797–806. 2001.

Tsikouris, J.P. and Cox, C.D. A Review of Class III Antiarrhythmic Agents for Atrial Fibrillation: Maintenance of Normal Sinus Rhythm. *Pharmacotherapy.*21(12):1514–1529. December 2001.

Tsuyuki, R. T. and Bungard, T. J. Poor Adherence with Hypolipidemic Drugs: A Lost Opportunity. *Pharmacotherapy.* 21(5)576–582. Mar 1, 2001.

Tuchmann-Duplessis, H. *Drug Effects on the Fetus.* 1975. Sydney, Australia: ADIS Press.

Tufts Center for the Study of Drug Development. November 30, 2001. *Tufts Center for the Study of Drug Development Pegs Cost of a New Prescription Medicine at $802 Million.* 192 South Street, Boston, MA.

Tyler, V. E. *The Honest Herbal: A Sensible Guide to the Use of Herbs and Related Remedies.* 3rd ed. 1993. New York: Pharmaceutical Products Press, Haworth Press, Inc.

United States Pharmacopeial Convention (USP) Dispensing Information 1997. Vol. 1: Drug Information for the Health Care Provider. 12th ed. Rockville, MD: United States Pharmacopeial Convention.

Urwin, R.E., et al. Investigation of Epistasis Between the Serotonin Transporter and Norepinephrine Transporter Genes in Anorexia Nervosa. *Neuropsychopharmacology.* 2003 May 14 (epub ahead of print).

Utian, W. H. *Menopause in Modern Perspective.* 1980. New York: Appleton-Century-Crofts.

Vacek, J.L., Rosamond, T.L., et al. Acute coronary syndromes A three-article symposium. *Postgraduate Medicine 2002;* 112(1).

Van Gelder, I.C., et al. A Comparison of Rate Control and Rhythm Control in Patients with Recurrent Persistent Atrial Fibrillation. *New England Journal of Medicine* 2002; 347(23):1834–1840.

VanWalraven, C., et al. A clinical prediction rule to identify patients with atrial fibrillation and a low risk for stroke while taking aspirin. *Archives of Internal Medicine 2003;* 163: 936–943.

Vasan, R.S., et al. Residual lifetime risk for developing hypertension in middle-aged women and men. *Journal of the American Medical Association 2002;* 287(8):1003–1010.

Vignola, A.M., et al. Efficacy and tolerability of anti-immunoglobulin E therapy with omalizumab in patients with concomitant allergic asthma and peristsent allergic rhinitis: SOLAR. *Allergy.* 59(7):709–17. July 2004.

Vinson, J.A., et al. Presentation: Cranberries: excellent source of polyphenol antioxidents. New Orleans, LA: American Chamical Society, 225th National Meeting, March 24, 2003. Abstract AGFD 65.

Volcheck, G.W. Which diagnostic tests for common allergies? *Postgraduate Medicine* May 2001; 109(5):71–85.

Volkow, N.D. and Swanson, J.M. Variables That Affect the Clinical Use and Abuse of Methylphenidate in the Treatment of ADHD. *Am J Psychiatry.* 2003; 160:1909–1918.

Vongpatanasin, W., et al. Differential effects of oral versus transdermal estrogen replacement therapy on C-reactive protein in postmenopausal women. *Journal of the American College of Cardiology.* 2003; 41:1358–1363.

Wallach, J. B. *Interpretation of Diagnostic Tests.* 6th ed. 1996. Boston: Little, Brown.

Watanabe, M.D. Antipsychotics in the Treatment of Schizophrenia. *The Rx Consultant.* X(5):1–7. 2001.

Ward, M.W., and Holimon, T.D. Calcium Treatment for Premenstrual Syndrome. *The Annals of Pharmacotherapy.* 33:1356–1358. 1999.

Ward, R.P., and Anderson, A.S. Slowing the progression of CHF. *Postgraduate Medicine.* 109(3):36–45. 2001.

Weimerskirch, P. R., and Ernst, M. E. Newer Dopamine Agonists in the Treatment of Restless Legs Syndrome. *The Annals of Pharmacotherapy.* 35:627–635. May 2001.

Weinblatt, M.E., et al. Adalimumab, a fully human anti-tumor necrosis factor alpha monoclonal antibody, for the treatment of rheumatoid arthritis in patients taking methotrexate: the ARMADA trial. *Arthritis Rheum. 2003;* 48:35–45.

Wenzel, R.P. and Edmond, M.B. Managing Antibiotic Resistance. *New England Journal of Medicine.* 343(26):1961–1963. December 28, 2000.

Willhite, L.A., and O'Connell, B. Urogenital Atrophy: Prevention and Treatment. *Pharmacotherapy;* 21(4):464–480.

Woerner, M.G., Clozapine as a First Treatment for Schizophrenia. *Am J Psychiarty 2003;* 160:1514–1516.

Wolf, M.M., et al. Gastrointestinal Toxicity of Nonsteroidal Anti-Inflammatory Drugs. *New England Journal of Medicine.* June 17, 1999:1888–1899.

Wolfenden, L.L., et al. Lower physician estimate of underlying asthma severity leads to undertreatment. Arch Intern Med. 2003; 163:231–236.

Wood, A.J.J., and Ito, S. Drug Therapy for Breast-Feeding Women. *New England Journal of Medicine*. 343(2):118–126. July 13, 2000.

Wood, A.J.J., et al. Diuretic Therapy. *New England Journal of Medicine*. 339(6):387–395. August 6, 1998.

Wood, A.J., DeSmet, P.A. Herbal Remedies. *New England Journal of Medicine 2002*. 347: 2046–2056.

Wood, M. J., and Cox, J.L. HRT to Prevent Cardiovascular Disease. What studies show, how to advise patients. *Postgraduate Medicine*. 108(3):59–72. Sept 1, 2000.

Worley, R. J., ed. Menopause. *Clinical Obstetrics and Gynecology*. 24(1):163–164. 1981.

www.cdc.gov/ncidod/flu/fluvac.htm Vaccine Information Influenza Vaccine. July, 2001.

www.fda.gov/cder/approval?index.htm: The Food And Drug Administration. June, 2001.

www.fda.gov/cder/drug/antidepressants/AntidepressanstPHA.htm created March 22, 2004.

www.fda.gov/cder/orange/docket/pdf: The Food And Drug Administration: CDERNEW6 June, 2001.

www.fda.gov/medwatch: The Food And Drug Administration: MedWatch various dates including 8/6/01, 2001, 2003, 2004.

www.fdanewsdigest@oc.FDA.GOC (FDA News Digest): The Food And Drug Administration. July, August, 2001.

www.medanews.com: MedAdNews. 20(5) May 2001.

www.naturaldatabase.com: The Pharmacist's Letter. 2002.

www.nlm.nih.gov/medlineplus/news/fullstory 2647. html: Herbal Medicines Pose Risk During Surgery: Report. July 11, 2001.

Wyse, D.G., et al. A Comparison of Rate Control and Rhythm Control in Patients with Atrial Fibrillation. *New England Journal of Medicine* 2002; 347(23):1825–1833.

Yashuda, J.M. and Chung, E.P. Diabetes Mellitus The New Insulin Analogs. *The Rx Consultant*. 11(2):1–8. 1999.

Yiu-Chung, Chan, et al. Atypical Antipsychotics in Older Adults. *Pharmacotherapy*. 19: 811–822. 1999.

Yki-Jarvinen, H., et al. Bedtime Insulin Plus Metformin Prevents Weight Gain and Reduces Frequency of Hypoglycemia in Type 2 Diabetes. *Annals of Internal Medicine*. 130: 389–396. 1999.

Young, D. S. *Effects of Drugs on Clinical Laboratory Tests*. 1991 supplement. Washington, DC: AACC Press.

Young, L. L., ed. *Nonprescription Products: Formulations and Features '96–97*. Washington, DC: American Pharmaceutical Association.

Yusuf, S., et al. Effects of an Angiotensin-Converting-Enzyme Inhibitor, Ramipril, on Cardiovascular Events in High-Risk Patients. *New England Journal of Medicine*. 342(3): 145–153. January 20, 2000.

Zametkin, A.J., and Ernst, M. Problems in the Management of Attention-Deficit-Hyperactivity Disorder. *New England Journal of Medicine*. 340(1):40–46. January 1999.

Ziccardi, P., et al. Reduction of inflammatory cytokine concentrations and improvement of endothelial functions in obese women after weight loss over one year. *Circulation 2002* accessed on line before print at *www.americanheart.org*.

Zonana-Nacach, A., et al. Damage in Systemic Lupus Erythematosus and Its Association with Corticosteroids. Arthritis & Rheu. 2000; 43(8):1801–1808.

Index

This index contains all the brand and generic drug names included in Section Two.

Brand names of drugs appear in italic type and are capitalized.

Each brand name is followed by its generic name. The generic name is the name under which you'll find the drug profile in Section Two.

The symbol [CD] indicates that the brand name represents a combination drug that contains other generic drug components; see the Drug Profile for details on other components present. To be fully familiar with any combination drug [CD], it is necessary to read the Drug Profile of each component.

The symbol ✤ before the brand name of a combination drug indicates that the brand name is used in both the United States and Canada but that the ingredients in the combination product in each country differ. The Canadian drug is marked with the symbol ✤ to distinguish it from the American drug with the same name.

A generic name with no page designation indicates an active component of a combination drug for which there is no Profile in Section Two. It is included to alert you to its presence, should you wish to consult your physician regarding its significance.

About the Author

JAMES J. RYBACKI, Pharm.D., was born in Oneonta, New York. He received his prepharmacy education at Creighton University and his Doctor of Pharmacy degree from the University of Nebraska Medical Center, College of Pharmacy, in Omaha. Dr. Rybacki has more than three decades of hospital and clinical experience that include early efforts in gas-liquid chromatography research characterizing human drug metabolites, and data collection for the College of American Pathologists to establish normal values for laboratory studies. He is a member of the clinical faculty at the University of Maryland School of Pharmacy and has provided clinical rounding and hospital experience for Pharm.D. and bachelor students. He presently teaches a Drug Information rotation for Pharm.D. students at The Clearwater Group. He is board certified in pain management at the Diplomat level by the American Academy of Pain Management, and he provides ongoing clinical pain management and medicine information nationwide. He is a guest lecturer and researcher at the Department of Family Medicine at the Georgetown University School of Medicine. He is a member of The National Council of Hospice Professionals. Dr. Rybacki is actively involved in the post marketing monitoring of medicines via The Drug Surveillance Network, a nationwide association of clinical pharmacists, and he is an approved External New Drug Application reviewer for the Canadian Drug Ministry. He lives in Maryland.

Dr. Rybacki's efforts in drug information and clinical pharmacy include many years of active practice, including infectious disease, pharmacokinetic, nutrition support, pain management, and pharmacological consultations. Through an Occupational Health Unit, he has offered independent pain management and pharmacological consultations nationwide. He has also advised the World Health Organization's Expert Committee regarding revisions as well as the selection of drugs to be listed in *The Use of Essential Drugs* and is an assistant editor for the Drugdex drug information system. His past role as a Vice President Clinical Services bought him added expertise in overseeing occupational health, physical medicines, laboratory services, imaging, cardiology, respiratory therapy, cancer programs, and continuing medical education. He served as conference coordinator for the first and second annual Dorchester General Hospital Pain conferences and as seminar coordinator for the eastern shore of Maryland for the "Take Control" physician and public pain education programs with Johns Hopkins.

Dr. Rybacki is now president of The Clearwater Group and the lead clinical consultant of the Medicine Information Institute—both headquartered in Easton, Maryland. He provides drug information support and clinical pharmacy services to physician groups, consumers, and employers; holds seminars and continuing education meetings on diabetes, cardiovascular disease, infectious disease, adherence, osteoporosis, pain management, women's health, and therapeutics; provides information support to insurance companies and HMOs; provides on-site hospital consulting on JCAHCO pain standards, optimizing use of medicines and other programs, produces educational tapes and television programming on medicines; designs clinical programs; and conducts independent pharmacological evaluations. He was on the Patient Education Committee of the American Heart Association on a national level, served as the first Pharm.D. committee member of the American Heart Association Pharmaceutical Roundtable and is actively designing research involving how, why, and when to enhance the way people take their medicines and decrease risk factors for cardiovascular disease. He is a strong advocate of a multilevel/interdisciplinary approach and is designing projects to involve pharmacists/physicians/PAs/nurses/nurse practitioners/cardiac rehab programs at the practice site itself in communicating risk factor reduction, medication adherence importance, and improving outcomes.

He was selected for full membership in the American College of Clinical Pharmacy, is a Certified Clinical Densitometrist (CCD) through the Society for Clinical Densitometry, and was asked by the governor of Maryland to join a state-wide Osteoporosis Task Force in Maryland (see *www.strongerbones.org*). He is a lifetime member of Who's Who in Global Business. Dr. Rybacki is director of clinical research, therapeutics, and outcomes at the Medicine Information Institute—an interdisciplinary consulting group. Dr. Rybacki has been a frequent guest on Comcast's *Family Talk* live television program as well as their new *Real Life TV*. He is now the writer and host of a patient education series called Medicines and Your Family with Dr. Jim Rybacki. You may have also heard him as the voice and writer of the Bayer Aspirin Pharmacist Report (a short-segment program on preventing a first heart attack). Catch Dr. Jim on TV, the Web, and on the radio (*www.medicinesandyourfamily.com*, *www.medicineinfo.com*, and *www. bayerasprin.com*)!

An active national speaker, Dr. Rybacki gave the keynote address at the 2004 Mended Hearts Leadership Conference, participates in numerous medical speakers bureaus, including Merck Pain Management and osteoporosis, Miles, Dupont Pharma and Glaxo. He has been a member of the Bristol-Myers Squibb Distinguished faculty in HIV faculty since 1994 and lectures across the country. He has jointly authored several articles in professional journals on use of medicines in infectious diseases, critical care, therapeutics, and cost containment and adherence. *The Essential Guide to Prescription Drugs*, first published in 1977, was co-authored by Dr. Rybacki since 1994, before he assumed full authorship in 1996. Dr. Rybacki leveraged his expertise on medicines to *The Medicine Man*, a nationwide live radio show, which was developed, written, produced, and hosted by Dr. Rybacki in 1995. He is the original writer and host of the American Pharmaceutical Association's *The Pharmacist Minute* radio program, and is the writer, producer, and host of *Medicines and Your Family with Dr. Jim Rybacki*.

Recently, Dr. Rybacki has created a new book supported by an unrestricted educational grant from the Bristol-Myers Squibb/ Sanofi Pharmaceuticals Partnership. The book is called *Medicines and Your Family, National Treatment Guidelines* and will be given away in the first edition by The Mended Hearts, Inc. (*www.mendedhearts.org*). Dr. Rybacki thinks that the best colleague any doctor can have is a more fully informed patient. Dr. Rybacki brings late-breaking information to people via popular sites on the World Wide Web at *www.medicineinfo.com* and *www.medicinesandyourfamily.com*.

Controlled Drug Schedules

Schedule I: These medicines have a high abuse and dependence potential. Typically, the only use for these drugs is for research purposes. Examples include LSD and heroin. A prescription cannot be legally written for these drugs for medicinal use.

Schedule II: These medicines have therapeutic uses and the highest abuse and dependence potential for drugs with medicinal purposes. Examples include pain medicines (analgesics), such as morphine (MS Contin). A written prescription is required, and refills are not allowed.

Schedule III: Medicines in this schedule have an abuse and dependence potential that is less than those in schedule II, but greater than those in schedule IV. These medicines have clear medicinal uses and include such medicines as codeine, or paregoric in combination. A common name is Tylenol Number 3 with codeine. A telephone prescription is permitted for medications in this class; however, it must be converted to a written form by a pharmacist. Prescriptions for these medicines may be refilled, but only five times in 6 months.

Schedule IV: This schedule contains medicines with less abuse and dependence potential than those in schedule III. Examples of medicines in this schedule include diazepam (Valium) and chlordiazepoxide (Librium). Prescriptions for these medicines may be refilled, but only five times in 6 months.

Schedule V: These medicines have the lowest abuse and dependence potential. Medicines in this class include diphenoxylate (Lomotil) and loperamide (Imodium). Drugs in this class that require a prescription are handled the same as any nonscheduled prescription medicine. Some drugs in this class do not require a prescription and can be sold only with the approval of a pharmacist. The buyer may be required to sign a logbook when the drug is dispensed. Examples include codeine and hydrocodone in combination with other active nonnarcotic drugs, sold in preparations that have limited quantities of codeine or hydrocodone for control of diarrhea or cough.

Pregnancy Risk Categories

Definitions of FDA Pregnancy Categories (many medicines carry A, B, C, D, or X labels at the time of this writing)

Category A: Adequate and well-controlled studies in pregnant women do not show risk (are negative) for fetal abnormalities. Basically, risk to the fetus is remote based on the studies that have been done.

Category B: Animal reproduction studies are negative for fetal abnormalities, and data from adequate and well-controlled studies in pregnant women are not available. Basically, no evidence of risk in humans.

OR:

Animal-reproduction studies are positive for fetal abnormalities. Adequate and well-controlled studies in pregnant women are negative for fetal abnormalities and fail to show a risk to the fetus.

Category C: Animal reproduction studies are positive for fetal abnormalities. Information from adequate and well-controlled studies in pregnant women is not available.

OR:

Information from animal reproduction studies and from adequate and well-controlled studies in pregnant women is not available. Basically, risk can't be ruled out—but potential benefits may outweigh potential risk in certain circumstances.

Category D: Studies in pregnant women and/or premarketing (investigational) or postmarketing uses show positive evidence of human fetal risk. The drug is only used in serious disease or in life-threatening situations where safer medicines will not work or cannot be used. These situations may make the medicine acceptable despite its risks. Basically, potential benefits may outweigh potential risk in certain circumstances.

Category X: Animal reproduction studies and/or human pregnancy studies are positive for fetal abnormalities.

OR:

Studies in pregnant women and/or premarketing (investigational) or postmarketing (Phase Four) experience show **positive** evidence of human fetal risk.

AND:

Potential fetal risks clearly outweigh possible benefits of the drug. These medicines should never be used in pregnancy.

The FDA adopted the original system in 1979. The Pregnancy Labeling Task Force started to revise this system in 1997 in order to create a system that is more clinically useful. An FDA subcommittee met in 2000 that would require all new drugs to have labeling that tells about clinical considerations (like past medical history and gestational age) versus risk information (such as case reports, pregnancy registries, and retrospective research). At the time of this writing, more specific recommendations and a final change have not been made.